Pediatric Neurology

EDITED BY

Thomas W. Farmer, M.D.

Sarah P. Graham Kenan Professor of Neurology, Department of Neurology,
University of North Carolina School of Medicine,
Chapel Hill, North Carolina

Pediatric

Neurology

THIRD EDITION

with 25 contributors

HARPER & ROW, PUBLISHERS

PHILADELPHIA

Cambridge
New York
Hagerstown
San Francisco

London
Mexico City
São Paulo
Sydney

1817

Acquisitions Editor: William Burgower
Sponsoring Editor: Richard Winters
Indexer: Julia B. Schwager
Art Director: Maria Karkucinski
Designer: Lawrence Didona
Production Assistant: Barney Fernandes
Compositor: Waldman Graphics, Inc.
Printer/Binder: Halliday Lithograph

3rd Edition

1   3   5   6   4   2

Library of Congress Cataloging in Publication Data
Main entry under title:
Pediatric neurology.
  Bibliography
  Includes index.
  1. Pediatric neurology.   I. Farmer, Thomas W.
RJ486.P33 1982   618.92'8   81-19280
ISBN 0-06-140802-6   AACR2

The authors and publisher have exerted every effort to ensure that drug selection and dosage set forth in this text are in accord with current recommendations and practice at the time of publication. However, in view of ongoing research, changes in government regulations, and the constant flow of information
relating to drug therapy and drug reactions, the reader is urged to check the
package insert for each drug for any change in indications and dosage and for
added warnings and precautions. This is particularly important when the recommended agent is a new or infrequently employed drug.

Printed in the United States of America

To my wife, Phyllis

Contributors

Arthur S. Aylsworth, M.D.

Associate Professor of Pediatrics,
Department of Pediatrics,
UNC School of Medicine,
Chapel Hill, North Carolina

Michael J. Bresnan, M.D.

Associate Professor of Neurology,
Department of Neurology,
Harvard Medical School and
The Children's Hospital Medical Center,
Boston, Massachusetts

Sidney Carter, M.D.

Professor Emeritus of Neurology and Pediat-
   rics,
Departments of Neurology and Pediatrics,
College of Physicians & Surgeons
   of Columbia University,
New York, New York

Harrie R. Chamberlin, M.D.

Professor of Pediatrics,
Division for Disorders of Development
   and Learning,
Department of Pediatrics,
UNC School of Medicine,
Chapel Hill, North Carolina

Enrique Chaves, M.D.

Assistant Professor,
Department of Neurology,
Eastern Virginia Medical School,
Norfolk, Virginia

Philip R. Dodge, M.D.

Professor of Pediatrics and Neurology,
Head, The Edward Mallinckrodt Department
   of Pediatrics,
Washington University School of Medicine,
St. Louis, Missouri

James E. Etheridge, Jr., M.D.

Professor and Chairman,
Department of Neurology,
Eastern Virginia Medical School,
Norfolk, Virginia

Thomas W. Farmer, M.D.

Sarah P. Graham Kenan Professor of Neurol-
   ogy, Department of Neurology,
UNC School of Medicine,
Chapel Hill, North Carolina

Gilbert B. Forbes, M.D.

Professor of Pediatrics,
Department of Pediatrics,
The University of Rochester Medical Center,
School of Medicine and Dentistry,
Rochester, New York

L. Matthew Frank, M.D.

Assistant Professor,
Department of Neurology,
Eastern Virginia Medical School,
Norfolk, Virginia

Arnold P. Gold, M.D.

Professor of Clinical Neurology and Pediatrics,
Departments of Neurology and Pediatrics,
College of Physicians & Surgeons
   of Columbia University,
New York, New York

Robert S. Greenwood, M.D.

Assistant Professor of Neurology
    and Pediatrics,
Department of Neurology,
UNC School of Medicine,
Chapel Hill, North Carolina

Faustino C. Guinto, Jr., M.D.

Associate Professor of Neuroradiology,
Department of Radiology,
The University of Texas Medical Branch,
Galveston, Texas

Colin D. Hall, M.D.

Professor of Neurology,
Department of Neurology, UNC School
    of Medicine,
Chapel Hill, North Carolina

James F. Hammill, M.D.

Professor of Clinical Neurology,
Departments of Neurology and Pediatrics,
College of Physicians & Surgeons
    of Columbia University,
New York, New York

E. M. Hicks, M.B., B. Ch., M.R.C.P.

Clinical Fellow in Neurology,
Department of Neurology,
Harvard Medical School and
The Children's Hospital Medical Center,
Boston, Massachusetts

Stephen G. Kahler, M.D.

Clinical Instructor and Fellow,
Department of Pediatrics,
UNC School of Medicine,
Chapel Hill, North Carolina

Chung S. Kim, Ph.D.

Research Assistant Professor of Neurology,
Department of Neurology,
UNC School of Medicine,
Chapel Hill, North Carolina

Kenneth L. McCormick, M.D.

Assistant Professor of Pediatrics,
Department of Pediatrics
University of Rochester Medical Center,
School of Medicine and Dentistry,
Rochester, New York

Robert L. McLaurin, M.D.

Professor of Surgery,
Department of Surgery,
Division of Neurosurgery,
University of Cincinnati Medical Center,
College of Medicine,
Cincinnati, Ohio

Charles E. Morris, M.D.

Professor and Chairman,
Department of Neurology,
University of Health Sciences,
The Chicago Medical School,
North Chicago, Illinois

Lorcan A. O'Tuama, M.D.

Professor of Neurology and Pediatrics,
Department of Neurology,
UNC School of Medicine,
Chapel Hill, North Carolina

Richard J. Schain, M.D.

Adjunct Professor,
Department of Neurology,
UCLA School of Medicine,
Los Angeles, California

Major Edwin A. Stevens, MC USAF

Wilford Hall, US Air Force Medical Center
    (SGHR),
Lackland AFB, Texas

Joseph J. Volpe, M.D.

Professor of Pediatrics, Neurology,
    and Biological Chemistry,
Department of Pediatrics,
Washington University School of Medicine,
St. Louis, Missouri

Ken R. Winston, M.D.

Assistant Professor of Surgery (Neurosurgery),
Department of Surgery,
Harvard Medical School and
The Children's Hospital Medical Center,
Boston, Massachusetts

Preface

Since the publication of the second edition of this text, many advances have been made in the diagnosis and treatment of children with neurologic disorders. These advances are integrated into this third edition. For example, a new chapter on neuroradiologic examination presents the major procedures available for the diagnosis of intracranial and spinal disorders, and applications of these new procedures are presented in subsequent chapters. These procedures include computed tomography—which has dramatically improved the physician's ability to diagnose many cerebral disorders; metrizamide myelography—which has improved greatly the diagnosis of brain stem and spinal cord lesions; and sector scans—which have greatly improved the evaluation and treatment of infants with neonatal intracranial disorders.

Other chapters, too, have been added or expanded. A new chapter on perinatal disorders includes the management of seizure disorders, cerebral hypoxia and ischemia, and intracranial hemorrhage occurring at birth. A new chapter on learning disorders presents the diagnosis and treatment of cerebral palsy, drug abuse, autism, hyperactivity with minimal brain dysfunction, developmental dyslexia, and other disorders of speech. And an extensive new chapter with detailed references on inherited metabolic diseases describes a clinical approach to the diagnosis of children with possible metabolic disorders; it includes a section on the principles of genetics.

In the chapter on paroxysmal disorders, seizures are presented in accordance with the new international classifications, the current treatment of febrile seizures is delineated, and the role of anticonvulsant blood levels in the drug therapy of different types of seizures is described. In the chapter on intoxications, many recently described toxic disorders are presented, as well as a thorough description of the current state of knowledge of Reye's syndrome and infant botulism. Chapters on intracranial infections and tumors, head injuries, and cerebrovascular diseases describe the important use of computed tomography in the early diagnosis of these disorders and the advances in therapy that have decreased mortality and morbidity in many of them. Finally, in the chapter on peripheral neuropathy, there are new sections on the clinical approach to peripheral nerve disease and on the interdisciplinary approach to treatment, as well as descriptions of new disorders.

The bibliographies at the end of each chapter have been greatly enlarged with the addition of current references, and a large number of new illustrations have been added throughout the text.

Seventeen new authors and nine of the previous authors have contributed to this edition. I wish to thank them all. I also wish to thank Mrs. Carolyn Reams and the other secretaries who have typed portions of the manuscript.

I am very grateful to the publisher and to his editorial staff.

Thomas W. Farmer, M.D.

From the Preface to the First Edition

New diseases and discoveries relating to the many known neurologic disorders in children are being described each year. Today a wide variety of these conditions is being investigated by the general physician and the pediatrician as well as the neurologist and the neurosurgeon, since neurologic and sensory disorders afflict 6% of children. Approximately 3% of all children are mentally subnormal; about 0.5% have convulsive seizures; and another 0.5% have cerebral palsy. Fortunately the many other neurologic diseases occur less frequently.

The purpose of this volume is to provide an up-to-date textbook of pediatric neurology for medical students, resident physicians, and those in practice who have felt the need, as I have, for a convenient reference work in this increasingly important area of medicine.

The organization of the book combines an etiologic and anatomic approach to neurologic disorders in children. Descriptions of common clinical syndromes, their differential diagnosis, their treatment, and their prevention are presented in detail, while rare disorders are mentioned briefly.

Pertinent information from the fields of neuroanatomy, neurophysiology, and neuropathology, as well as from biochemistry, microbiology, and genetics, are incorporated directly into these chapters. For more detailed information concerning these areas, appropriate reference lists are included as guides to the original literature.

The authors include pediatricians, neurologists, pediatric neurologists, neuroradiologists, and neurosurgeons who have drawn from their wide clinical experience to present a thoroughly up-to-date well-rounded text. In addition to clinical descriptions of neurologic disorders, current diagnostic laboratory procedures are presented fully and illustrated. Many tables of differential diagnosis are included. Therapy is discussed in detail, and a special effort has been made to incorporate the newest techniques of treatment—for example, included are the latest information on the dosage and toxicity of recommended chemotherapeutic and antibiotic drugs; the management of the retarded child; treatment of seizures; regulation of water and electrolytes; the newest radiologic techniques, nerve conduction studies, and screening tests for biochemical disorders.

I freely accept the responsibility for all omissions and errors. I also invite criticism from the reader.

I wish to thank the publishers of the books and journals who have permitted the reproduction of material from previous publications by me and others. I also am indebted to the many other writers upon whose work we have drawn. The selected bibliographies in the text do not permit annotation of the many additional sources of information which I wish to acknowledge.

Finally, I wish to thank my teachers in neurology, Drs. Derek Denny-Brown, H. Houston Merritt, and Raymond D. Adams.

T.W.F

Publisher's Note
Eponyms in this book follow the style established by
Dorland's Illustrated Medical Dictionary, 26th edition.

Contents

Neurologic History and Examination

Philip R. Dodge
Joseph J. Volpe

Approximately one-fourth of all children in large teaching hospitals suffer from a primary neurologic disease or a disturbance in the function of the nervous system secondary to a systemic medical or surgical disorder. In addition, chronic disease of the nervous system, exemplified by mental retardation and cerebral palsy, yearly disables thousands of children, many of whom spend their lives in institutions under the care of physicians. In caring for well infants the pediatrician also spends considerable time assessing the growth and maturation of the nervous system in order to determine if mentation, behavior, and other nervous activities are normal or pathologically deviant.

The general principles of clinical diagnosis developed in adult neurology also apply to the infant and child. The principal symptoms and signs are ascertained by history and examination, and their strict interpretation with respect to neuroanatomy and neurophysiology enables the medically trained person to localize disease in the nervous system and to suggest its cause. For example, a peculiar disorder of gait may be due to weakness, ataxia, or rigidity of the legs and trunk, each of which has a special signficance in relation to the anatomic locus of disease; or a transient loss of awareness and responsiveness may represent a seizure, a breath-holding attack, or a simple faint, each based on a special pathophysiologic mechanism. Anatomic localization ordinarily takes precedence over etiologic considerations in arriving logically at a specific diagnosis. Each illness is first judged according to whether it could be caused by a single lesion or whether it requires the prediction of multiple lesions at one or more levels of the nervous system. Starting from this vantage point the etiologic diagnosis based on the natural history of the disease and other medical data, particularly pertinent laboratory findings, follows in logical sequence.

However, certain special problems arise that hinder this orderly sequence of thought in pediatric neurologic diagnosis. First, infants or young children are incapable of describing precisely their own symptoms, so the physician must rely on the report of parents or some other person who can never know the subjective aspects of the illness. Second, the examination is hampered by the inability of the infant or young child to cooperate to a degree that is possible in an older child or adult. In fact, the direct and systematic approach to the neurologic survey used in adult neurology may result in complete negativism, making examination impossible. With infants and children a subtle, tangential approach is more likely to succeed.

Ideally the examination should be fun for both the examiner and the patient. This assures a relaxed atmosphere that is advantageous to everyone including anxious parents who may fear the child will balk at the entire examination. To avoid frightening the patient it is often preferable to shed the white hospital coat with which many children associate unpleasant medical experiences. If resistance is encountered early, then a new approach to this part of the examination should be employed or it should be left until later. A smile on the examiner's face, the humming of a nursery rhyme, and an occasional tickle are of great help. Many phy-

1

sicians are so reserved and self-conscious that it is difficult for them to adapt their examination to the infant, but failure to do so may prove a great handicap.

Simple observation of the patient at play may yield more information about the function of the nervous system than formal clinical tests. The manner in which he manipulates toys and his reactions to what is going on around him are particularly informative. Often maximal cooperation is obtained when the examiner sits on the floor and joins in the play. Usually ophthalmoscopy and direct visualization of the eardrum should be attempted only at the conclusion of the examination because they are usually frightening to the young child. The same is true of tests for pain perception.

Another problem, uniquely difficult in the neurology of children, is the decision about whether a given disorder of the nervous system represents a stationary sequel of some past disorder or a progressive disease of the nervous system. Not uncommonly this decision is critical to the diagnosis because once it is determined that a given disease is nonprogressive, the number of diagnostic possibilities materially narrow. The baseline of normality undergoes constant change throughout childhood and adolescence as the nervous system matures anatomically and physiologically, and the neurologic findings must always be considered in light of the expected level of normal or average development. The course of disease, whether progressive, stationary, or regressive, must be superimposed on the ascending trajectory of the growth curve, and the composite may be difficult to plot. Also, a number of nonneurologic factors such as poor nutrition, fever, disturbed attitude, and emotional state may temporarily alter the orderly processes of development so that the normal standards become obscured.

It may be confidently assumed that in cases in which the history gives undeniable evidence of progressive loss of previously acquired nervous functions, helpfully documented with a photograph or home movie, a disease of the nervous system is advancing. Conversely, a steady acquisition of developmental skills from birth or after the onset of symptoms leads to the conclusion that the disease is static. It must be remembered, however, that at times the course of a progressive neurologic disease may be slower than that of maturation, and the net result is a retardation or arrest of the developmental process rather than regression.

A problem of the same order relates to the fact that certain neurologic symptoms and signs of disease require that the nervous system function has somewhat matured before they become manifest. Choreoathetosis, for example, which may result from a disease that antedates birth, is seldom recognizable as a specific neurologic abnormality prior to 1 year of age and is often recognizable only considerably later than this. Similarly, diseases that derange structures that subserve language cannot be detected before the age when speech is normally acquired. Thus in pediatric neurology the onset of a disease may have occurred before the appearance of the first symptom.

HISTORY

PRESENT ILLNESS

The resourceful clinician, prepared to grasp every available item of value in the study of a disease, is never neglectful of the child's observations and reports. If properly approached by the physician, small children may give a surprising amount of valuable historical data relative to their own illnesses. This may be true even in children below 5 years of age, and of course older children can often describe their symptoms in a delightfully refreshing and naive manner.

Yet experience teaches us that children tend to live more in the present and future than do adults, and their recollection of past events is notably inaccurate. Below the age of 5 or 6 years the concept of time, as abstracted from a series of happenings, is not sufficiently well developed to permit the narration of a sequential history. Even adolescents often confuse the timing of past events, especially if they are somewhat dull, frightened, or overly anxious to please their doctor. The infant or very young child is, of course, completely unable to describe his own symptoms and their temporal relationship. One must turn to the parents.

As in all history-taking, the elicitation of reliable data is greatly facilitated if the examiner is able to create an atmosphere of relaxation and can arouse the confidence of the parents by his sympathetic interest; anxiety and fear may prevent quiet, reflective analysis. Precise historical data must be sought, but overzealousness in eliciting this may result in the parents' giving incorrect information.

It is often advantageous to interrogate both father and mother whenever possible because one parent's memory may complement that of the other. In general, fathers seldom can recall the times when the "milestones of development" were passed, yet their general impressions may be more objective than those of the mother. The latter can usually be trusted to give the precise details of the illness and mode of treatment up to that time. A conscientiously kept baby book serves to document the developmental status, especially when there are many children in the family. Unfortunately after the the first child most parents are less compulsive in keeping such a record.

A sound plan is to take a complete history before beginning the examination and then during the latter procedure return to the history in order to clarify certain points. The principal data on the observed effects of the present illness should be carefully documented. It is good to encourage the parents to relate the problem in their own language with only enough questions from the examiner to keep them to the point. Once the main sketch of the presenting problem is finished, its time of onset with respect to the life history of the patient is ascertained, that is, the time of departure from normal development and health. Subsequently, the developmental history is taken.

DEVELOPMENTAL HISTORY

Prenatal History

Development begins at the time of conception, and the maternal state of health during this period may be important. Any unusual incident during the first trimester may be significant because gross malformations of the nervous system usually date from this period, when embryogenesis and organogenesis proceed at a maximal rate. In other words, an infant or child with grossly dysplastic features or absence, malplacement, or excessive development of certain parts may be assumed to have a disease that originated at the time of conception or during the early weeks of intrauterine life. A knowledge of teratogenesis (origins of malformations) permits one to ascertain with a considerable degree of precision the time that certain developmental faults occur. Most of these may be dated to the first 3 weeks of prenatal life. By the end of that time the formation of the neural tube is essentially complete; by the end of 3 months it has been encased by the neural arch developing from the primitive notochord and related mesenchymal tissue elements. Developmental disorders of the neural tube and failure of the neural arch to close properly are attributed to pathologic processes at work during those periods. Numerous factors acting together over a period of time, however, may injure the developing brain, and the final form of the malformation may be considerably modified by compensatory growth of uninjured regions. The problem of malformations is dealt with further in Chapter 3.

The organogenesis of the nervous system has biochemical as well as structural aspects. These are just beginning to be appreciated. Certain enzyme systems become functional only at a certain time in intrauterine life, presumably influencing the possibility of disease. Also, many of the patterns of development are determined by these chemical changes.

During the first trimester of pregnancy the developing fetus is threatened in numerous ways. Should implantation of the ovum and formation of the placenta be improper, or the relative balance of hormones not be attained, the fetus may be expelled from the uterus. On the other hand, it may be retained but will have suffered permanent damage; under these circumstances the nervous system is more often affected than any other part. A history of even slight vaginal bleeding during this trimester may be a clue to a threatened abortion.

The mother should be queried about

exposure to or actual occurrence of infections during pregnancy. The risk to the embryo is maximal during the first months, and the deleterious effect on the embryo during this period of a maternal rubella infection with consequent cataract, deafness, heart disease, mental retardation, and seizures has become a familiar association. Toxoplasmosis and cytomegalovirus infection usually cause minimal symptomatology in the pregnant woman but can produce serious damage to the fetal brain. Other maternal viral infections must be considered as potential causes of similar aberrations in development, but surprisingly these relationships have not been well established. Excessive radiation to the fetus at this early stage of development is also known to harm the fetal nervous system seriously, so evidence of such exposure should be sought. Toxic substances and medicines represent other possible causes of disordered structure and function in the immature nervous system; for example, the harmful effect of the tranquilizer thalidomide is well established, and alcohol and certain anticonvulsive drugs can produce characteristic somatic abnormalities including those of the central nervous system.

Syphilis, toxemia, and diabetes mellitus in the mother also are associated with a high incidence of defective infants, including central nervous system abnormalities. Similarly, injury may result from accidents in which the abdominal wall is struck or in which there is a critical lowering of blood pressure, as from blood loss.

Fetal movement is generally detected by the mother between the fourth and fifth months of pregnancy, and observant multiparous women may report an excess or reduction of fetal movement. A history of weak fetal movement is particularly important in estimating the time of onset of Werdnig-Hoffmann disease. A change in activity pattern may be taken as an indication of the beginning of the disease.

Any anatomic or biochemical defect of the nervous system present at the time of birth is properly classified as congenital. This term has no causal implications, and its frequent misuse as a synonym for hereditable or genetic disorders has resulted in much confusion. Hereditary disorders may not manifest until years after birth.

Another mistake has been the attempt to establish a dichotomy in the etiology of disease with heredity on one side and environment on the other. The inadequacy of this concept was exposed by the fact that both factors may be involved in the determination of hereditable diseases; for example, inherited enzymatic defects of galactosemia and phenylketonuria fail to find expression in disease in the absence of ingested galactose and phenylalanine.

Birth History

The events surrounding the birth process are important. A mother who has received little or no medication may give an accurate description of parturition, whereas a heavily sedated mother must rely on remembered fragments and on the secondhand reports of physicians, nurses, and attendants who helped with the labor and delivery.

The duration of various stages of labor, the type of medication, and the details of delivery may prove to be significant. Birth weight, signs of injury, color of the infant, abnormalities of respiration, and methods of resuscitation immediately following birth should all be noted. It should be emphasized that skin pallor is at least as revealing as cyanosis in the newborn.

Data obtained from electronic fetal monitoring may provide important information about hypoxic–ischemic insults during labor. Thus, ominous patterns include late decelerations of fetal heart rate and loss of beat to beat variability (i.e., "fixed baseline" fetal heart rate). When these data are combined with other phenomena, for example, meconium-stained amniotic fluid or low Apgar scores, it is probable that the infant has sustained intrauterine asphyxia.

Prolonged labor and premature rupture of the membrane predispose to neonatal infection. Premature separation of the placenta always threatens the fetus. A history of one of these pathologic states is common in patients with cerebral diplegia, quadriparesis, choreoathetosis, and mental retardation. Twitching, convulsions, or periodic apneic spells during the neonatal period are other revealing signs of so-called birth injury. Reference to them is often omitted in histories obtained later in life. Conversely, such signs may have other meanings, resulting at times from antenatal pathologic processes. Premature birth is of particular importance in this regard with cerebral diplegia being the most common late sequela.

Jaundice within the first hours or days of life raises the question of kernicterus, which in itself may account for respiratory difficulty, unresponsiveness, rigidity or hypotonicity, seizures, and death; or in the event of recovery, a chronic neurologic syndrome including mental defect, choreoathetosis, and deafness may manifest later. Jaundice developing after the end of the first week of postnatal life never seems to lead to kernicterus, a fact that again emphasizes the importance of an accurate history.

Postnatal History

As a rough guide in this retrospective reconstruction of the developmental history, it may be said that an infant who leaves the hospital with his mother probably had no severe symptoms or signs of disease while in the newborn nursery. Failure of the child to leave the hospital with the mother may be of historical import.

The mother's observations of the child's movements, his ability to suck and swallow, and his pattern of sleep and wakefulness are other reliable indications of development. A normal child usually extends his head shortly after birth when in the prone position; smiles at 6 weeks to 8 weeks of age; has good control of his head in the vertical position by 16 weeks to 20 weeks; rolls from prone to supine by 20 weeks to 24 weeks, from back to abdomen by 24 weeks to 28 weeks; sits alone by 7 months to 8 months; stands by 9 months to 10 months; and walks by 16 months.

Equally as important as evidence of adequate functioning of the nervous system at any stage of maturation is the general responsiveness to parents and objects in the environment by vocal and other motor activity. The *a, ba, da-da,* and *ma-ma* sounds initially heard late in the first year of life represent the earliest developmental phase of the articulatory process and of communication but are usually without specific word meaning at this stage. The same sounds are uttered by Japanese, Swedish, Hottentot, and all other children of the world. During the first half of the second year of life the infant begins to associate simple words and sounds with objects around him. Usually phrases including nouns and verbs are first constructed during the second half of that year. The average child between the ages of 9 months to 15 months enjoys and readily learns simple nursery games such as peek-a-boo and patty-cake. The examiner should habitually inquire about all these details of speech and social development.

The acquisition of hand and arm movement toward a proffered object is another hallmark in the development of the child because it becomes not only a means of exploring his environment by touch but also of acting on or manipulating the world about him. The manner in which he seizes and the skill with which he examines, moves, and releases the object are also informative. These manual skills emerge in an orderly and sequential manner during the latter part of the first year of life. Lack of hand preference (*i.e.,* ambidexterity) is the rule during the first 2 years of life. An infant who shows an unequivocal preference before this time usually has some defect in the use of the other hand; this may be the first sign of infantile hemiplegia.

The general play activity of the child from age 2 until kindergarten, including his behavior when playing with other children, is usually very helpful in assessing development. Here are most clearly revealed some of the important facets of personality and social adaptation. Facile use of toys, scissors, crayons; throwing a ball; doing the hop-skip-jump; riding a tricycle; and dressing become possible only after the nervous system has matured to a certain point.

After the child is enrolled in school his learning ability and capacity for social adjustment are more systematically subjected to demanding tests. Special disorders of language function may first become obvious at this time. The nature of any such difficulty should be investigated with care. Often specific information must be obtained from teachers about school deportment, capacity to learn different sub-

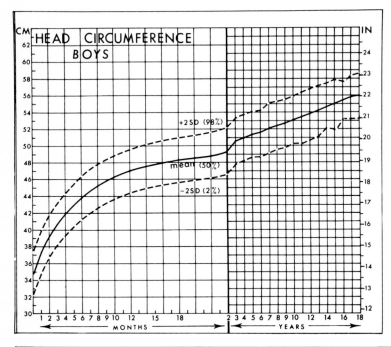

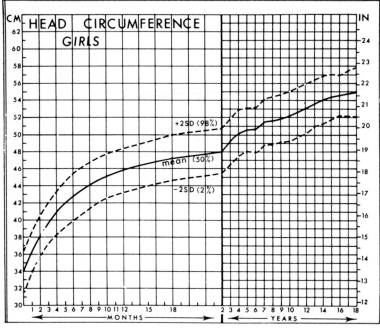

◀ FIG. 1-1. Head circumference; composites of international and interracial data. A. Males from birth through 18 years. B. Females from birth through 18 years. (From Nellhaus G: Pediatrics 41:106, 1968)

jects, adaptation to other students, and so on. Defects in learning, such as specific reading disability, should be suspected when there is a history of success in mathematics but a reading failure in the early grades of school.

REVIEW OF SYSTEMS

A review of systems completes the personal history. For example, attention should be paid to unusual growth or change in the size and shape of head, mannerisms suggesting head pain, curious ways of looking at objects, seizures and other paroxysmal attacks, prior infections of the meninges, episodes of delirium, severe head injuries, or periods of altered responsiveness. Symptoms reflecting dysfunction of other organ systems of the body that may be pertinent to the neurologic illness should also be noted.

FAMILY HISTORY

The family history should include the age of the parents, age and health of other siblings, history of previous pregnancies and miscarriages, the existence of familial diseases, and an inquiry about consanguinity.

EXAMINATION

PHYSICAL EXAMINATION

Neurologic diagnosis requires not only an assessment of nervous system function but also a complete physical examination. It obviously begins with a few moments of general observation in which the proportions of the body, nutritional status, and deportment in a strange situation are noted. Measurements of height, weight, circumference of the thorax at the zyphoid process, and the maximal circumference of the head

are taken and recorded for comparison with established norms and measurements at subsequent examinations. A disproportionately large head or extremities shortened in relation to the size of the trunk immediately brings to mind certain pathologic considerations such as hydrocephalus and chondrodystrophy.

The appearance, color, and texture of the skin and hair should be carefully noted. Cutaneous vascular malformations suggest a disorder such as Sturge-Weber syndrome. Subcutaneous nodules and pigmented or depigmented spots are characteristically found in neurofibromatosis or tuberous sclerosis. Abnormally cool, dry, yellowish and mottled skin in the lethargic and retarded child should lead the examiner to consider hypothyroidism.

It is important to inspect and palpate the midline of the back for evidence of a defect in closure of the neural or vertebral arch. A small dimple in the midline of the back from which black hairs emerge suggests a dermoid sinus tract. This may be in continuity with a large dermoid tumor within the spinal canal or in the cerebellum when it overlies the occipital region of the scalp. Such tracts may provide access to the meninges for bacteria. Recurrent attacks of meningitis always suggest the possibility of a dermoid sinus. Defects in the posterior vertebral arches can often be palpated and then confirmed by radiography. A comparison of the length and girth of the right and left extremities may establish the existence of hemihypertrophy or hemiatrophy. Tracing the size of the right and left feet with the patient standing facilitates comparison of the size of the two feet for significant differences. Similarly, a disparity in size of the thumbnails should alert the examiner to a somatic growth disturbance.

The infant's head should be examined with great care. In addition to bony defects, the general contour of the head may at once suggest the possibility of hydrocephalus or craniosynostosis. The head normally increases in size at a fairly predictable rate (Fig. 1-1). The speed of growth is greatest during the first months of life and is thought to reflect the rapid development of the brain during this period. In general, the circumference increases 1 cm/month during the first 6 months of life and 1 cm every 2 months

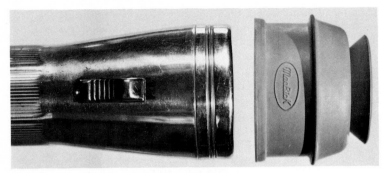

FIG. 1-2. Flashlight and rubber adapter used in transilluminating the heads of infants.

for the remaining 6 months of the first year. By the age of 3 years, 90% of the adult circumference can be expected.[11]

Assessment of head growth in the premature infant requires awareness that the standard charts of head growth are based on normal fetal head growth.[10] The premature infant with systemic illness exhibits a deviant pattern of head growth with three major phases. The first phase is a period of delayed head growth during the time of significant illness, when there is little or no change in head circumference. This period lasts for approximately 2 weeks to 4 weeks. Upon recovery from the systemic illness a second phase of head growth ensues, during which head circumference follows approximately the normal curve for fetal head growth. This phase is variable in duration but averages 6 weeks to 8 weeks. A third phase then evolves, characterized by growth of head and increase in weight and length that exceed the "normal" rates, that is, "catch-up" growth. This period continues for approximately 4 weeks to 8 weeks.

Three major deviations from the usual pattern of head growth in the sick premature infant should be recognized. Two that suggest hydrocephalus include the development of "normal" head growth too quickly, that is, during the early period when delayed head growth should be expected, or the development of accelerated, apparent "catch-up" head growth before the later, expected time for this phase. A third deviant pattern, which should suggest developmental or destructive disease of brain, is persistence of the early phase of delayed head growth.

Factors that lead to deformation of the skull are an abnormal thrust of the growing brain or intracranial mass against the inner table of the cranial bones, external compression, or a restricted capacity for expansion because of early fusion at cranial suture lines. Minor asymmetries of the skull are common during infancy, although their cause is not always apparent. At times, flattening in the posterior region on one side or the other is noted at or soon after birth. This deformity usually becomes less apparent as the child begins to sit and as the continued thrust of the growing brain produces a more symmetrical contour.

If, however, the child's development is retarded so that he fails to sit at the expected age, and particularly if he remains recumbent during the period of maximal cranial enlargement, the asymmetry may be quite pronounced and may persist into adult life. In addition to posterior flattening, there is always a prominence in the frontal region on that same side and in the occipitoparietal region on the opposite side (scoliosis capitus). This type of asymmetry of the skull, plagiocephaly, may result also from absence of a coronal or lambdoidal suture and from congenital torticollis.

Palpation of the suture lines may reveal remarkable ridging in craniosynostosis, particularly when the sagittal suture is involved. During the early weeks of life the various cranial bones barely approximate each other over the convexity and a large anterior fontanel is usual; the posterior fontanel is small or nonpalpable. This loose arrangement permits overriding of the cranial bones at the sutures, a condition that characteristically occurs with delivery. It may also appear during the early weeks of life as a consequence of severe dehydration or an encephaloclastic disease.

The presence of a fontanel in infancy affords a simple method of estimating the intracranial pressure. Normally the fontanel is somewhat depressed and pulsates slightly; the tension is of course altered by position. When a state of increased intracranial pressure is present, the fontanel may be extremely full and tense, and vascular pulsations may be absent. In the presence of increased intracranial pressure the veins of the scalp may be full and prominent.

The accessibility of the anterior fontanel as an indicator of intracranial pressure has led to the refinement of techniques that allow noninvasive, continuous monitoring of pressure from that site. The sensors that have been devised for application to the skin of the anterior fontanel rely on applanation or fiberoptic transducers. Excellent correlations of intracranial pressure measured by the anterior fontanel monitors with intracranial pressure measured by direct determination in the lumbar subarachnoid space or lateral ventricles have been obtained.

By auscultation of the head of infants and children in a quiet room, one may hear audible systolic bruits in 50% to 75% of infants and young children. They are uncommon beyond 6 years of age. These vascular sounds are most easily heard over the orbits but may be audible over all parts of the head, and the older child may report hearing them. Most of these bruits are of no clinical significance, and the manner of their production is obscure. Some are transmitted from murmurs at the base of the heart or from the great vessels in the neck and may be eliminated by compression of the carotid artery. When extremely loud, extending through diastole as well as systole, or when asymmetrical, an arteriovenous shunt should be considered. Bruits may be audible over the posterior fossa in tumors of the cerebellum in children. On occasion, breath sounds, normally transmitted to the head, are modified over a porencephalic cyst.

Transillumination of the head is another useful procedure in diagnosing certain major intracranial defects in infants. The technique is simple, requiring an ordinary flashlight to which is attached a rubber adapter (Fig. 1-2). The infant is brought into a dark room, and after 1 minute to 3 minutes for accommodation of the examiner's eyes the entire surface of the head is explored. Today a high-intensity light source ("Chun gun") requiring less dark adaptation is used extensively. Complete glowing of the head occurs in hydranencephaly or in hydrocephalus, when the cerebral mantle is reduced in total thickness to 1 cm or less (Fig. 1-3). Large unilateral porencephalic cysts are clearly delineated by this technique. Localized glowing well beyond the rim of the light source may be seen when the distance between the inner surface of the skull and the outer surface of the brain is increased, as occurs in subdural effusion, cerebral atrophy, and certain malformations. Extracranial fat or fluid within the scalp may at times give the false impression of an intracranial abnormality, but palpation of the scalp at the time of the examination should exclude these possibilities. In newborns a subperiosteal hematoma (cephalohematoma), which is usually limited to a single bone, and a subgaleal hemorrhage (caput succedaneum), which is not restricted in distribution to an individual bone, do not transilluminate. Increased transillumination is a normal characteristic of the pre-mature infant.[3]

FIG. 1-3. Transillumination of extreme thinning of the cerebral mantle in an hydrocephalic infant.

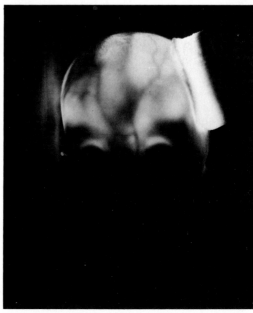

NEUROLOGIC EXAMINATION

It is obvious that the physician must adapt the examination procedure to the condition and reaction of his patient, and naturally enough it differs according to the patient's age. Examination of the older child differs in no essential way from that of the adolescent or adult. With younger children and infants, as already indicated, one must use a number of techniques that are not familiar to the physician who works only with older individuals.

Mental Status

Usually it is not difficult to carry out a complete mental status examination in the school-age child, inasmuch as he possesses adequate speech and comprehension of language. Of course impairment of either of these functions may reflect a general defect in intellect or a specific disorder of the language mechanisms. An obvious discrepancy between the levels of performance on verbal and nonverbal tests helps to differentiate between these two types of difficulty.

General behavioral patterns of patients, for example, hyperactive, hypoactive, autistic, excitable, apathetic, are meaningful, as are the degree of cooperation in the examination and the awareness and responsiveness to various stimuli. Orientation with reference to time, place, and persons is another useful indication of mental function and should be recorded. Memory of events that took place in the immediate and remote past, though difficult to apply to the younger child, may be readily assessed in the child of school age. Immediate retention may be tested by asking the child to recall something he was asked to remember minutes before or to recite forward or backward a series of different numbers given at 1-second intervals.

Achievement tests designed to assess the patient's fund of information, reading skill, and mathematical ability should take the child's school experience into account. Solving puzzles and learning new material depend little upon past school experience and can be used to test cognitive functions at various age levels. Subtraction of 3s or 7s from a hundred, and then serially from each successive remainder, is a useful test of the older child's ability to concentrate on a task, calculate, and remember for brief periods; it is rarely applicable to children less than 10 years to 12 years of age. Formal tests such as the Stanford-Binet or Wechsler Intelligence Scale for Children should be given whenever the clinical study indicates cerebral dysfunction.

The psychic function referred to as judgment is difficult to evaluate in the clinical situation. The family is usually better able to supply this information. An attempt to evaluate mood, especially a recent change in mood, is important in deciding whether a child is depressed or possibly manic. Unusual fears, nightmares, disturbed eating and sleeping patterns, compulsive behavior, obsessive thoughts, delusions, hallucinations and feelings of unreality, or excessive familiarity may be accurately reported by older children and may be used effectively as signs of neurologic and psychiatric diseases.

In examining the infant or young child with whom avenues of communication are limited, a great and perhaps inordinate importance must be attached to the child's repertoire of motor skills. This allows for considerable uncertainty about the significance of poor performance because it may reflect not only a general defect in intelligence but also a primary motor abnormality. Despite these limitations it is often possible to assess intelligence by using a variety of tests and comparing the patient's performance with norms established for infants and children of the same age (Table 1-1).[5,8]

Cranial Nerves

The anatomic locations of the cranial nerves are indicated in Figures 1-4 and 1-5.

Olfactory (I) Nerve. Suspicion of disease of structures seated in the anterior fossa or the patient's complaint of a disorder of smell or taste are the principal indications for testing olfactory nerve function. Testing for such simple odors as coffee, peppermint, and orange is satisfactory. Each nostril, which must be patent, is tested separately. It should be remembered that irritating vapors such as ammonia stimulate the trigeminal nerve and therefore should not be

(*Text continues on p. 14*)

TABLE 1-1. Summary of Milestones in Infant and Child Development

Age	Reflex Functions and Integrated Motor Activities	Specific and General Sensory Functions	Adaptive and Social Behavior
Newborn period	Strong sucking, rooting, swallowing, and Moro reflexes. Infantile grasping, hands and feet. Tonic neck reflexes variable. Plantars flexor. Knee jerks, biceps reflexes present, other tendon reflexes variable, abdominal reflexes difficult to elicit. Flexion postures predominate. Extension and flexion movement of limbs. Briefly extends neck in prone position. Reflex walking.	Blinks to light. Opticokinetic nystagmus. Startle to loud noise. Ocular pursuit variable.	
6 weeks	Tonic neck reflexes prominent. Tendon reflexes usually present. Unsustained ankle clonus not unusual. Plantars usually extensor. Asymmetrical postures usual. Extends and turns neck in prone position. Marked head lag when pulled to sit. Reflex walking usually lost unless facilitated by practice.	Improved fixation and following with eyes 45° to either side. Opticokinetic nystagmus easily elicited.	Smiles in response to play.
12 weeks (3 months)	Incomplete tonic neck reflexes. Infantile grasp and sucking reflexes variable and modified by volition. Slight head lag when pulled to sit. Head bobs in sitting position. Briefly holds object placed in hand. Better organized movement of individual extremities. Holds head above plane of body for long periods in prone position.	Watches movement of own hands. Rapidly fixes on objects and follows fully in all directions. Turns to object presented in visual field. May turn head to sound.	Ready smile and makes pleasant sounds when talked to.
16 weeks (4 months)	Hand grasp, sucking, and tonic neck reflexes subservient to volition and evident only when drowsy. Minimal head lag, holds head well and looks about when held in sitting position. Makes swimming movements when in prone position. Holds and shakes rattle, but cannot retrieve it if	All visual responses quicker and better developed. Turns rapidly to sound.	Laughs aloud. Shows pleasure when played with and at sight of food and friendly faces.

(Continued)

TABLE 1-1. Summary of Milestones in Infant and Child Development (*Continued*)

Age	Reflex Functions and Integrated Motor Activities	Specific and General Sensory Functions	Adaptive and Social Behavior
	dropped. Moro response absent or nearly so. Symmetrical attitudes of extremities predominate and precede two-hand reach (20 weeks).		
20 weeks (5 months)	Extends knees when soles of feet contact surface if held in standing position (positive supporting reaction). Some movements of progression. No head lag on pull to sit, maintains head posture when body pulled or pushed by examiner. Grasps objects with both hands. Holds on to bottle.	Discriminating with respect to food by this time at least. Vision said to be 20/400.	Primitive articulated sounds *ga-goo*. Regards self in mirror and smiles. Pulls cloth from over face in play.
24 weeks (6 months)	Beginning to grasp with one hand rather than with both hands. Sits with support. Supports upper parts of body on hands in prone position. Rolls from prone to supine. Grasps own feet and takes object with whole hand.		Range of sounds greater. Vocalizes spontaneously in social play. Tries to recover lost object. Extends arms in anticipation of being lifted. Expresses displeasure clearly.
28 weeks (7 months)	Sits with hands for support (tripod). Stands with support. Rolls supine to prone. Transfers object from hand to hand. Bangs object on table.		A, *ba*, *da*, *ga* sounds usually heard. Repeats sounds in imitative way. Refuses food or things he does not want. Feeds self a cracker. Responds to name. Mimics.
32 weeks (8 months)	Sits briefly without support. Supports weight and may stand holding on. Mounting of objects prominent.		Uses *da-da*, *ba-ba* sounds. Imitates sounds readily. Responds to "No."
36 weeks–40 weeks (9 months–10 months)	Sits well and pulls self to sitting position. Crawls using arms; grasps small object between thumb and forefinger. Beginning to release objects. Stands holding on. Sits well.		Nursery tricks, e.g., waves bye-bye and plays patty-cake on request. Seeks attention.
44 weeks–48 weeks (10 months–11 months)	Creeps well. Usually puts object into and removes it from container. Walks holding on.		Usually one or two words with meaning. Shakes head for "No." Responds to questions such as, "Where is daddy?" Releases object for examination on request. Plays peek-a-boo.
52 weeks (1 year)	Plantar reflexes flexor in 50% of children. Abdominal reflexes elicited easily.	Vision said to be 20/200 or better.	Two to four words with meaning. Assists in dressing. Often shy. May

Age	Motor	Language / Adaptive / Personal-Social	Special Senses
	Cruises and walks, one hand held. Dexterous in manipulating small objects. Throws objects. Less mouthing of objects.	kiss on request. Understands the name of several objects in environment.	
15 months	Walks by self, toddles. Falls easily. Can feed self clumsily if allowed. Scribbles with crayon.	Several intelligible words. Often babbles in communicating. Imitates family in play, may build tower of two to four blocks. Requests things by pointing.	
18 months (1½ year)	Walks up and down stairs holding on. May pull toy and carry objects. Seats self in chair. Throws ball. Removes shoes, socks, and unzips clothing. Uses spoon well.	Many intelligible words. Well developed jargon language. Points to two to three parts of body, common objects, pictures in books. Answers question, "Where is the . . . ?" Carries out simple commands, e.g., "Bring the ball."	
24 months (2 years)	Plantar reflexes flexor in 100% of normal children. Walks up and down stairs by self (2 feet per step). Bends over and picks up objects without falling. Runs, kicks ball, turns knob, washes hands, puts on shoes, socks, and pants.	Makes two- to three-word sentences. Uses I, me, and you. Asks for things by name. Imitates circle. Points to four to five parts of body. Organized play (e.g., puts doll to bed). Turns single pages of book. Builds tower of six to seven blocks. Toilet training often completed.	
30 months (2½ years)	Jumps both feet. Walks on tiptoes when requested.	Communicates well with simple sentences, asks questions. Knows full name. Helps put away toys. Holds pencil in hand. Builds tower of eight blocks. Can complete three-piece form board. Understands one to three colors. Tends to own toilet needs.	
36 months (3 years)	Can stand on one foot. Rides tricycle. Dresses self except for buttons. Confuses feet.	Constantly talking, asking "Why?" Uses pronouns accurately. Recites nursery rhymes. Copies circle. Often can identify five colors. Obeys commands, recognizing three prepositions. Dresses and undresses doll. Plays with others. Tells sex.	Visual acuity 20/20. May cooperate in testing of vibratory sensation and position sense.
48 months–54 months (4 years–4½ years)	Walks one foot to a step on stairs. Hops and skips on one foot. Throws ball overhand. Laces shoes.	Articulation no longer infantile. Tells fanciful stories. Copies cross and square. Counts three to four objects and answers "How many?" builds block building. Cooperates in play; boastful and critical.	

This table was modified from Gesell and Amatruda, *Developmental Diagnosis.* New York, Harper and Row, 1974. Also from Illingworth, *The Development of the Infant and Young Child. Normal and Abnormal.* New York, Churchill Livingstone, 1980.

FRONTAL

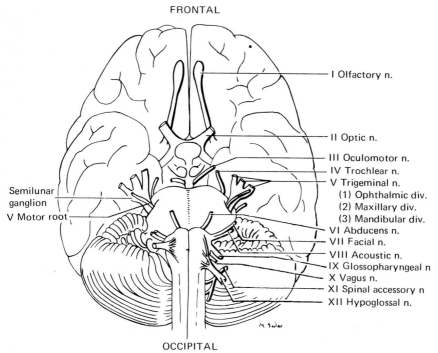

I Olfactory n.

II Optic n.

III Oculomotor n.
IV Trochlear n.
V Trigeminal n.
   (1) Ophthalmic div.
   (2) Maxillary div.
   (3) Mandibular div.
VI Abducens n.
VII Facial n.
VIII Acoustic n.
IX Glossopharyngeal n
X Vagus n.
XI Spinal accessory n
XII Hypoglossal n.

Semilunar
ganglion
V Motor root

OCCIPITAL

FIG. 1-4. Cranial nerves as viewed from the undersurface of the brain. (From Farmer TW: Cranial Nerves. In Cantor PD (ed): Traumatic Medicine and Surgery for the Attorney, Vol 4, p 445. Washington DC, Butterworth & Co, 1961)

used in testing olfaction, and that lacrimation thus provoked in an infant does not prove intact olfactory nerve function. A transient loss of smell commonly accompanies upper respiratory infections and may in some cases last several weeks or longer. A permanent loss frequently follows severe head injury, cranial operations, and diseases of the orbital parts of the frontal lobes. Unilateral loss of smell is characteristically seen with olfactory groove meningioma.

Optic (II) Nerve and Retina. The optic nerves, like the olfactory nerves, are direct extensions of the brain and are not peripheral nerves in a strict sense. Much can be learned from viewing the optic fundi, and ophthalmoscopy is an essential part of the neurologic examination of children. Since infants do not cooperate in funduscopy and may dislike it, a useful technique is to look at the fundi while the parent or assistant holds the child in his arms, fixing the head close to his own. Humming a nursery rhyme may distract the infant from the examination. Also, an interesting object held by an assistant may cause the patient to fix his gaze, thus facilitating the examination. If this is not successful, the patient should be restrained in the supine position. An exceptionally good view of the fundi may be had by examining the drowsy child. One should never omit examining the fundi because the child is uncooperative or the pupils are too small. If the examiner perseveres and, if necessary, instills a short-acting mydriatic, for example, 10% phenylephrine (Neo-Synephrine) or 1% cyclopentolate hydrochloride (Cyclogyl), the fundi can always be seen.

At birth and during the first few months of life the small vessels of the optic disk are poorly developed, so that normally they appear pale and gray, presenting an appearance similar to that of optic atrophy in later life. A deep cup of the optic nerve head, which appears white, may also be misinterpreted as optic atrophy at any age, but there is always a distinguishable rim of pinkness along the temporal margin. In myopia the choroid retracts from the temporal margin of the disk exposing the sclera. Deposits of pigment are frequently seen in this region (myopic crescents).

During childhood the disk margins are, compared with those of an adult, often indistinct and slightly elevated. This is especially the case in hyperopic eyes and may simulate papilledema. Other conditions that may be misinterpreted as papilledema include drusen, congenital maldevelopment of the disk, and medullated nerve fibers (Fig. 1-6).

In true papilledema, blurring of the disk margin is observed earliest on the nasal side and is associated with edema and streaking of the surrounding retina. Elevation of the nerve head (measured as the difference in diopters between the lenses used for visualizing vessels on the surface of the disk and those in the retina), progressive blurring of disk margins and of surrounding retina, obliteration of the optic cup, and distention and loss of pulsation of veins are seen in the more advanced stages of papilledema. Hemorrhages and exudates about

the optic disks are late signs of increased intracranial pressure except in cases of subarachnoid hemorrhage and in patients with primary vascular disease (Fig. 1-7). In the acute stages of optic neuritis the disk may appear normal, but if the pathologic process involves the nerve head itself (papillitis) the resultant ophthalmoscopic appearance may be indistinguishable from papilledema. The differential diagnosis is usually not difficult, however, because loss of visual acuity occurs early in optic neuritis and in the late stages of papilledema.

Retinal hemorrhages have been observed in 20% to 40% of all newborn infants. A relationship to vaginal delivery is apparent; in one study, 38% of infants delivered vaginally exhibited retinal hemorrhages versus 2.6% of those delivered by

FIG. 1-5. Base of the skull, illustrating the foramina through which the cranial nerves pass. (From Farmer TW: Cranial Nerves. In Cantor PD (ed): Traumatic Medicine and Surgery for the Attorney, Vol 4, p 445. Washington DC, Butterworth & Co, 1961)

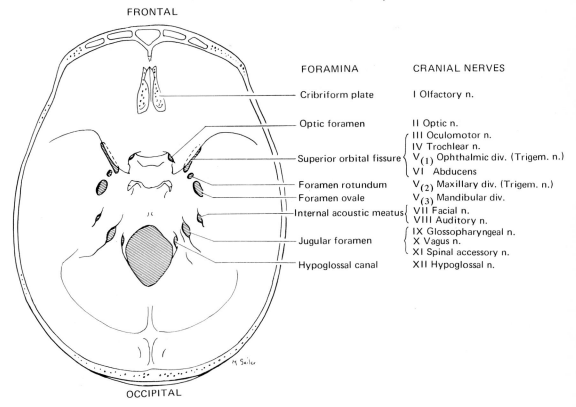

FRONTAL

FORAMINA	CRANIAL NERVES
Cribriform plate	I Olfactory n.
Optic foramen	II Optic n.
Superior orbital fissure	III Oculomotor n.
	IV Trochlear n.
	V(1) Ophthalmic div. (Trigem. n.)
	VI Abducens
Foramen rotundum	V(2) Maxillary div. (Trigem. n.)
Foramen ovale	V(3) Mandibular div.
Internal acoustic meatus	VII Facial n.
	VIII Auditory n.
Jugular foramen	IX Glossopharyngeal n.
	X Vagus n.
	XI Spinal accessory n.
Hypoglossal canal	XII Hypoglossal n.

OCCIPITAL

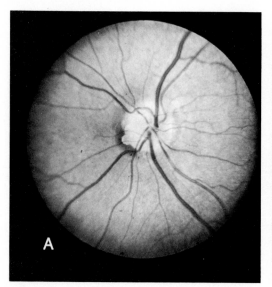
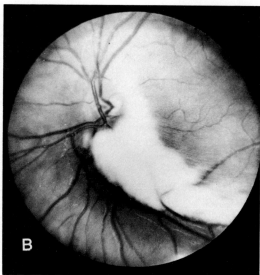

FIG. 1-6. Congenital defects of the optic disk that may be mistaken for papilledema. *A.* Drusen. *B.* Myelinated nerve fibers.

cesarean section. These hemorrhages generally resolve completely within approximately 4 days to 14 days.

The fundi should also be scrutinized for vascular lesions, colobomas, tumors, and degenerative changes. The macula is usually the site of maximal damage in congenital infections such as cytomegalic inclusion disease, toxoplasmosis, and syphilis. Perimacular deposition of lipoid in ganglion cells of the retina occurs in infantile cerebromacular degeneration (Tay-Sachs disease), the vascular macula appearing then to be a cherry-red spot surrounded by the whitish neurons.

Visual acuity can be tested in the older child by employing the standard test letters. Special cards picturing common toys and objects were developed by Allen for the preschool child.[1] A good estimate of visual acuity can often be obtained by watching the child at play. An infant who precisely picks a small crumb from the table obviously has reasonably good acuity. A comparison of visual acuity in the two eyes can be made by placing a patch over one eye at a time. Perfect alignment of the eyes and following movements are not seen during the first 3 months to 4 months of life, although even in the early weeks crude

fixation and the following of moving objects through a narrow range can usually be demonstrated. Even in the newborn there is sufficient fixation for the development of opticokinetic nystagmus in response to a rotating drum on the surface of which there are alternating vertical white and black stripes. Results of a number of techniques, such as varying the width of the vertical stripes on the opticokinetic drum, have led to the estimate that visual acuity approaches 20/20 sometime before 1 year of age.

Standard perimetry cannot be applied to the young infant, but his response in turning the head and eyes to a stimulus presented in one or the other visual field can be shown as early as 2.5 months to 3.0 months of age, and hemianopsia usually can be demonstrated conclusively by 4 months to 5 months of age. In testing visual fields in infants, brightly colored toys or a nursing bottle are particularly useful targets. Such objects are ideally presented from behind the patient (Fig. 1-8). Repeated testing on several occasions may be necessary to verify an asymmetry of responsiveness between sides.

A simple technique for testing opticokinetic nystagmus is to move slowly across the child's field of vision a piece of ordinary cloth on which a series of alternating animal figures or geometric patterns is printed on a plain background (Fig. 1-9). Normally the child fixes on each figure, follows it briefly, and then jerks his eyes back to follow the next figure. Adequate response requires that the child's attention be attracted to the figures, that there be sufficient visual acuity to see the objects, and that ocular movement be more or less intact. If opticokinetic nystagmus is asymmetrical, that is, more marked when the stimuli move away from a cerebral lesion, and absent or weak when the direction of movement is toward it, a disorder of visual attention on one side can be suspected. Opticokinetic nystagmus may also be absent when the stimulus is presented from a hemianopic field. It is similarly lost in parietal lobe lesions that do not affect visual field functions. Lesions of the brain stem may also interfere with the opticokinetic response.

Oculomotor, Trochlear, and Abducens (III, IV, VI) Nerves. Lateral and vertical movements of the eyes may be tested at the same time as visual fields. Ocular movement may also be tested by passively rotating, flexing, and extending the head (doll's head maneuver). During the early months of life it is normal for movements to be disconjugate at times, but generally the eyes move together in all directions. During this period ocular movements tend to be somewhat more jerky than is characteristic of those of the older child and adult.

Strabismus frequently occurs in children and is especially common in the age group 3 years to 6 years, when it is usually due to excessive convergence in association with hyperopia. The accommodative effort necessary to overcome the refractive error is accompanied by a turning in of one eye (esotropia). Since this frequently first becomes manifest in association with measles or other intercurrent disease, the strabismus is often erroneously attributed to the disease or to a muscle imbalance, whereas the more direct cause is a refractive error. At first intermittent, it may become constant, and the vision of the squinting eye may fail (amblyopia ex anopsia).

A functional strabismus may be differentiated from a paralytic strabismus because movements in the former are concomitant and full. With paralytic strabismus the dissociation of the eyes varies with the direction of gaze, and movement in the field of action of the paralyzed muscle is limited. Also, if full ocular movements are elicited in one eye when the other is covered, then a paralytic strabismus or ocular muscle palsy can be excluded. At times these maneuvers

FIG. 1-7. Early (A) and late (B) stages of papilledema. B. The edges of the disk are obscured in part by flame-shaped hemorrhages. Note also the extreme distention of the retinal veins.

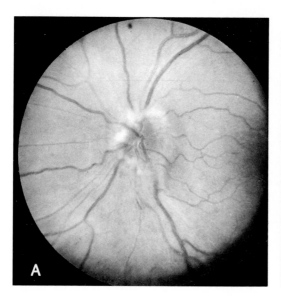

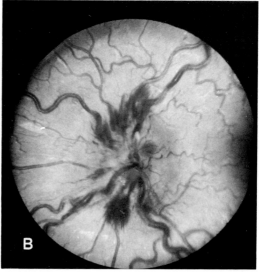

fail to induce movement in a nonparalytic strabismus and an erroneous diagnosis of paralytic strabismus is reached. In such a circumstance, putting a patch over the good eye should result in normal mobility of the affected eye within a matter of days. Binocular vision is acquired relatively late, and many children fix alternately with one or the other eye. This can often be demonstrated by covering and uncovering first one and then the other eye, with the recently uncovered eye fixing the target. If in this procedure one eye always fixes on the target and the other drifts away, it may be concluded that the eye that fixes is dominant. The young child who has not developed binocular vision does not close an eye or complain of diplopia even if he has a paralytic strabismus.

Adequate testing of extraocular muscle function requires a knowledge of the muscles' actions. For a comprehensive discussion of these, the reader is referred to Cogan.[2] A simplified, schematic summary

of the actions of the extraocular muscles and their nerve supply is presented in Figure 1-10.

In testing for extraocular muscle palsies in a child old enough to cooperate it is frequently useful to identify the images seen by each eye. This is easily done by placing a red glass over one and then systematically presenting a target light in the various fields of vision. The child is then asked to identify the relative position of the red and white images; normally a single red–white light is perceived. When an ocular palsy is suspected the degree of displacement and the directions of movements increasing and decreasing the separation of images are noted. Maximal displacement of images occurs in the field of action of the weakened muscle, the most peripherally seen image being that perceived by the eye with the paretic muscle. With either a medial or external rectus palsy, the image appears most lateral on horizontal gaze. If maximal displacement of images is demonstrated by vertical movement, the position of the eyes on the horizontal axis determines whether an oblique or rectus muscle is weak. In the adducted position an oblique muscle is primarily concerned with elevation and depression of the globe, and in the abducted position a rectus muscle is primar-

FIG. 1-8. Demonstration of a right visual field defect in a 10-month-old infant with a congenital lesion of the left cerebral hemisphere. *A.* She failed to turn to the toy hatchet when it was presented on the right side. *B.* She turned to hatchet in left visual field. Note also the attitude of the hemiparetic right hand.

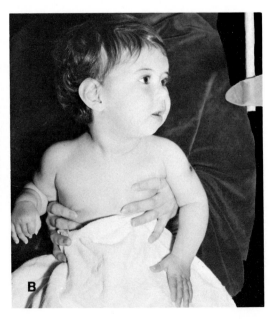

ily concerned. This method of analysis is obviously not applicable to the infant and young child in whom interpretations of an ocular palsy must be based on observation alone.

Sixth nerve palsies are probably most common, and a failure of abduction is usually easy to demonstrate (Fig. 1-11). The patient often rotates his head in the direction of the palsied lateral rectus muscle to compensate for the abducens weakness and to avoid diplopia. The combination of ptosis, a large pupil that is poorly reactive to light, and an outward, downward displacement of the eye with defective adduction and elevation are indicative of a third nerve palsy. With trochlear nerve involvement and weakness of the superior oblique muscle, the eye fails to move down when adducted and the head may be tilted away from the side of the paretic muscle.

Not infrequently an internuclear ophthalmoplegia (most often caused in childhood by brain stem tumor) may be confused with a medial rectus palsy. It is due to dysfunction of the medial longitudinal fasciculus, which carries nerve fibers from the abducens nucleus to the opposite oculomotor nuclear complex for adduction on volitional lateral gaze. There is an associated nystagmus in the abducting eye. Full adduction often occurs with convergence, but not from labyrinthine stimulation. Conjugate horizontal gaze palsies result from lesions of the cerebral hemisphere or brain stem. With unilateral hemisphere lesions, the eyes may deviate toward the side of the responsible lesion with the paralysis of gaze being to the opposite side. Unilateral seizure discharges cause conjugate deviation of the eyes to the opposite side. Such deviation is often intermittent, the eyes jerking rhythmically. Because of the decussation of the descending pathways for conjugate ocular movement, lesions of the brain stem cause deviation of the eyes to the opposite side and paralysis of gaze to the side of the lesion. Vertical gaze paralysis is always indicative of brain stem disease. Paralysis of upward gaze results from tectal region lesions and of downward gaze from periaqueductal lesions of the mesencephalon. Tumors of the pineal region and hydrocephalus are the most common causes of impaired upward

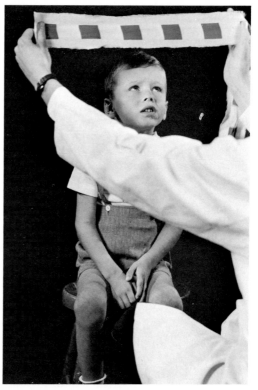

FIG. 1-9. Testing of opticokinetic nystagmus by moving a piece of printed cloth across the field of vision. Opticokinetic nystagmus was absent in this patient when the stimulus was brought in from the right side. He also had a right homonymous hemianopia and a supranuclear type of facial weakness, the latter of which is visible here. A hemorrhage into the left occipitoparietal region secondary to an antihemophilic globulin deficit was judged responsible. The deformed knees were the result of recurrent hemarthroses.

gaze in childhood. Gaze palsies of cerebral origin rarely persist for longer than a few days, whereas those due to brain stem disease are often permanent.

A Horner's syndrome from sympathetic nerve paralysis results in a mild ptosis, but in this instance there is also miosis and defective sweating over the face on the same side. When the syndrome is congenital a defect in pigmentation of the iris is usual: all or part of the iris remains blue. Ptosis may occur in primary disease of muscle or of neuromuscular transmission, as in muscular dystrophy, particularly of the myotonic variety, and in myasthenia gravis. In these conditions there is usually an associated weakness of the orbicularis oculi muscle as shown by weakness in closing the eye. In myasthenia gravis the weakness is aggravated by fatigue. Ptosis, which is influenced by motion of the jaw muscles (Marcus-Gunn phenomena), is usually noted first in childhood. This is probably the result of mixed innervation involving fibers of the fifth and third nerves. Aberrant regeneration within the third nerve complex resulting in abnormal association of movement such as opening the eyelid on downward gaze is occasionally seen in infants.

The size, regularity, and reactivity of pupils to light and in accommodation–convergence should be noted before mydriatics are used. Failure to record use of a mydriatic may give rise to much confusion. The effect of atropine may last for days.

A dilated pupil that fails to constrict in response to a bright light but does so when the other eye is illuminated (consensual response) implies that the afferent limb (retina or nerve) of the pupillary reflex is involved. In such a circumstance the eye is usually blind because the pupillary reaction is lost late in disease. Pupillary responses are normal in children with cortical blindness, and these children usually blink to a bright light. Involvement of the parasympathetic nerve fibers in the third nerve gives rise to a large pupil that reacts poorly or not at all to light (directly or consensually) or in accommodation.

A dilated pupil that reacts briskly in accommodation but only slowly in response to an intense light source is frequently referred to as a tonic or Adies pupil. Such a pupil constricts readily when a drop or two of 2.5% mecholyl is placed in the conjunctival sac. Absent ankle jerks are fre-

FIG. 1-10. Ocular muscles involved in conjugate movement of eyes in various directions of gaze.

RIGHT UPWARD GAZE

Rt. superior rectus III   Lt. inferior oblique III

LEFT UPWARD GAZE

Rt. inferior oblique III   Lt. superior rectus III

RIGHT LATERAL GAZE

Rt. external rectus VI   Lt. medial rectus III

LEFT LATERAL GAZE

Rt. medial rectus III   Lt. external rectus VI

RIGHT DOWNWARD GAZE

Rt. inferior rectus III   Lt. superior oblique IV

LEFT DOWNWARD GAZE

Rt. superior oblique IV   Lt. inferior rectus III

quently associated with an Adies pupil. A tonic pupil is also seen in familial dysautonomia (Riley-Day syndrome). A transient, unreactive enlargement of the pupil may follow direct trauma to the eye or may accompany a seizure; in the latter instance the pupil on the side of the seizure discharge is most often involved.

Small, irregular pupils that react in accommodation but not to light (Argyll Robertson pupils) occur in juvenile paresis and tabes dorsalis. The small pupil found in Horner's syndrome was alluded to earlier. Finally, a difference in pupillary size (anisocoria) without other abnormalities may be of no clinical importance.

The presence or absence of nystagmus in the primary position and in all four directions of gaze should be noted. The direction of the nystagmus is determined by the fast component.

Sustained jerk nystagmus indicates impaired vestibular function, which may arise from disease or dysfunction of the labyrinth or its central connections within brain stem and cerebellum. Elaborate schemes of localizing the site of disease by the form and direction of the nystagmus have been proposed, but most of these are of limited clinical value. Pure vertical nystagmus is always indicative of brain stem dysfunction, however. In cerebellar disease lateral nystagmus is usually coarser and of greater amplitude when the gaze is directed toward the side of the lesion. Rotatory nystagmus is seen with labyrinthine disease but is observed also when central vestibular mechanisms are affected. In labyrinthine disease the nystagmus is fine, often rotary, and maximal in a certain direction of gaze; it is associated with vertigo, nausea, and vomiting. Seesaw nystagmus, in which the eyes actually rise and fall alternately, is rare and cannot be localized to specific anatomic structures, but has been seen along with bitemporal hemianopia from suprasellar mass lesions that also extend along the clivus into the posterior fossa. In blind infants and children, irregular, oscillating, wandering, and searching eye movements of marked amplitude without a rapid jerk component are characteristic. In congenital nystagmus and in spasmus nutans of ocular origin to-and-fro, jellylike oscillations of one or both eyes are characteristic, and slow and

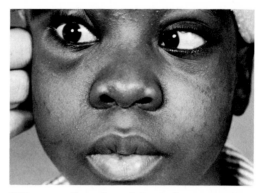

FIG. 1-11. Complete right sixth nerve palsy in a young boy. The asymmetrical reflections of light from the corneal surfaces are striking.

fast components of the nystagmus are usually not evident.

Trigeminal (V) Nerve. The motor division of this nerve supplies the muscles of mastication. Unilateral paralysis of these muscles is indicated by a deviation of the jaw to that side on opening the mouth and, if chronic, by atrophy of the temporal muscles revealed by hollowing of the temporal fossae. The latter finding associated with a constantly open mouth and malocclusion are characteristic features of myotonic dystrophy. The jaw jerk, a stretch reflex involving the masseter muscles, is elicited by a gentle downward tap of the reflex hammer on the examiner's finger resting on the chin. A brisk or accentuated jaw jerk indicates bilateral corticobulbar tract disease.

Disturbances of the sensory division of the fifth cranial nerve, which provides most of the face and scalp with all modalities of sensation, are manifested by numbness and paresthesias over the face or scalp. These may be complained of by the older child. The cutaneous distribution of its three divisions (ophthalmic, maxillary, and mandibular) are illustrated in Figure 1-12. All but a small pie-shaped inferior segment of the cornea, which is innervated by the second or maxillary division, is subserved by the ophthalmic division. A defective corneal reflex should be suspected when spontaneous blinking is slower and less complete on the affected side. This must be interpreted cautiously in very young infants because normally they may blink in

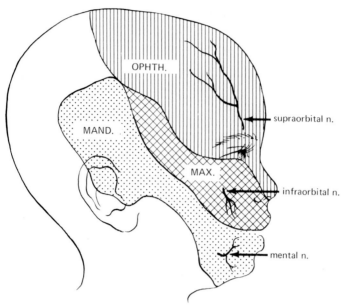

FIG. 1-12. Segmental innervation of the skin by the major sensory divisions of the trigeminal nerve. Note that the skin over much of the lower jaw is not innervated by this nerve but rather by the second cervical nerve. It is not clearly shown that a pie-shaped inferior segment of the cornea is supplied by the maxillary division. The posterior extent of the trigeminal innervation over the scalp and the innervation over the nose by the first and second divisions of the fifth cranial nerve are variable.

an asymmetrical fashion. In testing the corneal reflex, using a wisp of cotton, care should be taken to present the stimulus from the side to minimize the visual cue. Although impaired facial sensation may result from numerous causes, in childhood the most common one is probably tumor, usually a glioma of the brain stem or a neurofibroma, sarcoma, or undifferentiated tumor at the base of the skull or of the cerebellopontine angle.

Facial (VII) Nerve.   The facial nerve is divided into motor and sensory divisions; the former supplies the muscles of facial expression, and the latter, through the chorda tympani, innervates taste buds over the anterior two-thirds of the tongue. With disease of the facial nucleus or whole nerve trunk, facial weakness is usually severe, involving all muscles on the affected side. Facial asymmetry is striking, accentuated on

attempted movement, and often most obvious when the infant or child laughs or cries.

Corticobulbar weakness of facial musculature is manifested by a slightly widened lid slit and drooping lower angle of the mouth on the side opposite the anatomic or physiologic lesion (Fig. 1-9). This is usually accentuated on volitional innervation of facial muscles, retraction of the corner of the mouth being weaker than eye closure. Wrinkling of the brow, however, is typically normal. In contrast, during laughing or crying the facial expression is often normal without asymmetry. In bilateral corticobulbar facial weakness, tapping the corner of the mouth with a reflex hammer often demonstrates a heightened stretch reflex analogous to an exaggerated jaw jerk.

After noting the presence of asymmetry about the mouth in the very young infant, the inexperienced examiner may have difficulty deciding which side of the face is weak. Isolated weakness of the depressor and retractor of the lower lip is a common form of facial weakness during early childhood and is manifested by an excessive elevation of the corner of the lip on the unaffected side. The site of the lesion is unknown in such cases, but clearly it must be a peripheral one. A total lack of expression, even with crying and laughing, is a feature of the

Möbius syndrome. In this condition a peripheral type of bilateral facial paralysis is usually associated with weakness of abduction of the eyes and other congenital abnormalities. Impairment of peripheral facial nerve function during early infancy results in poor sucking. The older infant or child frequently drools on the side of the facial weakness. Tearing due to corneal irritation, a result of impaired closure of the eyelid, is frequent in peripheral facial palsies.

With disease of the facial nerve, proximal to the point where the chorda tympani joins it, there is impaired taste sensation. It is of course difficult to assess taste function in the infant or young child, although a defect may be suspected from a delayed response to placement of an unpleasant substance like quinine on the affected side, with the normal side acting as a control.

In the older child a response to salt, sugar, and quinine can be evaluated by grasping the tongue with a clean cloth and applying the test solution with a cotton swab. In testing taste the patient should not withdraw the tongue into the mouth until he has nodded a response to the question, "Do you taste something?" The tongue is then wiped clean and the patient permitted to withdraw it and identify the test solution. Practically speaking, it is necessary to evaluate taste sensation only when involvement of associated cranial nerves or brain stem is suspected.

Acoustic (VIII) Nerve. The auditory and vestibular nerves originate in the end organs in the cochlea and labyrinth and course together through the temporal bone to central nuclei in the brain stem.

Auditory Division. The physician is often called upon to evaluate a child's hearing. Hearing loss should be suspected when speech development is delayed or when a child does not respond to being called. Deafness in a single ear usually goes unrecognized until the child receives a routine hearing examination in school.

A valid impression of the intactness of hearing can usually be obtained by asking the mother if the young infant responds to soft music or the spoken voice. The parents often report that the deaf child is startled when, not having heard them approach, he first sees them at the bedside. A variety of crude methods may be used to assess hearing in the infant and young child. The examiner, by mimicking a cat, dog, or other familiar animal, or by softly calling the patient's name, may elicit a smile or response that leaves little doubt that the stimulus was perceived. A tuning fork, soft click, bell, or rattling of keys may evoke a response and give some idea of hearing localization. A negative response, for example, turning away the head when the examiner speaks, can be reasonably interpreted as indicating intact hearing. If one fails to elicit a response by these methods, it may be necessary to refer the patient for audiometric study. It is surprising how often a response to music or voice of low intensity can be evoked when presented through a loudspeaker into a soundproof room. This is particularly valuable in differentiating between a simple perceptual defect and a defect due to inattention, autism, or impairment of audition at a central level. Because hearing is registered bilaterally in the brain, deafness does not result from unilateral cerebral disease. For a proper evaluation of hearing in the older child, formal audiometric methods must be employed. Evoked potential brain stem audiometry is especially useful for testing the hearing of infants and uncooperative older children because drug-induced sleep does not interfere with the response.

Vestibular Division. Increased or decreased sensitivity of the labyrinth results in vestibular imbalance and its cardinal symptom, vertigo. This is not often encountered as a clinical problem in infants or young children, in contrast to its frequent occurrence in adults. The older child may experience acute labyrinthine vertigo with severe vomiting associated with acute disease of the middle ear. Associated tinnitus and deafness, common in the older patient, are often absent. The precise nature of this illness, sometimes called *acute toxic labyrinthitis,* is not clear.

Dizziness is a common complaint of adolescents, but on close questioning one finds that this is generally not of a vertiginous nature but a sensation of lightheadedness often precipitated by rapid assumption of the upright from the recumbent position.

The presence of intact vestibular function can be demonstrated even in the neonate by holding the infant under the arms and rotating him in one or the other direction. The eyes deviate in the direction of rotation with intermittent nystagmus to the opposite direction. Although the neonate's eyes remain closed much of the time, they nearly always stay open during rotation. An absence of response to rotation is strongly suggestive of impaired vestibular function in all but the neonate, in whom it is inconclusive. The labyrinth may be stimulated by a variety of other means, including instillation of cold water into the external auditory canal with the patient supine and the head flexed 30 degrees. This drives the eyes conjugately toward the stimulated ear with nystagmus developing in the opposite direction.

Glossopharyngeal and Vagus (IX, X) Nerves. The ninth and tenth nerves are generally tested together. Difficulty in swallowing and a change in the quality of the voice are common symptoms attributable to dysfunction of these nerves or of their nucleus of origin (n. ambiguus). In testing, the response of the soft palate to saying *ah* is noted. A palatal paralysis results in sagging of the palate on that side and failure to elevate when uttering the test sound. Regurgitation of liquid through the nose because the soft palate fails to obstruct the nasopharynx may occur during swallowing. The gag reflex is subserved by afferent and efferent portions of the vagus nerve and is examined by rubbing a cotton-tipped stick against the posterior wall of the pharynx. The responses of the two sides should be compared. Since there is normally great variation in activity of the gag reflex among people, only strikingly asymmetrical responses can be interpreted as definitely abnormal. Dysphagia and impaired palatal movement occur with supranuclear (pseudobulbar) weakness, but in this circumstance the palate elevates normally in response to sensory stimulation of the posterior pharyngeal wall. Asymmetry of the palate may result from removal of tonsils and adenoids and have no neurologic significance. Also, the uvula adheres so frequently to one side of the soft palate that its behavior in testing palatal function may be misleading.

The larynx must be examined by direct or indirect laryngoscopy. Normally the vocal cords are abducted during inspiration and adducted during phonation and coughing. Unilateral weakness of adduction is usually compensated for by movement of the healthy vocal cord across the midline toward the paralyzed side. When there is bilateral vocal cord paralysis, the cords tend to approximate one another and stridor results. Stridor occurs commonly in children with inflammation of the vocal cords and in tetany. It may also result from impaired coordination of the laryngeal muscles in patients with supranuclear lesions. In such instances breathing irregularities are common.

The dorsal efferent nucleus of the vagus gives rise to the parasympathetic fibers of the vagus nerve that innervate the heart and smooth muscle of the trachea, bronchi, bronchioles, and alimentary tract. These functions are not easily examined. The glossopharyngeal nerve provides taste sensation for the posterior third of the tongue, and both the ninth and tenth cranial nerves innervate small portions of the external auditory canal and pinna of the ear. This is usually of no clinical significance, although reflex coughing during otoscopic examination of the tympanic membrane is said to result from stimulation of these sensory nerve endings.

Spinal Accessory (XI) Nerve. The spinal accessory nerve supplies the sternocleidomastoid and upper portion of the trapezius muscles. The sternocleidomastoid is tested by having the patient forcibly rotate his head against resistance. The contracting muscle can be seen and felt during this maneuver. Torticollis in the young infant may result from hypertrophy and fibrosis of this muscle. This restricts neck motion and leads secondarily to scoliosis capitis and facial asymmetry. The torticollis of sternocleidomastoid fibrosis can be distinguished from torticollis determined by an imbalance of postural reflexes by permitting the neck to hyperextend passively while slowly lifting the infant's body off the examining table. The contractured muscle is usually obvious in this position and reflex torticollis disappears. The upper part of the trapezius muscle is tested by having the patient elevate his shoulder. The strength of movement and the bulk of muscle may be assessed by this maneuver.

Hypoglossal (XII) Nerve. The muscles of the tongue are supplied by the twelfth or hypoglossal nerve. Atrophy and fasciculation can be seen when the nucleus or nerve is diseased. On protrusion, the tongue deviates to the side of the weakness. In the infant or young child there is ordinarily a considerable amount of irregular movement of the tongue when it is slightly protruded or at rest, so that clinically significant fasciculations and choreoathetosis may be difficult to identify. Dysarthria and dysphagia result when tongue movement is impaired from any cause, but in pseudobulbar paralysis atrophy and fasciculations are absent.

In the infant an enlarged tongue is seen in various disorders including cretinism, mongolism, gargoylism, and macroglossia. In the older child tapping the tongue with a percussion hammer against a throat stick placed on the lower teeth is an excellent way of demonstrating myotonia (Fig. 1-13).

Motor System

Evaluation of tone and power of muscles in the premature infant must be made with an awareness of important developmental changes that occur. Thus, at 28 weeks of gestation there is minimal resistance to passive manipulation in all limbs, but by 32 weeks distinct flexor tone becomes apparent in the lower extremities. By term, strong flexor tone is apparent in all extremities. These changes in tone of limb muscles are accompanied by concomitant changes in power. In addition, neck extensor power becomes strong enough at 36 weeks of gestation to maintain the head in upright posture for a few seconds when the infant is held sitting. By term, neck extensor power is adequate to maintain the head in the same plane as the rest of the body for several seconds when the infant is held in ventral suspension.

The value of watching the spontaneous activity of an infant or observing an

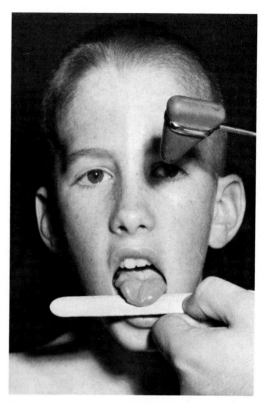

FIG. 1-13. Myotonic response of the tongue in a child with myotonic dystrophy. The right side was percussed with a reflex hammer a moment before this picture was taken. Note the lump caused by the prolonged contraction of muscle fibers.

older child at play cannot be overemphasized. Gross defects in movement and a lack of facility or coordination in carrying out certain skilled motor acts are readily detected. The unwanted movements of dystonia and choreoathetosis frequently can be analyzed in detail before the patient is aware that he is being examined. The mobility of a child must always be compared with what is average for the particular age. A slow, clumsy grasping of a proffered object is normal at 6 months to 7 months of age but is quite abnormal at a year. A tottering gait is to be expected at 15 months, but in a child of 3 years it is distinctly abnormal and suggests cerebellar or some other motor or sensory disorder.

One must be alert to obvious differences in motor function of various parts of the body. For example, an infant of 18 months who is facile with the use of fingers and hands, alert, and communicating well verbally for his age, yet scooting about the floor in the sitting position rather than walking, almost certainly has a defect in motor function of the lower extremities.

Although some normal children begin walking on tiptoes, persistence of this motor pattern always suggests spasticity or a contracture of gastrocnemius muscles. This is also seen as a presenting symptom in pseudohypertrophic muscular dystrophy. If in addition there is a scissoring motion of the legs in walking, there is almost certainly spasticity of the legs. Weakness of dorsiflexion of the feet with a constant flapping gait is common in polyneuropathies and is not uncommonly seen in lower leg paralysis resulting from congenital defects in the region of the cauda equina.

The school-age child who walks with a broad-based gait and is unable to walk tandem or hop on one leg or the other may have disease of the vermis of the cerebellum or of its connections. A combination of lordosis and waddling as the child walks with inability to climb stairs is characteristic of proximal muscle weakness and is particularly common in various myopathies (progressive muscular dystrophies and polymyositis). The association of extension of the fingers and flexion of the thumb at the metacarpophalangeal joints, pronation of the arm at the elbow, and progressive retroflexion of the arm at the shoulder during walking is pathognomonic of dystonia. Often there is a phasic reversal of this pattern with assumption of an attitude of flexion of these parts. This and associated writhing movements of face and trunk are the salient features of athetosis. Progressive twisting of the trunk, torticollis, inversion and plantar flexion of the foot that increases with effort, and an exaggerated lumbar lordosis with tendency for the thigh to flex on the abdomen while standing and walking are also features of the dystonic state.

If the examiner is patient during this preliminary period of observation, one after another of the various major muscle groups will be called into play in the normal random activity of an infant. It may be difficult to ascertain the strength of individual muscles and muscle groups in the infant or

TABLE 1-2. Code for Grading Muscle Power

Grade	Characteristic	Muscle Power (%)
0	No muscular contraction	0
1	Trace, visible contraction without motion of joint	10
2	Movement at joint but not against gravity	25
3	Full movement at joint against gravity, variable resistance	50
4	Resists opposing force of moderate strength	75
5	Maximal resistance	100

young child, however, and to do so taxes the ingenuity of the examiner. In the cooperative older child, testing motor power of specific muscle groups poses no real problem. Whenever disease of the lower motor neuron is suspected, muscles should be tested individually and their strength estimated (Table 1-2).

Considerable fat overlying the muscles of an infant usually precludes an adequate analysis of the muscle by palpation and obscures fasciculations; but at any age, whenever weakness is encountered along with atrophy and fasciculations, disease of the lower motor neurons is present. The belly of the muscle should be percussed with a reflex hammer, looking for the prolonged contraction of the muscle fibers that is characteristic of myotonia.

In addition to the above observations, the response of the muscles to passive manipulation and stretch should be tested. It often takes considerable time to achieve complete relaxation, but this is essential before a statement can be made as to basic muscle tone. Those muscles most affected by spasticity are the flexors of the upper extremities, flexors and adductors of the hips, extensors of the knees, and plantar flexors of the feet (Fig. 1-14). Rapid passive supination of the forearm at the elbow elicits a spastic reaction of the pronator muscles in even slight degrees of spasticity. Spasticity of the adductors of the hips explains why the mother of a child with spas-

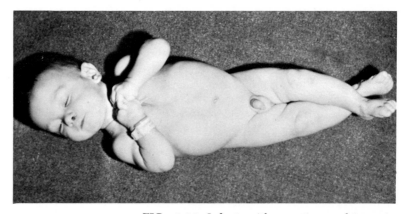

FIG. 1-14. Infant with spastic quadriparesis, demonstrating clenched fists, flexed arms, and extended legs. Marked spasticity of the adductors of the hips accounted for the "scissoring" or crossing of the legs. This is the same infant as in Figures 1-15 through 1-17.

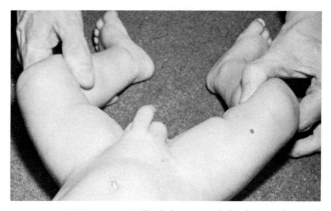

FIG. 1-15. Full abduction of the legs is limited by spasticity of the adductors of the hips. This is the same infant as in Figures 1-14, 1-16, and 1-17.

tic diplegia commonly complains of difficulty in passively abducting the legs at the hips during bathing and changing the diapers (Fig. 1-15). With an infant in the recumbent position, passive dorsiflexion of the foot at the ankle or gentle abduction of the legs at the hip meets with firm resistance if spasticity exists. If the examiner persists with steady pressure, the resisting muscles suddenly give way in a clasp-knife or lengthening reaction characteristic of all spastic muscle (Fig. 1-16). Often children

with severely damaged nervous systems suffer from a combined spastic and extrapyramidal rigidity. In rigidity of extrapyramidal origin the resistance to passive movement is more or less constant throughout a full range of movement, and the clasp-knife reaction is not encountered.

In contrast to infants with increased resistance to passive movement, the extremities of the hypotonic or floppy child may be flexed and extended about joints with ease. The head often lolls about when the infant is held upright, and when he is held under the arms it tends to slip through the examiner's hands. Such hypotonia is often congenital and may be related to a variety of central and peripheral neuro-muscular disorders. For example, it is striking in children with mongolism, spinal muscular atrophy, and various forms of myopathy. Hypotonia is a characteristic finding in the infant with atonic cerebral

diplegia, although spasticity supervenes as the child grows older. Similarly, the 3-year-old child with choreoathetosis and variable rigidity has usually been hypotonic as a young infant.

Coordination as related to gait was mentioned previously. Impaired coordination of breathing and speech mechanisms due to cerebellar disorder is frequently expressed in a rhythmic tremor of the voice with noticeable waxing and waning in volume as the patient attempts to sustain a note in singing.

Tests of cerebellar function requiring the performance of rapidly alternating movements are of limited value unless one appreciates the normal lack of facility most children display in carrying out such tasks.

FIG. 1-16. Testing resistance to passive stretch of the plantar flexors of the foot in an infant with a spastic quadriparesis. There was a history of jaundice and hypoxia in the neonatal period. *A.* Considerable resistance to lengthening of the muscle was encountered. *B.* This was accomplished suddenly, however (clasp-knife reaction). This is the same infant as in Figures 1-14, 1-15, and 1-17.

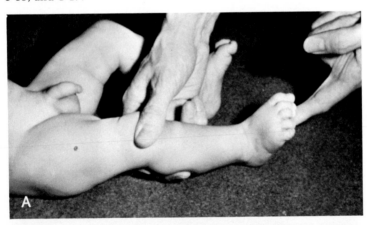

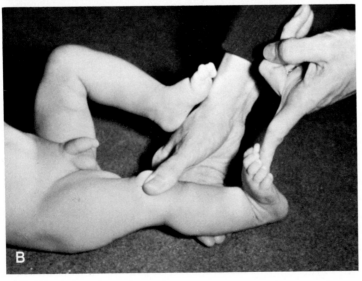

Ataxia with rhythmic tremor of extremities is demonstrable on finger-to-nose and heel-to-shin testing. The child who fails to cooperate in these tests can usually be coaxed into reaching for a marble or touching with finger or toe some small object such as the nose of a doll. Accentuation of the tremor as the patient approaches the target is characteristic of the cerebellar or intention tremor. Benign or essential tremor (sometimes called *action tremor*) has the same amplitude of excursion throughout an intended act. The anatomy of this tremor is poorly understood, although dysfunction of the red nucleus and its connections has been postulated.

Involuntary movements of athetosis and dystonia have been commented on in relation to disorders of gait because they are so accentuated by movement. All of their characteristics are visible in the sitting or recumbent positions, and reaching for objects or an attempted change in posture emphasizes this point. The increased writhing, grotesque postures, and attitudes on intention illustrate how a simple act is almost indescribably complicated by the involuntary activation of muscle groups unessential for the act. The unwanted participation of these muscles, a phenomenon referred to as *intention spasm*, impedes the success of the intended action. If complete relaxation can be achieved with the patient lying in the prone position, all involuntary movement may temporarily cease and the associated rigidity vanish.

In contrast to the writhing distortions of body parts characteristic of dystonia and athetosis, choreiform movement is rapid and displacement of body parts momentary, although another choreiform jerk may almost immediately draw the face, digit, arm, leg, or trunk in another direction. Breathing may be interrupted by a sudden expulsion of air and audible grunt. Such irregular jerks are unpredictable and do not occur in a definite sequence or pattern. Almost pure movements of this type are seen in Sydenham's chorea, whereas an admixture of chorea, athetosis, and dystonia occur in most other congenital and acquired extrapyramidal disease states. The so-called resting or parkinsonian tremor evoked by minimal sustained effort is rarely encountered in children with extrapyramidal disease.

Habit spasm or tic may at times be difficult to distinguish from involuntary movements. Simple and even complex tics, however, tend to be repeated in a stereotyped fashion and, more importantly, are controllable for brief periods. If the child is old enough, he always appreciates and reports that the tic movement is voluntary and that making the movement relieves tension or makes him "feel better." The patient has no control over the choreiform movement, and no relief of tension is afforded by it.

All tremors and involuntary movements disappear with sleep, with the exception of the myoclonic jerks and clonic seizures. Since irregular myoclonic jerks can be confused with other involuntary movements, their persistence during sleep may be an important diagnostic point. *Jitteriness* is the term that best describes the coarse tremulousness observed in the neonatal period. Jitteriness can be distinguished from seizure at the bedside if the following points are recalled: (1) in jitteriness there is no abnormality of ocular movement, whereas in seizure there almost always is; (2) the movements of jitteriness are exquisitely stimulus-sensitive but convulsive movements are not; (3) the rhythmic movements of jitteriness principally resemble tremor, that is, they are of equal rate and amplitude, whereas the clonic jerking of seizure exhibits a fast and slow component; and (4) the movements of jitteriness can be stopped with gentle passive flexion of the affected limb, whereas convulsive movements will not cease with that maneuver.

Sensory System

A proper sensory examination is most difficult at any age. It is particularly difficult in the infant or young child who is unable to describe his feelings adequately. One must then often be content to use the child's change in facial expression or withdrawal of a part in response to tickle (subserved by touch mechanisms) or to painful stimuli, usually applied as a pinprick, as evidence that the stimulus was perceived. In addition, it is often possible to condition an older infant or young child to smile in response to vibration, whereas the tuning fork applied without vibration elicits a different reaction. In a bright child as young as 3 years to 5 years, a surprisingly complete sensory examination, including position sense testing, recognition of objects placed in the hand, and touch localization, can often be carried out. The brandishing of a pin by the examiner is cause for alarm in most children. The author usually enlists cooperation in the testing of pain perception, even from a fearful child, by handing *him* the pin and having him test sensation over various parts of his body.

Reflexes

Certain reflex functions appear and evolve during fetal life. A considerable number of important reflexes are present at birth and should be examined routinely in the newborn. Absence or distortion of certain of these reflexes can usually be interpreted as evidence of significant dysfunction of the infantile nervous system, although it may be difficult to make a precise statement about the level or levels of disorganization. Most of the reflexes found in the neonate and young infant may be elicited in children lacking cerebral hemispheres, indicating that the brain stem and more caudal levels of the nervous system are sufficient to subserve them. Presumably our testing is concerned primarily with an evaluation of these parts.

The following may be considered among the more important reflexes that are not considered elsewhere in this chapter.

Sucking Reflex. The sucking reflex is prominent in the newborn once the effect of anesthesia used during delivery has worn off. The examiner's finger placed in approximation to the lips leads to a movement of the lips (cardinal points) in the direction of the stimulus, orienting the mouth in line with it. The reflexogenous zone may extend for a variable distance over the face. Most infants turn the head toward a light contactual stimulus applied to the cheek (rooting response). Once the finger enters the oral cavity, the lips of the infant close about it and produce rhythmic sucking movements, in which the tongue participates. The vigor of the response is some indication of the infant's potential effectiveness in nursing. In the premature infant or the term infant with neurologic disease, sucking may be extremely weak and pre-

clude effective oral feeding for a variable period of time. The concerted action of sucking, swallowing, and breathing necessary for oral feeding develops as early as 28 weeks of gestation. However, the ability to maintain synchrony of these motor functions to ensure productive oral feeding is not present until approximately 32 weeks to 34 weeks. It should be pointed out that the vigor of the suck and the persistence of sucking appear conditioned, at least in part, by the state of hunger or satiation of the infant. The sucking reflex persists for a variable period in childhood though it usually becomes more discriminating and modified by volition after the first few months of life. Reflex sucking may persist for a longer period in the drowsy normal infant and in the patient with congenital or acquired cerebral disease.

Grasp Reflex. If the examiner's finger or other object is placed within the palm of an infant, flexor tonus is enhanced and reflex grasping occurs. Tone is increased synergistically in other flexor muscles of the arm, and if facilitated by stretch, a full-term infant can at times be suspended by the object he is holding. Palmar grasp is clearly present at 28 weeks of gestation, is strong at 32 weeks, and is powerful enough and associated with enough spread to upper extremity muscles to allow the infant to be lifted from the bed at 37 weeks. In contrast to the grasp reflex seen with acquired cerebral disease of later life, a moving tactile stimulus is usually not necessary. An identical grasping response is demonstrable in the infant's foot, but for its elicitation, pressure applied to the ball of the foot is often required. Opening of the hand and release of the foot grasp can be elicited by tactile stimulation over the dorsum of these parts. The ease with which the grasp reflex can be elicited in the infant decreases over the first 2 months to 3 months of life as physiologic mechanisms subserving volitional grasping and prehension appear. Thus after the early weeks of life the examiner can no longer elicit the infantile type of grasp response in the hand, although it may persist normally in the foot well into the second year.

Moro Reflex. In the Moro reflex the patient's back is extended, the arms extended and abducted, and the hands and fingers held wide open. The arms are then brought forward over the chest with flexion at the elbows and wrists. Associated extension of the legs at the knees and hips is inconsistently present. This response can be elicited by a variety of means that have in common extension of the neck, but dropping of the head, held a few inches off the table with the examiner's hand supporting the body behind the shoulders, is most effective. The reflex undergoes a definable evolution with maturation. Thus, hand-opening is the principal manifestation at 28 weeks of gestation, followed at 32 weeks by extension and abduction of upper extremities with audible cry, and at 37 weeks by anterior flexion of upper extremities. Mild asymmetries and incompleteness of the response are difficult to evaluate, but total absence of movement is seen in infants with a generalized suppression of neural activity such as occurs in perinatal hypoxia. Local disease, such as a fractured clavicle or brachial plexus paralysis, may account for the failure of one arm to respond. An apparently normal Moro response is described in infants lacking both cerebral hemispheres. However, in such circumstances the reflex is stereotyped and does not habituate (*i.e.,* there is no response decrement with repeated elicitation of the reflex). The response is usually suppressed by 3 months to 4 months of age, although what are probably fragments of this reflex persist into childhood as a startle reaction.

Tonic Neck Reflexes. The tonic neck reflexes play an important role in the development of motor mechanisms. If the infant's head turns or is turned sharply to either side while he is in the recumbent position, extension of the arm and leg on the side to which the infant is looking and flexion of the opposite members occur. This pattern is reversed if the head is turned in the other direction. There may be a brief delay in assumption of the tonic neck posture in the newborn, but a more immediate reaction and a fuller response can be expected in the infant a few weeks of age. The variability of this reflex in the newborn dictates caution in its interpretation, although a striking asymmetry of response is usually abnormal. The mere absence of participation of an upper extremity does not constitute a pathologic response, or at least not an interpretable abnormality. These reflexes merge gradually into voluntary movement patterns, and by 4 months of life an obligatory tonic neck response should not be elicitable. Its persistence beyond this time is worrisome and frequently seen in children who are later noted to have severe motor disorders, especially of the extrapyramidal sort (Fig. 1-17). It should be pointed out, however, that fragments of the tonic neck response may normally be observed well into the second year of life as an alteration in flexor and extensor tone of the arms on turning the head.

FIG. 1-17. The posture of the infant shown here is determined by abnormally active tonic neck reflexes. This is the same infant as in Figures 1-14 through 1-16.

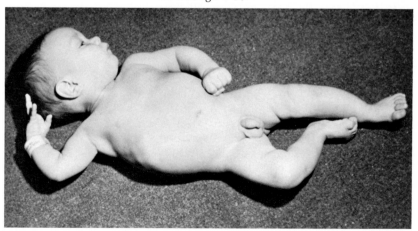

Plantar Reflex. The plantar reflex, one of the most important reflexes in neurology, is elicited by applying a noxious stimulus to the heel and drawing it forward along the lateral surface of the plantar aspect of the foot. Normally there is brisk plantar flexion of the toes, including the great one. Dorsiflexion of the great toe and fanning of the other toes (Babinski sign) are indicative of corticospinal tract disease. In normal babies the usual response is plantar flexion during the newborn period, but for the remainder of the first year of life dorsiflexion of the great toe is frequently observed.[7] By 1 year of age the response of plantar flexion obtains in approximately half of the normal infantile population and should be present in all children before the age of 2. Interpretation of what constitutes an abnormal plantar reflex during infancy may therefore be difficult. Nevertheless, an abnormal response can often be suspected when there is a slow movement of dorsiflexion limited to the great toe. A difference between the two sides may also lead the examiner to suspect an abnormal response. The infant with unilateral brain disease usually has more definite dorsiflexion on the side of the hemiparesis.

Abdominal Reflexes. The superficial abdominal reflexes are tested by stroking the skin with a pin in all four quadrants of the abdomen. Contraction of the underlying muscles should draw the umbilicus in the direction of the stimulus. Abdominal reflexes can always be obtained in the newborn if time is taken for their demonstration. On casual examination they are frequently difficult to elicit until 6 months to 12 months of life. Depression or absence of the reflex is seen on the side of acquired corticospinal tract disease. Curiously, the reflex is usually unimpaired in patients with congenital brain disease.

Tendon Reflexes. The tendon reflexes are muscle stretch reflexes obtained by sharply tapping the tendon of the muscle to be tested. A single synapse is interposed between the sensory and motor neurons so that there is only a short latency before the muscle contracts. Interference with the sensory or motor limb of the reflex arc results in lost or decreased activity of the tendon reflex. The spinal cord segments responsible for the various tendon reflexes are listed in Table 1-3. Increased activity of a tendon reflex, often with repetitive contractions alternating with relaxation of the muscle (clonus), is indicative of corticospinal tract disease except during the early weeks of life when unsustained ankle clonus is commonly obtained in normal infants. On the other hand, because of the predominance of flexor tone in the newborn, the inexperienced examiner may fail to elicit the tendon reflexes until the muscle of the reflex to be tested is properly positioned under optimal tension.

Autonomic Nervous System

The autonomic nervous system is concerned with regulation of body temperature, pupillary responses, and many glandular and visceral functions. The craniosacral or parasympathetic division of the autonomic nervous system has its preganglionic neurons within the brain stem and sacral portion of the spinal cord. Fibers from these neurons course with various cranial and pelvic nerves and synapse with neurons in or near the effector organs. Efforts to assess the integrity of most parasympathetic functions are rarely made in a routine examination. Others, such as the pupilloconstrictor fibers, are routinely examined in evaluating functions of the third

TABLE 1-3.   Segmental Level of Representation of Reflexes

Reflex	Segmental Level
Tendon reflexes	
Jaw jerk	Pons; fifth nerve
Biceps reflex	Cervical 5–6
Radial-periosteal reflex	Cervical 5–6
Triceps reflex	Cervical 6–7–8
Knee reflex	Lumbar 3–4
Ankle reflex	Sacral 1–2
Superficial reflexes	
Corneal reflex	Pons; fifth and seventh nerves
Pharyngeal reflex	Medulla; ninth and tenth nerves
Abdominal reflex	Thoracic 8–12
Cremasteric reflex	Lumbar 1–2
Plantar reflex	Lumbar 5, sacral 1–2

nerve. Disturbances in lacrimal and salivary gland function usually are not the consequence of neurologic disease, although excessive tearing without emotional provocation (crocodile tears) may be associated with lesions of the fifth and seventh cranial nerves. Abnormalities of cardiac rate and rhythm may result from disordered function of the parasympathetic fibers of the vagus nerve.

Cells of the intermediolateral portion of the sacral cord give rise to fibers that are carried through the second, third, and fourth sacral nerves to the pelvic nerves, synapsing with postganglionic neurons in proximity to the bladder and lower bowel. These nerves innervate the bladder, descending colon, rectum, anus, and genitalia. In the infant the reflex nature of bowel and bladder function is evident. Only with maturation of the cerebral hemispheres does voluntary control of the sphincters develop (18 months–30 months). In general, retarded children are slow in attaining control of the bowel and bladder, but since toilet training is dependent upon other factors, such as motivation and the child–parent relationship, it may not be a reliable index of intelligence.

Disease of the suprasegmental mechanisms concerned with bladder control generally leads to an irritable or spastic bladder of small capacity and to frequent voiding. Involvement of the sacral cord or plexus interrupts the reflex functioning of the bladder, and a large, hypotonic bladder results. A substantial amount of residual urine is characteristically obtained by catheterization after voiding.

The cells of origin of the thoracolumbar or sympathetic division of the autonomic nervous system arise from cells in the intermediolateral cell column of the thoracic and upper lumbar segments of the spinal cord. These fibers course with the spinal nerves to synapse in the paravertebral sympathetic ganglion chain or course through these to terminate in collateral thoracic and abdominal ganglia. The postganglionic fibers of this system innervate most of the viscera and the secretory glands. Fibers of the sympathetic nervous system also course along the major vessels of the body, supplying the terminal blood vessels and the sweat glands within the skin.

Abnormalities in function of the sympathetic division of the nervous system are manifested by disturbed functioning of the innervated organs. A common condition resulting from this is Horner's syndrome. Faulty temperature regulation may also result from a disturbance in function of the central or peripheral portions of the autonomic nervous system. This may be normal in the young infant, especially the premature infant who is relatively poikilothermic and at the mercy of his environment. As the autonomic nervous system matures, maintenance of the normal body temperature characteristic of the adult is seen. Congenital absence of sweating (anhydrotic ectodermal dysplasia) subjects the child to an extreme risk because hyperthermia may irreparably damage the cerebral and cerebellar cortex. Lack of sweat glands, rather than a defect in the autonomic nervous system, is responsible for this condition, however.

LABORATORY EXAMINATION

Determination of the cause and pathogenesis of a neurologic illness frequently depends upon specific laboratory data. The usefulness of a particular laboratory examination depends on the nature of the clinical syndrome. An electroencephalogram is of immense value in evaluating a seizure problem but is of no use in a patient with primary muscle disease. Laboratory tests are most helpful when they are well chosen to complement clinical data. They never serve as substitutes for a carefully taken history and examination.

CEREBROSPINAL FLUID

Cerebrospinal fluid (CSF) fills the cerebral ventricles and subarachnoid space around the brain and spinal cord. Despite intensive study, its full function remains to be elucidated. Cushioning of the brain and an exchange of substances between blood and brain have been ascribed to it. Although recent studies employing tracer substances indicate exchange of water and solutes between blood and CSF at various sites along the neuraxis, the concept of its formation by the choroid plexus and its absorption mainly through the arachnoid villi into the intracranial venous sinuses remains most useful clinically in understanding hydrocephalus and other states of disturbed intracranial pressure.

Lumbar Puncture

In most instances, the simplest and safest way to obtain CSF is by lumbar puncture. This may be carried out at any age. At times it is desirable to prepare the patient for this procedure by administering a sedative drug, but oversedation is to be avoided because hypoventilation may result in an artificially high CSF pressure reading.

Cooperation is seldom ideal in the infant and child, so it is usually necessary to restrain him. The patient is held in the lateral recumbent position by an assistant who maintains the spine maximally flexed by partially overlying him and holding him behind the head, neck, and knees. Following careful cleansing of the back with antibacterial solutions, the site to be anesthetized is infiltrated with an injection of procaine 2%. Local anesthesia may be omitted in the infant or young child. The second puncture, although painless, often evokes as much struggling as the first one did. In the infant a 4-cm to 6.5-cm 20-gauge to 22-gauge needle is better than the longer needles used in adults. In the newborn an ordinary 23-gauge, short-beveled scalp vein needle without stylet is less likely to produce a traumatic tap. Use of a needle attached to polyethylene tubing, such as is used for scalp vein infusions, has also been advocated.[6] The needle is inserted in the midline between the spines of the lumbar vertebrae and angled slightly upward. Any space below L_2 is satisfactory but the L_{3-4} or L_{4-5} interspace is usually used. If there is reason to suspect a malformation of the spinal cord with tethering to the base of the spine, the lowest possible interspace should be employed. Entry into the lumbar subarachnoid space usually can be predicted by feeling a sudden give of the posterior spinal ligaments followed by a similar feeling as the dura is pierced. At this point the stylet is withdrawn and a manometer attached by way of a three-way stopcock.

If an accurate pressure measurement is vital, an attempt should be made to lose

no CSF. At this point in the examination it is often possible to comfort the patient by talking or singing to him, and waiting several minutes before measuring the pressure. The cooperative older child may be partially released and the legs extended before recording the pressure because falsely high pressures may be obtained from pressing the knees against the abdomen. Free flow of fluid is reflected in the rapid rise and fall of CSF in the manometer with straining and respiration. Those maneuvers that tend to increase venous pressure also tend to increase the spinal fluid pressure.

Normally the CSF pressure is less than 180 mm water. It is lower in newborn infants. Measurements with anterior fontanel sensors (see above) in the newborn infant have led to a remarkable consistency of values for intracranial pressure, that is, 95 mm of water to 105 mm of water. No definite postnatal change can be discerned in the full-term infant, but a modest postnatal increase that peaks on the second day has been described in the premature infant. In the struggling, older child initial pressures of well over 300 mm water are found, but with most patients at least a transient fall to normal levels can be obtained. The Queckenstedt maneuver, in which the jugular veins are compressed bilaterally, is useful only in the demonstration of a spinal subarachnoid block and should be avoided in all other instances. Failure of the CSF pressure to rise on compression of the ipsilateral jugular vein is of questionable value in the diagnosis of lateral sinus and jugular vein thrombosis because of variations in the anatomy of the intracranial sinuses.

If examination of the fluid for cellular constituents is considered more important than an exact pressure recording, a few drops of spinal fluid are obtained prior to attempting a pressure measurement. In the struggling patient an initially clear fluid frequently becomes bloody from movement of the needle during the course of the procedure.

Determinations Made on Cerebrospinal Fluid

Fluid is permitted to drip slowly from the needle after pressure measurements are made. Normally CSF is crystal clear. In jaundiced patients the bilirubin concentration in the spinal fluid may be increased. Bilirubin is also responsible for the xanthochromia found with elevated protein concentrations, usually above 300 mg/dl. Deep xanthochromia frequently results from subarachnoid hemorrhage. Unless bleeding has been extreme, the supernatant fluid from a traumatic lumbar puncture is colorless, or nearly so, after centrifugation. In the early hours following subarachnoid hemorrhage, oxyhemoglobin gives the fluid an orange–red color. A few hundred white or red cells render the fluid faintly opalescent. Cloudy, white fluid usually indicates the presence of large numbers of white cells, as occurs in meningitis.

The cells in the fluid should be counted immediately. Normally there are fewer than five mononuclear and no polymorphonuclear leukocytes or red cells in the fluid. If there is an increase in cells, it is important to lyse the red cells with concentrated acetic acid and repeat the cell count. The addition of methylene blue or thionine to the acetic acid facilitates differential counting of the remaining cells. If a traumatic tap is suspected, a comparative cell count should be made between fluid collected in the first and third tubes. Whenever meningitis is suspected a Gram's stain should be done.

CSF is always collected under sterile precautions and should be cultured for bacteria and for fungi or viruses if appropriate. It should be recalled that although the white cells are usually present in the early stages of meningitis, they may be inconspicuous in fluids teeming with bacteria.

Difficulties in interpretation of the CSF in the newborn period arise most commonly when dealing with infants at greatest risk for intracranial disease, that is, infants in neonatal intensive care facilities. Recent careful studies of such populations indicate that, when instances of proven intracranial hemorrhage or bacterial meningitis are excluded, CSF values are not as different from those of older children as is often stated.[12] Thus, more than 30 red blood cells/mm^3 are unusual and the most frequent red blood cell (RBC) count, that is, the mode, is zero. In one large series of 117 high-risk infants, mean values for term and preterm infants were: for white blood cell (WBC) count, 8 and 9 cells/mm^3; for protein concentration, 90 and 115 mg/dl; for glucose concentration, 52 and 50 mg/dl; and

for the ratios of CSF to blood glucose, 81% and 74%, respectively. The points worthy of greatest emphasis are that combinations of abnormalities of CSF values are much more significant than single isolated abnormalities and that the CSF in the newborn must always be interpreted in the context of other clinical data.

The protein concentration is obtained routinely, and the glucose concentration determined whenever meningeal infection, tumor of the meninges, or hypoglycemia is suspected. Under ordinary circumstances the CSF sugar concentration is approximately two-thirds that of the blood level, although this implies that the blood glucose level has been stable for some time, that is, a steady state. Changes in the blood sugar concentration are reflected by appropriate changes in the CSF over a period of an hour or so.

At birth the cerebrospinal fluid protein is albumin, with the various globulin fractions making up the remainder. γ-Globulin is increased in specific diseases such as syphilis, multiple sclerosis, and subacute sclerosing panencephalitis.

The level of the spinal fluid protein gradually decreases during the first week of life, and after approximately 3 months of age a level of 10 mg/dl to 20 mg/dl is expected. The level then gradually rises throughout childhood until the adult figures of 20 mg/dl to 40 mg/dl are reached. The precise reason for these variations with age is not known.[14]

The ventricular fluid normally contains about half the protein concentration of the lumbar subarachnoid fluid, with cisternal fluid values lying midway between these figures. At times in the course of subdural puncture fluid is obtained from the subarachnoid space over the surface of the cortex. Examination of this fluid on numerous occasions has shown it to contain as much as twice the protein concentration of fluid obtained from the lumbar sac.

SUBDURAL FLUID

Whenever a subdural collection of fluid is suspected in an infant with open anterior fontanel and coronal sutures, a subdural puncture or tap should be carried out. In the supine position the infant is restrained securely in a sheet and held by an assistant. The infant's head is placed as near as possible to the edge of the bed. The hair and scalp are thoroughly washed and the hair shaved over the anterior half of the head. After preparing the scalp with antibacterial solutions, the scalp is anesthetized with procaine at the lateral angles of the anterior fontanel or at the adjacent coronal suture line.

A short (4 cm–6.5 cm) spinal needle with a 45 degree bevel is inserted perpendicularly through the procaine wheal. The dura can usually be felt to give after the needle has been inserted only a few millimeters. It is rarely necessary to insert the needle more than 1 cm. After the dura is pierced the stylet is removed. If after positioning the needle a few millimeters in one direction or another no fluid (or only a few drops of crystal clear fluid) is obtained, the tap may be considered negative and the needle removed. Subdural fluid or blood, when present, usually flows freely and is collected by gravity drip into sterile tubes for microscopic, chemical, and bacteriologic study. During the removal of fluid it is wise to clamp a hemostat on the needle close to the skin to prevent inadvertent slipping of the needle into the brain.

The volume of a subdural collection can be determined by injecting a known amount of Tc-labeled albumin into the subdural collection of fluid. After mixing and equilibration, a small sample of fluid is withdrawn and its radioactivity measured in a gamma counter. The volume can be calculated from the dilution of the original counts. Repeating such studies over time gives useful information about the course of the effusion and has proved valuable in the management of this condition. The distribution of the isotope can be ascertained by scanning techniques. The characteristics of subdural fluid and therapeutic subdural punctures are discussed in Chapter 12.

ULTRASONOGRAPHY

Ultrasound has been used to identify the location and width of the third ventricle. Some investigators find this method valuable as a screening procedure for ventricular displacement.

Real-time, gray scale ultrasonography of the cranial contents is of major value in the evaluation of the newborn infant.[13] Thus, intraventricular and intracerebral blood is detected readily, as are ventricular size and intraparenchymal cystic lesions. This technique has major advantages over other imaging techniques, for example, computed tomography, because the instruments are portable and can be used without disturbing the infant, the technique does not involve radiation, and it is not associated with any recognized risks.

ELECTROENCEPHALOGRAPHY

Maturation in structure and function of the cerebral cortex is paralleled by changes in the electroencephalogram. Electroencephalographic tracings must be interpreted in relation to what is normal for the patient's age. Well modulated "adult" activity is not usually seen until about the time of puberty. Asynchronous, irregular, slow waves of relatively low voltage characterize the electroencephalogram of the newborn. Over the ensuing months and years the rate increases gradually, synchronization between the two hemispheres develops, and an adult pattern is obtained (Fig. 1-18). Specific abnormalities of the electroencephalogram are discussed elsewhere in relation to epilepsy and specific disease processes.

ELECTRODIAGNOSTIC STUDIES IN NEUROMUSCULAR DISORDERS

The ability to amplify and record action potentials from muscle and nerve has led to the development of a variety of tests that are very useful in determining the site of involvement within the lower motor or first sensory neuron. Information about the degree of injury also may be obtained and is helpful in prognosis. These tests fall into three main groups: tests of neuromuscular excitability, electromyographic studies of motor unit or other muscle action potentials, and nerve conduction studies.

Tests of Neuromuscular Excitability

Nerve Trunk Stimulation. In normal subjects a brisk muscular contraction occurs

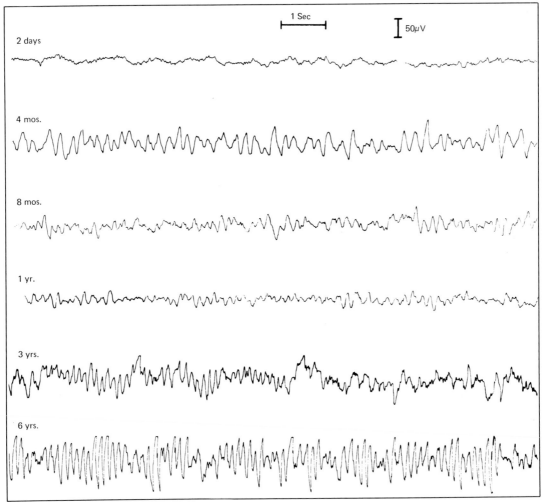

FIG. 1-18. Changes in the electroencephalographic pattern with age. All recordings were obtained from bipolar, occipitoparietal lead placements with the subject awake. The upper four strips are from a single infant; the bottom two are from different children. The activity becomes faster, better organized, and of higher voltage with increasing age.

when a brief electrical stimulus is applied to a motor nerve. Lack of a normal response indicates either defective conduction or actual degeneration of the nerve between the point of stimulus and the muscle. A reduced response also may be seen where there is severe muscle wasting from primary muscle disease such as muscular dystrophy. Preservation of a normal response despite the presence of clinical weakness may indicate that this weakness is due to lack of cooperation, lesions of the upper motor neuron, or a neurapraxia at the level of the anterior horn cell, motor root, or nerve proximal to the site of stimulation. This relatively crude test is still useful as a screening procedure.

Strength Duration Curves. This test assesses the response of muscle when electrical pulses of varying duration are applied to its motor point. Where nerve fibers are degenerating or have already degenerated, the muscle is stimulated directly and requires more current to produce a response with short duration pulses than in the normally innervated state. Although misleading normal results are sometimes obtained in states of partial denervation resulting from patchy disease of anterior horn cells, this test gives the earliest possible evidence of impending or actual denervation as opposed to a temporary conduction block (neurapraxia) when the lesion involves the peripheral nerve.

Electromyography

A concentric needle electrode inserted into muscle picks up the action potentials generated by volitional activity of neighboring motor units or subunits; these can then be amplified and displayed visually on an oscilloscope or aurally through a speaker.[9] Normal muscle at rest is electrically silent. With increasing volitional activity "motor unit" discharges appear in increasing numbers and with increasing frequency of discharge until the baseline becomes completely disrupted, producing a "full interference pattern" in which individual units can no longer be distinguished. Individual motor unit discharges represent the summated action potentials of a group of fibers all supplied by a single anterior horn cell and nerve fiber. The shape, duration, amplitude, and rate of discharge vary widely in normal people depending on such factors as age, choice of muscle, and the intensity of volitional activity. In general, normal motor unit discharges have two to four phases, last 5 msec to 15 msec, vary from 200 μV to 3000 μV in amplitude, and discharge at rates up to 50/sec. Variations from the normal occur in several ways.

1. There may be a reduction in the number of motor units or in the rate of discharge so that the interference pattern is incomplete or consists only of the rhythmic firing of a few discrete units. In complete denervation no units are seen on attempted volition. These variable degrees of reduction in interference pattern correlate approximately with the degree of lower motor neuron damage, but reduction can also occur in paresis of upper motor neuron origin, in conversion reaction, or from simple lack of cooperation. It may be possible to differentiate organic lesions from the others because the units that do fire will rapidly speed up with increased effort, although they will not do so if the reduction is due to conversion or lack of cooperation.

2. The amplitude or shape of individual units may be abnormal. In partial denervation due to anterior horn cell disease polyphasic potentials with increased amplitude and duration occur. In peripheral nerve lesions a proportion of units may be polyphasic of prolonged duration but have low to normal amplitude. In primary muscle disease the predominant pattern is of short duration, polyphasic motor units of low amplitude containing many brief spike-like components; however, these summate into a full interference pattern except in the late stages of the disease.

3. In addition to the discharges visible on volitional activity, spontaneous discharges may be seen or be provoked by mechanical stimulation. These may appear as normal or sometimes large complex, motor unit discharges (fasciculation potentials), or as brief (1 msec–3 msec), low voltage (100 μV–200 μV) fibrillation potentials. The latter originate probably from single muscle fibers. Fasciculation potentials are seen in a variety of conditions and may be rather nonspecific in significance. They are most common in anterior horn cell disease, quite common in certain stages of polyneuritis, occasionally are seen in compressive lesions of roots or peripheral nerves, and rarely occur in primary muscle disease. Fibrillation potentials, when they occur, persistently at rest, indicate denervation of at least 2 weeks' to 3 weeks' duration. They may, however, be seen in myopathic conditions, including inflammatory myopathies and some dystrophies in association with an interference pattern more suggestive of primary muscle disease than of neural atrophy. Rapid high frequency discharges of short duration, variable form, and wide distribution may be provoked by mechanical stimulation near the needle or by voluntary contraction in myotonia (Chap. 19). Brief runs restricted to very small areas, however, may be seen in various other conditions.

Electromyography requires a high degree of rapid subjective analysis and experience. Particularly in children where cooperation may be poor, it is of most use in confirming the presence of denervation. The multiple needle punctures sometimes necessary to assess the extent of involvement are not often well tolerated by young subjects.

Nerve Conduction Studies

Motor Conduction Studies. This is, in a sense, an elaboration of the simple nerve trunk stimulation test already described. Conduction rate is estimated by stimulating a nerve at two points and finding the latency between each stimulus and the ensuing muscular contraction. Subtraction of one latency from another gives the latency for the propagation of the nerve impulse between the two points stimulated, and hence conduction rate can be estimated. The nerves most commonly tested are the median, ulnar, peroneal, and posterior tibial. Patchy disease of anterior horn cells or involvement of a single motor root may show no abnormality by this means of testing. In peripheral nerve disease conduction is normal beyond the damaged segment unless wallerian degeneration has developed and progressed distally. Slowing of conduction rate is seen when the measurement is made over a locally damaged segment or in a diffuse peripheral neuropathy where the larger and therefore faster conducting fibers are selectively involved. Changes in nerve conduction rate in successive examinations may give a useful quantitative estimation of the course of the disease. Where the nerve can be examined in more than one segment, clear evidence of localization of damage may be obtained, for example, in ulnar nerve lesions at the elbow. Normal values are about 45 m/sec to 65 m/sec in children over the age of 5 years, but may be as low as 25 m/sec at birth rising to the low normal range by the age of 3 years.

H Reflex and F Wave Studies. The H reflex is recorded as a delayed muscle action potential following stimulation of the mixed motor-sensory nerve to that muscle. The response is due to an impulse being conducted proximally along the sensory fibers, synapsing in the spinal cord with the anterior horn cell, and being conducted down the motor nerve to the muscle. The F wave is a delayed muscle action potential following nerve stimulation that is due to an impulse being conducted antidromically up the motor nerve to the anterior horn cell. This results in firing of the anterior horn cell and an orthodromic impulse down the motor nerve that fires the muscle. Each of these phenomena may be used to study more proximal conduction in the nerve trunk.

Study of Evoked Potentials. The amplitude of the compound motor action potential obtained by stimulating a nerve and recording over the surface of the appropriate muscle may be reduced in conditions that lead to loss of motor axons, such as anterior horn cell disease or peripheral neuropathy. If the large myelinated fibers are unaffected, this may occur in the face of normal nerve conduction velocity. Evoked sensory potentials can be readily elicited from the larger fibers of the median and ulnar nerves at the wrist by application of a brief electrical stimulus to the appropriate digital nerves. Mixed motor and sensory potentials can be elicited from these nerves at the elbow or axilla by stimulating the mixed trunk distally (Fig. 1-19). Minor changes in conductivity in the lower motor or first sensory neurons very readily cause a temporal dispersion of the individual nerve fiber potentials forming these evoked potentials, and lead to a reduction in amplitude and increase in latency, or both. For this reason this method of testing is more sensitive than simple motor conduction rate estimation in detecting early evidence of peripheral nerve damage. The presence of definite clinical sensory loss with the preservation of normal evoked sensory potentials suggests either that the lesion is proximal to the posterior root ganglia or that there is a localized area of neurapraxia proximal to the segment examined. The latter may be the case in some patients with polyradiculoneuritis involving the sensory roots. In the more slowly developing neuropathies such as occur in diabetes, abnormalities in evoked potentials may be noted before clinical evidence of involvement is definite. Evoked potential studies require no needle insertions and are well tolerated by children.

No single method of electrodiagnostic testing is universally applicable, and all such tests must be carefully considered in relation to the clinical picture. Details of the techniques and their usefulness are well

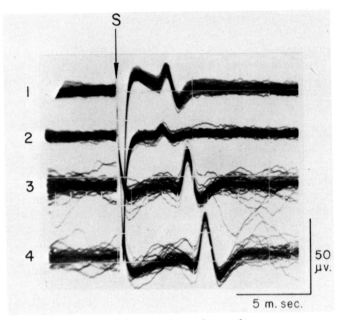

FIG. 1-19. Evoked potentials from the median and ulnar nerves in a normal subject. *1.* Stimulus applied to index, recording from median nerve above wrist. *2.* Stimulus to fifth finger, recording from ulnar nerve above wrist. *3.* Stimulus to median nerve above wrist, recording from above elbow. *4.* Stimulus to ulnar nerve above wrist, recording from above elbow. S. Point of application of stimulus. Multiple sweeps are superimposed at each site.

discussed by Licht.[9] Some of the findings to be expected in lesions at different sites are summarized in Table 19-1.

Brain Stem Auditory Evoked Response

The electrical events generated within the auditory pathways after stimulation by click or pure tone comprise the brain stem auditory evoked response. The complete response consists of seven components, generated by sequential activation of the major components of the auditory pathway. The technique is useful in the neonatal period, when the first (I) and fifth (V) waves are detected most readily. The former emanates from eighth nerve, and the latter principally from inferior colliculus. With maturation there is a decrease in latency and in threshold for these wave forms, with the sharpest change occurring at approximately 34 weeks of gestation.[4] Disease of peripheral structures, for example, the cochlea or eighth nerve, has been defined by prolonged latency and increased threshold of wave I in asphyxiated, acidotic infants. Disease of brain stem has been defined principally by prolonged conduction time between waves I and V in severely asphyxiated infants. This technique may prove valuable in detection of deleterious effects of certain insults, for example, hyperbilirubinemia, bacterial meningitis, intracranial hemorrhage, aminoglycoside therapy, and excessive ambient noise, all of which are capable of injuring various components of the auditory pathway.

REFERENCES

1. **Allen HA:** Testing of visual acuity in preschool children: norms, variables and a new picture test. Pediatrics 19:1093, 1957

2. **Cogan DG:** Neurology of the Ocular Muscles, 2nd ed. Springfield, Ill, Charles C Thomas, 1956

3. **Dodge PR, Porter P:** Demonstration of intracranial pathology by transillumination. Arch Neurol 5:594, 1961

4. **Galambos R, Despland PA:** The auditory brainstem response (ABR) evaluates risk factors for hearing loss in the newborn. Pediatr Res 14:159, 1980

5. **Gesell A, Amatruda CS:** Developmental Diagnosis, 3rd rev ed, edited by Knobloch H, Pasamanick B. Hagerstown, Harper & Row, 1974

6. **Greensher J, Mofenson HC, Borofsky LG, et al:** Lumbar puncture in the neonate: a simplified technique. J Pediatr 78:1034, 1971

7. **Hogan GR, Milligan JE:** The plantar reflex of the newborn. N Engl J Med 285:502, 1971

8. **Illingworth RS:** The Development of the Infant and Young Child. Normal and Abnormal, 7th ed. New York, Churchill Livingstone, 1980

9. **Licht SH:** Practical Electromyography, 4th ed, edited by Johnson EW. Baltimore, William & Wilkins, 1979

10. **Marks KH, Maisels MJ, Moore E, Gifford K, et al:** Head growth in sick premature infants—a longitudinal study. J Pediatr 94:282, 1979

11. **Nellhaus G:** Composite international and interracial graphs. Pediatrics 41:106, 1968

12. **Sarff LD, Platt LH, McCracken GH Jr:** Cerebrospinal fluid evaluation in neonates: comparison of high-risk infants with and without meningitis. J Pediatr 88:473, 1976

13. **Volpe JJ:** Evaluation of neonatal periventricular-intraventricular hemorrhage: A major advance. Am J Dis Child 134:1023, 1980

14. **Widell S:** On the cerebrospinal fluid in normal children and in patients with acute abacterial meningo-encephalitis. Lund, Berlingska Boktryckeriet, 1958

SUGGESTED READINGS

Bray PF: Neurology in Pediatrics. Chicago, Year Book Medical Publishers, 1969

Caffey J: Pediatric X-ray Diagnosis—A Textbook for Students and Practitioners of Pediatrics, Surgery and Radiology, 7th ed. Chicago, Year Book Medical Publishers, 1978

Clarke CA: Genetics for the Clinician, 2nd ed. Philadelphia, FA Davis, 1964

DeJong RN: The Neurologic Examination, 4th ed. Hagerstown, Harper & Row, 1979

Dekaban A: Neurology of Early Childhood. Baltimore, Williams & Wilkins, 1970

Denny-Brown D: Handbook of Neurological Examination and Case Recording, revised edition. Cambridge, Harvard University Press, 1957

Ford F: Diseases of the Nervous System in Infancy, Childhood and Adolescence, 6th ed. Springfield, Ill, Charles C Thomas, 1973

Gamstorp I: Pediatric Neurology. New York, Appleton-Century-Crofts, 1979

Hamilton WJ, Boyd JD, Mossman HW: Human Embryology, 4th ed. Cambridge, W Heffer & Sons, 1972

Hooker D: The Prenatal Origin of Behavior. Lawrence, University of Kansas Press, 1952

Menkes JH: Textbook of Child Neurology, 2nd ed. Philadelphia, Lea & Febiger, 1980

Paine RS, Oppé TF: Neurological Examination of Children. Clinics in Developmental Medicine numbers 20/21. London, Heinemann, 1966

Waelsch H (ed): Biochemistry of the Developing Nervous System. New York, Academic Press, 1955

Walsh FB, Hoyt WF: Clinical Neuro-ophthalmology, 3rd ed. Baltimore, Williams & Wilkins, 1969

Watson EH, Lowrey GH: Growth and Development of Children, 6th ed. Chicago, Year Book Medical Publishers, 1973

Volpe JJ: Neurology of the Newborn. Philadelphia, WB Saunders, 1981

Neuroradiologic Examination

2

Faustino C. Guinto, Jr.
Edwin A. Stevens

An array of neuroradiologic studies, ranging from simple plain film radiography to the more sophisticated computed or computer assisted tomography (CT) is available for the evaluation of maladies that affect the skull, brain, vertebral column, and spinal cord in children as well as adults. Skill in their interpretation demands not only familiarity with the procedures themselves but also an awareness of the advantages and the limitations inherent in each technique.

Because "a child is not a small adult," neuroradiologic procedures used in the pediatric age group are significantly dissimilar from those used in the approach to the adult patient.

A brief discussion of the conduct of the following modalities and their clinical applications will be given in this chapter: (1) plain skull radiography, (2) pneumoencephalography, (3) ventriculography, (4) carotid and vertebral angiography, (5) CT scanning, (6) plain film of the spine, and (7) myelography.

SKULL RADIOGRAPHY

Assessment of the pediatric skull requires careful selection of special views necessary to evaluate the particular clinical problems. The pediatric skull has a wide range of normal variations that can mimic pathologic conditions. A dynamically growing structure, the skull changes appearance notably during the first two years of life.

An abnormality of the skull may fall into one of the following categories: congenital, infectious, traumatic, neoplastic, or metabolic.

The following approach, in our experience, has proven to be useful in the evaluation of the skull. The face-to-cranium ratio is observed. The normal values at different ages, according to Gooding,[1] are: at birth, 1:4; at 2 years, 1:3; at 6 years, 1:2.5; and at adulthood, 1:1.5. In microcephaly the skull is unduly small. A large skull, on the other hand, may indicate either macrocephaly (large brain) or severe, generalized enlargement of the ventricles. As a rule, separation of sutures is due to increased intracranial pressure, which may be produced by (1) neoplastic (Fig. 2-1) or inflammatory masses with or without ventricular obstruction, (2) brain swelling, (3) neoplastic leptomeningeal infiltration, or (4) hypervitaminosis A. Suture separation is also observed during the active treatment of deprivation syndrome. Abnormal contour is commonly associated with premature closure of the sutures or hemiatrophy of the brain. Skull thickening may be caused by local or systemic processes (Fig. 2-2). Skull thinning may be secondary to erosive or pressure changes, but delayed ossification may at times mimic these findings. Lückenschädel is almost always associated with meningocele (Fig. 2-3). This pattern is ob-

(Text continues on p. 46)

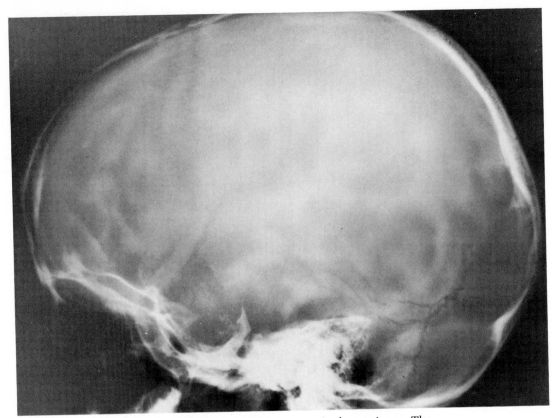

FIG. 2-1. Increased intracranial pressure due to a craniopharyngioma. The coronal suture is widened. Note erosion of sella turcica with suprasellar calcifications. CT of same patient is shown in Fig. 2-19.

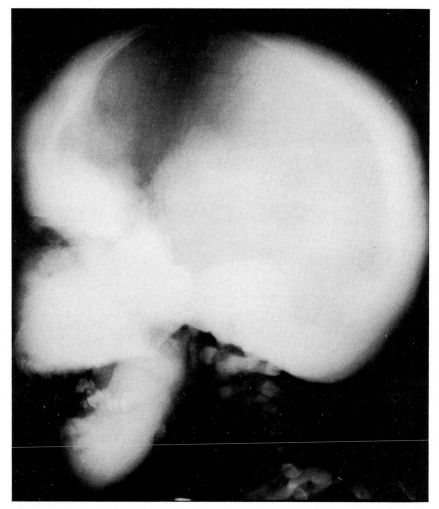

FIG. 2-2. Hyperostotic skull in a patient with craniometaphyseal dysplasia. The facial and mandibular thickening is also part of the systemic process. (Courtesy of Dr. R. McPherson)

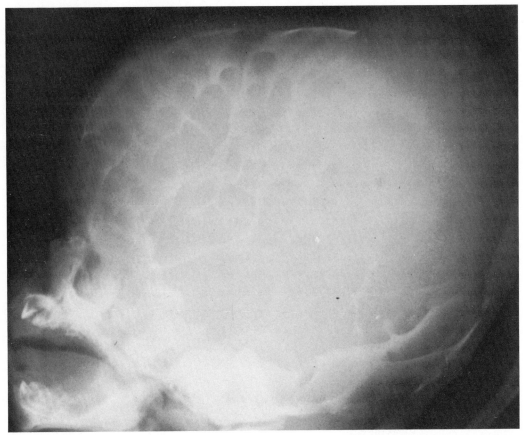

FIG. 2-3. Lückenschädel (craniolacunia). There are multiple lucencies representing deep pits separated by slender ridges of bone.

FIG. 2-4. Epidermoid. A lucent lesion with ▶ sclerotic margin is present in the left frontal bone.

FIG. 2-5. Histiocytosis X. Multiple well-defined ▶ lytic lesions are present throughout the calvarium.

served from birth to 6 months of age and should be differentiated from normal convolutional markings that are observed in the older child.

The presence of wormian bones can be a normal finding but other causes are cretinism, osteogenesis imperfecta, and cleidocranial dysostosis.

Localized increased densities are usually due to osteomas, but artifacts such as braids and electroencephalogram (EEG) conduction paste can simulate pathologic processes.

Localized lytic lesions have many etiologies. When midline and associated with a bulging soft tissue mass, a meningocele must be considered. Although most cranial meningoceles are occipital, some may bulge into the nasopharynx through a defect in the base of the skull. Parietal foramina regarded as normal variants are typ-

ically located in the posterior parasagittal region. Epidermoids characteristically present with sclerotic margins (Fig. 2-4), whereas eosinophilic granulomas have the typical "button sequestrum" appearance without sclerotic margins. Multiple lytic lesions are most likely caused by metastasis from a malignant neoplasm or lymphoma, but histiocytosis X cannot be excluded on

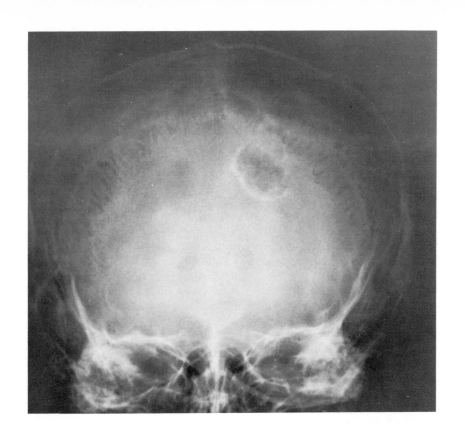

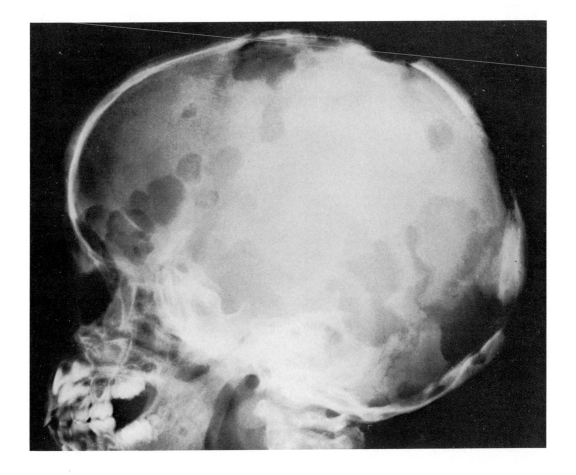

the basis of skull films alone (Fig. 2-5). Intracranial calcification in a child is a pathologic finding. Primary cerebral neoplasms that calcify include ependymoma, medulloblastoma, and lipoma of the corpus callosum. Calcification in the suprasellar region strongly suggests a craniopharyngioma. A calcified pineal body should indicate a pinealoma. Sturge-Weber syndrome presents with a characteristic "double tract" type of calcification (Fig. 2-6). Scattered parenchymal calcification is often seen in toxoplasmosis and cisticercosis, whereas periventricular distribution is suggestive of cytomegalic inclusion disease. The pattern of calcification of tuberous sclerosis is both parenchymal and periventricular.

Evaluation of the skull following trauma requires careful attention to the location and course of a linear or depressed fracture. The crossing of a fracture line over a meningeal artery groove or the presence of a depressed fracture overlying the superior sagittal sinus may be associated with

an epidural hematoma. In some types of congenital anomalies plain skull films are helpful in providing clues to their presence. A large posterior fossa, as determined by elevated sigmoid sinus grooves or torcular, is seen in Dandy-Walker malformation. A small posterior fossa, on the other hand, is a common finding in Arnold-Chiari anomaly.

PLURIDIRECTIONAL TOMOGRAPHY

This technique, which can provide a tomographic slice as thin as 1 mm, is useful in defining small bony structures such as the optic canal, sella turcica, and petrous bones. It is also very helpful in the evaluation of congenital bony anomalies occurring at the craniovertebral junction.

PNEUMOENCEPHALOGRAPHY

With the advent of CT scanning, pneumoencephalography has become a virtually

FIG. 2-6. Sturge-Weber. Serpiginous calcifications are present overlying the occipital cortex. The true extent of the calcifications is depicted by CT in Fig. 2-15.

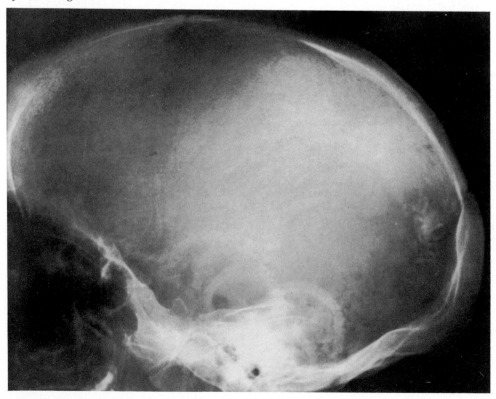

obsolete neurodiagnostic procedure. Its occasional application is limited to the evaluation of suprasellar lesions, where, in conjunction with pluridirectional tomography, it can provide a much clearer display, still unsurpassed by current CT scan technique, of small anatomic structures in this area. It is also useful in establishing the pattern of communication of certain cerebral cystic lesions in relation to the ventricles and other cerebrospinal fluid (CSF) spaces.

VENTRICULOGRAPHY

Ventriculography implies direct instillations of air or positive contrast materials into the lateral ventricles. Like pneumoencephalography, this procedure has been rendered unpopular by the introduction of CT scanning. Its occasional application is mainly in defining the nature and extent of an obstructing lesion of the third ventricle (Fig. 2-7), aqueduct of Sylvius, and the fourth ventricle.

CEREBRAL ANGIOGRAPHY

The primary indication of cerebral angiography is for the evaluation of potential vascular disease, that is, arteriovenous malformation, occlusive vascular disease, and aneurysm. It is of value in the preoperative assessment of meningoencephalocele (Fig. 2-8) and some brain tumors. The differentiation between massive subdural effusion and hydranencephaly and the diagnosis of certain types of congenital anomalies, such as agenesis of the corpus callosum and Dandy-Walker and Arnold-Chiari malformations, are readily made by cerebral angiography.

The approach in the interpretation of an angiogram in children is not greatly dissimilar from that of the adult. However, a few normal variations must be kept in mind. The arteries are generally straighter in children except for the internal carotid artery, which commonly presents as a localized kink in the neck just before it enters the

FIG. 2-7. Conray ventriculogram demonstrating a large pinealoma occupying and obstructing the third ventricle.

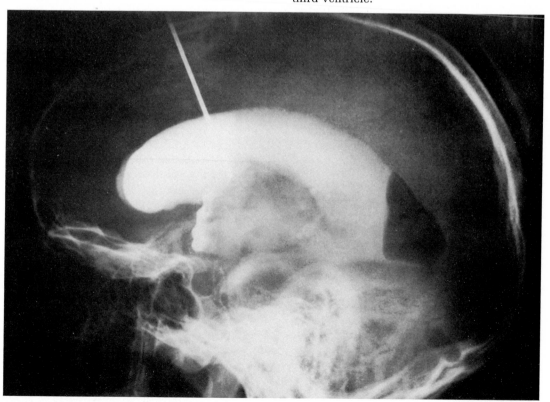

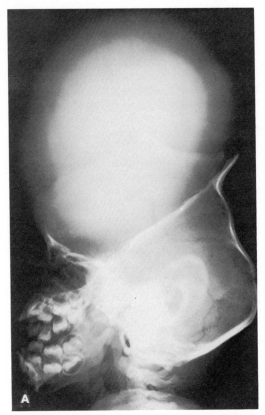
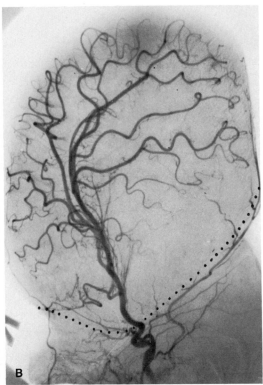

FIG. 2-8. *A.* Encephalocele protruding from a large frontoparietal cranial defect. *B.* Angiogram shows entire cerebral hemispheres contained within the encephalocele. *Dotted line* corresponds to edge of cranial defect.

carotid canal of the petrous bone. The axis of the sylvian vessels tends to be more vertically oriented in the very young child and approximates the adult configuration in the older child (Fig. 2-9). "Blushing" of the basal ganglia is a normal phenomenon in children and is apparently due to the relatively larger lenticulostriate arteries that nourish this structure. The vertebral and basilar arteries tend to be straighter and their configuration mimics an inverted Y when viewed in the frontal projection. Reflux of contrast material into the carotid system through the posterior communicating arteries during the course of cerebral angiography is a frequent, normal occurrence. The circulation time in younger children is comparatively faster than in the adult; hence, a more rapid filming sequence is employed.

SPINE

Plain film examination of the spine can be rewarding in many disease processes. With careful attention to detail, clues to the presence of congenital anomalies, neoplastic, inflammatory, and metabolic processes, and effects of trauma can be obtained from plain radiographs. Occasionally, tomography may be necessary to define more clearly structures that are ordinarily obscured by overlying soft tissue and bone, such as those at the craniocervical and cervical-thoracic junctions.

Like the skull, the pediatric spine can present with a wide range of normal variations. On the lateral projection, up to a 4-mm separation between the odontoid and anterior arch of C1 can be present in chil-

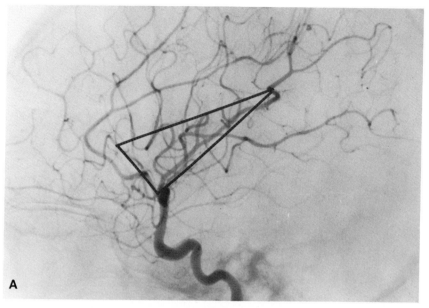

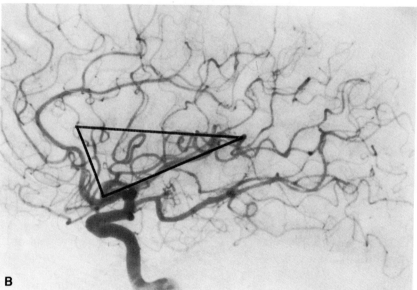

FIG. 2-9. Sylvian vessels. *A.* Lateral angiogram in a 2-year-old showing apparent elevation of the sylvian triangle, a normal variation at this age. *B.* Normal lateral angiogram in an adult, for comparison.

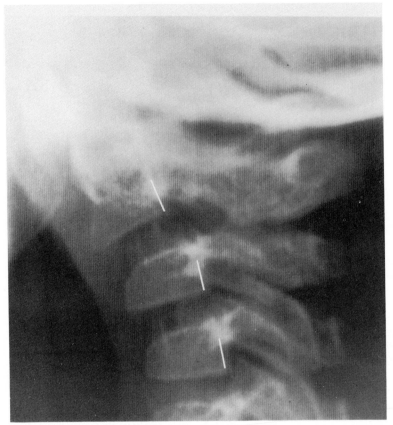

FIG. 2-10. Apparent subluxation of C_2 on C_3, a normal variation. *White lines* added to the film for clarification indicate posterior margins of vertebral bodies.

dren under 8 years of age. In flexion, forward subluxation of C2 on C3 to as much as 3 mm is considered normal (Fig. 2-10). Occipitalization of C1 can be normal but it should also be regarded as a clue to the possible presence of other anomalies occurring about the foramen magnum. The accessory ossicle of the odontoid, the os odontoideum (Fig. 2-11), should not be mistaken for a fracture.[3] Pedicular thinning at the thoracolumbar junction, a normal variant, can mimic erosive changes from an intraspinal mass lesion.

Among the clinically significant segmental congenital anomalies are various types of dysraphism, hemivertebrae, blocked vertebrae, Klippel Feil syndrome, and agenesis involving the ossification centers of the posterior elements. The latter can mimic a fracture, especially in the face of recent trauma. Tomography will usually reveal the unossified portion of the vertebrae.

Lytic processes involving the vertebral body are usually secondary to metastases from common pediatric malignancies such as Ewing's sarcoma or osteogenic sarcoma. Histiocytosis X can masquerade as a malignant process. Direct invasion of the vertebrae from an adjacent neuroblastoma can occur occasionally. Among the important osteoblastic processes that may involve the vertebral body are osteoid osteoma and lymphoma.

Unlike malignant processes, inflammatory lesions have special predilections for the disk space, a feature that differentiates the two entities.

Widening of the neural foramen is almost always secondary to a neurofibroma. Increased interpediculate distance may be seen in hydrosyringomyelia, large arterio-

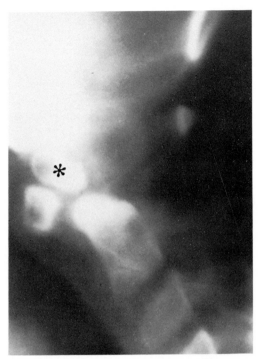

FIG. 2-11. Os odontoideum. A midline tomogram demonstrates a separate odontoid ossification center (*).

venous malformation, ependymoma, and astrocytoma of the spinal cord. Disk calcification is invariably traumatic in origin.

The spine can reflect generalized genetic and acquired diseases. This reflection is sometimes quite specific, such as that seen in the achondroplastic dwarf, or nonspecific, such as the osteoporosis of leukemia or Cushing's disease.

MYELOGRAPHY

Myelography is indicated when determining the nature and extent of an intraspinal lesion. It is considered mandatory in the preoperative workup for scoliosis patients, in whom a significant incidence of diastematomyelia has been discovered.[2] The procedure is best performed with the patient under general anesthesia because complete patient cooperation can rarely be obtained with heavy sedation. Since the conus ends

at a lower level in younger children, the spinal puncture must be made low and with care, to avoid piercing the spinal cord. Isophendylate (Pantopaque), a safe myelographic contrast material, is preferred by most investigators. Air or oxygen is reserved for special diagnostic situations such as the differentiation between hydrosyringomyelia and intramedullary tumors and the evaluation of the position and termination of the spinal cord in various types of dysraphism. Metrizamide (Amipaque), an ionic water-soluble contrast material, is widely used in Europe and Canada but has not received the approval of the Federal Drug Administration for routine use in children in this country.

The commonly encountered pathologic entites affecting the spine in children fall into two groups, namely, congenital conditions and acquired conditions, the latter consisting mostly of neoplastic processes.

The congenital anomalies are readily recognized by their characteristic myelographic features. In diastematomyelia there is a persistent central defect in the Pantopaque column corresponding to the fibrous or bony bar that splits the cord centrally (Fig. 2-12). In the tethered cord anomaly, the conus is low-lying and the thickened filum terminale is readily demonstrated by air or positive contrast myelography. In meningoceles there can be varying degrees of dilation of the arachnoid sac.

The traditional meylographic classification of the acquired lesions is (1) intramedullary, (2) intradural–extramedullary, and (3) extradural (Fig. 2-13). This classification is not only helpful in predicting the histologic diagnosis of the lesion but it also provides the clinician with invaluable information in planning therapy.

COMPUTED TOMOGRAPHY

The dramatic improvements in scanning time, slice thickness, and resolution have allowed fine anatomic evaluation of the pediatric brain and spine by computed tomography. Most invasive studies have been eliminated or reduced to supplementary diagnostic procedures.

(Text continues on p. 56)

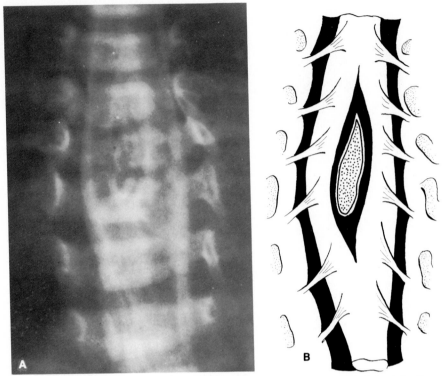

FIG. 2-12. Diastematomyelia. *A.* Myelogram. There is a central defect in the contrast column corresponding to the bony spur. *B.* Illustration of *A.*

FIG. 2-13. Myelographic classification of spinal tumors. *A.* Normal for comparison. *B.* Intramedullary. *C.* Intradural-extramedullary. *D.* Extradural.

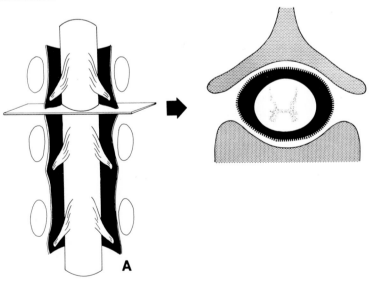

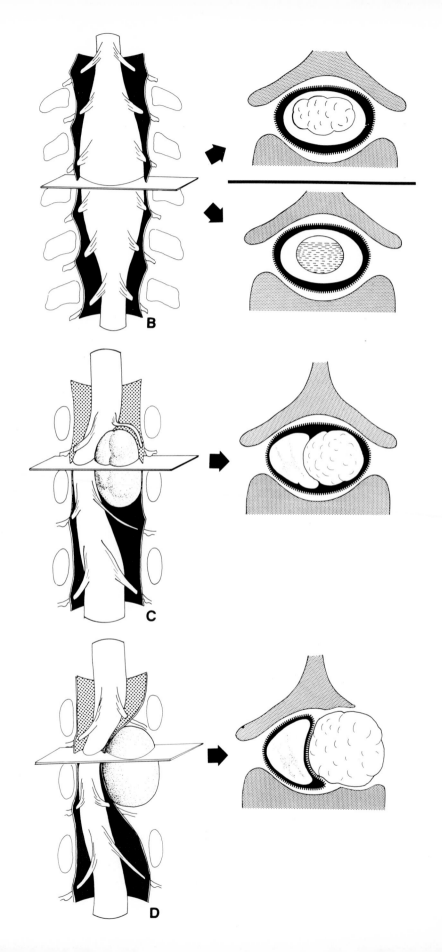

Congenital malformations such as Dandy-Walker, Arnold-Chiari, agenesis of the corpus callosum, and hydranencephaly have characteristic CT scan appearances (Fig. 2-14). The polygyria and agyria deformities are more difficult to identify with the current resolution capabilities. The periventricular calcifications of tuberous sclerosis and the cortical calcification of Sturge-Weber syndrome are much more extensive than those demonstrated by plain films (Fig. 2-15).

The enlarged head can easily be separated into megalencephaly or hydrocephaly. The etiology of hydrocephalus is readily defined and the resultant treatment followed by CT. Germinal matrix hemor-

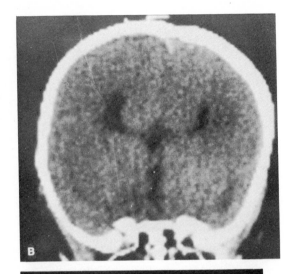

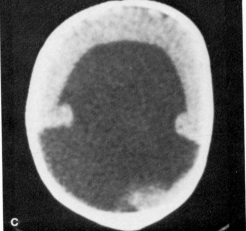

FIG. 2-14. Congenital malformation revealed by CT. *A* and *B.* Transverse and coronal views in agenesis of the corpus callosum. The separation of the lateral ventricles and high position of the third ventricle are characteristic findings. *C.* Holoprosencephaly. Basic findings are the absence of the interhemispheric fissure and a monoventricle. *D.* Dandy-Walker malformation. A large CSF-containing space occupies a large portion of the posterior fossa. The association of vermian agenesis and hypoplastic cerebellar hemispheres is a classical finding of the anomaly.

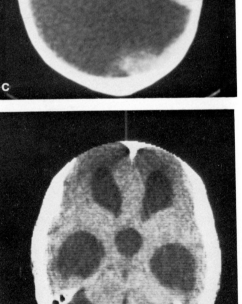

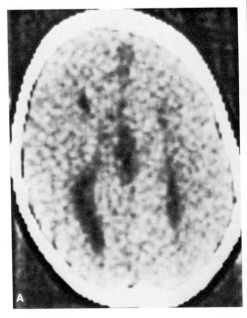

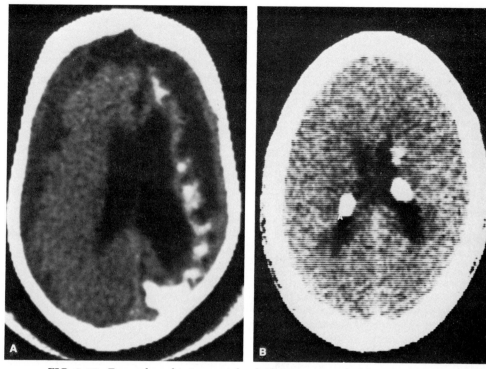

FIG. 2-15. Examples of intracranial calcifications revealed by CT. *A.* Sturge-Weber. Extensive calcification of the atrophic right cerebral hemisphere is present. Plain skull of same patient is shown in Fig. 2-6. *B.* Tuberous sclerosis. Periventricular calcifications are demonstrated. Skull films (not shown) failed to show the calcifications.

rhage in the premature infant under 1500 g occurs more frequently than previously appreciated.

CT has decreased the mortality of cerebral abscess from 30% to 60% to 0% to 5%. Precise localization and definition of multiloculated abscesses allow for improved surgical intervention (Fig. 2-16). If a positive blood, sinus, or mastoid culture can be obtained, surgical intervention may not be necessary.[4]

Many neurosurgeons now operate on childhood posterior fossa masses on the basis of CT alone. The typical midline location of the medulloblastoma, the lateral location of the cerebellar astrocytoma, and the calcifications of the ependymoma eliminate the necessity for angiography (Fig. 2-17). However, those patients suspected of

having Von Hippel-Lindau disease may harbor more hemangioblastomas than appreciated by CT. Angiography is indicated for these patients (Fig. 2-18). Craniopharyngiomas usually have suprasellar calcifications easily demonstrated by axial and coronal CT (Fig. 2-19).

Traumatic contusion, cerebral edema, frank hemorrhage, and subdural and epidural hematomas are best evaluated by CT (Fig. 2-20). The high density of blood is primarily due to the hemoglobin. As this protein breaks down, the density decreases by approximately 2 Hounsfield units per day until it is isodense at 2 weeks to 4 weeks. Care must be taken not to miss a clinically important lesion at this time.

Although angiography is the definitive procedure for the evaluation of vascu-

(*Text continues on p. 60*)

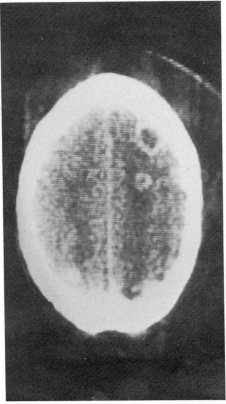

FIG. 2-16. Brain abscesses. CT following contrast infusion reveals two brain abscesses with well-defined enhancing rims in the right frontal lobe.

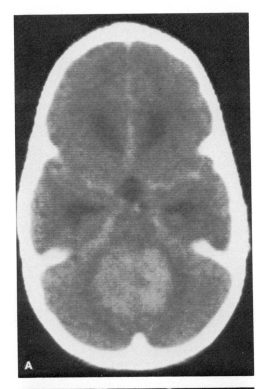

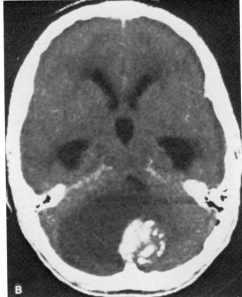

FIG. 2-17. Examples of posterior fossa tumors revealed by CT following contrast infusion. *A.* Medulloblastoma. Midline, contrast-enhancing mass with surrounding edema and without calcification is suggestive of the diagnosis. *B.* Cystic astrocytoma. A large cystic mass involving the right cerebellar hemisphere with an enhancing calcified nodule is a characteristic finding.

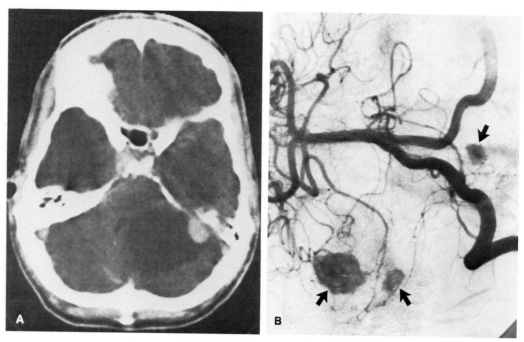

FIG. 2-18. Hemangioblastoma. *A.* CT following contrast infusion reveals a cystic mass with an enhancing nodule involving the right cerebellum. Multiple CT cuts (not shown) through the posterior fossa failed to show other enhancing nodules. *B.* Vertebral angiograms demonstrate 3 separate hemangioblastomas (*arrows*).

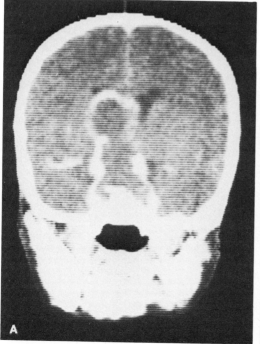

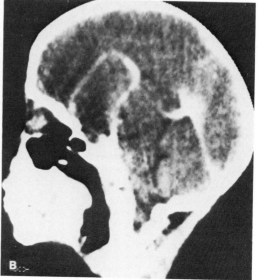

FIG. 2-19. Craniopharyngioma. *A* and *B.* Coronal and sagittal CT scans demonstrate true size and morphology of the tumor. Plain skull film of same patient is shown in Fig. 2-1.

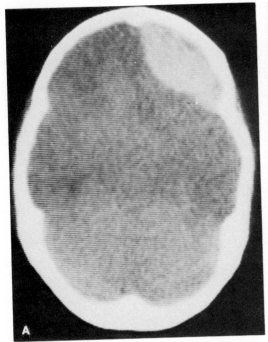
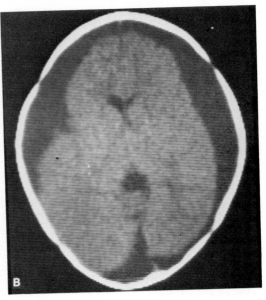
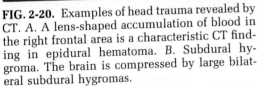

FIG. 2-20. Examples of head trauma revealed by CT. *A.* A lens-shaped accumulation of blood in the right frontal area is a characteristic CT finding in epidural hematoma. *B.* Subdural hygroma. The brain is compressed by large bilateral subdural hygromas.

lar lesions, CT can provide additional information not obtainable from arteriograms, such as the demonstration of blood in the subarachnoid space from a ruptured aneurysm, parenchymal hematoma from arteriovenous malformation, and edema resulting from arterial occlusive disease.

REFERENCES

1. **Gooding CA:** Skull Vault, Size and Shape. In Newton TH, Potts DG (eds): Radiology of the Skull and Brain: The Skull, Vol 1, Bk 1, p 141. St. Louis, CV Mosby, 1971

2. **Harwood-Nash DC:** Myelography in children. Semin Roentgenol 7:297, 1972

3. **McRae DL:** Skull Base, Craniovertebral Junction. In Newton TH, Potts DG (eds): Radiology of the Skull and Brain: The Skull, Vol 1, Bk 1, p 260. St. Louis, CV Mosby, 1971

4. **Stevens EA, Norman D, Kramer RA et al:** Computed tomographic brain scanning in intraparenchymal pyogenic abscess. Am J Roentgenol 130:111, 1978

Birth Defects and Developmental Disorders

3

James E. Etheridge, Jr.

VULNERABILITIES OF THE DEVELOPING NERVOUS SYSTEM

The multitude of processes in cerebral morphogenesis, appearing as a rapid succession of phases in the early embryo but continuing at a decelerating pace well into postnatal life, makes possible the full efflorescence of the human brain but also renders it vulnerable to many injurious agents. The susceptibility to damage during this prolonged period of growth and differentiation is reflected in the high incidence of congenital malformations of the central nervous system, in some countries approaching 1% of births. To these prenatal disorders must be added the injuries resulting from the special liabilities of the neonatal brain to events at birth and systemic biochemical disorders that may spring into prominence in the young infant no longer shielded by the filtrative protection of the maternal circulation. The continued growth, maturation, and myelination of the nervous system of the young child permits the expression of another set of diseases related to particular metabolic characteristics of neurons and glia.

In the embryonic brain the critical timing of morphogenetic events may determine the nature of the resulting malformation, irrespective of etiologic agent. Thus x-irradiation applied during the stage of the open neural groove may produce anencephaly, but much later in fetal life it may result mainly in cerebellar abnormalities. Some crucial stages of high vulnerability include the development and closure of the neural tube, differentiation of neurons and glia, evagination of paired vesicles from the neural tube, flexure formation, neuroblast migration from the germinal epithelium to the cerebral cortex, differentiation of the roof of the rhombencephalon, and laminar development of the cerebral cortex. In addition to these major growth processes, changes in cellular metabolism may determine the timing and limits of injury. Thus vitamin A deficiency in a pregnant experimental animal may so selectively affect the fetus as to produce only hydrocephaly, and brief anoxia may be without effect upon the fetal brain but can produce a characteristic encephalopathy in the newborn. In experimental animals a great number of agents are capable of producing cerebral maldevelopments including x-irradiation, virus infections, vitamin deficiencies, metabolic antagonists, hormonal alterations, and a variety of diverse toxic compounds. In human beings, however, with such prominent exceptions as x-irradiation or maternal rubella, incrimination of teratogens has been largely restricted to individual case reports. Placental and uterine pathologic processes remain a potential but still undefined source of fetal damage.

A major cause of developmental disorders of the brain consists of defects due to genetic or chromosomal alterations, and although the ponderous genetic legacy of man may have permitted the emergence of his brain, it has also rendered him susceptible to a vast number of metabolic errors. Such genetic factors may be operative in specific examples of almost all the major categories of cerebral malformations.

Although attempts to relate cerebral

malformations to precise times of injury during gestation are often misleading, it is possible to draw an approximate relationship to failure of certain general processes. After formation of the neural groove, the rostral extremity of the neural plate becomes greatly expanded. In the midportion of the primitive nervous system the margins of the groove approximate each other and fuse into a neural tube. Fusion then proceeds both cephalad and caudad. These proliferating cells are quite sensitive to many metabolic poisons as well as to x-irradiation. The latter acts upon germinal cells just before cell division or in postmitotic differentiation. Injury prior to tube closure may produce widespread necrosis resulting in total failure of tube formation with craniorachischisis. If damage is limited to the cephalic end, proliferation continues for a time but secondary cell disintegration ultimately leads to anencephaly.

With further differentiation the neural tube comes under two inductive processes. Spinal cord and lower brain stem are influenced by the notochord, and the forebrain and diencephalon by the prechordal mesoderm upon the dorsal lip of the foregut. There is evidence that these two systems may be damaged independently. The prechordal mesoderm also induces the development of parts of nose, upper lip, and related medial parts of the face. In both experimental as well as clinical situations there may be examples of severe forebrain and diencephalic malformation associated with midline facial deformities, but with an intact brain stem and spinal cord. In man this association is most commonly seen in the univentricular brain deformities.

As the primitive forebrain rapidly expands around the cavity that ultimately becomes the third ventricle, the walls of the diencephalon undergo a series of paired evaginations to produce the optic, cerebral, and olfactory vesicles. The delicate and precise growth patterns that permit these outpouchings of the forebrain are quite vulnerable to injury. Destruction at this time, even with replacement by the ever proliferating germinal epithelium, may nevertheless alter the timing or total quantity of cell components of one or more of these vesicles. The respective effects may be anophthalmia, microphthalmia, or bilateral ocular coloboma; failure of cerebral hemispheric development with univentricular cerebrum; or absence of the olfactory bulbs and tracts.

At about the time of vesicle formation, neural tubulation is finally completed at the caudal end of the primitive central nervous system with closure of the posterior neuropore. Interference with this process culminates in the common condition lumbosacral spina bifida. Both in human and experimental embryos prevention of posterior tube closure creates a local overgrowth of cells in the primitive spinal cord. In human and some experimental conditions an accompanying set of posterior fossa and cerebral malformations with secondary hydrocephaly is recognized as the Arnold-Chiari malformation. It is not yet known whether this complex of anomalies results from simultaneous action of an etiologic agent upon brain stem and cerebral development or whether early effects from the neural tube fistula or late results of fetal hydrocephaly may contribute to the morphogenetic process.

Following the appearance of the flexures of the developing brain and the forebrain vesicles, the cerebral vesicles rapidly enlarge and become recognizable hemispheres whose lateral ventricles are filled with a choroid plexus. During the second and third months there appears a process of major importance in the pathology of mental retardation. This consists of massive migration of waves of neuroblasts from the mantle zone about the lateral ventricles outward to the marginal zone for the formation of the cerebral cortex and its characteristic layers. Prevention or inhibition of this process produces characteristic abnormalities in the formation of cerebral gyri and cortical lamination. In the experiments of Hicks it was shown that rodent fetuses irradiated prior to neuroblast migration suffered necrosis of cells about the germinal epithelium. Irregular indentations of epithelium created multiple little rosettes that subsequently took up the replication of neuroblasts and glia. Many of the neuroblasts, however, now failed to attain the marginal zone but remained clustered around the rosettes ultimately to form neural heterotopias. The cerebral hemispheres remained abnormally small. In man similar consequences can be found after the action of teratogenic agents during the first 3 months of gestation. A severe form of this class of defects is the lissencephalic or agyric brain. Here the cerebral hemispheres are much reduced. The surface is smooth with absent or very shallow sulci. Surrounding the ventricles is a massive plate of heterotopic gray matter. Around this is a small zone of white matter beyond which is found a crude cerebral cortex containing neuroblasts that have attained the hemispheric surface but have failed to form a laminated cortex. In partial forms of this defect, portions of the hemispheres may reveal gyrus formation but large symmetrical areas are smooth and without sulcation and may be designated as *pachygyric*. The most common defect in cortical development is microgyria (Fig. 3-1) often associated with small cerebral hemispheres or microencephaly. Heterotopic islands of gray matter are commonly seen between cortex and ventricle (Fig. 3-2).

The development of the cerebellum takes place later than that of the forebrain. Thus cerebellar anomalies are more likely to be associated with defects of the already formed cerebral hemispheres than with the profound forebrain malformations of the first few weeks of gestation. From the lips of the developing rhombencephalon, bilateral thickenings push into the rhombencephalic roof, merge, and become the cerebellar hemispheres. Not until the fifth month of intrauterine life does the thickened tela choroidea just caudal to these processes undergo a differentiation in which a small locus of the membranous structure in the midline pushes outward as a diverticulum that ultimately disappears to leave the foramen of Magendie. At the same time in the anterior portion of the tela choroidea the thickening appears that forms the posterior portion of the cerebellar vermis. These two events may fail concomitantly, resulting in absence of the foramen of Magendie, cystic dilation of the roof of the fourth ventricle, and absence of the posterior cerebellar vermis.

During the last trimester of gestation, after the general outlines of all parts of the central nervous system are apparent and cerebral fissuration and sulcation is well under way, the brain once more shows new patterns of reaction to injury, including cavity formation and the process of cortical sclerosis termed *ulegyria*. The brain of the fetus approaching term has the capacity for a total parenchymatous dissolution of damaged loci. With focal injuries there may result the large porencephalic cavities of destructive origin. Another process seen in the late fetus or young infant consists of total destruction of central white matter and replacement by a series of large interconnected cystic cavities. In ulegyria there is an area of disturbance of cortical architecture often conforming to the territory of the cerebral blood vessels. The cortical surface may be retracted and irregular, or there may be extensive atrophy of whole convolutions most marked in the depths of the sulci and with preservation of the cortex at the crest of the gyral summit. The process differs from microgyria in that there is no abnormality of neuroblast migration or cortical lamina formation, but rather a secondary destruction with gliosis.

At term the neonatal brain becomes capable of reacting to ischemia in a manner resembling that of the adult brain with typical encephalomalacia. Furthermore, general asphyxia or cardiac arrest may evoke an encephalopathy similar to that of the

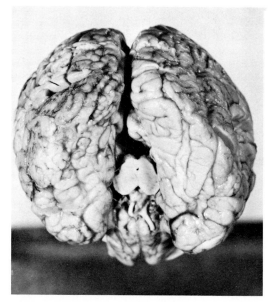

FIG. 3-1. Multiple areas of microgyria in the occipital and inferior temporal cortex.

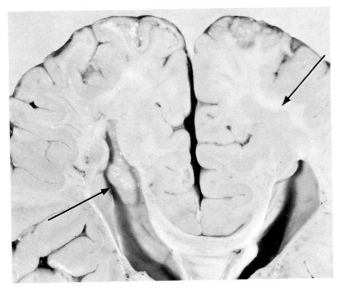

FIG. 3-2. Heterotopic gray matter. *Arrows* indicate subependymal masses and large islands within the central white matter.

mature brain, with cortical necrosis maximal in the middle and deeper cortical layers where respiratory enzymes are concentrated, in Ammon's horn, and in the thalamus.

During the neonatal period when the infant is freed from the maternal regulation of circulating substrate and removal of toxic intermediaries, some of the systemic errors of metabolism become fully developed. The brain may suffer a group of diffuse destructive processes resulting from the hypoglycemias, the disturbances of amino acid and protein metabolism, and some disorders of fluid and electrolyte regulation.

In the newborn's brain myelination is restricted to optic radiation, somatic sensory afferents, the cranial nerves, and most neural circuits of the brain stem. Myelination proceeds rapidly throughout infancy, continuing at a progressively slow rate in early childhood. This process seems to be dependent upon the interaction of axis cylinder and oligodendrocytes of the white matter, thereafter functionally united as an oligodendrocyte-myelin complex. The concentric lipid protein layers comprising the myelin coat have a characteristic molecular composition that includes among others the compounds cerebroside, sphingomyelin, plasmalogen, and cholesterol. Of central importance in the chemical pathology of myelin as well as neuronal lipid is the long-chain hydroxylated amine sphingosine. It is a component of the gangliosides of the neuronal cell body as well as the sphingomyelin, cerebroside, and sulfatide of the myelin. The metabolism of this compound affords another special site of vulnerability of the young brain. Many of the degenerative brain diseases of childhood are attributable to genetically determined biochemical errors of sphingolipids.

DEVELOPMENTAL DISORDERS CHIEFLY AFFECTING THE CEREBRUM AND CRANIUM

ANENCEPHALY

Anencephaly has been of pivotal importance in studying the responses of the embryonic nervous system to experimental teratogens. Although the condition is readily reproduced in laboratory animals by a variety of agents, the etiology of human examples is quite uncertain, only a single case having been reasonably attributed to the action of aminopterin. Nevertheless, this lethal anomaly is one of the most common of the congenital defects of the nervous system. The world incidence ranges between 0.5/1000 births to 3.7/1000 births, with especially frequent occurrence in Scotland and Ireland. The malformation is at least twice as frequent in female as in male infants, is more prone to occur in mothers over 40 years of age, and carries a 30-fold increased risk in parents having had a previous anencephalic infant.

Experimental studies on pathogenesis indicate an initial fusional failure at the anterior portion of the neural fold, with secondary dissolution of all forebrain neuroblasts. Epithelialization occurs, but the calvarium fails to develop, ultimately producing the familiar appearance of protuberant eyes and rudimentary supraorbital ridge sloping backward as a poorly formed cranial floor containing a few tissue masses of glial or vascular derivation. The sphenoid bone is malformed. In the posterior fossa a remnant of midbrain is succeeded by a small pons and cerebellum below which the neuraxis is relatively normal except for the absence of descending tracts. The pituitary is absent or vestigial, and the adrenal cortex hypoplastic.

A number of motor responses may be elicited in the anencephalic fetus. When undisturbed it usually lies quietly with infrequent slow movements. Cutaneous stimuli may produce head rotation, limb flexion, or complex movements of slow, stereotyped character. A partial Moro reflex may be obtained on passive head extension. Reflex sucking is possible in some cases, whereas sneezing, yawning, and crying may be absent. Some reflex facial counterparts of emotional expression may be elicited. The fetuses are subject to episodic attacks either of general extension or of the type resembling massive infantile spasms with flexion of neck and trunk.

CYCLOPIAS AND HOLOTELENCEPHALIES

In the cyclopias and holotelencephalies severe midline defects of eyes, nose, and palate are associated with univentricular cerebri. The frequent association of facial and cerebral anomalies suggests the possibility of pathogenetic mediation by the specialized prechordal mesoderm between the foregut and the anterior end of the neural tube, which influences forebrain development and induces some midline facial structures. It has been estimated that the most severe forms may result from an etiologic factor operative during the third week of gestation, whereas other cases may be related to a period just before the 30th day. Three such infants are now on record as having been born of diabetic mothers, one of whom was documented as having poor control during gestation, with episodes of hypoglycemia and ketosis.

Cyclopias are characterized by a single, fused, or rudimentary eye and absence of the nasal septum. The brain consists of a single ventricled chamber with absence of olfactory bulbs and corpus callosum and with poorly formed hippocampus and basal ganglia.

More frequent is that group designated as *arhinencephalies*, which, as pointed out by Yakovlev in his detailed analysis of the subject, should properly be called *holotelencephalies* because the limbic and "rhinencephalic" structures are indeed present.[56] Most cases are associated with striking defects such as absent nasal septum, failure of fusion of the maxillary processes, marked medial cleft lip and palate, broad nose, and closely spaced orbits. Microphthalmia, ocular coloboma, polydactyly, and visceral anomalies may also be present. These associated anomalies characterize patients with trisomy for chromosome group 13–15, as first reported by Miller and associates.[36] A familial distribution with normal chromosome complement was reported by DeMyer and associates.[12]

Brains of these patients are lacking in olfactory bulbs and exhibit gross failure in evagination and expansion of the cerebral ventricles. The usual appearance is that of a spherical object with a dorsal opening covered by a membranous derivative of the diencephalic roof. Along the dorsal border of the cerebral mass is a crescentic hippocampal formation, its two arches uniting anteriorly. The vesicles have failed to evaginate properly, to participate in the huge expansion of neocortex that produces the convoluted and opercularized hemispheres, and to effect the anterior-to-posterior rotation that results in the progressive shift of the hippocampus from its origin in the medial telencephalon to its ultimate inferior and medial position in the temporal lobe. In less severe examples partial interhemispheric fissuration develops posteriorly. Absent or hypoplastic are the corpus callosum, septum pellucidum, infundibulum, and mammillary bodies.

Most of these patients die at birth or in the neonatal period, a few surviving into early childhood. Such infants are severely defective in mental and motor behavior. They are unable to sit, walk, acquire language, or develop prehensile facility. Sucking is effective, and some may smile and show visual and auditory recognition. Massive myoclonic jerks or extensor seizures with head retraction are usually present. Poikilothermia is often noted. The electroencephalogram (EEG) is abnormal with spikes, periodicity, or hypersynchrony, and reduced voltage over fluid pools.

The malformation may be recognized in life by a characteristic group of facial anomalies (Fig. 3-3). The membranous dorsal roof of the brain and large pools of cerebrospinal fluid (CSF) may permit transillumination of a portion of the calvarium in some cases.

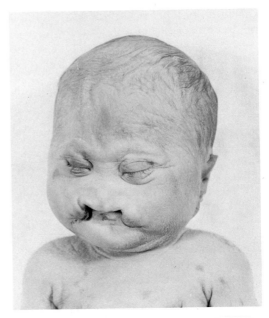

FIG. 3-3. Facial malformation in holotelencephaly.

SCHIZENCEPHALIES AND PORENCEPHALIES, DEFECTS CHARACTERIZED BY CLEFT FORMATION IN LOCALIZED AREAS OF TOTAL NEURONAL DESTRUCTION

Since its inception by Heschl in 1859 and its amplification by Kundrat, the term *porencephaly* has been used to describe a variety of lesions having in common the presence of one or more gross defects in the cerebral hemispheres. Some are cystlike and may communicate with the ventricle or subarachnoid space. Others consist of large gaps in the cerebral substance crossed only by a thin membrane. It is clear that both older and more recent descriptions include two distinctive categories that may be divided into the schizencephalies, considered to be developmental abnormalities occurring quite early in the cerebral morphogenesis, and the encephalomalacic porencephalies, which result from injurious agents acting on the formed brain in late fetal or neonatal life.[57]

Pathology. Yakovlev[56,57] demonstrated that the schizencephalies appear to result from injury to developing cerebral vesicles during the second month of intrauterine life. There is a total loss of neurons in restricted symmetrical zones of each developing hemisphere. In the wake of the neuronal destruction, ependyma and pia–arachnoid approximate one another and become fixed. With expansion of the surviving cerebral substance on either side of the pia–ependymal junction there results a streaming of ependyma back toward the ventricle and of pia toward the surface. On either side of the resulting cleft-shaped defects is evidence of subtotal injury to developing neuroblasts, with heterotopic islands of neurons entrapped in the white matter, trails of gray matter extending from basal ganglia into continuity with the cortex, and zones of focal microgyria. In examples of more massive neuroblast destruction over wider areas, there results a great defect in each hemisphere in which the cerebral tissue is reduced to a thin membrane composed of approximated sheets of pia and ependyma. About the edges of the defect may be found microgyria and heterotopic gray matter. Both the symmetrical clefts and the symmetrical porencephalies have been found in any lobe of the cerebrum, but the favored site is the central region, including Rolandic and Sylvian areas (Fig. 3-4).

The encephalomalacic porencephalies are dependent upon that property of the young brain that permits the rapid total dissolution of parenchyma after a necrotizing lesion, leading to a cavity or defect with sharply circumscribed borders. In the usual retrospective postmortem analysis, etiology can only be surmised but has variously been ascribed to vascular, traumatic, and infective lesions. The net result is a cavity or series of communicating cavities often restricted to one lobe or one vascular territory of the brain. Commonly the lesion is bordered not by microgyria and defects in cortical development but rather by shrunken discolored cystic gyri of the type encountered in known anoxic and ischemic disorders. The remainder of the brain may be entirely normal except for secondary degenerations in affected long tracts.

Clinical Characteristics. The extensive cortical maldevelopments of the schizencephalies are incompatible with any appreciable postnatal neurologic development. Those individuals who survive into late childhood or adulthood are at best moderate defectives with spastic double hemiplegias. Others are bedridden idiots who never walk or talk and who have tetraplegia with generalized rigidity. Seizures are common and in infants are similar to those associated with other severe forebrain defects, consisting of episodic general extension and head retraction. Reduction in head size need not be present, and indeed occasional patients may develop a coexistent hydrocephalus.

In the encephalomalacic porencephalies clinical effects depend entirely upon the extent and location of the porus and accompanying foci of encephalomalacia. Often there is a hemiplegia, cortical sensory defect, or hemianopia dating from birth (Fig. 3-5), frequently associated with seizures. Well circumscribed lesions may be compatible with normal mentality, but more often large lesions or those associated with scattered focal encephalomalacia produce mental deficiency accompanied by predominantly unilateral motor and sensory defects. Occasionally a cavity at the temporal or frontal pole may be entirely asymptomatic or attended only by a convulsive disorder.

Diagnosis. There are no characteristic facial or cranial features that serve to identify the schizencephalies. They are to be sought

FIG. 3-4. Weigert preparations of hemispheric sections from a patient with symmetrically placed schizencephalic defects. Large masses of heterotopic gray matter can be seen in the insular areas and can be traced microscopically to the ependyma.

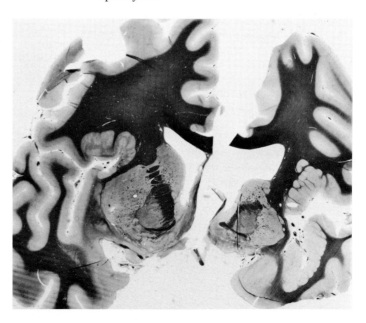

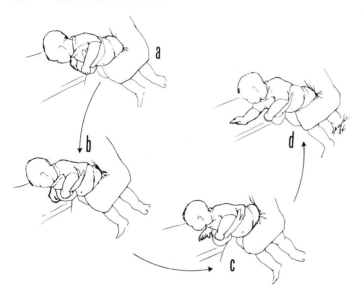

FIG. 3-5. Hemiplegia and unilateral failure of visual placing reaction of the left arm and hand in encephaloclastic porencephaly of right parietal area. As the arms are moved closer to the table in *a* through *d*, the placing reaction of the right arm and hand, but not the left, is completed.

among those patients with particularly profound neurologic abnormalities dating from birth and not ascribable to neonatal asphyxia. One may expect to identify a few of the larger symmetrical defects by demonstrating localized symmetrical transilluminable areas. On CT scan many show large lateral ventricles. Most cases, however, cannot be diagnosed in life and must be relegated to that heterogeneous group of congenital tetraplegias with idiocy, to which belong some of the other clinically occult developmental disorders and the cerebral atrophies of perinatal origin, and which merge imperceptibly into some of the categories of microcephaly. Encephalomalacic porencephaly may sometimes be suspected by demonstrating a unilateral localized transilluminable area of the infantile calvarium. CT scan may show a localized ventricular enlargement and sometimes communication with a cavity.

HYDRANENCEPHALY

To be distinguished from severe hydrocephaly and destructive cerebral disorders of the perinatal period is a class of malformations characterized by rather normal external appearance of the infant but with almost total absence of the cerebral hemispheres (Fig. 3-6). The basis of the disorder relates to the remarkable property of the immature brain to undergo rapid dissolution with removal of degraded cellular components following widespread or total cell death in the cerebral hemispheres.[10] The less damaged brain stem is capable of maintaining vital functions for extended periods. The rapid removal of necrotic cerebral tissue has been demonstrated experimentally in puppies by paraffin injection into cerebral arteries. Subsequently the ependyma and pia–arachnoidal layers merge together to form a thin membranous sac containing CSF.[56] In some cases a maintained rate of fluid formation in the presence of aqueductal scarring or impaired fluid resorption produces secondary expansion of the cranium.

Pathology. A number of pathologic entities can be described, evidently varying with etiology and with stage of development. Morphogenetic studies using associated defects in nervous system development for timing of the process indicate that the condition may begin as early as the end of the third month of gestation and until as late as the second postnatal year.[24] Postnatally the process, from onset to formation of the fluid-filled sac, has been observed in less than 3 months. One of the earliest developing varieties is a form of lissencephaly (agyric brain) with gross failure of neuroblast migration and cortex formation. In some of these cases layers of defective neuroblasts constitute a thin wall of cerebral tissue composing the central portion of the brain but trail off into a mere membrane laterally and superiorly. The cerebellum consists of a flattened arc of poorly foliated tissue. There is often an accompanying aqueductal stenosis. Subependymal deposits of minerals and lipofuscin are abundant, and in some cases grossly abnormal blood vessels have been found. Another early process is the condition of schizencephaly or bilateral symmetrical porencephaly. The injury evidently takes place after cerebral vesicle formation but before completion of neuroblast migration with highly selective destruction of symmetrically placed portions of the developing hemispheres. These become occupied by the usual approximated leaflets of ependyma and pia–arachnoid, but at the border of the membrane merging into surviving cerebrum is a zone of neuroblast arrest with heterotopias and microgyria extending from ependyma to cortex. The remaining cortex is normally formed but in many cases may consist only of remnants of occipital or temporal lobes. In other cases the process has clearly occurred later in prenatal life with remnants of undestroyed cerebrum showing normal architectural development. In infants dying early after birth considerable inflammatory reaction may be observed suggesting an infectious origin; cytomegalovirus was implicated in one such case. In still other examples the process is quite similar to that of multiple cystic encephalomalacia except that most of the cystic cavities have coalesced into the characteristic massive fluid-filled sacs. Cases of postnatal origin may reveal evidence of the causative process, such as fulminant postnatal meningitis.

Etiology.   It appears certain that there are multiple causes of hydranencephaly. The lissencephalic variety can be familial, presumably on a genetic basis. Intrauterine cytomegalovirus disease was implicated in one case. A number of authors favor prenatal occlusive disease of the internal carotid or cerebral arteries as the essential mechanism. This may well hold for a number of encephalomalacic varieties of later prenatal origin but cannot be invoked as a general cause in view of the symmetry of the hydranencephalic disorder, the common

FIG. 3-6. Hydranencephaly. The right half of the calvarium and dura is removed and the cerebrospinal fluid drained to show an empty cavity with a thin membrane adhering to the falx and inner aspect of the dura. There are remnants of basal ganglia and thalami and of occipitotemporal cortex.

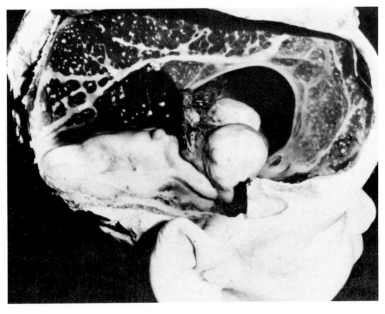

associated presence of schizencephalic deformities, the association of other neural malformations originating early in fetal life, the occasional presence of congenital anomalies elsewhere, and the probable onset of many cases prior to definitive development of cerebral blood vessels. Other prenatal events that have been implicated include maternal syphilis, toxoplasmosis, infectious hepatitis, listeriosis, influenza, attempted abortion, maternal trauma, anemia, and carbon monoxide poisoning. Evidence of postnatal herpes simplex infection has been found recently.

Clinical Characteristics. Infants with severe defects involving the diencephalon and midbrain show difficulties with sucking, respiration, and autonomic functions, and die within the first month. Many of the others appear robust at birth and of normal or even attractive physiognomy. The external appearance as well as the preservation of cranial nerve functions and the ability to suck, yawn, and cough may foster in the parents the illusion of normality during the first few months of the child's life.[58] Some relatively subtle defects, however, can be noted in the early months, and by 4 months to 6 months motor defects and other abnormalities of development are apparent.[24]

Early manifestations include a disorder in sleep and arousal cycle with a characteristic alternation between the two extremes of drowsiness or sleep on the one hand and alertness with loud monotonous crying on the other. The cry is limited to a narrow range of quality and intensity, and the variable vocalizations of infancy with gurgling or cooing do not appear. Disorders of tonus are commonly present from birth and consist of moderate spasticity of all limbs with clasp-knife phenomena, clonus and brisk reflexes, and sometimes a soft plastic rigidity. A useful sign is the failure of evolution of the neonatal grasp reaction. In the normal newborn a moving tactile stimulus on the palm elicits flexion of all fingers with flexion and abduction of the thumb. After 2 weeks the thumb begins to oppose with development of the normal infantile grasp reaction. In hydranencephalics the thumb never opposes, but rather remains in marked adduction and flexion as is commonly seen unilaterally in acquired infantile hemiplegias.

After the fourth month it can generally be recognized that other aspects of motor development fail and reactions remain limited and of neonatal form. Most of the spontaneous behavior consists of rhythmic stepping movements, fragments of the Moro reaction, or rhythmic pawing movements of the upper extremities similar to nursing behavior. Visual following reactions to not appear, and reaching for objects is never seen. Visual and tactile placing reactions, which are normally well developed by the third or fourth month, fail to appear or remain rudimentary. The Moro reaction often persists well past the age of normal suppression and may be elicited by a wide range of stimuli including not only quick extension of the neck, auditory stimuli, and slapping the bed but also brisk stroking of the abdomen or chest and passive extension of the limbs. The child does not sit and never crawls. When placed in the prone position, the limbs become generally flexed. Later more persistent dystonic postures either in flexion or bilateral hemiplegic position may develop. Stretch reflexes remain brisk, with clonus and extensor plantar responses. Rare evanescent smiling may occur, but laughter is absent. Although brief periods of quiet relaxation may be seen, usually the child alternates between sleep and crying. The children are often poikilothermic and show other defects in central thermal regulation. After several months of life convulsive seizures may appear, taking the form of massive infantile myoclonic attacks with neck flexion and extension of the arms or brief attacks of general extension with retraction of the head. In those cases in which hydrocephaly appears there is progressive general enlargement of the head with separation of sutures and upward retraction of the palpebral fissures.

The cranium may be of normal size during the neonatal period. Percussion, however, yields an abnormal note somewhat akin to that obtained upon tapping an overripe melon. The head, and occasionally the pupils, can readily be transilluminated throughout the entire vault, a red glow outlining persistent sagittal sinus and meningeal vessels (Fig. 3-7). In some, a sloping opacity may remain at the occipital or frontal pole.

In the case of complete transilluminability in a normal sized head, diagnostic

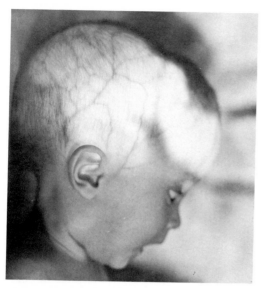

FIG. 3-7. Transillumination of the skull in hydranencephaly.

radiography is not necessary. With an enlarged head a diagnostic difficulty is encountered; not only may progressive obstructive hydrocephaly appear in hydranencephaly, but occasional examples of severe infantile hydrocephaly may transilluminate brilliantly. CT scan permits differentiation. Subdural hygroma may also transilluminate but usually is asymmetrical and over a rather limited field. Expansion of the head in this condition tends to be asymmetrical and to involve the temporal region. In some cases pneumography may be necessary to delineate the two. Destructive brain lesions producing cavitation (encephalomalacic porencephaly) may also transilluminate but over a more restricted area that is usually unilateral.

Prognosis. The disorder ends fatally with pneumonia or advancing hydrocephaly. Those infants surviving the neonatal period often linger 1 year to 3 years.

SMALL OR MALFORMED CRANIUM

The major division of patients with a small or malformed cranium must be between those having a primary reduction in brain volume and those with a surgically cor-

rectable primary craniosynostosis having characteristic head deformities. In the microcephalies secondary premature closure of sutures is common but is usually symmetrical and generalized and exists in the presence of an overall reduction of cranial capacity (Fig. 3-8).

Microcephalies

Within the mentally deficient population there is a general shift of the cranial dimensions below the normal distribution, a tendency particularly evident in mongolism, phenylketonuria, and kernicterus. The term *microcephaly*, however, is generally restricted to that group of diverse etiologies whose common characteristic is a cranium disproportionately small in relation to the rest of the body, and that constitutes an arresting physical feature of the disease.[3] For standardization microcephaly is arbitrarily defined by a cranial circumference less than three standard deviations below the normal for age and sex (Table 3-1). Defined in such a way the microcephalies comprise as much as 20% of consecutive admissions to hospitals for mentally defectives. Here it is convenient to consider these in three principal groups: those of genetic origin, those arising from intrauterine injury or disease, and those attributable to perinatal and postnatal disorders (Table 3-2).

FIG. 3-8. Secondary closure of cranial sutures in microcephaly.

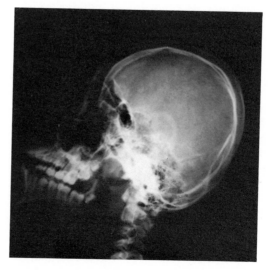

**TABLE 3-1.   Standards for Head
Circumference for
American Children
of North European Stock**

Age	Boys (cm)		Girls (cm)	
	Mean	Range (±3 SD)*	Mean	Range (±3 SD)*
Months				
0	35.3	31.7–38.9	34.7	31.7–37.7
3	40.8	37.2–44.4	40.0	36.4–43.6
6	44.0	41.0–47.0	42.9	39.3–46.5
9	45.8	42.8–48.8	44.7	41.1–48.3
Years				
1	47.1	43.8–50.4	45.9	42.0–49.8
1½	48.8	45.5–52.1	47.4	43.8–51.0
2	49.6	46.0–53.2	48.2	44.0–52.4
2½	50.1	46.5–53.7	49.0	44.8–53.2
3	50.4	46.8–54.0	49.3	45.4–53.2
3½	50.7	47.1–54.3	49.6	45.4–53.8
4	51.0	47.4–54.6	49.9	46.0–53.8
4½	51.2	47.6–54.8	50.2	46.0–54.4
5	51.3	47.7–54.9	50.3	46.4–54.2
5½	51.3	48.0–54.6	50.6	46.7–54.5
6	51.9	48.3–55.5	50.8	46.6–55.0
8	52.7	48.8–56.6	51.8	47.6–56.0
10	53.1	49.8–56.4	53.0	48.8–57.2

*Standard deviation.
Modified from Vickers and Stuart: J Pediatr 22:155, 1943

Genetic Microcephaly. Hereditary micro-cephaly is uncommon, probably account-ing for only 6% of institutionalized mi-crocephalies. Of the several varieties, all conform to recessive inheritance.

The first and most common variety in-cludes the cases of Penrose and the families investigated by Böök and associates.[2] The head is narrow with sloping forehead and marked reduction in the vertical dimension (Fig. 3-9). The face and ears are of normal size in contrast with the reduced vault. Al-though the condition may escape notice at birth, it becomes evident within 6 months. Mental capacity ranges from severely to moderately subnormal. Stature is short, but the body is otherwise well formed. Except for those few cases with severe idiocy and failure of motor development, motor func-tion is not profoundly altered in these pa-tients, but in some families mild spastic

paraparesis can be found. Radiographs of the skull during infancy commonly show premature ossification of cranial sutures. Detailed pathologic studies have been sparse, but in several instances there has been a small brain, its weight sometimes less than half of normal. Gyri are well formed, but there is general simplification of the convolutional pattern. The cortex may show a tendency toward columnar arrange-ment of neurons.

A second and quite rare type of in-herited microcephaly is that of familial liss-encephaly. The cerebrum is small with an agyric cortex and enlarged ventricles. Clin-ically there is not only reduction of head size but also gross neurologic disability. All are idiots and none acquire language. Some are able to walk by age 3 years to 5 years but show evidence of spastic diplegia with scissors gait. Others are bedridden, blind, and inaccessible. The latter are spastic at birth, but as in other examples of stationary severe forebrain defect, decerebrate postur-ing with head retraction gradually emerges during the first few months of life.

Familial microcephaly with calcifica-tion, (Cockayne's syndrome) is a rare dis-order with autosomal recessive inheri-tance. It follows the characteristic evolution of a degenerative rather than a develop-mental disease, that is, affected children may be normal at birth but during infancy or early childhood begin having seizures that recur frequently. Somatic features include dwarfism, beaked nose, and dermatitis in butterfly distribution.

Progressive deterioration of mentality appears, and motor accomplishments are lost with the appearance of symmetrical spastic paralysis and sometimes athetosis, pro-gressing eventually to a decerebrate state.[27] The head is small and round, and optic atrophy may be present. Pathologically the brain is generally reduced in volume, and ventricles are dilated. Mineralized deposits are distributed throughout the cerebral cor-tex, basal ganglia, dentate nucleus, sub-thalamus, and red nucleus. Nerve cell loss may be found in the cortex, thalamus, pu-tamen, and granular layer of cerebellum. Areas of bilateral demyelination and de-posits of an abnormal lipid are seen in the cerebral white matter. The mineral deposits are sufficiently dense to suggest that diagnosis could be made in life on radiography of the skull.

A hereditary type of microcephaly, described by Paine, follows a sex-linked recessive pattern of transmission. Affected infants feed poorly after birth, and development is retarded. With progression of the disease, by the second year there is microcephaly, spastic diplegia, opisthotonus, tonic neck responses, absent grasp and sucking reflexes, and pale optic disks. There is a general hyperaminoaciduria, and total amino acid nitrogen of the CSF is increased.

The rare acceptable instances of pro-

gressive degeneration of the cerebral gray matter (Alpers' disease) constitute an additional disorder that when occurring in infancy may result in microcephaly.[32] Characteristic symptoms are myoclonus, seizures, mental failure, and paralysis. The disease may occur in familial distribution.

Seckel's bird-headed dwarfism is an autosomal recessively inherited condition resembling the Penrose-Böök form in having marked microcephaly and moderate mental retardation but only minor motor disorder.[19] It differs, however, in being accompanied by multiple other anomalies including dwarfism, birdlike facies, low set ears, club foot, and multiple skeletal malformations.

The etiology of deLange's syndrome is uncertain but is probably genetic.[19] The head is microbrachycephalic. The face is characteristic with upturned nose, midline fusion of the eyebrows, micrognathia, and a small midline beak on the upper lip. Other

---

TABLE 3-2.   Etiologic Classification of the Microcephalies

Genetic
 Familial microcephaly (Penrose-Böök)
 Familial lissencephaly
 Familial microcephaly with calcification
   (Cockayne)
 Sex-linked microcephaly with aminoaciduria
 Bird-headed dwarf syndrome (Seckel)
 deLange's syndrome
 Smith-Lemli-Opitz syndrome
 Progressive cerebral cortical atrophy (Alpers'
   disease)
 Phenylketonuria
 Kinky hair disease
Chromosomal aberrations
 Mongolism
 Trisomy 17–18
 Chromosome 18 deletion
 Cri-du-chat syndrome
 Ring chromosome 18
 Fanconi's anemia
Intrauterine injuries and infections
 Radiation
 Rubella
 Toxoplasmosis
 Diabetes mellitus
 Cytomegalic inclusion disease
Perinatal and postnatal disorders
 Diffuse cerebral cortical atrophy
 Multiple cystic encephalomalacia
 Encephalitis (herpes simplex, Coxsackie group B,
   eastern and western equine)
 Incontinentia pigmenti
Unknown
 Happy puppet syndrome
 Beckwith's syndrome
 Rubinstein's syndrome

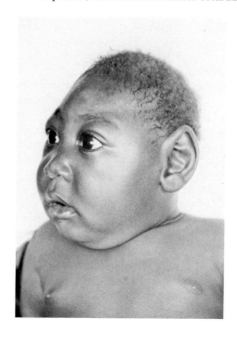

FIG. 3-9. Microcephaly conforming to the recessive type: prominent ears, normal somatic development, and minimal motor retardation.

anomalies include micromelia or phoco-melia, simian line, hirsutism, and cutis marmorata. The cry is a characteristic fee-ble, low-pitched growl.

The Smith-Lemli-Opitz syndrome is a rare condition probably of autosomal reces-sive inheritance and consisting of micro-cephaly, severe mental retardation, broad bridged and upturned nose, increased na-solabial space, epicanthal folds, and mul-tiple skeletal and genital anomalies.[19]

Fanconi's anemia, a condition asso-ciated with polyploidy and multiple chro-mosomal aberrations, is initially mani-fested by the effects of intractable pancytopenia.[38] Major symptoms appear between ages 4 and 10. Examination at this time reveals microcephaly in about one-half of cases, but with feeble-mindedness in only about one-fifth. Strabismus often occurs. There is a characteristic diffuse mottled pigmentation of the head and trunk that is either brown or slate colored (Fig. 3-10A). Stature is somewhat small, and hypoplasia of the thumb occurs regularly (Fig. 3-10B). Other chromosomal disorders, described elsewhere, are characterized by micro-cephaly (Table 3-2).

Microcephaly Acquired in Utero. To be contrasted with genetic microcephalies are the much more frequent instances in which clinical or pathologic evidence is indica-tive of intrauterine injury during the first trimester of pregnancy. Characteristically such cases do not show the sloping fore-head and decreased height of one of the ge-netic varieties, but rather a small, rounded skull sometimes with prominent occipital flattening. Neurologic abnormalities are al-most invariably present. Depending upon the severity of the disorder, these may vary from a decerebrate state to mild mental de-ficiency with exaggerated stretch reflexes.

Etiology. Relatively few etiologic agents of microcephaly acquired *in utero* have been identified, the most completely documented of these being ionizing radia-tion. From data on accidental or intended irradiation of the pelvis during pregnancy it has been found that central nervous sys-tem malformations are commonly pro-duced, the most frequent being micro-cephaly. In about three-fourths of reported instances of radiogenic microcephaly the mother received exposure during the first 2 months of gestation. During the early form-ative period radiation dosage need not be great, stimulating doses for the ovaries hav-ing been teratogenic. During the rest of the first trimester microcephaly has occurred only with doses in the therapeutic range. Microcephaly with severe mental defi-ciency has developed, however, with ex-posure as late as the sixth month of preg-nancy in an instance of implantation of radium in the cervix. The critical factors in producing malformation after atomic bomb radiation were gestational age of less than 15 weeks and a distance of less than 1500 m from the hypocenter.

Another established cause of micro-cephaly is maternal infection with rubella. As in other anomalies characteristic of the rubella syndrome, microcephalies are most likely to appear if the infection occurred within the first 3 months of gestation. A few microcephalic infants are born to diabetic mothers in whom control (during gestation) was poor and who had associated episodes of ketosis or hypoglycemia. Maternal tox-oplasmosis may be mild or inapparent but nevertheless can infect the fetal brain and result in either microcephaly or hydro-cephaly.

Pathology. Etiologic and pathologic information on microcephalies acquired *in utero* fail to converge, and it is not possible to describe morphologic patterns for all of the recognized etiologic varieties. In gen-eral, the prototype for this group of micro-cephalies is a small brain with generalized microgyria. There are recognizable lobes and fissures, but the normal convolutional pat-tern is replaced by an irregular pebbly sur-face due to small and excessive numbers of abnormal gyri (see Fig. 3-1). Microscopi-cally the cortex may be composed of four abnormal layers consisting of an outer zone corresponding to a molecular layer, a sec-ond layer containing abundant neurons of granular and pyramidal type, a zone of myelinated fibers composed of those hori-zontal bundles normally appearing in the deeper layers of cortex, and finally a layer of disorganized neurons trailing off into the subcortical white matter. Heterotopic gray matter (see Fig. 3-2) is frequently found in

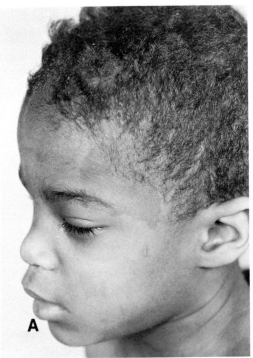

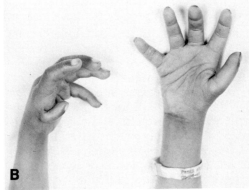

FIG. 3-10. Fanconi's anemia. *A.* Cutaneous pigmentation. *B.* Hypoplasia of thumbs.

the centrum ovale, and there may be such associated malformations as schizencephaly, absent olfactory bulbs, and a small corpus callosum. Toxoplasmosis produces characteristic disseminated foci, often in a periventricular distribution and consisting of granulomatous reaction with cavitation and calcification. In the few neuropathologic reports on the rubella syndrome small brains with hypoplasia or absence of the corpus callosum and other commissural structures were found.

Clinical Characteristics. In severe cases gross neurologic abnormalities are evident during infancy and may consist of lack of visual following, limited behavioral range, clasp-knife phenomenon, increased stretch reflexes, failure of evolution of the grasp reflex, presence of tonic neck responses, and blindness. If such infants survive into early childhood, the reduced size of the cranium becomes evident (usually within the first 4 months) and the appearance is that of a bedridden blind idiot with spastic tetraplegia, later developing into dystonic postures and paralysis in flexion. Less severe cases may display some slow acquisition of postural, prehensile, and am-

bulatory skills with but minimal spastic paralysis. Partial and generalized epilepsies are frequent in these patients and may be quite severe.

The finding of associated abnormalities may facilitate recognition of individual types of microcephaly. Microcephaly appearing as a complication of maternal rubella infection is often associated with ophthalmic abnormalities, deafness, and congenital heart defects. The most common ocular anomaly is bilateral congenital cataract, which may consist either of a uniform lenticular opacification or a central dense zone fading off toward the periphery. Microphthalmia is found in about one-third of children with the rubella syndrome. In addition there may be a fine perivascular pigmentation of the retina. Deafness is usually partial, most marked at the intermediate frequencies, and due to developmental failure of the organ of Corti. Main cardiac defects include patent ductus arteriosus and interventricular septal defect. Hemiplegia or diplegia may occur but are not common. The microcephaly and mental deficiency may escape notice during the neonatal period and can be identified with certainty only in late infancy.

Radiogenic microcephaly is associated with microphthalmia in about one-half of cases and with optic atrophy in a lesser number. Even though the mental defect may be severe, motor impairment is usually not profound.

In fetal toxoplasmosis the newborn may appear normal but in a few weeks or months develops feeding difficulties, loss of vision, ocular palsies, and developmental failures. In cases of toxoplasmosis with persisting active infection in the newborn period there is evidence in the neonate of a severe systemic disease with rash, hepatosplenomegaly, jaundice, and abnormalities of the CSF including xanthochromia, elevated protein, and a mononuclear pleocytosis. Subsequently microcephaly develops in about one-fifth of all instances of congenital toxoplasmosis. Cases seen in late infancy without a history of the characteristic active disease may be suspected on the basis of chorioretinitis, which is present in over 90% of cases. In the early stage this takes the form of white exudative patches around the macula and later appears as gray foci with prominent pigmentation. Vitreal opacities are common, and microphthalmus appears in about one-third of cases. Intracranial periventricular calcification usually develops within a few weeks after birth. Spastic paralysis, brain stem signs, and cranial nerve abnormalities occur frequently.

Microcephalies of Perinatal and Postnatal Origin. A major group of microcephalies can be shown to date from anoxic states or infection in the perinatal period or to develop gradually after birth in the course of evolution of certain nongenetic diseases. Documented examples of prenatal, intrapartum, and postnatal fetal anoxia are associated with two pathologic entities in which microcephaly may be a prominent physical finding. These are diffuse cerebral cortical atrophy and multiple cystic encephalomalacia. Less common instances of proved cerebral cortical atrophy appearing in infants with microcephaly and severe loss of cerebral function have followed

episodes of cardiac arrest and protracted status epilepticus.

Microcephaly developed in 14 of the 17 cases of proved cytomegalic inclusion disease of infancy described by Weller and Hanshaw.[55] The ultimate syndrome closely resembles that of congenital toxoplasmosis with associated mental deficiency, paralyses, seizures, intracranial calcification, and often chorioretinitis. Infection with the cytomegaloviruses produces an acute systemic illness during the neonatal period, although in some cases destructive involvement of the brain may have already been present for months *in utero*. Early symptoms include petechial hemorrhages with low platelet counts, and in the second week jaundice and hepatosplenomegaly. The neurologic sequelae usually develop after several weeks or months. Other viral infections known to cause microcephaly include herpes simplex and Coxsackie group B during the perinatal period and eastern and western equine encephalitis in the neonatal period.

Microcephaly is one of the complications of the dermatologic entity incontinentia pigmenti and may develop after birth, sometimes accompanied by spastic tetraplegia. Familial microcephaly with calcification, progressive degeneration of the cerebral gray matter, and sex-linked microcephaly with aminoaciduria all develop postnatally in the manner of degenerative diseases.

Microcephalies of Uncertain Cause. The "happy puppet" syndrome includes a small brachycephalic head, easily elicited paroxysms of laughter, protruding tongue, and jerky ataxic movements.[19] Under the term *Beckwith's syndrome* is included microcephaly, neonatal hypoglycemia, macroglossia, umbilical hernia, and hepatomegaly. Rubinstein's syndrome consists of microcephaly with severe retardation, broad thumbs and toes, beaked nose, and other anomalies.

Differential Diagnosis. When evaluating the microcephalic infant or child it is important to seek historical information not only of affected siblings and parental consanguinity but also of affected male antecedents in the case of sex-linked microcephaly, and of feebleminded or borderline microcephalic heterozygotes in the genetic microcephalies of the Penrose-Böök type. Relevant gestational data include evidence of rubella, exposure to radiation, badly controlled diabetes, intoxications, and attempted abortion. Associated abnormalities in the patient are helpful in the diagnosis of rubella, cytomegalic inclusion disease, toxoplasmosis, and Fanconi's anemia. The cutaneous pigmentation is highly characteristic for incontinentia pigmenti. Radiographs of the skull reveal a perivascular calcification in toxoplasmosis and cytomegalic inclusion disease, and one may expect to find diffuse cortical and basal ganglia calcification in familial microcephaly with calcification. In microcephaly after congenital toxoplasmosis dye test antibodies in high titer after the 4th month of life are of diagnostic significance, and in a patient under 2 years of age complement-fixing antibodies may be demonstrable. For cytomegalic inclusion disease the demonstration of intranuclear inclusions in exfoliative cytologic examinations of the urinary sediment is useful in early infancy, but demonstration of a viruria is of greater diagnostic significance. In the case of diffuse cerebral cortical atrophy and multiple cystic encephalomalacia it is generally impossible to distinguish these entities in life and is usually not of critical value. However, a CT scan may show dilated ventricles and excess subarachnoid fluid with cortical atrophy, and occasionally multiple cysts communicating with the ventricle in cystic encephalomalacia.

Prognosis. Almost all patients with the disorders discussed here are mental defectives, the severity being roughly proportional to the degree of reduction of cranial volume and the extent of associated neurologic deficits. Rarely, moderate microcephaly may be compatible with normal or slightly subnormal intelligence as in Fanconi's anemia and some instances of radiogenic microcephaly. In the rubella syndrome it is important to assess the relative contributions of visual and auditory defects to the apparent intellectual performance because surgical correction of the cataract and the application of hearing aids and speech therapy may permit some progress to be made in cases with minimal mental defect.

Craniosynostosis

Premature fusion of cranial bones may occur independently of cerebral growth resulting in increased intracranial pressure, deformities of the skull, and compression of neural structures. The combination in certain families of skeletal and cranial defects has led to eponymic subgroups such as Apert's syndrome (craniosynostosis with facial dysostosis and marked syndactyly) and Crouzon's disease (craniosynostosis with facial dysostosis).[19] Since the basic defect in membranous bone is the same in all types, there seems to be no justification for subclassifying the group into separate diseases. It was recently found that various types of hydrocephaly can coexist with craniosynostosis in some patients.

Etiology. Most cases appear sporadically, some probably representing new mutations. A smaller number of cases occur on a genetic basis, usually following a dominant transmission. There is a tendency for similar patterns of expression to remain constant in a given family; thus there are families on record in which dolichocephaly has been transmitted through three generations. In other cases brachycephaly may predominate. On the other hand, families with facial bone synostosis combined with multiple premature synostosis of the cranial bones may exist, even as Crouzon described. Syndactyly is a frequently associated anomaly in some families but has been attributed to a separate gene.

Pathology. There is histologic evidence attributing the premature bony fusion to absence of periosteum on that edge of the bone involved in the disease and suggesting that osseous union takes place because of failure of an opposing force.

Clinical Characteristics. In the course of normal development the metopic suture is obliterated at birth whereas others are open and associated with planes of active growth. Complex interdigitation of opposing cranial bones begins at about 2 years of age, but fusion does not take place until adulthood. Cerebral growth is extremely great throughout intrauterine development but continues at an ever declining rate through the first 5 years of life. Premature fusion of cranial bones within the first 2 years of life is liable to result in a gross distortion of cranial growth, often with intracranial pressure phenomena due to bony constraint of the expanding brain.

After 3 years no skull distortion is likely to appear, nor would any symptoms be expected. With premature fusion between two plates of cranial bone, growth is retarded in the direction perpendicular to the line of fusion, whereas excessive compensatory growth occurs parallel to the line. Thus in premature synostosis of the sagittal suture the head remains narrow but elongated in the anterior–posterior dimension. In obliteration of a single suture or part of one before the second year of life, the patient may escape with no or minimal neurologic symptoms. With multiple suture obliterations, however, there is likely to be a chronic increase in intracranial pressure during the growth period, with frequent appearance of visual loss, optic atrophy, mental deficiency, and convulsive disorder.

Obliteration of sagittal suture (dolichocephaly) is the most commonly encountered type. It is more common in males, and in the occasional inherited case is transmitted as a dominant. The affected infant shows a striking elongation of the cranium with reduction in width (Fig. 3-11A and B). Premature closure at the coronal suture is next in frequency. When the abnormality is bilateral, the skull is broad (brachycephalic) and rather high anteriorly, somewhat suggestive of a fireman's helmet. With unilateral involvement of a coronal suture or both coronal and squamosal, a decrease in volume of anterior fossa may be seen, with a relative downward and lateral expansion of the middle fossa. When all the sutures are involved, the skull shows an increase in its vertical dimension, particularly in the area of the anterior fontanel, thus producing a somewhat pointed appearance from which the designation acrocephaly is derived. Closure at both sagittal and coronal sutures produces a rather cylindrical restriction of the anterior part of the skull but with general increase in height of the cranium and expansion of the posterior half. With both sagittal and lambdoid sutures obliterated, the skull is high and broad. Fusion at the metopic suture occurring before birth can result in a narrow pointed forehead (trigonocephaly).

A number of associated abnormalities of orbital and facial structures may appear. With coronal synostosis the interocular distance may be excessively wide (secondary hypertelorism). With involvement of coronal or of multiple sutures the orbital plate tends to be vertical. The shallow orbits lead to exophthalmus and some divergent displacement of the eyes. Premature fusion of the bones of maxillary and nasal areas may produce considerable facial deformity, with depression of the upper part of the nose and a rather beak-shaped lower nose, depression of the maxillary areas with relative prognathism, choanal atresia, and a superior lip in the shape of an inverted V. These facial features with exophthalmus and acrocephaly have been designated the craniofacial dysostosis of Crouzon; however, facial deformities of this type may coexist in premature ossification at the coronal suture alone. Symmetrical syndactyly may also occur, particularly when there is complete involvement of all the cranial sutures.

During infancy there may be no symptoms other than the structural deformity of the pliable skull. Later, particularly in multiple synostosis, there may be retardation of motor development, mental deficiency, and episodes of headache and vomiting. Papilledema may at times be seen early in life, but it is more common to find reduced visual acuity and various grades of optic atrophy later in childhood. Seizures occasionally develop. With involvement of nasal bones, chronic obstruction of respiratory passages with mouth breathing, recurrent nasal infections, and anosmia occur. The course of the disorder shows considerable variation. Some families may exhibit mild deformities of the skull without other manifestations. Some individuals may have episodes of headache, nausea, and vomiting during early childhood that disappear, leaving the patient asymptomatic and with intelligence within normal range.

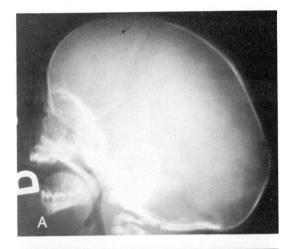

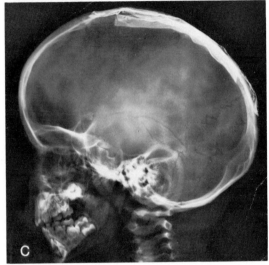

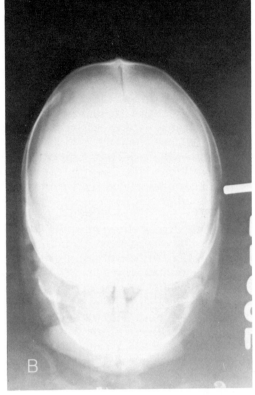

FIG. 3-11. Craniosynostosis involving sagittal suture. *A.* Preoperative films at age 6 weeks to show dolichocephalic deformity. *B.* Partial closure of the sagittal suture and a bony sagittal ridge. *C.* Appearance 2 years after parasagittal craniectomy and insertion of tantalum foil.

Others, however, may be severely affected to the point of requiring institutionalization for mental deficiency.

Radiographic Characteristics. Skull radiographs aid greatly in defining the skull deformity and indicating relative restrictions of the cranial fossae. The process initially appears as narrowing of the suture with osseous bridging (Fig. 3-11B) and later as a linear dense calcification replacing the suture. When increased intracranial pressure has been present, digital markings may be quite prominent. Some of the cranial venous foramina may be enlarged, such as the parasagittal parietal foramina. Posterior clinoids may be decalcified.

Differential Diagnosis. The principal conditions to be considered include microcephaly, mongolism, hydrocephaly, primary hypertelorism, fibrous dysplasia of bone, syphilis of the cranial bones, and gargoylism. Most of these may be readily distinguished upon careful inspection and x-ray examination.

A few conditions present special difficulties. In microcephaly premature fusion of cranial bones is symmetrical and associated with reduction in cranial volume. In some of the forms of microcephaly due to destructive brain diseases there may be considerable flattening in the occipitoparietal region with a tendency toward brachycephaly. The circumference of the skull, however, is clearly reduced, and ossification of the cranial sutures may not be complete until late in infancy when microcephaly is quite obvious. Furthermore, gross failure of evolution of motor pattern with variants of spastic tetraplegia are quite common in such microcephalies but are not seen as a part of primary craniosynostosis. *Primary hypertelorism* has been described as a marked increase in the interocular distance associated with excessive transverse growth of sphenoid and ethmoid bones, and sometimes with nasal cleft. Radiographs of the skull differentiate this from secondary hypertelorism associated with coronal suture obliteration.

Treatment.   To be effective, surgical treatment must be carried out early in life, preferably during the first 6 months. It is not possible to predict with accuracy the cases that will develop neurologic defects if untreated. In view of this fact as well as the uniform appearance of marked deformities and the low risk of surgery, early surgical treatment is indicated in all cases. When there is involvement of multiple or all sutures in infancy, then early surgery is imperative. Surgical treatment consists of linear craniectomy along the obliterated suture, or parallel to it in the case of sagittal suture. Polyethylene or tantalum strips are placed along the bone edge (Fig. 3-11C) to prevent recalcification and bridging of the defect. When the orbit has been shortened, orbital decompression is indicated. Most cases can be satisfactorily treated in this manner. Synostosis at the sagittal suture is liable to show particularly good results. Occasionally in other forms of the disorder mental deficiency may remain despite early treatment. In the case of trigonocephaly this is attributable in some instances to an associated arhinencephaly. The possibility of coexisting hydrocephaly should also be considered; if it is progressive then evaluation for ventricular shunting should be done.

HYPERTELORISM

An abnormally large interocular distance may be found in developmental abnormalities involving the anterior part of the floor of the skull and the nasal bones. This may occur secondarily in such recognized osseous disorders as Hurler's disease, the brachycephalic variety of craniosynostosis, mongolism, or median cleft fact syndrome. Increased interocular distance is also simulated in Waardenburg's syndrome, which includes heterochromia iridis, congenital deafness, and white forelock. In primary hypertelorism, however, there is no other recognized disease process. Overgrowth of the lesser wing of the sphenoid has long been cited as the basic defect; however, it may be stated more accurately that variable enlargement of the sphenoid bone may be present, but that there is a general abnormality in the frontal–nasal regions with widening of the lamina cribrosa and nasal bones and sometimes clefts in the nose, maxilla, or lip. Gross suggests that these anomalies could result from a fusional defect at the anterior neuropore.[21] Morphologic abnormalities of the brain have not been well-defined, but one autopsied case showed agenesis of the corpus callosum.

Etiology.   Although most reports are of sporadic cases, the disorder is a heritable disease. It may be transmitted either as an autosomal dominant or a recessive trait. Hyperaminoaciduria has been noted in some instances of hypertelorism with mental retardation.

Clinical Characteristics.   The bridge of the nose is flat and broad, whereas the eyes are widely spaced. Palpebral fissures may slope downward toward the outer canthi. Strabismus is often present. Infrequently there is a midline nasal groove or cleft.

Mentality can be entirely normal, but in some individuals mental deficiency or epilepsy may be present. Estimates of the frequency of mental deficiency in hypertelorism range from 20% to 45%. It is seldom of severe degree, is usually in the imbecile or moron range, and is compatible with a placid personality. Motor abnormalities are not characteristic features.

Laboratory Examinations. Skull radiographs may demonstrate an enlargement of the lesser wing of the sphenoid. The interorbital distance is increased, and the pyriform aperture is likely to be large and quadrilateral. The sella turcica may be long and deep.

HYDROCEPHALIES

In considering the hydrocephalies one must exclude destructive and atrophic diseases of the brain that produce passive ventricular dilatation as well as those profound cerebral malformations that allow the embryonic vesicular ventricles to persist. The term instead is restricted to those conditions that alter the normal relationships of pressure and volume movement within the interconnected compartments of the cerebrospinal fluid so as to cause an enlargement of the ventricles with progressive cranial distention in the heads of the young, but with prominent mechanical brain disturbances and alterations of cerebral circulation in older children.

Etiology. Cerebrospinal fluid is formed within the ventricles by an active process that determines the normal composition of the fluid. Sodium transport into the ventricles is dependent upon carbonic anhydrase. In normal animals the major contribution to the CSF appears to be from choroid plexuses, but another component of uncertain magnitude is derived from the ependyma. Normally only a small proportion of fluid is reabsorbed through the ependyma and choroid plexuses; hence the bulk flow is through ventricular orifices into the subarachnoid spaces. Total production rates in man have been measured at 0.35 ml/minute (about 500 ml/day).

Some absorption of CSF or its components can take place at the perineurial sheaths or through the subpial vessels; however, the major route of removal is by way of the arachnoidal villi of the large venous sinuses.

Most examples of hydrocephaly are due to partial obstruction within the ventricular channels or to failure of the absorptive processes. Particularly vulnerable sites

for obstruction include the foramen of Monro, the third ventricle, the aqueduct of Sylvius, and the foramina of Luschka and Magendie. Total obstruction of ventricular flow terminates fatally unless relieved. With subtotal obstruction the mean intraventricular pressure rises, fluid accumulates, and the ventricles distend due not only to active secretion by the choroid plexus and ependyma but also to the effect of pressure pulses originating in the choroid plexuses.[31] Later transependymal fluid absorption is greatly increased and fluid exchange stabilized at normal or slightly increased pressure levels.

Hydrocephaly caused by absorptive failure is usually of the communicating type, that is, air injected into the lumbar sac enters the ventricular system, and dye injected into the ventricles can be demonstrated in the lumbar fluid within 2 min to 12 min. Types that may reasonably be attributed to impaired absorption include granulomatous or fibrotic obliteration of large absorptive surfaces or subarachnoid blocks around the brain stem that may prevent access of cerebrospinal fluid to the cisterns, cerebral convexities, and arachnoidal villi.

Hydrocephaly due to excessive production of fluid in the absence of obstruction is of doubtful importance but appears to be one of the mechanisms involved in the hydrocephaly accompanying some intraventricular choroid plexus papillomas.[31]

Among specific etiologic agents, a large and ever increasing cause of hydrocephaly is arachnoidal fibrosis in the cisterns at the base of the brain and at the tentorium following bacterial meningitis, subarachnoid hemorrhage, and rarely, viral meningitis and sterile inflammatory reactions. Another large group is attributable to developmental disorders of early intrauterine life and includes the Arnold-Chiari malformation, atresia of the foramen of Magendie, and some anomalies of the aqueduct of Sylvius.[6] The only hereditary cause of hydrocephaly in man is stenosis of the aqueduct of Sylvius due to a sex-linked recessive gene. Obstruction of pathways by neoplasms or by aneurysm of the vein of Galen is a common mechanism of hydrocephaly. Vitamin A deficiency produces a reversible hydrocephaly in experimental animals and has been known to produce increased intracranial pressure in infants.

Pathology. Some general features are common to most categories of hydrocephaly. In cases developing during infancy with marked distention of the head there is massive enlargement of the brain with great saclike ventricles. In older, more acute cases in which enlargement of the cranium does not accommodate the rising intraventricular pressure, flattened gyri and less extensively enlarged ventricles appear. In general, with distal blockades in the cerebrospinal fluid pathways the lateral ventricles tend to enlarge first and to greatest degree followed by the third ventricle and only later by the fourth ventricle and aqueduct. As dilatation of lateral ventricles proceeds there may be rupture of the septum pellucidum. Stretching of the surrounding cerebral hemispheres may be unequally distributed with the parietal lobe and vertex bearing the maximal effect. There may then result particularly severe stretching of the long cortical efferent fibers deriving from the medial or leg areas of the Rolandic cortex, thereby accounting for the frequent appearance of spastic paraplegia. With severe or protracted cases there may be ballooning of some thin and vulnerable parts of the brain including the floor of the third ventricle, the supraoptic recess, and the suprapineal recess. The third ventricular dilatation may stretch the optic tracts and chiasma and lead to atrophy of hypothalmic nuclei, accounting for the occasional appearance of bitemporal visual field defects and hypothalmic disorders. Some patients develop diverticula of the ventricles, extending outward and occasionally rupturing into the subarachnoid pathways. Favored sites for these are the anterior horn and the medial aspect of the posterior portion of the lateral ventricles. Rarely after ventricular needling there may be passage of fluid into the subdural space with the creation of a complicating subdural hygroma. In late cases atrophy of the choroid plexuses and numerous ependymal granulations may be seen.

The Arnold-Chiari malformation exists in two forms, in each of which the essential feature is a characteristic deformity of the lower brain stem and cerebellum. The more benign of the two varieties is the Chiari type I malformation, in which there is elongation and caudal displacement of the medulla and a tonguelike extension of posterior vermis into the upper cervical canal. Although cervical syringomyelia and bony deformities of the foramen magnum may occasionally coexist, there is no association with spina bifida cystica or infantile hydrocephaly.

The Chiari type II defect, which by general usage is designated the Arnold-Chiari malformation, not only shares the medullary–cerebellar anomaly but is regularly associated with spina bifida cystica, infantile hydrocephaly, and other malformations of the brain and spinal cord.[40] Among the variants of spina bifida, the myelocele is most consistently attended by the Arnold-Chiari malformation, whereas the syndrome occurs but rarely with the meningocele. At the site of the myelocele the spinal cord is anchored and deformed and often shows adjacent malformations such as duplication of the cord, hydromyelia, and diastematomyelia. In this zone spinal roots course in a transverse instead of the usual caudad direction. The entire cord is not, however, fixed by the anchoring anomaly. On the contrary, it elongates with growth, and the normal caudad angulation of spinal roots is resumed only a few segments above the spina bifida. As the foramen magnum is approached, cervical spinal roots again show an abnormal angulation, coursing in a cephalad direction. This is not explainable by downward traction of the entire cord but rather by an independent displacement of medulla into the cervical canal. With elongation of the lower brain stem the caudally displaced fourth ventricle may empty into the subarachnoid space in the upper cervical canal. At the inferior tip of the fourth ventricle there is often a tuft of choroid plexus and a small knuckle of medulla, suggesting a buckling effect. The posterior vermis of cerebellum extends downward into the cerevical canal to lie just above the displaced fourth ventricle. In the forebrain may be found other defects, including microgyria, interdigitation of the medial-frontal convolutions across the midline, and enlargement of the massa intermedia. In many cases the site of obstruction is in the pathways about the brain stem and posterior cerebellum owing to the impaction of these structures at the foramen magnum or to adhesive arachnoidal thickening in the same area. Narrowing of the aqueduct of Sylvius occurs in about one-half of cases.

In postmeningitic or postinflammatory hydrocephaly there can be thickening of the arachnoid and obliteration of subarachnoid pathways at the cisterns about the tentorial opening, in the posterior fossa, and about the outlets of the fourth ventricle.[47] Very dense organized exudate remains in the basal and ambient cisterns after treatment in some cases of tuberculous meningitis. Less frequently encountered than subarachnoid obstructions are intraventricular blocks, such as gliosis of the Sylvian aqueduct following ependymitis developing in the course of pyogenic or tuberculous meningitis. Rarely, mycotic infection produces a chronic granulomatous ependymitis with obstructive hydrocephalus.

Narrowing of the aqueduct of Sylvius may result from several pathologic processes. Uncomplicated narrowing of the channel with no other distortion in its architecture characterizes simple aqueductal stenosis, which may exist as a hereditary disorder.[15] It is occasionally associated with fusion of the corpora quadrigemina. Another category consists of branching or forking of the aqueduct into dorsal and ventral channels, which may in turn break up into smaller channels, many of which may end blindly. A similar process has been produced experimentally in newborn rodents by infections with myxoviruses, reovirus, and arbovirus. There may be insufficiency of the aqueduct due to inflammatory ependymitis and to progressive periaqueductal gliosis, both of which are often acquired lesions.

With the disorder designated atresia of the foramen of Magendie, there is enlargement of the posterior fossa due to a conversion of the fourth ventricle into a huge membrane-lined sac that spreads apart the cerebellar hemispheres and displaces them forward (Fig. 3-12). The foramen of Magendie is absent, although in some cases the

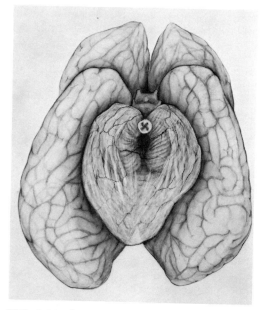

FIG. 3-12. Atresia of the foramen of Magendie. A large translucent sac replaces the fourth ventricle. The posterior midline cerebellar structures are defective.

foramina of Luschka may be present. The membrane is composed of a lining of ependyma and pia–arachnoid, and an intervening layer of vascularized tissue. At the anterior limit of the membrane a malformed and flattened posterior cerebellar vermis is layered over the ependyma.[4]

Tumors are common causes of hydrocephaly. In the pediatric age group one may encounter colloid cysts obstructing at the foramen of Monro or third ventricle, craniopharyngiomas and gliomas at the third ventricle, pinealomas compressing the aqueduct, and astrocytomas or glioblastomas narrowing the same structure. Ependymomas, medulloblastomas, and cerebellar astrocytomas compress the fourth ventricle, and astrocytoma or glioblastoma of the pons may cause narrowing of this ventricle or impaction of the posterior fossa subarachnoid pathways. Diffuse meningeal malignancies of glial or metastatic origin may widely obstruct subarachnoid pathways. Choroid plexus papilloma of the fourth ventricle may directly induce obstruction. Papillomas of lateral ventricles may produce hydrocephaly in the absence of demonstrable obstruction and in part at least by excessive secretion.

Clinical Characteristics. *General Features.* In hydrocephaly that develops very acutely during infancy or in cases appearing later in childhood when the skull is less pliable, attacks of nausea and vomiting are prominent and are accompanied by some intermittent head pain. Episodes of neck retraction and extensor rigidity of the limbs often occur, and papilledema may be present. With reduction in the level of consciousness in infants there is lethargy and loss of recently acquired motor achievements, and in older children drowsiness or confusion occur.

In the case of chronic obstructive disorders of less abrupt onset, enlargement of the head is usually quite evident; if untreated the head may become of massive size with enlarged fontanels and palpably separated sutures, thinned scalp, prominent scalp veins, upward retraction of the eyelids, inverted triangular appearance of the face, strabismus due to sixth nerve paralysis, and spastic paraplegia. In very severe cases in which dilatation of the lateral ventricles progressively thins the surrounding cerebrum to but a few millimeters, neurologic deficiencies may be profound and may approach those described for hydranencephaly, with failure of evolution of the grasp and of prehensile activity; inability to sit, stand, or walk; and generalized spasticity.

In milder and even more chronic instances, no severe neurologic abnormalities may be present and mental deficiencies may not be apparent until considerably later in life; hence enlargement of the head is a paramount clinical sign in early life. In such cases serial measurement of head circumference is imperative for clinical appraisal. Head circumference may enlarge in increasing disproportion to other bodily dimensions, or it may follow the course of appearing consistently above the ninety-fifth percentile but developing parallel to that of the expected normal. Compensatory factors may result in cessation of any progressive enlargement at 2 years to 3 years of age, but it is to be expected that most of these patients will reach a level of psychologic development below that which would have been expected from their native endowment.[30] Some may be jolly or euphoric and able to perform remarkable feats of rote memory, yet their initiative, comprehension, and ability to accomplish abstraction may be much impaired.

Certain secondary manifestations may appear owing to regional brain damage in severe hydrocephaly. Damage to the hypothalamic nuclei from distention of the floor of the third ventricle may account for some of the endocrinologic disorders occasionally encountered, including precocious puberty, obesity, genital atrophy, and diabetes insipidus. The same mechanism with pressure effects upon the optic chiasm may account for instances of bitemporal hemianopia. Ventricular diverticula burrowing through cerebral white matter may produce such focal signs as hemianopia or hemiplegia.

Arnold-Chiari Malformation. The Chiari type I anomaly does not usually become apparent until late childhood or adulthood, when after many years of latency there develops subacutely a syndrome associated with foramen magnum impaction and obstructive hydrocephaly. There appear signs of increased intracranial pressure including episodes of nausea, vomiting, headache, and sixth nerve palsy, together with cerebellar ataxia, nystagmus, and paralysis of the lower cranial nerves. The condition is frequently associated with bony anomalies about the foramen magnum, such as basilar impression, assimilation of the atlas, and the Klippel-Feil anomaly.

The Chiari type II (Arnold-Chiari) malformation is made evident from birth by the presence of myelocele. Simple meningocele occurs in less than 10% of cases of spina bifida cystica and is not associated with the Arnold-Chiari malformation. Some form of myelocele accounts for the rest, and hydrocephaly develops in over 80% of patients with this defect. If the myelocele includes the lumbar area and paraplegia is present, then the association with hydrocephaly is almost constant.

The hydrocephaly can be present at birth or become evident late in the first year of life. Repair of the spina bifida does not cause the hydrocephaly but may accelerate its rate of development. A small group of patients develop lower cranial nerve palsies within the first 6 months, usually beginning with laryngeal stridor. The severe spinal cord defect accompanying the myelocele accounts for the frequent appearance of paralysis and atrophy of the lower extremities, failure of sphincter control, and chronic cutaneous lesions due to sensory denervation. On skull radiographs a characteristic finding is craniolacunia, present in over one-half of cases and quite typical of the disorder (Fig. 3-13). The radiographic findings consist of multiple oval and rounded areas of radiolucency distributed over the skull. The defects are not attributable to increased intracranial pressure, and they differ from digital markings of chronically increased pressure by their sharp borders and their presence during the neonatal period when digital marking should not occur. Some of the mental and somatic neurologic abnormalities found in those who survive the Arnold-Chiari malformation cannot all be ascribed to the hydrocephaly but to associated malformations of the cerebral hemispheres as well.

Postinflammatory Hydrocephaly. This variety represents the most common type of hydrocephaly and has been seen with increasing frequency in recent years following late or inadequate antibiotic treatment of pyogenic meningitis. When hydrocephaly develops after severe or incompletely treated infantile pyogenic meningitis, especially in that due to *H. influenzae,* the clinical signs may be overshadowed by those resulting from irreversible cerebral lesions of the primary disease or from subdural effusion. After tuberculous meningitis, evidence of hydrocephaly often develops concurrently with signs of diencephalic and midbrain infarctions. Nevertheless, to the total clinical pattern hydrocephaly contributes the findings of progressive head enlargement, drowsiness, nausea, and poor feeding. Following less disastrous meningeal infections, hydrocephaly may gradually appear after a latent period and presents the usual signs of subacute or chronic hydrocephaly, according to the age of development. Most postmeningitic cases are of the communi-

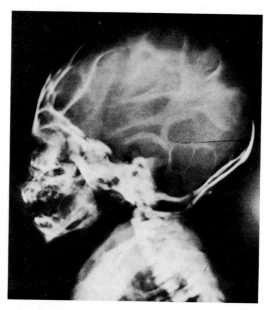

FIG. 3-13. Plain skull film with craniolacunia in child with Arnold-Chiari malformation.

cating variety, and on pneumoencephalography it may be possible to demonstrate filling of the ventricular system with failure of air to pass into the subarachnoid spaces of the cerebral hemispheres. Occasionally the hydrocephaly is noncommunicating, due to ependymitis at the aqueduct of Sylvius.

Many cases of congenital or early infantile hydrocephaly conform to the postinflammatory type on pathologic examination and have been ascribed to perinatal meningitis or to subarachnoid hemorrhage at birth. Postinflammatory infantile hydrocephaly should be suspected in instances of communicating hydrocephaly including the physical and radiographic signs of the Arnold-Chiari malformation.

Narrowing of the Aqueduct of Sylvius. Hydrocephaly from aqueductal narrowing may occur on the basis of several pathologic processes. All, however, present the clinical appearance of noncommunicating hydrocephaly in which there is impedance to the passage of air through the aqueduct either on pneumoencephalography or ventriculography, and slowing or prevention of the appearance of dye in the lumbar subarachnoid space upon ventricular injection. True aqueductal stenosis, a developmental malformation, may be severe producing congenital or neonatal hydrocephaly. Many cases, however, are relatively compensated with but slight enlargement of the head. Such patients may be subject to intermittent periods of decompensation in which headache, vomiting, and attacks of extensor rigidity appear. Aqueductal stenosis may be inherited as a sex-linked recessive trait. Some examples occur sporadically, and others appear in association with the Arnold-Chiari malformation. Congenital forking of the aqueduct and acquired aqueductal gliosis have no associated characteristics that permit their recognition in life, but together make up most of the remaining cases of hydrocephaly due to aqueductal insufficiency. Gliosis may arise sufficiently late in life to result in initial onset of symptoms during late childhood and maturity.

Atresia of the Foramen of Magendie (Dandy-Walker Syndrome). Although this condition may result in progressive hydrocephaly in infancy, it quite commonly remains compensated for long periods, resulting in the development of symptoms in late childhood or young adulthood. The abnormal membrane forming the greatly distended roof of the fourth ventricle may permit passage or absorption of some ventricular fluid, and in some cases the foramina of Luschka may be patent. Decompensation appears to occur after progressive fibrotic thickening of the membrane or occasionally following meningitis or trauma. In addition to an expanded head in infants and symptoms of increased intracranial pressure in older children, cerebellar ataxia may be present. The head is characteristically dolichocephalic. Plain x-ray films of the skull often reveal the diagnosis by showing upward displacement of the transverse sinuses, a marked increase in the A-P dimension, and a greatly enlarged posterior fossa. A CT scan confirms the diagnosis (Fig. 3-14).

Choroid Plexus Papilloma. These vascular tumors, when present in the lateral ventricles, may produce communicating hydrocephaly due at least in part to excessive secretion and recurring hemorrhage. The condition usually develops during

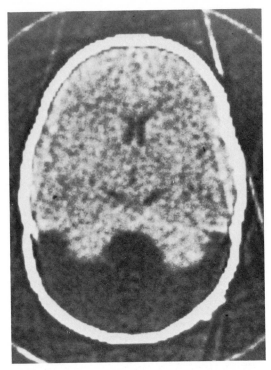

FIG. 3-14. CT scan demonstrates cystic enlargement in the posterior fossa.

the first year or two of life. Unlike hydrocephalies of infancy that are not of neoplastic origin, choroid plexus papilloma often produces papilledema. As a result of repeated bleeding, the CSF may be xanthochromic with elevated protein and cell content. If the physician is forewarned by papilledema or an acute onset, he should plan pneumography as a preliminary procedure to surgery. An adequate air study outlines the intraventricular mass.[31]

Hydrocephaly Associated with Achondroplasia. Most achondroplastics have enlarged brachycephalic heads, yet they are generally of normal intellect. Two cerebral abnormalities have been noted: megalencephaly and hydrocephaly; but mental deficiency, when it exists, may vary independently of either of these disorders.[13]

The megalencephaly is usually of the primary type, that is, an increase in brain mass without other detectable abnormality. Hydrocephaly may exist (Fig. 3-15A and B)

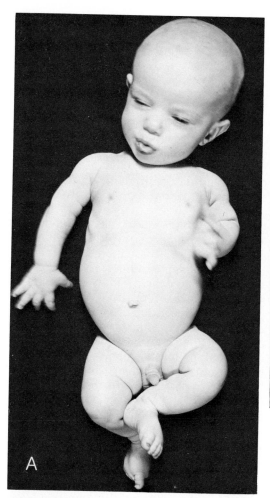

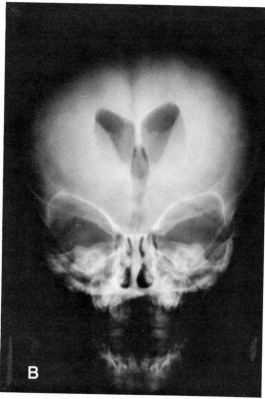

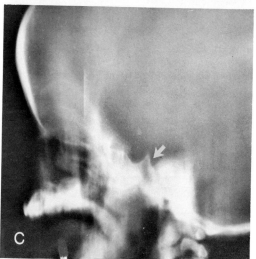

FIG. 3-15. Achondroplasia. *A.* Prominent head, short humeri and femurs. *B.* Moderate ventricular dilatation. *C.* Premature closure of sphenooccipital synchondrosis (*arrow*).

and attain moderate severity with enlarged head, greatly dilated ventricles, and reduced intelligence. For the most part, however, proved hydrocephaly advances very slowly and is rarely subjected to surgical treatment. The prevailing opinion holds that the condition may cease to progress in many cases. The pathogenesis is obscure; the posterior fossa tends to be small and the cerebellum and brain stem disproportionately large, but no obstructive mechanism has yet been demonstrated.

The clinical diagnosis of achondroplasia in the infant is usually evident. A characteristic radiographic sign on skull films is the obliteration during infancy of the sphenooccipital synchondrosis (Fig. 3-15C). Normally this does not occur before age 11. With no well established guides to the natural history of the disorder, one is obliged to approach the problem of hydrocephaly in the achondroplastic infant with caution. Clearly no surgical intervention should be contemplated unless unequivocal progress of the disorder can be demonstrated. Since significant hydrocephaly and concomitant mental defect occasionally occur, it may be possible to prevent this in selected cases with judicious shunting procedures.

Differential Diagnosis. In approaching the differential diagnosis of hydrocephaly (Table 3-3) it is convenient to group cases according to rapidity of evolution and age. There is one group of disorders that develops rather acutely during infancy and in the absence of spina bifida or preexisting hydrocephalus. In such infants there appears over a period of days or weeks such symptoms as irritability, poor feeding, vomiting, head-rubbing, convulsions, and loss of recently acquired motor performances. On examination one finds bulging fontanels, papilledema, or early cranial enlargement. Several types may develop this rapidly but do not usually cause papilledema; these include the aqueductal narrowings, atresia of the foramen of Magendie, and certain cases of postinflammatory hydrocephaly of occult origin.

One must particularly consider other conditions, however, including intracranial tumors of infancy, craniosynostosis, choroid plexus papilloma, lead encephalopathy, vitamin A deficiency, hypoparathyroidism, tetracycline therapy, hypophosphatasia, and subdural hematoma. Craniosynostosis is identified by inspection and radiographic examination. Lead poisoning is detected by the basophilic stippling of red cells, osseous lead line, urinary coproporphyrin excretion, and urinary lead content. Vitamin A deficiency has been observed in infants on milk substitute diets without adequate vitamin supplementation. In addition to bulging fontanels, lethargy, and increased cerebrospinal fluid pressure, there is xerophthalmia, gynecomastia, and other evidence of epithelial metaplasia. The symptoms promptly respond to vitamin A administration. Asymmetrical enlargement of the head, when present, suggests the possibility of subdural hematoma. With other disorders considered and excluded, it is then necessary to perform subdural diagnostic aspiration for subdural hematoma. This should be done as a neurosurgical procedure, to be followed if findings are negative by ventriculography for the identification of tumor and major types of hydrocephaly.

Cases of hydrocephaly present at birth or developing gradually during infancy constitute another group. One may expect to find examples of the Arnold-Chiari malformation, postinflammatory hydrocephaly, congenital hydrocephaly of clinically occult origins, narrowing of the aqueduct of Sylvius, atresia of the foramen of Magendie, and achondroplasia. Hydranencephaly must be differentiated, particularly because a complicating progressive obstructive hydrocephaly may develop after birth in this disorder. Intracranial tumors producing obstruction or massive displacement have to be considered. A rather rare condition that may be confused with hydrocephaly is megalocephaly in which the head is enlarged owing to increased cerebral mass, but without CSF obstruction. This condition may be seen in achondroplasia and a variety of endocrinopathies and familial conditions, as well as in several degenerative diseases including metachromatic leukoencephalopathy, late stages of Tay-Sachs disease, spongy leukoencephalopathy, and tuberous sclerosis.

In defining the diagnosis of chronic hydrocephaly, considerable information is gained from relatively simple examinations. Important in historical information is previous meningitis or evidence of a neonatal disease compatible with toxoplasmosis or cytomegalic inclusion disease. It is important to ascertain if severe neurologic symptoms antedated the onset of head enlargement. In the family history one seeks evidence of affected male antecedents and inquiries for those degenerative diseases that may produce megalocephaly. On general examination the presence of myelocele identifies the Arnold-Chiari malformation, and enlarged dolichocephalic head suggests the possibility of the Dandy-Walker syndrome. Total transillumination of the calvarium identifies hydranencephaly and renders contrast studies unnecessary. Chorioretinitis is evidence for toxoplasmosis or cytomegalic inclusion disease. The importance of adenoma sebaceum and achondroplastic limbs is self-evident. Enlargement of the head in Tay-Sachs disease always appears late and after the establishment of well-defined neurologic defects and retinal degeneration. In spongy degeneration there may be an enlarged head and increased cerebrospinal fluid pressure, but convulsions, progressive paralysis, and mental arrest antedate the enlargement. On plain skull films the presence of craniolacunia is evidence of the Arnold-Chiari malformation, and a high transverse sinus with large posterior fossa of the Dandy-Walker syndrome (see Fig. 3-13). Periventricular calcification is seen in toxoplasmosis and cytomegalic inclusion disease. Finally, by CT scan, it is possible to confirm ventricular enlargement and its extent, detect narrowing of the aqueduct, demonstrate a cystic fourth ventricle, or find evidence of tumor. In megalocephaly the ventricles are either small or but slightly enlarged.

In later childhood clinical patterns and causes of hydrocephaly are different. Because the head is no longer distensible, one encounters instead symptoms of recurring or progressive nausea, vomiting, irritability, drowsiness, diplopia, and visual loss. Papilledema may be present and skull x-ray films show diastasis of the cranial sutures and erosion of the sella turcica with digital markings as a less reliable finding. The Chiari type I malformation may be associated with hydrocephaly in late childhood and can be suspected in the presence of short neck, vertical nystagmus, gait ataxia, lower cranial nerve paralyses, and bony anomalies at the foramen magnum. Atresia of the foramen of Magendie may also decompensate in childhood and can be recognized by the characteristic radiographic abnormalities. Gliosis of the aqueduct of Sylvius must be defined by careful ventriculographic study. Mycotic infections usually require repeated cerebrospinal fluid investigations. Intracranial neoplasms constitute a major cause of obstructive hydrocephaly. Craniopharyngioma may be suspected clinically in cases of hydrocephaly with bitemporal hemianopia, diabetes insipidus, or precocious puberty. Many of these tumors in children, however, produce only ventricular obstruction with suprasellar calcification on plain films. Pinealoma commonly obstructs the aqueduct or posterior third ventricle and is occasionally calcified. It frequently produces prominent midbrain neurologic abnormalities including loss of pupillary light reflex, paralysis of upward gaze, and loss of convergence. Gliomas of the midbrain can produce aqueductal narrowing simulating gliosis at the aqueduct, but they become evident in time after displacement of parts of the ventricular system and progressive brain stem signs. The symptomatic courses of some cases of medulloblastoma and cerebellar astrocytoma may be identical with those of atresia of the foramen of Magendie and of Chiari type I malformations. These tumors usually produce progressively prominent cerebellar signs, however, and air or isophendylate (Pantopaque) ventriculography completes the diagnosis.

Finally, in older children one must consider nonobstructive causes of increased intracranial pressure and papilledema. Vitamin A intoxication may appear after the intake of about 100,000 units/day for several months. Increased intracranial pressure and papilledema appear, but the ventricles are not enlarged. General signs of diagnostic importance include alopecia, hypomenorrhea, and cracks about the corner of the mouth. Other causes of nonobstructive intracranial hypertension include dural sinus thrombosis and hypoparathyroidism.

Treatment.   In any considerations of therapy it is evident that the results must exceed the natural expectation of the disease. According to the series of Laurence, which included cases collected from 1938 to 1957 and were somewhat weighted for severity, a mortality of 49% may be expected in nontreated cases.[30] Of the survivors, it would be anticipated that 59% have an IQ below 85, and 67% would have some degree of physical handicap. In the past, surgical procedures produced results no better than these. With techniques now practiced, however, it is possible to obtain significant benefits.

The most important surgical therapy involves the various shunting procedures in which an artificial passage is created for the transfer of fluid from ventricle to cistern, mastoid, body cavity, or right auricle,

(*Text continues on p. 92*)

TABLE 3-3. Differential Diagnosis of Hydrocephaly

	Age of Onset	Clinical Characteristics	Head Shape	Skull Films	Communicating	Air Study or CT Scan
Arnold-Chiari malformation	Congenital or in infancy	Spina bifida	Hydrocephalic	Craniolacunia in infancy	Usually	General ventricular dilatation, cerebellar ectopia
Atresia, foramen of Magendie	Any	Cerebellar ataxia	Dolichocephalic	Large posterior fossa, elevated transverse sinus	No	Cystic fourth ventricle
Aqueductal stenosis	Any	May be sex-linked recessive	Hydrocephalic		No	Aqueductal block
Aqueductal forking	Infancy		Hydrocephalic		No	Aqueductal block
Aqueductal gliosis	Any		Hydrocephalic		No	Aqueductal block
Postinflammatory hydrocephaly	Any	Follows meningitis, subarachnoid hemorrhage	Hydrocephalic		Usually	Failure to fill cisterns or convexities
Toxoplasmosis	Congenital or in infancy	Rash, choriorentinitis, serologic tests	Hydrocephalic	Periventricular calcification	Sometimes	
Hydranencephaly	Congenital	Failure of mental development, transilluminable	Normal or hydrocephalic		Sometimes	Absence of cerebrum
Anomalies at foramen magnum	Childhood and adolescence	Ataxia, vertical nystagmus, short neck, headache	Normal or mild enlargement	Basilar impression, Klippel-Feil	Usually	Cerebellar ectopia
Subdural hematoma	Infancy	Developmental failure, vomiting, seizures	Often asymmetrical		Yes	Ventricular displacement, sulcal obliteration
Choroid papilloma	Infancy and childhood	Papilledema, CSF xanthochromic with elevated protein	Hydrocephalic		Yes	Intraventricular mass

Disease	Age of onset	Clinical features	Skull enlargement	Sella/sutures	Signs of increased pressure	Ventriculography/radiographic findings
Cerebellar tumor	Childhood	Ataxia, vomiting, headache, papilledema	No or little enlargement	Suture diastasis	Sometimes	Compression at fourth ventricle, aqueductal kink
Brain stem glioma	Late childhood	Cranial nerve disorders, headache, vomiting, papilledema	Variable enlargement	Suture diastasis	Usually	Posterior displacement of aqueduct and fourth ventricle
Craniopharyngioma	Any	Bitemporal hemianopia, optic atrophy, diabetes insipidus, hypopituitarism	Seldom enlarged	Suprasellar calcification	Yes	Third ventricular filling defect
Hurler's disease	Late infancy	Corneal opacity, hepatosplenomegaly, skeletal defects	Moderate enlargement frequent	Elongated sella	Yes	Failure to fill convexities
Achondroplasia	Infancy or childhood	Skeletal defects	Moderate enlargement frequent	Closure of sphenooccipital synchrondrosis	Yes	Ventricles normal or moderately dilated
Megalencephalies (degenerative)	Infancy	Severe neurologic deterioration	Slight enlargement		Yes	Ventricles normal or slightly dilated
Cerebral edema	Any	Convulsions, stupor or coma, acute onset	Normal	Normal or suture diastasis	Yes	Small ventricles
Lateral sinus thrombosis	Any	Headache, lethargy, symptomatic relief from lumbar puncture, papilledema	Normal	Normal or suture diastasis	Yes	Normal

or from subarachnoid space to ureter. In the absence of active intracranial infection, most cases of hydrocephaly should be subjected to one of the shunting procedures.

There are two main exceptions. The first includes instances in which hydrocephaly is so advanced or an associated cerebral defect so profound that treatment is of no avail. In evaluating this group one should not place major reliance upon the estimation of thickness of the cerebral wall at ventriculography because this is an undependable index of potential response. If, however, the remaining cerebral tissue is so thin that brilliant transillumination is possible throughout the entire calvarium, no treatment should be attempted. Furthermore, if the neurologic signs indicate an extremely severe maldevelopment or destructive process amounting virtually to decerebration, treatment is also to be avoided. The other possible exception is the mild case of hydrocephaly with spontaneous "arrest." There may be examples of this phenomenon with resolution of partial blocks or compensatory increase in transependymal absorption of ventricular fluid. More common are instances of mild hydrocephaly in which cephalic enlargement continues after age 2 or 3 but at a declining rate. In such cases, however, shunting procedures may actually reduce head size toward normal with some evidence of clinical improvement. The concept of compensation must therefore be viewed with caution and accepted only after careful ser-

ial head measurements and clinical appraisal.

None of the several possible shunting operations is applicable to all cases of hydrocephaly or likely to be attended by excellent results. At the present time, however, it seems reasonable to view ventriculoauriculostomy by means of the Holter or Heyer-Pudenz valves as most widely applicable.[8] The former device consists of a set of double fish-mouth valves arranged in tandem fashion and designed to open either at 10 or 50 mm water (Fig. 3-16). This arrangement prevents reflux of blood up the catheter from the auricle or jugular vein. With growth of the subject, the distal end of the catheter is drawn upward and requires surgical revision. The procedure should be avoided in cases of suspected chronic intracranial infection or any bacteremia. Otherwise, it may be used in any variety. The Torkildsen procedure of ventriculocisternostomy is of perennial usefulness but is indicated only in obstruction of the aqueduct or the fourth ventricle by tumor or other acquired disorder.

Even with technically superior operations one is unlikely to find more than 70% clinical improvement. In some, irreversible damage from hydrocephaly may already have occurred. In many, permanent damage to the brain may have occurred at the time of an original infection or there may be coincidental cerebral developmental defects. In the Arnold-Chiari malformation the hydrocephaly may be successfully treated, but permanent paraplegia and incontinence may remain as a result of the spinal

FIG. 3-16. Holter valve, with distal and right-angled central tubing.

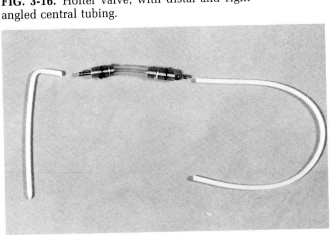

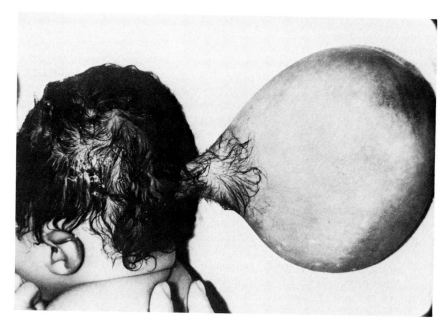

FIG. 3-17. Cranium bifidum and occipital meningocele. The posterior fossa contained abnormal neural rudiments.

cord defect. With current methods of treatment of this condition, 40% still die; about one-fourth are non-competitive, and only one-third competitive.

In special situations other procedures may be indicated. During acute obstructions and in the course of meningitis under treatment intermittent or continuous ventricular drainage may be necessary. Posterior fossa decompression combined with high cervical laminectomy has been useful in cases of Chiari type I malformation. In the Arnold-Chiari malformation repair of the myelocele is deferred until epithelialization has taken place unless there is an acute rupture. A shunting procedure is instituted at a later date. In the case of chronic leakage of CSF repair of the myelocele may be followed by an acute hydrocephaly; hence ventricular drainage should be planned or a preliminary shunt accomplished.

CRANIUM BIFIDUM

Localized cranium bifidum compatible with postnatal survival is much less common than spina bifida. Such fusional defects in the cranium are associated with cystic and often pedunculated masses containing meningeal and nervous tissue. Simple meningocele is uncommon, and more often there are abnormal neural rudiments or large cerebral hernias.

The most common site is the occipital region, this presentation being found in 74% of the cases of Ingraham and Matson.[26] Other sites include parietal, frontal, and nasal regions. Occipital encephaloceles are likely to be combined with the Arnold-Chiari malformation and hydrocephaly. Other cerebral abnormalities include microcephaly and cerebellar agenesis (Fig. 3-17).

Despite these many complications that may ultimately defeat surgical treatment, a number of cases can be successfully repaired and will develop normally. In occipital meningocele three-fourths of the patients survive and one-half are normal, whereas in encephalocele only 40% survive with 10% being normal.

CONGENITAL DERMAL CYST

Lengthy invagination of ectodermal tissue may pierce the cranium to end in a dilated cystic mass often residing within nervous tissue. These congenital sinuses are composed of dermis and epidermis as well as sebaceous and sweat glands, hair follicles, and adipose tissue. The centers usually contain sebaceous material and cholesterol.

If the sinus tract is obliterated during early development and continuity with the exterior lost, the cyst is likely to remain dormant for many years, presenting as a tumor in childhood or adult life. When a patent opening is maintained, however, the condition is made evident in infancy or early childhood by a chronic cutaneous discharge or by the onset of intracranial infection. The intracranial cysts have been reported in many locations, but by far the most common site is the posterior fossa, where the sinus tract is located in the midline and the cystic termination rests between the cerebellar hemispheres, in the fourth ventricle, or extending laterally into one cerebellar hemisphere.[35]

Clinical Characteristics. There are three principal clinical patterns. One consists only of chronic or irregularly recurrent drainage of sebaceous material from a sinus opening just beneath the occipital protuberance. If this is derived from an intracranial dermal cyst that is entirely extradural, there are usually no signs of central nervous system disorder and the mass can be removed without difficulty. If the tract leads to an intradural cyst, then meningitis or abscess can be expected in due course. A second presentation is that of acute pyogenic meningitis or of recurrent meningitis. The infecting organism is often *Staphylococcus aureus.*

The third syndrome is that of cerebellar cyst or abscess with fourth ventricular obstruction. In the infant there may be listlessness, poor feeding, vomiting, enlarging head, and suture diastasis. In older children gait ataxia, vomiting, and headache may be prominent, so that medulloblastoma is suspected. If a complete sinus tract is present, meningitis may be superimposed at any time.

Diagnosis. Congenital dermal sinus should be suspected in instances of *Staphylococcus aureus* meningitis in the absence of some other presumptive source of systemic or cranial infection. Recurrent meningitis always suggests this condition. Dermal cyst

or abscess is part of the differential diagnosis of posterior fossa tumors.

The initial diagnostic procedure is to shave the head in order to better search for a sinus. A pitted opening is seen usually at the summit of a local swelling beneath the occipital protuberance. Coursing caudad a few centimeters a cordlike tract may be palpated. Such a finding is present in a majority of cases in children, although in those cases manifesting as a posterior fossa mass the sinus may be absent.

Plain radiographs of the skull may be helpful. In the extradural cyst Logue and Till described a roughly circular radiolucent area in the midline of the occipital bone below the inion.[35] It penetrates the inner table and diploë and is bordered by a sclerotic margin. Intradural cysts may be associated with another characteristic finding. Located also in the midline is a radiolucent channel lined by a sclerotic border (Fig. 3-18), which may terminate caudally in a large oval groove. In instances of large posterior fossa cysts, ventriculography shows dilatation of lateral and third ventricles, with failure of fourth ventricular filling and sometimes kinking of the aqueduct.

Treatment. Surgical excision is required and should be carried out as soon as feasible after the diagnosis is made. Even those cases presenting only with a draining sinus should have neurosurgical exploration to prevent future intracranial infections.

CLINICALLY OCCULT CEREBRAL DEFECTS

Agenesis of the Corpus Callosum

Failure of the corpus callosum to develop is seen in a heterogeneous group of anomalies including the univentricular holotelencephalies, examples where frontal lobes fail to cleave with absence of corpus callosum, cases in which defects in midline structures and cortical development may be present with absence of corpus callosum as the most prominent anomaly, and finally, instances of complete or only partial absence of the corpus callosum with little or no accompanying defect. Cases other than the most severe of these anomalies, al-

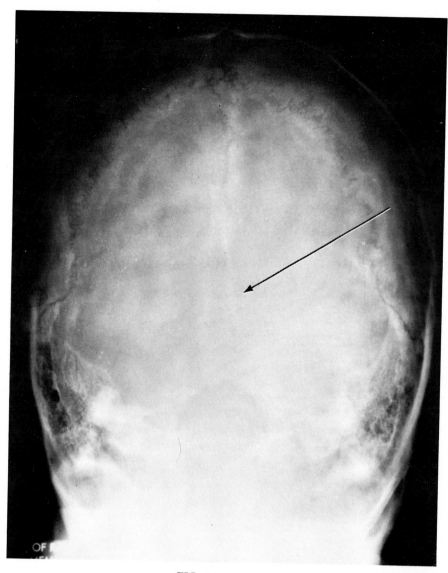

FIG. 3-18. Congenital dermal cyst. Plain radiograph of the skull. *Arrow* indicates midline channel with sclerotic margin.

though often accompanied by mental defect and epilepsy, are extremely difficult to recognize clinically and may be found only incidentally at autopsy.

Etiology.   The only known causes of lack of or incomplete development of the corpus callosum are those associated with gross forebrain anomalies or examples of microgyria and microcephaly resulting from genetic factors or maternal irradiation or infection.

Selective agenesis of the corpus callosum with little or no cortical defect has not been elucidated. The structure arises as a local thickening of the lamina terminalis toward the end of the third month, and one suggested morphogenetic mechanism has been that of a fusional error in the anterior neuropore, which is believed to give rise to the lamina terminalis.

Pathology.   In complete absence of the corpus callosum, the sagittal fissure extends down to the thin-walled roof of the

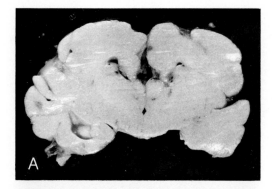

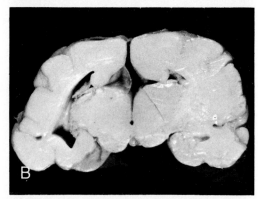

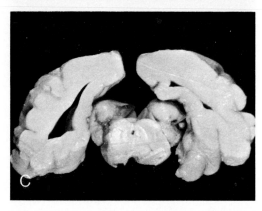

FIG. 3-19. Agenesis of the corpus callosum in an infant brain. Note the widely separated lateral ventricles, elongated foramen of Monro, and dorsal extension of the third ventricle on successive gross sections A, B, and C.

third ventricle. There is no septum pellucidum and often no hippocampal or anterior commissure. The third ventricle is often enlarged and rises to a greater than normal vertical height. The lateral ventricles are widely separated so that the interventricular foramen becomes elongated (Fig. 3-19).

Just medial to the bodies of the lateral ventricles there may be a prominent longitudinal callosal bundle probably representing aberrant callosal fibers. The posterior portion of the lateral ventricle is often greatly dilated. The medial aspects of hemispheres usually show radially arranged sulci with absence of the callosal gyrus. Associated cerebral abnormalities are often present and include failure of normal gyral pattern, abnormalities in the granular layers of the cortex, microgyria, absence of the fornices, and absence of olfactory nerves. Occasionally at the site normally occupied by the genu there is a lipoma or meningioma.

Clinical Characteristics.   There is no characteristic clinical syndrome, but neurologic abnormalities are common, including epilepsy and mental defect ranging from speechless idiocy to slight subnormality. The corpus callosum normally functions in the interhemispheric integration of some learned discriminations, and abnormalities of these functions have been found in an agenesis patient with alexia in the left field and inability to transfer motor acts from right to left hand. However, it is very likely that the most profound mental symptoms in this malformation are ascribed to the frequently associated defects in cerebral hemispheres. In more than half of the cases described in infants there has been mental retardation and epilepsy with either focal or generalized seizures. In some infants the head was noticeably abnormal, usually of a brachycephalic appearance or with wide interocular distance and the median cleft face syndrome. Occasionally there is overt evidence of increased intracranial pressure with tense fontanel or papilledema due to the appearance of a concurrent hydrocephaly. In some individuals there may be only epilepsy of later onset, or no overt manifestations at all, and a normal or slightly inferior mentality. Spastic diplegia is seen infrequently. Mirror movements of the hands have been reported in a few cases.

Diagnosis.   The diagnosis in life can be made only radiographically. In infants plain films of the skull may reveal wide separation of the frontal bones by a greatly expanded metopic suture. Pneumoencephalography (Fig. 3-20) reveals a characteristic set of findings including wide separation of the lateral ventricles, sharply angulated dorsal margins of the ventricles, concave medial walls of the lateral ventricles, dilatation of the posterior portion of the lateral ventricles, elongation of the interventricular foramen, and dorsal extension and dilation of the third ventricle. At times it may be possible to detect the radial arrangement of sulci on the medial aspects of the hemispheres and in some cases a marked enlargement of the cisterna magna.[25]

Treatment.   The seizures usually respond to anticonvulsive medication. No surgery is indicated unless a coexistent hydrocephaly intervenes.

Other Occult Cerebral Defects

In any group of children having serious mental deficiency and other neurologic incapacitations it is possible to describe but few according to etiology and pathogenesis. Yet one may assign a majority of these patients to useful clinical categories that although sometimes lacking in a foundation of causation, have relevance with respect to morphology, prognosis, and genetic transmission. Thus one may expect to identify most examples of the symptomatic and genetic microcephalies, hydrocephalies, developmental defects with identifying physical signs, mongolism and other chromosomal aberrations, known biochemical disorders, degenerative diseases, sequelae of infection, kernicterus, and the encephalopathies following documented asphyxia.

There remain a fraction of cases that defy all attempts at classificaton. Most of these are stationary disorders without evidence of progressive degenerative disease. There are no distinguishing physical characteristics. The known biochemical derangements are lacking. With respect to function, such patients range from paralytic idiots to mobile imbeciles. Autopsies on these individuals usually reveal definite morphologic abnormalities but of a type that cannot be detected in life. Some have minor expressions or localized distributions of defects in neuroblast migration and cortical lamination. Thus there may be scattered or symmetrical patches of microgyria, neural heterotopias, and zones of agyric

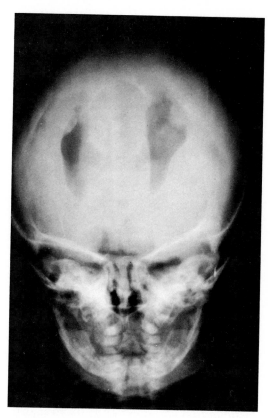

FIG. 3-20. Pneumoencephalograph in agenesis of the corpus callosum, showing wide separation, dorsal peaking, and concave medial borders of the lateral ventricles.

cortex. There are some examples of cortical atrophy and encephalomalacia suggesting old anoxic or vascular lesions. A few cases may show developmental defects restricted to the limbic system or simply cerebellar agenesis with apparently intact cerebri. Many display only a moderate reduction in brain size.

Within the realm of mildly subnormal cases, many of whom are not institutionalized, the problem of identifying the disease is even more difficult. Only an occasional patient can be given such diagnoses as phenylketonuria, hereditary ataxia with mental deficiency, rubella syndrome, birth injury, ichthyosis syndrome, or corpus callosum agenesis. Most individuals cannot be classified, and the view has been presented that disease need not be present but that such individuals comprise the tapering foot of an intelligence curve. However, a num-

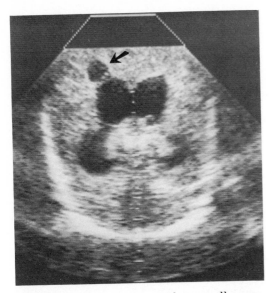

FIG. 3-21. Sector scan reveals a small porencephalic cyst in the paraventricular area (*arrow*) that developed following a previously visualized intracerebral hemorrhage in the same location.

ber of pieces of evidence suggest new areas for definition. In nine brains examined by Crome in individuals above the imbecile level, slight microencephaly was found in seven. Feeblemindedness frequently exists as a hereditary disorder in which the genetic mechanisms are complex or unclear. Benda noted several families having dolichocephaly and either imbecility or high grade mental deficiency in which postmortem examination showed morphologic defects, including asymmetries of paired structures of the nervous system, slight microencephaly, and disorders of cortical lamination. A potentially large and relatively unexplored area is that of mild expressions in herterozygotic form of disorders well recognized in the homozygotic state. One example of this is the genetic microcephalies of Böök in which heterozygotes were mildly defective.[2]

SECTOR SCAN

Real-time B-mode ultrasonography (sector scan) of the infant brain is a rapid, accurate, noninvasive technique for delineating normal and abnormal anatomy of the brain. Sector scans can be performed at the bed-side and the examination is particularly helpful in the neonatal nursery.[17]

Radiation exposure, sedation, and body cooling during transportation are the risks associated with computerized tomography and are eliminated by the use of sector scan. A major asset of this technique is the ability to obtain sequential studies of the infants for as long as the anterior fontanelle remains patent.[18]

The examination is exceedingly accurate in the evaluation of neonates with developmental abnormalities of the brain, including ventricular dilatation, porencephaly (Fig. 3-21), the Dandy-Walker anomaly, and other cystic anomalies of the brain.[22,33,50]

CEREBRAL DEFECTS WITH PROMINENT ECTODERMAL, VISCERAL, OR SKELETAL ABNORMALITIES

CHROMOSOMAL ABERRATIONS: MULTIPLE CONGENITAL DEFECTS

Defective separation of chromosomes during gametogenesis or the initial cell divisions of the fertilized zygote have been related to a large number of human developmental defects. Of particular neurologic interest are three major groups: (1) mongolism, (2) multiple congenital anomalies attended by cerebral defects, and (3) abnormalities in sex chromosomes accompanied by mental deficiency.[42]

Down's Syndrome (Mongolism)

The most common of these groups, mongolism, is a prototype of the multiple congenital abnormalities with developmental defects of nervous, cutaneous, osseous, ligamentous, cardiac, and hematopoietic tissues. The disorder is known to occur in all races and geographic areas. In Europe and America it has an incidence of 1 to 2/1000 births and accounts for 12.5% of defective infants.

Etiology. Mongolism is related to an excessive complement of material of chromosome 21, either in the form of a trisomy or a translocation involving the bulk of the chromosome. The common aberration in mongolism, trisomy 21, is believed to result from nondisjunction or failure of separation of a pair of daughter chromosomes during the second meiotic division of the ovum resulting in a gamete with two instead of one chromosome 21. After fertilization with a normal sperm, a zygote containing three chromosomes 21 is produced (Fig. 3-22). The likelihood of non-disjunction may increase with the age of the parent, thereby accounting for the marked increase in incidence of mongolism with advancing maternal age. The mean maternal age for mongoloid offspring is 37 years, and 64% of these defectives are born to women over 30.

A much less common form of the disorder is the familial type. Most of these cases are accounted for by chromosomal translocations that may be transmitted through several generations. In this aberration it is thought that the long arm of one chromosome 21 may mutually translocate with the short arm of another chromosome such as number 15 during the prophase of the first meiotic division (D/G translocation). The abnormal 21/15 chromosome then carries the bulk of genetic information of both individual chromosomes. After maturation of the gamete and fertilization, the possible viable zygotes include: (1) a normal chromosome complement; (2) two normal chromosomes 21, one normal 15, and one 21/15 chromosome, resulting in a mongoloid child; (3) one normal 21, a normal 15, and a 21/15 resulting in an individual who is phenotypically normal but who may produce a mongoloid offspring (Fig. 3-23). Familial mongolism probably accounts for no more than 1% of all cases. It may occur, however, in the offspring of young mothers and partly explains the increased likelihood of a second mongoloid child in women under 25. In these young mothers having one mongoloid child the likelihood of a second afflicted infant is about 50 times greater than the random risk.[7] Rarely mongolism coexists with Klinefelter's syndrome, in which case the karyotype includes trisomy 21 as well as the XXY combination.

Pathology. The mongoloid brain tends to weigh less than normal. Cerebellum and brain stem are disproportionately small. There is occipital flattening, and frontal lobes and superior temporal gyri tend to be small. There is general simplification of the convolutional pattern of the cerebral hemispheres. A decrease in neuronal population may be found in the cortical layers.

Clinical Characteristics. Most of the clinical features of mongolism are quite nonspecific, and individual stigmata at times occur in normal individuals. Some of the features may be seen in relatives of mongoloids who are otherwise normal, and rarely mosaicism (chromosomal aberration restricted to one or more stem lines) results in ectodermal or osseous defects but spares the nervous system. The diagnosis of mongolism is made by the concurrent appearance of multiple characteristic features in a mentally retarded individual having slow physical development. In the following description the characteristics mentioned occur in a third or more of cases.[34]

Mongoloids are small in stature. Although average weight at birth is 6.5 lb (2.2 kg), weight gain is quite slow during infancy. Development continues to lag through childhood, and at maturity height is usually under 5 ft (1.5 m).

The head tends to be brachycephalic with a flattened occiput. The skin, soft at birth, later becomes dry and the cheeks are red and roughened. The face is broad and the nasal bridge flat (Fig. 3-24A). The small round mouth may be constantly open, allowing an enlarged tongue with an irregular network of furrows to protrude. The lips may show transverse fissuring. Teeth are small and irregular, and the palate is high-arched. The ears may be large but often show an absence of the lobule. The eyes commonly show oblique slanting of the palpebral fissures and in about half of the cases have an epicanthal fold. Palpebral fissures are shortened in the horizontal dimension. Irises may be heterochromic or show a characteristic speckling (Brushfield spots), which takes the form of tiny white or cream-colored spots distributed along an arc just within the outer margin of the iris.

In the extremities, laxity of ligaments and hypotonia of muscles permit an unusual mobility of joints. Curious postures of repose may be maintained by the mongoloid child, such as a seated position on the floor with full flexion at the hips, and the chest and head resting upon the extended legs. The hands are particularly

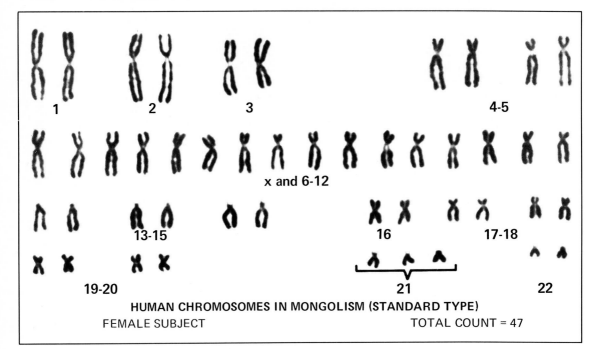

HUMAN CHROMOSOMES IN MONGOLISM (STANDARD TYPE)
FEMALE SUBJECT   TOTAL COUNT = 47

FIG. 3-22. Trisomy 21 in mongolism. (Courtesy of Dr. M. Neil MacIntyre, Western Reserve University, Cleveland, Ohio)

FIG. 3-23. Chromosomal translocation in familial mongolism. (Courtesy of Dr. M. Neil MacIntyre, Western Reserve University, Cleveland, Ohio)

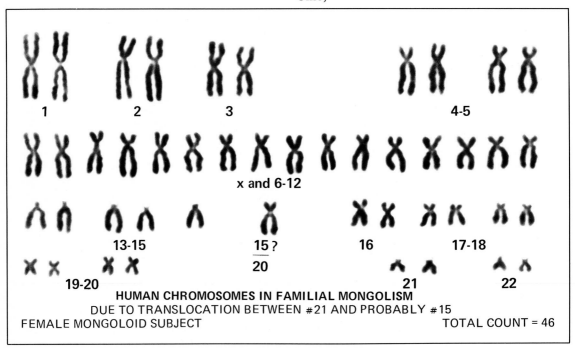

HUMAN CHROMOSOMES IN FAMILIAL MONGOLISM
DUE TO TRANSLOCATION BETWEEN #21 AND PROBABLY #15
FEMALE MONGOLOID SUBJECT   TOTAL COUNT = 46

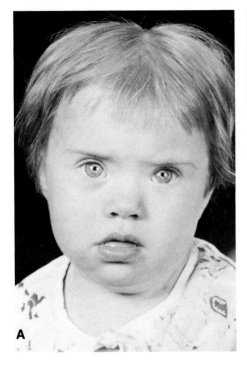

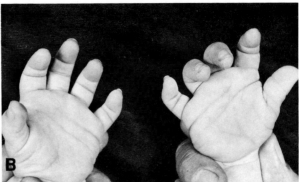

FIG. 3-24. Mongolism. *A.* Slanting palpebral fissures, epicanthal folds, Brushfield spots, protruding tongue, and brachycephaly. *B.* Prominent transverse palmar creases, small incurved fifth digits.

characteristic (Fig. 3-24B). They are short and broad, with shortened or tapering fingers. The fifth digit is disporportionately short and curves inward. The palmar dermatoglyphics are profoundly alerted.[53] The normal palmar creases may be replaced by a prominent transverse line. In Negroes heavy pigmentation may render this especially striking. The axial triradix (formed by the convergence of three lines in the midpalm just beyond the wrist) is displaced distally into the palm. On the feet there may be an abnormal gap between the first and second toes, and extending from this a linear plantar crease. On the sole proximal to the great toe, normal dermal markings usually consist of whorls and large loops, but in about half of mongoloids they consist only of arching of the dermal lines or very small loops.

The neck is broad and short. The abdomen may show *diastasis recti,* and the genitalia are hypoplastic. Congenital heart defects are found in about 40% of all cases. Particularly common are the atrioventricularis communis defect and the ventricular-septal defect. Less often encountered are patent ductus arteriosus, atrial-septal defect, tetralogy of Fallot, and isolated aberrant subclavian artery.

All developmental achievements are delayed. The average age for holding the head up is 6 months, for sitting 12 months, for walking 2 years, for initial dentition 12 months, and for first word 2 years. The intelligence quotient is usually in the range of 25 to 45. Mongoloids are notable for being cheerful and affectionate, and for having relatively good imitative abilities. Five percent to 10% develop seizures, which often occur late in the course of the disorder. An occasional late complication is paraplegia due to atlantoaxial or other cervical vertebral dislocation.

Laboratory Examinations. In mongolism there is a tendency for a shift toward immature forms of polymorphonuclear leukocytes in the peripheral blood. Acute leukemia occurs in a greater incidence in mongoloids than in normal children. The serum uric acid tends to be elevated.

Radiography discloses many characteristic features. There is moderate microcephaly with a brachycephalic configuration. Nasal bones and maxillas are hypoplastic. On the hands there may be hypoplasia of the middle and terminal phalanges of the fifth digits. The pelvic bones display important findings.[5] There is flattening of the acetabular slopes with marked reduction or obliteration of the angle between acetabula and a horizontal line. The iliac wings flare laterally. Later in infancy the ischial rami become hypoplastic and tapering.

Diagnosis. Diagnosis is especially difficult in the newborn when many of the characteristic features have not yet appeared. Findings that may be sought at this age include the small head, absent lobule, short and curved fifth digits, slanting eyes, flat bridge of nose, and the transverse palmar line. The radiographic changes in the pelvis are present at birth as are the dermatoglyphic patterns quantitated by Walker.

Certain cases of prenatal microcephaly associated with congenital heart disease may have to be differentiated from mongolism. Usually the resemblance is superficial, and on careful examination the cardinal features of mongolism are absent. Pseudohypoparathyroidism in children may produce small stature, short fingers, and mental deficiency, but often is also accompanied by basal ganglia calcification and lacks the characteristic stigmata of mongolism. Contrary to the usual statement, cretinism in the infant shows little resemblance to mongolism and may easily be differentiated by the low body temperature, puffiness of face and subcutaneous tissue, dry skin, harsh low-pitched voice, and by serum-free thyroxine index based on T_3 resin uptake and T_4 competitive protein binding.

Prognosis. About 25% of mongoloids die in infancy. During the neonatal period many of these deaths are attributable to gastrointestinal anomalies. During the first year of life most deaths are due to congenital heart disease and to infection. These two factors continue to produce a steady mortality throughout childhood. A small percentage of deaths are due to acute leukemia. Only 40% of mongoloids are alive at 5 years, but those surviving childhood may live to an advanced age.

Management. At present there is no treatment for this disorder other than institutionalization of survivors. Some prevention could be expected by counseling parents in reference to optimal age for childbearing. In a parent with known translocation, a cytogenetic diagnosis on cells from amniocentesis permits interruption of pregnancy.

Multiple Congenital Anomalies

Abnormalities in segregation of some of the small autosomes have been associated with mentally defective infants having deformities of many organ systems. One of the more common of these, the group D or 13–15 trisomy, was described under *Cyclopias and Holotelencephalies*.[36]

The trisomy 17–18 (group E) syndrome, which can also be caused by a translocation with another group E or D chromosome, is accompanied by severe mental retardation and microcephaly with prominent occiput.[54] Neural heterotopies are commonly found in the brain. Ears are low set and often malformed, the eyes may be small, and there is micrognathia. Of the abundant associated malformations, the following are the most common: congenital heart defects, horseshoe kidney, double ureter, Meckel's diverticulum, gastrointestinal malrotation, flexion contractures of extremities, syndactyly, hammer toes, short sternum, and rocker bottom feet.[52]

The cri-du-chat (cry of the cat) syndrome is attributable to deletion of a short arm in group 4–5.[19] Affected children are microcephalic and severely retarded. The characteristic cry is present during infancy. Other findings include hypertelorism, epicanthic folds, antimongoloid slant, low set ears, micrognathia, and rounded face.

In deletion 18 (partial deletion of long arm of chromosome 18) microcephaly and moderate mental retardation occur.[19] Hypertelorism and epicanthal folds are found. The ears are low set with prominent anthelix and antitragus. Other findings may include cleft lip and palate, genital hypoplasia, club feet, congenital heart defects, and hypotonia.

The same chromosome may undergo deletion and fusion in the ring chromosome 18 syndrome.[19] Characteristic features are severe mental retardation, microcephaly, hypertelorism, epicanthus, low set ears, high arched palate, syndactyly, club feet, rocker bottom feet, and congenital heart defects.

Translocation of chromosomes 13 and 22 has been associated with mental retardation and a language defect.[37] Trisomy 11 has been found with the combination of mental retardation, hypertelorism, and hypogonadism. Complete triploidy with 69 chromosomes produced syndactyly, small mandible, multiple lipomas, and severe mental defect.

Abnormalities of Sex Chromosomes

Although a wide variety of aberrations of sex chromosomes have been discovered, two are of particular interest in neurology. Klinefelter's syndrome is most commonly caused by the XXY configuration. The disorder is characterized by testicular atrophy with tubular sclerosis and Leydig cell hyperplasia. Patients may have an eunuchoid appearance, gynecomastia, and mental subnormality usually in the borderline or moron class. A buccal smear often reveals the presence of sex chromatin. This group constitutes approximately 1% of male mental defectives. The XYY pattern results in a tall male with mild mental retardation and may predispose to antisocial behavior.

Another disorder affecting females is the trisomy X syndrome, which may be associated with mental deficiency and epilepsy. The buccal smear usually reveals two sex chromatin bodies. The disorder is found in slightly less than 1% of female mental defectives.

In evaluating patients having both hypogonadism and mental deficiency it must be remembered that this association is found in many disorders other than chromosomal aberrations. It occurs regularly in the Laurence-Moon-Biedl syndrome and rarely in neurofibromatosis and craniopharyngioma. It appears in the syndromes of ichthyosis with dementia and xeroderma pigmentosa with dementia. In the ataxic family whose neurologic defects resembled the Roussy-Lévy syndrome, reported by Richards and Rundles, there was early deafness, mental deficiency, hypogonadism, and a possible block in androgen metabolism.[43]

CUTANEOUS DISORDERS

Tuberous Sclerosis

Tuberous sclerosis, a genetically determined disorder, comprises a characteristic set of hamartomatous growths involving many organs; although displaying some histologic manifestations of neoplasia, with but rare exceptions it lacks the invasiveness, autonomy, and rapid cell division of analogous malignant tumors. Although not tending toward metastases or local invasive erosion, these growths, by their multiplicity or occasional great size, may induce sufficient mechanical distortion or replacement of parenchyma to engender severe and even lethal functional failure of brain, heart, kidney, and lung.[20]

Genetics. The disorder is inherited as an autosomal gene whose expression is probably limited by the presence of an additional commonly occurring modifying gene.[22] Given a genotype capable of producing tuberous sclerosis, the presence of the modifying gene in homozygous form may prevent phenotypic expression of the disorder, whereas the modifier in heterozygous form may result in the mild syndrome. Absence of the modifying gene allows complete expression of the severe disease.

Pathology. Except in severe congenital cases, the brain shows normal development of its growth patterns but undergoes local distortion by abnormal glial masses. In the cerebral cortex are found local expansions of the crests of convolutions that are firm to the touch and on section show a pale homogeneous appearance obliterating the cortical markings and fading off into surrounding tissue. These are composed of chaotically arranged cells sometimes attaining giant size and having characteristics at times approaching astrocytes, but also resembling ganglion cells. Dense astrocytic gliosis accounts for the hardened texture. Similar masses of glial proliferation occur in white matter or basal ganglia but are particularly prevalent on the medial surface of thalamus projecting into the ventricular cavities and often containing calcification. Less common are areas of gliosis and nerve cell loss in cerebellum and brain stem. At times intraventricular masses may attain a large size, producing obstruction and having histologic characteristics of large cell astrocytomas. Rarely, massive areas of the brain such as an entire hemisphere may be replaced by proliferating glia, sometimes containing malformed ganglion cells.

The cutaneous lesions, adenoma sebaceum, shagreen patches, and ungual fibroma are all composed of proliferated connective tissue, richly vascular in the case of ungual fibromas, and sometimes containing excessive quantities of sebaceous glands in the facial excrescences. Small and often multiple kidney tumors, present in 80% of cases, are composed of mature adipose tissue and smooth muscle derived from vessel walls. Other lesions that may appear in childhood include cardiac rhabdomyoma, endocardial fibroelastosis (rare), fibrolipoma of the liver, and myomas of uterine and vaginal walls.

Clinical Characteristics. There may be recognized a fully developed form consisting of cutaneous lesions, mental deficiency, epilepsy, and visceral manifestations, as well as a milder form with limited manifestations and normal mentality.[39]

In the severe form, a few patients may be affected in infancy with large cardiac tumors producing congestive heart failure or sudden death, or with massive cerebral, often unihemispheric involvement with gross mental defect, failure of motor development, and seizures. Tuberous sclerosis may also declare itself in infancy in the form of recurrent infantile spasm.[45] Characteristic skin nodules are not present at this age, but an important diagnostic sign is the presence of multiple hypopigmented 0.5-cm to 1.0-cm macules over the trunk.

Much more commonly, the severe form becomes evident during early childhood with gradual expression of systemic involvement. Adenoma sebaceum, though rarely noted in infancy, usually appears at about 4 years, becoming progressively prominent. The lesions consist of crops of closely packed rounded excrescences, fine to the touch and of a pink or yellow coloration. They are particularly abundant at the nasofacial margins and extend onto maxillary areas, sparing the skin above the upper lip but occasionally involving the chin or forehead (Fig. 3-25). The anachronistic term *shagreen patch* refers to the resemblance of certain cutaneous lesions of the trunk to a variety of coarsely grained leather. These patches may also appear in early childhood and are commonly distributed over the dorsal or lateral aspects of the lumbar and lower thoracic regions. Often solitary, they range from coin size to greater than a hands breadth. They are often lightly pigmented and slightly raised, with an irregular surface containing many indentations. Some

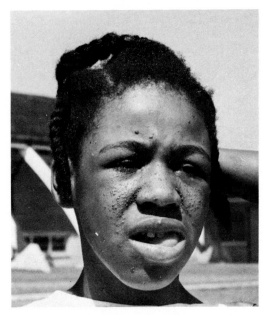

FIG. 3-25. Adenoma sebaceum in tuberous sclerosis.

of the involved skin may develop fine crinkling on compression.

Ungual fibromas appear later in childhood and consist of smooth masses originating from the nail bed or borders and expanding to cover the lateral portion of the nail. Less common skin findings include fibromas of the scalp and areas of depigmentation. Cerebral involvement is usually indicated first by lagging development with mental deficiency evidenced by 3 years. The level of defect is quite variable, ranging from borderline to severe subnormality. Some children with moderate mental impairment may in later childhood display an independent behavioral disorder with frequent screaming attacks and at times withdrawal into a detached state accompanied by frequent stereotyped hand and finger mannerisms.[9] Seizures rarely begin before age 2, and may be focal or more often general. Apart from those with severe mental deficiency, motor defects are uncommon and are limited to mild or incomplete hemiparesis. Occasionally a patient may develop evidence of increased intracranial pressure with papilledema and may have a tumorlike mass obstructing the third or lateral ventricles. The retinas are involved in about 15% of cases, with two types of abnormality. The more common consists of small, flat, white plaques smaller than a disk diameter and often multiple. The other lesion is larger, is usually on or near the optic disk, and has the appearance of a translucent grapelike cluster of protuberant tissue. The kidneys may contain palpable firm masses in about 8% of cases. Clinical involvement of the heart is usually evident only in children. Cystic or honeycombed lung is a rare complication.

A mild form may consist of minimal involvement with adenoma sebaceum or visceral involvement or epilepsy alone. Mental capacity may be average or slightly subnormal.

Laboratory Examinations. Radiographs of the skull often reveal one or more foci of light calcification in the intracranial cavity (Fig. 3-26A), usually in the region of the lateral ventricles. There may also be fluffy areas of increased density of the inner table of the skull especially in the parietal bone. Pneumoencephalography often outlines multiple glial masses, imparting the effect of dripping wax along the floor and lateral wall of the lateral ventricles. The CT scan is exquisitely sensitive in demonstrating intracerebral calcification. (Fig. 3-26B) Radiographs of the hands and feet frequently show small cystlike defects of trabeculation in the distal phalanges as well as irregular cortical thickening of metatarsals and metacarpals. Patchy sclerosis has also been described in the innominate bones and vertebral bodies.

Treatment. There is no means of treating cases with severe cerebral involvement and mental defect. Seizures usually respond well to anticonvulsant medication. An occasional patient not severely incapacitated may develop evidence of ventricular obstruction from glial masses. Such cases should receive surgical intervention that may prove much more successful than is usually to be expected with glioma surgery.

Prognosis. The mild form of the disorder need not shorten the life span, and some patients with widespread involvement may survive to old age. Death in infancy and childhood is usually attributable to cardiac

tumors. In later childhood and adolescence death may be due to tuberculosis or pulmonary infection. Less commonly, patients succumb to status epilepticus, ventricular obstruction, or operation for visceral tumor.

Neurofibromatosis

In the fully developed form of neurofibromatosis a multitude of peripheral subcutaneous neurofibromas coexist with neurofibromas of spinal and cranial nerves, meningiomas, and gliomas. Prominent involvement of the central nervous system, however, may occur in the presence of relatively inconspicuous peripheral neurofibromatosis. In most examples, inheritance is by simple autosomal dominance.

Pathology. Peripheral manifestations consist of neurofibromas distributed along the course of subcutaneous nerves, nerve trunks, and autonomic nerves and ganglia.[41] Occasionally these appear in malignant form as neurogenic sarcomas. Beneath areas of cutaneous pigmentation are thickened nerve terminals. Within the cranium and spinal canal, sensory nerves and roots are more commonly affected than motor nerves and roots, and the auditory nerves when affected are usually involved bilaterally. Oligodendrogliomas involving optic nerve and chiasm produce fusiform expansion of the nerve. About the walls of the third ventricle there arise well differentiated pilocytic astrocytomas that tend to involve the hypothalamus. In the spinal cord, central ependymomas are associated with syringomyelia. Scattered focal astrocytomas may occur in any part of the central nervous system, and multiple meningiomas are common. Less frequent are varieties of diffuse gliomatosis with mature astrocytic proliferation symmetrically distributed within thalami, limbic areas, and frontal lobes.

Clinical Characteristics. The subcutaneous tumors usually appear in childhood and may become prominent after puberty. They consist of nontender, soft, sessile, or pedunculated polyps. They occur in greatest numbers over the trunk and proximal parts of the extremities and are often heavily dis-

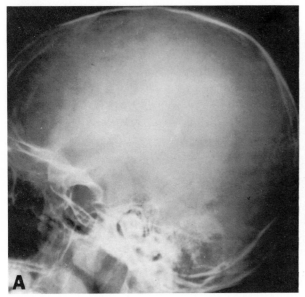
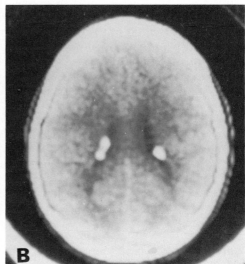

FIG. 3-26. Tuberous sclerosis with intracerebral calcification. *A.* Plain radiograph of the skull with intracranial calcifications. *B.* CT scan with bilateral calcifications.

tributed in the lumbosacral area, dorsal thorax, and posterior neck (Fig. 3-27A). The café au lait spots over trunk or limbs appear in the form of flat, angulated patches of a light brown color (Fig. 3-27B). It must be emphasized that these cutaneous stigmata may be minimal or absent in children with central neurofibromatosis. Scoliosis is commonly encountered.

Less frequent are plexiform neurofibromas producing diffuse thickening of multiple nerves and local hypertrophy of soft tissues. With plexiform neurofibromatosis of the orbit, buphthalmos appears. Congenital glaucoma with buphthalmos may also occur as an independent manifestation.

Mental deficiency occurs in about 8% of cases, and epilepsy is a common neurologic symptom. Optic nerve tumors as a manifestation of neurofibromatosis tend to appear in childhood and are characteristically slow-growing.[11] When arising in the orbital extension of the nerve, usual symptoms are painless progressive exophthalmos with reduction in vision and optic atrophy. Those arising or extending into the intracranial portion of the nerve produce gradual monocular amblyopia, with the addition of bitemporal hemianopia as the chiasm becomes involved (Fig. 3-27C). The astrocytomas of the third ventricle and the hypothalamus also occur in childhood and despite relatively large size may produce minimal symptoms. These may include diabetes insipidus, precocious puberty, and adiposogenital dystrophy.

Other syndromes encountered in childhood include syringomyelia and intramedullary tumor of the spinal cord. The retina may occasionally contain small, flat, pale masses. Unilateral pulsating exophthalmos may occur in neurofibromatosis as a result of a congenital defect in the wall of the orbit with transmission of the intracranial pulsations. No vascular murmur is present. Radiographically there is enlargement of the orbit and a sharply demarcated defect in the posterior orbital wall. The condition is generally benign. It is usually not until adolescence that the manifestations of acoustic nerve tumors and of diffuse gliomatosis appear. Coarctation of the aorta and renal artery stenosis can cause hypertension. Pheochromocytoma, associated with adult neurofibromatosis in at least 10% of cases, has not been recognized in affected children, nor has cystic lung disease.

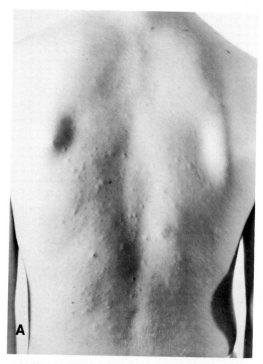

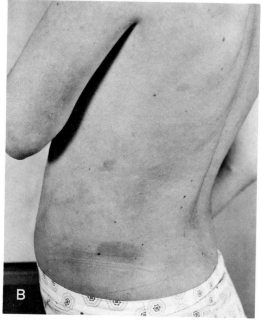

FIG. 3-27. Generalized neurofibromatosis in a child. *A.* Appearance of the inconspicuous cutaneous neurofibromas. *B.* Café au lait spots. *C.* Deformation of the anterior part of the third ventricle by a slowly growing glioma of the optic chiasm.

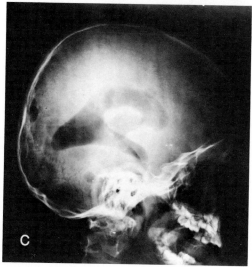

veals enlargement of the optic nerve as well as change in position or size of the ventricular system.

Treatment. Due to the general benign nature of the tumors, solitary involvement of spinal nerve roots, acoustic nerve, or optic nerve may be treated surgically with good results. Often, however, the ultimate outcome is defeated by appearance of multiple or inaccessible tumors elsewhere. For the spinal ependymomas and the astrocytomas of brain stem or diencephalon x-irradiation may be used, but dosage schedules should be quite conservative. At times hormonal replacement therapy is indicated, as in diabetes insipidus.

Polyostotic Fibrous Dysplasia (Albright's Syndrome)

The prominent osseous lesions of fibrous dysplasia may be combined with cutaneous pigmentation, precocious puberty, and rarely mental deficiency.[28] The pigmentation ap-

Laboratory Examinations. In the diagnosis of optic nerve and chiasmatic gliomas, radiographs of the skull may help by revealing an enlarged optic foramen or erosion of the anterior clinoid. Pneumoencephalography facilitates diagnosis of the diencephalic glioma with demonstration of a deforming mass or obliteration of part of the third ventricle. CT scan frequently re-

pears in childhood in the form of one or more large tan or brown areas with a jagged outline. Painless deformities with lateral bowing of the femurs and asymmetrical enlargement of the skull also commonly appear in childhood followed later by pathologic fracture. Precocious puberty is limited to females with development of secondary sexual characteristics and menstruation at an early age. Mental deficiency of varying severity has been reported in a few cases.

The pathogenesis of the sexual precocity is undefined. In a single detailed neuropathologic study of a severely defective male a small brain was found with atrophy in frontal and temporal regions.[28] There was a reduction in neuronal population of cerebral and cerebellar cortex, with giant neurons in the cerebral cortex.

Laboratory Examinations. Radiographic examination of affected long bones shows large multiple cystlike formations with thinning of the cortex and expansion of the shaft. In the head, areas of cystic radiolucency intermingle with regions of extensive new bone formation. Blood calcium and phosphorus are normal.

Differential Diagnosis. Albright's syndrome may be distinguished from hyperparathyroidism by the painless development of deformities, the local and asymmetrical bony lesions, and the normal calcium and phosphorus; and from neurofibromatosis by the absence of tumors, the large size and jagged outline of cutaneous pigmentation, and the characteristic bone lesions on x-ray films.

Inherited Dyskeratoses

Many physicians have noted the concurrence of ichthyosis and mental deficiency at a rate greater than could be expected from chance.[16] Two major syndromes have emerged.

Congenital Ichthyosis, Mental Deficiency, and Spastic Diplegia. This disorder, first identified in many pedigrees from one area of northern Sweden, consists of the uniform association of ichthyosis of the congenital type (ichthyosiform erythroderma) with oligophrenia and spastic diplegia.[48,49] The cutaneous disorder is present from infancy or early childhood with generalized scaliness including flexural areas. The mental defect is usually severe. The spastic disorder ranges from symmetrical spastic diplegia with maximal involvement in the legs to severe congenital paralysis with generalized flexion. In a few cases there has been retinal atrophy and enamel dysplasia. Epilepsy is not common. Elevations of blood histidine levels have been found in some cases and glutamine in one.

A case probably similar to this with severe mental defect, generalized paralysis, congenital ichthyosis, and retinal atrophy was examined pathologically by Stewart who found a small brain with poorly developed corpus callosum and frontal atrophy. There was numerical deficiency of neurons of the cerebral cortex, and the retina showed atrophy of all layers.

Congenital Ichthyosis, Mental Deficiency, and Epilepsy. Variants of this form reported originally by Rud and by van Bogaert have been recognized in Europe, England, and America.[16,51] The skin disorder is also of congenital type. Epilepsy may be present from infancy and usually takes the form of generalized motor seizures. The mental defect need not be profound, usually producing mild to moderate subnormality. Some cases have been associated with sexual infantilism.

Other Ectodermal Defects. Less common or well-defined cerebral disorders have been associated with anhidrotic ectodermal dysplasia and with xeroderma pigmentosa. In the original description of de Sanctis and Cacchione, three brothers with xeroderma pigmentosa were slow in development and underwent mental deterioration in early childhood.[14] Progressive paralysis was followed by flexion contractures. Stature was small, and there was hypogonadism. Autopsy in one case disclosed a small brain with severe neuronal loss in frontal and temporal cortex. In a recent case hyperaminoaciduria was reported.

Incontinentia Pigmenti

Incontinentia pigmenti produces characteristic dermatologic findings that become evident shortly after birth and that in some cases are associated with devastating involvement of the central nervous system.[46] The etiology is unknown. Although sometimes familial, a genetic origin has not been defined. There is a marked prevalence in female children. It has been reported in Caucasians, Negroes, and Orientals.

The disorder may be first recognized in the neonatal period when there may appear vesicles in linear cluster distribution, principally over the extremities. These recede leaving linear verrucous defects. Some months later there may appear the characteristic pigmentation that is especially prominent over the flanks and thighs. The color varies from gray-blue to brown and is distributed in irregular marbled or wavy lines (Fig. 3-28). Many cases have shown mental deficiency associated with spastic hemiplegia, tetraplegia, or seizures. Microcephaly occurs in about 10% of patients, and a few show optic atrophy. The few reported pneumoencephalographs have revealed dilated ventricles or communicating cystic cavities. Other abnormalities include dental defects, alopecia, corneal opacity, and cataracts. The neuropathologic features have not been described.

OPHTHALMIC DEFECTS

Pigmentary Degeneration of the Retina

The retinal neuroepithelium often shares in the hereditary afflictions of the central nervous system, and retinal degeneration may be found in amaurotic familial idiocy and in the hereditary ataxias. In classic retinitis pigmentosa about 4% of cases are afflicted with epilepsy, idiocy, or other severe neurologic disorders.

Laurence-Moon-Biedl Syndrome. Having neither well-defined pathologic characteristics nor any pathognomonic clinical or biochemical sign, this syndrome is recognized by the concatenation in familial distribution of obesity, mental deficiency, pigmentary degeneration of the retina, polydactyly, and hypogenitalism. Although the general pattern of the disease is well-defined, individual expressions are variable, one or more of the cardinal features usually being absent. Inheritance follows a well-defined autosomal recessive pattern.[29]

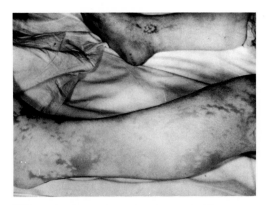

FIG. 3-28. Incontinentia pigmenti. Characteristic pigmentation.

Pathology. Within the retina there is a selective, profound loss of the photoreceptor cells, both rods and cones. Less prominent loss is seen in the bipolar and ganglion cell layers, and there is some pigment migration to a perivascular distribution. Changes in the brain vary considerably, but the most consistent findings include moderate cortical atrophy with narrowing of convolutions. There is a diffuse reduction in neuronal population of cerebral cortex with slight marginal and periventricular gliosis. There may be a reduction in cells of mammillary bodies and the subthalamic nuclei.

Clinical Characteristics. Obesity, mental defect, and retinal atrophy are the most constant findings. Adiposity develops in early childhood and is similar to that of Froehlich's syndrome, with distribution over abdomen, hips, chest, and the proximal portions of the limbs. The mental defect ranges from mild to moderate subnormality; it may progress very slowly, but more often remains constant throughout life. The retinal degeneration has its onset after age 4 with an initial symptom of night blindness followed later by progressive visual loss. The fundi usually do not give the appearance of typical retinitis pigmentosa but are more likely to show marked attenuation of vessels with optic atrophy. Pigment deposits may take the form of perivascular clumps in the retinal periphery but often are inconspicuous and limited to some stippling around the macula. The polydactyly most commonly consists of a supernumerary sixth digit existing either as a rudimentary tag or a fully formed member (Fig. 3-29). Both upper and lower extremities may be involved, and the disorder tends to be bilateral. Hypogenitalism is variably present. In the male the genitals may be evidently small in childhood with failure of development at puberty and with sparse body hair, often of female distribution. In the female the uterus, vagina, and external genitals are small. Occasional associated findings in some pedigrees include syndactyly, nerve deafness, nystagmus (due to early macular degeneration), and short stature. Rare associated findings include diabetes insipidus and anal atresia.

Laboratory Examinations. The urinary 17-ketosteroid excretion may be below normal.

Differential Diagnosis. The full developed form presents no diagnostic difficulty. In young children with only adiposity, mild or uncertain hypogenitalism, and mental deficiency of uncertain duration and without polydactyly or characteristic retinal findings, diagnosis may be extremely difficult, and the possibilities of exogenous obesity, idiopathic adiposogenital dystrophy, acquired hydrocephaly, central neurofibromatosis, Klinefelter's syndrome, Prader-Willi syndrome, and tumor of the pituitary or hypothalamus must be considered. The presence of the syndrome in a sibling, or fragmentary expressions of the disorder in relatives is helpful. Careful search for early visual abnormalities may reveal the presence of night blindness, or

there may be a diminished or absent response to light in the electroretinogram even in the absence of characteristic funduscopic abnormalities. On the other hand, hemianopic field defects such as may be found in tumor or neurofibromatosis do not occur in the Laurence-Moon-Biedl syndrome. Klinefelter's syndrome may include testicular atrophy, obesity, and mild mental deficiency, but gynecomastia is usually present and sex-chromatin bodies may be found in the buccal smear. The Prader-Willi syndrome (obesity, mental retardation, strabismus, hypogonadism, and hypotonia) does not show retinal degeneration or polydactyly.

The disorder can usually be distinguished without difficulty from other hereditary and degenerative diseases of the nervous system, but it should be recalled that pigmentary atrophy of the retina is seen in juvenile amaurotic idiocy, some hereditary ataxias, cases of ichthyosis with oligophrenia and spastic paralysis, Hallervorden-Spatz disease, Refsum's syndrome, and Kornzweig-Bassen syndrome.

Prognosis. The disorder is compatible with prolonged survival. Among reported deaths there is a high incidence of uremia attributed to a diversity of causes including obstructive nephropathy and pyelonephritis as well as vascular and glomerulonephritis.

Defects of Globe, Cornea, and Lens

Abnormalities of the lens and coverings of the eye contribute to the clinical pattern of many developmental and degenerative diseases of the brain. In most conditions the ocular manifestations are inconstant or are not of prime importance in diagnostic recognition; hence these diseases are more appropriately described elsewhere.

It is useful, however, to bear in mind the possible causes of the prominent ocular defects associated with mental deficiency and somatic neurologic deterioration. These relationships are summarized in Table 3-4. Microphthalmia usually appears in disorders of genetic or prenatal origin, including radiation damage, rubella syndrome, toxoplasmosis, trisomy 13–15, holotelencephalies, and hereditary microphthalmia.

FIG. 3-29. Polydactyly in the Laurence-Moon-Biedl syndrome with rudimentary extra digits.

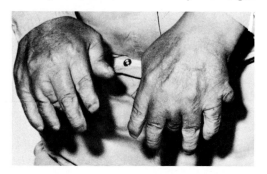

TABLE 3-4. Disorders Combining Neurologic and Ocular Defects

	Microphthalmia	Cataract	Corneal Opacity	Buphthalmos
Holotelencephaly	+			
Trisomy 13–15	+			
Trisomy 17–18	+			
Radiogenic microcephaly	+			
Toxoplasmosis	+			
Rubella syndrome	+	+		
Sex-linked microphthalmia	+	+	+	
Galactosemia		+		
Hypoparathyroidism		+		
Cerebrotendinous xanthomatosis		+		
Familial oligophrenia, ataxia, cataract		+		
Incontinentia pigmenti		+	+	
Mucopolysaccharidoses			+	
Oculocerebrorenal disease		+	+	+
Neurofibromatosis				+
Sturge-Weber disease				+

In oculocerebrorenal disease (Lowe's syndrome) a severe disorder in intraocular fluid dynamics brings about congenital glaucoma, buphthalmos, hydrophthalmos, corneal opacification, and cataract. Buphthalmos, usually unilateral, may also be found in neurofibromatosis and the Sturge-Weber syndrome. Corneal clouding is a characteristic feature of several types of the mucopolysaccharidoses. Cataract is commonly found in galactosemia. Older children with primary hypoparathyroidism may develop cataract.

In two rare hereditary disorders the ocular abnormalities are essential for recognition of the syndrome. The first is the Marinesco-Sjögren syndrome of cerebellar ataxia, oligophrenia, and cataract.[1] The disease is caused by a single autosomal recessive gene. Mental deficiency is moderate and does not seem to progress. Gait ataxia, limb ataxia, dysarthria, and nystagmus are present from infancy and become increasingly worse in maturity. Punctate cataracts develop in early childhood and progress to blindness.

Roberts reported a pedigree of 14 cases having a rare disorder inherited as a sex-linked recessive trait.[44] Microphthalmia is present from birth in affected males. Intraocular pressure is not increased, but the cornea and lens become opacified. Most of the involved members showed mental deficiency, ranging from feeblemindedness to severe idiocy.

DEGENERATIVE DISEASES OF WHITE MATTER

These familial diseases are probably inborn errors of metabolism affecting myelin but the nature of the defects is unknown. These diseases must be distinguished from the leukodystrophies, the disorders of myelin due to inborn errors of metabolism (see Chap. 9). The degenerative diseases of white matter include Pelizaeus-Merzbacher disease, spongy degeneration of the nervous system (Cannavan disease), and Alexander disease. All of these diseases begin in infancy and are progressive. Megalencephaly, ataxia, hypotonia, and psychomotor regression constitute the usual clinical presentation of these disorders. Infantile neuroaxonal dystrophy is also included among the degenerative diseases of white matter because the white matter is affected in this disorder. Gray matter involvement, however, is also prominent pathologically and clinically.

Pelizaeus-Merzbacher Disease

Pelizaeus-Merzbacher disease, a rare variety of leukodystrophy, is distinguished by its early onset in infancy with prominent nystagmus and cerebellar signs, its exceedingly slow rate of progression, and a characteristic pattern of inheritance. Its transmission generally follows the X-linked recessive mode. Some documented cases have been found in females that may represent random inactivation of one of the female X chromosomes.

Pathology. The characteristic morphologic feature of this disorder is a diffuse symmetrical demyelination involving both the cerebellar and cerebral white matter, but sparing isolated patches of myelinated fibers surviving in a perivascular distribution. The brain stem and spinal cord are irregularly and inconsistently involved. The only by-products of demyelination are relatively sparse collections of neutral fat in perivascular phagocytes.

Biochemistry. The cerebral white matter reveals a marked reduction in all the lipids characteristic of myelin without selective retention of sphingolipids as in other leukodystrophies, or cholesterol esters as in Schilder's disease and multiple sclerosis.

Clinical Characteristics. Characteristically Pelizaeus-Merzbacher disease begins in a male during infancy or early childhood. The prominent manifestations from the beginning consist of pendular oscillations of the globes in combination with titubation of the head. Achievement of erect posture and ambulation are delayed. Some infants never attain sitting ability, slumping to the bed when unsupported, and confined permanently to bed and chair. Others eventually stand and are able to walk until further progression of the disease incurs added deprivation of motor performance. Evident cerebellar signs appear in early childhood with ataxia, action tremor, and cerebellar dysarthria. Chorea has been noted as well as masklike facies. Vision is slowly impaired owing to optic nerve involvement. Late in childhood spastic diplegia gradually appears. Some patients develop seizures. Mental impairment is usually inconspicuous until late in the course when dementia occurs.

Atypical cases have been seen, such as the female in whom slow development was noted in early life with mental retardation being evident by age 7. Only in late childhood did there appear progressive spastic paralysis, chorea, and epilepsy.

Spongy Degeneration of the Nervous System

Although the first reported example of spongy degeneration of the nervous system was described as a case of Schilder's disease, it is now possible to distinguish the spongy type of leukodystrophy from other examples of diffuse sclerosis on both clinical and pathologic grounds. It is characterized by rapid progression and increasing head circumference. Inheritance is compatible with autosomal recessive transmission, and most cases appear in Jews of Eastern European origin.

Pathology. The brain is characteristically enlarged and soft, sometimes with flattened convolutions. There is widespread demyelination accompanied by a network of microscopic vacuolation presenting the characteristic spongy appearance. The abnormality may be limited to subcortical white matter with some extension into deeper cortical layers, or may be much more extensive with symmetrical diffuse involvement of all the cerebral white matter, corpus callosum, pyramidal tracts, cerebellar white matter, and optic tracts. Characteristically there is a band of vacuolation in the Purkinje layer of the cerebellar cortex.

Biochemistry. The cerebral white matter reveals a greatly increased water content with a marked uniform reduction in the myelin lipids.

Clinical Characteristics. The onset is typically early in infancy, between birth and 2 months. In some cases initial symptoms are vomiting, inability to suck, and failure to gain weight, associated with convulsions and followed by progressive paralysis. In others a motor defect is the initial manifestation with weakness of neck muscles and a progressive spastic diplegia. Later the infant becomes drowsy and suffers an arrest of mental development. Optic atrophy appears after several months with ultimate blindness. A characteristic clinical finding is enlargement of the head, which may begin between 2 and 5 months and progress for several months. Occasionally the anterior fontanel becomes tense. Spasticity gradually develops, with increased reflexes in the lower extremities and extensor plantar responses. After paroxysmal attacks of general rigidity, there appears terminally extensor rigidity in the lower extremities and flexor rigidity often with shoulder abduction in the upper extremities. The disorder is uniformly fatal, the patients terminating at an average age of 18 months.

Laboratory Examinations. The CSF may be under increased pressure in the phase of head enlargement but is otherwise normal. Radiographs of the skull may reveal separation of the sutures. Pneumoencephalograms may show that the ventricles are either normal or slightly enlarged.

Alexander's Disease (Megalencephalic Infantile Leukodystrophy)

Alexander's disease, a disorder of unknown pathogenesis, resembles spongy leukodystrophy with regard to early onset and enlargement of the head. It is also transmitted by autosomal recessive inheritance. The brain is enlarged and heavy, with reduction in stainable myelin. The major pathologic feature consists of large masses of fibrillary astrocytes with club-shaped Rosenthal fibers distributed along the boundaries of blood vessels, pial junctions, and ependyma.

Onset is during infancy with slowing of mental and motor development, weakness of the limbs, and spasticity. The head gradually enlarges by 6 months of age. Rigidity and opisthotonos appear. Death occurs at 2 years to 9 years of age.

Infantile Neuroaxonal Dystrophy

Neuroaxonal dystrophy, a rare degenerative disease of infancy, appears to be on a basis of recessive inheritance but predominantly appearing in females. There is a highly characteristic pathologic process involving the presence of iron-containing pigment in the globus pallidus and putamen resembling Hallervorden-Spatz disease. In addition, axonal spheroids are present in a widespread distribution including much of the gray matter of the spinal cord and lower brain stem. There is cerebellar atrophy, and loss of anterior horn cells may be seen.

The disorder begins in late infancy with loss of ability to walk and failure to develop normal speech. Progression is quite slow. Signs of upper motor neuron disease compete with those due to lower motor neuron deficit. Consequently there may be either spasticity or hypotonia and atrophy. Loss of pain sense has been reported. Atonic bladder may develop. Late in the course of disease there is nystagmus, blindness, and optic atrophy. Death tends to occur by age 12.

The electroencephalogram is normal early, but later shows diffuse fast activity with spikes and spike wave complexes. Electromyography may reveal evidence of partial denervation of muscles. There are no specific tests, and no treatment is available.

REFERENCES

1. **Alter M, Talbert OR, Croffead G:** Cerebellar ataxia, congenital cataracts, and retarded somatic and mental maturation. Neurology 12:836, 1962
2. **Böök JA, Schut JW, Reed SC:** Clinical and genetical study of microcephaly. Am J Ment Defic 57:637, 1953
3. **Brandon MWG, Kirman BH, Williams CE:** Microcephaly. J Ment Sci 105:721, 1959
4. **Brodal A, Hauglie-Hanssen E:** Congenital hydrocephalus with defective development of the cerebellar vermis (Dandy-Walker syndrome). J Neurol Neurosurg Psychiatry 22:99, 1959
5. **Caffey J, Ross S:** Pelvic bones in infantile mongoloidism. Am J Roentgenol Radium Ther Nucl Med 80:458, 1958
6. **Cameron AH:** Arnold-Chiari and other neuroanatomical malformations associated with spina bifida. J Pathol Bact 73:195, 1957
7. **Carter CO, Evans KA:** Risk of parents who have had one child with Down's syndrome (mongolism) having another child similarly affected. Lancet 281:785, 1961
8. **Carrington KW:** Ventriculo-venous shunt using the Holter valve as a treatment of hydrocephalus. J Mich Med Soc 58:373, 1959
9. **Critchley M, Earl CJC:** Tuberous sclerosis and allied conditions. Brain 55:311, 1932
10. **Crome L, Stern J:** The pathology of Mental Retardation. London, J&A Churchill, 1967

11. **Davis FA:** Primary tumors of the optic nerve (a phenomenon of Recklinghausen's disease). Arch Ophthalmol 23:735, 957, 1940

12. **DeMyer W, Zeman W, Palmer CG:** Familial alobar hydroprosencephaly (arrhinencephaly) with median cleft lip and palate. Neurology 13:913, 1963

13. **Dennis JP, Rosenberg HA, Alvord EC Jr:** Megalencephaly, internal hydrocephalus and other neurological aspects of achondroplasia. Brain 84:427, 1961

14. **Desanctis D, Cacchione A:** L'idiozia xerodermica. Riv Sper Freniat 56:269, 1932

15. **Edwards JH, Norman RM, Roberts JM:** Sex-linked hydrocephalus. Arch Dis Child 36:481, 1961

16. **Ewing JA:** Association of oligophrenia and dyskeratoses. Am J Ment Defic 60:98, 307,575, 1955–1956

17. **Frank LM:** Subdural collections and intracranial hemorrhage: precise identification by sector scan. Presented at the annual meeting of the Society for Computerized Tomography and Neuro-Imaging, San Juan, Puerto Rico, Jan 21, 1981

18. **Frank LM, Wirth FH, Karotkin EH:** Real-time B-mode ultrasonography (sector scan) of the infant brain. Presented at the annual meeting of the American Neurological Association, Boston, Sept 1980

19. **Gellis SS, Feingold M:** Atlas of Mental Retardation Syndromes. Washington, DC, Government Printing Office, 1969

20. **Gomez M,** editor: Tuberous Sclerosis. New York, Raven Press, 1979

21. **Gross H:** Der Hypertelorismus. Ophthalmologica 131:137, 1956

22. **Gunther M, Penrose LS:** Genetics of epiloia. J Genet 31:413, 1935

23. **Haber K, Wachter RD, Christenson PC, et al:** Ultrasonic evaluation of intracranial pathology in infants: a new technique. Radiology 134:173, 1980

24. **Halsey JH Jr, Allen N, Chamberlin HR:** The morphogenesis of hydroencephaly. J Neurol Sci 12:187, 1971

25. **Hankinson J, Amador IV:** Agenesis of the corpus callosum diagnosed by pneumoencephalography. Br J Radiol 30:200, 1957

26. **Ingraham FD, Matson DD:** Neurosurgery of Infancy and Childhood. Springfield, Ill, Charles C Thomas, 1954

27. **Jervis GA:** Microcephaly with extensive calcium deposits and demyelination. J Neuropathol Exp Neurol 13:318, 1954

28. **Jervis GA, Schein H:** Polyostotic fibrous dysplasia (Albright's syndrome): report of a case showing central nervous system changes. Arch Pathol 51:640, 1951

29. **Klein D, Ammann F:** The syndrome of Laurence-Moon-Bardet-Biedl and allied diseases in Switzerland. J Neurol Sci 9:479, 1969

30. **Laurence KM, Coates S:** Spontaneously arrested hydrocephalus. Dev Med Child Neurol 9 (Suppl)13:4, 1967

31. **Laurence KM, Hoare RD, Till K:** Diagnosis of the choroid plexus papilloma of the lateral ventricle. Brain 84:628, 1961

32. **Laurence KM, Cavanagh JB:** Progressive degeneration of the cortex in infancy. Brain 91:261, 1968

33. **Lees RF, Harrison RB, Sims TL:** Gray scale ultrasonography in the evaluation of hydrocephalus and associated abnormalities in infants. Am J Dis Child 132:376, 1978

34. **Levinson A, Friedman A, Stamps F:** Variability of mongolism. Pediatrics 16:43, 1955

35. **Logue V, Till K:** Posterior fossa dermoid cysts with special reference to intracranial infection. J Neurol Neurosurg Psychiatry 15:1, 1952

36. **Miller JQ, Picard EH, Alkan MK et al:** Specific congenital brain defect (arrhinencephaly) in 13–15 trisomy. N Engl J Med 268:120, 1963

37. **Moorhead PS, Melman WJ, Wenard C:** Familial chromosome translocation associated with speech and mental retardation. Am J Hum Genet 12:32, 1961

38. **Nilsson LR:** Chronic pancytopenia with multiple congenital abnormalities (Fanconi's anemia). Acta Paediatr 49:518, 1960

39. **Paulson GW, Lyle CB:** Tuberous sclerosis. Dev Med Child Neurol 8:571, 1966

40. **Peach G:** The Arnold-Chiari malformation: morphogenesis. Arch Neurol 12:527, 1965

41. **Penfield W, Young AW:** Nature of von Recklinghausen's disease and the tumors associated with it. Arch Neurol Psychiatry 23:320, 1930

42. **Redding A, Hirschhorn K:** Guide to human chromosome defects. Birth Defects 4(4):1, 1968

43. **Richards BW, Rundles AT:** Familial hormonal disorders associated with mental deficiency, deaf mutism and ataxia. J Ment Defic Res 3:33, 1959

44. **Roberts JAF:** Sex-linked microphthalmia sometimes associated with mental deficiency. Br Med J 2:1213, 1937

45. **Roth JC, Epstein CJ:** Infantile spasms and hypopigmented macules: early manifestations of tuberous sclerosis. Arch Neurol 25:547, 1971

46. **Rubin L, Becker SW Jr:** Pigmentation in the Bloch-Sulzberger syndrome (incontinentia pigmenti). Arch Dermatol 74:263, 1956

47. **Russell DS:** Observations on the pathology of hydrocephalus. Med Res Counc Spec Rep Ser (London) 265:1, 1949

48. **Selmarowitz VJ, Porter MJ:** The Sjögren Larsson syndrome. Am J Med 42:412, 1967

49. **Sjögren T, Larsson T:** Oligophrenia in combination with congenital ichthyosis and spastic disorders. Acta Psychiatr et Neurol Scand (Suppl 113) 32:1, 1957

50. **Skolnick ML, Rosenbaum AE, Matzuk T et al:** Detection of dilated cerebral ventricles in infants: a correlative study between ultrasound and computed tomography. Radiology 131:447, 1979

51. **Stewart RM:** Congenital ichthyosis, idiocy, infantilism and epilepsy-the syndrome of Rud. J Ment Sci 85:256, 1939

52. **Uchida IA, Bowman JM, Wang HC:** The 18-trisomy syndrome. N Engl J Med 266:1198, 1962
53. **Walker NF:** Use of dermal configurations in the diagnosis of mongolism. Pediatr Clin North Am 5:531, 1958
54. **Warkany J, Passarge E, Smith LB:** Congenital malformations in autosomal trisomy syndromes. Am J Dis Child 112:502, 1966
55. **Weller TH, Hanshaw JB:** Virologic and clinical observations on cytomegalic inclusion disease. N Engl J Med 266:1233, 1962
56. **Yakovlev PI:** Pathoarchitectonic studies of cerebral malformations. III. Arrhinencephalies (hototelencephalies). J Neuropathol Exp Neurol 18:22, 1959
57. **Yakovlev PI, Wadsworth RC:** Schizencephalies: study of the congenital clefts in the cerebral mantle. I. Clefts with fused lips. J Neuropathol Exp Neurol 5:116, 1946
58. **Yakovlev PI, Wadsworth RC:** Schizencephalies: study of the congenital clefts in the cerebral mantle. II. Clefts with hydrocephalus and lips separated. J Neuropathol Exp Neurol 5:169, 1946

Perinatal Disorders

4

Joseph J. Volpe

This chapter deals with the major neurologic disorders of the perinatal period with particular emphasis on those that are common and often associated with subsequent neurologic sequelae. The latter may take the form of nonprogressive motor disturbances, for example, spasticity, ataxia or choreoathetosis, and, as such, are included under the rubric, "cerebral palsy." Delays and ultimate deficits of intellectual development, that is, mental retardation, and seizure disorders are other important sequelae.

In the following discussion we review first the problem of neonatal seizures, particularly because most of the major neurologic disorders of the neonatal period may result in convulsive phenomena. This review is followed by a discussion of the major hypoxic–ischemic and hemorrhagic lesions that occur in newborn infants. Together the latter two processes account by far for most of the neurologic sequelae related to perinatal events.

NEONATAL SEIZURES

Seizures are the most frequent of the major manifestations of neonatal neurologic disorders. The frequency of neonatal seizures is usually seriously underestimated because many of the subtle manifestations of the convulsions escape detection. Recog- nition is critical, however, because the convulsive phenomena are usually related to significant illness, sometimes requiring specific therapy. Moreover, neonatal seizures may be sustained for considerable periods of time and may thus interfere with ventilation or supportive measures for associated disorders. In addition, seizures per se may be a cause of brain injury.

The following discussion reviews the clinical features, etiology, diagnosis, prognosis, and therapy of neonatal seizures.

CLINICAL FEATURES

Seizure phenomena in the newborn differ considerably from those observed in the older infant, and the phenomena in the premature infant differ somewhat from those in the full-term infant. Unlike older infants, newborns rarely have well-organized, symmetric, tonic–clonic seizures. Premature infants have even less well-organized spells than do full-term infants. The precise reasons for these differences must relate to the status of neuroanatomic and neurophysiologic development in the perinatal period (see reference 1 for a more detailed discussion).

In our experience five major varieties of seizures can be delineated in the neonatal period. These are, in order of decreasing frequency, subtle, generalized tonic, multifocal clonic, focal clonic, and myoclonic seizures.

Subtle

Subtle seizures are observed in both premature and full-term infants and are the most frequent seizure type. We have used the term *subtle* because the clinical phenomena are so readily and frequently overlooked.[1,34,35] These phenomena, the major manifestations of subtle seizures, include principally: tonic horizontal deviation of eyes with or without jerking of eyes; repetitive blinking or fluttering of eyelids; paroxysms of oral–buccal–lingual movements such as sucking, lip smacking, and drooling; peculiar "swimming" or "rowing" movements of upper limbs or "pedaling" of lower limbs; or an apneic spell. It should be emphasized, however, that apneic spells, especially in the premature infant, are much more likely to be related to a mechanism other than seizure. Indeed, when an apneic spell is a manifestation of seizure, the spell is almost always accompanied or preceded by one or more of the other subtle seizure phenomena. Subtle seizure phenomena are readily identified as seizures because of accompanying electroencephalogram (EEG) correlates and cessation with anticonvulsant medication.

Tonic

Tonic seizures are more common in premature than in full-term infants and are observed particularly in association with intraventricular hemorrhage. This seizure type is usually generalized and characterized by tonic extension of all limbs, occasionally by flexion of upper limbs and extension of lower limbs. As such, this seizure type may mimic decerebrate or decorticate posturing, respectively. Helpful distinguishing features include accompanying eye signs or occasional clonic movements.

Multifocal Clonic

Multifocal clonic seizures are observed more commonly in full-term than in premature infants and most frequently are associated with perinatal asphyxia with hypoxic–ischemic encephalopathy. This is a distinctive seizure type, characterized by clonic movements of one or another limb that migrate to another body part in a nonordered fashion (e.g., left upper extremity jerking may be accompanied by or followed by right lower extremity jerking). This non-Jacksonian migration is characteristic.

Focal Clonic

Focal clonic seizures are more common in full-term than premature infants and occur in most typical form in association with focal traumatic injury, for example, cerebral contusion. However, metabolic encephalopathy, such as hypocalcemia, may be associated with focal clonic seizures in the newborn. These episodes are characterized by well-localized clonic jerking and are not usually accompanied by unconsciousness.

Myoclonic

Myoclonic seizures are the least common of neonatal seizure types. The spells are characterized by single or multiple jerks of flexion of upper or lower limbs. In full form this seizure type is usually indicative of severe bilateral cerebral disease and may presage development of massive myoclonic spasms and a hypsarrhythmic EEG.

Jitteriness

Though not a type of seizure, *jitteriness* not infrequently is confused with seizure. The term refers to a striking movement disorder of newborns in which coarse tremulousness is the principal feature. Distinction from seizure can be made at the bedside if four essential points are remembered. Thus, jitteriness is not accompanied by abnormalities of gaze or extraocular movement, whereas seizures usually are. Jitteriness is exquisitely stimulus-sensitive but seizures are not. The dominant movement in jitteriness is tremor; the alternating movements are rhythmic, of equal rate and amplitude. The dominant movement in seizure is clonic jerking; the movements have a fast and slow component. The rhythmic movement of limbs in jitteriness usually can be stopped by flexion of the affected limb. Convulsive movements will not cease with this maneuver. The most consistently defined etiologies of jitteriness are hypoxic–ischemic encephalopathy, hypocalcemia, hypoglycemia, and drug withdrawal. The major features of jitteriness that distinguish it from seizure are summarized below:

No abnormality of gaze or eye movement
Movements exquisitely stimulus-sensitive
Predominant movement tremor
Cessation of movements with passive flexion

ETIOLOGY

Although many neonatal neurologic disorders may cause convulsive phenomena to occur, relatively few etiologies account for the vast majority of infants with seizures. These are listed in Table 4-1 in relation to the usual postnatal age when seizures are likely to accompany the specific etiologic process. This simple point, that is, the time of onset of seizures, is a very useful initial clinical clue to etiology.

Perinatal Asphyxia

Perinatal asphyxia results in hypoxic–ischemic encephalopathy, which is discussed in detail in the next major section. This is the most common cause of neonatal seizures in both full-term and premature infants. The spells characteristically occur in the first 24 hours of life. Indeed, in our series 60% of infants with seizures secondary to hypoxic–ischemic encephalopathy experienced the onset of spells within 12 hours of birth. Seizures with hypoxic–ischemic encephalopathy may be very difficult to control with anticonvulsant drugs, especially in the first 48 hours of life.

Intracranial Hemorrhage

Seizures may accompany all types of intracranial hemorrhage but are observed most commonly in association with intraventricular hemorrhage and primary subarachnoid hemorrhage. However, even in these settings, the incidence of seizures is quite low. Nevertheless, because of the relatively high frequency of these hemorrhages, they are relatively common causes of neonatal seizures. The seizures occur relatively early, particularly on the second and third postnatal days. Seizures with major intraven-

TABLE 4-1. Major Etiologies of Neonatal Seizure

Etiology	Time of Onset*	
	0–3 Days	>3 Days
Perinatal Asphyxia	+	
Intracranial Hemorrhage	+	
Intracranial Infection		+
Developmental Defect	+	+
Hypoglycemia	+	
Hypocalcemia†	+	+

*Age when seizures most likely to occur
†Two varieties of hypocalcemia are included (see text).

tricular hemorrhage are often of the generalized tonic variety and are difficult to distinguish from decerebrate or decorticate posturing. The frequently poor response of such seizures to therapy with anticonvulsant drugs suggests that posturing is commonly the more appropriate designation.[32]

Intracranial Infection

Intracranial infection accounts for approximately 10% to 15% of all cases of neonatal seizures. The most common time of occurrence of the seizures is the latter part of the first week and later. The infections involved include bacterial meningitis in the majority of cases. However, relevant nonbacterial infections are the various neonatal encephalitides, that is, toxoplasmosis, herpes simplex, Coxsackie B, rubella, and cytomegalovirus infection.

Developmental Defects

A wide variety of aberrations of brain development may be associated with neonatal seizures, which may begin at any time during the neonatal period. The common denominator of nearly all of these aberrations is a cerebral cortical dysgenesis, related most commonly to a disturbance of neuronal migration. Thus, the most frequent disorders responsible are lissencephaly, pachygyria, and polymicrogyria.

Hypoglycemia

Hypoglycemia may be associated with seizures in the newborn, as in older infants and children.[27] Hypoglycemia is most frequent in small infants, especially those small for gestational age or in infants of mothers who are diabetic or prediabetic. Neurologic phenomena, including seizures, are more common in small infants and relate to the duration of hypoglycemia and, particularly, the time before onset of adequate therapy. Seizures in this context occur most frequently on the second postnatal day. However, in such infants it is often particularly difficult to establish that hypoglycemia is the cause of the neurologic syndrome, because perinatal asphyxia, intracranial hemorrhage, intracranial infection or hypocalcemia are frequently associated.

Hypocalcemia or Hypomagnesemia

Deficiency of one or both of these divalent cations may cause seizures to occur in the newborn, as in older infants and children. Hypocalcemia has two major peaks of incidence in the newborn period. The first peak occurs in the first two to three days of life, especially in infants of low birth weight or of diabetic mothers. Not infrequently perinatal asphyxia is in the background. As with hypoglycemia, hypocalcemia in this setting is rarely the only potential etiologic factor when seizures occur. A therapeutic response to intravenous calcium is of value in determining whether the low serum calcium is etiologically related to the seizures. In our experience it is much more common for early hypocalcemia to be an association of neonatal seizures rather than the cause.

Later onset hypocalcemia, that is, hypocalcemia occurring later in the first week and into the second week of life, is associated most commonly with nutritional factors, such as consumption of a formula with a suboptimal ratio of calcium (and magnesium) to phosphorus (e.g., cow's milk). Classically these hypocalcemic babies are large, full-term infants avidly consuming a milk preparation of the type just noted. Hypomagnesemia is a frequent accompaniment or may be present without hypocalcemia.[7] The neurologic syndrome is consistent and distinctive, consisting primarily of hyperactive tendon reflexes, knee, ankle, and jaw clonus, and jitteriness, in addition to seizures. The convulsive phenomena are often focal, both clinically and electroencephalographically.

Other Metabolic Abnormalities

Other metabolic processes that uncommonly are associated with neonatal seizures include hyponatremia, hypernatremia, pyridoxine dependency, aminoacidopathy, organic acidopathy, hyperammonemia, intrauterine drug intoxication (e.g., local anesthetic), or postnatal drug intoxication (e.g., theophylline).

Hyponatremia occurs most commonly in our experience with inappropriate antidiuretic hormone (ADH) secretion, associated usually with bacterial meningitis or intraventricular hemorrhage. Hypernatremia results most commonly iatrogenically as a complication of overly vigorous use of hypertonic sodium bicarbonate for the treatment of acidosis. Seizures often occur during correction of the hypernatremia, especially if markedly hypotonic solutions are used or too rapid correction is attempted.[17] Pyridoxine dependency, a defect in pyridoxine metabolism, may produce severe seizures recalcitrant to all therapy.[2,19,31] Diagnosis is made best with a therapeutic trial of pyridoxine. Aminoacidopathy may result in neonatal seizures, and maple syrup urine disease is the most common of these. Of the organic acidopathies, those involving propionic acid and methylmalonic acid metabolism are most commonly associated with neonatal seizures. Hyperammonemia may complicate amino acid disturbances (e.g., urea cycle defects) or the organic acid disturbances just noted and result in neonatal seizures. Hyperammonemia may also occur in association with perinatal asphyxia (see next section) or in preterm infants without easily recognized cause.

Intoxication with local anesthetics may lead to neonatal seizures and occurs when the drug, usually mepivacaine, is injected inadvertently into the fetal scalp at the time of placement of paracervical or pudendal blocks.[16,24] Affected infants exhibit low Apgar scores, bradycardia, apnea, or hypoventilation, hypotonia and seizures, usually tonic, with onset in the first 6 hours. Fixed, dilated pupils and impaired eye movements with oculocephalic maneuver aid in differential diagnosis. Properly supported infants improve over the first 24 hours to 48 hours of life. Postnatal drug intoxication is a rare cause of neonatal seizures. Of commonly used drugs, theophylline has been associated with seizures as a toxic manifestation.

Drug Withdrawal

Although a generally uncommon cause of neonatal seizures, in some urban medical centers drug withdrawal is an important etiologic consideration. Such infants have been passively addicted to a drug consumed by the mother during pregnancy. The drugs particularly involved are narcotic–analgesics, sedative–hypnotics (especially shorter-acting barbiturates), and alcohol.

Narcotic–Analgesics. Narcotic–analgesics are the most commonly recognized drugs associated with passive addiction of the newborn. In this class only passive addiction to methadone is associated with neonatal seizures to a significant degree, occurring in nearly 10% of such infants.[15] The mean age of onset of seizures in such patients is 10 days.

Sedative–Hypnotics. Among the sedative–hypnotics shorter-acting barbiturates such as secobarbital have been associated with neonatal seizures.[4] In contrast to the situation with methadone, seizures in this setting occur usually in the first 48 hours of life.

Alcohol. Although the dysmorphic, so-called fetal alcohol syndrome is most common after maternal abuse of alcohol during pregnancy, neonatal seizures secondary to alcohol withdrawal have been described.[26] The seizures have occurred in the first 24 hours of life.

Familial Neonatal Seizures

An interesting syndrome of familial neonatal seizures has been recognized.[3,6,28] We observed a typical case with onset of frequent subtle and multifocal clonic seizures on the second postnatal day that responded to phenobarbital. Father and multiple paternal relatives had had neonatal seizures that had resolved after the first weeks of life in 80% of cases. The remainder of the family members continued to exhibit seizures of unknown cause into adulthood. Inheritance of this disorder is autosomal dominant and neurologic development is normal. Recognition requires specific questioning in the elicitation of the family history.

DIAGNOSIS

Consideration of the etiologic possibilities discussed above make it clear that a careful history and physical examination are the cornerstones of diagnosis in the newborn with seizures. Of the many laboratory tests that might be considered, the first to be done are directed against the two diseases that are especially dangerous but readily treated when recognized promptly, that is, hypoglycemia and bacterial meningitis. Thus, lumbar puncture and blood sugar determinations are performed urgently. In addition, blood should be drawn for determination of sodium, potassium, calcium, magnesium, and phosphorus. Other metabolic determinations, radiological and other studies are determined by the specific clinical features. EEG is useful, especially to determine to what extent the infant with subtle clinical phenomena is experiencing seizures, and to aid in estimating prognosis in the full-term infant (see below).[33] In neither instance does the EEG provide infallible information.

PROGNOSIS

Over the past 10 years to 20 years the outlook for infants with neonatal seizures has improved.[5,7,9–11,13,14,18,20,29] Mortality rates have decreased from approximately 40% to 50% to approximately 15% to 20%. The incidence of neurologic sequelae in the larger number of survivors has remained about the same, approximately 30%. The decrease in mortality rates relates to improvements in obstetric management and the advent of neonatal intensive care. However, these general figures are of little value to the clinician concerned with the outlook in a given infant. For a more precise determination of prognosis, the most useful approaches have used the EEG and the determination of the underlying neurologic disease.

EEG

In the full-term infant with seizures, determination of the interictal EEG may be of value in estimation of prognosis. Thus, in the large series of full-term infants with seizures studied by Rose and Lombroso, a normal interictal EEG was associated with an 86% chance for normal development at age 4 years, whereas an EEG with multifocal abnormalities was associated with only a 12% chance for normal development.[29] A smaller group of infants, approximately 10% in the series of Rose and Lombroso, demonstrated a striking, periodic, burst–suppression pattern.[29] The pattern consists of alternating periods of marked voltage suppression interrupted by bursts of high voltage, asynchronous, sharp activity, including spikes and slow waves. It bears a superficial resemblance to trace alternans of the normal newborn. However, the abnormal pattern just described is very strongly correlated with severe cerebral disease and a poor prognosis.[11,12] Nevertheless, some caution must be used in attributing a grave prognosis to abnormal paroxysmal patterns with long silent periods in young premature infants, especially those less than 33 weeks to 34 weeks of conceptual age. More important, at least 25% to 35% of full-term newborns with seizures will have EEGs that are either "borderline" or that demonstrate other less marked abnormalities, associated with an uncertain prognosis. In addition, no study to date has clearly demonstrated that the EEG is particularly valuable in establishing a prognosis for premature infants with seizures.

Underlying Neurologic Disease

The most valuable determinant of outcome with neonatal seizures is recognition of the underlying neurologic disease responsible for the seizures. Table 4-2 depicts the chances for normal neurologic development for the major etiologic categories of neonatal seizures when the neurologic disease is accompanied by sei-

TABLE 4-2.   Relation of Prognosis of Neonatal Seizures to Etiology

Etiology	Normal Development
Perinatal asphyxia	50%
Intraventricular Hemorrhage	<10%
Subarachnoid Hemorrhage	90%
Bacterial Meningitis	25%–65%
Developmental Defect	0
Hypoglycemia	50%
Hypocalcemia	
Early onset	50%
Later onset	100%

zures.[1,7,11,13,20,29,30,32] The outlook varies considerably with the nature of the responsible neurologic disorder. Thus, it is clear that the most critical task of the physician caring for the infant with seizures is to make as precise a determination of the neuropathologic process underlying the seizure, not only to institute appropriate therapy but also to provide as meaningful a prognostic statement as possible.

TREATMENT

The management of the infant with seizures should begin with the question of whether therapy is necessary at all. A few observers have suggested that in the absence of an obvious impairment of ventilation or perfusion, aggressive attempts to treat neonatal seizures are not indicated. Indeed, it is easy to ignore (or miss) frequent seizure activity in the newborn because the convulsive phenomena may be so subtle. We consider this an ill-advised approach because of the growing body of information that ascribes a harmful role to the seizures *per se.*[8,21–23,27,36]

Adverse Consequences of Neonatal Seizures

Potential adverse consequences of repeated neonatal seizures on the brain of the infant are shown in Table 4-3, together with the possible pathogenetic mechanisms. Hypoxic–ischemic brain injury might be expected to result (or be exacerbated) by hypoxemia, the latter occurring as a consequence of the hypoventilation that may accompany even subtle seizures. Studies with the transcutaneous oxygen electrode indicate that serious diminutions in PO_2 may result with seizures in the absence of clinically obvious hypoventilation (see section on hypoxic–ischemic encephalopathy). In addition, important substrates for energy metabolism, particularly glucose, may be seriously depleted by neonatal seizures and a fall in brain energy levels can be documented in the experimental situation.[36] An ischemic factor may become operative, secondary to diminished cerebral blood flow caused by hypoxic myocardial failure, a late complication of persistent hypoventilation or apnea. Intraventricular hemorrhage may result from neonatal seizures because of the increase in cerebral blood flow that has been well documented in animals undergoing seizures and that probably occurs in humans during seizures. The increase in cerebral blood flow may occur as a consequence of hypercapnia secondary to hypoventilation or apnea, an increase in arterial blood pressure, and the occurrence of lactic acidosis in the brain secondary to the accelerated cerebral metabolic rate and shift in the cytoplasmic redox state with seizures. The increase in arterial blood pressure has been well documented with even subtle neonatal seizures and would be expected to lead to an abrupt increase in cerebral blood flow because of the impairment of vascular autoregulation in human newborns (see sections on hypoxic–ischemic encephalopathy and intraventricular hemorrhage).

Acute Therapy

Our usual sequence of management when faced with a convulsing infant is to establish an intravenous line and to determine rapidly whether hypoglycemia is present by the use of a reagent strip, Dextrostix, on the first drops of blood. If hypoglycemia is present, 25% dextrose is given intravenously in a dose of 2 ml/kg to 4 ml/kg (0.5 g/kg–1.0 g/kg) and the baby maintained on intravenous dextrose at a rate as high as 0.5 g/kg per hr if necessary (this is approximately the maximal usable dose of glucose

TABLE 4-3. Potential Adverse Consequences of Repeated Seizures in the Newborn

Neuropathologic Consequences	Possible Mechanism(s)
Hypoxic–Ischemic Brain Injury	Hypoxemia secondary to hypoventilation or apnea. Decreased brain glucose and energy supplies secondary to accelerated cerebral metabolic rate. Decreased cerebral blood flow secondary to hypoxic myocardial failure (late).
Intraventricular Hemorrhage	Increased cerebral blood flow, as a consequence of: Hypercapnia secondary to hypoventilation or apnea. Increase in arterial blood pressure. Lactic acidosis in brain secondary to accelerated cerebral metabolic rate.

in the newborn period). The possibility of maintaining blood glucose at supranormal levels in all newborns with seizures should be considered, in view of the experimental demonstrations of the decline in brain glucose with seizures and the protective effect of pretreatment with glucose.[36]

If hypoglycemia is not present, we administer phenobarbital intravenously in a loading dose of 20 mg/kg, usually in two 10 mg/kg-increments, each administered over a period of 5 minutes to 10 minutes. Careful surveillance of respiratory effort is important under these circumstances. This dose is necessary to achieve a therapeutic blood level in the newborn over approximately 20 μg/ml.[25] In the unusual case in which the patient continues to exhibit active seizures after 20 mg/kg of phenobarbital, diphenylhydantoin is administered intravenously in a loading dose of 20 mg/kg, as described for phenobarbital. This dose has been shown to result in a therapeutic blood level in the newborn of approximately 15 μg/ml.[25] Cardiac rate and rhythm should be monitored during the infusion. We do not administer calcium routinely to all newborns during the initial seizure, except in the unusual instance of a classic presentation of later onset hypocalcemia. If hypocalcemia is found to be present, 5% calcium gluconate is given intravenously in a dose of 4 ml/kg (200 mg/kg). Electrocardiogram or at least cardiac rhythm by auscultation should be monitored during administration. It is important to recognize that phenobarbital can suppress the seizures of hypocalcemia. If hypomagnesemia is present, magnesium sulfate is best given intramuscularly as a 50% solution in a dose of 0.2 ml/kg. In this respect it should be recalled that approximately one-half of newborns with seizures secondary to later onset hypocalcemia also have hypomagnesemia.[7] The importance of treating these hypocalcemic infants with magnesium is emphasized by the following two facts: (1) the administration of calcium to such infants may increase renal excretion of magnesium, aggravate the hypomagnesemia and maintain the convulsive state; and (2) the administration of magnesium has been shown to correct both the hypocalcemia and the hypomagnesemia, perhaps by increasing movement of calcium from bone to plasma.[7] However, magnesium cannot be administered injudiciously because magnesium can produce a neuromuscular blockade.

Severe, recurrent seizures, not accompanied by any obvious associated findings that might aid in diagnosis, and that prove recalcitrant to the above modes of therapy, suggest the possibility of pyridoxine dependency. The best means of diagnosis is a therapeutic trial of pyridoxine administered intravenously in a dose of 50 mg, accompanied by simultaneous monitoring of the EEG. In the true case this trial is accompanied by cessation of seizure activity and normalization of the EEG within minutes.

Maintenance Therapy with Anticonvulsant Drugs

Administration of phenobarbital in a dose of 3 mg/kg per day to 4 mg/kg per day provides a blood level of approximately 20 μg/ml and maintenance of anticonvulsant action. If diphenylhydantoin was needed for treatment of the acute episode, it should also be used for maintenance in a dose of 3 mg/kg per day to 4 mg/kg per day. The maintenance doses are begun 12 hours following administration of the loading doses

and administered in divided doses every 12 hours. Intravenous, intramuscular, or oral administration is adequate for phenobarbital, although the parenteral routes should be used in the seriously ill infant. Only intravenous therapy is used for diphenylhydantoin because the drug is not absorbed reliably in the newborn after oral or intramuscular administration.[25]

Elimination rates for phenobarbital and diphenylhydantoin increase with increasing duration of therapy and thus dose requirements may increase. However, careful correlation of clinical state and blood level assessments is necessary for rational therapy of the newborn with seizures.

Optimal Duration of Therapy

This remains an unresolved issue. We attempt to discontinue diphenylhydantoin prior to discharge, usually when intravenous lines are discontinued. Duration of therapy with phenobarbital initially depends principally on evidence of neurologic disturbance, especially as judged by neurologic examination. The drug is discontinued prior to discharge from the nursery in the child who is clearly normal. In the more usual, equivocal case this judgment is made next at three months of age. If at that time there are no abnormal neurologic signs, phenobarbital is tapered over two weeks and discontinued. A similar approach is used at six and nine months of age. If at one year of age an infant is not normal from the neurologic standpoint but has been seizure-free, an EEG is obtained; if overt paroxysmal activity is absent, phenobarbital is tapered and discontinued over 4 weeks.

HYPOXIC–ISCHEMIC ENCEPHALOPATHY

Hypoxic–ischemic encephalopathy encompasses a spectrum of neuropathologic and neurologic features that comprise a major portion of neonatal neurology. This encephalopathy is the major cause of neurologic morbidity in the full-term infant. In the premature infant only periventricular–intraventricular hemorrhage results in more neurologic morbidity and, indeed, because many examples of periventricular–intraventricular hemorrhage arise as a complication of hypoxic–ischemic encephalopathy, it is clear that this encephalopathy probably accounts for more neurologic morbidity than any other in all infants.

In this section we review in sequence the biochemical, physiologic, neuropathologic, and clinical aspects of hypoxic–ischemic encephalopathy. We discuss these aspects in this sequence because the neuropathology is a consequence of the biochemical and physiologic effects of the hypoxic–ischemic insults, and the clinical aspects, a consequence of the topography of the neuropathology.

BIOCHEMICAL ASPECTS

Basic Deficit in Energy Production

The perinatal brain is dependent on oxygen for maintenance of function and structure. Deprivation of oxygen may occur by two basic pathogenetic mechanisms, that is, hypoxemia, which is a diminished amount of oxygen in the blood supply, and ischemia, which is a diminished amount of blood actually perfusing the brain. The central biochemical effect of oxygen deprivation is on glucose and energy metabolism and is shown below.

Energy Production Under Aerobic Versus Anaerobic Conditions

Aerobic: Glucose + 38 ADP + 38 P_i + $6O_2$ → $6 CO_2$ + $44 H_2O$ + <u>38 ATP</u>

Anaerobic: Glucose + 2 ADP + 2 P_i → 2 Lactate + $2 H^+$ + <u>2 ATP</u>

Thus, under normal aerobic conditions glucose is oxidized completely to carbon dioxide and water with the production of 38 molecules of ATP for every molecule of glucose. However, with oxygen deprivation and anaerobic conditions glucose is converted by anaerobic glycolysis only to lactate, with the formation of hydrogen ions and, more importantly, only two molecules of ATP for each molecule of glucose. Thus, an enormous difference in energy production results as a consequence of deprivation.

Major Biochemical Consequences

The major biochemical effects of oxygen deprivation in the brain are shown below.[54,79,80]

Major Biochemical Effects of Oxygen Deprivation in Brain
1. Glycogenolysis
2. ↑ Glycolysis
3. ↑ Lactate and ↓ tissue pH
4. ↓ Glucose
5. ↓ Phosphocreatine
6. ↓ ATP

The increased demand for glucose, caused by the 19-fold diminution in amount of ATP derived from its metabolism, is met in part by glycogenolysis. In addition, the rate of glucose use by glycolysis is accelerated greatly, approximately five-fold to ten-fold. Under anaerobic conditions this variety of glycolysis results, however, in an increased production of lactate and hydrogen ions. The consequence is a lowering of tissue pH. Initially this is beneficial because the local acidosis results in vasodilation with a consequent increase in substrate supplies. However, with severe falls in brain pH there is cellular injury and loss of vascular autoregulation (with the risk of hemorrhagic or ischemic lesions with abrupt increases or decreases in perfusion pressure). Because glucose supplies from blood and from endogenous stores (e.g., glycogen) cannot keep pace with the accelerated use, brain glucose levels fall.[38] The final result is a fall in the major energy store in brain, that is, phosphocreatine, and ultimately in ATP. Although changes in energy levels in the brain do not account for all of the deleterious effects of oxygen deprivation, it is not unexpected that deficient ATP levels will lead to failure of ion transport, neurotransmitter synthesis, and macromolecular synthesis. The ultimate result is impaired neuronal function and structural injury.

Hypoxemia and ischemia share the essential effects described immediately above. However, it should be emphasized that with ischemia certain biochemical changes will be more severe. Thus, blood glucose supplies will be deficient and, therefore, will restrict the ability of brain to respond to increased glucose demands. Moreover, defective perfusion will not allow clearance of tissue acids (derived from lactate and CO_2) nor provide the buffering systems in plasma.

When hypoxemia and ischemia occur with asphyxia, hypercapnia is an essential additional feature. Hypercapnia has deleterious biochemical effects in the brain by causing an increase in tissue acidosis. In addition, the generalized cerebral vasodilation caused by hypercapnia may result in an "intracranial steal" phenomenon in which blood flow to areas with marginal blood supply becomes deficient enough to cause infarction.[75] Moreover, the vasodilation may lead to intracranial hemorrhage by causing hyperperfusion to areas of perinatal brain, for example, the periventricular region, which is already susceptible to the development of hemorrhage.

PHYSIOLOGIC ASPECTS

Cerebral Blood Flow in Experimental Asphyxia

The most critical of the physiologic aspects of hypoxic–ischemic encephalopathy relate to changes in cerebral blood flow. Experimental production of perinatal asphyxia by a variety of techniques that impair gas exchange between the mother and fetus causes several important effects on cerebral blood flow.[38,42,46,47,56,64] Initially there is: (1) an alteration in the fetal circulation such that a larger proportion of the cardiac output is distributed to the brain; (2) an increase in cerebral blood flow; and (3) a loss of vascular autoregulation. These effects are followed by: (4) a diminution in cardiac output with the occurrence of systemic hypotension, and as a consequence, (5) a decrease in cerebral blood flow.

The first of these effects, that is, the redistribution of cardiac output such that a significantly larger proportion enters the brain (and the coronary circulation), is reminiscent of the diving reflex in aquatic animals. This alteration participates in the second effect, that is, an increase in cerebral blood flow. The latter is also related to an increase in arterial blood pressure, an early accompaniment of asphyxia. The increase in cerebral blood flow is most marked in brain stem but is also observable in cerebrum as well. The third effect, the loss of vascular autoregulation, probably relates to the increase in perivascular hydrogen ion

concentration related to increased lactate production and the effects of hypercapnia. This impairment of vascular autoregulation causes cerebral blood flow to be "pressure-passive" and, thus, at the mercy of arterial blood pressure. Therefore, the serious result of the fourth and later effect of perinatal asphyxia, that is, decreased cardiac output and decreased blood pressure, is understandable. These cardiovascular effects are principally secondary to the deleterious effects of hypoxemia and acidosis on the myocardium. The final consequence, the fifth effect, is a decrease in cerebral blood flow and ischemic brain injury. Certain areas of perinatal brain are particularly vulnerable to ischemic brain injury, that is, parasagittal regions in the full-term infant and periventricular regions in the premature infant, and are common sites of injury with perinatal asphyxia (see below).

Cerebral Blood Flow in the Human Newborn

Studies of cerebral blood flow in the human newborn in the past few years indicate that the lessons learned from the experimental work are applicable to the human infant. Thus, using the xenon clearance technique to measure cerebral blood flow, Lou and coworkers have shown that vascular autoregulation in the human newborn is very sensitive to perinatal asphyxia.[65] Indeed, infants who by most criteria would be considered to have sustained minimal or even no significant hypoxic–ischemic insult exhibited impaired vascular autoregulation. Thus, these recent data suggest that the human newborn is particularly susceptible to ischemic brain injury with only modest changes in arterial blood pressure. Initial follow-up of 15 of the infants with cerebral blood flow determinations in the first day of life indicates that impaired cerebral blood flow, that is, values of 20 ml/100 g/min or less, correlate with the subsequent occurrence of neurologic sequelae and evidence for brain injury by CT scan.[66]

NEUROPATHOLOGY

The biochemical and physiologic consequences of perinatal hypoxic–ischemic insults lead, in the human, to one (or more) of several major neuropathologic lesions. The major neuropathologic varieties of neonatal hypoxic–ischemic encephalopathy include: selective neuronal necrosis, status marmoratus, parasagittal cerebral injury, periventricular leukomalacia, and focal (and multifocal) ischemic brain necrosis.[39]

Selective Neuronal Necrosis

As the name implies, selective neuronal necrosis refers to injury, principally of neurons, in a characteristic distribution. The major sites of injury include neurons of cerebral cortex, diencephalon, basal ganglia, brain stem, and cerebellum.[59,72] In cerebral cortex, neurons of hippocampus (Sommer sector) are more vulnerable than those of supralimbic cortex. In diencephalon, neurons especially affected are in thalamus, hypothalamus, and lateral geniculate bodies. In basal ganglia, the caudate, putamen, and globus pallidus are vulnerable. Often neuronal injury in these regions is dominant and is considered best as a distinct entity, status marmoratus (see below). In brain stem, vulnerable neurons include those of the inferior colliculi, cochlear nuclei, motor nuclei of cranial nerves, and reticular formation. Impressive involvement of pontine nuclei and neurons of the subicular portion of hippocampus, that is, pontosubicular necrosis, has been shown to be especially characteristic of the premature infant who experiences perinatal hypoxia and acidosis, followed by hyperoxia.[40] In cerebellum, Purkinje cells are especially vulnerable to oxygen deprivation, although injury to neurons of the dentate and other roof nuclei is not unusual.

Status Marmoratus

Status marmoratus is a striking lesion of basal ganglia, especially caudate and putamen but also globus pallidus. Most cases exhibit similar involvement of thalamus and slightly more than one-half, of cerebral cortex.[69] The characteristic features are: neuronal loss, gliosis, and hypermyelination. It is the hypermyelination that is the hallmark of the injury, and this does not become clearly apparent until a year or more after the perinatal period. The abnormal myelin pattern imparts a marbled appearance to the affected nuclei, and thus the appellation, status marmoratus or état

marbré. Electron microscopic observations demonstrate that the abnormal myelin is around glial fibers and not axons.[43] Thus, there is a peculiar response to injury that appears to be related to the time of occurrence of the insult, that is, the perinatal period.

Parasagittal Cerebral Injury

Parasagittal cerebral injury refers to bilateral, usually symmetric areas of necrosis, located principally in superomedial aspects of the cerebral convexities, affecting posterior more than anterior cerebrum (Fig. 4-1). The lesion is observed most frequently in the full-term infant and because of its distribution appears to be related principally to ischemia. Thus, the areas of injury are in the border zones between the end fields of the major cerebral arteries, the anterior, middle, and posterior cerebral arteries (Fig. 4-2). These so-called "watershed" areas would be expected to be especially vulnerble to falls in perfusion pressure. The data reviewed above indicating the loss of vascular autoregulation in human newborn infants and the apparent susceptibility to ischemic injury with systemic hypotension are clearly relevant in this respect.[65,84]

Periventricular Leukomalacia

Periventricular leukomalacia is characterized by necrosis of the white matter just adjacent to the external angle of the lateral ventricle (Fig. 4-3). The lesion of periventricular white matter termed perinatal telencephalic leukoencephalopathy by Gilles and coworkers may be an early example of periventricular leukomalacia.[61,62,63] Periventricular leukomalacia is observed most commonly at the level of the occipital radiation, near the trigone of the lateral ventricles, and at the level of the white matter around the foramen of Monro.[78] These sites are border zones between penetrating branches of the middle cerebral artery and the posterior cerebral artery (occipital radiation) or the anterior cerebral artery (frontal white matter). The specific characteristics of the periventricular vascular border zones and end zones have been described in neonatal brain by DeReuck and coworkers.[48,49] Thus, these anatomic features, as well as consideration of the clinical phenomena and pathologic changes in

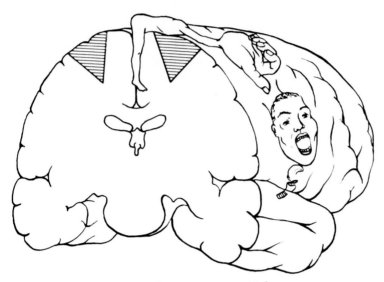

FIG. 4-1. Schematic   diagram—parasagittal cerebral injury. Distribution of the lesion is indicated by line-marked areas.

other organs in patients with periventricular leukomalacia, suggest that the lesion is an ischemic one. Again, the data reviewed above on the susceptibility of human infants to ischemic injury are relevant.[65,84]

Neuropatholic complications of periventricular leukomalacia include cavitation within cerebral white matter, with particularly severe lesions, and hemorrhage within the areas of leukomalacia. Hemorrhage in the latter context is usually small but in a few infants may be so severe as to suggest periventricular intraventricular hemorrhage emanating from the more usual site in the germinal matrix (see next section on periventricular–intraventricular hemorrhage).[37]

Focal (and Multifocal) Ischemic Brain Necrosis

Focal (and multifocal) ischemic brain necrosis refers to a pattern of necrosis of cerebral parenchyma, cortex, and subcortical white matter that resides within vascular distributions. The relative frequency of these lesions is emphasized by the recent work of Barmada and associates who observed also that the incidence of this lesion at postmortem examination varied with gestational age.[41] Thus, the incidence in infants less than 28 weeks of gestation was zero, approximately 5% for those between 28 weeks and 32 weeks, 10% for those between 32 weeks and 37 weeks, and fully 15% for those between 37 weeks and 40 weeks. Involvement of the middle cerebral artery occurred in approximately one-half of the affected cases. Single larger lesions were most common in full-term infants, and multiple smaller lesions, in premature infants.

The causes for such focal and multifocal sites of ischemia are not entirely understood. Thrombosis with disseminated intravascular coagulation and with vasculitis secondary to meningitis has been documented. Embolic phenomena from the placenta, involuting fetal vessels, have also been observed. Rarely, vascular maldevelopment is the causative substrate. However, in most cases the etiology is not clear.

The lesions may cavitate and result in porencephaly or even hydranencephaly. The larger cavitated lesions usually appear to relate to intrauterine insults, occurring well before the time of labor. Indeed, porencephaly within vascular distributions has been reproduced in the monkey by surgical occlusion of the internal carotid artery during the second trimester of pregnancy.[71]

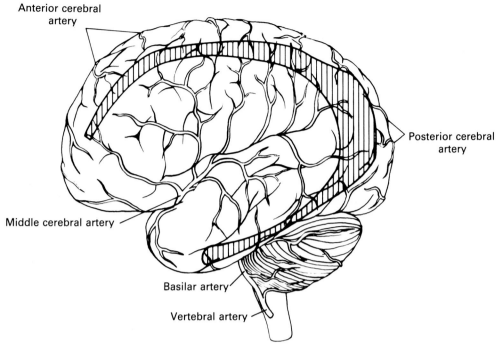

Anterior cerebral
artery

Posterior cerebral
artery

Middle cerebral artery

Basilar artery

Vertebral artery

FIG. 4-2. Schematic diagram—parasagittal cerebral injury. Major cerebral vessels are shown. Distribution of the lesion is indicated by line-marked areas.

FIG. 4-3. Coronal section of cerebrum—periventricular leukomalacia. Note white area of necrosis (*arrows*) just lateral to the external angle of the lateral ventricle.

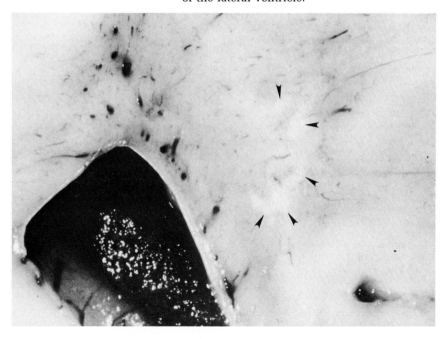

CLINICAL ASPECTS

The neurologic syndrome observed with neonatal hypoxic–ischemic encephalopathy occurs in association with clinical settings that have as a common feature deprivation of oxygen supply to brain. Serious hypoxemia is the result most commonly of (1) intrauterine asphyxia and the usual subsequent occurrence of respiratory failure at birth; (2) postnatal respiratory insufficiency, secondary to severe respiratory distress syndrome or recurrent apneic spells; and (3) severe right to left shunts, secondary to cardiac disease or persistent fetal circulation. Serious ischemia is the result most commonly of (1) intrauterine asphyxia with hypotension both *in utero* and at birth, (2) postnatal cardiac insufficiency secondary to severe congenital heart disease or recurrent apneic spells, and (3) postnatal cardiovascular collapse, secondary to sepsis, volume depletion, and so on.

Of these clinical settings, intrauterine asphyxia is the principal one in 90% of cases of neonatal hypoxic ischemic encephalopathy[82,83] Approximately one-half of these intrauterine cases have their onset prior to labor, and the other one-half during labor.

The major neonatal clinical features observed with hypoxic–ischemic encephalopathy are depicted below as a function of the time after a serious episode of intrauterine asphyxia.[1,82]

In the first 12 hours after birth the infant exhibits signs that we have attributed principally to bilateral cerebral hemispheral disturbance. Thus, there is deep stupor or coma, often with periodic breathing or respiratory irregularities akin to periodic breathing. Pupillary and oculomotor responses are intact, and distinct eye signs of brain stem disturbance are unusual at this time. When such signs are present, for example, fixed pupils or eyes not movable by doll's head maneuver or cold caloric stimulation, especially in the full-term infant, serious injury to brain stem is likely. There is minimal or no spontaneous or elicited movement, and the infant is usually markedly and diffusely hypotonic. Seizures occur in approximately 50% of infants within the first 12 hours after serious intrauterine asphyxia.

Over the latter one-half of the first day of life the infant's level of alertness may appear to improve slightly. However, the absence of other signs of higher level function makes it likely that this is apparent and not real improvement. Seizures become more frequent and severe, and overt status epilepticus is not unusual. This requires vigorous therapy (see below). Jitteriness occurs in approximately one-half of the infants, and apneic spells may be prominent in a similar proportion.[44] At this time weakness may be elicitable, particularly of proximal limbs (upper more than lower) in the full-term infant. This pattern relates to the parasagittal distribution of injury in such infants (see Fig. 4-1).

During the second and third days of life infants with severe insults will usually exhibit deep stupor or coma. Respiratory arrest may ensue and the brain stem oculomotor and pupillary abnormalities noted above become more common. Infants who are to die with hypoxic–ischemic encephalopathy usually do so at this time, especially if the criterion for death is so-called brain death. Premature infants who die with

Major Neonatal Clinical Features of Hypoxic—Ischemic Encephalopathy

Birth–12 Hours
  Deep stupor or coma
  Intact pupillary and oculomotor responses
  Hypotonia, minimal movement
  Seizures
12 Hours–24 Hours
  Apparent increase in level of alertness
  More seizures
  Jitteriness
  Weakness (proximal limbs—full-term)
24 Hours–72 Hours
  Deep stupor or coma
  Respiratory arrest
  Brainstem oculomotor disturbances
  Catastrophic deterioration (premature)
>72 Hours
  Persistent, though diminishing stupor
  Impaired sucking, swallowing, gag, tongue
    movements
  Hypotonia > hypertonia
  Weakness
    Proximal limbs—full-term
    Hemiparesis—full-term
    Lower limbs—premature

serious hypoxic–ischemic encephalopathy usually exhibit a catastrophic deterioration with major intraventricular hemorrhage (see next section).

Infants who survive past approximately day three usually show improvement in level of consciousness, although stupor persists to some degree, often for many days. Suck, swallow, gag, and tongue movements are impaired and feeding is consequently seriously disturbed. This disturbance relates to affection of neurons of cranial nerves 5, 7, 9, 10, and 12 (see selective neuronal necrosis above) and may require tube feeding for weeks. Hypotonia remains the dominant motor abnormality. Hypertonia of the spastic type does not become clearly apparent for months after the neonatal period. Patterns of weakness now become more commonly observable. In the full-term infant the proximal limb weakness of parasagittal cerebral injury may be prominent, or in infants with focal ischemic brain injury, hemiparesis may be recognized. In premature infants, weakness of lower limbs is more common and probably relates to periventricular leukomalacia.

DIAGNOSIS

Diagnostic procedures of value in establishing the presence, nature, and severity of neonatal hypoxic–ischemic encephalopathy include a careful history, neurologic examination, lumbar puncture, EEG, assessment of several metabolic parameters, technetium brain scan or CT scan and, in selected instances, other specific determinations. As with the evaluation of the infant with seizures, the history and neurologic examination form the cornerstones of the evaluation.

Careful historical questioning about maternal conditions associated with impaired placental function, for example, toxemia and diabetes, is important. Data obtained from electronic fetal monitoring should be elicited; particular attention should be paid to signs of fetal distress, such as late decelerations or loss of beat-to-beat variability of fetal heart rate, or passage of meconium. The duration of such signs prior

to "emergency" cesarean section is critical information, often difficult to determine precisely. Apgar scores provide useful data, especially if obtained for longer than just the first few minutes after delivery.

Careful assessment of the neonatal neurologic examination, as outlined in the previous section, provides critical insight into the severity and topography of injury. Specific neurologic features, for example, seizures, as well as the rapidity of neurologic improvement, also provide important diagnostic (and prognostic) information (see below).

Lumbar Puncture is a necessary component of the evaluation. Determinations of value include initial pressure, cell count, and protein and glucose contents. Preliminary data suggest a potential role for determinations of CSF lactate and lactate dehydrogenase levels.

Metabolic Parameters of interest include blood gases, glucose, calcium, and ammonia. Derangements of these parameters, secondary to the systemic consequences of asphyxia, may cause impressive neurologic abnormalities or exacerbate those caused by the original hypoxic–ischemic insult. Recent data suggest that hyperammonemia is a common and previously unrecognized cause of neurologic deterioration in infants with hypoxic–ischemic encephalopathy.[52]

The EEG exhibits a characteristic sequence of changes after hypoxic–ischemic insult.[76] The initial alteration is moderate voltage suppression and a decrease in frequency into the delta and theta ranges. Within a day a periodic pattern appears and, in the severe case, over the next day or so the ominous burst–suppression pattern may appear. The rate of recovery of EEG may be of prognostic value.

Technetium Brain Scan may demonstrate the site and severity of brain injury in neonatal hypoxic–ischemic encephalopathy.[73,81] Thus, on delayed images, selective neuronal necrosis may be accompanied by a diffuse increase in uptake of radionuclide, status marmoratus by uptake localized to basal ganglia and thalamus, parasagittal cerebral injury by uptake in superomedial cerebral convexities, especially in the posterior regions, periventricular leukomalacia by uptake in the periventricular regions, and focal and multifocal ischemic brain necrosis by uptake in regions within vascular distributions. More than one-half of infants with neonatal hypoxic–ischemic encephalopathy will exhibit an abnormal technetium brain scan.[73] The optimal time for obtaining the scan is 7 days to 10 days after the insult. In the majority of cases the abnormalities become much less obvious or disappear entirely after approximately 3 weeks to 4 weeks. Persistence of abnormality beyond this time is a poor prognostic sign.

CT Scan is useful especially in identification of complicating intracranial hemorrhage, particularly intraventricular hemorrhage in the premature infant, and of periventricular white matter injury. Focal and multifocal ischemic brain injury may also be recognized by CT scan several days or more after the responsible insult. We have found the technetium scan to be more valuable than the CT scan in the determination of parasagittal cerebral injury.

Other Neurodiagnostic Studies of value in the evaluation of the infant with neonatal hypoxic–ischemic encephalopathy include, particularly, the brain stem auditory evoked response. Initial data indicate abnormality in the cochlea as well as in the brain stem in affected infants.[51]

PROGNOSIS

Outcome of infants with hypoxic–ischemic encephalopathy will relate to a major degree to the severity of the insult(s). Because the most frequent severe insults occur *in utero*, assessment of severity has been particularly difficult, particularly with retrospective analysis. The advent of electronic fetal monitoring to assess the status of the fetus during labor may provide a better starting point for future systematic prospective studies of the outcome after perinatal hypoxic–ischemic insults. Initial data with relatively small numbers of patients suggest that this may be a fruitful approach.[74]

Useful overall prognostic data have been provided by several studies in the past decade, the most recently reported of which was derived from an analysis of over 38,000 consecutive deliveries in a single medical center between 1970 and 1975 (Table 4-4).[68,70] Asphyxiated infants were identified by a requirement for positive pressure ventilation of more than one minute prior to the onset of spontaneous respiration. That this requirement related to intrapartum asphyxia was presumed because of the absence of other causes of neonatal apnea, for example, maternal anesthesia or analgesia. The most notable findings included a sharp inverse relationship of mortality with gestational age. Thus, asphyxiated premature infants of less than 30 weeks' gestational age exhibited a mortality rate of 89% versus that of 19% for infants of more than 36

TABLE 4-4   Outcome in Neonatal Asphyxia* as a Function of Gestational Age

Gestational Age	Number of Infants	Outcome (%)		
		Normal	Major Sequelae	Dead
> 36 weeks	48	67	14	19
30 weeks–36 weeks	38	48	10	42
< 30 weeks	37	8	3	89

*Defined as requirement for positive pressure ventilation of > 1 minute prior to the onset of spontaneous respiration. (This requirement was presumed to be related to intrapartum asphyxia—see text.)
(Data adapted from Mulligan et al, 1980)

weeks' of gestational age. The incidence of neurologic sequelae among survivors varied little as a function of gestational age. Among the infants of more than 36 weeks' gestational age, who accounted for the largest numbers of survivors, approximately 17% exhibited neurologic sequelae.

Certain factors aid the clinician in the neonatal period in estimating prognosis. These include especially the occurrence of seizures as part of the neurologic syndrome and the rate of improvement of neurologic function. Thus, infants who exhibit seizures do less well than those who do not. In most series only approximately 50% of infants with hypoxic–ischemic encephalopathy with seizures are normal on follow-up. Those infants whose neurologic examination becomes normal by approximately 7 days of age have a good prognosis, and prolongation of neurologic deficits beyond 14 days of age is not likely to be followed by normal neurologic development.[50,76,77] Rates of improvement of the EEG and the technetium brain scan also have prognostic value, although more detailed data are needed to quantitate their roles.

NEUROLOGIC SEQUELAE AND CLINICOPATHOLIC CORRELATIONS

The long-term neurologic sequelae observed in infants with hypoxic–ischemic encephalopathy appear to relate clearly to the recognized neuropathology. The proven and probable neuropathologic correlations are displayed in Tables 4-5 through 4-9.

MANAGEMENT

Management of this devastating type of brain injury should begin with the question, "How could this have been prevented?" Prevention depends principally upon the prompt recognition of significant fetal hypoxia and ischemia, and upon immediate institution of appropriate intervention. Often the latter ultimately is a cesarean section. Management of the high risk pregnancy, labor, and delivery, a critical aspect of the management of neonatal hypoxic–ischemic encephalopathy, is an issue that is beyond the scope of this presentation.

TABLE 4-5 Selective Neuronal Necrosis: Long-Term Clinicopathologic Correlates

Distribution of Major Neuropathology	Neurologic Features
Cerebral cortex	Mental retardation
Thalamus	Seizure disorder
Cerebellar cortex	Spastic quadriparesis
Brain stem nuclei— inferior colliculi, cochlear nuclei, motor nuclei of cranial nerves	Ataxia Bulbar > psuedobulbar palsy
Reticular formation	Hyperactivity and impaired attention

Subsequent management of the infant who has sustained intrauterine asphyxia depends principally on diligent and vigorous supportive care. Particular attention must be paid to careful control of ventilation, perfusion, and metabolic homeostasis.

Maintenance of adequate ventilation is necessary to avoid the recurrence of hypoxemia or hypercapnia. Although hypoxemia may result obviously from overt hypoventilation or apnea, continuous transcutaneous oxygen monitoring indicates that these sick infants frequently exhibit serious hypoxemia with a variety of occurrences, for example, airway manipulations, crying, feeding procedures, and diagnostic procedures, not previously recognized to be associated with oxygen deprivation.[55,67] (Periodic sampling of arterial blood will miss these transient events.) The deleterious effects of such hypoxemia on an already compromised central nervous

TABLE 4-6 Status Marmoratus: Long-Term Clinicopathologic Correlates

Distribution of Major Neuropathology	Neurologic Features
Caudate, putamen, globus pallidus	Choreoathetosis, rigidity
Thalamus	Mental retardation
Cerebral cortex	Spastic quadriparesis

TABLE 4-7   Parasagittal Cerebral Injury: Long-Term Clinicopathologic Correlates

Distribution of Major Neuropathology	Neurologic Features
Cerebral cortex and subcortical white matter, superomedial (parasagittal) convexities, posterior > anterior cerebrum	Probable spastic quadriparesis, and hemiparesis Probable intellectual (questionable "perceptual") deficits

TABLE 4-8   Periventricular Leukomalacia: Long-Term Clinicopathologic Correlates

Distribution of Major Neuropathology	Neurologic Features
Periventricular white matter, including descending motor fibers, optic and acoustic radiations, and association fibers	Spastic diplegia Intellectual deficits

TABLE 4-9   Focal (and Multifocal) Ischemic Brain Necrosis: Long-Term Clinicopathologic Correlates

Distribution of Major Neuropathology	Neurologic Features
Cerebral cortex and subcortical white matter, in a vascular distribution, unilateral > bilateral, ± cavity formation	Spastic hemiparesis > quadriparesis Mental retardation Seizure disorders

system are obvious. Preliminary data obtained by transcutaneous CO_2 monitoring indicate a similarly high frequency of unexpected hypercapnia, heretofore undetected by periodic sampling of arterial blood.[53] The deleterious metabolic and vascular effects of hypercapnia were reviewed in the discussion of the biochemical and physiologic aspects of hypoxic–ischemic encephalopathy.

Maintenance of adequate perfusion is a major issue, particularly in view of the infant's impaired vascular autoregulation. Cerebral blood flow is exquisitely dependent on arterial blood pressure. Recent data indicate that myocardial failure is a frequent concomitant of perinatal asphyxia.[45,60] Vigorous therapy, including the use of inotropic agents, will cause rapid improvement in circulatory status in such infants and presumably prevent additional ischemic injury to brain.[45]

Metabolic parameters to be controlled carefully include particularly glucose, ammonia, and electrolytes. In part, these metabolites may be deranged because of concomitant asphyxial injury to liver and kidneys. Because of its prime importance in brain energy metabolism, glucose should be provided so as to avoid hypoglycemia. Controversy exists about a beneficial or deleterious role for supranormal levels of blood glucose in the infant with hypoxic–ischemic encephalopathy.[1] We recommend the administration of glucose supplements to maintain blood glucose between 75 and 100 mg/dl.

Seizures may result in brain injury (see previous section on neonatal seizures) and should be treated vigorously. We use phenobarbital in the doses discussed in the section on neonatal seizures. In fact, we administer anticonvulsant doses of phenobarbital to all full-term infants with neonatal hypoxic–ischemic encephalopathy even prior to the onset of seizures. Phenobarbital is discontinued after seven days to ten days if no seizures occur. The rationale for this approach relates to our clinical impression that the use of phenobarbital before the onset of clinical seizures reduces the likelihood of subsequent uncontrolled seizures and because of the experimental data suggesting a beneficial role of barbiturates (albeit at higher doses) in hypoxic–ischemic encephalopathy.[1]

Brain swelling, which may occur in full-term infants with serious tissue injury, should be contained by avoidance of fluid overload. This is particularly important in asphyxiated infants because of the frequent concomitant occurrence of inappropriate ADH secretion.[57] A role for more vigorous therapy, for example, glucocorticoids or hypertonic solutions such as mannitol, has not been established by systematic or controlled investigations.

INTRACRANIAL HEMORRHAGE

Intracranial hemorrhage is an important problem in neonatal neurology because of its high frequency of occurrence and the severity of many of the lesions. There are four major varieties of neonatal intracranial hemorrhage namely, subdural hemorrhage, primary subarachnoid hemorrhage, intracerebellar hemorrhage, and periventricular–intraventricular hemorrhage.[1,136,137,138,139] Subdural hemorrhage is usually a serious lesion but is uncommon. Primary subarachnoid hemorrhage is usually a benign lesion and is quite common. Intracerebellar hemorrhage is usually a serious lesion but its incidence is not entirely known. Periventricular–intraventricular hemorrhage is of the greatest importance because it is both a serious and a very common lesion.

In the following discussion we review briefly the problems of subdural hemorrhage, primary subarachnoid hemorrhage, and intracerebellar hemorrhage. Periventricular–intraventricular hemorrhage is discussed in more detail because of its preeminence among the major types of neonatal intracranial hemorrhage.

SUBDURAL HEMORRHAGE

Subdural hemorrhage, formerly a very frequent lesion, is now uncommon principally because of improvements in obstetric practice. Recognition of subdural hemorrhage is important because therapeutic intervention can be lifesaving.

Neuropathology

When considered in the context of the anatomy of the major veins and sinuses the neuropathology of subdural hemorrhage is readily understood (Fig. 4-4). There are four major varieties: (1) tentorial laceration with rupture of the sagittal sinus, transverse sinus, vein of Galen, or smaller infratentorial veins; (2) occipital osteodiastasis with rupture of the occipital sinus; (3) falx laceration with rupture of the inferior sagittal sinus; and (4) rupture of superficial bridging cerebral veins.

Tentorial laceration is usually associated with major infratentorial hemorrhage and an acute fatal evolution with brain stem compression.[91,102,104] Smaller lesions with subacute evolution have been described more recently.[90]

Occipital osteodiastasis, that is, traumatic separation of the cartilaginous junction between the squamous and lateral portions of the occipital bone, may result in posterior fossa subdural hemorrhage.[106,117,146] Laceration of cerebellum may be associated.

Falx laceration results in a subdural hematoma located between the cerebral hemispheres. Evolution of this now rare lesion is usually rapid.

Cerebral convexity subdural hematoma results from rupture of superficial cerebral bridging veins. This, the most common variety of subdural hemorrhage in the newborn, is commonly unilateral, in contrast to convexity subdural hematoma later in infancy.

Pathogenesis

Pathogenetic factors relevant to subdural hemorrhage are principally traumatic in nature and, in general, lead to excessive or unusual deformations of skull with resulting rupture of the dural veins described in the previous section.[1] These factors are considered best with respect to those aspects relative to the mother, the infant, the labor, and the delivery. Thus, subdural hemorrhage is most likely to occur in the primiparous or older multiparous mother, with a relatively rigid birth canal, or in a mother with a small birth canal. Factors relevant to the infant include large size or prematurity, the latter because of the particularly compliant, readily deformed skull. Subdural hemorrhage is most likely to occur in labors that are unusually brief, not allowing the fetal head to adapt to the birth canal, or unusually prolonged, subjecting the head to excessive stresses. Factors relative to the delivery include situations in which the infant's head is not adapted to the birth canal, for example, breech extractions or foot presentations, or is subjected

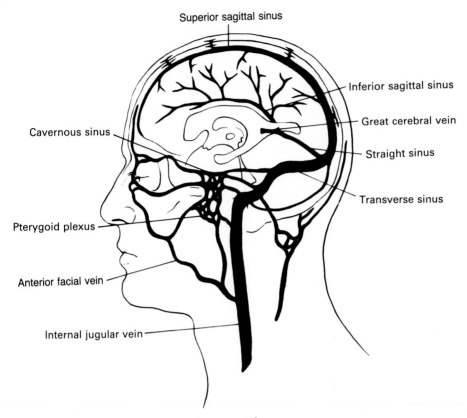

Superior sagittal sinus

Inferior sagittal sinus

Great cerebral vein

Cavernous sinus

Straight sinus

Transverse sinus

Pterygoid plexus

Anterior facial vein

Internal jugular vein

FIG. 4-4. Schematic diagram—major cranial veins and dural sinuses.

to unusual stresses, such as face or brow presentations, difficult forceps extractions, or difficult rotational maneuvers.

Clinical Aspects

Tentorial laceration with major infratentorial hematoma is characterized by neurologic features referable to upper brain stem compression. An additional helpful clinical feature, when present, is retrocollis or opisthotonus.[142] Evolution is usually measured in hours and diagnosis has been made almost exclusively at postmortem examination. Smaller lesions with an evolution over many hours to days have been described and raise the possibility of surgical intervention and salvage of affected infants.[90]

Occipital diastasis with posterior fossa subdural hemorrhage or cerebellar hemorrhage is characterized by rapid neurologic deterioration with signs referable to med-

ullary compression.[117,146] Diagnosis premortem has not been reported.

Falx laceration would be expected to present with bilateral cerebral signs, but no clear clinical descriptions are available. Diagnosis has been made at postmortem examination.

Cerebral convexity subdural hematoma, the most common of the four varieties, is characterized by three major clinical syndromes. The first is a lack of or minimal signs associated with a small lesion. The second is a focal cerebral syndrome with hemiparesis, focal seizures often leading to homolateral pupillary dilation and other signs of transtentorial herniation.[85,91,92,128,140] A third syndrome, still to be defined clearly, is the occurrence of chronic subdural effusion after undetected neonatal subdural hemorrhage.

Diagnosis

Diagnosis of neonatal subdural hemorrhage depends on a high index of suspicion, careful analysis of clinical signs, and demonstration by a definitive imaging technique, especially CT scan. Subdural tap may be useful in the diagnosis of convexity subdural hematoma, although CT scan is safer and preferable. Skull x-ray films will identify occipital osteodiastasis.

Prognosis

As indicated in the section on clinical features, the rapidity of evolution of major subdural hemorrhage secondary to tentorial laceration, occipital osteodiastasis, and falx laceration has been associated with fatal outcome in most cases. The possibility of improving outcome with early recognition of subacute tentorial laceration is real, especially with the advent of CT scanning for early diagnosis.

The prognosis with convexity subdural hematoma is relatively good. From 50% to 80% of infants are well on follow-up. The remainder are left with focal cerebral signs and occasionally hydrocephalus.

Management

The feasibility of early diagnosis by CT scan raises the possibility of surgical intervention for serious subdural hemorrhage secondary to tentorial laceration, occipital osteodiastasis, or falx laceration. Recent experience with surgical evacuation of posterior fossa subdural hemorrhage in the term newborn is encouraging.[123]

Cerebral convexity subdural hemorrhage is dealt with by surgical evacuation if the lesion is life-threatening. In stable infants serial subdural taps are recommended for two major indications: (1) to ameliorate signs of increased intracranial pressure, or (2) prevent the development of cranial cerebral disproportion.

PRIMARY SUBARACHNOID HEMORRHAGE

Primary subarachnoid hemorrhage refers to hemorrhage within the subarachnoid space that is not secondary to extension from subdural, intracerebellar, or intraventricular hemorrhage. The lesion is relatively common but usually not of major clinical importance. In a consecutive series of 76 newborn infants weighing less than 2000 g at birth who exhibited bloody cerebrospinal fluid in the first 3 days of life, 29% exhibited primary subarachnoid hemorrhage by CT scan.[112]

Neuropathology

The hemorrhage is located over the cerebral convexities and in the posterior fossa and is usually not of major proportions. The bleeding is venous in origin and, therefore unlike the dramatic arterial subarachnoid hemorrhage observed in older infants and children with arteriovenous malformations or aneurysms.

Pathogenesis

The pathogenesis of primary subarachnoid hemorrhage appears under certain conditions to be related principally to trauma, as described above for subdural hemorrhage. Under other circumstances the hemorrhage appears to be related to the alterations in cerebral blood flow and other factors associated with asphyxia and related events, as described below for periventricular–intraventricular hemorrhage.

Clinical Features

Clinical features associated with primary subarachnoid hemorrhage can be categorized into three major syndromes. First, and by far the most common, there are minimal or no clinical signs. Second, seizures may occur, especially on the second or third postnatal day.[125,136] In the interictal period the infant, usually a full-term one, often appears quite well. A related syndrome in premature infants may be the occurrence of recurrent apneic spells, which may or may not be the manifestation of seizure. Third, and least commonly, major hemorrhage may occur with a catastrophic neurologic deterioration, similar to that observed with major intraventricular hemorrhage (see below).

Diagnosis

Identification of primary subarachnoid hemorrhage is based on the finding of bloody cerebrospinal fluid and the demonstration by CT scan of blood in the subarachnoid space, observable most readily in the superior longitudinal fissure in the posterior portion of the cranium. Exclusion of the other major causes of neonatal intracranial hemorrhage, for example, subdural, intracerebellar, and periventricular–intraventricular hemorrhage, is necessary. In addition, certain rare causes for bleeding into the subarachnoid space in newborns should be considered, for example, arteriovenous malformation, aneurysm, hemorrhagic infarction (secondary to embolus or venous thrombosis), congenital tumor, or coagulation disturbance, such as thrombocytopenia or disseminated intravascular coagulation.[87,96,110,122,126,130]

Prognosis

The outlook for infants with primary subarachnoid hemorrhage is very good. If there are minimal or no neonatal neurologic signs, the prognosis is uniformly favorable. If neonatal seizures occur, approximately 90% of infants are well on follow-up. In the rare example of catastrophic deterioration, the infant either dies or is left with hydrocephalus or other serious neurologic residua.[133]

Management

Management is essentially that of posthemorrhagic hydrocephalus, as described below in the section on periventricular–intraventricular hemorrhage.

INTRACEREBELLAR HEMORRHAGE

Intracerebellar hemorrhage has been reported to be a relatively frequent lesion at postmortem examination of small premature infants. Thus, 15% to 25% of infants of less than 1500 g body weight or 32 weeks of gestation have been said to exhibit major intracerebellar hemorrhage.[103,113,118,131] The precise frequency in populations that include infants who survive is less clear. Thus, we have not observed a single case in over 150 cases of intracranial hemorrhage proven by computed tomography (CT) in small premature infants. The reason for such discrepancies between autopsied and living populations is unclear, and further definition of the recognition and clinical significance of intracerebellar hemorrhage in the small premature infant is needed.

Neuropathology

There are four major varieties of neonatal intracranial hemorrhage that may involve the cerebellum. These include: (1) traumatic laceration of cerebellum or rupture of major infratentorial veins or the occipital sinus, often with occipital osteodiastasis, (2) venous (hemorrhagic) infarction of cerebellum, (3) primary intracerebellar hemorrhage, and (4) extension into cerebellum of intraventricular or subarachnoid blood. The latter two varieties account for most of the recognized examples of "intracerebellar" hemorrhage in the small premature infant. The proportion of lesions that arise within the cerebellum versus those that arise from extension of blood into the cerebellum from the intraventricular or subarachnoid space is unclear, although in one report the latter mechanism was thought to account for approximately one-half of cases.[93]

Pathogenesis

The pathogenesis of intracerebellar hemorrhage in the small premature infant remains to be elucidated. The increase in frequency of the lesion with decreasing gestational age and with increasing duration of survival suggests that factors referable to the premature infant and to certain postnatal events are critical.

The relation of the hemorrhage to prematurity probably relates in part to the immaturity of the capillary bed in the rapidly developing cerebellum.[117] Such capillaries might be considered vulnerable to rupture. A second factor may relate to the extreme compliance of the premature skull. Deformations of the occiput have been considered important in the genesis of at least some of the cerebellar hemorrhages; such deformations can be produced by application of bands across the head (e.g., for holding face masks or other apparatus) or by such simple procedures as fixation of the head for various therapeutic or nursing procedures. A third factor relevant to the premature infant is the presence of germinal matrices in both the subependymal and subpial locations in the developing cerebellum. These regions may provide poor support for the small vessels residing within.

The relation to certain postnatal events,

especially asphyxial events, probably includes several factors referable to cerebral blood flow and the regulation thereof, as described in more detail below for periventricular–intraventricular hemorrhage.

Clinical Features

Little precise clinical information is available relative to intracerebellar hemorrhage of the small premature infant because the lesions has been recognized at postmortem examination only. Apnea and bradycardia and a catastrophic neurologic deterioration have been common and probably relate to brain stem compression by the hematoma. More detailed data on ocular and other cranial nerve functions are lacking.

Diagnosis

Intracerebellar hemorrhage has been identified in the full-term infant by CT scan.[124] Thus, with the small premature infant, particularly in the presence of any signs referable to the posterior fossa, intracerebellar hemorrhage should be a serious consideration and a CT scan obtained promptly. Whether there is danger from lumbar puncture with respect to cerebellar tonsillar herniation is not known, but we would consider the procedure ill-advised if intracerebellar hematoma is a serious consideration on clinical grounds.

Prognosis

Assessment of prognosis is not possible because all of the lesions in small premature infants have been observed at postmortem examination. Hydrocephalus has been reported as a sequel of intracerebellar hemorrhage in the full-term infant.[115,129]

Management

Management begins with a high index of clinical suspicion and prompt diagnosis by CT scan. Surgical intervention has been lifesaving in the full-term infant, although recovery without surgery has also been reported.[100] Careful clinical assessment with surgical evacuation at the early signs of deterioration would appear to be the best approach.

PERIVENTRICULAR–INTRAVENTRICULAR HEMORRHAGE

Periventricular–intraventricular hemorrhage is the most important variety of neonatal intracranial hemorrhage. This relates in part to its very high frequency of occurrence and in part to the serious neurologic morbidity that may result from the lesion. The enormous importance of this hemorrhage is linked in many ways to the advent of modern neonatal intensive care and, as a consequence, to the marked increase in survival rates for small premature infants. Because periventricular–intraventricular hemorrhage is characteristic of such infants, the lesion is the dominant neurologic disorder in most neonatal intensive care facilities.

The incidence of periventricular–intraventricular hemorrhage in modern neonatal intensive care facilities in infants of less than 1500 g body weight or 35 weeks of gestation is approximately 40% to 45%. These data are derived from two studies of a total of 237 infants subjected to routine CT scan in the first week of life.[86,119] Most examples of periventricular–intraventricular hemorrhage are observed in infants less than 32 weeks of gestation.

In the following discussion we review the neuropathology, pathogenesis, clinical features, diagnosis, prognosis, and management of periventricular–intraventricular hemorrhage and its complications. Of the latter, particular emphasis is placed on posthemorrhagic hydrocephalus.

Neuropathology

Periventricular–intraventricular hemorrhage emanates from small vessels, principally capillaries, in the subependymal germinal matrix.[105] In most infants the hemorrhage originates in the matrix at the level of the head of the caudate nucleus and foramen of Monro.[148] However, in particularly immature infants, for example, those less than 28 weeks of gestation, the lesion often originates at the level of the body of the caudate nucleus and in mature infants often from the choroid plexus.[117] Approximately 80% of cases of periventricular hemorrhage rupture through the ependyma and fill the ventricular system (Fig. 4-5).

Blood tends to collect in the posterior fossa and this may subsequently result in an obliterative arachnoiditis. In particularly severe lesions periventricular hemorrhage extends into the cerebral parenchyma, and such lesions are often followed by the development of a porencephalic cyst. Also, with severe lesions acute hydrocephalus may result.

Pathogenesis

The pathogenesis of periventricular–intraventricular hemorrhage relates to several factors concerned with the distribution and regulation of cerebral blood flow, intravascular pressure, vascular integrity, and the extravascular environment (see list below).

Major Pathogenetic Factors for Periventricular—Intraventricular Hemorrhage

A. Intravascular Factors: Distribution and Regulation of Cerebral Blood Flow (CBF); Intravascular Pressure
  1. Distribution of CBF to periventricular region
  2. Rate of CBF
  3. Autoregulation of CBF
  4. Arterial pressure
  5. Venous pressure

B. Vascular (Endothelial) Factors
  1. Intrinsic capillary integrity
  2. Endothelial cell injury

C. Extravascular Factors
  1. Subependymal germinal matrix
  2. Periventricular fibrinolytic activity

These several factors combine in the premature infant, particularly the infant subjected to an asphyxial insult, to result in periventricular–intraventricular hemorrhage.

Intravascular Factors of importance relate first to the distribution of cerebral blood flow to the periventricular region. Thus, prior to approximately 32 weeks to 34 weeks of gestation the relative prominence of the vascular supply to the subependymal germinal matrix and the deep regions of cerebrum versus the relatively undifferentiated

FIG. 4-5. Coronal section of cerebrum—periventricular-intraventricular hemorrhage. Note blood in both lateral ventricles. Hemorrhage into the germinal matrix is apparent on the right over the head of the caudate nucleus. Probe is in the foramen of Monro.

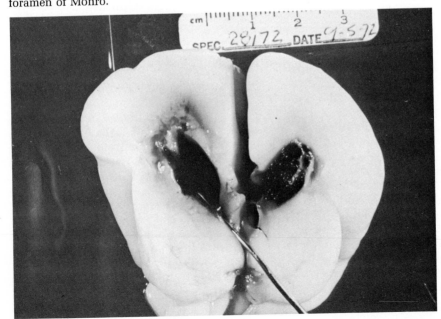

cerebral cortex suggests that a disproportionate amount of total cerebral blood flow enters the periventricular circulation.[117] Therefore, any factors causing an increase in cerebral blood flow in the small premature infant will tend to overperfuse preferentially the periventricular region. Such factors include asphyxial insults (because of hypercapnia and other factors discussed in the preceding section on hypoxic–ischemic encephalopathy) or rapid infusion of blood, colloid, or hypertonic solutions. Moreover, because autoregulation of cerebral blood flow is impaired in such infants (see preceding section on hypoxic–ischemic encephalopathy), blood flow to the periventricular region will be exquisitely sensitive to changes in arterial blood pressure. Elevations of arterial blood pressure or cerebral blood flow, in fact, have been observed in the first minutes after delivery, with motor activity (spontaneous or associated with handling), apneic spells, seizures, and asphyxia.[111] Experimental and clinical observations suggest an important pathogenetic role for raised or fluctuating blood pressure in periventricular–intraventricular hemorrhage.[97,99] Finally, elevations of pressure within the periventricular capillary bed may result from or be exacerbated by elevations in venous pressure. The latter may occur in the infant with myocardial failure secondary to perinatal asphyxia (see preceding section on hypoxic–ischemic encephalopathy). Additionally, elevated venous pressure may be more likely to occur in the periventricular region at the most vulnerable site for the occurrence of hemorrhage, that is, at the level of the foramen of Monro and the head of the caudate nucleus. This suggestion is based on the distinctive venous anatomy in this region, which is characterized by a U-turn in the direction of venous flow as the internal cerebral veins are formed from the confluence of the terminal, thalamostriate, and choroidal veins.

Vascular Factors of importance include the intrinsic integrity of the periventricular capillaries. Anatomic observations indicate that this is a relatively immature capillary bed and thus may be vulnerable to rupture.[117] Moreover, the metabolic activity of brain capillary endothelial cells suggests that these cells are dependent on oxidative metabolism and might be readily injured by hypoxic insult, so often found in the clinical background of periventricular–intraventricular hemorrhage.[116]

Extravascular factors of importance include the fact that the periventricular region is the site of the subependymal germinal matrix, a gelatinous region that provides very poor support for the small vessels that course through it. This matrix does not dissipate in the human until term; thus, again, the premature infant is especially vulnerable. Finally, the periventricular region of the human premature brain has been shown to contain an excessive amount of fibrinolytic activity, the source of which is not clear.[98,132] This factor may explain why a capillary hemorrhage may enlarge into a massive lesion that extends into the ventricles or the cerebral parenchyma.

Clinical Features

The clinical accompaniments of periventricular–intraventricular hemorrhage vary from a dramatic neurologic deterioration to an extremely subtle, perhaps even silent, presentation. Onset is recognized most commonly to be the second postnatal day. Indeed, in one large series in which intraventricular hemorrhage was timed by the use of chromium-50 labeled red blood cells, the median age of onset was 38 hours.[134] In more recent studies of living populations using serial ultrasonography, hemorrhage has been defined most frequently in the first day of life.[88]

Two basic clinical syndromes accompany the hemorrhage. The first is a catastrophic deterioration that usually occurs in the infant that does not survive the hemorrhage. The second is a more saltatory deterioration that usually occurs in the infant that does survive the hemorrhage.[135,136] The catastrophic deterioration is more common with major intraventricular hemorrhage, whereas the saltatory deterioration is more common with small lesions. Nevertheless, there is considerable overlap between these two clinical syndromes with respect to size of hemorrhage and likelihood for survival.

The catastrophic syndrome, dramatic in presentation, is characterized by evolution in minutes to hours of deep stupor or coma, respiratory abnormalities, "decerebrate" posturing, generalized tonic seizure, pupils fixed to light, eyes fixed to vestibular stimulation, and flaccid quadriparesis. The clinical distinction between tonic seizure and decerebrate posturing is very difficult in this setting; clinically overt seizures occur in the minority of patients. This neurologic syndrome may be accompanied by a falling hematocrit, bulging anterior fontanel, hypotension, bradycardia, temperature derangements, and abnormalities of glucose and water homeostasis.

The saltatory syndrome, more subtle in presentation, is characterized by a stuttering evolution over many hours to days. the most common presenting signs are an alteration in level of consciousness, a change in the quality and quantity of motility, hypotonia, and subtle aberrations of eye position, (e.g., skew deviation) and eye movement (e.g., vertical deviation of eyes, usually down). Respiratory disturbances may be additional concomitants.

The subtle phenomena of the saltatory syndrome are readily overlooked in many cases. Indeed, it can be argued effectively that clinically silent intraventricular hemorrhage may occur. Thus, in a prospective study of premature infants routinely subjected to CT scan in the first week of life, only approximately 50% of examples of periventricular–intraventricular hemorrhage were correctly predicted to have the lesion on the basis of clinical criteria.[109] The most reliable sign was an unexplained fall in hematocrit or a failure of hematocrit to rise after transfusion.

Diagnosis

Diagnosis must begin with recognition of the clinical setting, and in view of the high incidence of small premature infants in neonatal intensive care facilities, we believe that all such infants should be considered at high risk for the lesion. The most useful screening procedure in our hands in the past has been lumbar puncture. The presence of the cerebrospinal fluid (CSF) profile of hemorrhage, that is, an elevated number of red blood cells, elevated protein content, and xanthochromia (and later depressed glucose content), is an indication for a definite brain imaging procedure, for example, CT scan or ultrasonar scan. In a consecutive series of 76 infants (weighing less than 2000 g at birth) who had had a CT scan following the finding of the CSF profile of hemorrhage in the first three days of life, only six (8%) had a negative scan and fully 48 (63%) had periventricular–intraventricular hemorrhage (the remaining 22 [29%] had subarachnoid hemorrhage).[112]

CT Scan is the most definitive means of establishing the diagnosis of periventricular–intraventricular hemorrhage. The site and extent of the lesion are demonstrated very effectively (Figs. 4-6, 4-7). In addition, the size of ventricles, pattern of ventricular dilation, and presence of major white matter lesions (e.g., periventricular leukomalacia) may also be defined. However, despite the value of the CT scan, the procedure requires transport of an infant who is often in a precarious state with respect to maintenance of ventilation, perfusion, temperature, and metabolic status. Moreover, the long-term effects of the radiation exposure from multiple studies on brain, lens, and so on remain unknown.

Ultrasonic Scanning with modern, real-time, gray scale instrumentation has proven to be a highly useful, effective means of identifying periventricular–intraventricular hemorrhage in the premature infant (Fig. 4-8). Sector scanners with the transducer applied to the skin over the anterior fontanel provide excellent coronal and sagittal views. Transducers, particularly of the linear array type, applied to the side of the infant's thin skull, provide horizontal views, comparable to conventional CT scans. Ultrasonography also provides excellent data on the degree and distribution of ventricular dilation. The major advantages of ultrasonography are portability of instrumentation and apparent safety of the pulsed ultrasonic waves.

Prognosis

Prognosis of periventricular–intraventricular hemorrhage is considered best in relation to the short-term and long-term outlooks. Although all factors of importance in determining outcome are not clearly under-

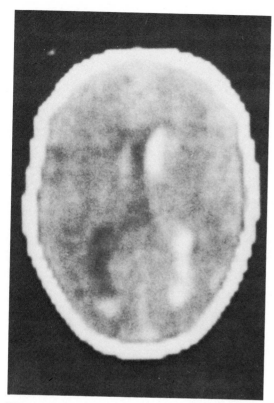

FIG. 4-6. CT scan—periventricular-intraventricular hemorrhage. Note blood in the subependymal regions over the heads of the caudate nuclei bilaterally and in the occipital horns of the lateral ventricles, especially on the right.

stood, there is a distinct relation between the severity of the hemorrhage and the prognosis.

The Short-Term Outcome of CT-proven periventricular–intraventricular hemorrhage is depicted in Table 4-10 with respect to the incidence of death and post-hemorrhagic progressive ventricular dilation in survivors.[1,86,107,112,119] These data indicate that with small lesions survival is the rule, and progressive ventricular dilation, rare. With moderate lesions, mortality rates are low, that is, approximately 10%, and the incidence of post-hemorrhagic progressive ventricular dilation also relatively low, approximately 20%. With severe lesions, the immediate outcome is unfavorable. The majority of affected infants die and most of the survivors develop progressive ventricular dilation.

Long-term Outcome depends upon a number of factors, most of which correlate with the severity of the original hemorrhage. Initial data with follow-up to 12 months to 36 months indicate a direct relation of outcome to the severity of hemorrhage.[108,121] Severe motor and intellectual deficits have been the rule in infants with marked hemorrhages and are rare in those with mild lesions. Longer follow-up data are needed.

The prognosis of periventricular–intraventricular hemorrhage relates directly to the mechanisms of brain injury as a sequel to the lesion. Currently recognized mechanisms include: (1) the hypoxic–ischemic insults that often precede the hemorrhage; (2) the marked increase in intracranial pressure and concomitant def-

FIG. 4-7. CT scan—periventricular-intraventricular hemorrhage. Note blood in the frontal horns contiguous with blood in the third ventricle. Hemorrhage is also prominent in both occipital horns.

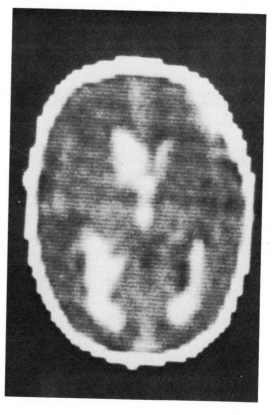

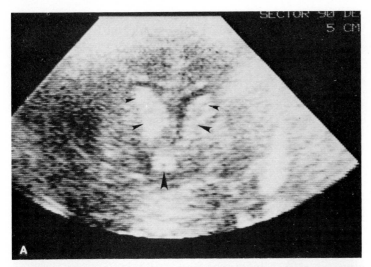

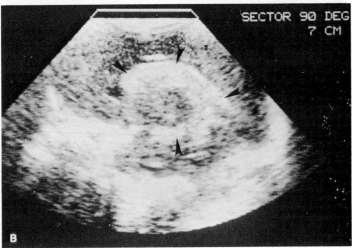

FIG. 4-8. Sonar scans—periventricular-intraventricular hemorrhage. *A.* Coronal view—note echogenic material, that is, blood, in lateral ventricles (*small arrowheads*) and third ventricle (*large arrowhead*). *B.* Sagittal view, same case—note blood in lateral ventricle, that is, frontal horn, body, occipital, and temporal horns (*arrowheads*).

icits in cerebral perfusion that occur at the time of the hemorrhage; (3) the destruction of periventricular white matter by the hematoma; (4) the destruction of germinal matrix with its glial precursors by the hematoma; (5) focal brain ischemia, perhaps secondary to vasospasm; and (6) the post-hemorrhagic hydrocephalus. The precise importance of each of these factors, of course, will vary depending upon the severity and locus of the hemorrhage.

Post-hemorrhagic Hydrocephalus

Hydrocephalus is a frequent sequel to periventricular–intraventricular hemorrhage, especially larger lesions. This complication is the most common treatable cause of neurologic morbidity. The impairment of CSF dynamics is caused usually by an obliterative arachnoiditis in the posterior fossa that either blocks the outflow of CSF from the fourth ventricle or the flow of CSF through the posterior fossa to the supratentorial space for reabsorption. A less common site of obstruction is at the aqueduct of Sylvius.

Temporal Features of the post-hemorrhagic ventricular dilation are distinctive and important to recognize.[1,136] Thus, although ventricular dilation may begin es-

TABLE 4-10   Short-Term Outcome of Periventricular–Intraventricular Hemorrhage as a Function of Severity of Hemorrhage*

Severity of Hemorrhage	Deaths (% of total)†	Progressive Ventricular Dilation (% of survivors)†
Mild	0	0–10%
Moderate	5%–15%	15%–25%
Severe	50%–65%	65%–100%

*Based on approximately 200 cases; nearly one-half were evaluated at St Louis Children's Hospital, and the remainder, at Emory University, University of New Mexico, and the Massachusetts General Hospital (see text for references).

†Values are ranges that encompass 75%–100% of cases.

sentially with the hemorrhage, especially with marked lesions, more often the process develops one week to three weeks after the hemorrhage. Most important, the traditional clinical criteria of evolving hydrocephalus, that is, rapidly enlarging head, full anterior fontanel, and separated cranial sutures, do not appear for days to weeks after ventricular dilation has already been present.[141] The reaons for the occurrence of impressive ventricular dilation prior to the development of rapid head growth must relate to the developmental state of the cerebrum in the human premature infant. The two most relevant features are: (1) the paucity of cerebral myelin and (2) the relative excess of water in the centrum semiovale. In experimental and human hydrocephalus the cerebral white matter is encroached upon and the central gray structures relatively spared. The paucity of myelin and the relative excess of water in the cerebral white matter of the human premature infant would serve to accentuate this general feature of hydrocephalus. This notion is supported by the disproportionate dilation of the occipital versus the frontal horns that is characteristic of infantile post-hemorrhagic hydrocephalus. A third contributory factor for the occurrence of ventricular dilation before rapid head growth is the relatively large subarachnoid space in the cranium of the premature infant.[117]

An important and still unanswered question is whether the "silent" ventricular dilation described above might be injurious to the developing brain. Experimental and clinical observations suggest that ventricular dilation per se may cause brain injury, but more data are needed.[94,114,127,143,144,145,147]

In view of the disproportionate involvement of occipital horns, careful assessment of higher visual function by clinical neurophysiologic (e.g., visual evoked responses) or more sophisticated techniques (e.g., positron emission tomographic determinations of blood flow and energy metabolism in occipital lobes) might be especially useful.

Management—Prevention

As with other neonatal neurological disorders, the primary goal in the management of periventricular–intraventricular hemorrhage is prevention. Consideration of the pathogenetic factors listed earlier indicates certain directions that may prove to be fruitful to accomplish prevention.

Those pathogenetic factors referable to the periventricular vascular anatomy and to the presence of the subependymal germinal matrix can be eliminated most decisively by prevention of premature birth. That complex topic is beyond the scope of this presentation.

Because periventricular–intraventricular hemorrhage in full form evolves after the first hours of life, it is reasonable to suspect that postnatal events are critical in pathogenesis. Many of these events should be susceptible to modification. Particular importance can be attributed to factors that alter periventricular intravascular pressure by effects principally on arterial pressure and flow, or perhaps less commonly, on venous pressure. Critical assessments of the relationship of occurrence of intraventricular hemorrhage to the management of the premature infant are needed with respect to such sophisticated aspects as the means of supporting ventilation and perfusion, as well as to some seemingly mundane aspects such as the amount of handling of the infant.

Acute Management

When faced with the infant who has experienced a periventricular-intraventricular hemorrhage, the physician must answer the critical initial question, should the infant be treated at all. Both clinical and CT data are important in making this determination. Those infants with a catastrophic clinical deterioration and severe intraventricular and intracerebral extension of hemorrhage on CT scan have a very poor outlook. In such cases we are dealing with an ethical issue that deserves detailed consideration in its own right.

If the infant is to be treated, the most important immediate task is to maintain cerebral perfusion. This requires maintenance of blood pressure, but because of impaired autoregulation this must be done cautiously. Lowering of intracranial pressure, for example, by ventriculostomy or lumbar puncture, may be indicated. Cerebral overperfusion may lead to extension of hemorrhage or provocation of new hemorrhage. Thus, factors causing abrupt increases in cerebral blood flow must be avoided; such factors include hypercapnia, hypoxemia, acidemia, rapid infusion of colloid, blood, or hypertonic solutions.

Ventricular size should be monitored by serial assessment with CT or ultrasonography. The latter is preferable. The aim is to detect ventricular dilation prior to overt clinical signs of increased intracranial pressure. Once detected, progressive ventricular dilation raises its own issues about management.

Management of Post-Hemorrhagic Ventricular Dilation

The therapeutic approach to the infant with post-hemorrhagic ventricular dilation is not yet based on decisive data. Several important questions remained unanswered. First, how often does such dilation resolve without therapy? Second, does transient or brief ventricular dilation cause any irreversible injury to developing brain? Third, do non-surgical modalities have any significant effect on the ventricular dilation? Research is under way in several centers, including our own, to provide information relative to these issues, but, obviously, design of such research is difficult.

The two basic approaches to the infant with post-hemorrhagic ventricular dilation depend upon the rate of progression of the ventricular dilation, its severity, and the intracranial pressure. In a general and somewhat oversimplified way infants can be divided into two categories, that is, first, those with slowly progressive dilation of ventricles that are slightly to moderately increased in size, and second, those with rapidly progressive dilation of ventricles that are moderately to severely increased in size. Evolution in the former group is usually measured in many days to weeks and intracranial pressure is usually normal, that is, approximately 100 mm of water. Rate of head growth is usually not excessive. Evolution in the latter group is measured over a few days and intracranial pressure is usually elevated. Also, the rate of head growth is usually excessive.

For infants with slowly progressive ventricular dilation, careful surveillance may be appropriate therapy (see below) because a significant though not clearly defined proportion will resolve spontaneously over weeks. Therapeutic maneuvers that have been considered beneficial include serial lumbar punctures or the administration of drugs that decrease CSF production, for example, carbonic anhydrase inhibitors such as acetazolamide and furosemide, or of osmotic agents, such as glycerol.[89,101,102,136] However, as of this writing no controlled studies of these measures have been reported. Currently we are evaluating these modalities in a controlled fashion. Compressive head-wrapping also has been advocated for the management of infantile hydrocephalus (see below).[95] We have had no experience with this approach and consider small premature infants with thin, fragile skin and easily deformed skulls poor candidates for such a therapeutic modality.

For infants with rapidly progressive ventricular dilation, prompt decompression is important to prevent brain injury. In infants who are not candidates for placement of ventriculoperitoneal shunt we have used external ventriculostomy. The catheter is left in place for approximately 5 days before removal (ventriculostomy in place for time periods in excess of approximately 7 days carries a rapidly increasing risk of infection). This usually serves as an effective temporizing procedure. Intracranial pressure and ventricular size decrease during the time the ventriculostomy is in place, and in a small minority of infants progression may not recur after removal of the ventriculostomy. However, most commonly, progression does begin again and either a second ventriculostomy may be inserted on the other side, or if the infant can tolerate the procedure, a ventriculoperitoneal shunt should be placed. The latter is probably the best initial step in an infant with rapidly progressive ventricular dilation who is of adequate size and otherwise well enough to be considered a suitable candidate for shunt placement.

Management of post-hemorrhagic ventricular dilation

A. Slowly progressive, slight-to-moderate ventricular dilation, normal intracranial pressure
  1. Careful surveillance only (?)
  2. Serial lumbar punctures (?)
  3. Acetazolamide and furosemide (?)
  4. Glycerol (?)
  5. Compressive head wrapping (?)

B. Rapidly progressive, moderate-to-severe ventricular dilation, elevated intracranial pressure
  1. Ventriculostomy
  2. Ventriculoperitoneal shunt

CONCLUSIONS

This chapter dealt first with the major sign of neurologic disorders in the newborn period, that is, seizures. The latter may take particularly subtle forms in the newborn and require careful clinical evaluation for recognition. Etiologic considerations include, principally, perinatal asphyxia and its complications, although intracranial infection, developmental disorders, and metabolic disturbances are also important causes. Prognosis is related primarily to the nature of the neuropathologic process causing the seizures. Management may require specific intervention, such as supplementation with a deficient metabolite, for example, glucose or divalent cation, but most commonly anticonvulsant drugs are used. Phenobarbital is the preferred of these drugs.

Hypoxic–ischemic encephalopathy encompasses 5 major neuropathologic states in the newborn period, namely, selective neuronal necrosis, status marmoratus, parasagittal cerebral injury, periventricular leukomalacia, and focal (and multifocal) ischemic brain necrosis. Certain of these are particularly more common in full-term (e.g., parasagittal cerebral injury) or in premature (e.g., periventricular leukomalacia) infants. Oxygen deprivation is presumed to be the critical pathogenetic factor. Ischemia is particularly important as the cause of this deprivation in the genesis of parasagittal cerebral injury, periventricular leukomalacia, and focal (and multifocal) ischemic brain necrosis. Careful neonatal neurologic assessment provides information of value in estimating the site and severity of injury and predicting outcome. Management is based principally upon diligent supportive care.

Intracranial hemorrhage in the newborn takes four major forms, namely, subdural hemorrhage, primary subarachnoid hemorrhage, intracerebellar hemorrhage, and periventricular–intraventricular hemorrhage. The latter is the most serious of these lesions because of its high frequency of occurrence and severity. The hemorrhage emanates from the germinal matrix in the subependymal region and relates to pathogenetic factors relevant to the maturation-dependent anatomy of cerebral blood vessels, the distribution and regulation of cerebral blood flow, the integrity of capillary endothelium, and the immediate extravascular environment. Clinical features include a catastrophic neurologic deterioration that is readily recognized but, more commonly, a saltatory deterioration that may be so subtle as to elude detection. Diagnosis is made best by a brain imaging procedure, such as CT or ultrasonar scan. Prognosis relates especially to the severity of the hemorrhage. Management includes careful control of cerebral perfusion and therapy for post-hemorrhagic ventricular dilation.

REFERENCES

GENERAL

1. **Volpe, JJ:** Neurology of the Newborn. Philadelphia, WB Saunders, 1981

SPECIFIC

Neonatal Seizures

2. **Bejsovec M, Kulenoa Z, Ponca E:** Familial intrauterine convulsions in pyridoxine dependency. Arch Dis Childh 42:201, 1967
3. **Bjerre I, Corelius E:** Benign familial neonatal convulsions. Acta Paediatr Scand 47:557, 1978
4. **Bleyer WA, Marshall RE:** Barbiturate withdrawal syndrome in a passively addicted infant. JAMA 221:185, 1972
5. **Brown JK, Cockburn F, Forfar JO:** Clinical and chemical correlates in convulsions of the newborn. Lancet 1:135, 1972
6. **Carton D:** Benign familial neonatal convulsions. Neuropädiatrie 9:167, 1978
7. **Cockburn F, Brown JK, Belton NR, et al:** Neonatal convulsions associated with primary disturbance of calcium, phosphorus, and magnesium metabolism. Arch Dis Childh 48:99, 1973
8. **Corsellis JAN, Meldrum BS:** Epilepsy. In Blackwood W, Corsellis JAN (eds): Greenfield's Neuropathology, pp 771–795. London, Edward Arnold, 1976
9. **Craig WB:** Convulsive movements in the first ten days of life. Arch Dis Childh 35:336, 1960
10. **Dennis J:** Neonatal convulsions: Aetiology, late neonatal status and long-term outcome. Dev Med Child Neurol 20:143, 1978
11. **Dreyfus-Brisac C, Monod N:** Electroclinical studies of status epilepticus and convulsions in the newborn. In Kellaway P, Peterson S (eds): Neurological and Electroencephalographic Correlative Studies in Infancy, pp 250–272. New York, Grune & Stratton, 1964
12. **Dreyfus-Brisac C:** Neonatal electroencephalography. Rev Perinatal Pediatr 3:397, 1979
13. **Eriksson M, Zetterstrom R:** Neonatal convulsions. Incidence and causes in the Stockholm area. Acta Paediatr Scand 68:807, 1979
14. **Harris R, Tizzard JPM:** The electroencephalogram in neonatal convulsions. J Pediatr 57:501, 1960
15. **Herzlinger RA, Kandall SR, Vaughan HG:** Neonatal seizures associated with narcotic withdrawal. J Pediatr 91:638, 1977
16. **Hillman LS, Hillman RE, Dodson WE:** Diagnosis, treatment, and follow-up of neonatal mepivacaine intoxication secondary to paracervical and pudendal blocks during labor. J Pediatr 95:472, 1979
17. **Hogan GR, Dodge PR, Gill SR, Master S et al:** Pathogenesis of seizures occurring during restoration of plasma tonicity in normal animals previously chronically hypernatremic. Pediatrics 43:54, 1969
18. **Keith HM:** Convulsions in children under three years of age: A study of prognosis. Mayo Clin Proc 39:895, 1964
19. **Lott IT, Coulombe T, Di Paolo RV et al:** Vitamin B_6-dependent seizures: Pathology and chemical findings in brain. Neurology 28:47, 1978
20. **McInery TK, Schubert WK:** Prognosis of neonatal seizures. Amer J Dis Child 117:261, 1969
21. **Meldrum BS, Brierley JB:** Prolonged epileptic seizures in primates: ischemic cell change and its relation to ictal physiological events. Arch Neurol 28:10, 1973
22. **Meldrum BS, Vigouroux RA, Brierley JB:** Systemic factors and epileptic brain damage. Prolonged seizures in paralyzed, artificially ventilated baboons. Arch Neurol 29:82, 1973
23. **Meldrum B:** Physiological changes during prolonged seizures and epileptic brain damage. Neuropädiatrie 9:203, 1978
24. **O'Meara OP, Brazie JV:** Neonatal intoxication after paracervical block. New Engl J Med 278:1127, 1978
25. **Painter MJ, Pippenger C, MacDonald H et al:** Phenobarbital and diphenylhydantoin levels in neonates with seizures. J Pediatr 92:315, 1978
26. **Pierog S, Chandavasu O, Wexler I:** Withdrawal symptoms in infants with the fetal alcohol syndrome. J Pediatr 90:630, 1977
27. **Plum F, Howse DC, Duffy TE:** Metabolic effects of seizures. In Plum F (ed): Brain Dysfunction in Metabolic Disorders, pp 141–157. New York, Raven Press, 1974
28. **Quattlebaum TG:** Benign familial convulsions in the neonatal period and early infancy. J Pediatr 95:257, 1979
29. **Rose AL, Lombroso CT:** Neonatal seizure states. A study of clinical, pathological and electroencephalographic features in 137 full-term babies with a long-term follow-up. Pediatrics 45:404, 1970
30. **Sarnat HB, Sarnat MS:** Neonatal encephalopathy following fetal distress. Arch Neurol 33:696, 1976
31. **Scriver CR:** Vitamin B_6-dependency and infantile convulsions. Pediatrics 25:62, 1960
32. **Seay AR, Bray PF:** Significance of seizures in infants weighing less than 2500 grams. Arch Neurol 34:381, 1977
33. **Tibbles JAR, Prichard JS:** The prognostic value of the electroencephalogram in neonatal convulsions. Pediatrics 35:778, 1965
34. **Volpe JJ:** Neonatal seizures. Clinics Perinatol 4:43, 1977
35. **Volpe JJ:** Neonatal seizures. New Engl J Med 289:413, 1973
36. **Wasterlain CG:** Neonatal seizures and brain growth. Neuropädiatrie (in press)

Hypoxic–Ischemic Encephalopathy

37. **Armstrong D, Norman MG:** Periventricular leucomalacia in neonates: complications and sequelae. Arch Dis Childh 49:367, 1974

38. **Ashwal S, Vain N, Macher J, Longo LD:** Patterns of fetal lamb regional cerebral blood flow (CBF) during and after prolonged hypoxia. Pediatr Res 13:522, 1979

39. **Banker BQ, Larroche J-C:** Periventricular leukomalacia of infancy. Arch Neurol 7:32, 1962

40. **Barmada MA, Moossy J, Painter M:** Pontosubicular necrosis and hyperoxemia. Pediatrics (in press)

41. **Barmada MA, Moossy J, Shuman RM:** Cerebral infarcts with arterial occlusion in neonates. Ann Neurol 6:495, 1979

42. **Behrman RE, Lees MH, Peterson EN et al:** Distribution of the circulation in the normal and asphyxiated fetal primate. Amer J Obstet Gynecol 108:956, 1970

43. **Borit A, Herndon RM:** The fine structure of plaques fibromyeliniques in ulegyria and in status marmoratus. Acta Neuropath 14:304, 1970

44. **Brown JK, Purvis RJ, Forfar JO et al:** Neurological aspects of perinatal asphyxia. Dev Med Child Neurol 16:567, 1974

45. **Cabal LA, Devaskar U, Siassi B et al:** Cardiogenic shock associated with perinatal asphyxia in preterm infants. J Pediatr 96:705, 1980

46. **Cohn EH, Sacks EJ, Heymann MA et al:** Cardiovascular responses to hypoxemia and acidemia in fetal lambs. Amer J Obstet Gynecol 120:817, 1974

47. **Dawes CS:** Foetal and Neonatal Physiology. Chicago, Year Book Medical Publishers, 1968

48. **DeReuck J:** The human periventricular arterial blood supply and the anatomy of cerebral infarctions. Europ Neurol 5:321, 1971

49. **DeReuck J, Chattha AS, Richardson EP Jr:** Pathogenesis and evolution of periventricular leukomalacia in infancy. Arch Neurol 27:229, 1972

50. **DeSouza SW, Richards B:** Neurological sequelae in newborn babies after perinatal asphyxia. Arch Dis Childh 53:564, 1977

51. **Galambos R, Despland P-A:** The auditory brainstem response (ABR) evaluates risk factors for hearing loss in the newborn. Pediatr Res 14:159, 1980

52. **Goldberg RN, Cabal LA, Sinatra RF et al:** Hyperammonemia associated with perinatal asphyxia. Pediatrics 64:336, 1979

53. **Hansen TN, Tooley WH:** Skin surface carbon dioxide tension. Pediatrics 64:942, 1979

54. **Holowach-Thurston J, Hauhart RE, Jones EM:** Anoxia in mice: reduced glucose in brain with normal or elevated glucose in plasma and increased survival after glucose treatment. Pediatr Res 8:238, 1974

55. **Huch R, Lucey JF, Huch A:** Oxygen: noninvasive monitoring. Perinatal Care 2:18, 1978

56. **Johnson GN, Palahniuk RJ, Tweed WA et al:** Regional cerebral blood flow changes during severe fetal asphyxia produced by slow partial umbilical cord compression. Amer J Obstet Gynecol 135:48, 1979

57. **Kaplan SL, Feigin RD:** Inappropriate secretion of antidiuretic hormone complicating neonatal hypoxic–ischemic encephalopathy. J Pediatr 92:431, 1978

58. **King LJ, Lowry OH, Passonneau JV et al:** Effects of convulsants on energy reserves in the cerebral cortex. J Neurochem 14:599, 1967

59. **Larroche JCL:** Developmental Pathology of the Neonate. Amsterdam, Elsevier, North Holland, 1977

60. **Lees MH:** Perinatal asphyxia and the myocardium. J Pediatr 96:675, 1980

61. **Leviton A, Gilles FH:** An epidemiologic study of perinatal telencephalic leucoencephalopathy in an autopsy population. J Neurol Sci 18:53, 1973

62. **Leviton A, Gilles F, Neff R et al:** Multivariate analysis of risk of perinatal telencephalic leucoencephalopathy. Amer J Epidemiol 104:621, 1976

63. **Leviton A, Gilles FH, Vawter GF:** The thymus in infants with perinatal telencephalic leukoencephalopathy. Arch Neurol 35:377, 1978

64. **Lou HC, Lassen NA, Tweed WA et al:** Pressure passive cerebral blood flow and breakdown of the blood–brain barrier in experimental fetal asphyxia. Acta Paediatr Scand 68:35, 1979

65. **Lou HC, Lassen NA, Friis-Hansen B:** Impaired autoregulation of cerebral blood flow in the distressed newborn infant. J Pediatr 94:118, 1979

66. **Lou HC, Skov H, Pedersen H:** Low cerebral blood flow as a risk factor in the neonate. J Pediatr 95:606, 1979

67. **Lucey J, Peabody J, Phillip A:** Recurrent undetected hypoxemia and hyperoxia. Pediatr Res 11:537, 1977

68. **MacDonald HM, Mulligan JC, Allen AC et al:** Neonatal asphyxia. I. Relationship of obstetric and neonatal complications to neonatal mortality in 38,405 consecutive deliveries. J Pediatr 96:898, 1980

69. **Malamud N:** Status Marmoratus: A form of cerebral palsy following either birth injury or inflammation of the central nervous system. J Pediatr 37:610, 1950

70. **Mulligan JC, Painter MJ, O'Donoghue PA et al:** Neonatal asphyxia. II. Neonatal mortality and long-term sequelae. J Pediatr 96:903, 1980

71. **Myers RE:** Brain pathology following fetal vascular occlusion: an experimental study. Invest Ophthalmol 8:41, 1969

72. **Norman MG:** Perinatal brain damage. Perspect Pediatr Pathol 4:41, 1978

73. **O'Brien MJ, Ash JM, Gilday DL:** Radionuclide brain-scanning in perinatal hypoxia/ischemia. Dev Med Child Neurol 21:161, 1979

74. **Painter MJ, Depp R, O'Donoghue MN:** Fetal heart rate patterns and development in the first year of life. Amer J Obstet Gynecol 132:271, 1978

75. **Pape KE, Wigglesworth JS:** Haemorrhage, Ischaemia and the Perinatal Brain. Philadelphia, JB Lippincott, 1979

76. **Sarnat HB, Sarnat MS:** Neonatal encephalopathy following fetal distress. Arch Neurol 33:696, 1976

77. **Scott H:** Outcome of very severe birth asphyxia. Arch Dis Childh 51:712, 1976

78. **Shuman RM, Selednik LJ:** Periventricular leukomalacia. A one-year autopsy study. Arch Neurol 37:231, 1980

79. **Siesjö BK, Plum F:** Pathophysiology of anoxic brain damage. In Gaull GE (ed): Biology of Cerebral Dysfunction, Vol 1, pp 319–372. New York, Plenum Press, 1973

80. **Vannucci RC, Plum F:** Pathophysiology of perinatal hypoxic–ischemic brain damage. In Gaull GE (ed): Biology of Brain Dysfunction, Vol 3, pp 1–45. New York, Plenum Press, 1975

81. **Volpe JJ, Pasternak JF:** Parasagittal cerebral injury in neonatal hypoxic–ischemic encephalopathy: Clinical and neuroradiologic features. J Pediatr 91:472, 1977

82. **Volpe JJ:** Observing the infant in the early hours after asphyxia. In Gluck L (ed): Intrauterine Asphyxia and the Developing Fetal Brain, pp 263–283. Year Book Medical Publishers, 1977

83. **Volpe JJ:** Perinatal hypoxic–ischemic brain injury. Pediatr Clin North Amer 23:383, 1976

84. **Volpe JJ:** Cerebral blood flow in the newborn infant: Relation to hypoxic–ischemic brain injury and periventricular hemorrhage. J Pediatr 94:170, 1979

Intracranial Hemorrhage

85. **Abroms IF, McLennan JE, Mandell F:** Acute neonatal subdural hematoma following breech delivery. Amer J Dis Child 131:192, 1977

86. **Ahmann PA, Lazzara A, Dykes FD et al:** Intraventricular hemorrhage in the high-risk preterm infant: Incidence and outcome. Ann Neurol 7:118, 1980

87. **Baird WF, Stitt DG:** Arteriovenous aneurysm of the cerebellum in a premature infant. Pediatrics 24:455, 1959

88. **Bejar R, Curbelo V, Coen RW et al:** Early diagnosis of intraventricular and germinal layer hemorrhage (IVH/GLH) by ultrasound. Pediatr Res 14:629, 1980

89. **Bergman E, Epstein M, Freeman J:** Medical management of hydrocephalus with acetazolamide and furosemide. Ann Neurol 4:189, 1978

90. **Blank NK, Strand R, Gilles FH et al:** Posterior fossa subdural hematomas in neonates. Arch Neurol 35:108, 1978

91. **Craig WS:** Intracranial haemorrhage in the newborn. Arch Dis Childh 13:89, 1938

92. **Deonna T, Oberson R:** Acute subdural hematoma in the newborn. Neuropädiatrie 5:181, 1974

93. **Donat JF, Okazaki H, Kleinberg F:** Cerebellar hemorrhages in newborn infants. Amer J Dis Child 133:441, 1979

94. **Ehle A, Sklar F:** Visual evoked potentials in infants with hydrocephalus. Neurology 29:1541, 1979

95. **Epstein F, Hochwald GM, Ransohoff J:** Neonatal hydrocephalus treated by compressive head wrapping. Lancet 1:634, 1973

96. **Friede RL:** Developmental Neuropathology. New York, Springer-Verlag, 1975

97. **Fujimura M, Salisbury DM, Robinson RO et al:** Clinical events relating to intraventricular haemorrhage in the newborn. Arch Dis Childh 54:409, 1979

98. **Gilles FH, Price RA, Kevy SV et al:** Fibrinolytic activity in the ganglionic eminence of the premature human brain. Biol Neonate 18:426, 1971

99. **Goddard J, Lewis RM, Armstrong DL et al:** Moderate, rapidly induced hypertension as a cause of intraventricular hemorrhage in the newborn beagle model. J Pediatr 96:1057, 1980

100. **Goldstein GW:** Spontaneous resolution of a neonatal cerebellar hemorrhage. Child Neurology Society Abstracts, 1977

101. **Goldstein GW, Chaplin ER, Maitland J et al:** Transient hydrocephalus in premature infants: treatment by lumbar puncture. Lancet 1:512, 1976

102. **Grontoft O:** Intracranial haemorrhage and blood–brain barrier problems in the newborn. Acta Pathol Microbiol Scand 100 (Suppl)100:1, 1954

103. **Grunnet ML, Shields WD:** Cerebellar hemorrhage in the premature infant. J Pediatr 88:605, 1976

104. **Haller ES, Hesbitt RE Jr, Anderson GW:** Clinical and pathologic concepts of gross intracranial hemorrhage in perinatal mortality. Obstet Gynecol Survey 11:179, 1956

105. **Hambleton G, Wigglesworth JS:** Origin of intraventricular haemorrhage in the preterm infant. Arch Dis Childh 51:651, 1976

106. **Hemsath FA:** Birth injury of the occipital bone with a report of thirty-two cases. Amer J Obstet Gynecol 27:194, 1933

107. **Krishnamoorthy KS, Fernandez RA, Momose KJ et al:** Evaluation of neonatal intracranial hemorrhage by computerized tomography. Pediatrics 59:165, 1977

108. **Krishnamoorthy KS, Shannon DC, DeLong GR et al:** Neurologic sequelae in the survivors of neonatal intraventricular hemorrhage. Pediatrics 64:233, 1979

109. **Lazzara A, Ahmann P, Dykes F et al:** Clinical predictability of intraventricular hemorrhage in preterm infants. Pediatrics 65:30, 1980

110. **Lee YJ, Kandall SR, Ghali VS:** Intracerebral arterial aneurysm in a newborn. Arch Neurol 35:171, 1978

111. **Lou HC, Lassen NA, Friis-Hansen B:** Is arterial hypertension crucial for the development of cerebral haemorrhage in premature infants? Lancet 1:1215, 1979

112. **Mantovani JF, Pasternak JF, Mathew O et al:** Failure of daily lumbar punctures to prevent hydrocephalus following intraventricular hemorrhage. J Pediatr 97:278, 1980

113. **Martin R, Roessmann U, Fanaroff A:** Massive intracerebellar hemorrhage in low-birth weight infants. J Pediatr 89:290, 1976

114. **Milhorat TH, Clark RG, Hammock MK et al:** Structural, ultrastructural, and permeability changes in the ependyma and surrounding brain favoring equilibrium in progressive hydrocephalus. Arch Neurol 22:397, 1970

115. **Oedku EL, Adcock KJ:** Neonatal hydrocephalus due to intracerebellar hematoma. Int Surg 51:302, 1969

116. **Oldendorf WH, Cornford ME, Brown WJ:** The large apparent work capability of the blood-brain carrier: a study of the mitochondrial content of capillary endothelial cells in brain and other tissues of the rat. Ann Neurol 1:409, 1977

117. **Pape KE, Wigglesworth JS:** Haemorrhage, Ischaemia, and the Perinatal Brain. Philadelphia, JB Lippincott, 1979

118. **Pape KE, Armstrong DL, Fitzhardinge PM:** Central nervous system pathology associated with mask ventilation in the very low birth weight infant: a new etiology for intracerebellar hemorrhages. Pediatrics 58:493, 1976

119. **Papile LA, Burstein J, Burstein R et al:** Incidence and evolution of subependymal and intraventricular hemorrhage: a study of infants with birth weights less than 1,500 gm. J Pediatr 92:529, 1978

120. **Papile LA, Burstein J, Burstein R et al:** Post-hemorrhagic hydrocephalus in low-birth-weight infants: Treatment by serial lumbar puncture. J Pediatr 97:273, 1980

121. **Papile LA, Munsick G, Weaver N et al:** Cerebral intraventricular hemorrhage (CVH) in infants < 1500 grams: Developmental follow-up at one year. Pediatr Res 13:528, 1979

122. **Pickering LK, Hogan GR, Gilbert EF:** Aneurysm of the posterior inferior cerebellar artery. Amer J Dis Child 119:155, 1970

123. **Ravenel SD:** Posterior fossa hemorrhage in the term newborn: report of two cases. Pediatrics 64:39, 1979

124. **Rom S, Serfontein GL, Humphreys RP:** Intracerebellar hematoma in the neonate. J Pediatr 93:486, 1978

125. **Rose AL, Lombroso CT:** Neonatal seizure states. A study of clinical, pathological, and electroencephalographic features in 137 full-term babies with long-term follow-up. Pediatrics 45:404, 1970

126. **Rothman SM, Nelson JS, DeVivo DC et al:** Congenital astrocytoma presenting with intracerebral hematoma. J Neurosurg 51:237, 1979

127. **Rubin RC, Hochwald GM, Tiell M, Mizutani H et al:** Hydrocephalus: I. Histological and ultrastructural changes in the pre-shunted cortical mantle. Surg Neurol 5:109, 1976

128. **Schipke R, Riege D, Scoville W:** Acute subdural hemorrhage at birth. Pediatrics 14:468, 1954

129. **Schreiber MS:** Posterior fossa (cerebellar) haematoma in the newborn. Med J Austral 2:713, 1963

130. **Schum TR, Meyer GA, Grausz JP et al:** Neonatal intraventricular hemorrhage due to an intracranial arteriovenous malformation: a case report. Pediatrics 64:242, 1979

131. **Shuman RM, Oliver TK Jr:** Face masks defended. Pediatrics 58:621, 1976

132. **Takashima S, Tanaka K:** Microangiography and fibrinolytic activity in subependymal matrix of the premature brain. Brain Develop 4:222, 1972

133. **Towbin A:** Central nervous system damage in the premature related to the occurrence of mental retardation. In Angle CR, Bering EA Jr (eds): Physical Trauma as an Etiologic Agent in Mental Retardation, pp 213–239. Washington, DC, U.S. Government Printing Office, 1979

134. **Tsiantos A, Victorin A, Relier JP et al:** Intracranial hemorrhage in the prematurely born infant: timing of clots and evaluation of clinical signs and symptoms. J Pediatr 85:854, 1974

135. **Volpe JJ:** Neonatal intracranial hemorrhage: iatrogenic etiology? New Engl J Med 291:43, 1974

136. **Volpe JJ:** Neonatal intracranial hemorrhage: pathophysiology, neuropathology, and clinical features. Clinics Perinatol 4:77, 1977

137. **Volpe JJ:** Neonatal periventricular hemorrhage: past, present and future. J Pediatr 92:693, 1978

138. **Volpe JJ:** Intracranial hemorrhage in the newborn: current understanding and dilemmas. Neurology 29:632, 1979

139. **Volpe JJ:** Intraventricular hemorrhage in premature infants. Pediatrics in Rev 2:145, 1980

140. **Volpe JJ, Manica JP, Land VJ et al:** Neonatal subdural hematoma associated with severe hemophilia A. J Pediatr 88:1023, 1976

141. **Volpe JJ, Pasternak JF, Allan WC:** Ventricular dilation preceding rapid head growth following neonatal intracranial hemorrhage. Amer J Dis Child 131:1212, 1977

142. **von Reuss A:** Diseases of the Newborn. London, MG, 1920

143. **Weller RO, Shulman K:** Infantile hydrocephalus: Clinical, histological, and ultrastructural study of brain damage. J Neurosurg 36:255, 1972

144. **Weller RO, Wisniewski H, Ishii N et al:** Brain tissue damage in hydrocephalus. Dev Med Child Neurol (Suppl 20)11:1, 1969

145. **Weller RO, Wisniewski H, Shulman K et al:** Experimental hydrocephalus in young dogs: histological and ultrastructural study of the brain tissue damage. J Neuropathol Exp Neurol 30:613, 1971

146. **Wigglesworth JS, Husemeyer RP:** Intracranial birth trauma in vaginal breech delivery: the continued importance of injury to the occipital bone. Brit J Obstet Gynaecol 84:684, 1977

147. **Wozniak M, McLone DG, Raimondi AJ:** Micro- and macrovascular changes as the direct cause of parenchymal destruction in congenital murine hydrocephalus. J Neurosurg 43:535, 1975

148. **Yakovlev PI, Rosales RK:** Distribution of the terminal hemorrhages in the brain wall in stillborn premature and nonviable neonates. In Angle CR, Bering EA Jr (eds): Physical Trauma as an Etiologic Agent in Mental Retardation, pp 67–78. Washington, DC, U.S. Government Printing Office, 1970

Mental Retardation

Harrie R. Chamberlin

Mental retardation is the common characteristic of a large and heterogeneous collection of chronic disorders encountered in children. Although it is the concern of professionally trained individuals in many disciplines, the study of a retarded child is not complete without appraisal by a physician thoroughly experienced in developmental evaluation and versed in the neurologic, biochemical, and genetic factors that play etiologic roles in the deficits of many of these patients.

DEFINITION

Mental retardation may be defined as intellectual inadequacy that originates during the developmental period and that may impair independent social adjustment at maturity. It is a symptom of a large group of disorders of many types. The term encompasses many conditions in which the mental and often the physical development of the patient have been retarded from birth. In addition it includes a much smaller group of persons who, following a period of normal early development, suddenly acquire brain damage or suffer from one of the cerebral degenerative diseases. Several hundred disorders associated with mental retardation have now been defined. Yet for a large proportion of the retarded the underlying etiology is still not understood.

Synonyms for the term mental retardation include *mental subnormality* and *mental deficiency*. The latter, as defined by the World Health Organization, specifically excludes emotional and sociocultural causes. When central nervous system pathology is clearly present, neurologists often use the term *static encephalopathy*. Older terms, now rarely used, include *feeble-mindedness, oligophrenia,* and *amentia*.

Mental retardation constitutes a major segment of the spectrum of the so-called *developmental disabilities*. The latter term in recent years has been promoted by federal and state governments for purposes of planning and of funding. It encompasses a broad range of frequently overlapping handicapping conditions, including epilepsy, the cerebral palsies, autism, and mental retardation. Determination of the presence or absence of a developmental disability by the federal definition is based upon an assessment of the degree of functional handicap.

PREVALENCE

The prevalence of mental retardation is generally considered to be approximately 3%, at present equivalent to some seven million persons in the United States alone. This figure, however, is based upon IQ levels. If "adaptive behavior" is considered to be one of the determinants in the definition of mental retardation, in addition to cognitive ability, the figure is considerably lower because the majority of the mildly retarded, by far the largest subgroup, when finally out of school, are able to adapt and to function within their surroundings in at least a marginal way.[127]

But more than 3% of persons in certain age ranges are involved when one includes all those who are actually functioning at a retarded level. Retarded performance may be secondary to emotional or sociocultural factors in a person whose innate cognitive potential is normal. Thus the prevalence of mental retardation may appear to vary considerably with age. An extensive study carried out some years ago in Onondaga County, New York, effectively illustrates this point. When an attempt was made to identify all the retarded residing in the county (by less sophisticated methods than are generally used today) the following prevalence rates were reported: birth to 1 year, 0.2%; 1 year to 2 years, 0.4%; 3 years to 4 years, 0.6%; 5 years, 2%; 6 years, 4%; 10 years to 13 years, 8%; 17 years, 2%.[88] During the first 4 years of life the mildly retarded were generally not identified by those who had contact with them. The identification of retarded functioning reached a peak during the period of maximum competition in school, where emotional and environmental factors play a major role. Following school, many of the mildly retarded merged imperceptibly into the overall society. Although modern emphasis on early screening and detection of developmental handicaps would doubtless raise these figures somewhat for the younger age groups, the differences continue to be striking.

in the range of 70 to 84. This borderline category has now been eliminated to avoid labeling those in the group who would be thus classified as a result of sociocultural deprivation alone.[49] The categories of mental retardation proper are: mild retardation, IQ 55 to 69, comprising about 90% of the retarded; moderate retardation, IQ 40 to 54, comprising about 6% to 7% of the retarded; severe retardation, IQ 25 to 39; and profound retardation, IQ below 25. The last two categories taken together constitute about 3% of the retarded.[1] The category boundaries in the above classification according to intelligence level correspond to successive standard deviations below the mean in the normal distribution curve for intelligence, the particular IQ numbers defining these boundaries differing somewhat depending upon the test used as the basis of classification.

In educational terminology mildly retarded children plus some of the more able moderately retarded are referred to as "educable." The remainder of the moderately retarded and many of the more able severely retarded are classified as "trainable." Those below this level are occasionally designated as "custodial." The synonymous terms moron, imbecile, and idiot are no longer used.

CLASSIFICATION

Mental retardation may be classified on the one hand by the predominating etiologic factor or, on the other, by intelligence or functional level. On occasion the specific major etiologic factor is known, but more often it is possible only to classify the etiology more generally as prenatal (including genetic), perinatal, or postnatal. Frequently no etiologic classification can be made. When classification is by intelligence level it has become conventional to use the categories suggested by the American Association on Mental Deficiency, which formerly included the extremely large group of persons with borderline intelligence, with IQs

ETIOLOGY

In spite of the many known causes of mental retardation, the exact defect in the majority of individual patients is still unknown. It is usually possible, however, to arrive at a rough determination of the role of prenatal, perinatal, and postnatal factors. Although it is impossible to achieve any accurate determination of the quantitative importance of each of these factors, it is generally agreed that prenatal elements probably account for as much as 90% of the total mentally retarded population if one omits from consideration the late effects of a socioculturally depressed postnatal environment.

Etiologic Classification of Mental Retardation

Prenatal
Genetic factors
  Conditions derived from polygenic causes
    Physiologic or cultural–familial group (postnatal environment usually also a factor)
  Conditions due to mutant genes
    Autosomal dominant
      Example: Neurocutaneous syndromes
      Others
    Autosomal recessive or X-linked
      Example: Inborn metabolic errors (majority of)
      Others
  Conditions associated with chromosomal abnormalities
    Involving autosomes
      Down's syndrome and other trisomies
      Translocations and deletions
    Involving sex chromosomes
      Example: "Fragile X" syndrome
    Mosaicism
External factors affecting the fetus
  Radiation
  Maternal infection
  Conditions occasionally associated with maternal malnutrition
    Toxemia
    Prematurity
    Probable direct effect (especially third trimester)
  Maternal ingestion of drugs
    Examples: Fetal hydantoin syndrome
              Fetal alcohol syndrome
  Maternal diabetes
  Maternal thyroid deficiency
  Maternal phenylketonuria
  Others
Unknown prenatal factors
Perinatal
Asphyxia
Intracranial vascular injury
Hyperbilirubinemia (in part prenatally determined)
Postnatal
Central nervous system infections and their sequelae
Postimmunization encephalopathies
Cerebral trauma
Severe hypernatremic dehydration in infancy
Poisonings
Severe protein malnutrition in infancy (probable)
Others

PRENATAL CAUSES

The large group of retarded resulting from prenatal causes may be separated into three major divisions: cases due to genetic factors, those due to external factors that impair fetal development, and a large remaining portion of cases of clearly prenatal but otherwise unknown etiology.

Genetic Factors

The division comprising genetic factors may in turn be separated into three distinct segments: conditions derived from polygenic causes, conditions due to mutant genes, and conditions associated with chromosomal aberrations.

Conditions Derived from Polygenic Causes. This, the largest of the three segments and sometimes called the *cultural-familial group*, is comprised of persons who may be classified as "physiologic" examples of mental retardation. They include the bulk of the mildly retarded, and it has been estimated that they account for 60% to 80% of all retarded individuals. They are thought by most to constitute the lower segment of the normal distribution of intelligence (Fig. 5-1).[29,94] It is clear that a poor socioeconomic environment, with its meager opportunities for learning, contributes further to the substandard abilities of many of this group, especially because one or both parents may have similar handicaps. These persons therefore do not suffer from a single genetic defect. They are considered by many to have inherited multiple genes that determine their limited intelligence, and to be entirely separate from the remainder of the retarded who suffer from one or more of a wide variety of specific defects of the central nervous system.

In most instances it is virtually impossible to separate from this physiologic group persons believed to function at a mildly retarded level solely because of years of living in a depressed socioeconomic environment. Theoretically these persons should have normal intellectual potential, but prolonged inadequate stimulation may have left such a mark that even years of careful guidance in an improved environment may not fully bring out this potential. Hence experts are often at odds over the

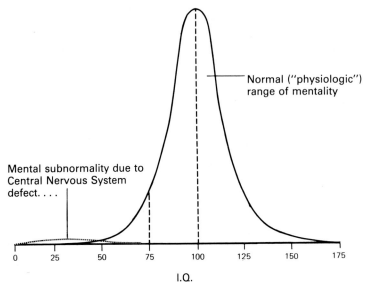

Normal ("physiologic") range of mentality

Mental subnormality due to Central Nervous System defect. . . .

0   25   50   75   100   125   150   175

I.Q.

FIG. 5-1. Distribution of human intelligence (hypothetical). According to this model the mentally retarded portion of the population may be classified into two groups: (1) a group, beneath the solid line, which may be designated as "physiologic" and which comprises the lower segment of the distribution of intelligence for persons with no actual defect of the central nervous system; and (2) a much smaller group, beneath the dotted line, of persons who are mentally retarded due to any of many possible defects of the central nervous system.

role of heredity versus environment in describing this largest group of the retarded. Inferior heredity clearly becomes associated with an inferior environment. On the other hand, inferior environment may lead to inadequate prenatal care, prematurity, and resultant central nervous system damage in offspring. Indirect evidence, moreover, strongly suggests that severe protein malnutrition, either during pregnancy or in infancy, can produce at least mild impairment of intellectual potential.[30] Rather than argue the importance of heredity as against that of environment in considering the millions of the mildly retarded, it would seem more fruitful to study the mechanisms whereby these two factors become inextricably entangled and the means by which their intellectual functioning may be brought closer to actual potential.

It should be recognized that both polygenic inherited factors and environmental factors are also in part responsible for the considerable individual variation seen among persons who represent any one of the more specific etiologies of mental retardation.

Conditions Due to Mutant Genes. This important group of the retarded is represented by many dozens of specific diseases or well-defined syndromes, each caused by a single mutant gene or pair of mutant genes at a single locus. Many others are strongly suspected to fall into this category. Some of these conditions, such as the two neurocutaneous syndromes, tuberous sclerosis and neurofibromatosis (the second of which is only occasionally associated with retardation), are transmitted as autosomal dominant traits with marked variation in expressivity. In the recent past it was thought that a major proportion of cases in this category were the result of de novo mutations because of an apparent lack of family history. Careful clinical study of parents, however, indicates that such mutations are far less frequent than was once supposed and underscores the variability of the expression of most autosomal dominant conditions.

The majority of forms of mental retardation resulting from the inheritance of mutant genes, including a majority of the responsible inborn errors of metabolism thus far identified, follow the laws of autosomal recessive inheritance. Examples of disorders of amino acid metabolism in this group are phenylketonuria, maple syrup urine disease, nonketotic hyperglycinemia, and methylmalonic acidemia (some cases are vitamin B_{12}-dependent and respond to large doses of this vitamin).[58] Inborn errors of carbohydrate or polysaccharide metabolism associated with mental retardation and involving autosomal recessive inheritance include galactosemia and the various mucopolysaccharidoses. The latter are still often identified by eponyms, such as Hurler syndrome for mucopolysaccharidosis IH. For each mucopolysaccharidosis the specific enzymatic defect has been identified.

Abnormalities of lipid metabolism in this category include Tay-Sachs, Niemann-Pick, and infantile Gaucher diseases, and metachromatic and globoid cell (Krabbe) leukodystrophy. Each of these is the result of a known specific enzymatic defect in the metabolism of sphingolipids.[9] All known forms of nonendemic goitrous cretinism are the result of specific enzymatic disorders, also due to autosomal recessive inheritance.

As identification of the specific enzymatic defect is accomplished for a rapidly growing number of inborn errors of metabolism, and as it becomes possible to measure the activity levels of these enzymes with fair accuracy in the laboratory, it has also frequently become possible to detect the defect in the normal-appearing heterozygous relatives. In general the enzymatic activity level in a heterozygote falls between levels in the normal individual and those in the homozygote. Due to overlapping levels, however, the results of such studies are often misleading. In diseases involving autosomal recessive inheritance the frequency of these heterozygotes is great in comparison to the small number of affected individuals. Mucopolysaccharidosis IH or Hurler syndrome (α-iduronidase deficiency), for example, has been estimated to occur in roughly only 1:100,000 people, yet it can easily be calculated that, to achieve even this, the heterozygote frequency must be greater than 1:160.[62] But to screen a large population for heterozygotes, even for a small number of specific autosomal recessive diseases, would be extremely costly and

totally impractical. By contrast, when a specific autosomal recessive enzyme defect is relatively common in a small identifiable population, such screening, for purposes of genetic counseling, can become extremely important. The screening of Ashkenazi Jews for carriers of Tay-Sachs disease is a prominent example; in this group the prevalence of heterozygotes may be as high as 1:25 and the disease, without counseling, appears in roughly 1:2500 births.

Several inborn metabolic errors associated with mental retardation have been identified that are inherited by an X-linked genetic mechanism, with transmission of the abnormal gene through a normal female carrier and the affected offspring almost invariably being male. Because there frequently is no family history, it is felt that many cases in this category are de novo mutations. Examples are the Lesch-Nyhan syndrome, a disorder of purine metabolism involving extrapyramidal symptoms and a tendency to self-mutilation with functional but not always true mental retardation, and mucopolysaccharidosis II (Hunter syndrome). Epidemiologic studies on large populations of the moderately and severely retarded clearly indicate that X-linked inheritance is also responsible for a significant fraction of otherwise unexplained cases of mental retardation, through the demonstration of a considerable preponderance of males after other potential causes for this finding have been ruled out. It is now known that a significant proportion of these males have an abnormality on one of the long arms of their X chromosome.[46]

New diseases secondary to inborn metabolic defects, many of them associated with mental retardation, are constantly being described. Presumably most of these depend upon autosomal recessive inheritance, although in many instances so few cases have been recognized that the genetic mechanism has not been conclusively determined.

There are many syndromes characterized by multiple congenital defects in which no specific inborn metabolic error has been discovered or for which the cause is unlikely to be the deficiency of a specific enzyme, and yet their existence appears to depend upon Mendelian laws of inheritance. Examples are the oculocerebrorenal syndrome of Lowe, determined by an X-linked mechanism, and the Laurence-Moon-Biedl syndrome, an autosomal recessive condition. Some forms of mental retardation associated with cranial defects may be genetically determined. Some cases of isolated microcephaly, for example, are the result of autosomal recessive inheritance. Occasional cases of craniosynostosis also appear to be autosomal recessive in character, whereas others are autosomal dominant. Certain cases of congenital hydrocephalus may be transmitted by X-linked genes. Many other unclassified forms of mental retardation that appear in siblings of an otherwise normal family probably result from recessive genes. This view is reinforced by the observation that otherwise unexplained forms of mental retardation occur with significantly higher incidence in offspring from incestuous matings.[3]

Conditions Associated with Chromosomal Aberrations. Remarkable advances have been made in the association of various combinations of congenital defects with specific chromosomal aberrations in the years since 1959 when Lejeune demonstrated the presence of 47 chromosomes in Down's syndrome, due to trisomy of chromosome 21. Once thought, though probably incorrectly, to occur in approximately one in every 600 births in the United States, more recent calculations suggest that the incidence of Down's syndrome may now be closer to one in 1000, or even 1100 births, primarily due to increased use of various approaches to the prevention of pregnancy in older women.[90] Although the trisomy most commonly results from meiotic nondisjunction during oogenesis, it is now evident that the extra chromosome has a paternal origin in a significant proportion of cases.[59,78] A small proportion of cases of Down's syndrome have the normal complement of 46 chromosomes but are associated with a translocation. This process involves a fusion of the extra chromosome 21 onto another chromosome, usually from the D group (13–15) or from the G group (21–22). This is the mechanism in some 8% of all Down's syndrome patients born of mothers under 30 and in about 2.5% of those born of older mothers.[81] This difference is due to the rapid increase in the frequency of

nondisjunction with maternal age, in contrast to the less variable frequency of translocation. It has now been demonstrated that paternal age, after approximately 55, also makes some contribution to the increase in nondisjunction.[124] In roughly half of the cases of Down's syndrome due to translocation, the translocation is inherited.[80] In this situation one of the normal parents and often other relatives show a balanced translocation with only 45 chromosomes, including the fused one derived from the translocation.

In addition to Down's syndrome, trisomies of other autosomes are well recognized, particularly of 13 (D trisomy) and 18 (E trisomy), which appear to occur in roughly 0.4/1000 and 0.2/1000 live births, respectively. Each shows a characteristic combination of congenital defects, including severe to profound mental retardation. These trisomies may rarely result from translocation rather than nondisjunction, as in the case of Down's syndrome.

Some abnormalities of the sex chromosomes may also be associated with mental retardation. Persons with XXY (Klinefelter syndrome) and XXX karyotypes are occasionally mildly retarded, although most are of normal intelligence. The far more rare XXXX, XXXXX, XXXY, and XXXXY karyotypes are almost always associated with mental retardation and often with a variety of physical defects. A combination of several surveys of newborn infants, involving over 46,000 subjects, revealed a major sex chromosome abnormality in approximately one of every 400 male neonates. About 1:1000 newborn males had either an XXY (Klinefelter) or an XYY karyotype. Approximately 1:700 newborn female infants possessed a major sex chromosome defect, of whom about 1:1000 were XXX.[55] Although mental retardation may not occur with significantly increased frequency in males with the XYY karyotype, some are of borderline intelligence and this group has been the subject of considerable controversy due to the discovery of a few of these individuals in early surveys of prisons and psychiatric wards. That this condition may predispose to psychopathic personality has now been shown to be a misconception, although careful behavioral studies do suggest that temper tantrums, other forms of impulsive behavior, and poor long-term planning are more common among those with this karyotype.[85] The rarer, more complex karyotypes in this group (e.g., XXYY, XXXYY, XXXXYY) are generally associated with retardation.

Only an occasional patient with gonadal dysgenesis (Turner syndrome), with only 45 chromosomes in an XO pattern, is mildly retarded, but a characteristic cluster of cognitive processing deficits is often present, particularly involving directional sense, visual–motor coordination, visual memory, and motor learning.[137] Although the incidence of the XO karyotype in the neonate is relatively low in comparison with several other chromosomal abnormalities (about 1:8000 among female newborns in the above combination of surveys), this karyotype is present in approximately 5% of aborted fetuses.[55,72] If we assume a 15% spontaneous abortion rate for conceptuses that implant, the karyotype of approximately 0.75% (or 1:133) of all implanted conceptions must be assumed to be XO. This observation underscores a point that deserves emphasis, namely that the gestational period is highly effective in selecting against major chromosomal abnormalities, 90% to 95% of which are lost prior to birth.[55]

The recent recognition of an X-chromosome marker, known as a "fragile site," in approximately one-third of families handicapped by X-linked mental retardation is of considerable importance. The marker is characterized by a thin segment that can easily break, near the end of one of the long arms of the X chromosome, though it is difficult to demonstrate this site without specific culture media. When this marker is present in males it is usually associated with a few subtle phenotypic features, the most obvious and characteristic being enlargement of the testes to several times their normal size. This macro-orchidism, however, may not become evident until fairly late in puberty. Screening of females with otherwise unexplained mild mental retardation has revealed that a small percentage also have the fragile X site, with no accompanying gross physical abnormalities. In one study, evaluation of the female heterozygous relatives of this small group suggests that close to one-third are mildly retarded.[46] Half the sons of these hetero-

zygotes, whether their mothers are mildly retarded or not, will typically be significantly retarded, usually with eventual macro-orchidism. The significant differences among females who possess fragile X sites is felt to be due to Lyonization, whereby only one of the X chromosomes is fully functional. It has been estimated that next to trisomy 21 (Down's syndrome) the fragile X syndrome is the most common of the causes of mental retardation that can be specifically diagnosed.[46]

Mosaicism, the presence of two or more cell lines, each with a different karyotype, occurs in some 2% to 3% of persons with Down's syndrome. The combination of a normal cell line with a Down's syndrome cell line will usually tend to blunt the characteristic features of the syndrome.[38] A wide variety of other mosaic patterns has been described, frequently associated with mental retardation and other defects. Mosaicism is far more common for the sex chromosomal than for the autosomal abnormalities. It occurs most commonly in patients with gonadal dysgenesis, where it has been estimated that as many as 30% show mosaicism of various types, the most frequent being XO/XY and XO/XX.[98]

Structural defects of individual chromosomes other than translocations are characteristic of certain syndromes that are often associated with severe degrees of mental retardation. These may take the form of deletions of parts of specific chromosomes, isochromosomes, or ring chromosomes. Deletion is the most common karyotypic abnormality in this group, one of the best known examples being the cri-du-chat syndrome, characterized by partial deletion of the short arm of a chromosome 5. Many other deletion syndromes are now well described and modern banding techniques are greatly accelerating the rate of discovery of new ones.[9] It has been shown that relatives of these patients may occasionally prove to be balanced translocation carriers.

External Factors Affecting the Fetus

The central nervous system is unique with respect to the long period required for the basic organization of its intricate structure. This, as well as its complexity, renders it especially vulnerable to environmental insults during gestation, particularly during the first trimester. It has long been recognized that excessive radiation to the maternal pelvis during the first third of pregnancy may damage the nervous system of the embryo.[106] In experimental animals specific defects of the brain can be produced by predetermined doses of radiation on specific days of gestation, and atomic warfare provided a grim demonstration of the effects of radiation on the human fetus.[83]

Infection in pregnant experimental animals by a variety of agents has resulted in defective offspring. Nevertheless, although viruses appear to be the most likely infectious agents to attack the fetus, only three thus far qualify with certainty as teratogens in man: rubella virus, cytomegalovirus, and herpes simplex virus.[40] Among nonviral infectious diseases other than syphilis, only toxoplasmosis has conclusively been shown to damage the fetus.[28] It is likely that this limited number of clearly proven teratogenic infections in man will eventually be expanded.[13,64,115]

The syndrome resulting from maternal rubella early in pregnancy includes congenital heart disease, cataracts, microphthalmia, deafness, and mental retardation, singly or in any combination. The high incidence of mild defects (e.g., high frequency sensorineural hearing loss, retinitis or chorioretinitis) following rubella in pregnancy is now recognized.[133] The virus also produces an acute neonatal illness, the symptoms of which include thrombocytopenic purpura and hepatosplenomegaly. If the infant survives, the virus may persist for many months. Indeed, the rare occurrence, usually in the second decade, of a progressive rubella panencephalitis, superimposed upon the original cluster of congenital defects, has now been described.[131] It appears that the risk of a live-born, seriously impaired infant is as high as 45% to 50% when maternal rubella occurs during the first 4 weeks of gestation, with an overall risk of at least 25% for rubella in the first trimester and some degree of risk as late as the fourth or fifth month.[24] Serologic studies during the neonatal period suggest that the vast majority of fetuses actually infected by the rubella virus *in utero* will show at least some of the characteristics of the rubella syndrome if they survive to be born

alive.[100] The incidence of spontaneous abortions and stillbirths is considerably increased, although figures vary greatly from study to study.

An acute neonatal illness and prolonged subsequent survival of the infectious agent, often with continuing central nervous system damage if the infant does not succumb, also characteristically follow prenatal toxoplasmosis, cytomegalic inclusion disease, and, though probably rarely, herpesvirus infection. Immunoglobulin M (IgM) antibody studies on cord sera from a large consecutive series of newborns, with subsequent follow-up of the infants with elevated levels, suggest that intrauterine infections may be a more important cause of unclassified congenital brain damage than was suspected in the past, particularly among depressed socioeconomic groups.[76,101,126]

The role of maternal nutritional deficiency in the production of mental retardation in humans, despite a variety of research studies, has been difficult to assess because of the problem of separating it from the effects of many closely associated variables. These include depressed socioeconomic status, generally poor prenatal care, and an inadequately stimulating postnatal environment. Whereas specific congenital malformations can clearly be produced in experimental animals by the absence or marked deficiency of a particular nutritional element in the material diet, this has not been shown in human beings. In recent years, however, research on malnutrition has underscored the fact that the period during which we have been most concerned about the potential effects of serious protein deficiency (from approximately midpregnancy to one and a half or two years postnatally) corresponds closely to the "growth spurt" in human brain development, when synaptogenesis and the development of overall dendritic circuitry are occurring at the most rapid rate.[30] Yet the presumed increased vulnerability of the developing brain to external insults at this stage appears to be somewhat shielded by a remarkable degree of plasticity. Severe human protein malnutrition is likely to prevent conception or to produce miscarriage. A consensus appears to have been reached that, although research is not conclusive, severe maternal protein malnutrition can also probably directly depress intellectual potential in surviving infants, particularly if continued through the critical infancy period. Lesser degrees of maternal malnutrition, however, probably do not directly impair the developing brain, although they are likely to be linked with subsequent inadequate stimulation of the infant and an overall depressed environment, definite handicaps to future cognitive development. Additional research is needed to clarify these problems.

Protein malnutrition during pregnancy may also lead to a small-for-gestational-age neonate, to true prematurity, or to a combination of the two, as well as to toxemia. Among potential complications of toxemia is neonatal hypoglycemia that, when severe, presumably introduces some risk for damage to the central nervous system.[50] The actual situation, however, is clouded by the demonstration that symptomatic neonatal hypoglycemia may in many instances be the result of preexisting brain damage, rather than the cause of it.[57] Moreover, follow-up studies of children with a history of uncomplicated mild-to-moderate hypoglycemia usually reveal no subsequent mental or motor deficit. It seems fairly certain, however, that if hypoglycemia is severe enough for a long enough period of time brain damage does result. Still more research is needed to determine the role of severe neonatal hypoglycemia in the etiology of subtle degrees of brain malfunction that could lead to selective learning disabilities or possible behavioral disorders.

Low birth weight, when other variables are taken into account, is clearly frequently associated with cognitive and neurologic handicap. There is, however, general agreement that the incidence of major handicaps in this group has declined in recent years, presumably due to improved prenatal and perinatal care of mothers and to improved postnatal care of their infants.[31] In a two-year follow-up study in Cleveland of very low birth weight infants born in 1975 and 1976, only 18% of those under 1500 g and 22% of those under 1000 g were found to have develomental quotients below 80, gross neuromotor deficits, or both.[51] In most studies small-for-gestational-age infants are not separated out from the larger group, but, when this is done, the potential morbidity for the former appears to be somewhat different from that for infants of corresponding birth weights who are solely premature. In a long-term follow-up study of 96 small-for-gestational-age infants, full-term but with birth weights at least 30% below the expected normal, major neurologic defects were at a minimum and the IQ average was normal; but, in contrast to their siblings, 25% had many of the symptoms characteristic of what is often called *minimal brain dysfunction* (hyperactivity, short attention span, learning difficulties, poor fine motor coordination, hyperreflexia, and an increased incidence of electroencephalographic abnormalities) and nearly half were performing poorly in school.[39] There is evidence that when a low birth weight infant is both preterm and small-for-gestational-age, morbidity may be especially high. In a prospective two-year follow-up study of 71 such infants born in 1974 and 1975, 49% proved to have either a major neurologic defect, a Bayley developmental index below 80, or both.[23] There has been inadequate time to assess potential learning and attentional deficits, too subtle in degree to demonstrate clearly in the preschool years, in very low birth weight school-aged survivors who have received the benefit of the most recent impressive advances in neonatology. But the extent of the overall problem is still evident when one considers that at least 15,000 infants with birth weights under 1500 g survive annually in the United States.[114]

The importance of adequate prenatal care is emphasized by the fact that reported prematurity rates for socioeconomically deprived populations in the United States are 10% to 20% (as high as 25.7% in one study for blacks who had received no prenatal care), whereas they are only 4% to 8% among economically secure groups (3.8% in the same study for the Caucasian group in which the mothers had had 16 or more years of education). Multivariate analyses on the data collected in this study indicated that the most important factor correlating with a high prematurity rate was lack of prenatal care, with a previous pregnancy loss, an excessively short interpregnancy interval, and out-of-wedlock delivery showing the next strongest correlations.[32]

Maternal diabetes, including the prediabetic state, is not only responsible for a greatly increased frequency of spontaneous

abortions, miscarriges, stillbirths, and neonatal deaths, but also is often associated with
perinatal complications that produce a significant increase in neurologic abnormalities among surviving offspring.[123]

The role of ingestion of drugs and of
certain environmental pollutants during
pregnancy in the genesis of congenital defects in humans was first highlighted by the
tragic production of phocomelia in several
thousand babies by the drug thalidomide,
principally in Germany in 1961 and 1962.
Although a broad spectrum of these agents
has long been recognized as potentially teratogenic in experimental animals when ingested during the first trimester of pregnancy, in recent years several have become
clearly implicated in man and many others
are strongly suspect. For the majority of these
teratogens the central nervous system is included among the several organ systems involved, usually leading to varying degrees
of psychomotor retardation. The timing and
amount of the agent ingested by the mother
during embryogenesis, in addition to the
nature of the agent itself, are important factors in the determination of the character
of the resultant defects in the neonate.

Among the first industrial wastes
shown to produce congenital abnormalities, methylmercury, after prolonged release into Japan's Minamata Bay, was found
in the mid-1960s to be producing serious
mental and motor deficits, often including
convulsions, the result of maternal ingestion of heavily contaminated fish.[128] Other
outbreaks have since been observed, including a carefully studied set of cases in
Iraq.[4] Recent demonstrations of significantly elevated blood lead levels in neonates born of mothers with moderate lead
burdens, combined with highly suggestive
evidence that such levels can impair the
eventual cognitive performance of the developing brain, underscore the potential
long-term risk to the fetus of moderate maternal exposure to this agent.[104,116]

Among drugs, folic acid antagonists,
as a result of their use in attempted abortion, were the first, in 1952, that were found
to be teratogenic in man.[129] More recently
oral anticoagulants such as warfarin, when
ingested during pregnancy, have been implicated as the potential cause of a variety
of congenital defects, including midface

hypoplasia and mental retardation, the
combination of defects varying considerably with the gestational timing of exposure.[125] Two groups of anticonvulsants, the
oxazolidinediones (trimethadione and
paramethadione) and the hydantoins, are
now clearly recognized as teratogens. The
risk of serious malformations following *in
utero* exposure to the oxazolidinediones
appears to be especially high. The pattern
of malformation includes an unusual facies
with frequent upslant of the eyebrows, occasional cleft palate, cardiac defects, uro-
genital abnormalities, and, frequently, delayed mental and physical development.[35]
The fetal hydantoin syndrome, more important because of the frequency with which
phenytoin is still prescribed, consists of a
variable pattern of craniofacial abnormalities, distal phalangeal hypoplasia, prenatal-
onset growth deficiency, and occasional mild
mental retardation. It appears that the infants of approximately 10% of mothers taking hydantoins in pregnancy will be seriously affected and that those of perhaps
another 30% will display some features of
the syndrome.[56]

It now seems probable that maternal
alcoholism during pregnancy is the most
frequent known teratogenic cause of mental
retardation, at least in the Western World.[19]
Although this relationship has been suspected since antiquity, a distinct pattern of
dysmorphic features among offspring of alcoholic mothers became evident only in the
late 1960s and early 1970s, a pattern that
has made it possible to separate the fetal
alcohol syndrome from the commonly accompanying effects of environmental disruption. The features most frequently seen
are pre- and postnatal growth retardation,
short palpebral fissures, a hypoplastic upper lip with thinning of the vermilion border, a diminished to absent philtrum, microcephaly, and varying degrees of mental
retardation. The frequency of the syndrome
has been estimated to be between one and
two per 1000 live births, with the frequency
of partial expression at three to five per 1000
live births.[19] If these figures are correct, the
incidence at birth of the fetal alcohol syndrome has now surpassed that of Down's
syndrome in the United States. Of the first
126 patients with fetal alcohol syndrome
described in the literature who received

standardized psychometric tests, 85% were found to have IQs below 70 and normal mental ability was found to be rare.[19] Recent studies suggest, however, that more subtle manifestations of central nervous system dysfunction may have been overlooked. In one university-based learning disorders clinic, comprising 87 school-aged children whose IQs ranged from 82 to 113, 15 of the mothers were retrospectively found to have a history of alcoholism during pregnancy. In contrast to the remaining 72 children, the 15 so identified demonstrated at least two of the characteristic dysmorphic facial features of the fetal alcohol syndrome in addition to a tendency to mild growth retardation.[113] Data of this sort suggest that maternal alcoholism during gestation not only may be important among the many etiologies of mental retardation but also may be primarily responsible for the deficits that characterize some of the vast number of children with various forms of learning disability. Although there is evidence that approximately three ounces a day of the equivalent of absolute alcohol (generally six drinks) constitute a major risk to the fetus, as little as one ounce to two ounces daily appear to carry a risk in some instances and no clearly safe level of alcohol consumption during pregnancy has as yet been established.[118]

Whereas the number of drugs and environmental pollutants that have been shown conclusively to be capable of damaging the nervous system of the developing human fetus still remains relatively small, it appears certain that the number will grow. Potential agents are constantly discussed in both the professional literature and the lay press, but despite impressive individual case reports, good statistical data with respect to the human fetus is inconclusive for most of these agents. A variety of substances have been reported to contribute to low birth weights and increased fetal and perinatal deaths, with those agents absorbed during cigarette smoking probably being the most common examples. Even here dissenters point to a variety of confounding variables, but the data appear relatively conclusive.[71] It is clear that lowered birth weights and increased perinatal difficulties increase the risk of central nervous system deficit in surviving infants.

The role of other external factors that might affect the fetus can only be conjectured. Among these are heat stress, hypoxia, and possibly even severe maternal emotional stress. Although there is suggestive evidence that severe maternal hyperthermia may rarely produce malformations, including central nervous system defects, in the human fetus, data in most of these areas are inadequate to provide any conclusions on the possibility of causal relationships.[20]

The external fetal environment is not always able to compensate for the deficiency of thyroid hormone in congenital hypothyroidism. Thus, because adequate amounts of maternal thyroid hormone may not reach the fetus through the placenta, a degree of brain damage may have occurred in these infants prior to delivery.[43] Such damage presumably accounts for the occasional failure of exogenous thyroid hormone to prevent mild retardation even when therapy is begun during the neonatal period. In such cases central nervous system damage may be considered secondary to a faulty fetal environment. This is true regardless of the specific cause of the congenital hypothyroidism.

Unknown Prenatal Factors

The large segment of the prenatally determined mentally retarded for whom the etiology is unknown is second in size only to the cultural–familial group. It includes a large proportion of the moderately to severely retarded. These persons cannot otherwise be classified and reflect our continued ignorance of the causes that underlie the disabilities in a large share of the mentally handicapped. Although they present no consistent clinical picture, the deficit is considered to be prenatally determined because of a high incidence of associated congenital defects and the frequent demonstration of cerebral malformations at autopsy. Occasional cases present a similar enough constellation of features to be considered the result of similar mechanisms, for example, the Rubinstein-Taybi or Cornelia de Lange syndromes, although they are almost always sporadic and have no apparent genetic pattern or other etiology. Our steadily increasing knowledge of genetics and teratology promises continued gradual clarification of the mechanisms responsible for many of these defects.

PERINATAL CAUSES

Although the prevalence of severe brain damage following perinatal asphyxia and trauma appears to have diminished considerably in recent decades, presumably due to major advances in obstetric and neonatal care, these factors are nonetheless of great importance because they are theoretically in large measure preventable.[41,109] Thus this volume contains an entire chapter on perinatal encephalopathy, to which the reader is referred for more detail.

Perinatal asphyxia leads not only directly to potentially damaging central nervous system hypoxemia, but also indirectly if there is accompanying severe bradycardia or transient cardiac arrest leading to ischemia. A variety of secondary factors also contribute to the production of damage, including accumulation of metabolites, gross disturbance of pH, and disruption of overall homeostatic mechanisms. Correlations of Apgar scores with subsequent status are rather poor, unless the former, particularly the five-minute scores, are impressively low. Several factors may account for this. First, the resistance of the nervous system of the neonate to hypoxemia, at least with respect to major morbidity, is remarkably great. Second, the asphyxic event may have occurred in utero, just prior to actual delivery, and the period of maximal stress may thus be largely over by the time the one-minute Apgar score is obtained. Third, most follow-up studies tend to focus on evidence of significant neurologic and cognitive disability and are not carried on long enough to document possible later attentional and learning disorders. It must also be recognized that failure of the newborn to establish respiration promptly is occasionally the result of preexisting abnormality. Subsequent evidence of brain injury may be wrongly ascribed to perinatal asphyxia rather than to the underlying congenital defect.

Prolongation of perinatal asphyxia beyond a critical level results either in death or permanent brain damage. Initiating conditions include premature separation of the placenta, prolapse of the cord, prolonged labor secondary to dystocia, depression of the respiratory center from excessive anesthesia or other causes, and obstruction of the respiratory airway. Gestational age at the time of delivery has considerable influence on the character of the later clinical manifestations of asphyxic brain damage. Periventricular leukoencephalopathy, leading to spastic diplegia, is particularly characteristic of asphyxic damage in premature infants, although, with improved care, its prevalence is now decreasing.[52] Although spasticity of the lower extremities predominates, when the leukoencephalopathy is extensive spasticity in the upper extremities also becomes prominent and associated mental retardation will generally be more marked.[136] A wider variety of neurologic deficits is seen following perinatal asphyxia in term neonates due to considerable variation in the resulting neuropathology. These features may include spastic tetraplegia, seizures, severe mental retardation, occasional accompanying ataxia, and late onset choreoathetosis.

The potential role of lesser degrees of perinatal asphyxia in the etiology of more subtle deficits that might fall into the poorly defined category of minimal brain dysfunction has been less well studied. It seems evident, however, that there is a "continuum of casualty," ranging from combinations of severe motor dysfunction and mental retardation to more mild handicaps characterized by attentional and behavioral disorders, learning deficits, and possible mild neurologic abnormalities. Birth in human beings occurs during the extended process of dendritic spine formation in cortical pyramidal neurons and there is good evidence that this process may be disrupted, presumably to varying degrees, by asphyxic insult.[96]

The incidence of intracranial vascular injury at birth has likewise been greatly reduced by modern obstetric methods, although it still occurs, particularly in association with prematurity or dystocia. Subarachnoid hemorrhage is probably the most common problem in this category. Fortunately the prognosis is usually benign, in striking contrast to the more serious outlook for older children and adults, but mild neurologic damage, seizures, and even secondary hydrocephalus occasionally result. Subdural hematoma is more likely to be seen in large full-term babies, especially when they are firstborn or the result of breech delivery, although this form of intracranial hemorrhage has now become a fairly uncommon birth injury. With prompt and adequate treatment the outlook is frequently good, but especially with inadequate management, continued seizures, mental retardation, hemiparesis, or tetraparesis may develop. Intracerebral hemorrhage is fairly rare and may as often be the indirect result of anoxia as of trauma. Intraventricular and subependymal hemorrhages are the most common forms of intracranial hemorrhage in the small premature infant. Again, anoxia, along with other factors, plays a significant etiologic role. A frequent cause of death in these infants, intraventricular hemorrhage was usually felt to be massive. Recent studies using computed tomography scans, however, have demonstrated its presence in over 40% of infants under 1500 g with close to half of these surviving.[93] In the majority of the survivors these hemorrhages were clinically silent. Initial follow-up evaluations of those survivors who lack apparent impairment in the neonatal period are encouraging, although adequate long-term studies are still needed.[69] It seems probable that ultrasonography will largely replace computed tomography in the near future for studies of this sort. New ultrasound technology is now essentially as effective as computed tomography in picking up intracranial hemorrhage in the neonate, with the exception of subarachnoid hemorrhage. In addition to eliminating exposure to radiation, it has the advantage of being cheaper than computed tomography and a mobile ultrasound unit can be taken directly to the nursery.

Hyperbilirubinemia of the newborn, potentially leading to kernicterus, is still another hazard of the perinatal period. Whereas isoimmunization due to blood group incompatibility between mother and infant is often the etiology of neonatal hyperbilirubinemia, undue elevations of indirect bilirubin may result from any factor leading to excessive intravascular hemolysis or impaired hepatic conjugation. Among

these factors are neonatal sepsis, prematurity, and a variety of drugs. The last may promote further hemolysis or compete for the serum albumin binding sites that are available to free indirect bilirubin. The drugs so incriminated include excessive vitamin K, sulfonamides, salicylates, diazepam (Valium), and gentamycin. Although uncommon, on occasion breast-feeding may contribute to excessive indirect bilirubin, possibly due to the presence of an unusual steroid in the mother's milk that competes for the conjugating activity of glucuronyl transferase that is essential to adequate bilirubin metabolism in the infant. This situation is not by itself adequate to produce kernicterus and is easily reversed by temporary cessation of breast-feeding for several days.[79]

Although the exact pathogenesis of kernicterus is still poorly understood, the serum level of indirect bilirubin is clearly an important factor.[74] Whereas it is generally considered safe to allow this level to approach 20 mg/dl in term infants before a risk of brain damage is encountered, there is some evidence that clinical abnormality may develop in small premature infants whose maximal levels are as low as 10 mg/dl to 14 mg/dl.[111] Moreover, kernicteric staining of basal ganglia is occasionally seen in small premature infants who fail to survive and whose indirect bilirubin does not surpass 6 mg/dl to 10 mg/dl.[132] The possible roles, in such circumstances, of hypoxia with acidosis, variations in albumin-binding capacities, greater permeability of brain barriers, or other mechanisms are still unclear, but it is known that the presence or absence of brain damage correlates far better with the degree to which an infant's serum proteins are saturated with bilirubin than with the serum bilirubin concentration.[91]

The eventual clinical picture of kernicterus results from selective damage to basal ganglia and various other areas of the brain, including tectal and auditory nuclei. Clinically there is gross retardation of the development of postural motor patterns, hypotonia with hyperreflexia, and a gradual onset of athetosis. By contrast, the majority of patients appear to have normal or low-normal intelligence. Indeed, some feel that there is as yet no good evidence that long-term cognitive function is impaired, although proof of this is elusive because of the cluster of other deficits so frequently associated with kernicterus.[105] Besides extrapyramidal cerebral palsy with accompanying oral motor dysfunction, these deficits may include sensorineural hearing loss, auditory receptive aphasia, paralysis of upward gaze, and overlying environmental deprivation resulting from the extreme difficulty of establishing adequate communication with persons who are thus afflicted. Such a combination easily leads to an erroneous diagnosis of mental retardation. Fortunately, modern understanding of the risk of even mild hyperbilirubinemia in small premature infants, the use of phototherapy to counteract rising indirect bilirubin levels, the use of exchange transfusions when necessary, and the introduction of hyperimmune Rh γ-globulin to prevent maternal Rh sensitization have impressively reduced the prevalence of this condition.[11]

POSTNATAL CAUSES

The many causes of postnatally acquired brain damage are far better recognized and understood than the many prenatal etiologies. The sequelae of central nervous system infections are an important subdivision of this group. These infections include the inadequately treated meningitides, among them tuberculous meningitis, which is fortunately now becoming relatively uncommon in the United States. They also comprise a wide range of encephalitides and encephalomyelitides, including those associated with measles and varicella; herpesvirus encephalitis and other viral encephalitides; pertussis encephalopathy; the encephalomyelitides that in rare instances follow the use of pertussis or rabies vaccines; and many of unknown etiology.

Postnatal cerebral trauma, which can result from falls and automobile accidents, may result in varying degrees of mental retardation, as well as in seizures, aphasia, and motor deficits. Thrombosis of a cerebral vessel may occur in severe dehydration of infants, in sickle cell disease, or secondary to the increased viscosity of blood in cyanotic congenital heart disease. In the latter, a cerebral embolus is also an occa-sional cause of postnatal brain damage. Hypertonic dehydration during infancy may produce multiple hemorrhages, including subdural hematomas. Severe hypoglycemia may cause seizures and progressive cerebral deterioration, although it may prove to be secondary to a preceding central nervous system deficit.[57] Other etiologies of postnatal brain damage include cerebral neoplasms and a variety of poisonings. Among the latter, lead poisoning is especially prominent. Although the damaging results of acute lead encephalopathy are well known, it is now evident that chronic lead burdens in young children with blood levels as low as 40 μg/dl to 50 μg/dl can lead to mild impairments of cognitive, and probably behavioral, functioning.[86,108] Although difficult to prove positively in humans because of inadequate control of the many variables, it is virtually certain that severe protein malnutrition during the critical first two years, when brain growth and dendritic differentiation are progressing rapidly, can produce at least mild impairment of future mental ability.[34] Evidence for this is best, however, when the severely malnourished infant and an adequately nourished but otherwise matched control are both from a socioeconomically depressed background.[102]

It is clear that there are many known causes of postnatal brain damage. Yet, at least in areas where protein malnutrition is uncommon and when consideration is limited to organic factors, all perinatal and postnatal etiologies combined are responsible for a mere fraction (probably no more than 10%) of the mentally retarded population.

EVALUATION

Early evaluation of the retarded infant or young child is all important. On occasion, though rarely, this results in the identification of a metabolic defect at an early age and may lead to improvement or correction with specific therapy. More commonly it furnishes an opportunity for early manipulation of the environment, allowing the child to make the fullest possible use of his limited capabilities. Early evaluation also occasionally leads to much needed early genetic counseling for the parents.

Many retarded children are evaluated primarily by the family physician or pediatrician with help from a psychologist, particularly as the child approaches school age. A few are seen in consultation by a neurologist. Despite the apparent lack of a hearing deficit, audiometric assessment is important. A social worker, or occasionally a psychiatrist, is sometimes sought when assistance is needed in aiding the parents to cope with their feelings and reactions. Other professionals, such as a physical therapist, will at times be required. This form of evaluation and the resultant guidance given can be adequate in many instances when the physician uses a broad approach, has some relevant genetic and biochemical knowledge, and can set aside the time needed for continuing support of the family.

When the situation is complex the most thorough and effective evaluation calls for a team of persons trained in a variety of disciplines, including pediatrics, neurology, psychology, audiology, speech and language, physical therapy, social work, and nursing. The team is joined, as needed, by persons from other fields: occupational therapy, special education, psychiatry, pedodontics, nutrition, ophthalmology, orthopaedics and genetics.[17] A single individual, not necessarily the team physician, must coordinate the findings and recommendations of the group. Many such developmental evaluation teams, particularly in medical centers and large urban areas, have been organized in recent years. In some states a dozen or more such teams, primarily supported by state funds, are widely distributed. Yet the vast numbers of the mentally retarded make it impossible for all families with a child thus handicapped to receive this extensive consultation.

HISTORY

The techniques of history-taking have been covered in Chapter 1. Certain areas of the history require emphasis, however, when evaluating the mentally retarded infant or child.

Knowledge of the child's home envi-

ronment is important. How far did the parents go in school? How is the child managed at home and is there adequate cognitive stimulation? If an interdisciplinary team is involved in the evaluation, a preliminary home visit by a team member can make a significant contribution. Or it may be possible and appropriate to arrange this through a local public health nurse.

An especially searching family history is indicated, including a check for possible consanguinity. Was conception difficult? Have there been frequent miscarriages? Thorough detail on the character of the pregnancy, particularly the first trimester, and of the delivery should be obtained from the obstetrician. Were there unusually low Apgar scores? How did the infant behave during the neonatal period? Was there significant neonatal jaundice?

In addition to a detailed review of the usual developmental milestones, certain less usual questions may prove of value. When did the first consonants appear? When was the pincer grasp first noted? When did the infant first play peek-a-boo and patty-cake, and wave bye-bye? When did such accomplishments as adequate management of a tricycle and coloring between the lines first appear? If the child attends a day care center, a preschool program, or a regular or special education class in school, a detailed letter from a staff person or teacher can be of considerable value. A wide range of questions unrelated to developmental progress may be indicated. Has there ever been an exceedingly high fever? Were neurologic symptoms ever associated with a childhood exanthem, such as varicella? If there have been seizures, were they of a type, such as infantile spasms, which may be associated with progressive retardation? Is there any evidence of chronic exposure to lead? Carefully developed parent and teacher questionnaires, to be completed before the evaluation, can be most useful.

Considerable experience on the part of the historian may be required to gain insight into the role of emotional factors, which almost invariably complicate the situation for any family with a retarded child. Are there feelings of guilt, however unwarranted? Is there an undercurrent of parental hostility and unconscious rejection? Is the child infantilized or overprotected? Or in their desire to promote as normal a level of achievement as possible are the parents pushing too hard? Is there resultant frustration on the child's part, possibly resulting in rebellion and a functional level well below his true potential? An attempt should be made to assess the emotional status of the total family, including the effect of the retarded child on the ability of the parents to meet the needs of the siblings. The impact of a retarded child upon some parents can threaten the entire course of their marriage, particularly if it is already unstable.

When the child's behavior includes autistic features, and particularly when they are prominent, questions about very early behavior are especially pertinent. Was the infant a "colicky" baby who cried for long periods and did not respond to attention? Was there inadequate responsiveness, with little or no smiling or giggling on stimulation? Was the child normally cuddly or was there a tendency to resist or draw away? If there was none of the expected response to the parents' love and attentiveness, it is important to learn how they reacted to this and how the combination of resultant severe parental emotional stress and the child's continued bizarre behavior influenced the character of the present parent–child relationship. At times this becomes seriously distorted. It was this distortion that often led psychiatrists in the past to conclude that the child's autistic behavior was primarily the product of the family environment. It is now generally agreed that this behavior is probably triggered by serious inherent deficits in perceptual or integrative central nervous system function.[107] It constitutes a behavioral syndrome that is usually accompanied by parallel cognitive deficits, so that most of these children are also seriously retarded. Skilled history-taking is most important in the analysis of situations of this sort.

PHYSICAL EXAMINATION

A thorough physical examination of a retarded child includes observation of behavior, a search for contributory physical characteristics, and a detailed neurologic evaluation. Certain points warrant emphasis. For more detail on the techniques of the neurologic examination the reader is referred to Chapter 1.

Observation of Behavior

In evaluating a potentially retarded child, the physician should observe the general level of activity, reactions to external stimuli, persistence, and the degree of accomplishment in a variety of tasks. A short attention span associated with apparent hyperactivity may be appropriate to the child's developmental level, though not to his chronological age. On occasion this general category of behavior appears to have a "driven," uncontrollable quality, seemingly more inherent in nature than a mere response to the environment. Often called the *hyperkinetic behavior syndrome* in the past, this complex of symptoms has now been officially designated as "*attention deficit disorder (ADD) with hyperactivity*" by the American Psychiatric Association. This picture, which appears to vary significantly among different children rather than to be a homogeneous syndrome, is commonly seen among retarded youngsters as well as among otherwise normal youngsters, particularly boys.[73] It may respond dramatically to certain stimulants, such as methylphenidate. The use of such medications, however, must be carefully monitored, partly because of a frequent placebo effect. In addition, their use should constitute only a portion of the overall therapeutic management and guidance of the child and the family. This syndrome must be distinguished from the more common hyperactive behavior of many emotionally disturbed children, which tends to disappear when their interest is finally gained.

During the interview one may also observe the character of the parent–child interaction. Its nature during the latter phases of a long evaluation when both child and parents are becoming fatigued may be most revealing. The adequacy of the parents' responses to the real needs of such children is basic in the attempt to train the latter to take as full advantage as possible of the capabilities that they do possess.

Some mentally retarded children show varying degrees of autistic behavior. The typical child with severe autism, with which mild-to-severe mental retardation usually but not always appears to be associated, presents a combination of symptoms that include severe language delay, stereotyped and repetitive motor activity, and marked perceptual deficits with apparent inadequate awareness of the identity of self or of others.[27] Eye contact is poor or absent and people may be treated as inanimate objects. Echolalia and repetition of words or phrases out of context are common. There is striking resistance to change. Bizarre behavioral patterns are frequent, such as tendencies to walk on tiptoe, to turn round and round, to ignore loud but familiar sounds, or to stare intently at constant movements of the hands and fingers or at spinning objects. As in the case of mental retardation itself, with which this symptom complex generally overlaps, autistic behavior presumably results from a broad range of etiologies. It is thus not surprising that symptoms of this sort, usually called *autistic characteristics* and usually less intense than in the fully developed picture of childhood autism, are seen in some retarded children, particularly among the more markedly retarded. Generally, however, the retarded child will relate adequately to the examiner and shows an awareness of his surroundings appropriate to his mental age.

Physical Signs

A wide variety of physical signs is distributed among the diseases and syndromes associated with many of the prenatally determined forms of mental retardation. So many of these signs and syndromes have now been described that it is no longer appropriate to attempt to list even the more important ones in a single table. The reader, on encountering a possible but unrecognized syndrome, should refer to one of the several excellent texts now available on this subject.[45,48,60,117] Occasionally such signs, especially when they appear in a particular combination, contribute directly to arrival at a specific etiologic diagnosis. More frequently they suggest a prenatal origin for the accompanying central nervous system defect. Certain physical signs may lead one to suspect a damaging perinatal or postnatal event.

Basic physical measurements are an important part of a thorough examination. They are especially helpful when earlier measurements are available for comparison. Although a gradual falling away from normal growth channels may lead to consideration of hypothyroidism, severe brain damage alone often results in retarded growth.

Serial head circumference measurements should be obtained on all infants and on all retarded young children. Macrocephaly, certain forms of which demand prompt neurosurgical intervention, and microcephaly are thus detected in their early stages. The shape of the head should be observed. Asymmetrical flattening of the occipital region in the older infant is often due to lying constantly in one position. Transillumination of the infant's skull may demonstrate advanced hydrocephaly, hydranencephaly, chronic subdural hematoma, occasional porencephaly, and often cortical atrophy.

In some disorders (such as Down's syndrome, most of the mucopolysaccharidoses, or the Laurence-Moon-Biedl syndrome) there are characteristic physical signs that are diagnostic when the classic picture is present, although there is marked variability from patient to patient and there are several forms of some of these conditions. Many of the signs, such as simian palmar creases or lenticular cataracts, may be present in otherwise normal persons. Certain other physical findings may be almost pathognomonic for specific central nervous system disorders: marbled pigmentation of the skin for incontinentia pigmenti, adenomata sebacea for tuberous sclerosis, and a macular cherry-red spot for certain of the sphingolipidoses, most notably Tay-Sachs disease (GM_2 gangliosidosis). Research on dental enamel and crown morphology has demonstrated that dental markers can occasionally be detected that may be helpful in dating certain etiologic events. The study of these markers, known as *odontoglyphics*, has shown that enamel defects are more common in neurologically impaired children, in cohorts of children with learning, behavior, and language disorders, and in situations involving a low socioeconomic status.[21]

Certain organs, such as the skin and the eye, are especially prone to show variations from normal in persons with central nervous system defects.[16] The discovery of one physical variant during the examination should lead the physician to check carefully for others. He should be familiar with the combinations of physical signs in specific diseases or syndromes characterized by mental retardation.

Neurologic Evaluation

The neurologic examination of the retarded child includes documentation of definite abnormal neurologic signs, a search for more subtle signs of brain dysfunction, and observation, especially in infants and younger children, of the developmental level of primitive and postural reflex patterns.

The demonstration of overtly abnormal neurologic signs can be useful in differential diagnosis. One would not expect such evidence of nervous system abnormality in a mildly retarded child judged to belong to the large "physiologic" or cultural–familial group. Definite neurologic abnormalities, beyond mere retardation of the development of normal neurologic findings, are frequently associated with specific motor deficits that, though they should be classified more exactly, fall under the general rubric of cerebral palsy (or, in the terminology of many neurologists, static or nonprogressive encephalopathy). The overlap of this group of conditions with some of the many forms of mental retardation is well recognized. Although only a small portion of the retarded have cerebral palsy, 50% to 70% of the cerebral palsied can be shown to have some degree of mental retardation.[135]

Among the cerebral palsies, the spastic forms, associated with corticospinal tract involvement, are the most common and include the spastic hemiplegias, the spastic tetraplegias or quadriplegias, and the spastic diplegias. Over half of the hemiplegias seen in the pediatric age group are congenital in origin, many of them perinatally acquired. The remainder are acquired acutely during infancy or childhood. Few of the congenital hemiplegias are recognized in early infancy, although careful observation of the symmetry of spontaneous movement in the early weeks may lead to their detection. They should become evident through the observation of asymmetrical placing reflexes at several months of age or when definite handedness has developed during the first year. Intelligence is better preserved in patients with congenital hemiplegias than in those with other forms of congenital spastic cerebral palsy, but over a third of the former will prove to have some degree of cognitive deficit.[25] Totally in contrast to the prognosis when hemiplegia is acquired as a child or adult, the side of the lesion in congenital hemiplegia appears to have a minimal effect on the rate of speech development, although there is now evidence to suggest that a somewhat greater degree of hemispheric specialization for language is present at birth than was previously recognized.[25] Approximately half of the persons with congenital hemiplegia will have at least a few ipsilateral seizures, approximately two-thirds will have some degree of associated sensory deficit, and a fifth to a quarter will show an associated homonymous hemianopsia. Although they are important considerations in planning treatment, both these sensory deficits and visual field defects can easily be overlooked in infants and young children if the evaluation is not done with considerable care.

When the neurologic examination reveals bilateral spasticity, the likelihood that it is associated with mental retardation is considerably greater. This is particularly true for the occasional bilateral hemiplegias, in which there is a significant difference in the degree of spasticity on the two sides of the body, and for the spastic tetraplegias, which show relative symmetry. In these forms of cerebral palsy, in which there is considerable involvement of the arms as well as the legs and microcephaly is common, mental retardation is almost always present and is often of severe or profound degree.[25] In spastic diplegia, symmetrical involvement of the legs predominates and that of the arms, though present, is slight. Here the degree of intellectual impairment varies greatly and intelligence is frequently normal when the motor impairment is mild. As previously indicated, this is by far the most common motor deficit following perinatal asphyxia during premature delivery, but presumably as a result of improved perinatal care, its incidence appears to be decreasing.[52] A small but significant proportion of infants with diplegia tend to be hypotonic rather than spastic, though the supporting reaction is often exaggerated and deep tendon reflexes are usually brisk. In addition the clinician may see various intermediate states, such as a combination of relatively spastic hip adductors with excessive mobility and floppiness at the ankles.

If the neurologic examination reveals only extrapyramidal cerebral palsy, the chances are great that mental development will be normal, or at least borderline. As mentioned earlier, however, its assessment may be exceedingly difficult. Clinically there is a gradual evolution from diffuse hypotonia with hyperreflexia to choreoathetosis. The latter typically becomes evident at one to three years but on occasion may not be obvious until the child is five or six years old. Along with the overall reduction in the prevalence of cerebral palsy among young children in recent years, the reduction has been most dramatic for the extrapyramidal group, primarily because of the impressive advances in the prevention of severe kernicterus. It has been shown that today in Sweden the typical athetotic child has only a mild motor handicap, is of normal intelligence, and was born at term with a history suggesting perinatal asphyxia, sometimes combined with a moderately elevated indirect serum bilirubin.[53]

A purely ataxic form of cerebral palsy, unaccompanied by other motor deficit, is relatively rare. Progressing from a picture of hypotonia with delayed motor milestones in infancy, the picture becomes one of a wide based, unsteady gait with considerable truncal ataxia. A mild intention tremor may also be present. The underlying cerebellar dysgenesis is also often associated with cerebral malformations, so that significant mental deficit is frequently present.

Experience with cerebral palsied children quickly reveals that mixed forms of cerebral palsy are common, usually as a combination of spasticity and extrapyramidal signs. An example is the mild degree of athetotic posturing frequently seen in association with spastic hemiplegia. Spastic tetraplegia associated with athetosis or rigidity and severe retardation may be secondary to perinatal asphyxia. Estimates of the proportion of mixed forms among a series of cerebral palsied patients range from 15% to 40%.[84]

On occasion the neurologic examination of an infant with a delay in both motor and mental development reveals little more than hypotonia. On follow-up the hypotonia persists without the appearance of either extrapyramidal signs or ataxia. This combination of hypotonia and mental retardation, which cannot be classified among the cerebral palsies, is a fundamental characteristic of Down's syndrome and is seen in the early stages of some degenerative conditions, such as Tay-Sachs disease, but it is also characteristic of the clinical findings in a variety of otherwise unclassifiable retarded children.

More subtle suggestions of abnormality on the neurologic examination may still suggest brain dysfunction. Findings of this sort are commonly called *soft signs* because of their indefinite character and the uncertainty of their significance. It is clear that most soft signs indicate abnormality only after a certain age because they are normally found in younger children and thus represent an abnormal persistence of immature responses.[66] By contrast, hard neurologic signs are those that are abnormal at any age. Soft signs are thus apt to be present in children who are developmentally slow, either in all areas, as in mental retardation, or in selected areas, as in abnormally awkward children or in some children with learning disabilities. Accordingly, adequate evaluation of such signs requires knowledge of the average age at which each becomes abnormal. There are many reviews of appropriate tests for the demonstration of soft signs, including the age at which failure of each may become significant.[95,97,130] They generally include a series of tests for gross and fine motor function, subtle sensory deficits, visual–motor abilities, and a variety of conceptual abilities. They overlap and often extend far into areas more typically considered the domain of the psychologist, special educator, speech pathologist, or occupational therapist because they frequently include tests of such abilities as reading, auditory and visual word association, or imitation of body postures.

It is important to stress that many neurologists have grave concerns about the term "*soft signs*" or their use in arriving at a diagnosis.[6,63] Among their arguments is the point that one may be using rather vague and poorly quantitated tests of one system (neurologic function) to appraise the status of another system (neuropsychologic function) if, as is often the case, one is applying this approach to the assessment of a child with learning disabilities or an attention deficit disorder. Because the majority of so-called soft signs do indeed depend upon demonstration of a lag behind the usual time of accomplishment of a given function, it seems more appropriate for the pediatrician or pediatric neurologist to think in these terms and to be familiar with the average timing of some of these accomplishments.

Examples of tests for level of accomplishment in the areas of posture and gross motor functioning include horizontal extension of the arms and hands (significant pronation of the arms and spooning of the fingers is abnormal over 5 years of age), balancing on one leg (for at least 10 seconds by 5 years–6 years), and forward and backward tandem gait (by 5 and 6 years, respectively). Tests of fine motor functioning include serial apposition of thumb and fingers and alternating pronation and supination of the hands (both normally done slowly and with little or no rhythm at 3 years but deliberately and with slow rhythm by 5 years), and absence of mirror movements (synkinesia) in the opposite hand with these tests after a maximum of 9 years.[97] Among tests of subtle sensory functioning are graphesthesia (the average child should be able with his eyes closed to identify single arabic numbers traced on his palms by age 9–10) and double simultaneous touch (by 5 years–6 years a normal child identifies with closed eyes two areas touched simultaneously on his face and hands). Visual–motor functioning is best initially tested by observation of the ability to scribble (18 months–24 months) and to copy a circle (2.5 years–3 years), crossed straight lines (3 years), a square with sharp corners (5 years), a triangle (5 years–6 years), and a vertical diamond (7 years). Other tests for soft signs include those for right–left orientation (a child should be able to name his right and left eye, ear, hand, and foot by 7 years–8 years) and for finger gnosis (by 7 years–8 years the average child can tell with his eyes closed how many fingers there are between two touched simultaneously).[97] Eye, hand, and foot dominance should also be determined, although the role of mixed dominance as a cause of reading and writing difficulties was probably exaggerated in the past. At least several developmental lags should clearly be present to be of significance in judging a child's overall functioning. It should be remembered, moreover, that significant gross and fine motor delays may be present with no significant defects in cognitive functioning.

Documentation of the developmental level of a variety of primitive and postural reflexes in infants is another important phase of the neurologic examination for that age group (see Chap. 1). This requires a thorough knowledge of the normal ages of appearance and possible disappearance of such signs as the Moro reflex, the asymmetrical tonic neck reflex, the palmar and plantar grasp reflexes, placing reflexes, weight-bearing, the parachute reaction, and many others.[15,140] Observation of these reflex patterns provides a new set of developmental milestones in infancy parallel to the usual motor and mental milestones more generally familiar to pediatricians. In addition, a check for possible abnormal persistence of primitive reflexes is an important screening tool in the early diagnosis of cerebral palsy.

DEVELOPMENTAL SCREENING

Pediatricians or pediatric neurologists who are well versed in developmental assessment should be able to arrive at rough estimates of developmental age, although their awareness of potential pitfalls is enhanced by their experience. These estimates are derived from developmental data in the history and from an assessment of the maturity of gross and fine motor patterns, language development, and overall adaptive and social behavior. The examiner may observe any of a wide variety of activities appropriate to the child's age, including preference for handling large versus small objects, manipulation of routine examining instruments such as the measuring tape, use of blocks, reaction to a picture book handed to the child upside down, and use of a pencil or crayons. The ability to draw a person has become the basis of a standardized psychologic test, the Goodenough draw-a-person test. Even without resorting to detailed standards, the experienced physician can ascertain much from observing such a drawing.

Among developmental screening tests for children under 6, the popular Denver Developmental Screening Test (DDST) is probably the most useful.[42] Like the Gesell Developmental Schedule, widely used in the recent past and (now updated) still of considerable value, it divides overall assessment into four areas: personal–social, fine motor–adaptive, language, and gross motor.[67] The proper techniques for its administration can be learned relatively easily, although it is important to have studied the accompanying manual. It takes only 15 minutes to 25 minutes to administer, depending upon the age of the child. Although it is merely a screening test, it shows a relatively good correlation with both the Bayley Scales of Infant Development and the Stanford-Binet Intelligence Scale. Instruction on how to administer the DDST is now generally incorporated into the curricula for pediatric and public health nurses, nurse practitioners, and students of other disciplines dealing with child development. Many pediatric house officers are now also learning the proper techniques of its administration, although it is probable that those who go into practice, because of their busy schedules, will delegate it to a nurse or some other professional in their office. It is essential, however, that the physician take the responsibility to see that the test is being administered in the standardized fashion. Routine developmental screening, using the DDST, is now carried out, often on two or three occasions, on all infants in the practices of many pediatricians and family practitioners. The growing use of the DDST in the field is making a valuable contribution toward much needed earlier detection of infants and children with developmental problems. It must be emphasized, however, that a screening test can never be used to make a diagnosis, but can be used only as the basis for possible referral of a "questionable" infant or child for more definitive study.

Despite the popularity of the DDST, a broad variety of other developmental screening tests is now available.[122] An easily learned screening test for children up to 10 or 12 years, based on an interview of a parent or anyone who knows the child well, is the Alpern-Boll Developmental Profile.[10] This test is intended to assess academic achievement, in addition to physical, self-help, personal–social, and communication skills, and yields a chronological age level in each area. Further validation studies would contribute to the usefulness of the test, but it is one of the few instruments available that can be used to screen general development through the middle childhood years and that includes standardization data on minority as well as Caucasian children.[122] Some tests focus on only one facet of development. Physicians with experience in child development frequently use the Developmental Test of Visual–Motor Integration, produced by Beery and Bukenica. This test, for children from 5 years to 15 years, involves the copying of progressively more difficult figures and can be scored with ease to give a rough level of perceptual–motor function.

PSYCHOLOGIC TESTING

For more sophisticated developmental testing and whenever mental retardation is suspected, a psychologist with expertise in developmental assessment should share in the evaluation. Even when the child is severely or profoundly, and hence obviously, retarded, psychological evaluation can be valuable for documentation of baseline observations. It can also aid in the detection or raise the question of possible contributing factors, such as a specific perceptual deficit or handicapping environmental elements. The psychologist may choose from a wide variety of well standardized individually administered tests.[75] These comprise IQ tests to measure mental development, including tests for special populations (such as the severely physically handicapped, the hearing impaired, and the visually impaired), tests to evaluate academic achievement, and tests of adaptive ability to evaluate personal–social and self-help skills. Only the first and the last of these three forms of assessment will be discussed here.

The most widely used tests for evaluation of overall mental development in children are the Stanford-Binet Intelligence Scale Form L-M, the Wechsler Intelligence Scale for Children-Revised (WISC-R) and, for infants, the Bayley Scales of Infant Development (which provide both mental and motor indices). The Stanford-Binet Intelligence Scale is applicable from two years of age on into adulthood but is primarily used for the preschool years and for severely retarded older individuals because its items require increasingly verbal responses above the five year level. The WISC-R, applicable from 6 years to 16 years, yields a verbal IQ, a performance IQ, and a full-scale IQ. It is preferred by most psychologists over the Stanford-Binet test after a child has achieved a developmental level of 6 years because it permits a better assessment of differential abilities, particularly verbal versus nonverbal abilities, in addition to a total IQ score. A newer test, the McCarthy Scales of Children's Abilities, for assessment of mental ability between 2.5 and 8.5 years, is preferred by some psychologists over the Stanford-Binet test because it gives a clearer outline of strengths and weaknesses. It is most widely used for children in the 4 year to 6 year developmental range and is less useful above and below that. Other psychologists are hesitant to use it to label children as mentally retarded because it tends to give lower estimates of cognitive ability than the Stanford-Binet or WISC-R tests, particularly for learning disabled children.

The Bayley Scales of Infant Development have proved to be extremely useful in the detailed assessment of infants, from birth to 30 months. Although there are both mental and motor scales, even the mental scale is necessarily laden with motor items. Thus their predictive capacity is somewhat impaired in that they do not discriminate between average and bright children, but they do discriminate between those children who will have significant mental deficit and those who will not; also, their predictive capacity increases among infants with lower developmental quotients. Although one is on tenuous ground in making any, even a rough, prediction of an infant's future, at least one good study suggests that test scores are better predictors than are the estimates of pediatricians, although the predictions are even better when the two are combined.[139]

The two tests used most frequently to assess adaptive behavior, which comprises personal–social and self-help skills, are the Vineland Social Maturity Scale and the Adaptive Behavior Scale of the American Association on Mental Deficiency.[49] The Alpern-Boll Developmental Profile does include some aspects of adaptive behavior but is really a screening test of general development. Both the Vineland, which yields a social quotient (SQ), and the AAMD Adaptive Behavior Scale, which categorizes the child with respect to degrees of adaptive impairment, are based upon the parents' or caretaker's description of the child's accomplishments rather than upon direct assessment of the child. Neither should be used in lieu of direct testing of cognitive development or to arrive at a diagnosis, but they are most useful as supplements to direct testing by providing a better picture of the overall situation.

A wide variety of tests of cognitive development in special populations is available and new ones continue to appear. When a child is unable to make an adequate verbal response, as in extrapyramidal cerebral palsy with associated oral motor dysfunction, the Peabody Picture Vocabulary Test permits assessment of auditory receptive vocabulary. Administration of this test is relatively simple and can be carried out after a minimum of practice. Other tests for severely physically handicapped children include the Columbia Mental Maturities Test and the Pictorial Test of Intelligence. The severely hearing impaired are best assessed with the Leiter International Performance Scale or the Hiskey Nebraska Test of Learning Aptitude. A modification of the Stanford-Binet is available for the severely visually impaired and the Reynell-Zinkin Developmental Scales for Young Visually Handicapped Children have recently become available.

The IQ obtained on psychologic testing must never be considered as constant or absolute. These scores may change from one testing to the next, sometimes by considerably more than merely a few points, because the tests lack precision, the child's responsiveness varies, there may be some variability among examiners, and one test is never quite comparable to another. As the young severely retarded child grows older, his IQ typically appears to drop somewhat, in part because earlier tests are apt to depend to some degree on motor elements, whereas those given some years later can focus more sharply on cognitive function alone. For these reasons many professionals prefer to withhold actual quantitative scores, when this is possible, in interpreting their findings to parents, and to describe the child's functioning in a more general way. A single quantitative figure can tend to stick in a parent's mind, never to be forgotten. But detailed psychologic testing is invaluable in the overall evaluation of the retarded child, both for gaining as clear a picture as possible of the current situation and for informed planning for the future.

EVALUATION BY OTHER DISCIPLINES

Whereas a skilled interdisciplinary team can doubtless provide the most comprehensive and truly effective approach to the evaluation of patients with complex developmental problems, these teams frequently have excessively long waiting lists or are not easily available. However, knowledge on the part of the experienced physician of what professionals in other disciplines have to offer and a judicious choice of those available can often prove to be adequate.[17,70] The importance of sharing with a psychologist who is well versed in developmental assessment has already been stressed. At times a home visit by an able public health nurse or social worker will provide valuable information on parent–child interaction and background for effective guidance of the parents. For especially complicated overlying behavioral problems or severely distorted parent–child relationships, evaluation of the situation by a child psychiatrist, possibly in a local mental health clinic, may be needed. A psychologist skilled in behavior modification techniques can judge the potential effectiveness of that approach. Developmental information gleaned from psychological and achievement tests is frequently difficult to convert into practical educational suggestions without a background in both curriculum and classroom procedures. A special educator can be especially valuable in bridging this gap.

Adequate evaluation of both vision and hearing is important. Hearing deficits in particular tend to be missed because the child often can still respond to the sounds used in gross testing by the physician. Yet significant hearing loss may still be present, or the sounds heard may be so distorted that speech development is seriously impaired. Thus every retarded child and every child with apparent communication problems should have a thorough audiometric evaluation. Analysis of speech and language abilities by a knowledgeable communicative disorders specialist is needed prior to guidance of the parents in the techniques of speech stimulation or the initiation of formal speech and language therapy.

The occupational therapist can carry the analysis of fine motor and perceptual–motor dysfunction well beyond that of the pediatrician and even of most pediatric neurologists. Identification of the greatest weaknesses and the latent strengths in these areas is important in planning appropriate therapeutic programs. The physical therapist may make a similar contribution with respect to gross motor functioning, in addition to documenting the baseline motor status of a patient prior to the initiation of special activities designed to improve posture and locomotion or, in cerebral palsy, to inhibit primitive tonic reflexes and prevent contractures. Evaluation by a nutritionist or a pedodontist occasionally may be indicated, including a check for possible dental markers.

Those in most of these professions, somewhat in contrast to the physician, not only play a valuable role in the evaluation process, but also by their nature are deeply committed, when indicated, to subsequent direct involvement in long-term therapeutic regimens.

Yet it should be reemphasized that, although it is far preferable to have representatives of these various professional disciplines at hand, the experienced physician, with the help of a psychologist and access to an audiologist, can on his own accomplish fairly effective evaluations of many retarded children, though he is ill-equipped to plan the details of extended therapeutic management.

LABORATORY EXAMINATION

A wide variety of laboratory studies can be used in evaluating retarded children. Only a few, however, should be used routinely and at times none may be indicated. If an inborn metabolic error is suspected, a wider range of biochemical investigations is necessary. In each case they should be selected with respect to the possible etiology suggested by the clinical evaluation.

Routine skull roentgenograms are usually normal. They are of course indicated for all suspected cranial defects or when conditions associated with intracranial calcifications are considered, such as cytomegalic inclusion disease, toxoplasmosis, cerebral angiomatosis, or tuberous sclerosis.

An electroencephalogram will usually contribute very little. When there is no history suggesting seizures it may be normal, nonspecifically abnormal, or simply show an immature pattern. In a suspected degenerative encephalopathy an electroencephalogram may serve as an objective baseline that can be used to detect deterioration. It is indicated if there is any suggestion of a convulsive disorder, such as head dropping in an infant, which may signal an early stage of infantile spasms. Moreover, certain types of seizures, such as psychomotor epilepsy or petit mal status, may be misinterpreted as symptoms of a behavioral disorder, and the chance to diminish the child's handicap with specific anticonvulsant therapy is lost if the seizures are not suspected and confirmed by electroencephalography. If hypoglycemia is to be ruled out as the underlying cause of seizures, the blood sugar level should be measured soon after the onset of an episode, if at all possible, in view of the risk of ascribing too much significance to the ordinary fasting blood sugar level.

The advent of computed tomography scanning techniques has made a dramatic contribution to the evaluation of certain conditions that may be associated with mental retardation or may become associated with it. Examples are situations that may call for prompt neurosurgical intervention, such as a rapidly enlarging head or progressive focal neurologic signs. It is also used in suspected intracranial hemorrhage in the neonate and in the study of families of children with tuberous sclerosis to allow more accurate genetic counseling. When it is used in conjunction with a contrast medium such as metrizamide, it generally appears to be as useful as the pneumoencephalogram, or nearly so, in the evaluation of hydrocephalus, cystic intracranial lesions, and similar problems, and has been rapidly replacing that procedure. Because of the expense of computed tomography, however, it has little place in the assessment of chronic static encephalopathies, such as most forms of mental retardation or cerebral palsy, where it is unlikely to alter treatment plans; it should, however, be considered in the unusual situation in which it may contribute to a better understanding of prognosis or of genetic factors.[36] Cerebral angiography may occasionally be indicated for the definition of vascular abnormalities, but, again, the need for this procedure among the retarded population would be infrequent. The brain scan is usually more appropriate for the localization of acute nervous system disease. Recent rapid advances in ultrasound technology have already been discussed with respect to the detection of intracranial hemorrhage in the neonate. Because of its avoidance of radiation, reduced cost, and greater mobility of equipment, ultrasonography is already taking the place of computed tomography in many areas of intracranial imaging.

The routine study of any mentally retarded child would generally include basic hematologic and urinary examinations unless they have been done recently. Urinary screening for reducing substances should not employ a method specific for glucose because galactosemia may then be overlooked. If there is even a most remote possibility of phenylketonuria (cases of which very rarely still elude neonatal screening programs), a fresh urine specimen should be tested for phenylpyruvic acid using ferric chloride or by a specific paper tape method; if either test is positive, it should be followed by the dinitrophenylhydrazine test. These procedures will also detect maple syrup urine disease, often already suspected due to the characteristic urinary odor.

Although urinary screening with cetylpyridinium chloride (CPC) or cetyltrimethylammonium bromide (CTAB) was once considered the primary approach when one of the mucopolysaccharidoses was an etiologic possibility, the use of such urinary screening alone is now recognized as hazardous. In early infancy, before suspicious clinical signs would generally have appeared, these tests may be falsely positive. More important, for certain of the many forms of the mucopolysaccharidoses, these urine screening tests may give false negative results in older infants even after suggestive clinical signs have become evident. The newer acid albumin turbidity test occasionally gives false positives.[62] Far more emphasis must therefore be placed on a high index of suspicion during the clinical evaluation than on any laboratory screening test for this group of metabolic diseases. When the possibility is present, skeletal roentgenograms to detect characteristic changes are indicated, as is a search for excessive amounts of abnormal mucopolysaccharides in the urine and for metachromatic granules in white blood cells and in bone marrow plasma cells. For a specific diagnosis, however, which can make later prenatal diagnosis and accurate genetic counseling possible, the specific enzyme deficiency must be identified, usually in cultured fibroblasts.[62]

Thus, whereas several of the inborn metabolic errors with associated mental retardation may be detected or confirmed by relatively simple laboratory procedures, confirmation of others can be carried out only in special laboratories. Screening for aminoacidurias is performed routinely in a few centers. This can be accomplished by unidimensional high voltage electrophoresis with long runs. The yield, however, is extremely low when either electrophoresis or the much more expensive column chromatography is used routinely on all children with unexplained mental retardation. Moreover, interpretation of an apparent aminoaciduria is fraught with hazard. Any debilitating condition with muscular wasting, for example, may produce a generalized increase in amino acids. Much can be said about the poor cost-effectiveness of routine screening, in contrast to a careful choice of laboratory studies based upon specific indications in the differential diagnosis.[119]

The yield from amino acid screening of apparently retarded infants and young children is far greater when it is applied in the presence of specific findings: vomiting, unexplained acidosis or hyperammonemia, growth failure, odd smelling urine, or a similarly affected sibling. Such findings in a sick neonate with ketosis may prove, upon a check of urinary amino acids, to be the result of propionic acidemia (ketotic hyperglycinemia) or methylmalonic acidemia. In the absence of ketosis, the appearance of lethargy, hypotonia, and convulsions in the neonatal period should still lead to a check of urinary and serum glycine levels because of the possibility of nonketotic hyperglycinemia.

If the clinical picture in a neonate raises the possibility of an intrauterine infection, serum IgM antibody studies are indicated, although this test, unfortunately, is sometimes falsely negative.[112] If the suspicion is strong, specific serologic studies for antibodies to rubella virus, cytomegalovirus, herpesvirus, and toxoplasmosis should be obtained.

When cretinism or hypothyroidism are considered and have not been thoroughly ruled out by a neonatal hypothyroid screening program, a blood specimen for determinations of thyroxine (T_4) and of thyrotropin (TSH) should be submitted. Roentgenograms for bone age are also indicated, but it should be recognized that many moderately to profoundly retarded persons with normal thyroid function are small in stature and retarded in bone age. In relation to height, however, this retardation of bone age is generally not as striking as in cretinism.

If Lesch-Nyhan syndrome is a possibility, as in a male who displays unexplained extrapyramidal signs and, particularly, self-mutilation, the urinary uric acid–creatinine ratio should be determined. Reliance on a serum uric acid assay can be misleading because it is not necessarily constantly elevated in this condition.

Determination of the karyotype is indicated in the patient with multiple unexplained congenital abnormalities, which raise the question of a cytogenetic defect. Karyotyping of all cases of Down's syndrome is most important, even when no further siblings are anticipated, in order to detect those cases due to translocation and, if translocation is present, to determine, by karyotyping each parent, whether one parent is a balanced translocation carrier. When Down's syndrome proves to have been inherited by this mechanism, it is important that relatives of the involved parent be made aware that they may also be balanced translocation carriers. Thus a letter, to be kept in the family files, should be sent to the parents of every Down's syndrome child, indicating the child's karyotype and the risks of recurrence among close relatives, particularly if translocation is present. The degree of risk of recurrence in a later sibling is greatly influenced by the type of translocation. It is approximately 15% in Group D/Group G translocations when the mother is a balanced translocation carrier, about 5% in this same situation when the father is the carrier, approximately 6% when a parent carries a 21/22 balanced translocation, and a full 100% in the rare situation in which a parent is a 21/21 balanced translocation carrier.[14,54] Approximately half of Down's syndrome cases due to translocation, however, prove to be sporadic, both parents having normal karyotypes. These figures contrast with the 2% risk of recurrence in a sibling when nondisjunciton is the etiologic mechanism. The physician must also be alert to the possibility of translocation in any of the other autosomal trisomies, in which a similar need to detect balanced translocation carriers is present. Karyotyping is also essential to the detection of other cytogenetic abnormalities, including the many variations in the number of sex chromosomes and conditions due to a partial chromosomal deletion, such as the cri-du-chat syndrome. The use of banding techniques now allows demonstration of subtle variations in the karyotype and has led to the detection of an increasingly large number of recognized syndromes.

The development of diagnostic amniocentesis and its use in high risk pregnancies for the prenatal detection of certain metabolic diseases and of chromosomal abnormalities in cultivated amniotic fluid cells has revolutionized the field of genetic counseling and has extended the use of both karyotyping and measurements of specific enzyme levels to as early as the third or fourth month following conception. These techniques have already made possible the prenatal detection of virtually all fetal cytogenetic aberrations, certain major structural defects of the central nervous system such as anencephaly and meningomyelocele, and close to a hundred different inborn errors of metabolism, a figure that is rapidly growing.[82,134]

DIFFERENTIAL DIAGNOSIS

There are several conditions that may lead to an erroneous diagnosis of irreversible mental retardation. Inadequate environmental stimulation or deprivation of an infant or young child may result in delay of both motor and mental development. A complete change in the environment, particularly if accomplished at an early age, may show this to be largely a reversible process, though far less so if the deprivation has been severe and prolonged. Children who are able to gain their needs by pointing and grunting or by tugging at their mothers and leading them to what they want, or who are not exposed to appropriate speech models or reinforced for their speech attempts, may show delayed expressive language skills. Such children must be carefully watched if there is any concern that receptive skills also may not be within normal limits, and their parents should be encouraged to stimulate their language development.

A variety of physical handicaps may be misleading. Hearing disorders, including high frequency sensorineural losses that may be overlooked unless audiometric studies are carried out, must always be excluded as a cause of language delay. It is probable that prolonged serous otitis media during a critical developmental period can also delay language development.[99,141] On occasion, when hearing deficits are unrecognized, behavioral problems may also arise and further complicate the question of retardation. In school even a visual handicap may occasionally be misinterpreted by the teacher as evidence of mental impairment.

Some forms of emotional disturbance in older children may eclipse all initiative and result in a thoroughly inadequate performance, especially in school.

It is important to distinguish between the child who is primarily autistic and the child who is primarily retarded but who has some associated autistic behavior. In accordance with the theory that both autism and retardation are largely rooted in dysfunction of the central nervous system, there is considerable overlap between them, with varying combinations of symptoms ranging all the way from the child in whom autistic behavior is dominant to the child in whom retardation predominates.[108] Because children from the two ends of this spectrum show striking differences in their interaction with other persons and with their overall environment, the therapeutic approach to each group, though multifaceted, must be entirely different in emphasis.

Severe motor handicaps secondary to one of the several forms of cerebral palsy may give the impression that mental retardation is present when frequently it is not. An appearance of severe retardation may be seen in fully developed kernicterus, characterized by marked extrapyramidal movements, hearing impairment, and oral motor dysfunction. Yet it can be shown through careful speech therapy and an intensive education program, coupled with physical therapy and often with behavioral management, that the intelligence of these patients is often in the borderline or low normal range.

Several specific illnesses can produce moderate-to-marked retardation of motor development with no involvement of the brain. If there is complicating environmental deprivation, the potential for normal mental development may not be appreciated. Among these illnesses are infantile spinal muscular atrophy (Werdnig-Hoffmann disease), the more marked examples of the poorly defined syndrome of benign congenital hypotonia, and the rare case of infantile polyneuritis or uncomplicated congenital muscular dystrophy. Any chronic, debilitating illness in an infant, with associated wasting of musculature, may give a similar impression.

Frequent, uncontrolled convulsions may suggest gross retardation. When adequate anticonvulsant control is established, this apparent retardation occasionally proves to have been the result of almost continuous ictal and postictal states. Petit mal seizures, when exceptionally frequent, may so constantly interrupt a schoolchild's mental processes that his performance is seriously retarded. Excessive doses of certain anticonvulsants may also give the impression of retardation.

The various forms of learning disorders that impair reading and writing, abilities that our society places at a premium, produce handicaps that, when inadequately studied, are occasionally misdiagnosed as borderline cognitive deficit or mild mental retardation. When learning impairments due to environmental or educational deprivation or to emotional disturbance have been excluded, there remain many children with problems of inherent inability to maintain attention ("attention deficit disorder" or ADD), with selective cognitive deficits, or with a combination of the two. Children handicapped by selective cognitive deficits, which are usually designated as learning disabilities, present strikingly varied findings. Characteristically they show a marked unevenness or scatter in their performance on tests of the many abilities that combine to constitute normal mental functioning. In many cognitive areas they perform normally and sometimes above the average range. Only when these children's abilities are consistently depressed in essentially all performance areas may they instead be classified as borderline or as mildly retarded. The complexity and importance of the learning disorders are so great that the next chapter in this volume is entirely devoted to them.

TREATMENT

SPECIFIC THERAPY

Only a few of the conditions associated with mental retardation are amenable to specific therapy. One of these is hypothyroidism, in which nervous system damage, already presumably often present to a slight degree at birth, may be prevented or prevented from advancing beyond this minimal level with exogenous thyroid hormone. In addition, there are certain diseases that result from inadequate metabolism of components in the regular diet. The brain damage that occurs in galactosemia usually, though not always, is minimized when a galactose-free diet is instituted early.[111] Initiation soon after birth of a carefully controlled diet low in phenylalanine usually allows the development of a phenylketonuric infant to continue within the normal range. Recently data from several studies have strongly suggested that this low phenylalanine diet cannot be terminated at the age of 4 years, as has been the traditional practice, without considerable risk of an IQ drop of as much as 10 or 15 points.[61,120] This view, however, remains controversial and a long-awaited collaborative study of the problem is still not complete. A synthetic diet free of the branched-chain amino acids and begun during the neonatal period theoretically allows infants with maple syrup urine disease to develop normally. Its maintenance, however, is extremely difficult, and in most cases success has been limited.[26] Infants afflicted with a variety of other inborn metabolic errors involving amino acid metabolism, such as propionic acidemia and methylmalonic acidemia, often seem to benefit from low protein diets.[89,103]

It appears likely that approaches other than the use of diets in the amelioration of metabolic errors will eventually become progressively more available. Massive doses of specific vitamins have already been shown to be effective in vitamin B_6 (pyridoxine)-dependent seizures in infants and in those cases of methylmalonic acidemia that prove to be vitamin B_{12}-dependent.[58] Induction of enzyme systems with such drugs as phenobarbital, phenytoin, and the steroids appear to hold promise. Actual enzyme replacement therapy for some of the inborn metabolic errors that lead to retardation may someday become feasible. Provision of an endogenous source for missing enzyme through eventual success with liver transplants or the use of viruses to supply missing genetic information are both possibilities.

Neurosurgery may prevent the chronic brain damage that might otherwise result from a subdural effusion or hematoma and rarely from extensive premature closure of multiple cranial sutures. It is frequently effective in controlling hydrocephaly.

The use of stimulant drugs, such as methylphenidate, to counteract severe inherent attention deficits or hyperactivity has already been discussed. These symptoms, far exceeding what might be expected in relation to actual developmental level, are seen in both retarded and normal children. If stimulant drugs are ineffective and some kind of medication seems essential, less specific drugs such as thioridazine (Mellaril) may be of some aid, although the long-term consequences, such as tardive dyskinesia, of neuroleptic drugs should limit their application to only the more severe cases. For the vast majority of the retarded, no dietary, drug, or surgical therapy is now available.

INTERPRETIVE COUNSELING AND GUIDANCE

The hardest job for the physician may begin when the clinical and laboratory studies are completed. The challenge lies in how he informs the parents of his findings and in his ability to give continuing help and guidance. Despite markedly improved understanding in recent years of appropriate assessment and management approaches to the retarded, many physicians remain insecure with respect to differential diagnosis, uncertain about how to organize suitable evaluation and therapeutic programs that involve several professional disciplines and community resources, and unable to provide real and lasting support for the parents.

The realization that they have a retarded child is a tremendous blow to a family. It frequently produces a more severe and lasting wound than would the death of a child. In preparation for the interpretive conference following the evaluation, a portion of the physician's assessment should include, when possible, a careful, sensitive discussion with the parents of their perceptions of the child's developmental level and of their expectations for the child. The approach to be taken in the conference will depend on many factors: the degree of rapport and trust thus far established between the physician and the family; the character of the family structure and environment; the degree of the child's retardation; the extent of the associated physical handicap; the child's behavioral status; the degree of understanding that the parents already have of the problem; the parents' current attitude towards and interaction with the child; the accessibility of appropriate community services; the apparent inner strengths of the nuclear family; and the amount of support available from the extended family.

Even initial interpretive counseling often requires more than one conference. Both parents should, of course, be present and sessions should be scheduled at an hour when neither interruptions nor the pressure of time are factors. Emotional support and gentle honesty are guidelines. If the parents are helped to express their fears and these are accepted, they may gain some emotional preparation for the physician's confirmation of the fact that the child is retarded. Unless some groundwork of this sort has been carried out, any further discussion beyond this confirmation during the initial conference may largely fall upon deaf ears. In an occasional instance it may even be wise to avoid the use of the word "retarded" during the initial interview, speaking only about delayed development unless asked directly. Appropriate terms must be introduced eventually, however, and the interpretive process cannot be considered as complete until this has been accomplished. Occasionally, when rapport has not been firmly established and no preliminary groundwork has been laid, a defensive parent may develop a suggestion of transient hostility toward the physician, but if the latter manages these situations well, such parents will return. It is important that inexperienced physicians in this situation realize that an irrational affect of this sort is not directed towards them as individuals but as symbols of the reality of the parent's position.

The physician must be alert to the possibility of deep feelings of guilt on the part of one or both parents and must attempt to lead them into expressing it. Occasionally parents with fundamentalist religious beliefs will have become convinced that their child is handicapped because they were not "right with God." When possible, there should be a frank discussion of what did cause, or may have caused the problem and,

equally important, of factors that may be of concern to the parents that did not cause it. Unwarranted reassurance must be avoided. Hopefully the physician will be able to state convincingly that nothing that the parents did or failed to do was responsible. If the strain on either parent is especially severe or the future of an already insecure marriage is in jeopardy, counseling by an able social worker, or possibly a psychiatrist, may be needed.

The physician should be aware of the emotional responses of handicapped children themselves to their evaluation. For children with mental ages of roughly 6 years or above, individual interpretive conferences designed specifically for them can be important.[22]

Genetic counseling, when it is indicated and particularly when new siblings are a possibility, should be the next step in the physician's discussions with the parents. It is important that every physician develops a certain minimal degree of competence in this area because it is logistically impossible to refer all families that need this guidance to a genetic clinic or center. The ability to arrive at an appropriate differential diagnosis is vital for such counseling, far more so than for the therapeutic management of a retarded infant or child. The physician outlines the potential risks and possible special diagnostic steps, such as the use of amniocentesis, which could be taken. The lifelong nature of the handicap in question is emphasized, so that the parents can be better equipped to arrive at a decision with respect to the options available to them. It is a fundamental rule that families are never told what they should do; the decision is totally theirs, based on the information that the physician has given. If the situation is complex or the differential diagnostic possibilities uncertain, referral may, of course, be made to a specialized genetic counseling center. Indeed, in some instances this is essential.

The physician who has elected to hold the reins himself in the evaluation and management of his retarded patient, rather than to refer the family to a developmental evaluation clinic or similar interdisciplinary team, should now turn his attention to management counseling. This is a long-term and gradually evolving task because the needs of the retarded child change with age. Often this counseling, and certainly the therapeutic management of the child, are shared with professionals from other disciplines and with facilities in the community. It is important, however, that physicians monitor these contacts and that, unless another professional such as a psychologist, special educator, or social worker is clearly so designated, they be overall coordinators. The structure and socioeconomic status of the family are important factors when considering management approaches. The increasing number of one parent families, particularly those for which there are no supportive relatives nearby, has added to the proportion of particularly stressful situations. Families of low socioeconomic status, especially those in which neither parent completed school, will need special help in gaining access to appropriate facilities and to sources of financial aid.

A practical discussion of systematic habit training may be useful. Constant repetition is needed to teach the moderately retarded child techniques of self-care, such as washing, dressing, buttoning, and the

management of eating utensils. Guidance of the parents in the fundamental techniques of behavior modification may be particularly helpful, based on rewarding positive behavior and making sure that negative behavior is not unwittingly rewarded. Appropriate discipline should be determined according to the child's developmental rather than chronologic age. It may be helpful to draw a graph for the parents, illustrating a curve for the range of development of normal children alongside a hypothetical curve for their child (Fig. 5-2). Although in most instances this is an oversimplification, in this way they come to understand that the child cannot later be expected to catch up to the normal developmental range. It is essential that the physician realize that this technique should never be used unless one is certain of the presence of permanent retardation. For an infant under 12 months of age, particularly if premature, and often even for those under 18 months to 24 months, such predictions can be hazardous unless the retardation is relatively marked.

Suggestions for reading on mental retardation are usually given to the parents. Most should be told of the value of joining local and national parents' groups. Much support and satisfaction may be gained by meeting with other parents and by working through these groups on community services for the retarded. These may include preschool programs, an expansion of special education programs in the schools, camp and cub scout programs for the retarded and physically handicapped, Special Olympics, and other recreational programs.

During initial conferences with parents of a newly diagnosed retarded infant or very young child, it is generally unwise to discuss more than the immediate future in any detail unless they urge this. At later visits, as appropriate, preschool and schooling possibilities may be reviewed, along with the role of sheltered workshops, and opportunities for prevocational and vocational training.

The advent of Public Law 94-142, the Education for All Handicapped Children Act, which went into effect in 1977, has strongly stimulated the proliferation of many kinds of preschool programs for the retarded and otherwise handicapped.[92] All states now require public school programs

FIG. 5-2. A graph of this sort is often useful in the guidance of parents. Although an oversimplification, it illustrates that the developmental progress of a retarded child does not imply that he will eventually achieve normal ability. The upper curve represents the range of normal development with increasing age. The lower curve, which may be drawn at any appropriate level, represents the hypothetical future development of the child.

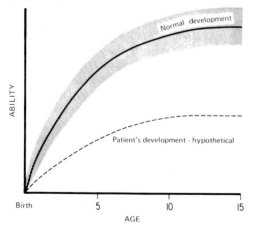

for the handicapped from age 5 onwards. In addition, the states have been mandated to provide educational services for far younger handicapped children once they have been identified and "individualized education plans" have been prepared. Partly as a result of this impetus, more handicapped infant groups, developmental day care centers, local interdisciplinary teams to guide parents in better management and stimulation of their children at home, and other similar programs are constantly appearing.

The child whose IQ is 50–70 is defined as educable. Whereas until recent years such a child was likely to attend an educable mentally retarded (EMR) class in the public schools, during the 1970s the concept of "mainstreaming" most of these youngsters into regular classrooms gradually became dominant and the number of EMR classes dropped precipitously. A variety of models of this approach have been used. In general either a special education teacher consults and provides services within the classroom or the child goes to a resource room for these special services for a short period of time each day. All of this fits the concept of education in the least restrictive environment, another goal of Public Law 94-142. The results thus far have been highly controversial.[8,18,139] For some of the mildly retarded mainstreaming appears to have been extremely valuable; for others it is said to be almost a disaster. Far more research on this sudden and drastic change in schooling for the handicapped is needed.

Children with IQs below 50 but above 25–30 are classified as trainable. Although special classrooms for the trainable mentally retarded (TMR classes) have long been a part of most school systems, there has recently been a considerable increase in their number. Here any attempt to teach the usual school curriculum is limited and emphasis is on self-care and meaningful activities, such as learning colors, recognizing numbers, printing the first name, boarding a bus, or making a bed. Supplementary speech or language therapy, as well as physical therapy, are usually available. There is considerable evidence that the developmental potential of many TMR children has been underestimated in the past. Some of them can clearly learn and are able to retain and use rudimentary academic skills. These skills add much to their potential for later quasi-independent living or, at the least, will make them highly successful residents of group homes. The majority of the trainable mentally retarded, which includes most children with Down's syndrome, later perform adequately in sheltered workshop settings and a few are even able to graduate to certain competitive types of employment.

Little in the way of academic skills can be taught to children whose IQs are below 25. They are more apt to have an associated motor deficit or recurrent convulsions. Here behavioral shaping techniques usually prove to be valuable because only a small proportion of these children are so retarded that they can scarcely learn at all. Indeed, it has been shown that a few can be taught rudimentary functional work skills with these techniques.[7] Management is otherwise largely a matter of sensitive, basic care, including as much interaction with the child as possible. For the most severely retarded, eventual institutional care is commonplace.

Even for the most profoundly retarded child it is usually best to wait for the parents to ask about residential programs, should they be inclined to do so. The years when larger and larger residential institutions were built, seemingly due to a belief that society needed protection from mentally retarded persons, have long since passed. The peak of approximately 215,000 institutionalized retarded in the United States was reached in about 1960 and, despite our increasing population, has since dropped by at least 20%.[87] Pressures for so-called deinstitutionalization have been especially strong since the early 1970s. As a result of both government and private efforts, this pressure has been accompanied by an impressive proliferation of group homes, halfway houses, and supervised independent living programs. In parallel with these changes, there has been a great increase in the degree of acceptance of the retarded in the community by large segments of the public, although certainly not by all of it. Yet it remains true that occasional early placement away from the family may be clearly indicated, such as when a child is so retarded that he can never be expected to communicate or even to roll over, or when he is so uncontrollably destructive that the home is constantly disrupted.

Placement in a residential center directly from the newborn nursery or during early infancy should generally be discouraged, except in the presence of the most profound retardation. Not only may this deprive the infant of the best chance for some degree of love and emotional security, but it may also produce strong guilt feelings on the part of the parents. Although the presence of a young retarded child in the family may become difficult for siblings as they mingle increasingly with their peers, if the emotional attitudes of the parents are healthy and the siblings' concerns are handled in a sensitive manner, it is unlikely that this will produce any lasting problem. The parents of a retarded child should be cautioned, however, to balance their time as much as possible among all their children.

It is obvious that, since only a small fraction of the retarded can ever be placed in regional residential centers, mental retardation is primarily a problem for the home and the community. If the parents can eventually come to realize that their goal should be the establishment of an atmosphere of acceptance and happiness for their child, much will have been accomplished.[2,44]

PREVENTION

Although our understanding of the etiology of many forms of mental retardation remains limited, already available knowledge has resulted in substantial approaches to prevention and the extent of this knowledge is growing rapidly.

Advances in the science of genetics and in the role of genetic counseling have been especially impressive. Careful family histories can lead to the identification of carriers of specific conditions associated with mental retardation, such as persons with balanced translocations. Such family histories would thus allow appropriate genetic counseling prior to a pregnancy. When a child is born with a recognizable genetic defect, the physician is legally responsible for seeing that the parents are given adequate genetic guidance with respect to possible later siblings. The advent of techniques of prenatal detection of many inherited metabolic diseases and of cytogenetic abnormalities has further revolutionized genetic counseling and has placed additional responsibility on the physician to arrive, when possible, at exact diagnoses.[33,82] Prenatal detection of a specific metabolic defect, with the possibility for subsequent therapeutic abortion of an involved fetus should the parents desire this, cannot be accomplished without the knowledge of exactly what metabolic abnormality is being sought.

Amniocentesis, used to detect cytogenetic abnormalities, particularly Down's syndrome, in the fetuses of older pregnant women, can make a significant contribution to the prevention of such abnormalities. It has been estimated that if amniocentesis could be used routinely when pregnancy occurs in the later childbearing years, to check for both cytogenetic and neural tube defects (see below), the risk of bearing an infant with a severe birth defect would be reduced by 28% for pregnant women from 35 through 39 years of age and by 56% for those from 40 years to 44 years of age.[47]

Detection of either phenylketonuria or hypothyroidism during the neonatal period allows the appropriate specific therapy to be instituted early. Although these therapies do not prevent the diseases, they do prevent, or at least markedly alleviate, the retardation that would rapidly develop without such therapy. For this reason statewide screening programs for phenylketonuria were set up throughout the United States in the mid-1960s and, once the technology had been developed, similar programs for congenital hypothyroidism were put in place in the late 1970s.[37]

Any young woman with classic phenylketonuria should be advised of the risks involved in becoming pregnant, even though, because she received early dietary treatment, she has no mental handicap and has the potential to be an adequate wife and mother. Although her fetus would usually be only heterozygous for phenylketonuria, its exposure from the very start to high maternal phenylalanine levels is likely to result in a combination of severe congenital defects, including microcephaly, cleft palate, congenital heart abnormalities, and either early neonatal death or severe mental and motor handicaps. Although a carefully controlled maternal diet during pregnancy presumably can prevent this, it is apt to be too late if begun after the first missed period.[121] When such women do plan to take the risk involved in having a child, it would seem wise to have them return to a low phenylalanine diet as soon as they discontinue contraception. It is sobering to recognize that inadequate maternal dietary control during pregnancy could lead to the birth of a highly defective but viable infant who might otherwise have been aborted had there been no attempt at all to employ a diet. Because early dietary treatment of infants with phenylketonuria first became established in the 1960s, in parallel with the setting up of comprehensive screening programs for that disease, it seems probable that we can expect, during the 1980s, the birth of significant numbers of severely handicapped infants of phenylketonuric mothers who will not be placed on low phenylalanine diets until after they are discovered to be pregnant.

Another major area of screening during pregnancy, for neural tube defects, is now in the large-scale pilot stage and may become universal throughout the United States during the 1980s.[68,77] Dependent upon the detection of slight elevations of α-fetoprotein in maternal serum, followed by ultrasound studies and then by amniocentesis when indicated, this endeavor is far more complex and requires careful avoidance of more pitfalls than does screening for either phenylketonuria or hypothyroidism. Unlike either of those neonatal screening programs, prenatal screening for anencephaly and spina bifida can lead only to a most difficult decision when abnormality is found: either therapeutic interruption of the pregnancy or the facing of an extremely serious medical problem. The choice can only be made by the family after careful counseling on the alternatives. More research is needed, not only to make this screening as foolproof as possible but also to determine the effects of the psychological stresses on mothers who are carrying a defective fetus and must participate in such

a choice. For some families a harsh ethical dilemma is involved. Yet the incidence of these problems at birth in the United States (roughly in the vicinity of 1:1000 for anencephaly and about the same for the spina bifidas, each similar to the incidence of Down's syndrome) demands that they be faced. All too often a surviving infant with meningomyelocele and complicating hydrocephalus, despite several neurosurgical procedures, will ultimately be a severely multihandicapped, retarded child.

As mentioned earlier in this chapter, the screening of Ashkenazi Jews for heterozygote carriers of Tay-Sachs disease is a good example of an approach to prevention that focuses on a high risk population. In this particular population this autosomal recessive disease occurs roughly a hundred times more frequently than in other races.[65] In women the serum level of the specific enzyme (hexosaminidase A) is preferably checked before pregnancy because the findings may be distorted during gestation. When both partners are found to be carriers, amniocentesis is carried out at the 14th to 16th week of pregnancy, enzyme levels are measured on amniotic fluid cell cultures, and therapeutic abortion is offered in the 25% of such pregnancies in which there is marked enzyme deficiency. Thus a simple blood test now makes possible complete prevention of a tragic genetic disease in a high risk group and at the same time enables couples, even if genetically at risk, to have unaffected children.

It should be recognized by physicians who give genetic counseling that there are unforeseen dangers of which they must be aware. As already stressed, it is particularly important to be certain that the retarded relative has been given a correct diagnosis. On the surface, for example, it might be easy to confuse mucopolysaccharidoses IH and II (the Hurler and Hunter syndromes); the first is an autosomal recessive condition, whereas the second is X-linked.

All pregnancies should be reported early and optimal prenatal care initiated promptly. Excessive radiation and unnecessary drugs should be avoided during gestation. Ideally a woman should abstain from all medications at this time, with the exception of vitamins and iron. Cigarette smoking should be minimized or eliminated, as should the ingestion of alcoholic beverages with the possible exception of infrequent small amounts. A history of pregnancy complications, such as diabetes, toxemia, or prematurity, should identify a pregnancy as high risk and ensure particularly careful monitoring, including careful follow-up of the resulting infant well into the postnatal period. Excessive anesthesia and analgesia should be avoided at delivery and manipulation leading to possible trauma minimized. The development of regionalized perinatal care programs should do much to promote prevention during this period.

Postnatally the infant, particularly the premature, should be watched for hyperbilirubinemia, occasionally anticipated by the previous history and by prenatal laboratory tests. Excessive use of vitamin K and other medications that can enhance hyperbilirubinemia should be avoided. All Rh-negative mothers should receive Rh-immune globulin following the birth of an Rh-positive infant, an abortion, or amniocentesis.[11] At least 36 hours after the first milk feeding the usual filter paper blood specimens should be obtained and sent to the appropriate central laboratory to be screened for phenylketonuria, galactosemia, and hypothyroidism. Screening for two or three other metabolic diseases from the same blood specimens is carried out in several states.

During the early infancy period any suggestion of cretinism should be promptly investigated on the assumption that it might have eluded a neonatal hypothyroid screening program; if the diagnosis proves correct, therapy should be initiated immediately to minimize nervous system damage. The growth of the cranium should be followed, using serial head measurements, for early detection of hydrocephalus as a part of the routine well-baby examination.

During infancy the hazard of dehydration, particularly hypertonic dehydration, should be avoided. Immunization against rubeola and pertussis, illnesses that can lead to brain damage, is important. For protection of members of the next generation, rubella immunization should be given universally to children before puberty. Constant emphasis on the education of physi-

cians in the early diagnosis of bacterial meningitis during infancy is needed to reduce the incidence of brain damage resulting from inadequate treatment of this condition. Continued vigilance against tuberculosis, with possible attendant meningitis, must be maintained, although tuberculous meningitis has fortunately now become relatively uncommon in the United States. Plastic bags should be kept away from infants and young children. Care should be taken to avoid acute or chronic exposure to poisons such as lead.[86,107] Efforts should be made by the many professions concerned with children to minimize the problem of child abuse, which is commonly associated with deliberate head trauma. Appropriate infants' and children's restraints, seat belts, and harnesses should be used in automobiles.[5]

Physicians should join forces with professionals from other disciplines in backing state and local programs that aim at the earliest possible detection of developmental problems in infants and children, thus increasing the likelihood of reversal or amelioration of these deficits, depending upon their nature. Likewise, in line with the mandate of P.L. 94-142, they should support programs that seek a thoroughly adequate evaluation of any child who is performing poorly in school, to be certain that children with adequate basic intelligence but with hearing, visual, or selective cognitive deficits or serious behavioral problems are not mislabeled as mentally retarded.

Finally, an overall attack is required against the ignorance and poverty present in our urban slums and in many rural areas. Such an effort, if effective, would result in better prenatal care and reduced prematurity, and, through improved education and living conditions, would create a lessening of many of the hazards already mentioned. Severe protein malnutrition, still seen occasionally in the United States and presumably damaging to the developing brain during pregnancy and early infancy, would thus also be avoided. Moreover, by reducing the number of homes that lack supportive adults and appropriate environmental stimuli, the proportion of apparently mildly retarded or inadequate persons would be decreased, owing to a rise in their functional ability to a level closer to that of their actual endowment.

REFERENCES

1. **Abramowicz HK, Richardson SA:** Epidemiology of severe mental retardation in children: community studies. Am J Ment Defic 80:18, 1975

2. **Adams M:** Social aspects of medical care for the mentally retarded. N Engl J Med 286:635, 1972

3. **Adams MS:** Incest: genetic considerations. Am J Dis Child 132:124, 1978

4. **Amin-Zaki L, Majeed MA, Elhassani SB et al:** Prenatal methylmercury poisoning. Am J Dis Child 133:172, 1979

5. **Baker SP:** Motor vehicle occupant deaths in young children. Pediatrics 64:860, 1979

6. **Barlow CF:** "Soft signs" in children with learning disorders. Am J Dis Child 128:605, 1974

7. **Bellamy GT (ed):** Habilitation of the Severely and Profoundly Retarded: Reports from the Specialized Training Program. College of Education, Center on Human Development, University of Oregon, Eugene, 1976

8. **Blatt B:** A drastically different analysis. Ment Retardation 17:303, 1979

9. **Bocian M, Mohandas T:** Recent cytogenetic advances and implications for pediatric practice. Pediatr Clin North Am 25:517, 1978

10. **Boll TJ, Alpern GD:** The developmental profile: a new instrument to measure child development through interviews. J Clin Child Psychol 4:26, 1975

11. **Bowman JM:** Suppression of Rh isoimmunization. Obstet Gynecol 52:385, 1978

12. **Brady RO:** Sphingolipidoses. Ann Rev Biochem 47:687, 1978

13. **Bray PF, Hackett TN:** Multiple birth defects in a newborn exposed to mycoplasma pneumoniae in utero. Am J Dis Child 130:312, 1976

14. **Buckton KE, Newton MS, Lauder IJ et al:** Familial transmission of a (21q22q) translocation. Cytogenet Cell Genet 15:103, 1975

15. **Capute AJ, Accardo PJ, Vining EPG et al:** Primitive Reflex Profile. Baltimore, University Park Press, 1978

16. **Chalhub EG:** Neurocutaneous symdromes in children. Pediatr Clin North Am 23:499, 1976

17. **Chamberlin HR:** The interdisciplinary team: contributions by allied medical and nonmedical disciplines. In Gabel S, Erickson MT (eds): Child Development and Developmental Disabilities, pp 435–470. Boston, Little, Brown & Co, 1980

18. **Childs RE:** A drastic change in curriculum for the educable mentally retarded child. Ment Retardation 17:299, 1979

19. **Clarren SK, Smith DW:** The fetal alcohol syndrome. N Engl J Med 298:1063, 1978

20. **Clarren SK, Smith DW, Harvey MAS et al:** Hyperthermia—a prospective evaluation of a possible teratogenic agent in man. J Pediatr 95:81, 1979

21. **Cohen HJ, Diner H:** The significance of developmental dental enamel defects in neurological diagnosis. Pediatrics 46:737, 1970

22. **Colley TE:** Interpretation of psychological test data to children. Ment Retardation 11:28, 1973

23. **Commey JOO, Fitzhardinge PM:** Handicap in the preterm small-for-gestational age infant. J Pediatr 94:779, 1979

24. **Cooper LZ:** Rubella: a preventable cause of birth defects. In Bergsma D (ed): Birth Defects: Original Article Series, IV, No. 7, pp 23–35. New York, The National Foundation, 1968

25. **Crothers B, Paine RS:** The Natural History of Cerebral Palsy. Cambridge, Harvard University Press, 1959

26. **Dancis J, Levitz M:** Abnormalities of branched chain amino acid metabolism. In Stanbury JB, Wyngaarden JB, Fredrickson DS (eds): The Metabolic Basis of Inherited Disease, 4th ed, pp 397–410. New York, McGraw-Hill, 1978

27. **DeMyer MK, Barton S, Alpern GD et al:** The measured intelligence of autistic children. J Autism and Child Schizophrenia 4:42, 1974

28. **Desmonts G, Couvreur J:** Cogenital toxoplasmosis: a prospective study of 378 pregnancies. N Engl J Med 290:1110, 1974

29. **Dingman HF, Tarjan G:** Mental retardation and the normal distribution curve. Am J Ment Defic 64:991, 1960

30. **Dobbing J:** The later development of the brain and its vulnerability. In Davis JA, Dobbing J (eds): Scientific Foundations of Paediatrics, pp 565–577. Philadelphia, WB Saunders, 1974

31. **Drillien CM, Thomson AJM, Burgoyne K:** Low-birthweight children at early school-age: a longitudinal study. Dev Med Child Neurol 22:26, 1980

32. **Eisner V, Brazie JV, Pratt MW et al:** The risk of low birthweight. Am J Pub Health 69:887, 1979

33. **Epstein CJ, Golbus MS:** Prenatal diagnosis of genetic diseases. Am Scientist 65:703, 1977

34. **Evans D, Bowie MD, Hansen JDL et al:** Intellectual development and nutrition. J Pediatr 97:358, 1980

35. **Feldman GL, Weaver DD, Lovrien EW:** The fetal trimethadione syndrome. Am J Dis Child 131:1389, 1977

36. **Ferry PC:** Computed cranial tomography in children. J Pediatr 96:961, 1980

37. **Fisher DA:** Screening for congenital hypothyroidism. Hosp Practice 12:73, 1977

38. **Fishler K, Koch R, Donnell GN:** Comparison of mental development in individuals with mosaic and trisomy 21 Down's syndrome. Pediatrics 58:744, 1976

39. **Fitzhardinge PM, Steven EM:** The small-for-date infant. Part II. Neurological and intellectual sequelae. Pediatrics 50:50, 1972

40. **Florman AL, Gershon AA, Blackett PR et al:**

Intrauterine infection with herpes simplex virus: resultant congenital malformations. JAMA 225:129, 1973

41. **Franco S, Andrews BF:** Reduction of cerebral palsy by neonatal intensive care. Pediatr Clin North Am 24:639, 1977

42. **Frankenburg WK, Goldstein AD, Camp BW:** The revised Denver Develomental Screening Test: its accuracy as a screening instrument. J Pediatr 79:988, 1971

43. **French FS, Van Wyk JJ:** Fetal hypothyroidism. J Pediatr 64:589, 1964

44. **Gayton WF:** Management problems of mentally retarded children and their families. Pediatr Clin North Am 22:561, 1975

45. **Gellis SS, Feingold M:** Atlas of Mental Retardation Syndromes. Washington, DC, Department of Health, Education and Welfare, Rehabilitation Services Administration, Division of Mental Retardation, 1968

46. **Gerald PS:** X-linked mental retardation and an X-chromosome marker. N Engl J Med 303:696, 1980

47. **Goldberg MF, Edmonds LD, Oakley GP:** Reducing birth defect risk in advanced maternal age. JAMA 242:2292, 1979

48. **Gorlin RJ, Pindborg JJ, Cohen MM:** Syndromes of the Head and Neck, 2nd ed. New York, McGraw-Hill, 1976

49. **Grossman HJ (ed):** Manual on Terminology and Classification in Mental Retardation. American Association on Mental Deficiency Special Publication Series No. 2, pp 4–5, 19–33. Baltimore, Garamond/Pridemark Press, 1973

50. **Gutberlet RL, Cornblath M:** Neonatal hypoglycemia revisited, 1975. Pediatrics 58:10, 1976

51. **Hack M, Fanaroff AA, Merkatz IR:** The low-birth-weight infant—evolution of a changing outlook. N Engl J Med 301:1162, 1979

52. **Hagberg B, Hagberg G, Olow I:** The changing panorama of cerebral palsy in Sweden 1954–70. Part I. Analysis of the General Changes. Acta Paediatr Scand 64:187, 1975

53. **Hagberg B, Hagberg G, Olow I:** The changing panorama of cerebral palsy in Sweden 1954–70. Part II. Analysis of Various Syndromes. Acta Paediatr Scand 64:193, 1975

54. **Hamerton JL:** Robertsonian translocations. In Jacobs PA, Price WH, Law P (eds): Human Population Cytogenetics, pp 64–80. Baltimore, Williams & Wilkins, 1970

55. **Hamerton JL, Canning N, Ray M et al:** A cytogenetic survey of 14,069 newborn infants. Clin Genet 8:223, 1975

56. **Hanson JW, Myrianthopoulos NC, Sedgwick MA et al:** Risks to the offspring of women treated with hydantoin anticonvulsants, with emphasis on the fetal hydantoin syndrome. J Pediatr 89:662, 1976

57. **Haworth JC:** Neonatal hypoglycemia: how much does it damage the brain? Pediatrics 54:3, 1974

58. **Hillman RE:** Megavitamin responsive aminoacidopathies. Pediatr Clin North Am 23:557, 1976

59. **Holmes LB:** Genetic counseling for the older pregnant woman: new data and questions. N Engl J Med 298:1419, 1978

60. **Holmes LB, Moser HW, Halldorsson S et al:** An Atlas of Diseases with Associated Physical Abnormalities. New York, Macmillan, 1972

61. **Holtzman NA, Welcher DW, Mellits ED:** Termination of restricted diet in children with phenylketonuria: a randomized controlled study. N Engl J Med 293:1121, 1975

62. **Horwitz AL:** The mucopolysaccharidoses: clinical and biochemical correlations. Am J Ment Defic 84:113, 1979

63. **Ingram TTS:** Soft signs. Dev Med Child Neurol 15:527, 1973

64. **Johnson RT:** Effects of viral infection on the developing nervous system. N Engl J Med 287:599, 1972

65. **Kaback MM, O'Brien JS:** Tay-Sachs: prototype for prevention of genetic disease. Hosp Practice 8:107, 1973

66. **Kinsbourne M:** Minimal brain dysfunction as a neurodevelopmental lag. Ann NY Acad Sci 205:268, 1973

67. **Knobloch H, Stevens F, Malone AF:** Manual of Developmental Diagnosis. Hagerstown, Harper & Row, 1980

68. **Kolata GB:** Prenatal diagnosis of neural tube defects. Science 209:1216, 1980

69. **Krishnamoorthy KS, Shannon DC, DeLong GR et al:** Neurologic sequelae in the survivors of neonatal intraventricular hemorrhage. Pediatrics 64:233, 1979

70. **Kugel RB, Koch R (eds):** The Pediatrician and the Child with Mental Retardation. Evanston, IL, Committee on Children with Handicaps, American Academy of Pediatrics, 1971

71. **Landesman-Dwyer S, Emanuel I:** Smoking during pregnancy. Teratology 19:119, 1979

72. **Lauritsen JG:** Genetic aspects of spontaneous abortion. Danish Med Bull 24:169, 1977

73. **Levine MD, Oberklaid F:** Hyperactivity: symptom complex or complex symptom? Am J Dis Child 134:409, 1980

74. **Levine RL:** Bilirubin: worked out years ago? Pediatrics 64:380, 1979

75. **Louick D, Boland TB:** Psychologic tests: a guide for pediatricians. Pediatr Annals 7:849, 1978

76. **MacDonald H, Tobin JO:** Congenital cytomegalovirus infection: a collaborative study on epidemiological, clinical and laboratory findings. Dev Med Child Neurol 20:471, 1978

77. **Macri JN, Haddow JE, Weiss RR:** Screening for neural tube defects in the United States: a summary of the Scarborough Conference. Am J Obstet Gynecol 133:119, 1979

78. **Magenis RE, Overton KM, Chamberlin J et al:** Parental origin of the extra chromosome in Down's syndrome. Hum Genet 37:7, 1977

79. **Mathis RK, Andres JM, Walker WA:** Liver disease in infants. Part II: Hepatic disease states. J Pediatr 90:864, 1977

80. **Mikkelsen M:** Down's syndrome at young maternal age: cytogenetical and genealogical study of eighty-one families. Ann hum Genet 31:51, 1967

81. **Mikkelsen M:** Down's syndrome: current stage of cytogenetic research. Humangenetik 12:1, 1971

82. **Miles JH, Kaback MM:** Prenatal diagnosis of hereditary disorders. Pediatr Clin North Am 25:593, 1978

83. **Miller RW:** Delayed effects occurring within the first decade after exposure of young individuals to the Hiroshima atomic bomb. Pediatrics 18:1, 1956

84. **Molnar GE, Taft LT:** Cerebral palsy. In Wortis J (ed): Mental Retardation and Developmental Disabilities, Vol V, pp 85–112. New York, Brunner/Mazel, 1973

85. **Money J, Annecillo C, Van Orman B et al:** Cytogenetics, hormones and behavior disability: comparison of XYY and XXY syndromes. Clin Genet 6:37, 1974

86. **Needleman HL, Gunnoe C, Leviton A et al:** Deficits in psychologic and classroom performance of children with elevated dentine lead levels. N Engl J Med 300:689, 1979

87. **Nelson RP, Crocker AC:** The medical care of mentally retarded persons in public residential facilities. N Engl J Med 299:1039, 1978

88. **New York State Department of Mental Hygiene, Mental Health Research Unit:** Technical Report: A Special Census of Suspected Referred Mental Retardation. Onondaga County, New York. Syracuse, Syracuse University Press, 1955

89. **Nyhan WL, Fawcett N, Ando T et al:** Response to dietary therapy in B_{12} unresponsive methylmalonic acidemia. Pediatrics 51:539, 1973

90. **Oakley GP:** Impact of prenatal diagnostic studies on disease prevention. Symposium on Developmental Disabilities, Johns Hopkins University School of Medicine, Baltimore, Maryland, June 1978

91. **Odell GB, Storey GNB, Rosenberg LA:** Studies in kernicterus. Part III. The saturation of serum proteins with bilirubin during neonatal life and its relationship to brain damage at five years. J Pediatr 76:12, 1970

92. **Palfrey JS:** Commentry: P.L. 94–142: The Education for All Handicapped Children Act. J Pediatr 97:417, 1980

93. **Papile L-A, Burstein J, Burstein R et al:** Incidence and evolution of subependymal and intraventricular hemorrhage: a study of infants with birth weights less than 1,500 gm. J Pediatr 92:529, 1978

94. **Penrose LS:** Measurement in mental deficiency. Br J Psychiatry 116:369, 1970

95. **Peters JE, Romine JS, Dykman RA:** A special neurological examination of children with learning disabilities. Dev Med Child Neurol 17:63, 1975

96. **Purpura DP:** Dendritic differentiation in human cerebral cortex: normal and aberrant developmental patterns. Adv Neurol 12:91, 1975

97. **Rabe EF:** Neurological evaluation. In Minimal Brain Dysfunction in Children, Phase Two: Educational, Medical and Health-Related Services, Appendix A, pp 69–71. Washington, DC, US Public Health Service, Publication No. 2015, 1969

98. **Race RR, Sanger R:** Quoted in Hecht F, MacFarlane JP: Mosaicism in Turner's syndrome reflects the lethality of XO. Lancet 2:1197, 1969

99. **Rapin I:** Conductive hearing loss: Effects on children's language and scholastic skills. Otitis Media and Child Development. Ann Otol Rhinol Laryngol (Suppl 60) 88(No 5, Part 2):3, 1979

100. **Rawls WE, Desmyter J, Melnick JL:** Serological diagnosis and fetal involvement in maternal rubella. JAMA 203:627, 1968

101. **Reynolds DW, Stagno S, Stubbs KG et al:** Inapparent congenital cytomegalovirus infection with elevated cord IgM levels: causal relation with auditory and mental deficiency. N Engl J Med 290:291, 1974

102. **Richardson SA:** The relation of severe malnutrition in infancy to the intelligence of school children with differing life histories. Pediatr Res 10:57, 1976

103. **Rosenberg LE:** Disorders of propionate, methylmalonate, and cobalamin metabolism. In Stanbury JB, Wyngaarden JB, Fredrickson DS (eds): The Metabolic Basis of Inherited Disease, 4th ed, pp 411–429. New York, McGraw-Hill, 1978

104. **Routh DK, Mushak P, Boone L:** A new syndrome of elevated blood lead and microcephaly. J Pediatr Psychol 4:67, 1979

105. **Rubin RA, Balow B, Fisch RO:** Neonatal serum bilirubin levels related to cognitive development at ages 4 through 7 years. J Pediatr 94:601, 1979

106. **Rugh R:** X-irradiation effects on the human fetus. J Pediatr 52:531, 1958

107. **Rutter M:** Diagnosis and definition. In Rutter M, Schlopler E (eds): Autism: A Reappraisal of Concepts and Treatment, pp 1–25. New York, Plenum Press, 1978

108. **Rutter M:** Raised lead levels and impaired cognitive/behavioral functioning: a review of the evidence. Dev Med Child Neurol 22 (Suppl)42:1–26, 1980

109. **Sabel K-G, Olegard R, Victorin L:** Remaining sequelae with modern perinatal care. Pediatrics 57:652, 1976

110. **Scheidt PC, Mellits ED, Hardy JB et al:** Toxicity to bilirubin in neonates: infant development during first year in relation to maximum neonatal serum bilirubin concentration. J Pediatr 91:292, 1977

111. **Segal S:** Disorders of galactose metabolism. In Stanbury JB, Wyngaarden JB, Fredrickson DS (eds): The Metabolic Basis of Inherited Disease, 4th ed, pp 160–181. New York, McGraw-Hill, 1978

112. **Sever JL:** Immunoglobulin determinations for the detection of perinatal infections. J Pediatr 75:1111, 1969

113. **Shaywitz SE, Cohen DJ, Shaywitz BA:** Behavior and learning difficulties in children of normal intelligence born to alcoholic mothers. J Pediatr 96:978, 1980

114. **Siegel E:** Personal Communication

115. **Siegel M:** Congenital malformations following chickenpox, measles, mumps, and hepatitis: results of a cohort study. JAMA 226:1521, 1973

116. **Singh N, Donovan CM, Hanshaw JB:** Neonatal lead intoxication in a prenatally exposed infant. J Pediatr 93:1019, 1978

117. **Smith DW:** Recognizable Patterns of Human Malformation, 2nd ed. Philadelphia, WB Saunders, 1976

118. **Smith, DW:** The fetal alcohol syndrome. Hosp Practice 14:121, 1979

119. **Smith DW, Simons FER:** Rational diagnostic evaluation of the child with mental deficiency. Am J Dis Child 129:1285, 1975

120. **Smith I, Lobascher ME, Stevenson JE et al:** Effect of stopping low-phenylalanine diet on intellectual progress of children with phenylketonuria. Brit Med J 2:723, 1978

121. **Smith I, Macartney FJ, Erdohazi M et al:** Fetal damage despite low-phenylalanine diet after conception in a phenylketonuric woman. Lancet 1:17, 1979

122. **Stangler SR, Huber CJ, Routh DK:** Screening Growth and Development of Preschool Children: a Guide for Test Selection. New York, McGraw-Hill, 1980

123. **Stehbens JA, Baker GI, Kitchell M:** Outcome at ages 1, 3, and 5 years of children born to diabetic women. Am J Obstet Gynecol 127:408, 1977

124. **Stene J, Fischer G, Stene E et al:** Paternal age effect in Down's syndrome. Ann Hum Genet 40:299, 1977

125. **Stevenson RE, Burton OM, Ferlauto GJ et al:** Hazards of oral anticoagulants during pregnancy. JAMA 243:1549, 1980

126. **Stray-Pedersen B:** Infants potentially at risk for congenital toxoplasmosis: a prospective study. Am J Dis Child 134:638, 1980

127. **Tarjan G, Wright SW, Eyman RK et al:** Natural history of mental retardation: some aspects of epidemiology. Am J Ment Defic 77:369, 1973

128. **Tatetsu S, Harada M:** Mental deficiency resulting from intoxication in the prenatal period. Adv Neurol Sci (Tokyo) 12:181, 1968

129. **Thiersch JB:** Therapeutic abortions with a folic acid antagonist, 4-aminopteroylglutamic acid, administered by the oral route. Am J Obstet Gynecol 63:1298, 1952

130. **Touwen BCL:** Examination of the Child with Minor Neurological Dysfunction, 2nd ed. Spastics International Medical Publications, Philadelphia, JB Lippincott, 1979

131. **Townsend JJ, Baringer JR, Wolinsky JS et al:** Progressive rubella panencephalitis: late onset after congenital rubella. N Engl J Med 292:990, 1975

132. **Turkel SB, Guttenberg ME, Moynes DR:** Lack of identifiable risk factors for kernicterus. Pediatrics 66:502, 1980

133. **Ueda K, Nishida Y, Oshima K et al:** Congenital rubella syndrome: correlation of gestational age at a time of maternal rubella with type of defect. J Pediatr 94:763, 1979

134. **United States Department of Health, Education and Welfare, National Institutes of Health:** Antenatal Diagnosis, rev ed: Part I. Predictors of Hereditary Disease or Congenital Defects. Washington, DC, NIH Publication No. 80–1973, 1979

135. **Vining EPG, Accardo PJ, Rubenstein JE et al:** Cerebral palsy: a pediatric developmentalist's overview. Am J Dis Child 130:643, 1976

136. **Volpe JJ:** Perinatal hypoxic–ischemic brain injury. Pediatr Clin North Am 23:383, 1976

137. **Waber DP:** Neuropsychological aspects of Turner's syndrome. Dev Med Child Neurol 21:58, 1979

138. **Warren SA:** What is wrong with mainstreaming? A comment on drastic change. Ment Retardation 17:301, 1979

139. **Werner EE, Honzik MP, Smith RS:** Prediction of intelligence and achievement at ten years from twenty months pediatric and psychologic examinations. Child Dev 39:1063, 1968

140. **Wilson J:** A developmental reflex test. In Vulpe SG: Vulpe Assessment Battery, 2nd ed, pp 335–364. Toronto, Institute on Mental Retardation, 1977

141. **Zinkus PW, Gottlieb MI:** Patterns of perceptual and academic deficits related to early chronic otitis media. Pediatrics 66:246, 1980

Learning Disorders

6

Richard J. Schain

The usual meaning of the term "*learning disorder*" refers to a child who, given an opportunity to enter into the teaching–learning process, is not learning at a rate commensurate with his intellectual abilities. The position adopted in this chapter is that a learning disorder is a clinical symptom arising from diverse and often multiple causes rather than a specific cognitive deficit affecting academic skill acquisition.

There are many social and cultural reasons why children fail to adequately take advantage of learning opportunities. It is the responsibility of the neurologic consultant to review thoroughly medical, neurologic, and psychological factors in a child with a learning problem. If this is done in an appropriate manner, parents, teachers, psychologists, and other professionals concerned with the child's learning performance will be in a better position to deal effectively with the child's educational difficulties.

NEUROLOGIC EVALUATION—HISTORY

The neurologic approach toward the child with a learning problem must contain a different emphasis than that toward a patient with conventional neurologic symptoms. It is advantageous to question parents and child separately to facilitate the free flow of confidential information.

Details of the developmental, behavioral, and school history are essential. Symptoms of importance are delayed or disordered speech, poor speech comprehension, hyperactive behavior, enuresis, pica, sleepwalking, conduct disorders, and motor difficulties in sports or home activities. The initial manifestations of the school difficulties should be ascertained. These may have been quite different from the presenting problem. Details of the child's classroom experiences will provide a more rounded picture of the child's problem.

The current grade status and academic performance should be determined to the extent possible. In particular, problems in learning should be distinguished from conduct disorders in the classroom. The presence of other behavioral problems unrelated to the classroom should be determined. Inquiry should be made into the presence of associated somatic complaints such as seizures, headaches, abdominal pains, or visual problems.

Establishing the occurrence of brain damaging events is often of key importance in determining etiologies. These include first trimester pregnancy illnesses, birth injuries or premature deliveries, neonatal illnesses, major head injuries, meningitis, encephalitis, prolonged seizures, and drug intoxications. Recurrent ear infections may be of significance.

There are few areas in child neurology in which it is more important to evaluate family circumstances. Initially, the composition of the family household should be determined. The educational history of parents and siblings should be noted along with evidence of learning problems. It is not infrequent to discover that a child's learning difficulties recapitulate the past educational experience of a parent. Parents who have surmounted classroom learning problems will usually be more tolerant of them than a parent who has always been a high achiever in the classroom.

The history of the family, along with overt disruptions or psychiatric disorders in family members, should be sensitively investigated. Any interest on the part of the physician in family dynamics may unleash a torrent of complaints and evidence of chaotic conditions in the family. Such interchange may be discomforting to the neurologic consultant but is often essential in placing a learning problem in proper perspective. A certain degree of home stability is necessary for children to function successfully in classroom environments.

The physician should inquire about medication history because this information may not always be volunteered. Dosage as well as identity of medications prescribed in the past should be determined. Inquiry into possible drug abuse habits should be made with pubertal children. This should be done separately with child and parent.

NEUROLOGIC EVALUATION— EXAMINATION

The examination of a school-age child should be approached in a circumspect manner. The white coat is best discarded in order to avoid unpleasant associations. The child may be initially engaged in conversation about an appropriate topic, perhaps the nature of the problem that has brought him to the neurologic consultant. After a relationship has been established, the child will be more inclined to cooperate for the neurologic examination. A casual and friendly demeanor should be cultivated by the examiner.

Certain aspects of the examination are of particular importance in learning disorders. These are enumerated below:

Height, weight, and head circumference plotted on standard growth curves
Inspection for evidence of unusual facial or cranial configuration
Inspection of skin for cutaneous lesions suggestive of neurocutaneous syndromes
Evaluation of mental status including recognition of thought disorders, autistic behavior, attentional difficulties, and estimation of level of intelligence
Evaluation of speech patterns
Estimation of visual and hearing abilities
Motor functions including incoordination, hypertonia, movement disorders
Screening of reading, spelling, and arithmetical skills

SPECIAL PROCEDURES

Electroencephalogram

There is much variation of opinion over the value of the routine electroencephalogram (EEG) in the diagnosis of learning disorders. Its main value is in the confirmation of the presence of atypical seizure disorders. The EEG may be helpful at times in the early recognition of brain tumors or degenerations. It provides an objective, if limited, picture of one aspect of cerebral activity that is of value in assessment of brain function. A normal EEG may be reassuring to a parent who fears that her child may have brain damage. In general, obtaining an EEG is justified in a child with a chronic learning or behavioral problem of unknown origin.

Psychometrics

A standard measure of intelligence is often helpful. The Wechsler Intelligence Scale for Children (WISC) is most often used. Analysis of subtest scores may be of interest but rarely establishes the origin of the learning problem. The value of the WISC lies in determining the child's current level of cognitive functioning.

The Bender Gestalt and Frostig tests are instruments used to assess visual perceptual and motor skills. Poor performance of perceptual motor tasks frequently is associated with but not necessarily etiologically related to learning difficulties. The translation of performance "profiles" into educational remediation is a task for the special educator.

Pure tone audiometry, measures of visual or auditory acuity, chromosomal studies, or urine screening for metabolic defects may be indicated in selected cases. A CT scan is indicated if a structural lesion is suspected.

BRAIN DAMAGE SYNDROMES

There are a number of brain damage syndromes with which learning disorders are frequently associated. Recognition of the presence of these disorders along with appropriate management may greatly aid the child in the task of classroom adjustment.

CEREBRAL PALSIES

By definition, the presence of a cerebral palsy syndrome indicates the presence of brain damage. One of the most important aspects of cerebral palsy is that affected children are often multiply handicapped. Learning problems are common in children with cerebral palsy.[17] Visual, hearing, and speech problems are additional complicating factors found in many of these children.

Borderline forms of cerebral palsy present greater difficulties with diagnosis than overt forms. Clumsiness, involuntary movements, gait disturbances, and muscular hypertonia are findings that often give rise to suspicions of cerebral palsy. It must be remembered that there is a wide variety of normal variations of motor behaviors in young children. The diagnosis of cerebral palsy should be made only in the presence of unequivocal evidence of motor, coordination, or muscle tone abnormalities.

The presence of cerebral palsy does not in itself automatically account for a learning disorder in an affected child. Associated problems involving vision, hearing, or speech may be interfering with the learning process. Some degree of mental retardation is commonly but not invariably found in cerebral palsied children. Frank motor deficits may produce serious psychological as well as physical impediments to classroom adjustment. Finally, problems in family attitudes toward a child may interfere with the child's motivation to function in a classroom setting. It should be remembered that handicapped children are more vulnerable than normal children to difficulties in family relationships.

EPILEPSY

A substantial number, perhaps the majority, of children with chronic seizure disorders exhibit significant learning problems.[16,51] The occurrence of seizures often overshadows the presence of serious behavioral and learning problems. It is important for the neurologist not to permit treatment programs to narrowly focus on anticonvulsant therapy but also to encourage a comprehensive management approach that includes evaluation of school performance.[26]

There are three main reasons why children with epilepsy often manifest learning disorders. First, the frequent occurrence of seizures tends to interfere with mental processes and impair learning. Focal spike discharges from the left hemisphere are most likely to be associated with learning problems.[44] Second, anticonvulsant agents, especially those with strong sedative properties such as phenobarbital and primidone, diminish alertness and attentive abilities.[34,35] Ethosuximide and clonazepam are also anticonvulsants that tend to produce sedation in therapeutic doses. Lastly, psychological pressures produced by exaggerated reactions to seizures often result in the epileptic child withdrawing from classroom activities. The neurologic consultant should act whenever possible against the tendency toward emotional isolation that occurs in children with epilepsy. This may include support of the child's participation in most sport and exercise activities and encouragement of the school to permit the child to attend classes in spite of occasional seizures.[9a] The practice of immediately sending a child home after a seizure is not justified in the majority of cases.

MENTAL RETARDATION

This term refers to a condition of global developmental delay and diminished intelligence that leads to adaptive difficulties in social life. By convention, intelligence quotients obtained with a standard measure of intelligence that are under 70 are usually regarded as indicating mental retardation. Scores of 70 to 84 may be considered in the borderline range. However, the diagnosis of mental retardation cannot be based on psychometric testing alone but must also include consideration of developmental, social, and cultural factors.

Many parents of children with mild but global retardation syndromes prefer to regard their children as having specific learning disabilities. Some retarded children are trained in verbal skills far beyond their actual abilities in judgment and performance. Excessive pressure for academic achievement often leads to reactive behavioral disturbances and psychogenic disorders such as tics or compulsive verbosity.

The developmental history of retarded children generally yields evidence of delayed motor and language development. Persistent inability to develop peer relationships is suggestive of mental retardation. Conversation with a child will often suggest the presence of a lag in the acquisition of mental abilities.

Administration of one of the standard psychometric measures of intelligence is essential if mental retardation is suspected. The most commonly used measure is the Wechsler Intelligence Scale for Children (WISC), which has the virtue of division into verbal and performance sections. In spite of the undeniable influence of cultural and environmental factors upon test performance, intelligence tests are valuable aids to the clinician and usually the only objective measure of mental abilities.

The diagnosis of mental retardation should be based upon a judicious consideration of developmental and historical information, data from psychometrics and the neurologic examination, and consideration of familial and cultural factors. If uncertainty exists, diagnosis should be delayed pending further evaluation. It is important, however, to distinguish the child with a mild global retardation syndrome from one with a selective learning disorder who is otherwise capable of functioning in a normal manner.

PROGRESSIVE NEUROLOGIC DISORDERS

There are degenerative disorders of the brain in which the onset of symptoms is first noted as disturbances in classroom performance.

These disorders are rare but their recognition is an important responsibility of the neurologic consultant. Slow but steady progression of symptoms is the hallmark of a degenerative disorder. Genetic counseling is essential for the family of affected children. Brain degenerations are reviewed elsewhere (Chapter 9). This discussion will be limited to early manifestations of certain degenerative disorders that may present as learning problems.

Huntington's Disease, one of the common dementias, may manifest itself by clumsiness, emotional lability, and restlessness for years before the presence of an organic disorder is recognized. Onset of symptoms in childhood is a frequent occurrence with difficulties noted principally in classroom behavior. In the absence of a family history, establishment of the diagnosis may require prolonged observation. Eventually the appearance of characteristic motor disturbances and muscular hypertonia will clarify the clinical picture.

Early recognition of Wilson's Disease (hepatolenticular degeneration) is especially important because of the value of dietary and drug therapy in all stages of the disease. Intellectual or emotional disturbances may be the first manifestations of this disease. Muscle rigidity, masklike facies, and movement disorders are later manifestations of Wilson's Disease.

The first symptoms of subacute sclerosing panencephalitis (SSPE) may be mild intellectual impairment and coordination difficulties. After a variable time period, but usually within one year, myoclonic seizures and evident dementia make clear the organic basis of the disorder.

Hemispheric brain tumors in children may produce subtle signs of impaired cortical functions for years prior to the appearance of florid symptoms. Listlessness, indifference, and a tendency to withdraw from group activities are characteristic behavioral changes. The presence of persistent, severe headaches in children with recent personality alterations should alert the examiner to a possible brain tumor. Repeated examination of the optic discs should not be neglected in children with persistent headaches. The occurrence of a seizure may be the first obvious sign of a structural lesion.

PSYCHIATRIC DISORDERS

A number of psychiatric disorders may be first recognized through deterioration of learning performance in the classroom. Recognition of any of these problems is an indication for referral to a psychiatrist.

DRUG ABUSE

An older child or adolescent who manifests unexplained evidence of mental deterioration with alteration of prior personality patterns may be self-administering drugs. Failure to recognize drug abuse in a patient will obviously delay appropriate therapeutic measures.

The chronic user of barbiturates seems sluggish and slow of speech, and exhibits poor memory and faulty judgment. Specific neurologic signs include dysarthria, nystagmus, tremor, vertigo, and incoordination. Sudden withdrawal may result in seizures.

Individuals who ingest large doses of amphetamines or related stimulants may manifest hallucinations that are difficult to distinguish from schizophrenic reactions. Continuous chewing movements, lip licking, and teeth grinding occur in amphetamine addiction.

Phencyclamine (PCP) usage may result in circumscribed but profound memory deficits. Violent mood swings as well as memory difficulties are seen in PCP and lysergic acid diethylamide (LSD) users. Prolonged psychotic reactions can occur in certain cases. The long-term consequences of recurrent usage of major hallucinogens have not been carefully evaluated.

Marijuana usage is widespread at even the elementary school level. Recurrent usage may be associated with failing school work for a variety of reasons. The effect of prolonged marijuana usage on mental abilities is an unsettled issue.

The screening of urine for toxic compounds should be performed if there is persistent suspicion of drug abuse.

SCHOOL PHOBIA

Children who refuse to attend school are usually seen by the neurologic consultant because of somatic complaints such as recurrent headaches, dizziness, syncopal episodes, abdominal pains, or visual symptoms. The information that the child is not attending school may not be provided unless the physician specifically asks about school attendance. The diagnosis becomes evident when it is established that symptoms only occur when pressure is placed upon the child to go to school. It is often difficult to determine if the child is consciously feigning the symptoms or if they represent an unconscious reaction to the stress of leaving home for school.

There is evidence that an important aspect of many school phobias is separation anxiety provoked by leaving the mother or other caretaker rather than any special problem with school.[37] The symptom is usually observed in elementary school children. Adolescents manifesting school phobia should be considered as exhibiting a severe psychiatric disturbance.

CHILDHOOD AUTISM

Children with childhood autism manifest early personality and behavioral disturbances characterized by lack of affect, stereotyped activities, and language deficits. There may be continuous activity that superficially resembles the behavior of severely hyperactive children but differs from the latter condition in that the autistic child is deficient in the ability to form relationships. Many of these children become severely retarded functionally whereas others develop sufficient school and language abilities to adapt to classroom situations. Hyperlexia or precocious mathematical skills can occur in certain autistic children without the judgment or comprehension to use theseskills effectively.[52]

It has been suggested that autism should be regarded as a "learning disability" involving the ability to form interpersonal relationships.[26] There is evidence that the symptoms of autistic children are associated with global perceptual disturbances.[26]

The odd behavior of autistic children may perplex teachers and result in referral for suspected neurologic disease or minimal brain dysfunction. Little can be done to alter the personality of autistic children. However, recognition of the underlying syndrome can result in more realistic expectations of the child. Seizures commonly occur in the course of autistic disorders.

CHILDHOOD HYPERACTIVITY (MINIMAL BRAIN DYSFUNCTION, ATTENTION DEFICIT DISORDER)

CLINICAL PICTURE

Hyperactivity is a behavioral disorder commonly found in children with learning problems. It is often the presence of a hyperactive behavior disorder that results in referral of a child to a physician because it is a more disruptive symptom than the failure to learn on the part of a child. Hyperactive children are unable to sit still and to concentrate. Their hyperactivity may result in classroom disturbances that are often highly distressing to the teacher. Incessant shifts of attention and wandering activity interfere with the child's own performance as well as that of classmates. Other personality traits often found in hyperactive children are explosive behavioral outbursts, negativistic behavior, and unpredictable mood changes. These behavioral patterns are variable and may be seen only in certain settings such as classrooms or other group activities. The Conners rating scale is a widely used measure for quantifying the behavioral disturbance seen in hyperactive children.[42]

Hyperactive behavior problems usually are noted in prepubertal children; after puberty the problem may disappear, to be transformed into learning or conduct disorders. There is a male preponderance in hyperactive children as high as 90%. Hyperactivity appearing in adolescence or as a sudden personality change should prompt consideration of specific organic etiologies such as hyperthyroidism or Sydenham's Chorea.

Recently, emphasis has been placed on the difficulty of sustaining attention that is exhibited by hyperactive children. The third edition of the American Psychiatric Association Manual of Mental Disorders (DSM-III) has adopted the term *attention deficit disorder* to include children previously labeled as hyperactive or as having minimal brain dysfunction, minimal brain damage, and so forth. Attention deficits profoundly influence a child's capacity to conform to group activities, develop motor and perceptual skills, and to acquire basic learning abilities such as reading and writing.

PATHOGENESIS

Brain Damage

Like learning disorders, the symptom of hyperactivity may occur in various clinical contexts. Brain damaged children may exhibit severe and persistent behavior problems. The concept of a brain damage behavioral syndrome gained popularity in the 1920s when it was recognized that children recovering from epidemic encephalitis lethargica often exhibited personality changes characterized by restlessness, irritability, distractibility, and affective disturbances.[10] Choreiform movements, tremors, and tics were the motor accompaniments of this postencephalitic behavior disorder. Subsequently, it was recognized that a wide variety of brain damaging events could lead to this behavioral syndrome. A distinction was made between behavior disorders following brain damage and the global intellectual deficit found in primary mental retardation syndromes.[45] Encephalitis, meningitis, postnatal brain injuries, cerebrovascular accidents, lead encephalopathy, and status epilepticus are some of the brain damaging events that may lead to hyperactive behavior disorders.

The concept of a brain damage behavioral syndrome later evolved into the notion that many hyperactive children, although not presenting with evidence of frank brain damage, exhibit constellations of minor, borderline or soft neurologic signs that suggest the presence of minimal brain dysfunction. The history of the development of this concept has been reviewed elsewhere.[34]

Environmental Factors

Labeling a child as hyperactive implies that he adapts poorly to his environment. Some environments are so ill-suited for children that some type of abnormal response may be expected. A child who is anxious and fearful because of adverse family or school circumstances will not be able to learn to curtail impulsive behavior and to adapt to classroom requirements. Many hyperactive children live in seriously disturbed home environments.

The frequency with which classroom hyperactivity and learning disorders occur in disadvantaged populations has produced feelings that the needs of minority children are concealed by applying labels that imply neurologic dysfunction. There can be little doubt that social and economic circumstances may influence motivation in ways that result in hyperactive behavior in the classroom. The physician should be cautious in attributing hyperactivity to intrinsic causes in children from minority cultures or disadvantaged environments. However, intrinsic factors and adverse environments may both contribute to the genesis of a hyperactive behavior disorder. This is probably often the case.

Developmental Hyperactivity

The majority of hyperactive children brought to a physician will not exhibit any clear evidence of brain damage by history or physical examination. Attention was first focussed by the Bakwins on the developmental nature of hyperactivity in many children.[1] The essential element of developmental hyperactivity is its presence dating from early life in a child who is otherwise mentally and neurologically intact.[48] Parents may regard restless, inquisitive behavior of their child as a sign of a vigorous personality, but this trait becomes a handicap for a child expected to conform to usual classroom restrictions.

The classic study of Thomas, Chess, and Birch has described how hyperactivity may be a temperamental trait, constitutional in origin and evident during the earliest months of infancy.[46] Hyperactive children normally manifest high activity levels with relative delay in the development of impulse control. When this personality trait is incompatible with the way in which home or classroom activities are organized, symptoms of adjustment problems arise. There is a deleterious effect on the social

or academic progress of the child. The anatomic or biochemical basis of hyperactivity as a temperamental trait is unknown. Little is to be gained by labeling such children as cases of minimal brain dysfunction. In spite of disclaimers in the literature, this expression implies a morbid disorder of the brain to most parents and school personnel.

DEVELOPMENTAL DYSLEXIA

Neurologists have long been interested in the developmental basis of specific reading disorders of childhood. The definition of *developmental dyslexia* formulated by the World Federation of Neurology in 1968 is as follows: "A disorder manifested by difficulty in learning to read despite conventional instruction, adequate intelligence and sociocultural opportunity. It is dependent upon fundamental cognitive disabilities which are frequently of constitutional origin."[9]

Characteristic spelling and handwriting errors have been regarded as the central sign of dyslexia. These include persistent reversals of groups of letters (e.g., god for dog, was for saw) and rotations of individual letters into mirror opposite letters (e.g., d and b, p and q). Associated speech disturbances commonly occur. Familial manifestations of dyslexia are well documented from twin and pedigree studies.[12]

It has been suggested that some forms of dyslexia may represent a developmental Gerstmann Syndrome (dysgraphia, dyscalculia, right–left disorientation, finger agnosia).[15,20] Boder has divided dyslexia into three subgroups: dysphonetic, dyseidetic and a combination of both.[3] The value of such formulations for educational therapy has not yet been established.

The problem of dyslexia as a neurologic entity lies in the lack of objective signs of brain dysfunction and the assumption, often poorly founded, of adequate opportunity for classroom learning. The term *dyslexia* has little prognostic or therapeutic implications beyond indicating reading and spelling difficulties. There is an increasing tendency to abandon its use in favor of expressions that are less likely to generate assumptions of organic disorder.

COGNITIVE STYLES

The concept of cognitive styles has been an important development in educational therapy.[19] It refers to individual differences or styles by which children attend to environmental stimuli and process sensory input. Certain constructs have been elaborated to define cognitive styles in children. The impulsivity–reflection construct developed by Kagan and associates refers to the tendency of some children to respond rapidly to novel situations (impulsive style) and of others to respond deliberately (reflective style).[18] Hyperactive children demonstrate an impulsive style of responding although this does not imply a disordered form of cognition and may be a more appropriate response in certain situations.

Another dimension of cognition is the global–analytic construct evolved by Witkin.[53] Global modes of perception are characterized by holistic, relational approaches to information acquisition, whereas analytic modes involve verbal, categorizing styles of learning. Overall, the analytic style of learning tends to be more successful with conventional classroom tasks although global styles may be more relevant in many life situations. There is a widespread belief among educators that educational programs should be individualized so as to be congruent with a child's cognitive style. However, application of this concept to actual educational practice has been limited.

Analytic styles of learning have been attributed to left cerebral hemisphere dominance and global styles to right hemisphere dominance.[24] Emphasis on "right brain" personality attributes is stylish at the time of this writing. However, such neurologic assignments add little to the fundamental problem of the relationship of cognitive style to learning and are best avoided when dealing with a child exhibiting an essentially educational problem.

MANAGEMENT OF LEARNING DISORDERS

The problem of assisting a child with a learning disorder requires that the physician be oriented toward family and community processes. Insofar as a neurologic consultant wishes to be of help to the child and his family, he must go beyond simple clarification of neurologic issues and develop the attitudes of a family-oriented physician. This may lead him far afield from neurologic diagnosis but he will be strengthened by recollecting that helping the patient in all aspects of life is in the oldest tradition of Hippocratic medicine. In addition, the neurologic consultant is in a better position than many others to evaluate the varied strands leading to a learning problem and to help the parents to develop a productive approach to the problem.

PARENT COUNSELING

The first task of the physician is to explain what has been learned from his evaluation. If there is no evidence of overt neurologic deficits, this should be clearly stated. EEG findings should be described to the parents. It can be explained that borderline EEG abnormalities are of no clinical relevance. If the child is of normal intelligence, this should be stated even if it appears self-evident. Diagnostic terms that may have been applied to the child such as *dyslexia, perceptual deficit, minimal brain dysfunction, fine motor coordination*, and so on should be discussed. The essentially descriptive nature of such terminology should be emphasized.

Attention to principles of child rearing are of special importance in counseling families of children with learning disorders. The initial interview with the parents should have as a primary goal the elucidation of the social biography of the child. This may bring out environmental factors that have an important role in the learning disorder. This approach will uncover at different times all of the ills of society that adversely affect children: hostile family separations, economic difficulties, disruptive family relocations, overbearing siblings or grandparents, angry or depressed parents, inadequate educational environments, minority problems, and rigid family or school attitudes. The physician will be able to solve few of these problems but helping the family to face them directly and consider their impact upon the child may have unforeseen benefits. Frank discussion of such issues may lead a family to mobilize resources in a more effective manner than had previously been the case.

If the psychological climate of the family appears to be seriously disturbed, the examiner should consider referral to a family-oriented therapist. He should be aware that family psychological systems may operate to the detriment of one family member.[54] Such systems may be relatively subtle but may undermine a child's ability to develop a receptive psychic state for learning. Psychological intervention may need to be focused on the disturbed family interaction rather than exclusively on the symptomatic child.

It is often helpful to spend time discussing the learning problem with the child himself. The child is usually treated as a passive object of numerous test procedures with little regard to his own thoughts and fears about the meaning of these tests. The examiner should reassure the child that there is usually no medical problem present and, when appropriate, that there is nothing wrong with his brain.

There are a number of conventional instructions that may be helpful in the management of the hyperactive child. A consistent daily routine should be adhered to and home activities should be relatively well structured. Hyperactive children do not easily tolerate frequent variations in daily activities. Firmness and consistency should be stressed but uncontrolled punitive reactions of parents should be avoided. Rewards for good behavior and restrictions for bad behavior (e.g., time out in an isolated area) should be prompt and without excessive lecturing of the child. Parents should be alert to signs of fatigue or excessive stimulation. Overstimulation before bedtime is especially to be avoided. A room of one's own is desirable for any child but may be particularly important for one with a hyperactive behavior problem. Much will depend upon the parent's own mental equilibrium and ability to tolerate the behavior of a restless child.

EDUCATIONAL CONSIDERATIONS

Few physicians possess the knowledge of school systems required to make specific recommendations about educational placement of a child with a learning problem. It is best for the physician to review options with parents and to refer them elsewhere for educational advice when necessary.

Individual tutorial instruction offers the most flexible means of supplementing classroom activities. A skilled tutor may do a great deal to increase a child's motivation for learning. Parents are usually poor tutors. Parents should be advised to avoid the tutorial role because it may conflict with the parental role and adversely affect the parent–child relationship.

Specialized resources or programs within many schools offer special assistance to children with learning problems. A major emphasis for handicapped children at the present time is *mainstreaming*, that is, maintaining children with learning problems in regular classes, with supplemental assistance. The parent is the child's most important advocate with respect to special instruction. The physician may provide advice but should avoid attempting to give directives to school personnel.

There has been a great increase in the number of private schools for children with learning problems. Some of these are based upon unproven theories of selective training of perceptual or motor deficits purportedly present in learning disabled children. Evaluation of private facilities usually reveals that a common denominator is a markedly reduced pupil–teacher ratio compared to public or parochial schools. Large classes often result in rejects from the learning–teaching process so that special schools are beneficial for children incapable of adapting to usual class sizes. Physicians who are asked about the advisability of transferring a child to a special school must consider their knowledge of the school, the severity of the problem, the financial impact upon the family, and the impact of educationally segregating the child. The decision is rarely obvious and the ultimate responsibility must be left with the parents.

STIMULANT DRUGS AND HYPERACTIVE BEHAVIOR

In 1937, Charles Bradley reported in a now classic paper that many children with behavioral disturbances manifested improvement of behavior following daily administration of amphetamine.[4] Since that time it has been repeatedly noted that children with hyperactive behavior frequently exhibit both improvement of attention span and calmer behavior when receiving stimulant drugs.[2]

Effects and Mode of Action

The locus of action of stimulants in the treatment of hyperactivity is entirely in the realm of speculation. Since the reticular formation of the brain is an area intimately involved in attentional mechanisms, interest has been focused on reticular arousal and cortical inhibition as possible physiological loci of effects of stimulants in hyperactivity.[32] Abnormal catecholamine metabolism has been reported in children with minimal brain dysfunction, providing a possible biochemical substrate for the action of stimulants.[38,40] However, there is no convincing evidence presently available that establishes a selective effect of stimulants on neurophysiological systems in hyperactive children. The justification for their use lies exclusively on empirical clinical grounds.

The key behavioral aspect of the stimulant drug effect is in the improvement of the ability to sustain attention.[5] Children become calmer, more attentive, and easier to handle in group situations. Speech and handwriting may improve in clarity.[21,33] Classroom teachers are relieved by the change in behavior that permits them to work with the child. This is particularly true of children with inherently good cognitive abilities that have been concealed because of hyperactive behavior.

Clinical Use

There is great variation of attitudes toward the use of stimulant drugs in the treatment of hyperactivity. Many psychiatrists use stimulants as a central part of the treatment program for indefinite time periods. Some clinicians are philosophically opposed to the use of such agents in children.[43] The issue is essentially one of use of drugs for personality alteration for the purpose of better adaptation in the home or classroom.

It should be stressed that the numerous short-term studies demonstrating behavioral improvement from stimulants are not matched by evidence of long-term benefit in academic performance or social development.[29,47,50] The greatest improvement in behavior of children receiving stimulants is seen during the early months of treatment. Effects of medication tend to lessen with prolonged therapy even though rebound phenomena may occur upon sudden withdrawal of drugs.[6] It is the writer's view that stimulant drugs should be used only as part of a short-term crisis intervention in order to deal with the severe maladaptive situations in which hyperactive children are often found. However, continuation of drugs for prolonged time periods may set into motion a subtle dependence on these agents for adjustment of the child to his social milieu.

Virtually all of the evidence supporting use of stimulants is based on studies of children 6 years to 12 years of age. Use of stimulants in preschoolers is not likely to result in behavioral improvement.[36] In older children hyperactive behavior usually gradually subsides after puberty. Nevertheless, administration of stimulants to adolescents has been advocated in order to improve ability to attend to learning tasks.[31] Perhaps a more relevant objection to the use of stimulants in adolescence is that teenagers resent compulsory medication and compliance is difficult to obtain.

The stimulants most often used for treatment of hyperactivity are methylphenidate (Ritalin) and dextroamphetamine (Dexedrine). There is some evidence that the former is preferable because of fewer side-effects.[23] Careful adjustment of dosage is essential in the use of stimulants. A common error is to prescribe a single dose and then judge results. The range of dosage for methylphenidate is 0.3 mg/kg per day to 1.0 mg/kg per day in one or two divided doses. Higher doses may produce undesired apathetic behavior (the "zombie" effect). The dosage range of dextroamphetamine is 0.2 mg/kg per day to 0.5 mg/kg per day.

Onset of stimulant drug action is rapid, appearing within an hour. These agents tend not to accumulate in tissues which leads to a rapid disappearance of drug effects (4 hours–6 hours). If hyperactivity recurs before the end of the day, a noon dosage can be added. Later doses should be avoided because of interference with sleep. Once an effective dose is reached, regular administration of the drug is recommended. In some situations, it may be acceptable to withhold medications during weekends or school holidays.

Although behavioral responses are usually used for dose adjustment, there is evidence that optimal learning performance occurs at doses much lower than those used for behavioral improvement.[41,42] In general, clinicians tend to use higher doses of psychopharmacologic agents than are necessary.[49] It is probably best to use lower dosage levels, which do not excessively reduce drive and activity.

As previously stated, it is the writer's opinion that discontinuation of stimulants should be attempted after several months in order to avoid development of dependence on the drug for social acceptance. This should be done gradually to minimize rebound behavioral effects that result in parental pressures for drug resumption. Many children will continue to exhibit behavioral improvement after discontinuation of stimulants.[6]

Adverse Effects

There are contradictory reports of stimulants suppressing or not suppressing linear growth.[25,30] If prolonged administration of stimulants is undertaken, height and weight increases should be regularly followed on growth curves. It is also advisable to monitor heart rate and blood pressure during administration of these agents.

Abdominal discomfort may be a minor adverse effect of stimulant drugs. This can be counteracted by giving medications with breakfast. Anorexia or insomnia are rarely major problems if dose schedules are appropriate.

The main adverse effect of stimulant agents is personality change characterized by social withdrawal. It has been described as zombielike behavior. This symptom may occur at any dose but is more commonly noted in higher doses, over 1 mg/kg per day. Methylphenidate hallucinosis has been reported.[22] Occasionally, stimulants may aggravate hyperactivity. Reduction or withdrawal of medication is mandatory if these types of adverse behavioral reactions occur.

OTHER PSYCHOTROPIC DRUGS

Tricyclic agents have been shown to exert beneficial effects in hyperactive behavior disorders.[28] Imipramine (Tofranil) is the most commonly used tricyclic agent. Dosage range is 10 mg to 150 mg daily given in two divided doses. Blood pressure should be routinely monitored.

Magnesium pemoline (Cylert) is a stimulant with a slower onset of action but longer-lasting effects. Its tendency to accumulate in tissues makes the issue of side-effects more worrisome than with shorter-acting stimulants. Long-term studies of the use of this drug are not available.

Phenothiazines have been used in the treatment of hyperactivity. Thioridizine (Mellaril) is the preferred agent. Doses over 1.0 mg/kg per day are often used but are likely to cause drowsiness and loss of alertness. There is evidence that prolonged use of phenothiazines depresses cognitive abilities in children.[14]

Phenobarbital is contraindicated in children with hyperactivity because of its notorious tendency to exacerbate this condition. If a seizure disorder is present in a hyperactive child, some other anticonvulsant should be used. In general, phenobarbital and its close chemical relative primidone (Mysoline) tend to aggravate behavioral and learning problems in school-age children.

OTHER THERAPIES

Training Programs

The concept that training in activities not specifically directed toward the learning process will improve learning has yet to be convincingly established. This applies to patterning, optometric programs, sensory integrative therapy, and perceptual training. Many training programs provide individual attention and establish relationships that are beneficial to the child's self-image and consequently may improve his performance in areas of weakness. However, these often require expenditure of time, energy, and resources that might be better directed specifically toward educational remediation.

Nutritional Programs

A nutritionally adequate diet is important for mental and physical development of children. Children who are hungry or malnourished are unable to attend to academic tasks. Beyond these basic generalizations, there is no scientific basis for recommending special diets to children with learning disorders. Megavitamin therapy (massive multivitamin dosage) has been used in the treatment of schizophrenia, autism, and learning disabilities.[8] Evidence for its value is entirely anecdotal.[39] The same is true for dietary treatment of presumed hypoglycemia in the absence of supporting laboratory data.

Feingold has asserted that the ingestion of artificial food additives is an important factor in the genesis of hyperactivity.[11] Diets eliminating food additives require major changes in the eating habits of families. The inconclusive evidence presently available does not justify widespread recommendation of the Feingold diet.[7,13]

REFERENCES

1. **Bakwin H, Bakwin RM:** Behavior Disorders in Children, 4th ed. Philadelphia, WB Saunders, 1972
2. **Barkley RA:** A review of stimulant drug research with hyperactive children. J Child Psychol Psychiat 18:137, 1977
3. **Boder E:** Developmental dyslexia: a diagnostic approach based on three atypical reading–spelling patterns. Dev Med Child Neurol 15:663, 1973
4. **Bradley C:** The behavior of children receiving benzedrine. Am J Psychiatry 94:577, 1937
5. **Charles L, Schain RJ, Zelniker T et al:** Effects of methylphenidate on hyperactive children's ability to sustain attention. Pediatrics 64:412, 1979
6. **Charles L, Schain R, Guthrie D:** Long-term use and discontinuation of methylphenidate with hyperactive children. Dev Med Child Neurol 21:758, 1979
7. **Connors CK, Gayett CH, Southeick DA et al:** Food additives and hyperkinesis: a controlled double-blind study. Pediatrics 58:154, 1976
8. **Cott A:** Orthomolecular approach to the treatment of learning disabilities. Schizophrenia 3:95, 1971
9. **Critchley M:** The Dyslexic Child, 2nd ed, p 26. Springfield, Illinois, Charles C Thomas, 1970
9a. **Dreisbach M, Ballard M, Russo DC et al:** Educational intervention for children with epilepsy: A challenge for collaborative service delivery. J Spec Ed 16:112, 1982
10. **Ebaugh FG:** Neuropsychiatric sequelae of acute epidemic encephalitis. Amer J Dis Child 25:89, 1923
11. **Feingold B, German DF, Braham RM et al:** Adverse reaction to food additives. Presented at the annual convention of the American Medical Association, New York, June, 1973
12. **Hallgren B:** Specific dyslexia (congenital word blindness). A clinical and genetic study. Acta Psychiatr et Neurologica Scand (Suppl)65:1, 1950
13. **Harley JP, Ray RS, Tomasi L et al:** Hyperkinesis and food additives: testing the Feingold Hypothesis. Pediatrics 61:818, 1978
14. **Helper MM, Wilcott RC, Garfield SL:** Effects of chlorpromazine on learning and related processes in emotionally disturbed children. J Consult Psychol 27:1, 1963
15. **Hermann K, Norrie E:** Is congenital word-blindness a hereditary type of Gerstmann syndrome? Psychiatr Neurol 136:59, 1958
16. **Holdsworth L, Whitmore K:** A study of children with epilepsy attending ordinary schools. Part I. Their seizure patterns, progress and behavior in school. Dev Med Child Neurol 16:746, 1974
17. **Holt KS, Reynell JK:** Assessment of Cerebral Palsy. Part II. Vision, Hearing, Speech, Language, Communication and Psychological Functioning. London, Lloyd-Luke, 1967
18. **Kagan J:** Impulsive and reflective children; significance of conceptual tempo. In Krumboltz JD (ed): Learning and the Educational Process, pp 609–628. Chicago, Rand McNally, 1965
19. **Keogh BK:** Perceptual and cognitive styles: implications for special education. J Spec Ed 1:83, 1973
20. **Kinsbourne M, Warrington E:** Developmental factors in reading the writing backwardness. Br J Psychol 54:145, 1963
21. **Lerer RJ, Lerer MP, Artner J:** The effects of methylphenidate on the handwriting of children with minimal brain dysfunction. J Pediatr 91:127, 1977
22. **Lucas A, Weiss M:** Methylphenidate hallucinosis. J Am Med Assoc 217:1079, 1971
23. **Millichap JG:** Drugs in management of minimal brain dysfunction. Ann NY Acad Sci 205:321, 1973
24. **Milner B:** Interhemispheric differences in the localization of psychological processes in man. Br Med Bull 27:272, 1971
25. **Oettinger L Jr, Majovski LV, Gauch RR:** Maturation and growth in children with MBD/LD before and after treatment with stimulant drugs. In Oettinger L Jr (ed): The Psychologist, the School, and the Child with MBD/LD. New York, Grune & Stratton, 1978
26. **Ornitz EM, Ritvo ER:** Perceptual inconsistency in early infantile autism. Arch Gen Psychiatry 18:76, 1968
27. **Paine RS, Werry JS, Quay HC:** A study of minimal brain dysfunction. Dev Med Child Neurol 10:505, 1968
28. **Rapoport JL, Quinn PO, Bradbard G et al:** Imipramine and methylphenidate treatments of hyperactive boys. Arch Gen Psychiatry 10:789, 1974

29. **Riddle KD, Rapoport JL:** A 2-year followup of 72 hyperactive boys: classroom behavior and peer acceptance. J Nerv Ment Dis 162:126, 1976

30. **Safer DJ, Allen RP:** Factors influencing the suppressant effects of two stimulant drugs on the growth of hyperactive children. Pediatrics 51:660, 1973

31. **Safer DJ, Allen RP:** Stimulant drug treatment of hyperactive adolescents. Dis Nerv Syst 36:454, 1975

32. **Satterfield JH, Cantwell DP, Lesser LI et al:** Physiological studies of the hyperkinetic child: Part I. Amer J Psychiatry 128(11):1418, 1972

33. **Schain RJ, Reynard CL:** Observations on effects of a central stimulant drug (methylphenidate) in children with hyperactive behavior. Pediatrics 55:709, 1975

34. **Schain RJ:** Neurology of Childhood Learning Disorders, 2nd ed. Baltimore, Williams & Wilkins, 1977

35. **Schain RJ, Ward J, Guthrie D:** Carbamazepine as an anticonvulsant in children. Neurology 27:476, 1977

36. **Schleifer M, Weiss G, Cohen N et al:** Hyperactivity in preschoolers and the effect of methylphenidate. Am J Orthopsychiatry 45:38, 1975

37. **Schmitt BD:** School phobia—the great imitator: a pediatrician's viewpoint. Pediatrics 48:433, 1971

38. **Shaywitz BA, Cohen DJ, Bowers MB:** CSF monoamine metabolites in children with minimal brain dysfunction: Evidence for alteration of brain dopamine. J Pediatr 90:67, 1977

39. **Silver LB:** Acceptable and controversial approaches to treating the child with learning disabilities. Pediatrics 55:406, 1975

40. **Snyder SH, Meyerhoff JL:** How amphetamine acts in minimal brain dysfunction. Ann NY Acad Sci 205:310, 1973

41. **Sprague RL, Sleator EK:** Effects of psychopharmacologic agents on learning disorders. Pediatr Clin North Am 20:719, 1973

42. **Sprague RL, Sleator EK:** Methylphenidate in hyperkinetic children: Differences in dose effects on learning and social behavior. Science 198:1274, 1978

43. **Sroufe LA, Stewart MA:** Treating problem children with stimulant drugs. New Engl J Med 289:407, 1973

44. **Stores G, Hart J:** Reading skills of children with generalized or focal epilepsy attending ordinary school. Dev Med Child Neurol 18:705, 1976

45. **Strauss AA, Lehtinen LE:** Psychopathology and Education of the Brain-injured Child. New York, Grune & Stratton, 1947

46. **Thomas A, Chess S, Birch EG:** Temperament and Behavior Disorders in Children. New York, New York University Press, 1968

47. **Weiss G, Kruger E, Danielson V et al:** Effects of long-term treatment of hyperactive children with methylphenidate. Can Med Assoc J 112:159, 1975

48. **Werry JS:** Developmental hyperactivity. Pediatr Clin N Am 14:581, 1968

49. **Werry JS, Aman MG:** Methylphenidate and haloperidol in children. Arch Gen Psychiatry 32:790, 1975

50. **Walen CK, Henker B:** Psychostimulants and children: a review and analysis. Psychol Bull 83:1113, 1976

51. **Whitehouse D:** Behavior and learning problems in epileptic children. Behav Neuropsychiatry 7:23, 1976

52. **Wing J (ed):** Early Childhood Autism: Clinical Educational and Social Aspects 2nd ed. London, Pergamon Press, 1976

53. **Witkin A:** Individual differences in case of perception of embedded figures. J Pers 19:1, 1950

54. **Zuk GH, Boszormenyi-Nagy I:** Family Therapy and Disturbed Families. Palo Alto, Science and Behavior Books, 1967

Paroxysmal Disorders

7

Thomas W. Farmer
Robert S. Greenwood

SEIZURES AND EPILEPSY

DEFINITIONS

Seizures are one of the most common neurologic problems in childhood, perhaps second only to psychomotor retardation in frequency.[94] The scope of seizures is implied by the definition; a *seizure* is the clinical manifestation of abnormal neuronal hyperactivity. Usually the neuronal hyperactivity involves cerebral cortical neurons, primarily or secondarily, and is manifested in a manner dependent upon the extent and location of the neuronal hyperactivity. Phenomena such as segmental myoclonus, cerebellar fits, or paroxysmal chorea are also clinical symptoms of neuronal hyperactivity but are not generally considered seizures. Seizures are symptoms of underlying disease and as such can be the mode of expression for a vast array of diseases. Although important diagnostic clues can be gleaned from a seizure, rarely is a seizure disease specific.

Terms that are often used by patients for seizures include: *fits, convulsions, spells,* or *epileptic attacks.* The distinctions among the terms *seizures, epilepsy,* and *convulsions,* however, should be clearly understood by physicians dealing with these patients because these terms have different epidemiologic, legal, financial, and social implications. *Epilepsy* is a chronic condition of recurrent seizures. *Convulsions* refer to seizures with motor manifestations; thus we speak of grand mal convulsions but not sensory convulsions.

INCIDENCE AND PREVALENCE OF SEIZURES

Several epidemiologic studies of specific seizure types in childhood are available. Unfortunately, most of these studies suffer some deficiency such as lack of complete case ascertainment, poor definitions, uninterpretable, outmoded classification schemes, or use of inappropriate population. Perhaps the most complete and recent epidemiologic study of seizures is that done by Hauser and Kurland.[99] Although their clinical classification scheme is of their own design, they have partially equated their definitions with those of the widely used International League Against Epilepsy (ILAE) classification.[75] These investigators delineated four seizure categories: (1) recurrent seizures, (2) single seizures without known cause, (3) single or recurrent seizures temporally related to an active illness known to produce seizures, and (4) febrile seizures.[99] They found that the lifetime seizure risk for a resident of Rochester, Minnesota was 8%. Two percent of children less than 5 years of age had febrile seizures. One half of the patients with afebrile seizures had single seizures. The (category 1) epilepsy incidence rate for 1955–1964, the epilepsy prevalence rate in 1965, and the (categories 2 and 3) isolated seizure incidence rate for 1955–1964 are shown in Table 7-1.[99] During this same period, 1955–1964, the incidence rate for febrile seizures was 440 per 100,000 population less than 5 years old. During childhood (0–20 yr old), therefore, the overall incidence rate of seizures would be 530 per 100,000.

TABLE 7-1. Incidence and Prevalence of Seizures

Age (yr)	Epilepsy Incidence 1955–1964				Epilepsy 1965 Prevalence		Isolated Seizures Incidence 1955–1964	
	No.	Pop.	Rate[a]		No.	Rate[b]	No.	Rate[a]
<1	15	1,084	138.4		—	—	8	73.8
1–9	48	7,863	61.0		39	3.30	15	19.1
10–19	30	6,195	48.4		36	4.40	10	16.1
	93	15,142	58.8		75	3.85	33	21.8

[a]Mean annual per 100,000 population.
[b]Per 1000 population.
(Adapted from Hauser AW, Kurland LT: Epilepsia 16:1, 1975)

PATHOPHYSIOLOGY OF EPILEPSY

The components of the epileptic process are considerable in number and complexity. These components include: heredity, systemic endocrine and metabolic factors, nervous system pathology, normal and abnormal neurophysiological mechanisms, anatomic alterations, connections, and relationships, and biochemical and neurotransmitter changes. Since seizures are a symptom, they can be a manifestation of many quite different disease processes. The role of the various components listed above varies according to the nature of the underlying pathology. For example, in pyridoxine dependency the seizures seem clearly related to a deficiency in gamma-aminobutyric acid (GABA), an inhibitory neurotransmitter synthesized from glutamate by a process requiring pyridoxal phosphate as a cofactor. The seizures, usually appearing in the neonatal period or infancy, are readily controlled by administration of pyridoxine. Pyridoxine, however, does not have anticonvulsant properties in other types of seizures, for example, post-traumatic seizures. In pyridoxine-dependent seizures, GABA-mediated inhibition is deficient because of inadequate GABA synthesis. In post-traumatic seizures, however, deficient GABA synthesis is not critically important. We do not wish to suggest, however, that these two seizures do not share any or even most of the same mechanisms. Indeed, at a

neuronal level most seizures probably are quite similar. The neuronal processes, individual and aggregate, and related events underlying most seizures can be conveniently divided into those characterizing interictal discharge of a seizure focus, interictal to ictal transition, ictus, seizure spread, termination of ictus, and the postictal period.

Focal or Partial Seizures

The seizure focus can be viewed as the portion(s) of the brain in which the neuronal activity is abnormally excessive at the start of the seizure. This may be the majority of the brain in the case of seizures induced by a systemic convulsant or it may be a microscopic focus buried within the temporal lobe. Animal models have been developed to study each of several types of seizures. These models differ phenomenologically in their longevity and the extent of brain involvement. Much of the following description will deal with events in acute focal seizures, especially the topical penicillin model, because these have been studied extensively. At the neuronal level, however, many of these models have been shown to behave quite similarly.

During the periods between clinically evident seizures, the interictal period, the focus is characterized electrographically by the epileptic spike.[191] As recorded from the scalp as the electroencephalogram (EEG) or from the cortical surface as the electrocorticogram (ECOG) the spike is a relatively rapid, high voltage event. The duration of the epileptic spike in an EEG is about 60 milliseconds; its amplitude is in the range of 50 μV to 200 μV. Characteristically the spike is positive in polarity but may also be negative or biphasic. The spike is often followed by a slow wave.

Neurophysiology of the Seizure Focus

Neuronal events within the focus have been studied in several models by extracellular macro- or microelectrode recordings and intracellular microelectrode recordings. Extracellular microelectrode recordings in experimental and human seizure foci reveal stereotyped, high-frequency bursts of unit activity during interictal spiking.[10,31,162,223] Intracellular recordings made in penicillin foci reveal that interictal spike activity is associated with a prolonged (50 msec–100 msec), high amplitude (20 mV–30 mV) neuronal membrane depolarization, and a high-frequency burst of spike activity; this phenomenon has been labeled the *paroxysmal depolarizing shift* (PDS).[161,162] The PDS is often followed by a large hyperpolarizing potential. The origin of these neuronal abnormalities has been a question of intense interest. Various authors have suggested that the PDS reflects an abnormality of synaptic transmission, an intrinsic neuronal membrane abnormality, or both.[8,201,202,223] Evidence for the synaptic origin of the PDS in the penicillin focus includes the graded behavior of the PDS, the presence of a conductance increase, the enhancement of excitatory postsynaptic potentials, and the reduction of inhibitory presynaptic and postsynaptic potentials.[8,47,258] Several features of the PDS suggest a primary neuronal membrane abnormality. In some instances the PDS can be elicited by an intracellular current pulse, and the PDS seems to behave as if it had a refractory period, as one might expect if the mechanism of the PDS was similar to that of the action potential.[126,127,202] Histologic studies of alumina foci and human epileptic foci have revealed neuronal changes, especially in dendrites.[221,222,255] Recent studies of pyramidal cells in the *in vitro* hippocampal slice preparation also suggest

that the PDS may be related to neuronal membrane alterations. Pyramidal cells in this preparation as well as in the cerebellum have been shown to generate calcium spikes in their dendrites.[148,226,262] These calcium spikes were found normally only in Cornu Ammonis (CA)3 pyramidal cells but appear in CA1 pyramidal cells when the slice is exposed to penicillin. Prince has hypothesized that the calcium spike mechanism may in some way be related to the PDS.[202]

Other factors in the focus that may be important in abnormal neuronal behavior are the ionic changes that occur during interictal and ictal activity. Ion-sensitive microelectrode recordings in several seizure models have noted substantial rises in extracellular potassium concentration and decreases in extracellular calcium concentration during interictal and ictal activity.[104,117,203,239] Prior to these observations, it had been suggested that alterations in extracellular ion concentrations could result in epileptogenesis.[90] In addition, perfusion of the hippocampus with solutions of high potassium concentration can produce seizure activity.[185,269] Considering the wide range of effects of ionic changes upon synaptic and nonsynaptic function, an influence of these changes on epileptogenesis is quite probable.[177]

In focal seizure models another abnormality is the occurrence of antidromic spikes in neurons sending axons to the focus. The origin of these spikes is unclear at this time. The influence of these spikes, if subsequently conducted orthodromically, however, would be profound. If such spikes occurred in axon collaterals of neurons in the focus, this could help generate the burst activity observed in neurons in the focus. Antidromic spikes generated in neurons of nuclei with extensive arborization, for example, the thalamus, would also serve a potent synchronizing function that would encourage interictal to ictal transition and seizure spread.

Seizure Spread

Although the focus is the driving force of seizures, seizure spread from the focus to remote or surrounding brain is usually the event that brings the seizure to light. In the cortex around the penicillin focus the majority of neurons are inhibited during the interictal discharge, thus preventing seizure spread outside this so-called inhibitory surround.[204] Seizure spread to the surrounding cortex is associated with a diminution of this inhibitory surround. This decrease in inhibition appears to be an important alteration leading to seizure spread. Diminution of inhibition prior to seizure initiation or spread has been observed in many different pathways during repetitive stimulation.[184,205,220] The mechanism accounting for this change is unclear. Extracellular potassium changes similar to those in the focus do precede the decrease in inhibition and subsequent seizure spread.[103,239] The physiological phenomenon of post-tetanic potentiation may also be involved in seizure propagation. Post-tetanic potentiation is an enhancement of excitatory postsynaptic potentials (EPSPs) during rapid, repetitive stimulation. The burst activity of neurons in the focus would be expected to elicit this phenomenon at its synaptic terminals. Finally, as noted above, antidromic spikes should be a powerful synchronizing force leading to seizure propagation.

Various subcortical nuclei and the cerebellum have been shown to have a profound effect upon cerebral cortical seizure activity. In general, stimulation of subcortical structures or the cerebellum inhibit, with a few exceptions, cortical seizure activity and seizure spread.[4] A discussion of the routes of spread available for seizure activity will not be attempted here. The reader can find a full description of these routes in the reference listed above. Seizure spread seems to occur more readily from particular areas of the brain, for example, associative cortex, and by routes dictated by anatomic connections, such as from one temporal lobe tip to the other by way of the anterior commissure.

Seizure Termination

Perhaps the least understood phase of a seizure is that in which the seizure ceases. Following a seizure the structures involved become electrically inactive and temporarily refractory to further seizure evocation. Several events occur in this period and may be involved with seizure cessation. Activation of a sodium pump could lead to neuronal membrane repolarization and a reversal of the disturbances in ion distribution wrought by the seizure.[9] This is likely to be an active energy-requiring process, as suggested by studies of cerebral blood flow, cerebral energy metabolism, and cerebral fluorometric studies.[39,53,123,184,197,216] Potassium ion-sensitive electrode recordings during seizures also reveal that the extracellular potassium concentration falls below resting levels after the termination of a seizure.[103,156,177] At present it is not known whether this undershoot in potassium reflects a redistribution of potassium through glial cells, an active pumping mechanism (glial or neuronal), or both.[103] This undershoot, however, is certain to have important influence on seizure activity.

Biochemical Studies

Cerebral energy metabolism is dramatically altered by seizure activity.[53,197,216] The magnitude of the alteration is dependent upon seizure type and duration. In the unparalyzed animal a tonic–clonic seizure induces substantial changes in body temperature, blood pressure, blood pH, glucose concentration, and oxygenation.[170,171,197,244] During seizures brain glucose and oxygen use and brain lactate production increase, whereas high-energy phosphate compounds decrease.[17,39,53,171,216] Even in paralyzed artificially ventilated animals prolonged seizures can result in requirements for energy substrates that cannot be met.[53] The cerebral demands for glucose during prolonged seizures may exceed the capacity of the blood–brain barrier glucose transport mechanism.[53] In the paralyzed, ventilated, normothermic baboon with prolonged seizures neuronal changes still occurred in the telencephalon and diencephalon, an observation consistent with a detrimental effect of seizure activity independent from that produced by the systemic alterations.[172] These results are most relevant to status epilepticus and frequent seizures and suggest that the seizure activity even in the absence of systemic alterations can be injurious to the brain.

The brain function requiring the greatest energy expenditure is ion homeostasis.

The importance of ion homeostasis in seizures was first suggested by the observations that ouabain applied to the cortex could induce seizures.[85,142] Ouabain inhibits active transport of sodium and potassium by binding to sodium-potassium adenosine triphosphate.[5] Additional biochemical observations supporting a role for faulty ion homeostasis in epileptogenesis include the observations that tissue from epileptic cortex has a deficient adenosine triphosphatase level, that it has a diminished ability to reaccumulate potassium after depolarization, and that synaptosomes from epileptic foci do not transport sodium and potassium normally.[55,56,207,243] These alterations in pump mechanisms could result in a less stable membrane potential and alterations in intracellular or extracellular ion concentrations.

Amino acid and neurotransmitter changes have also been suggested as important factors in epileptogenesis. Decreased GABA, aspartic acid, glutamic acid, and taurine have been found in human or experimental epileptic foci.[218,248] The severity of the seizures correlated with the extent to which the amino acids deviated from normal.[247] The deficiency of taurine is of particular interest because of the presumed role of taurine as a modulator of membrane excitability.[13] Administration of taurine in some animal models of epilepsy can ameliorate the seizures but the amino acid abnormalities lag behind the clinical improvement, returning toward normal at a time when the EEG is also becoming normal.[32,61,125,246] Unfortunately, there is not complete agreement about the reduction in taurine in epileptic cortex or its anticonvulsant effect.[71,72,193] The anticonvulsant effect of taurine may be a result of the return towards normal of the ratio of the relative concentrations of the excitatory amino acid, glutamic acid, to the inhibitory amino acid, GABA.[13]

The importance of GABA and the pathways involved in GABA metabolism in epilepsy have become increasingly apparent.[169] The biochemical and pharmacologic data supporting the importance of GABA in epilepsy include the following: (1) GABA arrests seizure activity when applied to cortex with seizure. (2) Some infantile seizures are a result of dietary vitamin B_6 deficiency or dependency. Administration of vitamin B_6 to these infants stops the seizures and returns the EEG back to normal. Vitamin B_6 as a coenzyme, pyridoxal phosphate, is required for the synthesis of GABA. (3) Inhibitors of GABA synthesis are potent convulsants. (4) Postsynaptic blockers of GABA-mediated inhibition, picrotoxin and bicucullin, are potent convulsants. (5) Inhibitors of GABA metabolism, such as aminooxyacetic acid and valproic acid, are anticonvulsants.[169] (6) Penicillin, another potent convulsant, blocks GABA-mediated inhibition.[157] (7) Many of the widely used anticonvulsants enhance GABA-mediated inhibition.[158] Other neurotransmitters have been implicated in the pathogenesis of epilepsy. Acetylcholine, an excitatory neurotransmitter, can induce seizures when applied directly to the brain, and inhibitors of acetylcholine esterase can produce seizures.[63,233,235] More recently enkephaline, a neuropeptide, has been found to be epileptogenic.[105]

The role of other substances such as the cyclic nucleotides in seizures is as yet unclear. Alterations in brain cyclic adenosine monophosphate (cyclic AMP) and cyclic guanosine monophosphate (cyclic GMP) levels accompany seizures and, in one in-vitro seizure model, microiontophoresis of cyclic GMP induced epileptiform activity.[42,108] Some of the changes in cyclic nucleotides, however, are probably secondary to the seizure activity.[64]

Secondary or parallel changes constitute a large portion of the changes associated with seizures. One should not conclude, however, that this necessarily negates the importance of these changes. One of the secondary changes accompanying tonic–clonic seizures is an increase in blood–brain barrier permeability accompanying seizures.[196] Considering the importance of the blood–brain barrier a change such as this is not likely to be without substantial effect.

EPILEPSY AND SEIZURE CLASSIFICATION AND CHARACTERIZATION

The evolution of seizure and epilepsy classifications has been dependent in large part on advances in our knowledge of basic anatomy and physiology and on technical advances that allow better seizure characterization. As our knowledge has become more complete we have been able to describe the patient, the disease, and the seizure more accurately and in greater detail.

The first classification scheme naturally focused on the clinical features of the seizure.[160] Since then we have come to realize that seizures can be symptomatic of disease, either within or outside the nervous system. We have also learned that the seizure is a reflection of neuronal overactivity and that the character of the seizure may reflect the location of the abnormal neuronal activity. The advent of the EEG has allowed further descriptions of interictal activity and ictal activity during the various seizures. Further advances in electronics have been followed by seizure descriptions based on long-term simultaneous monitoring of the EEG and video images. During this same period our knowledge of basic neuroanatomy and neurophysiology has allowed some speculative interpretations of our observations.

This tremendous increase in our knowledge has necessitated a continuous reclassification of seizures and epilepsy. The most current and comprehensive classifications of seizures and epilepsy are those formulated by the International League Against Epilepsy (ILAE) and approved by the World Federation of Neurology, the World Federation Neurosurgical Society, and the International Federation of Societies for Electroencephalography and Clinical Neurophysiology.[75,173]

Epilepsy Classification

Epilepsies are subdivided into two basic types, generalized and partial, corresponding to the subdivision of seizures. Partial epilepsies are viewed as symptomatic of structural brain lesions that also produce other neurologic abnormalities. Generalized epilepsies, however, are subtyped into primary, secondary, or undetermined. Primary generalized epilepsies are what, in the past, was called *idiopathic epilepsy*. The seizures that occur in patients with primary generalized epilepsy are absences, massive myoclonus, or tonic–clonic seizures alone or in combinations. These patients tend to be neurologically normal and very responsive to treatment. Patients who have secondary generalized epilepsy usually are neurologically abnormal and may have delayed psychomotor development. Patients with secondary generalized epilepsy often have several types of seizures, especially of the minor motor group (see below). Whereas patients with primary generalized epilepsy begin having seizures in late childhood or adolescence, those with secondary generalized epilepsy have their first seizures in infancy and early childhood. Diffuse or multifocal cerebral lesions are typical in children with secondary generalized epilepsy. The frequency of the various types of epilepsy in a large clinic is shown in Table 7-2.

Seizure Classification

The ILAE seizure classification has recently been revised.[45] This revised scheme of seizure classification is shown in Table 7-3. The classification subdivides seizures on the basis of the clinical features of the seizures and the ictal and interictal electroencephalographic features. The ILAE classifications have achieved the goal of providing greater uniformity in diagnostic terms and, thereby, have allowed better comparison of cases and improved communication.

The ILAE classification conforms to the widely accepted division of seizures into two basic types, partial and generalized. *Partial seizures,* as the name suggests, begin in only a portion of the brain. The term *partial* was first used by Pritchard and revived by Gastaut. Gastaut felt that the term *focal* was misleading because subcortical structures were also involved in this seizure type, making it multifocal.[160] Generalized seizures, in contrast, are propagated by way of brain region(s) with connections to most of the cerebral cortex; therefore, most of the cerebral cortex is involved at the onset. The distinction between generalized and partial seizures is not always discernible clinically and may require an EEG. The EEG in generalized seizures reveals essentially simultaneous onset of epileptic discharge in all leads, whereas in partial seizures the epileptic discharge begins in only some of the leads and may or may not spread to the other regions.

TABLE 7-2. Distribution of 6000 Epileptics as a Function of Age Based on the Classification of the International League Against Epilepsy

Classification	All Ages	Above Age 15	Below Age 15
Total no. of cases	6000	2978	3022
No. of unclassifiable cases	1409 (23.5%)	548 (18.4%)	861 (28.5%)
No. and distribution of classifiable cases	4591 (76.5%)	2430 (81.6%)	2161 (71.5%)
Generalized epilepsy	1731 (37.7%)[a]	543 (22.3%)[a]	1188 (55.0%)[a]
Primary generalized epilepsy, mainly or wholly	1306 (28.4%)[a]	496 (20.4%)[a]	810 (37.5%)[a]
grand mal seizures	517 (11.3%)[a]	292 (12.0%)[a]	225 (10.4%)[a]
petit mal absences	453 (9.9%)[a]	69 (2.8%)[a]	384 (17.8%)[a]
myoclonus	187 (4.1%)[a]	107 (4.4%)[a]	80 (3.7%)[a]
other (clinic seizures, unilateral clonic seizures, etc.)	149 (3.2%)[a]	28 (1.2%)[a]	121 (5.6%)[a]
Secondary generalized epilepsy	425 (9.3%)[a]	47 (1.9%)[a]	378 (17.5%)[a]
Lennox-Gastaut syndrome	235 (5.1%)[a]	15 (0.6%)[a]	220 (10.2%)[a]
West's syndrome	61 (1.3%)[a]	0 (0.0%)	61 (2.8%)[a]
Other	129 (2.8%)[a]	32 (1.3%)[a]	97 (4.5%)[a]
Partial epilepsy, with	2860 (62.3%)[a]	1887 (77.7%)[a]	973 (45.0%)[a]
elementary symptomatology	459 (10.0%)[a]	299 (12.3%)[a]	160 (7.4%)
complex symptomatology (± equivalent to temporal lobe epilepsy)	1821 (39.7%)[a]	1359 (55.9%)[a]	462 (21.4%)[a]
secondarily generalized seizures	580 (12.6%)[a]	299 (9.4%)[a]	351 (16.2%)[a]

[a]Percentage of classifiable cases.

(Gastaut H, Gastaut JL, Goncalres-Silva GE, et al: Epilepsia 16:457, 1975)

Partial Seizures

Partial seizures are the manifestation of a focal cortical epileptic discharge. A focal discharge may remain localized. If the involved region has an associated function that is sufficiently distinctive to the patient or an outside observer, then abnormal focal discharge of more than fleeting duration will not pass unnoticed. Our ability to detect such a discharge is frequently dependent upon elicited subjective symptoms. In a child this is usually difficult and may be impossible. Nevertheless, listing specific symptoms and asking the child if he or she has had these, will maximize the detection.

The route of seizure spread may also determine the sequence of symptoms in partial seizures. Spread of seizure activity to the opposite hemisphere may be associated with a loss of consciousness or a generalized seizure such as a grand mal seizure. A partial seizure that spreads rapidly to produce a generalized seizure may effectively obscure the clinical signature of the focal onset. In this case, the focal origin may become apparent only in the EEG.

In accordance with the variations in cortical location, the extent and route of seizure spread, the ILAE classification has subdivided partial seizures into three basic types: simple partial seizures, partial seizures with complex symptomology, and partial seizures with secondary generalization.

Simple Partial Seizures. Simple partial seizures arise from a single cortical region and produce sensory, motor, autonomic, or psychic symptoms. These seizures are not associated with impairment of consciousness. Simple partial seizures with motor symptoms commonly are manifested by focal clonic twitching involving the face or the hand on the side contralateral to the focal discharge. As Penfield and Jasper (1954) and others have shown, the face, especially the lips and adjacent regions, and the thumb and forefinger have a cortical representation that is disproportionately large for their anatomic size.[191] Possibly for this reason these body parts are more likely to be involved in focal motor seizures. When the focal discharge spreads from its origin

TABLE 7-3. ILAE Seizure Classification

	Clinical Seizure	Ictal EEG	Interictal EEG
I.	Partial Seizures		
A.	Simple partial seizures (focal seizures) and without loss of consciousness	Contralateral discharge, often a spike-and-slow-wave localized according to cortical representation	Localized contralateral discharge
	1. Motor symptoms (Focal, sequential, Jacksonian, versive, postural, phonatory)		
	2. Sensory (Somatosensory, visual, auditory, olfactory, gustatory, vertiginous)		
	3. Autonomic		
	4. Psychic (Dysphasic; dysmnesic, eg., déjà vu, déjà-véçu, jamais vu; cognitive, eg., forced thinking; affective, eg., fear, anger; illusions; complex hallucinations)		
B.	Partial with complex symptomatology and loss of consciousness	Focal or diffuse discharge, if focal often bilateral temporal or fronto-temporal	Asynchronous bilateral or unilateral discharge most commonly temporal
	1. Simple partial onset followed by impaired consciousness and with or without automatisms		
	2. Impaired consciousness at onset with or without simple partial symptoms or automatisms		
C.	Partial with secondary generalization	The discharge above becomes generalized.	Either of the above
	1. Simple, complex, or simple and complex evolving to a tonic–clonic seizure		
II.	Generalized Seizures		
A.	Absence seizures	2.5 cps–3.5 cps spike-and-slow-wave, synchronous and generalized from the start	Background activity normal. Spike-and-slow-wave or polyspike-and-slow-wave, brief and generalized
	1. Atypical absence	EEG is much more variable, 1 cps–2 cps. Spike-and-slow-wave often asymmetric. Bilateral 8 cps–10 cps rhythmic low voltage discharge	Background activity abnormal. Sharp and slow discharges often asynchronous, irregular, and asymmetric
B.	Myoclonic seizures		
	1. Myoclonic jerks (isolated, slow, or irregular)	Spike-and-wave Polyspike-and-wave Sharp and slow waves	Spike, polyspike, or sharp and slow waves
C.	Clonic seizures	Fast and slow waves, spike-and-wave patterns	Spike-and-wave or polyspike-and-wave
D.	Tonic seizures	Reduced amplitude High frequency low voltage activity that slows and grows in amplitude 10 cps negative sharp waves	Sharp and slow waves more or less rhythmic, sometimes asymmetrical. Background is often abnormal for age
E.	Tonic–clonic seizures	Prodrome. Isolated generalized spike-and-wave discharge	Generalized polyspike-and-waves, spike-and-wave, or

TABLE 7-3. ILAE Seizure Classification (*Continued*)

Clinical Seizure	Ictal EEG	Interictal EEG
	Tonic phase. Desynchronization and low voltage fast activity then 10 cps recruiting rhythm	sharp and slow wave discharge
	Clonic phase. Decrescendo polyspike and wave initially, at 4 cps	
	Postictal phase. Flat EEG then diffuse slow waves	
F. Atonic seizures	Polyspikes-and-wave, flattening, or low-voltage fast activity.	Polyspike, spike-and-wave, or sharp and slow waves
III. Unclassified Seizures		

(Modified from the Commission on Classification and Terminology of the International League Against Epilepsy: Proposal for revised clinical and electroencephalographic classification of epileptic seizures. Epilepsia 22:489, 1981)

to involve adjacent cortex an anatomic "march" will ensue, the so-called *Jacksonian march*. A Jacksonian seizure, for example, may begin with twitching of the thumb followed, in succession, by twitching of the hand, forearm, upper arm, and shoulder.

Simple partial seizures are unusual in childhood. One notable exception is the entity variously labeled *benign Rolandic epilepsy, Sylvian seizures,* and *mid-temporal spikes,* or *benign epilepsy of children with centrotemporal EEG foci.*[16,21,152] This is a common syndrome accounting alone for some 16% of all epileptic seizures in one population, a population in which it was also four times more common than absence seizures.[100] These seizures tend to begin in late childhood and disappear at or just after adolescence. They are quite recognizable by the clinical characteristics of onset during sleep of brief facial clonus, salivary pooling, and anarthria.[16,21,152] The seizure frequently awakens the patient, and unless the seizure becomes generalized, consciousness is preserved. These seizures are often preceded by somatosensory phenomena involving the tongue or mouth.[152] Facial clonus may slowly spread in a Jacksonian manner to become generalized or it may abruptly become generalized. Sensory marches may also occur.[152] The interictal EEG shows midtemporal spike foci with

normal background activity.[152] These patients are usually quite normal otherwise.[16,21,101,152] Genetic studies reveal a family history of seizures in 40% of the relatives of children with this disorder. Among siblings of patients with benign Rolandic epilepsy, 15% had seizures and Rolandic discharge, whereas 17% had Rolandic discharges alone. Eleven percent of the parents of these same children had seizures in childhood but only 3% had Rolandic discharges.[102] Based upon this information, it was concluded that this disorder was inherited in an autosomal dominant manner but with age-dependent penetrance.[103] These patients respond readily to any of the drugs for tonic–clonic seizures.

Focal motor seizures in adults often have an ominous implication because they are more frequently associated with tumors, cerebrovascular accidents, or traumatic head injury. In children this is less true because children with benign Rolandic epilepsy represent a substantial portion of the children with partial seizures with elementary motor symptoms. Loiseau and Orgogozo have also suggested that partial seizures with elementary symptoms beginning in adolescence may at times be a benign condition.[151] Additional studies will be necessary, however, before accepting this conclusion. Recent reports of cranial computerized scanning of children with seizures suggest that those with partial seizures with elementary symptoms do have more structural abnormalities than children with tonic–clonic or partial complex seizures.[78,266]

Simple partial seizures with sensory symptoms are notably infrequent in childhood. In studies of somatosensory seizures, onset of seizures after 20 years of age was more common.[164] As noted above, this may relate in part to the child's inability to communicate these symptoms to others. This problem of communication is frequently compounded by confusion and amnesia, a consequence of secondary seizure generalization. In adults simple somatosensory seizures are also often associated with cortical tumors, head injury, or cerebrovascular accidents.[164] Since the occurrence of these processes is relatively infrequent in childhood, this too may influence the frequency of sensory seizures in childhood. Typical simple partial seizures and their lobes of origin include tingling or numbness, parietal lobe; flashing lights or scotoma, occipital lobe; odors (usually disagreeable), hippocampus; and buzzing sound or vertigo, temporal lobe.

Simple autonomic partial seizures are rare. More commonly, autonomic symptoms, especially abdominal pain, are auras of a partial complex seizure. The temporal lobe and adjacent structures are the usual cerebral location to which the autonomic symptoms are attributed.

The revised ILAE classification has also included seizures with disturbance of higher cortical function in the simple partial seizure category. The impetus for this inclusion of seizures with disturbance of higher cortical function in the simple partial seizure category was the recognition that in these seizures, as in those with elementary symptoms, the patient remains aware or conscious. Prolonged EEG and video monitoring studies have shown that loss of awareness implies bilateral hemisphere involvement, whereas retention of awareness indicates focal, unilateral hemisphere discharge.

The potential variations of psychic simple partial seizures is as vast as the repertoire of human behavior itself. Most of the seizures, however, share one common feature, that is, the symptoms are subjective. The subgroups are listed in Table 7-3 and will be discussed briefly below.

Dysphasia implies an inability to produce speech sounds. Dysphasic simple partial seizures have been characterized to date by pallilalia or aphasia of a Wernicke's type. Epileptic discharge occurs in the supplementary motor region or dominant superior temporal region, respectively.

Dysmnesic seizures are those with psychosensory symptoms such as déjà vu, jamais vu, depersonalization, and other vague global disturbances of perception. *Déjà vu* refers to the feeling of familiarity when the perception of unfamiliarity is appropriate. *Jamais vu* is the inverse of déjà vu. Not surprisingly, these highly subjective and vague symptoms are rarely elicited in the young child. Their localizing value is uncertain. Cognitive symptoms are also unusual symptoms in childhood and also of doubtful localizing value. The most common affective symptom in simple partial seizures is fear accompanied by the usual body and facial reactions to this perception. Anger may occur as a seizure manifestation but is usually clearly a behavior out of context and poorly directed.

Psychosensory disturbances, illusions, and hallucinations are occasional manifestations of partial seizures. As is true of the disturbances of primary sensation, these perceptual events are recognized as bogus. Children rarely spontaneously complain of these symptoms. Formed hallucinations are frequently associated with parietal or temporal lobe epileptic foci. Illusions are usually visual and auditory. They are distinguished from hallucinations by the presence of an appropriate sensory stimulus that is misinterpreted.

Complex Partial Seizures.   Although complex partial seizures begin locally in one or both hemispheres, they are associated at some point with altered consciousness. Often there is bitemporal discharge associated with the altered consciousness. Symptoms may precede the onset of the altered consciousness. When these are a manifestation of a focal ictal discharge we refer to them as an *aura*. The symptoms in an aura can be equated with those seen in simple partial seizures. (See above for descriptions.)

Psychomotor symptoms or automatisms are a common and well known manifestation of partial complex seizures. Studies of automatisms as part of absence seizures suggest that several different types of motor behavior occur including (1) continuation of motor activity initiated prior to the onset of a seizure; (2) motor activity in response to environmental stimuli; and (3) released motor behavior normally repressed.[41,193] The patient is unaware of or amnestic for the behavior during automatisms. Common automatisms of the third type include scratching, fingering of clothes, lip smacking, chewing, and other activities normally performed without thought. Escueta has studied automatisms in partial complex seizures and has distinguished three types.[44,57] In the first type there are three phases: motionless stare, stereotyped automatisms, and reactive automatisms. These patients often have focal temporal epileptic discharges during nasopharyngeal or depth recordings. The second type has two phases: first, stereotyped automatisms, then reactive automatisms. A focal onset in the electroencephalogram of patients with the second type of automatisms was not seen. The third type consists of only a drop attack termed *temporal lobe syncope*.[44] Although there are relatively few autonomic changes (e.g., heart rate), the patient falls to the floor and is completely flaccid and unresponsive for several minutes. Following this the patient remains confused and may have reactive automatisms for several minutes. Importantly, these seizures seem to respond poorly to the usual drugs for partial seizures.[44] Bilateral synchronous medial temporal paroxysms precede the seizure onset and are followed by diffuse slowing.

Complex partial seizures must be differentiated from absence attacks. In both absence and complex partial seizures consciousness is lost and automatisms may or may not be seen. The automatisms are the same in both complex partial and absence seizures. The following are some useful features that allow these seizures to be distinguished clinically: (1) The mode of onset in partial complex seizures is less abrupt than in absence seizures and may begin with aura. (2) The duration of partial complex seizures is generally longer than that of absence seizures. The usual duration of a partial complex seizure is several minutes, whereas absence seizures are characteristically brief, 10 seconds or less. Clustering of absence seizures, however, may obscure this brevity. (3) Postictal confusion and lethargy occur in partial complex seizures but not in absence seizures.[45,194]

Generalized Seizures

Generalized seizures refer to abnormal neuronal discharge that is bilateral, and synchronized from the start. Clinically, therefore, no symptoms referable to a single anatomic or functional system occur. In the revised ILAE classification (see Table 7-3) there are six subtypes of generalized seizures: absence, myoclonic, clonic, tonic, tonic–clonic, and atonic.

Absence Seizures. Our knowledge of absence seizures was greatly expanded by continuous monitoring of patients with absence seizures. These studies, since their beginning, have revealed that absence seizures are quite variable clinically and electroencephalographically.[224] The term *absence* was coined in 1924 by Calmeil and is used in the revised ILAE classification as a term for those generalized seizures that are nonconvulsive.[30] As Table 7-3 shows, two types of absence seizures are recognized, simple and atypical. The essential clinical feature of these seizures is the loss of awareness and responsiveness. The relationship between the electroencephalographic epileptic discharge and behavior has been extensively studied, but the results have not been entirely consistent. Some investigators have noted that clinical manifestations precede the spike and wave discharge and others have not.[20,87,174,186,228] The variable results relate in part to the different measurements used to detect behavioral changes. Changes in eye movement associated with absence attack preceded the spike–wave discharge in one study, and followed the onset in another.[20,186] The studies do suggest several general points about behavior in absence attacks.[87] Long (greater than 3 sec) spike–wave discharges are more likely to be associated with changes in behavior. The variability of the behavioral effect of spike–wave discharge was greater among individuals than among bursts in a single individual. Complex tasks are more likely to be disturbed than simple tasks.

Electroencephalographic telemetry has allowed study of patients during their normal daily activities. These studies have revealed several important relationships between electrical discharge and clinically identifiable seizure activity. First, although the numbers of electroencephalographic discharges decrease with age, their duration, the number associated with clinical manifestations, and the influence of environment on the frequency of discharges increases.[82] Second, the environment influences the percentage of electroencephalographic discharges that are associated with clinical manifestations but not in a simple manner. In general, activities that are not interesting, enjoyable, and demanding (i.e., requiring full attention) for the patient are associated with increased numbers of electroencephalographic discharges and percentage of discharges clinically evident.[82,91] Sleep or rest are often associated with increased numbers of discharges and an increased percentage of discharges clinically symptomatic. This important information has therapeutic implications and is probably relevant even for patients with partial seizures. Prolonged monitoring of monkeys with experimental aluminum seizure foci reveals that the frequency of seizures even in this model of partial epilepsy is influenced by activity and attention.[264]

Simultaneous video and electroencephalographic monitoring has brought to light the considerable variability in absence seizures. Simple absence seizures consist only in variable disturbances of consciousness. However, absence seizures may also entail motor or autonomic symptoms. These seizures have been called *complex absence seizures*.[75]

Simple absence seizures or "petit mal" seizures are characterized by brief episodes of unawareness, lasting less than 10 seconds, with complete or nearly complete unresponsiveness. These attacks occur without warning and usually interrupt ongoing activity. The patient has complete amnesia for the event and may only know of its occurrence by the discontinuity of events and memory. Often a parent or teacher will complain of inattentiveness or daydreaming at home or school. No motor activity occurs during this type of seizure except eye-blinking or mild myoclonus. Just before or at the time of the termination of the abnormal discharge the patient resumes his prior activity, usually at the point where he left off. Postictal behavioral changes do not occur. Simple absence seizures infrequently are the only absence seizures. In one study only one patient out of 48 patients was found to have only simple absence seizures.[194] Forty percent of the patients in this study, however, had at least one simple absence seizure. The relative frequency of the various absence seizures types in the 374 seizures recorded by Penry is shown in Figure 7-1.[194]

As noted in Figure 7-1, more than 50% of the absence seizures studied by Penry and associates were characterized by automatisms alone or in combination with other components.[193] Other common manifestations were mild clonic movements and decreased postural tone. Absence seizures with these phenomena are termed *complex ab-*

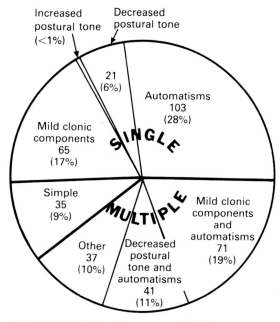

FIG. 7-1. Relative frequency of different types of 374 absence seizures. Penry JK, Parker RJ, Dreifuss FE: Simultaneous recordings of absence seizures with video tape and electroencephalography. Brain 98:427, 1975

sence.[75] Complex absence seizures generally are more difficult to treat than simple absence seizures.[50,76]

The automatisms in absence seizures are not qualitatively different from those occurring in partial seizures.[193] In general, automatisms are more likely to occur the longer the abnormal discharge lasts.[195] Both perseverative and *de-novo* automatisms occur during absence seizures.[193] The head, face, and upper extremities are the usual body parts involved in these automatisms.[194]

Electroencephalographically, absence seizures are divided into those with a "typical" petit mal pattern and those with an atypical pattern (see Table 7-3). The typical petit mal pattern consists of a recurring spike and wave pattern of 3 cycles per second (cps) of maximal amplitude over the frontocentral region. The background activity is usually normal. The interictal record may show isolated generalized spike and wave but is otherwise normal.

In atypical petit mal, abnormal diffuse slow waves are more common during the resting, awake EEG and are associated with a greater likelihood that seizures will persist. Many patients with atypical absence seizures have complex rather than simple absence seizures.[219] Ictal atypical absence EEG patterns are of two types: (1) low-voltage fast activity arrhythmic discharge at 10 or more cps , and (2) semirhythmic, 1 cps to 2 cps, sharp and slow wave discharge, often asymmetric but synchronous. The second EEG pattern has been called the *petit mal variant pattern.*[84]

The Lennox-Gastaut syndrome slow spike-and-wave pattern is associated not only with simple absence but also with myoclonic absence, tonic seizures, and neurologic impairment.[81,139] This syndrome is important because prognosis for development and seizure control are poor. Moreover, cerebral computerized tomography, when used in patients with this syndrome, often reveals abnormalities.[78,135,268] In this syndrome seizures usually begin during the first 2 years of life. Generalized seizures of all types occur in these patients, most often several types together.[22,36,81,139,159,182]

The coexistence of myoclonic, atonic, akinetic, and tonic seizures in the same patient is common not only in the Lennox-Gastaut syndrome but also in other children with encephalopathy and seizures and has given rise to the term "minor motor seizures." Minor motor seizures originally included infantile spasms as one of the seizure types.[146] The term *minor motor seizures* has also been used as a general term for all generalized seizures of childhood excluding simple absence and tonic–clonic seizures.[146] Minor motor seizures in the Lennox-Gastaut syndrome often coexist with tonic–clonic and absence seizures.

The majority of patients with Lennox-Gastaut syndrome have an array of neurologic and intellectual deficits.[159,268] Variable features of the Lennox-Gastaut syndrome that portend a bad prognosis are early onset of seizures, presence of neurologic abnormality, tonic seizures, and delta activity in the EEG.[22] Children with Lennox-Gastaut syndrome often reach early milestones at the appropriate times but then appear to fall behind in the last half of early childhood.[22] An etiology for this syndrome can be established in from one-fourth to three-fourths of patients with the Lennox-Gastaut syndrome.[78,135,268] Perinatal insults account for many of the identifiable causes but insults occurring in late infancy or childhood including progressive degenerative or metabolic diseases, can also be associated with this syndrome.[22,36,81,159] There is often a history of seizures in the families of patients with these seizures.[22] A close relationship between this clinical syndrome and syndromes associated with hypsarrhythmia or multifocal spike discharges is likely. Syndromes associated with these EEG abnormalities are caused by bilateral cerebral disease and include similar clinical abnormalities. Moreover, the EEG abnormalities found in these syndromes may coexist or occur serially.[81,159]

Tonic–Clonic Seizures. The tonic–clonic or grand mal seizure is another generalized seizure type. This seizure represents the ultimate in the sequence of motor behaviors during seizures. The tonic–clonic sequence is organized at the spinal level. As such it is possible in the high spinal cat to elicit the entire tonic–clonic sequence merely by applying an electrical stimulus at the point of spinal cord section.[58] Tonus in this spinal preparation occurs when the magnitude of the stimulus is increased. A grand mal seizure, therefore, is probably merely a reflection of the magnitude of the activity impinging on the spinal cord. Infant animals, including human infants, generally do not have tonic–clonic seizures, a reflection perhaps of the generally reduced neuronal excitability and relatively unmyelinated state of their nervous systems.[249]

The tonic–clonic seizure is only considered to be of the generalized type if it begins without a focal signature, for example, an aura. If defined in this manner and not as a symptomatic seizure, the *grand mal seizure* is usually part of a relatively well-defined syndrome.[76] Sexes are equally affected and in two-thirds of cases seizures begin in adolescence. The association of myoclonus and grand mal seizures in adolescence has been cited as a specific syndrome.[45,77,183] This so-called *myoclonic syndrome* of adolescence is characterized by early morning proximal upper extremity myoclonus at times followed by tonic–clonic seizures. These patients are, most often, otherwise normal females with a strong family history of seizures. The EEG reveals diffuse 4 Hz to 6 Hz multi-spike-wave complexes. Such patients are usually easily controlled with anticonvulsants. This group of patients and those patients with tonic–clonic and simple absence seizures account for the characteristics considered typical of patients with primary generalized epilepsy. These characteristics include high frequency of positive family history for seizures, low rate of neurologic abnormality, good response to anticonvulsants, and lack of an identifiable etiology.[183,245]

Tonic–clonic seizures are often preceded by generalized myoclonic jerks. These may occur as a prodrome in as much as 50% of patients with grand mal. Myoclonic jerks are not inevitably followed by the grand mal seizure. The frequent antecedent generalized myoclonus just before the tonic–clonic seizure, however, suggests that myoclonus is a manifestation of a partially controlled corticoreticular discharge that can progress to the uncontrolled discharge of the tonic–clonic seizure. Other premonitory symptoms are common before a grand mal seizure, especially in older patients who have experienced enough grand mal seizures to establish a pattern. Headaches, irritability, anxiety, and personality changes are among these.

The tonic phase of a tonic–clonic seizure actually consists of two phases. In the first phase tonic flexion predominates so that the patient assumes a "hands up" position and flexes the lower extremities. This phase is followed by tonic extension that at its peak is characterized by an opisthotonic posture. It is in this phase of tonus that an epileptic cry and sudden mouth closure occur. The total duration of the tonic phase usually is from 10 seconds to 20 seconds. Tonus blends into clonus that is characterized by approximately 30 seconds of flexor contractions separated by relaxation. The periods of relaxation gradually increase in duration until, in a decrescendo fashion, the seizure stops. Tongue-biting may also occur in the clonic phase.

A vast array of autonomic changes accompany the tonic–clonic seizure including mydriasis, profuse sweating, increased heart rate and blood pressure, increased urinary bladder pressure, perspiration, and piloerection. Respiration ceases with the tonic phase and may not begin again until well into the postictal period. Incontinence does not occur until the period of atonia, which follows the clonic phase. The total duration of the postictal phase is 5 minutes to 15 minutes excluding amnesia, mild changes in consciousness, and lethargy.

Considerable variation in the seizures can occur among patients or even among seizures in a single patient. The relative duration of tonic–clonic seizures can vary and is notoriously influenced by anticonvulsants. The existence of a clonic–tonic–clonic generalized seizure has also been documented through prolonged video and electroencephalographic monitoring.[45] These patients, too, often present in adolescence as a myoclonic syndrome. It is noteworthy that many of the patients with tonic–clonic seizures are photosensitive and indeed this may be the sole trigger for their seizures.[76,183]

Tonic Seizures. Tonic seizures are another of the generalized seizures. Although the term *tonic* might suggest that this seizure type is but a version of the tonic–clonic seizure, this is not so. Tonic seizures are especially common in the Lennox-Gastaut syndrome and imply a poor prognosis in this syndrome.[22,36,81,159,182] Tonic seizures are of three types, depending on the topography of involvement; (1) axial, characterized by fixed head position and tonic facial expression associated with respiratory changes; (2) axorhizomelic, characterized by additional shoulder shrug and upper arm abduction and elevation; or (3) global, in which the arms and hands assume a position similar to the defensive arm position of a boxer. The tonus in tonic seizures is distinguished from that occurring in the tonic–clonic seizure by a shorter seizure duration (15 sec versus 1 min), absence of tonic extension or prolonged clonus seen in tonic–clonic seizures, and relatively mild postictal depression. In addition, tonic seizures occur predominantly in young children, whereas tonic–clonic seizures are more common in adults and adolescents. Tonic seizures occur predominantly at night (see discussion above) and often in clusters.

Other clinical states in which tonus is important include myoclonus (generally much briefer, 1 sec–2 sec), adversive seizures (asymmetric tonus is characteristic), syncopal seizures, cerebellar seizures, and toxic tonic spasms. Cerebellar seizures are distinguished by an occurrence in patients with other posterior fossa symptoms and signs, long duration (2 min–10 min), slow progression of symptoms, opisthotonic posturing, and absence of any type of generalized corticoreticular EEG discharge.[118] Toxic tonic spasms occur in tetanus, strychnine intoxication, or rabies and are characterized by the preservation of consciousness, a normal EEG during the spasm, and the stimulus-sensitive nature of these spasms.[80] Tonic seizures can be seen in some progressive disorders such as Unverricht–Lundborg disease, Ramsay Hunt dentatorubral degeneration, and other degenerative diseases.

Myoclonic Seizures. In the revised ILAE classification, myoclonic seizures include both myoclonic jerks and clonic seizures. Myoclonus refers to an involuntary contraction of one muscle or, more commonly, several muscles. Myoclonus may be rhythmic or nonrhythmic. Alternate contraction of agonist and antagonist muscles, a feature of tremor, is not seen in my-

oclonus thus accounting for the brisk movement in one direction followed by a slow movement in the opposite direction. The underlying mechanism of myoclonus is probably a deficiency of inhibitory mechanisms. Myoclonus may represent abnormality at a spinal or higher level. Since myoclonus is such a nonspecific symptom, the diseases associated with myoclonus are both numerous and diverse. At least one form of myoclonus, myoclonus when one is falling asleep, occurs in almost everyone at some time. Myoclonus, therefore, is common and may be a manifestation of a variety of motor system abnormalities.

Halliday has divided myoclonus into three types on the basis of the relationship between electroencephalographic and electromyographic observations.[96] The pyramidal type is characterized by brief, irregular shocklike muscle contractions that follow a positive–negative EEG spike by a fixed interval. Evoked responses are often enhanced in this type of myoclonus. The extrapyramidal type is characterized by slower muscle contractions that are variable in their relationship to the EEG spike, often following the spike by a long latency or even occurring without the spike. The segmental type of myoclonus is usually more rapid, rhythmical, bilateral, and predominantly flexor. No electroencephalographic abnormality accompanies this type of myoclonus. Clinical conditions associated with the pyramidal myoclonus include seizure disorders, progressive myoclonic epilepsy, encephalitis, and many other diseases. Extrapyramidal myoclonus is often part of subacute sclerosing panencephalitis. Segmental myoclonus is the principal manifestation of subacute myoclonic spinal neuronitis.

Aigner has divided patients with myoclonus into four categories: (1) those with myoclonus, seizures, and neurologic or mental abnormalities; (2) those with myoclonus and seizures; (3) those with only myoclonus; and (4) those with myoclonus and neurologic or mental abnormalities.[3] Twenty-eight percent of their patients were in the first category. These patients most often were infants or young children who had massive myoclonic spasms and hypsarrhythmic EEGs. Forty-eight percent of the patients in the second category were older children or adolescents with grand mal seizures, 20% of their patients had essential myoclonus, category 3, and 4% were in category 4. Myoclonus then seemed to be commonly associated with seizures and in many younger children presented as infantile spasms. In older children or in adolescents, myoclonus, as discussed above, can precede tonic–clonic seizures in as many as one-third of patients.[77] When presenting in early childhood, myoclonus can occur alone or in combination with other generalized seizures and is associated with an EEG showing a fast spike-and-wave pattern.[2] Many of these patients are photosensitive. Additional manifestations include fatigue, awakening, and eye closure.

Clonic Seizures. Clonic seizures are another form of generalized seizure largely restricted to children. These seizures usually begin with loss of consciousness followed by hypertonus or hypotonus, which is then followed by a series of generalized, though often asymmetric, muscle twitches. Many of the clinical features of clonic seizures are quite similar to those occurring in myoclonus; therefore, clonic seizures have been included with myoclonic seizures in the past.

Infantile Spasms. Infantile spasms are massive myoclonic jerks usually beginning in infancy. These seizures were first described by West.[254] His name has become associated with a more restricted clinical entity, West's syndrome. This syndrome is characterized by infantile massive myoclonic spasms, retardation, and an EEG pattern termed *hypsarrhythmia*. The exact definition of *infantile spasms* has varied widely among authors.[133] Massive myoclonic spasms and hypsarrhythmia have sometimes been considered necessary components for the diagnosis of infantile spasms.[2] It is not clear, however, that patients with hypsarrhythmia are a group with distinctive etiology, prognosis, inheritance, or response to therapy. Other authors have suggested that age or duration of the myoclonic spasms be used to define infantile spasms.[12,134,145] Neither of these criteria, however, seems to define a unique group of patients.[133]

Infantile spasms seem to be phenom-

ena related in part to age or stage of development. Infantile spasms begin before 1 year of age in 86% of patients and in less than 6% after age 2 years.[119] Peak age of onset usually falls between 2 and 7 months.[133] Myoclonus is often the earliest manifestation of infantile spasms. The myoclonus usually begins abruptly and is bilateral and symmetric. Flexor spasms are most common but mixed or extensor spasms may occur alone or in combinations. Although the flexor spasm has been considered typical, a recent monitoring study revealed that mixed spasms are the most common form of infantile spasms.[130] In flexor spasms there is abrupt flexion of the neck and trunk and flexion–adduction of either all of the extremities or of the lower extremities and flexion–abduction of the upper extremities. In this study, 34% of the spasms were flexor, 22% extensor, and 42% mixed.[130] Extensor spasms were characterized by extension of neck and trunk and extension and adduction or abduction of the lower extremities. These same authors confirmed that head-nodding can be a form of infantile spasms.[130] In general, considerable variability in spasms occurred among patients or in a single patient. Clustering of seizures occurs in more than three-fourths of patients, often with variation of seizure intensity within a cluster.[130] Typically, the seizure frequency increases upon awakening but not while going to sleep.[130] Seizures, especially after large clusters, can be followed by lethargy. Other types of seizures, usually generalized, can accompany myoclonus.[51,119] Infantile spasms tend to increase in frequency, then decrease and finally stop, being replaced by other seizures (tonic–clonic) in about half of the cases.[120] In one study, 50% of patients stopped having spasms by 2 years of age, and 89% by 5 years of age.[120] The typical interictal EEG pattern, hypsarrhythmia, will be discussed in the section on laboratory diagnosis. This pattern may follow or precede the onset of the spasm and can be seen in patients without infantile spasms.[133]

Infantile spasms are generally thought of as nonfamilial but a recent study suggests that this may not be entirely accurate.[11] Infantile spasms are often symptomatic seizures (see list, Conditions Associated with Infantile Spasms).

Conditions Associated with Infantile Spasms

I. Developmental Defects
   Neurocutaneous syndromes
      Tuberous sclerosis
      Neurofibromatosis
      Sturge-Weber syndrome
   Chromosomal abnormalities, for example,
      Down's syndrome
   Agenesis of the corpus callosum
   Aicardi syndrome
   Hydrocephalus
   Hydranencephaly
   Happy puppet syndrome
II. Prenatal and Perinatal Insults
   Eclampsia
   Small for gestational age
   Intracranial hemorrhage
   Hypoxic-ischemic insult
   Kernicterus
   Trauma at delivery
III. Metabolic Disorders
   Aminoacidurias
      Phenylketonuria
      Histidinemia
      Maple syrup urine disease
      Carnosinemia
   Leucine-induced hypoglycemia
   Urea cycle defects, for example,
      hyperornithinemia
   Lipidoses, for example, Tay Sachs disease
   Pyridoxine dependency or deficiency
IV. Infectious Diseases and Postimmunization
      Reaction
   Intrauterine infections
      Toxoplasmosis
      Syphilis
      Cytomegalovirus
   Meningitis
   Encephalitis
      Rubeola
      Varicella
   Postimmunization reactions
      Pertussis
V. Cerebrovascular Accidents
VI. Tumors, for example, choroid plexus papilloma

In a review of the literature, infantile spasms were idiopathic in from 25% to 50% of patients.[133] In a recent study of infantile spasms in Finland, the percentage of idiopathic cases seemed to decrease each year.[211] This decrease in idiopathic cases is probably related to advances in diagnostic techniques and neonatal care. The impact of cerebral computerized tomography is likely to further reduce the idiopathic category, a possibility supported by recent observation.[79] The Finnish study also documented a sig-

nificant drop in symptomatic cases secondary to perinatal insult during the period between 1960 and 1976.[11] The annual incidence of all types of infantile spasm in this study, however, remained relatively constant (0.38–0.42/1000 live births) because cases associated with infection and developmental defects increased.

The prognosis for normal development in this syndrome is quite poor. A review of follow-up studies of patients with infantile spasms revealed that only 13% to 20% of patients were developmentally normal.[133] Good prognostic features are normal development before the onset of infantile spasms, absence of an etiology, and a short period of spasms.[37,120,232] As many as 37% of patients with these criteria may attend regular schools.[120]

Atonic Seizures. These nonconvulsive, generalized seizures are also seizures of childhood. Atonic seizures are characterized by sudden loss of postural tone lasting for several seconds. These seizures are associated with falls when the patient is standing and, for this reason, can be confused with myoclonic seizures and tonic seizures. It may be quite difficult to clinically differentiate these seizures, especially because atonic seizures can accompany myoclonic seizures. Lennox labeled the association of absence, myoclonic, and atonic seizures, the *petit mal triad*.[138] This is an unfortunate term because it is often confused with petit mal or simple absence seizures but is only remotely related to either. Atonic spells can be either brief (epileptic drop attacks) or long. Long atonic seizures can be of two etiologic types, a relatively benign early childhood type triggered by metabolic disturbances, especially fever, and a variety of adult types associated with a more ominous prognosis owing to the fact that these patients often have focal progressive brain lesions.[67,213]

ETIOLOGY

Epilepsies of Unknown Etiology

The large group of convulsive disorders with no known etiology has also been classified as *idiopathic, cryptogenic,* and *primary epilepsy.* In approximately half of the children with convulsive disorders careful study fails to reveal evidence of a specific cerebral lesion or of an extracerebral cause for the attacks. It is most likely that there is a biochemical defect that results in the periodic seizure activity. Although the etiology is not known, the electrophysiologic cerebral activity that accompanies these seizures is well established.

Genetic Factors

The most definite genetic factors in epilepsy relate to identical twins, both of whom may have petit mal epilepsy. The EEG patterns are almost identical in twins with petit mal epilepsy. The incidence of seizures in the families of children with idiopathic epilepsy is approximately 2.5% in contrast to an incidence of 0.5% in the total population.

Approximately one-third of children with nonfebrile convulsions and one-half of children with febrile seizures have a family history of convulsions in siblings, parents, or other relatives. The incidence of febrile convulsions among the parents and siblings of children with febrile seizures is 9%. Transmission is probably by a single dominant gene with incomplete penetrance.[68] The tendency to develop epileptic symptoms may be in part genetically controlled.

Epilepsy with Known Contributory Factors

Convulsive seizures associated with a known cerebral or extracerebral cause are classified as *symptomatic, organic,* or *secondary epilepsy.* A wide variety of cerebral and extracerebral disorders may result in convulsive seizures in children.

Developmental and Degenerative Disorders

In the course of fetal development malformations involving the cerebral cortex may occur. These may result from chromosomal defects, maternal infections occurring during early pregnancy such as German measles (rubella), or x-irradiation. Some malformations may be the result of occluded cerebral vessels. Convulsive seizures and other neurologic symptoms and signs in the infant are frequently associated with these disorders. Perinatal hypoxia and kernicterus may be associated with convulsive attacks.

Various degenerative disorders associated with biochemical defects in protein, lipid, and carbohydrate metabolism may frequently be associated with convulsive seizures, as well as with other neurologic findings. Degenerative disorders of unknown etiology, such as tuberous sclerosis, are frequently associated with seizures.

Infection

Febrile Convulsions and Systemic Infections. Febrile convulsions are seizures occurring in association with extracerebral systemic illnesses, of which 70% are acute infections of the upper respiratory tract. Acute pharyngitis, tonsillitis, otitis media, exanthem subitum, and pneumonia are the most common systemic infections associated with febrile convulsions. Approximately 40% of shigella infections of the intestinal tract in children are associated with convulsions.

The skin of these patients is often pale and dry at the time of a seizure. A rapid increase in body temperature produces a rapid rise in metabolic rate with an increase in cerebral oxygen requirements. If the individual's seizure threshold is reached, a seizure occurs.

Febrile convulsions appear most commonly in children between 6 months and 4 years of age. At 3 years, the cerebral circulation comprises 65% of the total body circulation. This is in contrast to the adult in whom 15% of the total circulation goes to the brain.

Febrile seizures usually are generalized clonic seizures that last less than 20 minutes and are associated with temperatures in the range of 104°F (40°C). Males have a higher incidence of febrile seizures than females in a ratio of 1.4:1.0. White children have a higher incidence than black children.

Complicated febrile seizures include those lasting more than 15 minutes, those recurring within 24 hours, or those with focal features.

It is very important to distinguish true

febrile convulsions from syncope and seizure secondary to anoxia associated with fever. In the anoxic group, ocular compression results in abnormal asystole lasting 4 seconds or longer. This test is of value in differentiating between anoxic and true febrile convulsions.[234]

Infections of Meninges and Brain. Acute infections of the central nervous system in infants and children are frequently associated with convulsive seizures. Focal or generalized convulsions may occur with meningitis, encephalitis, or brain abscess. Recurrent convulsions may occur subsequent to an acute central nervous system infection.

Congenital toxoplasmosis is associated with chorioretinitis, hydrocephalus, and retarded mental and intellectual development, as well as convulsive seizures. Cytomegalic inclusion disease may be accompanied by recurrent convulsions. Neurosyphilis, occurring rarely in children, may be associated with epileptic seizures.

Metabolic and Toxic Etiologies

Disturbances of Water and Electrolytes. Seizures are a prominent feature of water intoxication. This is due to hypotonicity of body fluids and consequent brain-swelling. The hyponatremia and hypochloremia seen in water intoxication may be due to an inadequate oral intake of salt, improper parenteral fluid therapy, an excessive loss of electrolytes either through the gastrointestinal tract in association with diarrhea or through the skin owing to excessive sweating, or to retention of water as a result of excessive secretion of antidiuretic hormone.

Hypertonicity due to a marked elevation in serum sodium may also be associated with twitching and seizures. Hypernatremia may be due to excessive sodium intake, decreased water intake, or sodium retention in excess of water.

Hypocalcemia. With a marked drop in the ionizable serum calcium, spontaneous muscle twitchings appear, and these may become generalized. The total serum calcium is usually below 7 mg/dl. Generalized or focal convulsions may occur with severe hypocalcemia. Hypocalcemia may also result from hypoparathyroidism, rickets, steatorrhea, celiac disease, or pseudohypoparathyroidism.

Hypoglycemia. With a marked drop in the level of blood glucose to the range of 20 mg/dl to 40 mg/dl, the child develops autonomic disturbances including sweating, nausea, pallor, and palpitation. This is followed by vomiting, tremor, mental confusion, unconsciousness, and sometimes convulsive seizures. Attacks may be related to insulin overdosage in children with diabetes mellitus, idiopathic hypoglycemia, ketotic hypoglycemia or rarely, hyperinsulinism, hypopituitarism, adrenocortical insufficiency, or glycogen storage disease.

Hypoglycemia in infants of diabetic mothers may be due to islet cell hyperplasia with hyperinsulinism. Functional islet cell adenomas occur rarely during the neonatal period and childhood.

Hepatic Disease. Convulsions occur with hepatic encephalopathy and Reye's syndrome. Children who develop acute hepatitis may become disoriented with a coarse flapping tremor, convulsions, and other evidence of encephalopathy. The EEG usually shows high-voltage slow wave activity. The early symptoms of Reye's syndrome, which include repetitive vomiting, lethargy, and confusion, may be associated with seizures. Convulsions occur more frequently in younger children than in older children.

Deficiency of Vitamin B_6, Pyridoxine. Infants may develop deficiency of pyridoxine manifested by convulsions if their diets contain less than 0.1 mg to 0.5 mg vitamin B_6 daily. This occurred in the United States between 1950 and 1954. Investigations revealed that the common dietary factor in these affected infants was a brand of liquid infant feeding mixture that, due to the changes in the autoclaving procedures, contained only 0.060 mg pyridoxine per quart. Deficiency of pyridoxine has also been observed in a few infants who were fed breast milk low in vitamin B_6 when no additional vitamin supplements were given. On this limited intake of pyridoxine, symptoms consisting of hyperirritability, increased startle responses, and convulsions were observed. The age of onset of seizures varied from 3 days to 10 months. Grand mal as well as minor seizures developed. Only a small percentage of all the infants who received the proprietary milk preparation that was low in vitamin B_6 developed convulsive seizures. It is known that certain enzyme systems in the brain are vitamin-B_6-dependent, so that seizures may reflect altered cerebral metabolism of specific amino acids.[250]

Although rare, neonates may have seizures related to pyridoxine dependency with a daily requirement of vitamin B_6 that is several times normal. It appears likely that these infants are suffering from an inborn error in pyridoxine metabolism.

After the first 6 months of life there is an increase in the variety of food and a resultant increase in the intake of vitamin B_6. Most foods, including cereals, pasteurized milk, and meat, contain significant amounts of vitamin B_6. Inadequate intake of vitamin B_6 has not been observed as a cause of convulsions in children. With large doses of isoniazid a conditioned deficiency of pyridoxine may result in convulsions.

Phenylketonuria and Other Disorders of Amino Acid Metabolism. Phenylketonuria is associated with mental retardation and convulsive or minor nonconvulsive seizures in about 15% of cases. It is related to a disorder in the metabolism of the amino acid phenylalanine, secondary to a deficiency of the enzyme phenylalanine hydroxylase. Seizures are also a common manifestation of other disorders of amino acid metabolism (see Chapter 9).

Metals, Chemicals, and Drugs. Lead intoxication may be associated with convulsive seizures as may poisoning with thallium, alkylphosphate, chlorophenothane (DDT), and salicylates. Antipertussis vaccination may also be associated with convulsions. Therapy with steroids or phenothiazine derivatives, which are used as tranquilizing drugs, can result in seizures.

Renal Disease. Convulsions may occur with severe renal disease and renal failure due to chronic renal insufficiency, chronic glomerulonephritis, chronic pyelonephritis, the nephrotic syndrome, or acute glomerulonephritis with hypertensive encephalopathy.

Physical Factors. Some children are sensitive to ordinary light intensities. This sensitivity may be to particular portions of the light spectrum and may trigger convulsive seizures. The television picture may produce epileptic discharges. Pattern-sensitive epilepsy occurs in about 1 in 400 patients with epilepsy. The epileptic activity produced by line patterns arises from the visual cortex. Voluntary eye closure also may trigger seizures. Many of these patients have a form of primary generalized epilepsy.

Cerebral Neoplasms

The incidence of cerebral neoplasms in infants and young children is very low. When neoplasms do develop they may be associated with focal or generalized seizures. Tumors of the posterior fossa may also produce seizures.

Cerebrovascular Disease

Convulsions may occur in association with thrombosis or embolus to cerebral arteries. Cerebral embolus may be secondary to bacterial endocarditis. Angiomatous malformations of the cerebral circulation are frequently associated with seizures. Focal convulsions may occur with thrombosis of cerebral veins.

Head Trauma

Birth Injury. At the time of delivery there may be direct injury with contusion or laceration of the brain of the newborn with subsequent convulsive seizures.

Postnatal Trauma. Head injury is frequent during infancy and childhood. Seizures may develop immediately following the injury or after an interval of 6 months to 3 years. Early seizures occur within 4 days after injury. The longer the duration of coma the higher the incidence of early seizures, half of which are focal and half of which are generalized attacks. If seizures occur early after head injury there is an 8% chance of recurrent late seizures during the first year after injury. Late seizures may occur 6 months to 3 years after head injury occurs and are usually generalized. Since minor head injuries are common in children, it is frequently difficult to relate a remote history of head injury to the subsequent appearance of a convulsive disorder. If there has been localized injury to the skull and intracranial contents with the subsequent development of focal seizures related to the same area, then the relationship is clear, but if there has been no localized head injury and the seizures are generalized, the relationship is difficult to establish with certainty.

Examination

If the physician has an opportunity to observe a seizure, the clinical manifestations are carefully recorded by him and he is able to document the fact that the child has had a tonic–clonic seizure, a petit mal attack, or some form of partial seizure (see list, Approach to Studying the Child with Seizures).

Examination of a child after a seizure may reveal an elevated temperature and evidence of an acute systemic infection, such as tonsillitis, pharyngitis, otitis media, or pneumonia. Fever of 102°F to 106°F (39°C to 41°C) and systemic infection in association with a seizure in a child 6 months to 4 years of age suggest the clinical syndrome of febrile convulsions, 85% of which are generalized and 15% are focal. Neurologic examination shortly after a febrile convulsion is usually normal. Follow-up of the child with a febrile seizure is essential to observe whether seizures recur. If they do, then it is essential to determine whether they are always associated with systemic febrile illnesses.

It is important to examine the scalp, trunk, and extremities for evidence of injury. If a child is examined shortly after a focal seizure there may be transient focal neurologic deficits, such as dysphasia, hemiparesis, or asymmetry of reflexes. Postictal focal signs usually disappear within a few minutes to a few hours. The presence of transient, focal neurologic signs after an attack is of value in determining the location of the abnormal neuronal discharge.

If the child is examined in the interval between seizures it is important to search

Approach to Studying the Child with Seizures

Present Illness
Age at onset of seizures
  Time of occurrence
  Precipitants
  Inhibitors
Description of seizure
  Aura
    Abdominal symptoms
    Headache
    Special senses
  Manifestations
    Generalized or focal
    With or without loss of consciousness
    With or without tongue-biting or incontinence
  Duration
  Postictal phenomena
  Frequency
    Number per day, week, or month
    Clusters
History of exposure to chemicals, drugs, or physical factors
    Lead, DDT, thallium
    Treatment with phenothiazine derivatives, steroids

Past History
Developmental history
Prior use of anticonvulsant drugs
Predisposing factors including dietary deficiency, head injury, diabetes mellitus treated with insulin, encephalitis, meningitis, perinatal insult, metabolic disorders

Family History
Seizures in siblings, parents, or other relatives
Familial neurologic disorders

Examination
Growth parameters
Dysmorphic features
Fever, evidence of systemic infection or other organ involvement, for example, visceromegaly
Developmental and mental status
Injury to the head or body, laceration of the tongue
Cutaneous vascular lesions of scalp or face, kinky hair, depigmental or hyperpigmental macules
Skull circumference and symmetry, fontanels, bruits
Stiff neck, papilledema, retinal abnormalities, Chvostek's and Trousseau's signs
Focal neurologic signs
Hyperventilation to induce absence seizure

Laboratory Examination
EEG
Radiographs of the skull, long bones
Urinalysis, ferric chloride test of urine for phenothiazine, amino acid analysis
Blood tests for urea nitrogen, fasting sugar, calcium, phosphorus, alkaline phosphatase; glucose tolerance test; serologic tests for toxoplasmosis; liver function tests; amino acid analysis
Cerebrospinal fluid
Selected procedures
  Computerized tomography
  Cerebral angiography

systematically for any physical signs that may be a clue to the etiology of the seizure disorder. The skin of the scalp and face is examined for evidence of cutaneous vascular malformations that may be associated with cerebrovascular malformations. The circumference of the skull is measured for evidence of micro- or macrocephaly and evidence of asymmetrical development. The fontanels are carefully examined. The arms and legs are compared for asymmetry of muscular and skeletal development. The neck is examined for limitation of flexion. The eyegrounds are carefully visualized for evidence of papilledema or chorioretinitis. The cranial nerves are examined systematically, as are the motor, sensory, and reflex systems. Speech and mental development are evaluated. Chvostek's and Trousseau's signs are checked for evidence of tetany. If the history suggests that the child has absence seizures, a period of hyperventilation for 2 minutes to 3 minutes may precipitate an attack and establish this diagnosis (see list, Approach to Studying the Child with Seizures).

Laboratory Findings

Electroencephalogram. The EEG is useful as a diagnostic aid in patients with suspected seizure disorders because it frequently shows evidence of a paroxysmal electrical dysrhythmia.[83,132] In addition, it may provide evidence about the lateralization and localization of a focal cerebral disorder associated with seizures. If a seizure occurs during the EEG recording, a record of the paroxysmal electrical dysrhythmia is obtained. If the child has a history of some type of spells that have not been observed, the recording of the electrical activity accompanying a seizure may establish for the first time the fact that the child has a convulsive disorder; it may also indicate its clinical type. However, the EEG is usually recorded during an interseizure period. Initially a record is obtained while the child is awake; this may show a paroxysmal dysrhythmia in approximately half of the children with seizures. In some children with normal waking EEGs, paroxysmal dysrhythmias may be recorded with the use of hyperventilation, photic stimulation with eyes closed, and spontaneous or in-

duced sleep recordings. With these supplemental procedures 75% to 85% of children who have convulsive seizures have paroxysmal abnormalities in the EEG. In children with photogenic seizures who show a paroxysmal dysrhythmia with photic stimulation, the relative sensitivities of various portions of the light spectrum are determined. Red is more productive of abnormal patterns than blue or green.

Paroxysmal dysrhythmias in the EEG are found in approximately 3% of school-age children with no history of epileptic seizure and no neurlogic findings. In the vast majority of these asymptomatic children the electroencephalographic abnormalities disappeared later in childhood or in adolescence. Only 5% of children with paroxysmal electroencephalographic abnormalities and no prior history of seizures subsequently developed epilepsy.[33]

During a tonic–clonic seizure the EEG is characterized by high voltage fast waves or spikes (see Table 7-3). After the seizure there is marked depression of cortical activity. In a child with tonic–clonic convulsions the record between seizures may show a brief paroxysmal dysrhythmia of a generalized nature (Fig. 7-2). This may consist of a burst of high voltage spikes occurring at a rate of 20 to 30/second for a period of 2 seconds to 4 seconds. Discharges of a seizure type occur in about 20% of interseizure records, and an additional 60% of records show abnormal patterns of slow or fast waves.

Abnormalities may be present in the EEG immediately after a febrile convulsion. However, if the EEG is recorded more than 1 week after the disappearance of fever it is usually normal, although seizure discharges have been reported in as many as one-fourth of these children.

During a partial complex seizure the EEG reveals a 2 to 4/second high voltage pattern predominantly in the temporal leads. In the intervals between attacks, spike discharges from the temporal lobes may be seen. Also bursts of slow 2 to 4/second high voltage waves may appear in the temporal lobes for a period of 1 second to 4 seconds (Fig. 7-3). Pharyngeal or tympanic leads may at times show spikes when slow waves appear over the convexity of the scalp. Temporal lobe spike or slow wave discharges are seen in 35% to 50% of the records of children with partial complex seizures, and slow or fast waves appear in an additional 35%.

During an absence seizure the electroencephalographic pattern is characterized by a 3/second spike-and-wave discharge (Table 7-3; Fig. 7-4). This rhythmic spike-and-wave pattern appears simultaneously throughout all leads and may last for 1 second to 30 seconds. In children with absence seizures a prolonged record reveals the spike-and-wave pattern occurring paroxysmally in approximately 80% of patients. Hyperventilation is frequently of value in precipitating this pattern in children with absence seizures. This primary bilateral synchrony is to be distinguished from the secondary bilateral synchrony following cortical spikes that are recorded in children with partial seizures.

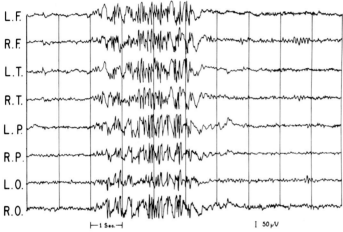

FIG. 7-2. Abnormal electroencephalogram with generalized paroxysmal dysrhythmia. The recording during the waking, interseizure state shows the simultaneous onset in all leads of paroxysmal, high amplitude (150–200) μV), sharp spikes, and fast activity lasting 3 seconds. This generalized dysrhythmia was not associated with any observed seizure. The dysrhythmia is followed in 2 seconds by the return to a pattern of normal amplitude (50–75 μV) and normal rhythm (10 cycles per second). This 12-year-old child had recurrent, generalized, tonic–clonic convulsions. L, left. R, right. F, frontal. T, temporal. P, parietal. O, occipital.

FIG. 7-3. Abnormal electroencephalogram with focal paroxysmal dysrhythmia. This recording during the waking state reveals high-voltage slow waves of 4 cycles per second occurring paroxysmally with a focal onset from leads overlying the left cerebral hemisphere in the temporoparietal area. This 14-year-old child had recurrent focal attacks classified clinically as complex partial seizures. L, left. R, right. F, frontal. T, temporal. P, parietal. O, occipital.

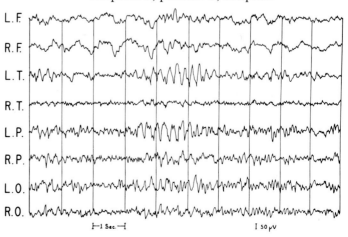

In children with infantile spasms the electroencephalographic pattern of hypsarrhythmia is seen in 85% of cases (Fig. 7-5). This consists of high voltage random slow waves and spikes in all cortical areas. It is almost continuous and appears while awake and asleep. At times the cortical activity may be generally decreased between bursts of seizure activity.

Attacks of paroxysmal headache, abdominal pain, and vomiting may be associated in some children with an electroencephalographic abnormality characterized by a pattern of 14 and 6 cps. This pattern may be noted at the beginning of sleep and is localized in the two temporal–occipital regions.

The EEG of children with myoclonic seizures may reveal polyspike-and-wave discharges (see Table 7-3). Table 7-3 details

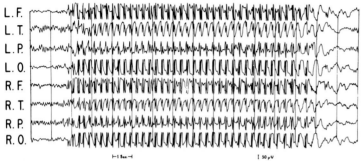

FIG. 7-4. Abnormal electroencephalogram with generalized paroxysmal dysrhythmia. In all leads a high voltage spike and slow wave pattern at a frequency of 3 cycles per second simultaneously appears, continues for 12 seconds, and then disappears within 2 seconds. During the paroxysmal discharge this 8-year-old child did not respond to questions. However, immediately after this rhythm ceased he was conscious and alert. The child had brief absence seizures. *L,* left. *R,* right. *F,* frontal. *T,* temporal. *P,* parietal. *O,* occipital.

FIG. 7-5. Hypsarrhythmia in a 2-year-old boy with infantile spasms and progressive psychomotor retardation. *A,* Initial electroencephalogram reveals numerous synchronous and asynchronous, single and multiple spikes with high-voltage slow waves of 2–5 cycles per second. *B,* After 1 month of therapy with corticotropin, the repeat electroencephalogram is improved, with less frequent spikes and slow waves. *L,* left. *R,* right. *F,* frontal. *T,* temporal. *P,* parietal. *O,* occipital.

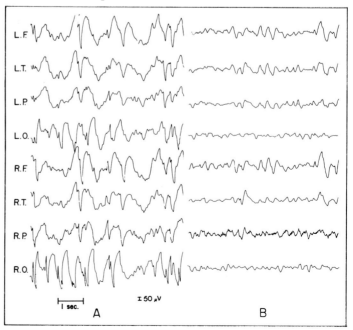

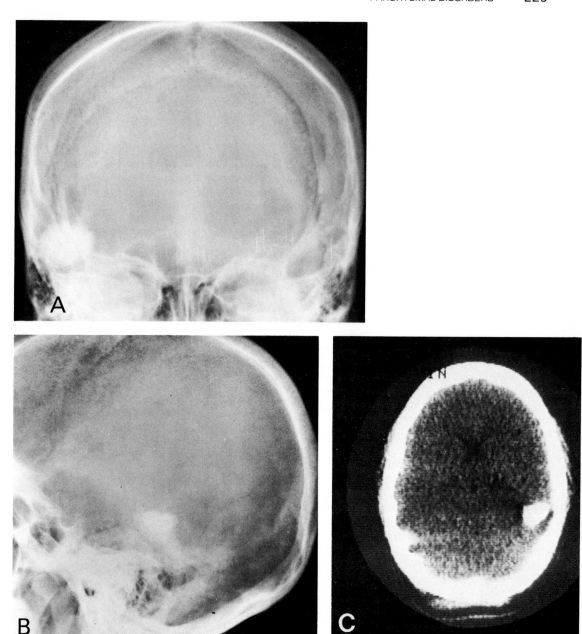

FIG. 7-6. *A* and *B*, Frontal and lateral radiographs of the skull show a 2 by 3 cm calcified mass in the right temporal area. *C*, CT scan shows right temporal area of increased density. These studies were obtained on a 16-year-old boy who had had left partial complex seizures with secondary generalization for 9 years. Electroencephalogram revealed a right posterior temporal delta wave focus. Pathological examination of the excised tumor revealed an astrocytoma.

the electroencephalographic features of other seizure types.

Roentgenograms.   In the majority of children with convulsive disorders skull radio-graphs are normal, although in some they may be of diagnostic value. There may be evidence of fracture, separation of the sutures, abnormal calcification (Fig. 7-6), or abnormalities in the size or shape of the skull. Thus skull radiographs may give definite evidence of hydrocephalus, toxoplasmosis, trauma, vascular malformation, or an expanding intracranial lesion. Radioisotopic brain scans are normal in children with seizures without other manifestations of neurologic disease.[200] The head CT scan is an extremely valuable procedure in those children in whom a partial cause for seizures is being considered. The unenhanced CT scan is a relatively safe, noninvasive test that provides information about the ventricles, cisterns, subarachnoid space, and parenchyma of the brain. An enhanced CT scan will provide additional information with the minimal risk of possible hypersensitivity of the child to the intravenously injected contrast. Since more than half of children with seizures have idiopathic epilepsy and since many of the known causes of epilepsy are not associated with abnormalities visible on the CT scan, abnormal CT scans will be seen in a minority of the total number of children with epilepsy. One-third of all children with seizure disorders will have abnormalities on the CT scan. However, two-thirds of children with seizures that began as neonates and that are associated with abnormal neurologic findings or with focal slowing on EEGs have abnormal CT scans. In contrast with this group, abnormal CT scans are seen in less than 3% of children with generalized seizures associated with a normal neurologic examination and a normal EEG. It is recommended that a noncontrast scan be performed first. If the unenhanced CT scan is normal, a contrast-enhanced CT scan does not usually furnish additional information. However, if an arteriovenous malformation or an isodense tumor without ventricular displacement is strongly suspected, then an intravenous contrast study is done.

In children with partial or generalized seizures who develop focal neurologic signs or signs of increased intracranial pressure, or who have an abnormality on the skull roentgenogram or CT scan that requires further delineation, cerebral angiography, pneumoencephalography, or ventriculography may be indicated because of a possible diagnosis of brain abscess, cerebral neoplasm, or subdural hematoma.

When lead intoxication is being considered as a possible cause of convulsive seizures, radiographs of the long bones may show dense lines at their ends owing to impregnation with metallic ion, and radiographs of the abdomen may demonstrate radiodense material in the bowel.

Examination of Cerebrospinal Fluid. In children with convulsions related to infection it is important to examine the cerebrospinal fluid for evidence of meningitis or encephalitis. In infants meningitis may be present in the absence of stiff neck, Brudzinski's sign, bulging fontanel, and depressed sensorium.[217] In children meningeal signs may be minimal early in the course of infection. Thus, in the patient with an acute febrile illness and convulsions, lumbar puncture is indicated to determine whether the child has meningitis or possibly benign febrile convulsions associated with a systemic infection.

When evaluating a child with a suspected focal cerebral lesion in association with seizures, CT scan is obtained first. Additional information may be obtained from skull x-ray films or skull roentgenograms and electroencephalography. If these studies do not establish a diagnosis and if it is decided that further diagnostic information might be obtained from examination of the cerebrospinal fluid, a lumbar puncture is then performed.

Urine, Blood, and Stool Studies. An initial evaluation of renal function with urinalysis and blood urea nitrogen is indicated to exclude uremia as a cause of seizures in selected children. Serologic tests for syphilis are performed. Fasting blood sugar and glucose tolerance curves are essential in the evaluation of possible hypoglycemia. To exclude hypocalcemia, serum calcium, phosphorus, and alkaline phosphatase determinations are performed. Rarely serologic tests for congenital infections are indicated. An analysis of urine for heavy metals, other toxins, and drugs may be helpful in selected patients. If seizures are associated with colitis, fresh stool cultures or cultures from swabs of ulcerations of the rectum or sigmoid colon are made in an effort to isolate shigella organisms. In kinky hair syndrome, which is due to an inherited defect in copper absorption, low levels of serum copper and ceruloplasmin are found during infancy.[43]

DIFFERENTIAL DIAGNOSIS

In each child with a convulsive disorder a thorough search is made for a specific cause for the seizures (see list, Approach to Studying the Child with Seizures). The age of onset of seizures may be of importance in etiologic considerations. Newborns may have seizures because of a cerebral malformation, hypocalcemia, anoxia, trauma, infection, kernicterus, or hypoglycemia. Infants with pyridoxine deficiency or dependency have seizures beginning at 3 days to 10 months of age. Hypocalcemia is probably the most common cause of seizures during the first 2 weeks of life.[214] Symptomatic neonatal hypoglycemia is increasingly recognized as a cause of neonatal convulsions, particularly in infants of low birth weight for gestational age. Over 50% of these infants are born after pregnancies complicated by toxemia. Seizures occur between 2.5 hours and 7 days of age.[225]

One-third of patients with phenylketonuria have seizures, which may occur during the first month of life; in maple syrup urine disease they occur in infancy. An infant born of a mother who is a morphine or heroin addict may show a withdrawal syndrome with an isolated generalized convulsion. Neonatal seizures may be due to trauma at the time of delivery, with intracerebral bleeding, or to intrauterine infection.

Infantile spasms usually occur first between 1 month and 6 months of age, whereas breath-holding attacks are most common between 6 months and 1 year of age. Febrile convulsions occur most often between 6 months and 4 years of age. Recurring seizures before 2 years of age may be associated with structural lesions of the brain or with metabolic disturbances. Most children with absence seizures have the onset of attacks between 4 years and 10 years of age.

It is of primary importance to obtain from the parents of the child, or from whoever has witnessed an attack, an accurate history of the spells and an adequate description of their manifestations, variations, and durations. This frequently enables one to distinguish seizures from breath-holding spells, syncope, narcolepsy, or psychologically determined attacks.

The child's description of the aura preceding the attack may furnish information about the anatomic localization of the initial seizure discharge. Initially there may be olfactory, gustatory, visual, or auditory phenomena.

A recent history of exposure to lead, thallium, or DDT, or of therapy with steroids or phenothiazine derivatives may establish a precipitating cause for seizures. A past history of dietary deficiency, previous head injury, previous meningitis, or a history of diabetes mellitus may be of significance. A developmental history may reveal retarded progress or regression. A history of the previous use of anticonvulsant drugs should be obtained and a family history of seizures elicited.

Neurologic examination or laboratory studies occasionally offer clues to the etiology of seizures. However, in the vast majority of children with recurrent seizures, careful history, examination, and laboratory study do not reveal a focal cerebral lesion or a specific extracerebral cause for the convulsive disorder. In following a child with recurrent convulsive seizures of unknown etiology, the physician should reexamine the child periodically and repeat selected laboratory procedures in order to diagnose as early as possible a specific cause for the seizures.

TREATMENT

Emergency Management of Neonatal Seizures

If a child begins to have a convulsion during the first few days of life, a blood specimen for determinations of calcium, glucose, magnesium, and sodium is obtained. An intravenous infusion is started so that intravenous injections can be given on an emergency basis. Initially pyridoxine hydrochloride, 20 mg to 50 mg, may be given intravenously to determine its effect upon seizures and upon the electroencephalographic record, if available on an emergency basis. If there is no effect in 2 minutes to 5 minutes, then an intravenous injection of 2% magnesium sulfate is given. If this has no effect, 5% calcium gluconate is administered. The injections of calcium and of magnesium are given slowly while monitoring the heart rate. Cessation of seizures after administration of magnesium is presumptive evidence of hypomagnesemia; cessation after the injection of calcium is presumptive evidence of hypocalcemic tetany. If pyridoxine, magnesium, and calcium injections do not alter the seizures, then 5 ml to 10 ml of a 20% solution of glucose is injected. If one of these injections controls seizures, the diagnosis is then confirmed by the laboratory findings and appropriate therapy instituted. If none of these infusions gives a definite therapeutic response, diazepam, 0.2 mg to 1.0 mg, is slowly injected intravenously. If seizures recur, a total dose of 2 mg to 3 mg diazepam may be given. If this does not control seizures, then phenobarbital is used.[214]

Therapeutic levels of phenobarbital are obtained in the newborn by the intravenous or intramuscular administration of 16 mg to 23 mg/kg of phenobarbital.[149] After control of seizures, 3 mg to 5 mg/kg of phenobarbital are given daily. The dose is adjusted by frequent blood levels. Phenytoin may also be administered if necessary. The dose should be 15 mg to 20 mg/kg given intravenously. If maintenance with phenytoin is necessary, this should be by the intravenous route as well.

Initial Management

During the convulsion it is essential to maintain an open airway and prevent aspiration by placing the child in the semi-prone horizontal position because cerebral anoxia may be a precipitating factor in the attack. Take care that his nose and mouth remain uncovered. Protect the child from falling in order to prevent bodily injury during the period of unconsciousness. If it is available, and if there is sufficient time before tonus occurs, a throat stick padded with gauze should be placed between the molar teeth to prevent tongue-biting. If the convulsion persists or recurs, it should be controlled with an anticonvulsant drug administered intravenously.

After a seizure the child is studied in search of a cause for the seizure (see list, Approach to Studying a Child with Seizures). If a specific etiologic factor is determined and there is a mode of therapy for

this condition, then treatment of the underlying disorder is carried out (Table 7-4). This therapy alone may prevent the recurrence of seizures in some types of disorder, for example, hypocalcemia. In other types of disorders the etiologic factor may require specific therapy, but the child may also have recurrent seizures that require treatment with anticonvulsant drugs. In still other types of disorders of known etiology that are associated with seizures, no specific therapy is available. In these disorders therapy with anticonvulsant drugs is the major initial form of treatment. Also, in children with seizures of unknown etiology the initial treatment is related chiefly to efforts to control them with drug therapy. After seizures have been controlled, management of the child's subsequent social development is of great importance. Very rarely neurosurgical treatment is indicated to control seizures.

Specific Therapy for Convulsive Seizures of Known Etiology

If the child has evidence of a disorder of water or electrolyte metabolism associated with convulsions, this is corrected (see Chap. 8).

Febrile Convulsions. If a young child is seen after a single, brief, generalized convulsive seizure related to high fever, and if a tentative diagnosis of febrile convulsion is made, the child is followed carefully and no anticonvulsant medications are used. With the subsequent development of acute systemic infections, antipyretic drugs and early specific antibiotic therapy or chemotherapy to control bacterial infections, if present, are prescribed (Table 7-4). One-third of children with febrile seizures have a second seizure, and only one in ten have three or more recurrences. The age of onset is a factor in the frequency of recurrences. One-half of children under 1 year of age who have a febrile seizure will have recurrent febrile seizures, in contrast to one-third of the total group of children under 7 years of age with febrile seizures.[180] Neither death nor persisting hemiplegia occur as sequelae of febrile seizures. A prospective study comparing a group of children with febrile seizures with their unaffected siblings has

TABLE 7-4. Therapeutic Approaches to Convulsive Seizures of Known Etiology

Etiology	Therapy
Infections	
Systemic infections including tonsillitis, otitis media, pneumonia, enterocolitis	Salicylates, antibiotics, chemotherapy
Meningitis	Antibiotics, chemotherapy
Cerebral abscess	Neurosurgical treatment, antibiotics, chemotherapy
Metabolic and Toxic Disorders	
Hyponatremia, hypernatremia	Correction of water and electrolyte disorder
Hypocalcemia	Calcium, parathyroid hormone
Hypoglycemia	Glucose, diazoxide, surgical treatment of islet cell tumor
Pyridoxine deficiency and dependency	Pyridoxine
Phenylketonuria	Low phenylalanine diet
Lead	Edathamil (Versenate)
Thallium	Dimercaprol (BAL)
Kernicterus	Replacement transfusions
Therapy with steroids or phenothiazine derivatives	Discontinuance of these drugs
Photogenic seizures	Glasses to filter light
Hypertensive encephalopathy with acute glomerulonephritis	Hypotensive drugs
Inherited defect of copper absorption	Parenteral copper
Head Trauma	
Subdural and extradural hematoma	Neurosurgery
Cerebrovascular Disease	
Cerebral embolus related to endocarditis	Antibiotics
Vascular malformations	Surgery in selected cases
Cerebral Neoplasms	
Benign neoplasms	Neurosurgery
Malignant neoplasms	Neurosurgery, radiotherapy

shown that febrile seizures have no effect upon intelligence quotient or early academic performance.[180] There are three factors that statistically increase the risk of children subsequently developing epilepsy after febrile seizures: a family history of afebrile seizures, preexisting neurologic abnormality, and complicated initial seizures. Only 1% of children in whom none of these risk factors is present develop epilepsy by 7 years of age. However, if two or more of these risk factors are present, then 10% develop epilepsy.[180]

If a child has a second febrile seizure and has none of the risk factors for epilepsy, it is reasonable that the child not be treated with daily phenobarbital because the risk of subsequent epilepsy is only 1%. This is only slightly increased over the risk in the general population. If a child has a recurrence of febrile seizures and is in the high risk group, then daily anticonvulsant therapy with phenobarbital is considered.

The major goals in considering daily phenobarbital therapy are reviewed with the parents. There are two potential goals. The first is a reduction of, or prevention of, the recurrence of febrile seizures, and the second is the prevention of subsequent afebrile seizures. Daily anticonvulsant therapy with the maintenance of an adequate plasma level above 15 µg/ml will decrease the frequency of recurrent febrile seizures.[259] However, hyperactivity and behavioral abnormalities develop in four of ten children treated with phenobarbital daily over a period of months for febrile seizures. These behavioral changes are sufficiently disturbing to the child and the parents so that medication is discontinued in one of five children.[260] Thus, it is explained to the parents that although daily phenobarbital medication may prevent possible recurrence of febrile seizures, the decision to treat the child with phenobarbital should be based further on the possible behavioral complications of the daily medication. Intermittent treatment with phenobarbital is of no value in the prevention of febrile seizures. Phenytoin does not prevent febrile seizures in children under 3 years of age.[168]

The second potential goal of treatment with phenobarbital for febrile seizures in the high risk group is the possible prevention of subsequent afebrile seizures that will occur in 10% of the children. However, there is currently no evidence that such treatment will prevent the eventual development of afebrile seizures. Therefore the physician and the parents must balance the risk of daily therapy against the unknown value of daily phenobarbital in the prevention of afebrile seizures.

If daily treatment with phenobarbital is administered either for the prevention of febrile seizures or for the possible prevention of subsequent afebrile seizures in children with high risk factors, it should then be continued for either 2 years or 1 year after the last febrile seizure, whichever is longer.

Children with a history of febrile seizures who subsequently develop afebrile seizures should be treated with anticonvulsant drugs.

Convulsions associated with shigella infections are treated initially with tetracycline (Achromycin) or with sulfadiazine. If a diagnosis of meningitis is made, appropriate antibiotic or chemotherapy is immediately instituted. Cerebral abscess is treated with appropriate neurosurgical and antibiotic therapy. Seizures secondary to hypocalcemia are treated with proper dietary control including supplemental calcium or parathyroid hormones, depending upon the etiology of the hypocalcemia. Seizures secondary to hypoglycemia are treated initially with intravenous glucose. A sensitivity to fasting with consequent hypoglycemia is the commonest type of hypoglycemia. Occasionally hypoglycemia may be associated with administration of excessive amounts of insulin in the treatment of diabetes mellitus, and rarely it is due to hyperinsulinism associated with an islet cell tumor of the pancreas.

Phenylketonuria is treated with a low phenylalanine diet. If seizures are associated with lead poisoning, chelation treatment is begun. If seizures are related to treatment with phenothiazine derivatives or steroids, these drugs are discontinued. Photogenic seizures may be prevented by the use of glasses that filter out the wavelengths of light to which the individual is photosensitive (see Table 7-4).

A child with seizures associated with subdural or extradural hematoma, brain abscess, or subdural empyema is treated with appropriate neurosurgical procedures. Seizures associated with acute glomerulonephritis and hypertensive encephalopathy may be improved by the use of hypotensive drugs. In some children with cerebrovascular malformations, surgical treatment may be indicated. In the occasional child in whom convulsive seizures are associated with the presence of a cerebral neoplasm surgical therapy is required. In addition to these specific therapies, anticonvulsant drugs may also be necessary.

Therapy with Anticonvulsant Drugs

In the majority of children with epilepsy no specific cause for the paroxysmal disorder is found. Complete control of seizures is the main initial goal, and anticonvulsant therapy is the chief means toward this end. Because one child's history and findings are different from those of another, each patient is managed according to the specific circumstances although there are a few general principles that can be applied. If a child is seen after a single convulsion and the physician can be certain from the history that the attack was a seizure, he may place the child on anticonvulsant therapy. If this is done, it should be explained to the family that the medication is to be continued daily for a prolonged period of time unless toxic symptoms from the drug require that it be discontinued. A reasonable minimal period of treatment without recurrence of seizures is 2 years. The chief reason for treating a child after a single seizure is to prevent the emotional and possible physical injury associated with a recurrent seizure. If there is some doubt about the clinical features of a single attack, if the attack may have been some form of anoxic convulsion, or if it was associated with fever or other unusual features, then it may be reasonable to observe the child without daily treatment. The reasons for this decision should be explained to the parents, and they should be instructed to report any behavior of the child that might suggest seizure activity. If a second attack occurs it usually clarifies the clinical problem and therapy is then instituted. All children who have recurrent seizures require anticonvulsant therapy.

The ideal anticonvulsant drug would be effective in patients with all different types of recurrent seizures, as well as patients in status epilepticus. It would be long-acting, require infrequent intake, and be nontoxic and nonsedative. All of the medications now available are limited in their effectiveness in various types of seizures. The anticonvulsant effect from a single dose is of relatively short duration. All of the drugs have occasional minor toxic effects, and some may produce severe, even fatal, reactions.

The anticonvulsant drugs available at the present time are divisible into the following groups: derivatives of hydantoin, dibenzoazepine, barbituric acid, valproic acid, succinimide, benzodiazepine, oxazolidine, carbonic anhydrase inhibitor, and amphetamines. Table 7-5 presents a summary of the drugs used, preparations available, the dosages, and the minor and major complications of these drugs. The drugs recommended for controlling various clinical types of seizures are given in Table 7-6.

The type of seizure is determined by history, examination, electroencephalography, and other investigations. The drug that is least toxic and most effective in controlling this type of seizure is then administered in the proper dosage for the child's body weight. Records of seizures are kept by the family. Medication is increased to the point of complete therapeutic effect or toxic reaction.

If only a partial therapeutic effect is obtained at the toxic level of the first medication administered, then the second most effective medication is added and the dose increased to its toxic level. In occasional cases the addition of a third drug may result in more complete control of seizures than that obtained with two medications. Trials of different medications are frequently required. Although an average dose of a single anticonvulsant drug may frequently be effective, adequate control in many cases requires close follow-up and individual care. Administration of new anticonvulsant drugs should be limited to those patients who do not respond to adequate dosages of well established drugs.

The therapeutic plasma levels of the commonly used anticonvulsant drugs are listed in Table 7-7. Factors that alter plasma levels are patient compliance, laboratory variability, concurrent medications, differences in metabolism, and variability in bioavailability among various pharmaceutical preparations.

Plasma levels are frequently of tremendous value in management. The indications for obtaining plasma levels of anticonvulsant drugs in children are as follows: (1) A plasma level will determine whether a therapeutic level has been obtained after the child with infrequent seizures has been on a therapeutic dose of anticonvulsant drug for several weeks. (2) The plasma level is also of definite value if seizures are not controlled on medication. If the level is therapeutic, then the child is taking his medication regularly. However, if the level is quite low then either there is poor compliance, rapid drug metabolism, or altered absorption. (3) If symptoms of possible toxicity develop it is important to know whether or not these symptoms are related to a toxic plasma level of the drug. (4) After an additional drug has been added to control seizures, it is important to determine whether drug interaction has altered the plasma levels. (5) If the child develops a gastrointestinal, hepatic, or renal disease, it is important to monitor the plasma level because of possible changes in absorption and metabolism of the drug.

The plasma half-life of the different drugs is important in the planning of therapy (Table 7-7). The total daily dose of drugs with a plasma half-life of more than 12 hours can be given as a single dose in the morning or evening to obtain better compliance than may be obtained with divided doses. However, drugs with a short plasma half-life must be given in divided doses to maintain therapeutic levels through each 24-hour period.

The doses of anticonvulsant medications for children are prescribed in proportion to the child's weight. Small children frequently require and are able to tolerate relatively more medication on a milligram

TABLE 7-5. Drugs Used in the Treatment of Epilepsy

Drug	Dose[a] mg/kg per day	Complications
Phenytoin sodium (Dilantin) Capsules (30 mg, 100 mg) Tablets (50 mg) Suspensions (30 mg/5 ml or 125 mg/5 ml) Ampules (50 mg/ml)	4–7	Nausea, vomiting, nervousness, skin rash, overgrowth of gums, nystagmus, diplopia, ataxia, hypertrichosis, lymphadenopathy, exfoliative dermatitis, hepatitis, psychosis, macrocytic anemia, lymphosarcomalike disorder, Raynaud's phenomenon, polyneuropathy, lupus erythematosus, osteomalacia
Carbamazepine (Tegretol) Tablets (200 mg)	20–30	Drowsiness, dizziness, diplopia, ataxia, nausea, vomiting, rash, edema, fever, sore throat, easy bruising, jaundice, aplastic anemia, agranulocytosis, thrombocytopenia
Phenobarbital Tablets (16 mg, 32 mg, 64 mg, 100 mg) Elixir (16 mg/5 ml)	3–5	Drowsiness, irritable behavior, skin rash, exfoliative dermatitis, delirium, hyperpyrexia, hyperactivity, osteomalacia
Mephobarbital (Mebaral) Tablets (32 mg, 100 mg, 200 mg)	4–15	Drowsiness, skin rash
Primidone (Mysoline) Tablets (50 mg, 250 mg)	10–25	Nausea, vomiting, drowsiness, minor psychic disturbances, ataxia, vertigo, rash, macrocytic anemia
Valproic acid (Depakene) Capsules (250 mg) Syrup (250 mg/5 ml)	15–60	Nausea, vomiting, diarrhea, skin rash, loss of hair, hepatitis, pancreatitis, encephalopathy, stupor, thrombocytopenia, prolonged bleeding time, leukopenia, appetite changes, tremor
Ethosuximide (Zarontin) Capsules (250 mg) Syrup (250 mg/5 ml)	20–30	Headache, dizziness, nausea, rash, drowsiness, agranulocytosis, leukopenia, lupus erythematosus, abnormal renal or liver function, hiccups
Methsuximide (Celontin) Capsules (150 mg, 300 mg)	5–20	Drowsiness, ataxia, vomiting, diplopia, skin rash, periorbital hyperemia, dizziness, aplastic anemia, psychosis
Diazepam (Valium) Tablets (2 mg, 5 mg, 10 mg)	0.1–1.0	Drowsiness, ataxia, rash, dysarthria, vertigo, neutropenia, jaundice
Clonazepam (Clonopin) Tablets (0.5 mg, 1 mg, 2 mg)	0.1–0.2	Drowsiness, ataxia, vertigo, nystagmus, hair loss, rash, edema, nausea, anemia, leukopenia, thrombocytopenia
Trimethadione (Tridione) Capsules (300 mg) Tablets (150 mg)	10–25	Skin rash, photophobia, nausea, drowsiness, alopecia, hemeralopia, aplastic anemia, agranulocytosis, nephrosis, hepatitis, exfoliative dermatitis, lupus erythematosus
Acetazolamide (Diamox) Tablets (125 mg, 250 mg)	10–20	Drowsiness, disorientation, paresthesias, agranulocytosis, thrombocytopenia, decreased renal function
Amphetamine sulfate (Benzedrine) Tablets (5 mg, 10 mg)	0.2–0.4	Insomnia, agitation
Dextroamphetamine sulfate (Dexedrine) Tablets (5 mg) Elixir (5 mg/5 ml)	0.2–0.4	Insomnia, agitation

[a]Method for determining percentage of adult dosage according to weight. From the age of 1 year, children should be given (1.5 × weight in kilograms + 10) percent of the dose for an adult or (0.7 × weight in pounds + 10) percent of the dose for an adult. This corresponds closely with the dosage per square meter of body area.

TABLE 7-6. Drugs Recommended for Controlling Clinical Types of Seizures

Types of Seizures	Drug Treatment	
	Major Drugs	Alternative Drugs
Partial		
Simple and Complex	Phenytoin Carbamazepine Phenobarbital	Primidone Valproic Acid Methsuximide
Generalized		
Absence	Ethosuximide Valproic Acid Clonazepam	Trimethadione Acetazolamide
Tonic–Clonic	Phenobarbital Phenytoin	Primidone Carbamazepine Valproic Acid
Myoclonic, Tonic, Atonic, Akinetic	Valproic Acid Clonazepam	Phenytoin Phenobarbital Acetazolamide
Infantile Spasms	ACTH	Valproic Acid Clonazepam Diazepam

per kilogram basis than adults. This is due to the fact that these drugs are eliminated from the body more rapidly in children than in adults.

Adolescent girls with well controlled epilepsy prior to conception usually do not have an increase in the frequency of seizures during pregnancy. However, when seizure frequency before pregnancy is greater than one seizure per month, more than one-half of women will have some deterioration in the control of seizures especially during the first trimester. This is associated with a decrease in plasma levels of anticonvulsant drugs in spite of a constant oral dose of medications. This is attributed to several factors including an increase in hepatic metabolic rate, intestinal malabsorption, and placental transfer and fetal elimination of the drugs. In these patients plasma levels are obtained at monthly intervals during pregnancy and in the postpartum period. If necessary, the dosage of drugs is increased to maintain therapeutic levels.[176]

Phenytoin. Phenytoin was first used clinically in 1938, and it has been a major anticonvulsant drug for the past 40 years. It

TABLE 7-7. Therapeutic Plasma Level and Plasma Half-life of Anticonvulsant Drugs

Drug	Therapeutic Plasma Concentration (μg/ml)	Plasma Half-life (hr)
Phenytoin	10–20	7–42
Carbamazepine	4–10	12–17
Phenobarbital	15–40	48–144
Primidone	6–12	3–12
Valproic Acid	50–100	6–18
Ethosuximide	40–100	36–72
Methsuximide	10–40	28–57
Clonazepam	0.013–0.072	18–50
Trimethadione	6–41	12–24

is available in 30-mg and 100-mg capsules. Phenytoin produces less gastric irritation if it is taken after meals than before. A 50-mg preparation of phenytoin (Infatab) is the best preparation for young children. A liquid suspension containing 30 mg phenytoin/5 ml diluent is also available for infants and young children, but crushed tablets are preferred to the suspension. Because the phenytoin is not dissolved in the suspension it is essential to instruct the parents to shake the suspension well before use to avoid variation in dose. If a suspension is prescribed, it is essential to make certain with the pharmacist that the 30 mg phenytoin/5 ml diluent suspension is dispensed because a suspension containing 125 mg phenytoin/5 ml diluent is also available. Rarely, reduced seizure control may be due to damage to phenytoin capsules produced by exposure to high temperatures exceeding 45°C and high humidity in excess of 85%. Discolored capsules should not be used.[38]

The method of action of phenytoin is probably related to prevention of the spread of seizure activity rather than to abolition of the primary focus of seizure discharges. It stabilizes but does not raise the normal seizure threshold.

Phenytoin is the least toxic of the hydantoinates. Symptoms of toxicity include nystagmus, ataxia with unsteadiness in walking, nausea, vomiting, and occasionally nervousness and drowsiness. Toxic psychosis may occur with large doses. These symptoms disappear when the dosage is decreased. Dermatitis occurs within 2 weeks of the onset of treatment in approximately 5% to 10% of patients. The rash is morbilliform and may be associated with fever. Upon withdrawal of phenytoin, the rash usually disappears. If treatment is reinstituted and rash recurs, then further use of phenytoin is contraindicated.[98]

Rarely, exfoliative dermatitis, blood dyscrasias, and hepatitis occur with phenytoin medication, and several fatal reactions have been reported.[187] Hypertrophy of the gums often develops in children treated with phenytoin; this can sometimes be controlled with good oral hygiene and daily massage of the gums. If gum hypertrophy has become excessive, excision of gum tissue by a dentist may be necessary. Hyper-

trichosis is a fairly frequent toxic manifestation of phenytoin. The emotional disturbance produced in adolescent girls by the development of hypertrichosis may be sufficient reason to replace the drug with another anticonvulsant medication.

Osteomalacia may occur in children taking phenytoin over many years, and this may result in bone fractures. The diagnosis is based on low blood calcium and phosphate associated with elevated alkaline phosphatase and appropriate roentgenographic changes.[95,242]

Rarely, a patient on phenytoin therapy develops macrocytic anemia associated with a megaloblastic bone marrow. This complication is related to a disturbance in nucleoprotein metabolism. The macrocytic anemia is corrected with folic acid, and phenytoin may be continued to control seizures.

Enlargement of lymph nodes, liver, and spleen with associated fever infrequently occurs with phenytoin therapy. This clinical picture suggests lymphosarcoma; furthermore, lymph node biopsy reveals the pathologic changes seen in lymphosarcoma (hyperplasia of the reticulum cells, pleomorphism, and focal necrosis). If these changes occur it is imperative that phenytoin therapy be stopped, not only to establish the diagnosis of this sensitivity reaction but also to prevent a possible fatal termination.[6] Phenytoin rarely produces Raynaud's phenomenon, polyneuropathy, drug-induced lupus erythematosus, and periarteritis nodosa. Cerebellar degeneration has been reported in association with chronic, high-dose phenytoin therapy.[166] Phenytoin rarely produces choreoathetosis in children.[35]

Phenytoin plasma concentrations are determined in children with a gas-liquid chromatographic assay technique and radioimmunoassays. The availability of these determinations is a major advance in the management of children whose seizures are not controlled on the prescribed dosage of phenytoin. With an average daily dose of 5 mg/kg, the average blood level is 10 μg/ml to 20 μg/ml. The toxic level is above 20 μg/ml. If a therapeutic level is not obtained with the prescribed daily dose of 5 mg/kg, the child may not be receiving his medication regularly. This possibility should then be reviewed with the parents. If an abnormally high plasma level is obtained with a dose of 5 mg/kg per day, there is probably a defect in hydroxylation by the liver. Normally 60% of phenytoin is degraded to 5-(p-hydroxyphenyl)-5-phenylhydantoin. In children with a congenital phenytoin parahydroxylation deficiency, less than 50% of the metabolite is excreted in the urine. As a result a smaller than usual dose of phenytoin produces a therapeutic plasma level.

Approximately 10% of the plasma concentration of phenytoin is free and 90% is bound to plasma proteins. The plasma concentration of free phenytoin represents the therapeutically significant measure of the active drug. Thus, a therapeutic concentration of 1.5 µg/ml to 2.0 µg/ml of free phenytoin is present when the total concentration is 15 µg/ml to 20 µg/ml.[163] Phenytoin concentration in saliva is similar to the concentration of free phenytoin in plasma.[23]

Studies of plasma levels of phenobarbital and phenytoin in children who are taking both medications show that phenobarbital does not significantly accelerate phenytoin metabolism.[29] Combined therapy with these two drugs, when indicated, frequently improves seizure control.

Severe intoxication with phenytoin is associated with coma, hypotension, unresponsive pupils, hyperglycemia, and rarely, permanent neurologic disability. Exchange transfusions have been used with severe intoxication. The hyperglycemia is reversible. With acute overdosage plasma levels of 40 µg/ml to 100 µg/ml or more occur, and the plasma half-life of phenytoin is prolonged to 40 hours to 60 hours in contrast with a half-life of 24 hours at a therapeutic level of 10 µg/ml.[109] Death due to overdosage is related to respiratory depression and apnea.

The metabolism of phenytoin is inhibited by isoniazid to some degree in almost all patients who are slow inactivators of isoniazid. Toxicity to phenytoin develops in about 10% of patients who are initially on therapeutic doses of the drug and who are then placed on isoniazid therapy for tuberculosis. Therefore if a child is receiving phenytoin, and isoniazid therapy is planned, it should first be determined whether the child is a slow inactivator of isoniazid. If he is, the plasma level of phenytoin can be measured when he is taking isoniazid and the dosage of phenytoin reduced if necessary, to maintain a therapeutic level and avoid toxicity.[24] Phenytoin concentrations in the plasma may also be elevated by coumadin, chloramphenicol, and ethosuximide.

In adolescent girls of childbearing age who are taking phenytoin for recurrent seizures, the potential risks of teratogenesis are important. A fetal syndrome characterized by dysmorphic facial features and digits along with retarded mental and physical growth occurs with an increased incidence in children exposed in utero to phenytoin. Phenytoin has also been associated with an increased incidence of other malformations including cleft palate, cleft lip, and central nervous system or cardiac defects in children exposed in utero to phenytoin.[97,106] The cause of this increased incidence of anomalies is not known. Although phenytoin probably is the cause, several other maternal factors may also be involved including heredity, the epileptic disorder itself, anoxia due to seizures during pregnancy, and so on.

Carbamazepine. Carbamazepine has been used as an antiepileptic drug since 1961. This drug is chemically unrelated to other anticonvulsant drugs, but it is related to the tricyclic antidepressants. It is metabolized in the liver and three-fourths of it is excreted in the urine. Carbamazepine is available in a 200-mg tablet. Prior to its use, complete blood, platelet, and reticulocyte counts as well as liver function studies and urinalysis are obtained. Any significant abnormalities will rule out the use of this drug.

An initial dose of 100 mg is given, and the dose is increased gradually at the rate of 100 mg daily to a maximal daily dose of 20 mg/kg per day to 30 mg/kg per day. During treatment the same blood studies are repeated at weekly intervals for the first 3 months and then at monthly intervals for 2 or 3 years. The drug should be stopped if any evidence of bone marrow depression develops. This includes a hematocrit of less than 32%, hemoglobin less than 11 g/dl, a leucocyte count of less than 4000/mm³, a reticulocyte count of less than 20,000/mm³, or a platelet count of less than 100,000/mm³.

Liver function studies and urinalysis are done at regular intervals, and the drug is discontinued if evidence of hepatic or renal damage occurs.

The patient's family should be advised to notify their physician immediately if a child develops fever, sore throat, ulcers in the mouth, easy bruising, or petechial or purpuric hemorrhages. If toxic symptoms develop the drug is discontinued. Other toxic effects of the drug include drowsiness, diplopia, dizziness, ataxia, nausea, rash, and edema. Severe toxicity may result in aplastic anemia, agranulocytosis, and thrombocytopenia. Because of the necessity of frequent blood tests for potentially serious side-effects, carbamazepine is not recommended as the drug of first choice in seizure disorders. It should not be used in children with a history of previous bone marrow depression or known sensitivity to any of the tricyclic antidepressant drugs.

The therapeutic plasma level is 4 μg/ml to 10 μg/ml. Carbamazepine will produce palatal defects in the offspring of pregnant mice when the drug is fed to pregnant mice between days 8 and 13.[189]

Phenobarbital. Phenobarbital was first used for the treatment of seizures in 1912. It is a relatively nontoxic drug that has been used extensively for the treatment of seizure disorders in children for a period of many years. It is available both in tablets and liquid form. The usual dose is 3 mg/kg per day to 5 mg/kg per day. Since the usual half-life of the drug is from 2 days to 6 days, it may be given as a single dose at bedtime. It may also be given in divided doses two or three times daily. The therapeutic plasma concentration is 15 μg/ml to 40 μg/ml. Drowsiness may be noted during the first week of medication, after which it diminishes. On a constant dosage schedule the plasma level reaches a plateau in 10 days to 14 days. After this the frequency with which the medication is given during the course of a single day changes the serum level of phenobarbital very slightly. If seizures are not completely controlled with the initial daily dosage of medication, the dose is gradually increased until seizures are controlled or toxic symptoms appear. Excessive drowsiness during the day is the symptom that usually limits the maximal

dosage of phenobarbital that can be prescribed for a particular child.

Infrequently an allergic reaction with a generalized skin eruption may occur with phenobarbital; usually the rash is mild and subsides rapidly when the drug is withdrawn. Very rarely hyperpyrexia, delirium, and exfoliative dermatitis may develop. In some children phenobarbital produces hyperactivity and learning problems of sufficient severity to require the replacement of phenobarbital with another anticonvulsant drug. Osteomalacia may develop when the drug is continued over a period of years.[242]

Mephobarbital. Mephobarbital may also be given as an initial medication; some children appear to tolerate it better than phenobarbital. The absorption of mephobarbital from the gastrointestinal tract is more variable than that of phenobarbital. Mephobarbital is demethylated to phenobarbital in the body. The daily dose is 4 mg/kg to 15 mg/kg. Mephobarbital, like phenobarbital, may produce drowsiness and skin rash.

Primidone. Primidone, a barbituric acid derivative, was first used in 1951. It is available in 50- and 250-mg tablets. An initial daily dose of 5 mg/kg is given at bedtime for the first week. After 1 week the daily dosage may be increased to 10 mg/kg, and after 2 weeks to 15 mg/kg in divided doses. If necessary to control seizures, the daily dose may be further increased to as much as 25 mg/kg. If toxic symptoms develop at any of these levels, the dosage should be decreased to a nontoxic level. The gradual increase in dosage often prevents undesirable sedation.

Primidone is converted to two major metabolites, phenobarbital and phenylethylmalonamide. Thus when a child is treated with primidone alone, serum levels of both primidone and phenobarbital develop. Clinical evidence suggests that not only the tissue level of phenobarbital but also the tissue level of unchanged primidone contributes to the anticonvulsant properties of orally administered primidone. The mean phenobarbital to primidone ratio is 1 with wide variability.[65] If a child is treated with both primidone and phenobarbital, then both drugs contribute to the resultant serum level of phenobarbital. If phenytoin is used in conjunction with primidone, the mean phenobarbital to primidone ratio is above 4 because phenytoin promotes the induction of an enzyme system responsible for the oxidation of primidone. As a result, toxic levels of phenobarbital may result from combined treatment with primidone and phenytoin unless drug levels are monitored to prevent toxicity. The therapeutic plasma level of primidone is 6 μg/ml to 12 μg/ml. The plasma half-life of primidone is 3 hours to 12 hours.

Primidone may produce nausea, vomiting, drowsiness, ataxia, vertigo, and minor psychic disturbances. Minor toxic reactions appear in approximately 20% of patients. The dosage must be maintained beneath the level of toxic reaction. Prolonged treatment with primidone is frequently associated with a subnormal serum level of folic acid but without anemia.[121] Rarely macrocytic anemia develops in patients taking this drug. The anemia is readily reversible by folic acid therapy. No fatal reactions have been reported. Prolonged treatment may also be associated with reduced serum calcium levels and raised serum alkaline phosphatase.[116] In a few cases clinical osteomalacia has occurred.[46] Primidone causes induction of hepatic microsomal enzymes, which alter the metabolism of vitamin D in the liver with a resultant increased requirement for that vitamin.

Valproic Acid. Valproic acid is an eight-carbon branched-chain fatty acid, which was discovered in 1882. Its anticonvulsant effect was first described in 1963. The initial clinical trials of valproic acid in 1971 have been followed by extensive use of this anticonvulsant drug.[209,229] Valproic acid is not chemically related to other drugs used to treat seizure disorders. It may raise the level of GABA in certain regions of the brain. It decreases the amount of epileptiform activity on the EEG, which correlates with a decreased frequency of clinical seizures.[1]

Valproic acid is supplied in 250-mg capsules. A syrup containing 250 mg/5 ml of sodium valproate is also available for infants and young children. Blood counts and liver function tests should be done prior to the institution of therapy. An initial daily dose of 15 mg/kg is given for the first week. The dosage can then be increased at weekly intervals by 5 mg/kg per day to 10 mg/kg per day until seizures are controlled or until side-effects develop. Medication is given three times daily. The maximal recommended dose is 60 mg/kg per day. If toxic symptoms develop at any level, the dosage should be decreased to a nontoxic level. The half-life of valproic acid in children varies from 6 hours to 18 hours. Therefore, it is important to administer this drug at 8-hour intervals.

Valproic acid is metabolized in the liver and is excreted in the urine. The therapeutic plasma level is 50 μg/ml to 100 μg/ml. On a constant dose, plasma levels vary widely in relation to the time interval between the last dose and the time of sampling due to the short plasma half-life.

Nausea, vomiting, diarrhea, and drowsiness may occur with valproic acid therapy. It is recommended that valproic acid be taken after meals to avoid nausea. The symptoms may subside with a decrease in dosage. Skin rash and transient loss of hair have also been reported. Hepatitis and pancreatitis have been reported very infrequently.[15,237] A few fatalities have been reported. There may be low plasma fibrinogen concentration, low platelet count, prolonged bleeding time, elevated serum transaminase, and leukopenia.[238] Acute toxic encephalopathy with confusion and hallucinations may occur with high doses of valproic acid.[34] Tremor of the benign essential type has been observed.[117] In children being treated with valproic acid, liver function tests, platelet counts, and bleeding time determinations are performed every 2 months. The drug should be discontinued if systemic symptoms of toxic hepatitis appear or if the serum enzyme levels exceed three times the upper limit of normal.[27] Parents should be warned to watch their child for easy bruising or bleeding. They should also be told of possible effects of aspirin and valproic acid on coagulation. If a child taking valproic acid is planning to have an operation, clotting factors, platelet counts, bleeding time, and platelet function should be thoroughly evaluated prior to surgery.

Stupor may occur as a result of drug interaction after the addition of valproic acid to a therapeutic regimen of other antiepileptic drugs.[215] The effect of valproic acid on the plasma levels of phenytoin and phenobarbital is variable, so that it is necessary to monitor the plasma levels of all the drugs being administered to children who are on multiple drug therapy. The plasma phenobarbital level is usually increased from 20% to 50%. The total plasma phenytoin level is decreased because valproic acid displaces phenytoin from protein-binding sites. However, the percentage of free plasma phenytoin is increased from 10% to 20%.[163] Valproic acid does not induce liver enzymes. In children taking primidone, the addition of valproic acid causes a rise in primidone and phenobarbital plasma levels.

Animal studies have shown dose-related teratogenesis with valproic acid. However, no human studies are available.

Ethosuximide. Ethosuximide is an effective drug in controlling absence seizures. The usual daily dosage range is 20 mg/kg to 30 mg/kg. If seizures are not controlled with an initial daily dose of 20 mg/kg, the dosage is gradually increased at weekly intervals until seizures are controlled or until the following toxic symptoms develop: skin rash, anorexia, headache, nausea, vomiting, ataxia, or drowsiness. White blood cell counts are done every 2 weeks to 4 weeks. If leukopenia develops, the drug is discontinued. Agranulocytosis and lupus erythematosus occur rarely. Because liver and kidney toxicity have been reported, periodic urinalysis and liver function studies are performed. Ethosuximide raises the convulsive threshold of the central nervous system and suppresses the paroxysmal spike-and-wave pattern. The therapeutic level of ethosuximide in the plasma is 40 μg/ml to 100 μg/ml.

The available clinical evidence suggests that the incidence of congenital anomalies in the offspring of women treated with ethosuximide during pregnancy is low. This is in contrast with a higher incidence of associated congenital anomalies in the offspring of pregnant women treated with trimethadione.

Methsuximide. Methsuximide has been used since 1955 for treating seizure disorders. The daily dosage range is 5 mg/kg to 20 mg/kg. Methsuximide may produce drowsiness, ataxia, vomiting, diplopia, skin rash, periorbital edema, and, rarely, aplastic anemia. The plasma half-life of methsuximide is usually 1 or 2 days. The therapeutic plasma concentration is 10 μg/ml to 40 μg/ml.[199]

Diazepam. Diazepam is an anticonvulsant drug available in tablets of 2 mg, 5 mg, and 10 mg and is also available for intravenous administration in the control of prolonged motor seizures. The daily dose of diazepam is 0.1 mg/kg per day to 1.0 mg/kg per day. Toxic symptoms observed with the oral preparation include drowsiness, ataxia, rash, dysarthria, vertigo, neutropenia, and jaundice. Diazepam given orally has limited use as an adjunct in the treatment of seizure disorders. Intravenous diazepam is frequently of value in the treatment of prolonged motor seizures in children. The initial dose is 0.1 mg/kg to 0.2 mg/kg. Since intravenous diazepam may cause severe respiratory depression, it should be used with adequate precautions.

Clonazepam. Clonazepam is used in the treatment of absence and atypical absence seizures in children. It suppresses the spike-and-wave discharges in absence seizures and decreases the spread of discharge in atypical absence seizures.[26] The initial dose is 0.01 mg/kg per day to 0.03 mg/kg per day given in two or three divided doses. Dosage should be increased by no more than 0.25 mg to 0.5 mg every third day to a maximal dose of 0.1 mg/kg per day to 0.2 mg/kg per day. It should not be used in children with a history of sensitivity to benzodiazepines or a history of liver disease. The drug is excreted in the urine. Drowsiness occurs in about one-half of patients and ataxia is common. Drowsiness and ataxia are usually dose related and can be reduced by a reduction in the dosage. However, in some patients these symptoms persist so that the drug must be discontinued. Behavioral disturbances including hyperactivity, irritability, and aggressive behavior occur in about 15% of patients. Other occasional toxic symptoms include thick speech, salivation, and bronchial hypersecretion. Periodic blood counts and liver function tests are performed for possible toxicity. The concomitant use of clonazepam and valproic acid may produce absence status.

Trimethadione. Trimethadione was first used in 1944. An initial dose of 5 mg/kg is administered in the morning, then every 3 days the dosage is increased by 5 mg/kg until the seizures are controlled or until a maximal dose of 25 mg/kg is reached. The plasma half-life of the original trimethadione is 12 hours to 24 hours. Trimethadione is demethylated in the body. The plasma level of demethylated trimethadione continues to rise for 4 weeks to 6 weeks after institution of therapy until the rate of excretion is equal to the rate of absorption. When trimethadione is discontinued, a significant plasma level of demethylated trimethadione may remain for 1 month.

The toxic effects of trimethadione are occasionally severe or even fatal in children, so caution must be exercised in its use. It may produce generalized morbilliform or urticarial skin eruption, photophobia, drowsiness, or nausea. The drug is withdrawn when the skin reaction appears. If it is reinstituted after the rash clears, it should be given in small dosage and the child observed closely. Photophobia does not usually develop until 1 week or more after initiation of therapy. The child notices that all brightly lighted objects appear white, and he avoids this unpleasant sensation. Photophobia may be controlled with dark glasses. Drowsiness and nausea usually disappear with continuation of therapy. Rarely trimethadione produces partial alopecia. Withdrawal of the drug is followed by regrowth of scalp hair. Severe and sometimes fatal reactions are due to agranulocytosis, aplastic anemia, and nephrosis with albuminuria. When children are placed on trimethadione therapy, blood count and urine examinations should be made at 2-week intervals during the first 2 months of therapy and thereafter at monthly intervals. If the blood count reveals a definite decrease in leukocytes (below 3000/mm^3) or in erythrocytes, or if urinalysis reveals albuminuria or erythrocytes, the drug should be discontinued. Parents should be instructed to notify their physician at once if their child develops malaise, rash, fever, sore throat, loss of appetite, or an upper respiratory infection. Blood counts should then be repeated because these symptoms may indicate the development of a blood dyscrasia. In addition, hepatitis, exfoliative dermatitis, or lupus erythematosus may occur.

In adolescent girls trimethadione therapy poses a risk of congenital anomalies in the fetus if the patient becomes pregnant. The fetal trimethadione syndrome includes developmental delay, speech difficulty, cleft palate, V-shaped eyebrows, low-set ears, and occasionally other anomalies.[267]

Acetazolamide. Acetazolamide was first recommended for use as an anticonvulsant in 1952. It inhibits brain carbonic anhydrase and has acidifying and dehydrating properties. The initial dose, 10 mg/kg to 15 mg/kg, may be increased to 20 mg/kg per day. Large doses may produce drowsiness and paresthesias of the face and limbs. Agranulocytosis, thrombocytopenia, and renal lesions have been reported. The drug is sometimes useful as an adjunct to other therapies.

Amphetamine Sulfate and Dextroamphetamine Sulfate. Amphetamine sulfate or dextroamphetamine sulfate is sometimes added to the anticonvulsant drugs used to reduce the frequency of seizures and to control drowsiness. An initial dose of 0.2 mg/kg per day may be increased to the point of toxicity, with symptoms that include overstimulation, anorexia, and insomnia.

Ketogenic Diet

In some children, the ketogenic diet is of value in the control of seizures.[144] This diet is designed to produce ketosis, and its administration must be systematic and closely supervised. It is used in children who have not been controlled on anticonvulsant medications. Sustained ketosis with a high fat diet is a factor in raising the convulsive threshold. The ketogenic diet may be used along with anticonvulsant drugs to improve seizure control.[49]

Use of Anticonvulsant Drugs in Different Types of Seizures

Simple and Complex Partial Seizures. The major drugs for the treatment of simple and complex partial seizures are phenytoin, carbamazepine, and phenobarbital (see Table 7-6). Treatment is initiated with one of these drugs and the dosage is increased to a therapeutic level. If complete control is not obtained with a single drug, then a second drug is added and, if necessary, a third drug. The drugs that may also be added to control partial seizures in some patients include primidone, valproic acid, and methsuximide. With the use of these relatively nontoxic medications in doses demonstrated by plasma levels to be in the therapeutic range, approximately 60% of children obtain complete control of seizures. An additional 20% demonstrate marked improvement. In approximately 20% the seizures are not satisfactorily controlled with any one or any combination of these medications.

Generalized Absence Seizures. Ethosuximide is the most effective drug in controlling absence seizures. Fifty percent of children with absence seizures treated with ethosuximide will have 90% to 100% control of their attacks. Some decrease in frequency of attacks occurs in 95% of children.[28] If seizures are not controlled with ethosuximide, valproic acid therapy is instituted. Approximately one-half of children have either marked improvement or complete control of seizures on adequate doses of valproic acid. Clonazepam is effective in controlling absence seizures in about one-third of children. Trimethadione and acetazolamide are alternative drugs for the control of absence seizures.

Absence status occurs in rare instances. This is treated with the same drugs used to control periodic absence seizures.

Sixty percent of children with absence seizures subsequently develop generalized tonic–clonic seizures. For this reason phenobarbital may be used along with ethosuximide or other drugs used for the control of absence seizures.[147] Since phenytoin may increase absence seizures, it is not used in these children.

Children who initially develop absence seizures alone have a better outcome for eventual cessation of seizures than do children with both absence and generalized tonic–clonic seizures.[219]

Generalized Tonic–Clonic Seizures. The two major drugs used in the treatment of tonic–clonic seizures are phenobarbital and phenytoin. Initially a therapeutic level of phenobarbital is obtained. If this completely controls seizures, no additional medication is needed. If only partial control of seizures is obtained with phenobarbital, then phenytoin is added to obtain more effective control. Alternate drugs of value in controlling tonic–clonic seizures in children who are not completely controlled on therapeutic levels of phenobarbital and phenytoin are primidone, carbamazepine, and valproic acid.

Generalized Myoclonic, Tonic, Atonic, and Akinetic Seizures. The major drugs used to treat these types of generalized seizures are valproic acid and clonazepam. Clonazepam is effective in controlling myoclonic seizures in approximately one-half of children, and it is effective in controlling tonic and akinetic seizures in approximately one-fourth of children. Additional drugs of value in controlling myoclonic, tonic, atonic, and akinetic seizures in children include phenytoin, phenobarbital, and acetazolamide. In addition the ketogenic diet is of value in some children.

Infantile Spasms with Hypsarrhythmia. If this disorder is related to pyridoxine deficiency or dependency, hypoglycemia, lead encephalopathy, phenylketonuria, or intracranial neoplasm, then therapy that is appropriate for that particular disorder is instituted. If infantile spasms are associated with a disorder for which no therapy is available or if the clinical picture is not associated with any specific disorder, then the major therapy consists in efforts to control seizures. Steroid therapy has been used successfully to reduce the frequency of seizures with a resultant return toward normal of the EEG in 25% to 50% of infants (see Fig. 7-5). However, in most infants there is not an associated improvement in subsequent psychomotor development. Steroid therapy, with both adrenocorticotropic hormone (ACTH) and prednisone, has been used. Several different schedules of ACTH therapy have been recommended. In one schedule ACTH is administered intramuscularly in a dose of 20 units daily for 20 days. This course may then be repeated after 2 weeks to 4 weeks if necessary. Groups of children have been treated with 80 units of ACTH given intramuscularly every other day for 10 months.[230] Prednisone in a dose of 2 mg/kg per day administered for 4 weeks produces control of seizures in 25% of infants serially monitored.[115] Either valproic acid or clonazepam in therapeutic doses controls infantile spasms in approximately one-fourth of infants. In some infants diazepam is effective in the control of infantile spasms.

Status Epilepticus or Prolonged Motor Seizure Activity

In children who develop frequently recurring or constant seizures persisting for many hours it is imperative that this continuous epileptic state be controlled to avoid a fatal outcome. Status epilepticus may be treated with diazepam, sodium phenobarbital, sodium diphenylhydantoinate, paraldehyde, or ether (Table 7-8).

Initially intravenous diazepam is used because it penetrates the brain more rapidly than phenobarbital or phenytoin. Phenobarbital and phenytoin are used to maintain seizure control because the clearance of these drugs from the brain is slow in contrast with the rapid clearance of diazepam.[206]

Diazepam is the initial drug of choice to control prolonged motor seizures. It is administered slowly intravenously in a dose of 0.1 mg/kg to 0.2 mg/kg. This usually results in a rapid cessation of seizures, the control persisting at least 15 minutes.[181] If seizures recur within the first few hours after injection, additional diazepam is administered intravenously. Subsequently oral or parenteral administration of anticonvulsants, such as phenobarbital or phenytoin in therapeutic doses, is necessary to sustain the control of seizures.

If diazepam is not effective, sodium phenobarbital is given slowly intravenously in an initial dose of 5 mg/kg. If seizures are only partially controlled after 15 minutes to 20 minutes, an additional dose of 3 mg/kg is given intravenously. Subsequent doses of sodium phenobarbital are given intramuscularly until the child is able to take oral medications. The risk of respiratory depression must be carefully considered when using sodium phenobarbital in large doses.

If sodium diphenylhydantoinate is used to control continuous seizures, it may be administered intravenously in an initial dose of 15 mg/kg to 20 mg/kg. The preparation for intravenous administration, which contains sodium diphenylhydantoinate, ethanol, and propylene glycol, is highly alkaline. It is injected intravenously at a rate not exceeding 50 mg/min. It should not be given in the scalp veins because of the risk of subcutaneous perivascular infiltration with subsequent local irritation and infection of the skin and subcutaneous tissue. After an initial injection of sodium diphenylhydantoinate a second intravenous dose of 2 mg/kg may be given after 15 minutes to 30 minutes. Intravenous sodium diphenylhydantoinate may produce fatal ventricular fibrillation, cardiac arrest, or respiratory arrest.

Paraldehyde in a dosage of 0.3 ml/kg may be given by rectum to control seizures. If diazepam, sodium phenobarbital, sodium diphenylhydantoinate, and paraldehyde are not successful in decreasing the frequency of seizures, inhalation anesthesia with ether may be required. Repeated suction and rarely tracheostomy may be needed to maintain an adequate airway. Oxygen therapy may prevent cerebral anoxia. With prolonged seizures, adequate fluid intake is maintained with parenteral fluids.

TABLE 7-8. Drugs Used in the Treatment of Status Epilepticus

Drug	Route of Administration	Initial Dose
Diazepam	Intravenous	0.1 mg/kg–0.2 mg/kg
Sodium phenobarbital	Intravenous, intramuscular	15 mg/kg–20 mg/kg
Sodium diphenylhydantoinate	Intravenous	15 mg/kg–20 mg/kg
Paraldehyde	Rectal	0.3 ml/kg (4% in oil)
Ether	Inhalation	Light anesthetic dose

After the continuous epileptic state has been partially controlled with these emergency measures, oral anticonvulsant medications are administered in therapeutic dosage. Serum drug levels are obtained frequently to maintain a therapeutic level of each drug.

Management of Social Development

The nature of the epileptic disorder should be carefully explained to parents to free their minds of misinformation, unfounded fears, shame, and a desire for secrecy. It is helpful to discuss the seizure disorder or epilepsy as a symptom of brain disease. An analogy with the symptoms of cough has proved useful in practice. Parents are told that just as cough may be a symptom of a cold, aspiration, pneumonia, tuberculosis, trauma, or tumor, so may seizures result from a great many disease processes. However, often a specific cause is not discovered, and this is referred to as *cryptogenic* or *idiopathic epilepsy*. It is pointed out that the capacity for sudden, excessive, and disorderly discharge of neurons is inherent in the brains of all people, as evidenced by the universal response to electroshock therapy. It is acknowledged that some individuals are more susceptible than others. The necessity for prolonged therapy is stressed. Parents are reassured that the drugs being used are not "dope," which is a common misconception. It is allowed that the child may eventually "outgrow" the tendency to seizures, but the parents are told that patience is necessary. The parents and patients are warned that control of seizures may take several trials of medications, and they are urged not to become discouraged. The dangers of sudden withdrawal of drugs are emphasized. The door should be left open for both patient and parents to ask any questions that bother them at any time.

After seizures have been controlled on medication an opportunity must be provided for the child to live a normal life. Small children should enjoy their play activities with friends and neighbors. With few exceptions the usual physical activities to which the child is accustomed at his age level should be continued. It is important to explain to the parents the risks involved in a child's swimming, particularly without supervision. With effective supervision children whose seizures are controlled should be encouraged to swim because the absolute risk of drowning is low. Epileptic children who swim are four times more likely to drown than normal children, so therefore they should never swim alone.[190]

Children with epilepsy should not bathe in a tub alone because most immersion deaths in these children occur in the bathtub.[190] Epileptic children should also not take showers alone, particularly if standing in a glass- or plastic-enclosed stall, because of the risk of injury. It is recommended that they sit on a chair in a shower and use a hand-held showering instrument controlled by finger pressure. If the seizures are not completely controlled, the risk of a sport such as horseback riding should be mentioned. If the child is of school age and the attacks are partly or completely controlled, then he should continue in school. A sympathetic attitude on the part of the teacher and appropriate explanations to the other pupils and their parents are important in the child's adjustment in his school life. As a child approaches adolescence it is important that he better understand the nature of his disorder and the reasons for taking daily medication. Children's questions to the physician should be answered simply and honestly. Adolescents frequently ask whether they may learn to drive an automobile. This is a legal and a medical problem, and the circumstances vary in each case. An individual whose seizures are not controlled cannot safely drive an automobile; the patient should be on medications and free of seizures for a period of 1 year to 2 years before the risk of driving is considered. The patient must adhere to the laws governing the licensing of epileptics. After a period of 2 years without a seizure on medication there is an 8% chance that a person will subsequently have a seizure. If the person drives an automobile 2 hours of a 24-hour period, then there is 1 chance in 12 that this possible seizure will occur while driving. Half of the seizures that occur while driving cause accidents, and one-fourth of these accidents cause death or serious damage.

Surgical Therapy

Removal of Epileptogenic Tissue. Cortical scars may be present due to head injury at birth or during infancy or childhood. It has been shown by electrocorticography that brain tissue adjacent to a scar may act as a focus for seizure discharges. Rarely in selected children who have not been controlled with anticonvulsant medications, surgical excision of epileptogenic tissue is indicated in an effort to control seizures. This is a highly specialized neurosurgical procedure for which only a few neurologic and neurosurgical centers are adequately equipped. It requires facilities for electrocorticography as well as personnel trained in clinical neurophysiology and a neurosurgeon who has had special experience in this field. In the procedure all of the cortex that shows electrical abnormality in the area of the scar is excised. After surgery anticonvulsant medication is continued. Excision of cerebral scars in patients with uncontrollable convulsive seizures has resulted in a definite decrease in the frequency of seizures in one-third of patients.

Hemispherectomy. In children with hemiplegia resulting from birth injury or developmental defect there may be recurrent focal and generalized seizures not controlled with anticonvulsant drugs. Hemispherectomy is performed in some of these patients with little increase in neurologic deficit and frequently with better control of seizures than prior to surgery.[257]

Anterior Temporal Lobectomy. If partial complex seizures are not controlled with medications initially it is advisable to defer surgical therapy for as long as possible because improvement may subsequently occur with other combinations of medications. Rarely, temporal lobectomy is indicated in children.[59,60] In patients with temporal lobe seizures associated with unilateral electroencephalographic foci recorded over the temporal lobes and in whom attacks were not controlled by anticonvulsant drugs, convulsive seizures were controlled after the excision of the epileptogenic foci in 64%. In patients with elec-troencephalographic evidence of bilateral foci in the anterior temporal lobes 23% were controlled after operation. Anticonvulsant drugs are usually required after surgery.

PROGNOSIS

The prognosis for infants who have had convulsions during the first month of life depends upon the cause of the seizures. One-fourth of them die during the first 3 months of life. They have a variety of cerebral lesions including absence of the corpus callosum, hydrocephalus, and areas of agenesis or destruction. Many of those who survive are mentally retarded with neurologic deficits.[225] However, about half of the infants have a good prognosis. The vast majority of those neonates who have seizures associated with a normal EEG develop normally.[214] Of the children who have an initial seizure during a febrile illness, 3% to 10% subsequently develop recurrent seizures not associated with fever, and in 5% of these, convulsions recur frequently.

Seizures occurring in association with meningitis, encephalitis, and acute head trauma usually do not recur after recovery from the acute illness. However, recurrent seizures may develop, and these require anticonvulsant therapy. Seizures observed in association with cerebral abscess, tumor, and vascular lesions of the cerebral hemispheres usually recur after treatment and require prolonged therapy with anticonvulsant drugs.

In children with epilepsy of unknown etiology who are not treated with anticonvulsant drugs the frequency of seizures may remain relatively constant from one month to the next, or there may be marked variation in the frequency of attacks. Absence seizures usually stop or become less frequent during adolescence, but they are often replaced by tonic–clonic or mixed seizures in adult life. A child with combined absence and tonic–clonic seizures may cease to have absence attacks during adolescence but the tonic–clonic attacks may persist.

The effectiveness of anticonvulsant drugs in the control of epilepsy of unknown etiology varies with the individual patient and with the types of seizures. Approximately one-half of children obtain complete control of seizures and an additional one-fourth of them obtain partial control with the drugs currently available. The effectiveness of anticonvulsant drugs of a given dosage in an individual child usually remains constant, although variations in the therapeutic effect may occur over a period of months or years. If variations do occur, then a change in the dosage or type of medication is required in an effort to control the seizures completely.

If therapy with anticonvulsant drugs results in the complete control of seizures, the importance of maintaining daily medications is emphasized to the parents and the child. After a child on medication has been completely free of tonic–clonic or partial seizures for 4 years, the need for continued treatment should be reviewed. Approximately one-fourth of children whose seizures have been completely controlled on medication for 4 years have a recurrence of seizures if their medications are discontinued. This incidence of recurrence is based on a follow-up period of 5 years to 10 years after withdrawal.[113] The risks of gradually withdrawing medication are reviewed with the parents, and a decision is then made. If it is decided to reduce medications, a slow withdrawal program is followed to determine whether the child requires continued anticonvulsant medication. If the child is taking a single anticonvulsant drug, this is withdrawn in three stages of decreased dosage over a period of 9 months. If two or more drugs are being administered, then only one is discontinued at a time. Each is decreased in three steps at 3-month intervals. Nearly two-thirds of children with seizure recurrence following gradual withdrawal of medication have the attacks within the first year after beginning withdrawal. The best prognosis for successful withdrawal of medication is in children with controlled tonic–clonic seizures. The relapse rate is highest in children with partial seizures and in those with multiple seizure types.[113]

Children free of absence seizures who have been on medication for 1 year may have their medication dosage for absence attacks reduced over a 3-month period, but phenobarbital is continued for an additional 3 years. If a seizure recurs during or after the withdrawal of medication, the drugs are resumed in the previous dosage. If the medication can be gradually discontinued without recurrence of seizures, then the child is followed carefully without medications. The EEG is not of prognostic value with reference to the need for continued anticonvulsant medication in patients whose seizures have been controlled with anticonvulsant drugs.

The mortality rate of children with status epilepticus is dependent upon the therapy administered. However, in spite of vigorous efforts to control seizures with anticonvulsant drugs, approximately 5% of such children die. In addition, occasional unexplained deaths in children with seizures may be the result of severe anoxia during a prolonged seizure. Death may result from an accidental consequence of seizures, for example, drowning, suffocation, head trauma, aspiration of food, or severe burns. Approximately 3% of deaths due to drowning are caused by seizures.[190] Occasional deaths are due to suicide. Rarely children with epilepsy probably die from acute disruption of brain stem, cardiac, or respiratory functions secondary to seizure discharge.[107]

OTHER PAROXYSMAL DISTURBANCES OF CONSCIOUSNESS

It is not possible to consider all of the conditions that potentially can produce disturbances of consciousness. We will instead restrict the discussion to those conditions that typically produce recurrent episodes of alterations of consciousness. These conditions are the most difficult to differentiate from seizures and yet they are some of the most treatable and, in some instances, the most potentially devastating disorders. The disorders that produce complete loss of consciousness characterized by unresponsiveness and unawareness should be distinguished from those with partial preservation of awareness or responsiveness. In the former group are included partial complex seizures of certain types, generalized seizures, syncope, metabolic disturbances such as hypoglycemia, and other miscellaneous conditions in which the mechanisms are not entirely understood. Conditions that can produce partial disturbance of consciousness include partial seizures, acute confusional migraine, cyclic metabolic disturbances, and hysteria. Those conditions that occur commonly include seizures, acute confusional migraine, cyanotic breath holding spells, and vasovagal syncope and postural hypotensive syncope.

SYNCOPE

Syncope is characterized by a transient complete loss of consciousness due to inadequate blood or oxygen supply to the entire brain or brain stem. (See list on some of the causes of syncope in childhood.) The most common form of syncope is vasovagal syncope. The sequence of events in this form of syncope is characteristic. The presentation in the pediatric patient usually occurs in adolescence. The circumstances surrounding this form of syncope usually entail a significant degree of fear, anxiety, or pain. Other predisposing factors include intercurrent illness, vasodilation, hypovolemic states, use of drugs with autonomic side-effects, anemia, bedrest, and inactivity. The patient usually is aware of impending syncope when nausea, vomiting, lightheadedness or vertigo, diaphoresis, a feeling of warmth, blurred vision, visual scotoma, or weakness occur. As a response to these warnings the patient will often seek a recumbent position or at least will be able to avoid an injurious fall. During unconsciousness the patient will appear pale and may have bradycardia and hypotension. Vasovagal syncope occurs only in the upright position. If the head remains above the level of the body after the onset of the hypotension a generalized clonic convulsion may occur.

One can usually clinically distinguish cardiac syncope from vasovagal syncope. In cardiac syncope the precipitating event is absent or often different from that in vasovagal syncope. Exercise is a common precipitant in aortic insufficiency, aortic stenosis, and the prolonged Q–T interval syndrome and fright or pain in pallid breath-holding spells. In most types of cardiac syncope there is no warning prior to loss of

Mechanisms and Etiology of Recurrent Syncope in Infants and Children

I. Reduced Peripheral Vascular Resistance
  A. Vasodepressor (vasovagal) effect
  B. Orthostatic hypotension
    1. Primary dysautonomia[7]
    2. Neuropathic, drugs, prolonged bedrest, hypovolemia, hyperbradykininism[236]
II. Reduced Cardiac Output
  A. Obstructed outflow
    1. Idiopathic hypertrophic subaortic stenosis[69]
    2. Discrete membranous subaortic stenosis[129]
  B. Reduced venous return; cyanotic breath-holding spells[153]
  C. Increased right-to-left blood shunting
    1. Tetralogy of Fallot[165]
    2. Pulmonic stenosis[155]
  D. Dysrhythmias
    1. Vagal
      Pallid infantile syncope[153]
      Excessive vagal tone[208]
      Mitral valve prolapse syndrome[137]
      Swallow syncope[252]
    2. Ventricular fibrillation
      Aortic stenosis, primary[69]
      Pulmonary hypertension[241]
      Secondary pulmonary hypertension[231]
      Pulmonary stenosis[69]
      Hypomagnesemia[150]
      Hypokalemic periodic paralysis[141]
      Hyperkalemic periodic paralysis[143]
      Aberrant coronary artery[124]
      Paroxysmal familial ventricular fibrillation[167]
    3. Long Q–T interval
      Hereditary with deafness or without deafness[122,251]
      Hypokalemia, hypomagnesemia, drugs[150]
    4. Disorders of cardiac conduction
      Congenital heart disease[212]
      Post cardiac surgery[265]
      Congenital heart block[179]
      Myocarditis[11,265]
      Rheumatic fever[140]
      Sarcoidosis[198]
      Mitral valve prolapse syndrome[25,263]
      Sick sinus syndrome[227]
III. Others of Uncertain Mechanism
  A. Cough syncope; pertussis
  B. Arnold Chiari type 1[48]
  C. Hyperventilation syndrome[54]

consciousness. Palpitations, a symptom that adults may recognize prior to cardiac syncope, is an unusual complaint in childhood. Loss of consciousness in cardiac syncope is usually abrupt and may even occur in the recumbent position. During unconsciousness the patient appears pale and cyanotic. The pulse is usually slow or irregular and the blood pressure is low. As in vasovagal syncope, brief generalized convulsions may occur, especially in the prolonged Q–T interval syndrome. Return of consciousness after cardiac syncope is rapid. An electrocardiogram (EKG) during an attack will often allow definite diagnosis. Between spells the routine EKG may also be abnormal. It may be necessary, however, to use special procedures to elicit the abnormality on EKG. These procedures include carotid sinus or ocular compression in pallid breath-holding spells, exercise in the prolonged Q–T interval syndrome, and Holter-monitoring in the mitral valve prolapse syndrome.[122,153,263] Cardiac exam is essential in these patients because cardiac murmurs or abnormalities of cardiac sounds or size may be obvious. Other clues may be helpful as well. Patients with prolonged Q–T interval may also be deaf.[122] The family history is important because prolonged Q–T interval with deafness is inherited in an autosomal recessive fashion and the isolated prolonged Q–T interval syndrome is inherited in an autosomal dominant fashion.[253] Diagnosis of these conditions is imperative because treatment of some of them is effective in avoiding sudden death.

CYANOTIC BREATH-HOLDING SPELLS

Lombroso and Lerman distinguished two forms of breath-holding spells occurring in infancy and early childhood: cyanotic and pallid.[153] The pallid breath-holding spell is a form of cardiac syncope characterized by asystole that often can be elicited by vagal stimulation. Pallid and cyanotic breath-holding spells tend to occur in the same age group, children less than 5 years of age. They begin between 6 and 18 months in most children and cease by 6 years in 90% of children.[153] Together these two types account for most of the syncope occurring in infancy and early childhood, occurring in perhaps as many as 5% of children. Pallid breath-holding spells are differentiated from cyanotic breath-holding spells on the basis of precipitating event, presence or absence

of cyanosis during the spell, and the response to vagal stimulation, (a positive response being asystole longer than 2 sec).[153] Cyanotic breath-holding spells are far more common than pallid breath-holding spells. Typically, the child with cyanotic breath-holding spells begins to cry after frustration, anger, or injury. Shortly after beginning to cry the child abruptly stops breathing in inspiration, becomes cyanotic, loses consciousness, becomes limp, and then develops, in sequence, opisthotonus and clonus.[136,153] As in most syncope, consciousness returns quickly. Incontinence may occur usually when opisthotonus occurs.[136] Children with cyanotic breath-holding spells are otherwise normal. Moreover, no apparent ill effect accrues despite attacks that may occur daily.[153] Breath-holding spells usually resolve spontaneously by 5 years of age, although in some children recurrent syncope may persist into adolescence.[153] Treatment of cyanotic breath-holding spells is unnecessary but parents should be reassured and encouraged not to pay undue attention to the spells. Breath-holding spells may occur in more than one member of the family.[153] Anemia has been reported in some patients with breath-holding spells and treatment of the anemia may improve the spells.[112,153] The EEG between episodes is normal and during the spell shows nonspecified slowing.[153]

OTHER CAUSES OF COMPLETE LOSS OF CONSCIOUSNESS

Occasionally metabolic disturbances such as hypoglycemia will present as recurrent loss of consciousness with or without seizures. The loss of consciousness, however, usually lasts long enough that the patient is taken to a medical facility where a blood glucose determination may be performed. Diabetic children requiring daily insulin are particularly likely to have recurrent hypoglycemia, often of short duration. The early symptoms of hypoglycemia, including diaphoresis, tremulousness, and hunger, as well as the prompt response to glucose, are helpful clinical clues in the diagnosis of hypoglycemia.

Sudden increases in intracranial pressure can also produce recurrent, sudden and complete loss of consciousness. A condition in which this occurs is Arnold-Chiari type 1.[48] Activity that increases intracranial pressure can in this condition lead to recurrent, brief loss of consciousness. Cranial nerve abnormalities, signs compatible with syrinx, and an appearance characterized by a short neck and low hairline are common features of this syndrome that should suggest the diagnosis. Rarely a tumor of the third ventricle, usually a colloid cyst, can act in a "ball valve" fashion to obstruct the foramen of Monro, thus producing a rapid increase in intracranial pressure.[192] Symptoms in this case are intermittent headache and loss of consciousness associated with opisthotonic posturing. Typically, patients with this tumor sleep with their head down and their buttocks up, apparently to prevent the obstruction of the foramen of Monro by the tumor.

EPISODIC PARTIAL DISTURBANCES OF CONSCIOUSNESS

The common causes of episodic partial disturbances of consciousness include seizures, partial or generalized, and acute confusional migraine. Most metabolic disturbances produce extended periods of disturbed consciousness characterized by acidosis, hyperammonemia, or hypoglycemia. These conditions will be considered in the chapter on metabolic diseases.

Bickerstaff called attention to a disturbance of consciousness in patients with migraine.[19] He described three adolescent girls who had episodes of loss of awareness and partial unresponsiveness. He noted that the disturbance of consciousness was curiously slow in onset and never complete. These same patients often had features of what has come to be called *basilar artery migraine* (see below).[18] On recovery they had throbbing occipital headaches associated with vomiting. These patients and patients like them who have what has been called *acute confusional migraine* usually have more typical migraine headaches at other times.[74] The confusion is often characterized by agitation.[74] As in other types

of migraine there is generally a strong family history of migraine. During the attack the EEG reveals diffuse or focal slowing.[74] The EEG between attacks is frequently abnormal with posterior slowing.

NARCOLEPSY

Narcolepsy and the frequently associated conditions of cataplexy, hypnagogic hallucinations, and sleep paralysis are often confused with other disturbances of consciousness. These disorders can occur alone or in combinations of two, three, or all four of the above symptoms. In a review of sleep disorders in childhood, the peak age of onset of narcolepsy was between 15 and 25 years.[92] Narcolepsy is characterized by a rapid transition from alertness to slow wave or rapid eye movement (REM) sleep. Narcoleptic attacks can occur in unusual circumstances often without warning. The patient sleeps only for short periods of time and is arousable during the narcoleptic attack. Children with narcolepsy may also have microsleep episodes, especially if napping is prohibited.[92] If the microsleep episodes occur frequently the child may develop an "automatic behavior syndrome" with amnesia.[93] These episodes are characterized by deterioration in performance and amnesia similar to that seen in the adult syndrome, transient global amnesia. Behavior may have an automatic quality, and therefore, be ill-adapted to environmental changes. Obviously, such behavior could be difficult to distinguish from that occurring in partial complex seizures. Narcolepsy can be confused with hypersomnia, which differs from narcolepsy in that the episodes of sleep are of long duration and the patient is difficult to arouse. The latter condition can be seen in a variety of conditions including the Klein-Levin syndrome and as one of the components of the sleep apnea syndromes. An EEG aids in the diagnosis of narcolepsy because it can reveal the rapid transition from waking to REM sleep.

Cataplexy is associated with narcolepsy in approximately 88% of patients.[92] Patients with this disorder have abrupt loss of muscle tone, often generalized, and resulting in a fall, but no loss of consciousness. These attacks occur when the patient is frightened, surprised, or laughing, the last of these being the most common precipitant.

Hypnagogic hallucinations are auditory or visual perceptions that are usually vague in quality. These often appear at the onset of sleep paralysis and are, therefore, even more frightening. Sleep paralysis usually occurs just before going to sleep or just before awakening. These attacks are quite frightening to the patient because he can breathe and move his eyes but is otherwise unable to move. Even slight cutaneous or auditory stimuli can end the paralysis, which otherwise usually lasts seconds.

Narcolepsy is a familial problem.[131] Its incidence in families is 5%. Inheritence, however, appears to be nonMendelian. The problem persists into adulthood, often becoming less frequent. Treatment consists of reassurance, frequent short naps, and methylphenidate or amphetamines in large doses. Imipramine is useful in treating sleep paralysis, cataplexy, and hynagogic hallucinations.

PSEUDOSEIZURES

The frequent confusion between organic seizures and pseudoseizures has a long history.[86] This confusion is not surprising considering the array of behavior observed in seizures.[42] The distinction is complicated by the frequent occurrence of pseudoseizures in patients with real seizures and the recognized influence of psychogenic factors on seizure frequency.[89,111,256] Pseudoseizures are common in childhood, most commonly occurring in adolescent females. Pseudoseizures can take a variety of forms but are typically characterized by altered consciousness that may be complete or partial, and by headaches or abnormal movements.[66] Incontinence, physical injury, and postictal changes are uncommon in pseudoseizures. Pseudoseizures often have an element of combativeness and occur in relation to stress.[111] Pseudoseizures usually fail to respond to anticonvulsants. Perhaps the most useful technique for separating pseudoseizures from organic seizures is si-

multaneously recording the EEG, ECoG, or nasopharangeal or sphenoidal EEG, and the patient's video image.[111,210] Psychiatric evaluation of patients suspected of having pseudoseizures should be obtained. The Minnesota Multiphasic Personality Inventory, when used in such patients, often reveals significant psychopathology.[66] Psychotherapy may be indicated in patients with suspected pseudoseizures because this therapy may also be beneficial in refractory seizure patients with psychogenically triggered organic seizures.[256]

HEADACHE

Headache is a common symptom in young children and adolescents; it is often associated with nausea or vomiting and may be preceded in a small percentage of children by an aura, usually a visual disturbance.[70] Migraine is a form of recurrent, throbbing, usually unilateral headache that occurs in 2% of children. *Tension headache* refers to a bilateral, frequently nonthrobbing, headache associated with emotional disorder.[69]

ETIOLOGY

Headache occurs commonly in association with a wide variety of systemic diseases. Acute febrile illnesses are frequently accompanied by headache. Infections of the ears and mastoids are associated with local head pain and headache. In older children sinusitis is a common cause of headache. A tumor or osteomyelitis involving the skull also produces head pain. A wide variety of neurologic disorders also cause headache, including meningitis, brain abscess, subdural empyema, encephalitis, cerebral neoplasms, vascular malformations, and acute head injuries.

Migraine headache is related to vasodilatation in the external carotid system. The extracranial arteries usually involved are the superficial temporal, maxillary, lingual, and posterior auricular arteries.[261] A genetic factor may be present in migraine, since in approximately one-half of children with migraine a history of similar headaches is elicited in other members of the family.

Tension headache may be precipitated by stressful situations in the child's environment.

PATHOLOGY

If the headache is associated with a systemic disorder or with a neurologic disorder of known etiology, the pathologic findings are those of the fundamental disorder. In other forms of recurrent headache no pathologic findings are observed.

SYMPTOMS

Headache associated with acute febrile illnesses in children is usually a generalized, bilateral pain that may be throbbing or nonthrobbing. If the pain is extremely severe, it may be associated with nausea. Ear and mastoid infections frequently produce unilateral, severe head pain. The pattern of pain associated with sinusitis varies with the sinuses involved and frequently follows a diurnal pattern. Localized frontal head pain, either unilateral or bilateral, suggests frontal sinusitis. With maxillary sinusitis, pain over the cheek is common. The severity of the pain is frequently related to the progress of the infection, and the headache is relieved when the sinus is adequately drained.

Meningitis and encephalitis are usually associated with generalized headache. Pain from a brain abscess or a subdural empyema may be unilateral or bilateral. Headache associated with vascular malformation in one cerebral hemisphere may be of a throbbing, unilateral type. Cerebellar neoplasms are often accompanied by occipital and suboccipital head pain, although headache may be referred to the frontal region. Tumors of the cerebral hemisphere are usually associated with frontal, parietal, or temporal headache that may be unilateral or bilateral and that may be worse in the morning than in the evening.

Approximately 2% of children develop symptoms of migraine during the first 10 years of life, and one-third of these complain of headache in the first 4 years. Cyclic vomiting is the dominant feature of migraine in small children. In girls the onset of migraine frequently coincides with the onset of menses at 12 years to 15 years of age. At least half of all migraine begins before the age of 16. Attacks frequently begin in the morning and may awaken the child from sleep, although they can occur at any time of the day.[14] In 10% of children, scotomas develop as the initial aura of a migrainous attack. Scotomas are noted by children over 10 years of age; they usually consist of jagged lines moving across one-half of the visual field, or they may appear throughout the visual field. Vision may become blurred to one side, and sometimes there is transient loss of vision on one side. Less frequent auras include numbness and tingling, weakness or paralysis of one side of the body, and dysphasia. These focal manifestations are rare and may suggest other etiologic bases for the symptoms. Usually the migrainous attack begins with the severe onset of a throbbing headache that is usually unilateral but may be bilateral. Unilateral headaches tend to recur on the same side, although most patients with migraine eventually do have attacks involving the opposite side of the head, as well as bilaterally. The duration of the headache varies from an hour to several days. Photophobia, nausea, and vomiting are common accompaniments of severe headache. When the headache subsides the child feels well. In the rare instances in which a migrainous attack is associated with a focal neurologic deficit, this deficit usually disappears within a few hours. Migraine may produce an acute confusional state in children.[74]

EXAMINATION

Headache associated with sinus infection may be quite localized and related to tenderness on percussion over the frontal sinus or on firm pressure over the maxillary sinus. Localized mastoid tenderness may be present, or visualization of the eardrum may reveal acute inflammation.

Cerebral disorders associated with headache may produce focal neurologic deficits. With a vascular malformation a bruit may be heard over the orbit or skull, but bruits in children must be interpreted with caution (see Chap. 1). Scalp tenderness may be present in association with migrainous headaches. Firm pressure over the common carotid artery in the neck on the same side as the headache or pressure over the superficial temporal artery may produce a decrease in headache.

LABORATORY EXAMINATION

In children with headache associated with systemic or neurologic infections the laboratory examinations indicated are those relating to the primary infection. When there is a suspected neurologic disorder lumbar puncture and roentgenograms of the skull may be indicated.

During the interval between headaches, one of ten children with periodic migrainous headaches has a spike dysrhythmia on the EEG, and three of ten have slow or paroxysmally slow recordings. Thus four of ten children with migraine have abnormal EEGs. These abnormalities occur most frequently in children between the ages of 5 and 13 years. Rarely EEGs recorded during the prodromal period of a migrainous headache associated with scotomas may show focal occipital slowing.

DIFFERENTIAL DIAGNOSIS

In children with persistent or recurrent occipital headache the possibility of neoplasm in the posterior fossa must be excluded. Headache may be associated with periodic vomiting. Examination may reveal unsteadiness in gait. The optic disks should be carefully examined for evidence of early papilledema. Roentgenograms of the skull may reveal separation of the sutures in young children or demineralization of the sella turcica in older children. Frontal, parietal, or temporal headache may rarely be an early symptom of a cerebral hemisphere neoplasm. Examination may reveal lateralizing signs. Roentgenograms of the skull, CT scan, EEG, and lumbar puncture may furnish additional information of value in diagnosis. The diagnosis of migraine is based on the recurrent nature of similar throbbing headaches frequently associated with nausea and vomiting and occasionally preceded by an aura. Similar periodic headaches may also occur with vascular malformations involving one cerebral hemisphere. CT scan or carotid angiography may be required to establish this diagnosis.

TREATMENT

The treatment of systemic infections and neurologic disorders associated with headache is related to the therapy of the primary disorder. The treatment of migraine is directed toward prevention of recurrent attacks and also toward control of individual attacks. During an acute attack the child is permitted to rest in a quiet, darkened room. Analgesic drugs are of greatest value in the treatment of acute migrainous attacks in children. Acetylsalicylic acid in a dose of 5 mg/kg to 10 mg/kg may be repeated at 3-hour to 4-hour intervals if needed. With severe, prolonged headache not relieved by salicylates, codeine sulfate in a dose of 1 mg/kg may be required.

In addition to analgesic drugs, derivatives of ergot are of value in controlling headache in some children by producing vasoconstriction of dilated vessels in the external carotid system.[110] Ergot drugs used in the treatment of migraine attacks are listed in Table 7-9. A variety of ergot preparations is available for different routes of administration. In the use of such preparations it is important that the medication be given at the onset of an attack with the hope of aborting a portion of it. In an older child 100 mg of caffeine and 1 mg of ergotamine tartrate is given after the onset of the initial symptoms. This dosage of one tablet may be repeated every 30 min for a total of three doses if necessary to relieve headache. In small children the dose is correspondingly smaller. If the attack is associated with vomiting after a short interval, sufficient time may not be available for absorption of an oral preparation prior to vomiting, and thus the medication is of no value. In some individuals headache is controlled by the use of suppositories. In an adolescent child one suppository containing 2 mg of ergotamine tartrate and 100 mg of caffeine is given rectally at the onset of the first symptoms. In young children with migraine one-half of a suppository is given at the onset of an attack. This may be repeated in 1 hour if necessary. Absorption of the oral and rectal preparation occurs over a period of 15 minutes to 1 hour. A sublingual tablet containing 2 mg of ergotamine tartrate is of particular value in some patients. The tablet is placed under the tongue, and the ergotamine is absorbed through the buccal mucosa. Relief of headache may be noted in 10 minutes to 15 minutes. One-half tablet is advised for children. The dosage may be repeated at 30 and 60 minutes if necessary, up to a total of three doses. Ergotamine is also available in an oral inhaler, the drug being absorbed through the respiratory tract. Each puff from the inhaler expels 0.36 mg of ergotamine. Ergotamine taken sublingually or by inhalation has the advantage of providing adequate absorption in spite of gastrointestinal symptoms. Occasionally it may be necessary to give ergotamine by intramuscular injection to relieve a severe headache. Dihydroergotamine mesylate is given intramuscularly in a dose of 0.5 mg to 1.0 mg at the onset of a severe headache. This dosage may be repeated after an interval of 1 hour, and a third injection may be given after another hour if necessary.

Most children obtain partial or complete relief from an attack of severe migraine with one of these preparations of ergotamine. The efficacies of the routes of administration differ with the individual. Slight variations in the amount of the initial dose and the number of repeat doses required are noted. It is important that in a single attack of migraine the child does not take more than two or three doses of the preparation being used. For this reason the drug is prescribed with careful directions and in small quantities, for example, a prescription for 12 tablets. Symptoms of intoxication with ergot include headache, nausea, vomiting, diarrhea, and dizziness. A severe overdosage produces confusion, ataxia, convulsions, paralysis, and psychotic symptoms. Very rarely circulatory disturbances lead to gangrene in the extremities. The margin of safety between the therapeutic doses of ergot-containing compounds and the toxic doses is quite wide, so that with the recommended doses intoxication does not occur.

Mild sedation with phenobarbital may be of additional value. Dimenhydrinate administered by injection or by suppository may control vomiting and produce sedation.

The major therapeutic effort in migraine should be directed toward the prevention of recurrent attacks. Studies have shown that the personality pattern in patients with recurrent migraine is that of an ambitious, perfectionistic, energetic individual, but this is not always the case. The physician may help the child in understanding the nature of the attacks, which represent the triggering of a sensitive physiological mechanism. The elimination of possible precipitating factors is important.

In the occasional child with migraine who has a spike focus in the EEG and whose headaches are not controlled by derivatives of ergot, salicylates, or sedatives, a thera-

TABLE 7-9. Derivatives of Ergot Used in the Treatment of Migraine

Preparation	Form	Route of Administration	Initial Dose
Ergotamine tartrate 1 mg, caffeine 100 mg (Cafergot)	Tablet	Oral	1 tablet
Ergotamine tartrate 1 mg (Gynergen)	Tablet	Oral	1 tablet
Ergotamine tartrate 2 mg, caffeine 100 mg (Cafergot suppositories)	Suppository	Rectal	½ suppository
Ergotamine tartrate 2 mg (Ergomar sublingual)	Tablet	Buccal mucosa	½ tablet
Ergotamine 0.36 mg in each puff (Ergotamine inhalant)	Inhalator	Respiratory	1 puff
Dihydroergotamine mesylate 1 mg/ml (DHE 45)	Ampule	Intramuscular	0.5 ml to 1.0 ml

peutic trial of phenytoin or phenobarbital may be given. This is recommended on the assumption that occasional migrainous attacks represent epileptic equivalents. Other prophylactic drugs that may be used include propranolol (10 mg twice daily) and amitriptyline (10 mg twice daily). These drugs are approved for children over 12 years of age.

PROGNOSIS

Migraine attacks may recur with great frequency for a period of months or several years and then become much less severe or even disappear, although the majority of children with recurrent migraine have persistent headaches in adult life.

NEONATAL APNEA

Apnea in the newborn can be defined as a cessation of respiration lasting longer than 20 seconds, or if briefer, accompanied by bradycardia, cyanosis, or pallor.[240] Apnea and periodic breathing appear to occur commonly in premature infants.[188] In term infants apnea exceeding 10 seconds is unusual and is generally seen only in the first week of life.[40,114] Apnea exceeding 15 seconds in the term infant and 20 seconds in the premature infant are probably always pathologic.[114] In general, apnea duration and frequency decrease with increasing gestational age. In infants of all ages central apnea and periodic breathing are most common during active or indeterminant sleep.[88,114,175] Obstructive apnea in infants, however, may be more common during quiet sleep.[93]

Apnea is a common symptom of a variety of disorders occurring in the newborn that include metabolic derangements (hypoglycemia, hypoxia, hypocalcemia, hyponatremia), serious infections, anemia, gastroesophageal reflux, congestive heart failure, central nervous system malformations, and seizures.[154]

The mechanisms responsible for apnea in infants can include an apneic response to hypoxemia, abnormal or hyperactive respiratory reflexes, decreased afferent input to the medullary respiratory center, and primary medullary respiratory hyporesponsiveness related to prematurity and genetic factors.[128]

Recurrent apnea in the neonatal period implies a very poor prognosis; in one study 58% of premature infants and 44% of term infants with apnea expired.[178]

Treatment of apnea has been generally aimed at diagnosis and treatment of the underlying disorder. Should this prove impossible, other measures can be tried such as a reduction of ambient temperature, stimulation, administration of stimulants, (caffeine, aminophylline), avoiding apnea reflexes, nasal continuous positive airway pressure and, as a last resort, mechanical ventilation.[128]

Apnea is an infrequent manifestation of neonatal seizures. Apneic seizures can be distinguished by the other manifestations of seizure activity, by the absence of the accompanying bradycardia and the simultaneous occurrence of EEG abnormalities.[52,62]

REFERENCES

1. **Adams DJ, Luders H, Pippenger C:** Sodium valproate in the treatment of intractable seizure disorders: A clinical and electroencephalographic study. Neurology 28:152, 1978
2. **Aicardi J, Chevrie JJ:** Myoclonic epilepsies of childhood. Neuropediatrie 3:177, 1971
3. **Aigner ER, Mulder DW:** Myoclonus: Clinical significance and an approach to classification. Arch Neurol 2:600, 1960
4. **Ajmone-Marsan C, Gumnit RJ:** Neurophysiological aspects of epilepsy. In Vinken PJ, Bruyn GW (eds): Handbook of Clinical Neurology, Vol 15, The Epilepsies. New York, American Elsevier Publishing Company, 1974
5. **Albers RW, Koval GJ, Seigel GJ:** Studies on the interaction of ouabain and other cardioactive steroids with sodium-potassium-activated adenosine triphosphate. Molec Pharmacol 5:324, 1968
6. **Anthony JJ:** Malignant lymphoma associated with hydantoin drugs. Arch Neurol 22:450, 1970
7. **Axelrod FB, Nachtigal R, Dancis J:** Familial dysautonomia diagnosis, pathogenesis and management. Adv Ped 21:75, 1974
8. **Ayala GF, Dichter M, Gumnit RJ et al:** Genesis of epileptic interictal spikes. New knowledge of cortical feedback suggests a neurophysiological explanation of brief paroxysms. Brain Res 52:1, 1973
9. **Ayala GF, Matsumoto H, Gumnit RJ:** Excitability changes and inhibitory mechanisms in neocortical neurons during seizures. J Neurophysiol 33:73, 1970

10. **Babb TL, Crandall PH:** Epileptogenesis of human limbic neurons in psychomotor epileptics. Electroenceph Clin Neurophysiol 40:225, 1976

11. **Bairan CC, Cherry JD, Fagan LF et al:** Complete heart block and respiratory syncytial virus. Am J Dis Child 127:264, 1976

12. **Baird HW:** Convulsions in infancy and childhood. Conn Med 23:149, 1959

13. **Barbeau A, Inoue N, Tsukada K et al:** The neuropharmacology of taurine. Life Sci 17:669, 1975

14. **Barlow CF:** Migraine in childhood. Res Clin Stud Headache 5:34, 1978

15. **Batalden PB, Van Dyne BJ, Cloyd C:** Pancreatitis associated with valproic acid therapy. Pediatrics 64:520, 1979

16. **Beaussart M:** Benign epilepsy of children with Rolandic (centro-temporal) paroxysmal foci: A clinical entity study of 221 cases. Epilepsia 13:795, 1975

17. **Beresford HR, Posner JB, Plum F:** Changes in brain lactate during induced cerebral seizures. Arch Neurol 20:243, 1969

18. **Bickerstaff ER:** Basilar artery migraine. Lancet 1:15, 1961

19. **Bickerstaff ER:** Impairment of consciousness in migraine. Lancet 2:1057, 1961

20. **Bickford RG, Klass DW:** Eye movement in the electroencephalogram. In Bender MB (ed): Ocular Motor System, pp 263–302. New York, Harper & Row, 1964

21. **Blom S, Heijbel J, Bergfors PG:** Benign epilepsy of children with centro-temporal EEG foci. Prevalence and follow-up study of 40 patients. Epilepsy 13:609, 1972

22. **Blume HT, David RB, Gomez NR:** Generalized sharp and slow wave complexes associated clinical features and long term follow-up. Brain 96:289, 1973

23. **Bochner F, Hooper WD et al:** Diphenylhydantoin concentrations in saliva. Arch Neurol 31:57, 1974

24. **Brennan RW, Dehejia H, Kutt H et al:** Diphenylhydantoin intoxication attendant to slow inactivation of isoniazid. Neurology 20:687, 1970

25. **Brown LM:** Mitral valve prolapse in children. In Barness LA (ed): Advances in Pediatrics, Vol 25, pp 327–348. Chicago, Year Book Medical Publishers, 1978

26. **Browne TR:** Clonazepam. New Engl J Med 299:812, 1978

27. **Browne TR:** Valproic acid. New Engl J Med 302:661, 1980

28. **Browne TR, Dreifuss FE et al:** Ethosuximide in the treatment of absence (petit mal) seizures. Neurology 25:515, 1975

29. **Buchanan RA, Allen RJ:** Diphenylhydantoin (Dilantin) and phenobarbital blood levels in epileptic children. Neurology 21:866, 1971

30. **Calmeil LF:** De L'épilepsie, étudiée sous le rapport de son siège et de son influence sur la production de l'aniénation mentale. Thèses de Paris 68:371, 1824

31. **Calvin WH, Sypert GW, Ward AA Jr:** Structural timing patterns within bursts from epileptic neurons in undrugged monkey cortex. Exp Neurol 21:535, 1968

32. **Carruthers-Jones DI, Van Gelder NM:** Influence of taurine dosage on cobalt epilepsy in mice. Neurochem Res 3:115, 1978

33. **Cavazzuti GB, Cappella L, Nalin A:** Longitudinal study of epileptiform EEG patterns in normal children. Epilepsia 21:43, 1980

34. **Chadwick DW, Cumming WJK, Livingstone L et al:** Acute intoxication with sodium valproate. Ann Neurol 6:552, 1979

35. **Chalhub EG, Devivo DC, Volpe JJ:** Phenytoin-induced dystonia and choreoathetosis in two retarded epileptic children. Neurology 26:494, 1976

36. **Chevrie JJ, Aicardi J:** Childhood epileptic encephalopathy with slow spike-wave: A statistical study of 80 cases. Epilepsia 13:259, 1972

37. **Chevrie JJ, Aicardi J, Thieffrey S:** Traitement hormonal de 58 cas de spasmes infantiles, resultats et prognostic psychique a long terme. Arch Cranc Pediat 25:263, 1968

38. **Cloyd JC, Gumnit RJ, Lesar TS:** Reduced seizure control due to spoiled phenytoin capsules. Ann Neurol 7:191, 1980

39. **Collins RC:** Metabolic response to focal penicillin seizures in rats: Spike discharge vs. after discharge. J Neurochem 27:1473, 1976

40. **Daily WJR, Klaus M, Meyer HBP:** Apnea in premature infants: Monitoring incidence, heart rate changes, and effects of environmental temperature. Pediatrics 43:510, 1969

41. **Daly DD:** Ictal clinical manifestations of complex partial seizures. In Penry JK, Daly DD (eds): Advances in Neurology, Vol 11, pp 57–83. New York, Raven Press, 1975

42. **Daly JW:** Cyclic neucleotides in the nervous system. New York, Plenum Press, 1977

43. **Danks DM, Campbell PE, Stevens BJ et al:** Menkes' kinky hair syndrome: An inherited defect of copper absorption with widespread effects. Pediatrics 50:188, 1972

44. **Delagado-Escueta AV:** Epileptogenic paroxysms: modern approaches and clinical correlations. Neurology 29:1014, 1979

45. **Delgado-Escueta AV:** How EEG findings correlate with the international classification of seizures. In American Academy of Neurology Special Courses #1-7, Vol 1, 1979

46. **Dent CE, Richens A, Rowe DJF et al:** Osteomalacia with long-term anticonvulsant therapy in epilepsy. Br Med J 4:69, 1970

47. **Diesz RA, Aickin CC, Lux HD:** Decrease on inhibitory driving force in crayfish stretch reception: a mechanism of the convulsant action of penicillin. Neurosci Letters 11:347, 1979

48. **Dobkin BH:** The adult chiari malformation. Bull L.A. Neurol Soc 42:23, 1977

49. **Dodson WE, Prensky AL, Devivo DC et al:** Management of seizure disorders: Selected aspects, part II. J Pediatrics 89:695, 1976

50. **Dreifuss FE:** Prognosis of petit mal epilepsy. In Epidemiology of Epilepsy, a Workshop. NINDS Monograph 14, pp 129–131. Washington, U.S. Government Printing Office, 1972

51. **Druckman RD, Chao DH:** Massive spasms in infancy and childhood. Epilepsia 4:61, 1955

52. **Duel RK:** Polygraphic monitoring of apneic spells. Arch Neurol 28:71, 1973

53. **Duffy TE, Howse DC, Plum F:** Cerebral energy metabolism during experimental status epilepticus. J Neurochem 24:925, 1975

54. **Enzer NB, Walker PA:** Hyperventilation syndrome in childhood. J Ped 70:521, 1967

55. **Escueta AV, Appel SH:** Brain synapses: an in vitro model of seizures. Arch Intern Med 129:333, 1972

56. **Escueta AV, Reilly EL:** The effects of diphenylhydantoin on potassium transport within synaptic terminals of epileptic foci. Neurology 21:418, 1971

57. **Escueta AV, Kunze U, Waddell G et al:** Lapse of consciousness and automatisms in temporal lobe epilepsy: A videotape analysis. Neurology 27:144, 1977

58. **Esplin DW, Laffan RJ:** Determinants of flexor and extensor components of maximal seizures in cats. Arch Int Pharmacodyn Ther 113:189, 1957

59. **Falconer MA:** Mesial temporal (Ammon's horn) sclerosis as a common cause of epilepsy. Aetiology, treatment, and prevention. Lancet 2:767, 1974

60. **Falconer MA:** Significance of surgery for temporal lobe epilepsy in childhood and adolescence. J Neurosurg 33:233, 1970

61. **Fariello RG, Lloyd KG, Hornykiewicz O:** Cortical and subcortical projected foci in cats: Inhibitory action of taurine. Neurology 25:1077, 1975

62. **Fenichel GM, Olson BJ, Fitzpatrick JE:** Heart rate changes in convulsive and nonconvulsive neonatal apnea. Ann Neurol 7:577, 1980

63. **Ferguson JH, Jasper HH:** Laminar DC studies of acetycholine-activated epileptic form discharge in cerebral cortex. Electroenceph Clin Neurophysiol 30:377, 1971

64. **Ferrendelli JA, Kinscherf DA:** Cyclic nucleotides in epileptic brain: effects of pentylenetetrazol on regional cyclic AMP and cyclic GMP levels in vitro. Epilepsia 18:525, 1977

65. **Fincham RW, Schottelius DD, Sahs AL:** The influence of diphenyhydantoin on primidone metabolism. Arch Neurol 30:259, 1974

66. **Finlayson RE, Lucas AR:** Pseudoepileptic seizures in children and adolescents. Mayo Clin Proc 54:83, 1974

67. **Fisher CM:** Transient paralytic attacks of nonconvulsive seizure paralysis. J Cand Neurol Sci 5:267, 1978

68. **Frantzen E, Lennox-Buchthal M, Nygaard A et al:** A genetic study of febrile convulsions. Neurology 20:909, 1970

69. **Freidberg CK:** Syncope: Pathological physiology: differential diagnosis and treatment. Modern Concepts Cardiovasc Med 15:55, 1971

70. **Friedman AP, Harms E:** Headaches in children. Springfield, Ill., Charles C Thomas, 1967

71. **Frigyesi TL, Lombardini JB:** Lack of correlation between taurine levels in 16 brain regions and paroxysmal discharges in the thalmocortical circuit. Neurosci Letters 7:213, 1978

72. **Frigyesi TL, Lombardini JB:** Augmentation of thalmo-motor cortico-cerebellar epileptogenesis by taurine and its antagonism by diphenylhydantoin. Life Sci 24:1251, 1979

73. **Gabriel M, Albani M, Schultz FJ:** Apneic spells and sleep states in preterm infants. Pediatrics 57:142, 1972

74. **Gascon G, Barlow C:** Juvenile migraine presenting as an acute confusional state. J Pediatr 45:628, 1970

75. **Gastaut H:** Clinical electroencephalographic classification of epileptic seizures. Epilepsia 11:102, 1970

76. **Gastaut H, Broughton R, Roger J et al:** Generalized convulsive seizures without local onset. In Vinken PJ, Bruyn GW (eds): Handbook of Clinical Neurology, Vol 15, The Epilepsies, pp 107–129. New York, American Elsevier Publishing Company, 1974

77. **Gastaut H, Broughton R, Roger J et al:** Generalized non-convulsive seizures without local onset. In Vinken PJ, Bruyn GW (eds): Handbook of Clinical Neurology, Vol 15, The Epilepsies, pp 130–144. New York, American Elsevier Publishing Company, 1974

78. **Gastaut H, Gastaut JL:** Computerized transverse axial tomography in epilepsy. Epilepsia 17:325, 1976

79. **Gastaut H, Gastaut TL, Regis H et al:** Computerized tomography in the study of West's Syndrome. Develop Med Child Neurol 21:21, 1978

80. **Gastaut H, Roger J, Ouachi S et al:** Electroclinical study of generalized epileptic seizures of tonic expression. Epilepsia 4:15, 1963

81. **Gastaut H, Roger J, Soulayrol R et al:** Childhood epileptic encephalopathy with diffuse slow spike-waves (otherwise known as "petit mal variant") or Lennox Syndrome. Epilepsia 7:139, 1966

82. **Geier S:** A comparative tele-EEG study of adolescent and adult epileptics. Epilepsia 12:215, 1971

83. **Gibbs FA, Gibbs EL:** Atlas of electroencephalography, Vols 1–3. Reading, Addison-Wesley Press, 1964

84. **Gibbs FA, Gibbs EL, Lennox WG:** Cerebral dysrhythmias of epilepsy. Measures of their control. Arch Neurol Psychiat (Chicago) 39:298, 1938

85. **Glaser GH:** Experimental derangements of extracellular ionic environment. In Purpura DP, Penry JK, Tower DB et al (eds): Experimental Models of Epilepsy—A Manual for the Laboratory Worker, pp 317–345. New York, Raven Press, 1972

86. **Glaser GH:** Epilepsy, hysteria and "possession." J Nervous Mental Dis 166:268, 1978

87. **Goode DJ, Penry A, Driefuss FE:** Effects of paroxysmal spike–wave on continuous visual motor performance. Epilepsia 11:241, 1970

88. **Gould JB, Lee HFS, James O et al:** The sleep state characteristics of apnea during infancy. Pediatrics 59:182, 1977

89. **Gowers WG:** Epilepsy and Other Chronic Convulsive Disorders, 2nd ed. London, J & A Churchill, 1901

90. **Green JD:** The hippocampus. Physiol Rev 44:561, 1964

91. **Guey J, Vureau M, Dravet C et al:** A study of the rhythm of petit mal absences in children in relation to prevailing situations. Epilepsia 10:441, 1969

92. **Guilleminault C, Anders TF:** The pathophysiology of sleep disorders in pediatrics. Adv Pediatr 22:137, 1976

93. **Guilleminault C, Ariagno R, Korobkin R et al:** Mixed and obstructive sleep apnea and near miss for sudden infant death syndrome: Part 2. Comparison of near miss and normal control infants by age. Pediatrics 64:882, 1979

94. **Hagberg B:** Pre-, peri- and postnatal prevention of major neuropediatric handicaps. Neuropediatrie 6:331, 1975

95. **Hahn TJ, Avioli LV:** Anticonvulsant osteomalacia. Arch Intern Med 135:997, 1975

96. **Halliday AM:** The electrophysiological study of myoclonus in man. Brain 90:241, 1967

97. **Hanson JW, Myrianthopoulos NC, Sedgwick MA et al:** Risks to the offspring of women treated with hydantoin anticonvulsants, with emphasis on the fetal hydantoin syndrome. J Pediatr 89:662, 1976

98. **Haruda F:** Phenytoin hypersensitivity: 38 cases. Neurology 29:1480, 1979

99. **Hauser AW, Kurland LT:** The epidemiology of epilepsy in Rochester, Minnesota, 1935 through 1967. Epilepsia 16:1, 1975

100. **Heijbel J, Blom S, Bergfors PG:** Benign epilepsy of children with centro-temporal EEG foci: A study of incidence rate in outpatient care. Epilepsia 16:657, 1975

101. **Heijbel J, Bohman M:** Benign epilepsy with centro-temporal EEG foci: Intelligence, behavior, and school adjustment. Epilepsia 16:679, 1975

102. **Heijbel J, Blom S, Rasmuson M:** Benign epilepsy of childhood with centro-temporal EEG foci: A genetic study. Epilepsia 16:285, 1975

103. **Heinemann U, Lux HD:** Undershoots following stimulus-induced rises of extracellular potassium concentration in cerebral cortex of cat. Brain Res 93:63, 1975

104. **Heinemann U, Lux HD, Gutnick MJ:** Extracellular free calcium and potassium during paroxysmal activity in the cerebral cortex of the cat. Exp Brain Res 27:237, 1977

105. **Henriksen SJ, Bloom FE, McCoy F et al:** B-Endorphin induces nonconvulsive limbic seizures. Proc Natl Acad Sci 75:5221, 1978

106. **Hill RM, Verniaud WM, Horning MG et al:** Infants exposed in utero to antiepileptic drugs. Am J Dis Child 127:645, 1974

107. **Hirsch CS, Martin DL:** Unexpected death in young epileptics. Neurology 21:682, 1971

108. **Hoffer B, Seiger A, Freedman R et al:** Electrophysiology and cytology of hippocampal formation transplants in the anterior chamber of the eye. Part II. Cholinergic mechanisms. Brain Res 119:107, 1977

109. **Holcomb R, Lynn R, Harvey B Jr et al:** Intoxication with 5.5-diphenylhydantoin (Dilantin). J Pediatr 80:627, 1972

110. **Holguin J, Fenichel G:** Migraine. J Pediatr 70:290, 1967

111. **Holmes GL, Sackellaris JC, Ragland M et al:** Pseudoseizures in childhood: a clinical appraisal using prolonged electroencephalographic telemetry and videotape monitoring. Ann Neurol 6:186, 1979

112. **Holowach J, Thurston DL:** Breath-holding spells and anemia. New Engl J Med 268:21, 1963

113. **Holowach J, Thurston DL, O'Leary J:** Prognosis in childhood epilepsy follow-up study of 148 cases in which therapy had been suspended after prolonged anticonvulsant control. N Engl J Med 286:169, 1972

114. **Hoppenbrouwers T, Hodgman JE, Harper RM et al:** Polygraphic studies of normal infants during the first six months of life: Part III. Incidence of apnea and periodic breathing. Pediatrics 60:418, 1977

115. **Hrachovy RA, Frost JD Jr, Kellaway P et al:** A controlled study of prednisone therapy in infantile spasms. Epilepsia 20:403, 1979

116. **Hunter J, Maxwell JD, Stewart DA et al:** Altered calcium metabolism in epileptic children on anticonvulsants. Br Med J 4:202, 1971

117. **Hyman NM, Dennis PD, Sinclair KGA:** Tremor due to sodium valproate. Neurology 29:1177, 1979

118. **Jackson HJ:** Case of tumor of the middle lobe of the cerebellum—cerebellar paralysis with rigidity (cerebellar attitude)—occasional tetanus-like seizures. Brain 29:425, 1907

119. **Jeavons PM, Bower BD:** Infantile spasms: a review of the literature and a study of 112 cases. Clinics in Dev Med No 15. London, Spastics Society and Heinemann, 1964

120. **Jeavons PM, Bower BD, Dimitrakoudi M:** Long-term prognosis of 150 cases of "West Syndrome." Epilepsia 14:153, 1973

121. **Jensen ON, Olesen OV:** Subnormal serum folate due to anticonvulsive therapy: A double-blind study of the effect of folic acid treatment in patients with drug-induced subnormal serum folates. Arch Neurol 22:181, 1970

122. **Jervell A, Nielsen FL:** Congenital deaf-mutism, functional heart disease with prolongation of the Q-T interval and sudden death. Am Heart J, 54:59, 1957

123. **Jobsis FF, O'Connor M, Vitale A et el:** Intracellular redox changes in functioning cerebral cortex. Part I. Metabolic effects of epileptiform activity. J Neurophysiol 24:735, 1971

124. **Jokl E, McClellan JT, Williams WC et al:** Congenital anomaly of the left coronary artery in young athletes. Cardiologia 49:253, 1966

125. **Joseph MH, Emson PC:** Taurine and cobalt induced epilepsy in the rat: A biochemical and electrocorticographic study. J Neurochem 27:1495, 1976

126. **Kao KI, Crill WE:** Penicillin induced segmental myoclonus. Part I. Motor responses and intracellular recording from motorneurons. Arch Neurol (Chicago) 26:156, 1972

127. **Kao KI, Crill WE:** Penicillin induced segmental myoclonus. Part II. Membrane properties of cat spinal motorneurons. Arch Neurol (Chicago) 26:162, 1972

128. **Kattwinkel J:** Neonatal apnea: pathogenesis and therapy. J Ped 90:342, 1977.

129. **Katz NM, Mortimer JB, Liberthson RR:** Discrete membranous subaortic stenosis: report of 31 patients, review of the literature and delineation of management. Circ 56:1034, 1977

130. **Kellaway P, Hrachovy RA, Frost JD et al:** Precise characterization and quantification of infantile spasms. Ann Neurol 6:214, 1979

131. **Kessler S, Guilleminault C, Dement WC:** A family study of 50 REM narcoleptics. Acta Neurol Scand 50:503, 1974

132. **Kooi KA, Tucker RP, Marshall RE:** Fundamentals of electroencephalography. Hagerstown, Md., Harper & Row, 1978.

133. **Lacy JR, Penry JK:** Infantile Spasms. New York, Raven Press, 1976

134. **Ladwig HA, Vanslager L, Thomas J et al:** Infantile spasms with hypsarrhythmia. Nebr Symp Motiv 47:614, 1962

135. **Lagenstein D, Kuhne D, Stanowsky HJ et al:** Computerized cranial transverse axial tomography (CTAT) in 145 patients with primary and secondary generalized epilepsies: West Syndrome, myoclonus–astatic petit mal, absence epilepsy. Neuropadiatrie, 10:15, 1979

136. **Laxdal T, Gomez MR, Reiher J:** Cyanotic and pallid syncopal attacks in children. (Breath-Holding Spells). Develop Med Clin Neurol 11:755, 1969

137. **Leichtman D, Nelson R, Gobel F et al:** Bradyarrhythmia in familial mitral valve prolapse syndrome. A potential mechanism of sudden death. Circ 52 (Supp 2): II-92, 1975

138. **Lennox WG:** The petit mal epilepsies. Their treatment with tridione. JAMA 122:1069, 1945

139. **Lennox WG, Davis JP:** Clinical correlates of the fast and slow spike-wave electroencephalogram. Pediatrics 5:626, 1950

140. **Lenox CC, Zuberbuhler JR, Park SC et al:** Arrythmias and Stokes-Adams attacks in acute rheumatic fever. Pediatrics 61:599, 1978

141. **Levitt LP, Rose LI, Dawson SM:** Hypokalemic periodic paralysis with arrythmia. N Engl J Med 286:253, 1972

142. **Lewin E:** Epileptogenic cortical foci induced with Ouabain: sodium, potassium, water content, and sodium-potassium-activated ATPase activity. Exp Neurol 30:172, 1971

143. **Lisak RP, Lebeau J, Tucker SH:** Hyperkalemic periodic paralysis. Neurology 22:810, 1972

144. **Livingston S:** Comprehensive Management of Epilepsy in Infancy, Childhood and Adolescence. Springfield, Ill., Charles C Thomas, 1972

145. **Livingston S:** Diagnosis and treatment of childhood myoclonic seizures. Pediatrics 53:542, 1974

146. **Livingston S, Eisner V, Pauli L:** Minor motor epilepsy: diagnosis, treatment, and prognosis. Pediatrics 21:916, 1958

147. **Livingston S, Torres I, Pauli LL et al:** Petit mal epilepsy: results of a prolonged follow-up study of 117 patients. JAMA 194:227, 1965

148. **Llinas R, Hess R:** Tetradotoxin-resistant dendritic spikes in avian Purkinje cells. Proc Natl Acad Sci USA 73:2520, 1976

149. **Lockman LA, Kriel R, Zaske D et al:** Phenobarbital dosage for control of neonatal seizures. Neurology 29:1445, 1979

150. **Loeb H, Raymond J, Gunnar R:** Paroxysmal ventricular fibrillation in two patients with hypomagnesemia. Circ 37:210, 1968

151. **Loiseau P, Orgogozo JM:** An unrecognized syndrome of benign focal epileptic seizures in teenagers. Lancet 2:1070, 1978

152. **Lombroso CT:** Sylvian seizures and midtemporal spike foci in children. Arch Neurol 17:52, 1967

153. **Lombroso CT, Lerman P:** Breathholding spells (cyanotic and pallid infantile syncope). Pediatrics 39:563, 1967

154. **Lucey JF, Kattwinkel J (eds):** Apnea of Prematurity: Report of the 71st Ross Conference on Pediatric Research. Columbus, Ohio, Ross Laboratories, 1977

155. **Luke MJ:** Valvular pulmonic stenosis in infancy. J Ped 68:90, 1966

156. **Lux HD:** The kinetics of extracellular potassium: relation to epileptogenesis. Epilepsia 15:375, 1974

157. **MacDonald RL, Barker JL:** Specific antagonism of GABA-mediated postsynaptic inhibition in cultured spinal cord neurons: a common mode of convulsant action. Neurology 28:325, 1978

158. **MacDonald RL, Bergey GK:** Valproic acid augments GABA-mediated postsynaptic inhibition in cultured mammalian neurons. Brain Res 170:558, 1979

159. **Markand O:** Slow spike-wave activity in EEG and associated clinical features: often called 'Lennox' or 'Lennox-Gastaut' Syndrome. Neurol 27:746,1977

160. **Masland RL:** The classification of the epilepsies: a historical review. In Vinken PJ, Bruyn GW (eds): Handbook of Clinical Neurology, Vol 15, The Epilepsies, pp 1–29. New York, American Elsevier Publishing, 1974

161. **Matsumoto H:** Intracellular events during the activation of cortical epileptiform discharges. Electroenceph Clin Neurophysiol 17:294, 1964

162. **Matsumoto H, Ajmone-Marsan C:** Cortical cellular phenomena in experimental epilepsy: interictal manifestations. Exp Neurol 9:286, 1964

163. **Mattson RH, Cramer JA, Williamson PD et al:** Valproic acid epilepsy clinical and pharmacological effects. Ann Neurol 3:20, 1978

164. **Mauguiere F, Courjon J:** Somatosensory epilepsy: a review of 127 cases. Brain 101:307, 1978

165. **McCord MD, van Elk J, Blount SG:** Tetralogy of Fallot. Clinical and hemodynamic spectrum of combined pulmonary stenosis and ventricular septal defect. Circ 16:736, 1957

166. **McLain Jr LW, Martin JT, Allen JH:** Cerebellar degeneration due to chronic phenytoin therapy. Ann Neurol 7:18, 1980

167. **McRae JR, Wagner GS, Rogers MC et al:** Paroxysmal familial ventricular fibrillation. J Ped 85:515, 1974

168. **Melchior JC, Buchthal F, Lennox-Buchthal M:** The

ineffectiveness of diphenylhydantoin in preventing febrile convulsions in the age of greatest risk, under three years. Epilepsia 12:55, 1971

169. **Meldrum BS:** Epilepsy and gamma aminobutyric acid-mediated inhibition. Int Rev Neurobiol 17:1, 1975

170. **Meldrum BS, Brierley JB:** Prolonged epileptic seizures in primates. Ischemic change and its relation to ictal physiologic events. Arch Neurol 28:10, 1973

171. **Meldrum BS, Horton RW:** Physiology of status epilepticus in primates. Arch Neurol 28:1, 1973

172. **Meldrum BS, Vigouroux RA, Brierley JB:** Systemic factors and epileptic brain damage. Prolonged seizures in paralyzed, artificially ventilated baboons. Arch Neurol 29:82, 1973

173. **Merlis JK:** Proposal for an international classification of the epilepsies. Epilepsia 11:114, 1970

174. **Mirsky AF, Van Buren JM:** On the nature of the "absence" in centrencephalic epilepsy: a study of some behavioral electroencephalographic and autonomic factors. Electroencephalogr Clin Neurophysiol 18:334, 1965

175. **Monod N, Curzi-Doscalova L, Guidasci S et al:** Pauses respiratoires et sommeil chez le nouveau—ne et la nourrism. Rev EEG Neurophysiol 6:105, 1976

176. **Montouris GD, Fenichel GM, McLain Jr LW:** The pregnant epileptic. Arch Neurol 36:601, 1979

177. **Moody W, Futamachi K, Prince DA:** Extracellular potassium activity during epileptogenesis. Exp Neurol 42:248, 1974

178. **Naege R:** Neonatal apnea: underlying disorders. Pediatrics 63:8, 1979

179. **Nakamura FF, Nadas AS:** Congenital heart block in infants and children. N Eng J Med 270:1261, 1964

180. **Nelson KB, Ellenberg JH:** Prognosis in children with febrile seizures. Pediatrics 61:720, 1978

181. **Nicol CF, Tutton JC, Smith BH:** Parental diazepam in status epilepticus. Neurology 19:332, 1969

182. **Niedermeyer E:** The Lennox-Gastaut Syndrome: a severe type of childhood epilepsy. Z Neurol 195:263, 1967

183. **Niedermeyer E:** The Generalized Epilepsies: A clinical electroencephalophic study, pp 14–17. Springfield, Charles C Thomas, 1972

184. **Oakley JC, Sypert GW, Ward AA Jr:** Conductance changes in neocortical propagated seizures: seizure initiation. Exp Neurol 37:287, 1972

185. **O'Conner MJ, Herman CJ, Rosenthal M et al:** Intracellular redox changes preceding onset of epileptiform activity in intact cat hippocampus. J Neurophysiol 35:471, 1972

186. **Orren MM, Mirsky AF:** Relation between ocular manifestations and onset of spike-and-wave discharges in petit mal epilepsy. Epilepsia 16:771, 1975

187. **Parker WA, Shearer CA:** Phenytoin hepatotoxicity: a case report and review. Neurology 29:175, 1979

188. **Parmelee AH, Stern E, Harris MA:** Maturation of respiration in premature and young infants. Neuropediatrie 3:294, 1972

189. **Paulson RB, Paulson GW, Jreissaty S:** Phenytoin and carbamazepine in production of cleft palates in mice. Arch Neurol 36:832, 1979

190. **Pearn JH:** Epilepsy and drowning in childhood. Br Med J 1:1510, 1977

191. **Penfield W, Jasper H:** Epilepsy and functional anatomy of the brain. Boston, Little, Brown & Co, 1954

192. **Pennybacker J:** Pituitary, pineal and third ventricular tumors. Postgrad Med J 25:141, 1950

193. **Penry JK, Dreifuss FE:** Automatisms associated with absence of petit mal epilepsy. Arch Neurol (Chicago) 21:142, 1969

194. **Penry JK, Porter RJ, Dreifuss FE:** Simultaneous recording of absence seizures with video tape and electroencephalography; a study of 374 seizures in 48 patients. Brain 98:427, 1975

195. **Perry TL:** A brain aminoacid possibly important in neurological and psychiatric disorders. In Usdin E, Hamburg DA, Barchas JD (eds): Neuroregulators and Psychiatric Disorders, pp 391–399. New York, Oxford University Press, 1977

196. **Petito CK, Schaefer JH, Plum F:** Ultrastructural characteristics of the brain and blood-brain barrier in experimental seizures. Brain Res 127:251, 1977

197. **Plum F, Posner JB, Troy B:** Cerebral metabolic and circulatory responses to induced convulsions in animals. Arch Neurol (Chicago) 18:1, 1968

198. **Porter FH:** Sarcoid heart disease. N Eng J Med 263:1350, 1960

199. **Porter RJ, Penry JK, Lacy JR et al:** Plasma concentrations of phensuximide, methsuximide, and their metabolites in relation to clinical efficacy. Neurology 29:1509, 1979

200. **Prensky AL, Swisher CN, DeVivo DC:** Positive brain scans in children with idiopathic focal epileptic seizures. Neurology 23:798, 1973

201. **Prince DA:** Electrophysiology of 'epileptic neurons.' Electroenceph Clin Neurophysiol 23:83, 1967

202. **Prince DA:** Neurophysiology of epilepsy. Ann Rev Neurosci 1:395, 1978

203. **Prince DA, Lux HD, Neher E:** Measurement of extracellular potassium activity in cat cortex. Brain Res 50:489, 1973

204. **Prince DA, Wilder BJ:** Cortical mechanisms in cortical epileptogenic foci—Surround inhibition. Arch Neurol (Chicago) 16:194, 1967

205. **Purpura DP, Shofer RJ, Musgrove FS:** Cortical intracellular potentials during augmenting and recruiting responses. Part II. Patterns of synaptic activities in pyramidal and nonpyramidal tract neurons. J Neurophysiol 27:133, 1964

206. **Ramsay RE, Hammond EJ, Perchalski RJ et al:** Brain uptake of phenytoin, phenobarbital, and diazepam. Arch Neurol 36:535, 1979

207. **Rapport RL, Harris AB, Friez PN et al:** Human epileptic brain: Na,K ATPase activity and phenytoin concentrations. Arch Neurol 32:549, 1975

208. **Rasmussen V, Haunso S, Skagen K:** Cerebral attacks due to excessive vagal tone in heavily trained persons. Acta Med Scand 204:401, 1978

209. **Redenbaugh JE:** Sodium valproate: pharmacokinetics and effectiveness in treating intractable seizures. Neurology 30:1, 1980

210. **Remick RA, Wada JA:** Complex partial and pseudoseizure disorders. Am J Psychiatry 136:320, 1979

211. **Riitman R, Donner M:** Incidence and aetiology of infantil spasms from 1960 to 1976: a population study in Finland. Develop Med Child Neurol 21:333, 1979

212. **Roberts NK, Gelband H. (eds):** Cardiac Arrythmias in the Neonate, Infant, and Child. New York, Appleton-Century-Crofts, 1977

213. **Roger J, Soulayrol R, Bureau M et al:** Etude electroclinique des crises d'epilepsie apoplectiques—a propos de 5 cas recents. J Med Lyon 1:1, 1967

214. **Rose AL, Lombroso CT:** Neonatal seizure states: a study of clinical, pathological, and electroencephalographic features in 137 full-term babies with a long term follow-up. Pediatrics 45:404, 1970.

215. **Sackellares JC, Lee SI, Dreifuss RE:** Stupor following administration of valproic acid to patients receiving other antiepileptic drugs. Epilepsia 20:697, 1979

216. **Saktor B, Wilson JE, Tiekert CG:** Regulation of glycolysis in brain, in site, during convulsions. J Biol Chem 241:5071, 1966

217. **Samson JH, Apthorp J, Finley A:** Febrile seizures and purulent meningitis. JAMA 210:1918, 1969

218. **Saradshizhvili P, Vatrogon F, Okudzhara V:** Changes in levels of gamma aminobutyric, glutamic and aspartic acids and glutamine in the primary and "mirror foci" of epileptic activity. Z Neuropatol Psikhiat, S.S. Karsakov 70:1771, 1970

219. **Sato S, Driefuss FE, Penry JK:** Prognostic factors in absence seizures. Neurol 26:788, 1976

220. **Sawa M, Maruyama N, Kaji S:** Intracellular potential during electrically induced seizures. Electroenceph Clin Neurophysiol 15:209, 1963

221. **Scheibel ME, Crandall PH, Scheibel AB:** The hippocampal-dentate complex in temporal lobe epilepsy. Epilepsia 15:55, 1974

222. **Scheibel ME, Scheibel AB:** On the nature of dendritic spines. Report of a workshop. Communic Behav Biol 1:231, 1968

223. **Schmidt RP, Thomas LB, Ward AA:** The hyperexcitable neuron. Microelectrode studies of chronic epileptic foci in monkey. J Neurophysiol 22:285, 1959

224. **Schwab RS:** Method of measuring consciousness in petit mal epilepsy. Arch Neurol Psychiat (Chicago) 41:215, 1939

225. **Schwartz JF:** Neonatal convulsions: pathogenesis, diagnostic evaluation, treatment and prognosis. Clin Pediatr 4:595, 1965

226. **Schwartzkroin PA, Slawsky M:** Probable calcium spikes in hippocampal neurons. Brain Res 135:157, 1977

227. **Scott O, Macartney FJ, Deverall PB:** Sick sinus syndrome in children. Arch Dis Child 51:100, 1976

228. **Sellden U:** Psychotechnical performance related to paroxysmal discharges in EEG. Clin Electroenceph 2:18, 1971

229. **Sherard Jr ES, Steiman GS, Couri D:** Treatment of childhood epilepsy with valproic acid: results of the first 100 patients in a 6-month trial. Neurology 30:31, 1980

230. **Singer WD, Rabe EF, Haller JS:** The effect of ACTH therapy upon infantile spasms. J Pediatrics 96:485, 1980

231. **Skully RE, Galdabini JJ, McNeely BU:** Case records of the Massachusetts General Hospital Case, 21–1979. N Engl J Med 300:1204, 1979

232. **Sorel F:** 196 cases of infantile myoclonic encephalopathy with hypsarrhythmias (IMEH: West Syndrome) treated with ACTH. Danger of synthetic ACTH (abstr). Electroenceph Clin Neurophysiol 32:576, 1972

233. **Spehlmann R, Chang CM:** Acetycholine sensitivity of partially deafferented cortex. Epilepsia 10:419, 1969

234. **Stephenson JBP:** Two types of febrile seizure: anoxic (syncopal) and epileptic mechanisms differentiated by oculocardiac reflex. Br Med J 2:726, 1978

235. **Stone WE:** Action of convulsants: neurochemical aspects. In Jasper HH, Ward AA, Pope A (eds): Basic Mechanisms of the Epilepsies. pp 184–193. Boston, Little, Brown & Co, 1969

236. **Streeten DHP, Kerr LP, Kerr CB et al:** Hyperbradykininism: a new orthostatic syndrome. Lancet 2:1048, 1972

237. **Suchy FJ, Balistreri WF, Buchino JJ et al:** Acute hepatic failure associated with the use of sodium valproate. N Engl J Med 300:962, 1979

238. **Sussman NM, McLain Jr LW:** A direct hepatotoxic effect of valproic acid. JAMA 242:1173, 1979

239. **Sypert GW, Ward Jr AA:** Changes in extracellular potassium activity during neocortical propagated seizures. Exp Neurol 45:19, 1974

240. **Task Force on Prolonged Apnea, American Academy of Pediatrics:** Prolonged Apnea. Pediatrics 61:651, 1978

241. **Thilenius OG, Nadas AS, Jockin H:** Primary pulmonary vascular obstruction in children. Pediatrics 36:75, 1965

242. **Tolman KG, Jubiz W, Sannella JJ et al:** Osteomalacia associated with anticonvulsant drug therapy in mentally retarded children. Pediatrics 56:45, 1975

243. **Tower DB:** Problems associated with studies of electrolyte metabolism in normal and epileptogenic cerebral cortex. Epilepsia 6:183, 1965

244. **Tower DB:** Neurochemical mechanisms. In Jasper HH, Ward Jr AA, Pope A (eds): Basic Mechanisms of the Epilepsies, pp 611–638. Boston, Little, Brown & Co, 1969

245. **Tsuboi T, Christian W:** Epilepsy: a clinical, electroencephalographic and statistical study of 466 patients. Berlin, Springer-Verlag 1976

246. **Van Gelder NM:** Antagonism by taurine of cobalt induced epilepsy in cat and mouse. Brain Res 47:157, 1972

247. **Van Gelder NM, Courtais A:** Close correlation

between changing content of specific amino acids in epileptogenic cortex of cats and severity of epilepsy. Brain Res 43:477 1972

248. **Van Gelder NM, Sherwin AL, Rasmussen T:** Amino acid content of epileptogenic human brain: focal versus surrounding regions. Brain Res 40:385, 1972

249. **Vernadakis A, Woodbury DM:** Maturational factors in development of seizures. In Jasper HH, Ward AA, Pope LA (eds): Basic Mechanisms of Epilepsies. pp 535–541. Boston, Little, Brown & Co, 1969

250. **Waldinger C:** Pyridoxine deficiency and pyridoxine dependency in infants and children. Postgrad Med 35:415, 1964

251. **Ward OC:** A new familial cardiac syndrome in children. J Ir Med Assoc 54:103, 1964

252. **Weiss S, Ferris EB:** Adams-Stokes syndrome with transient complete heart block of vasovagal reflex origin: mechanisms and treatment. Arch Intern Med 54:931, 1934.

253. **Wennevold A, Kringelbach J:** Prolonged Q–T interval and cardiac syncopes. Acta Pediatr Scand 60:239, 1971

254. **West WJ:** A peculiar form of infantile convulsions. Lancet 1:724, 1841

255. **Westrum LE, White Jr LE, Ward Jr AA:** Morphology of the experimental epileptic focus. J Neurosurg 21:1033, 1964

256. **Williams DT, Spiegel H, Mostofsky DI:** Neurogenic and hysterical seizures in children and adolescents: differential diagnostic and therapeutic considerations. Am J Psychiatry 135:82, 1978

257. **Wilson PJE:** Cerebral hemispherectomy for infantile hemiplegia: a report of 50 cases. Brain 93:147, 1970

258. **Wilson WA, Escueta AV:** Common synaptic effects of pentylenetetrazol and penicillin. Brain Res 72:168, 1974

259. **Wolf SM, Carr A, Davis DC et al:** The value of phenobarbital in the child who has had a single febrile seizure: a controlled prospective study. Pediatrics 59:378, 1977

260. **Wolf SM, Forsythe A:** Behavioral disturbances, phenobarbital, and febrile seizures. Pediatrics 61:728, 1978

261. **Wolff HG:** Headache and Other Head Pain, 3rd ed, revised by DJ Dalessio. New York, Oxford University Press, 1972

262. **Wong RKS, Prince DA:** Dendritic mechanisms underlying penicillin-induced epileptiform activity. Science 204:1228, 1979

263. **Woodley D, Chambers W, Starke H et al:** Intermittent complete atrioventricular block masquerading as epilepsy in the mitral valve prolapse syndrome. Chest 72:369, 1977

264. **Wyler AR, Lockard JS:** Seizure severity and acquisition of an operant task in a monkey model. Epilepsia 18:109, 1977

265. **Yabek SM, Jarmakani JM:** Sinus node dysfunction in children, adolescents and young adults. Pediatrics 61:593, 1978

266. **Yang PJ, Berger PE, Cohen ME et al:** Computed tomography and childhood seizure disorder. Neurology 29:1084, 1979

267. **Zackai EH, Mellman WJ, Neiderer B et al:** The fetal trimethadione syndrome. J Pediatr 87:280, 1975

268. **Zimmerman AW, Niedermeyer E, Hodges FJ:** Lennox-Gastaut syndrome and computerized axial tomography findings. Epilepsia 18:463, 1977

269. **Zuckerman EC, Glaser GH:** Hippocampal epileptic activity induced by localized ventricular perfusion with high-potassium cerebrospinal fluid. Exp Neurol 20:87, 1968

Disturbances of Water and Electrolytes

8

Gilbert B. Forbes
Kenneth L. McCormick

Evolutionary theory holds that life originated in a watery, salty medium: the sea. When animals became terrestrial they took this environment with them, and protoplasm continued to function on land in the same milieu in which it had evolved. In higher animals this particular environment is maintained inside the body and is known as the body fluids. Two of the great achievements of modern biology are the discovery of the constancy of the *milieu interieur* during health, and the elucidation of the mechanisms by which this stability is assured.

It has now been established that cell function is dependent on a proper ionic environment, that the function can be altered by changes in the composition or volume of body fluids, and that these functional alterations are often accompanied by clinical signs and symptoms. In the case of the nervous system, the signs and symptoms may simulate those of organic brain disease. In turn, the brain is one of the organs that regulates the volume and composition of body fluids, and hence abnormal activity of the brain can lead to aberrations in body fluid physiology.[22]

DEFINITIONS, CLASSIFICATION, FUNCTIONAL ASPECTS

The body fluids are divided into a number of compartments: blood plasma and interstitial fluid, which together make up the extracellular fluids; intracellular fluid; and certain specialized fluids, such as cerebrospinal fluid, synovial fluid, and the aqueous humor of the eye.

BODY FLUID VOLUME

Body fluid volume can be measured (approximately) in the intact subject by the *dilution principle*, that is, the volume of distribution of a particular injectate. Plasma volume can be determined with Evans blue dye or labeled serum albumin; extracellular fluid with inulin, bromide, thiocyanate, or sucrose; and total body water with deuterium, tritium, or urea. Intracellular fluid volume is calculated by subtracting plasma and extracellular fluid volumes from total body fluid volume.

The infant has a relatively larger extracellular fluid volume and total water content than the adult, whereas plasma volume is about the same as that in the adult on a body weight basis (Fig. 8-1). Many of the materials used to measure extracellular fluid volume do not readily penetrate into cerebrospinal fluid.

In dealing with tissue samples extracellular fluid (ECF) volume is commonly equated with the chloride "space." For liver and muscle the calculated chloride space corresponds to extracellular space as determined by histologic methods. In the case of brain the criteria for estimation of ECF volume are not so well established, because the microscopically visible ECF space is but a small fraction of that determined by chloride analysis. The possibility exists that microglia occupy much of the chemically determined chloride space of the brain.

Infants have a much higher rate of water turnover than adults and thus have a reduced tolerance for water deprivation (Fig. 8-1). Cutaneous water losses are relatively higher (greater surface area/weight ratio) and renal conservation of water less efficient in infants than in adults.

CONSTITUENTS OF BODY FLUIDS

The concentrations of the various body fluid constituents are set forth in Table 8-1. Interstitial fluid concentrations (derived from muscle) can be calculated by multiplying the plasma concentration by the reciprocal of the plasma water content and the appropriate Donnan factor after due allowance for plasma protein binding in the case of Ca^{2+} and Mg^{2+}.

The young infant differs from the adult in that the former's plasma Cl^- and phosphate levels are higher and his bicarbonate and protein levels lower. Cerebrospinal fluid (CSF) protein in the very young infant is two to three times higher than in the adult and approaches the adult range by age 3 months.

With certain notable exceptions (*i.e.*, higher content of Mg^{2+} and Cl^-, and lower HCO_3^- level) CSF appears to be a transudate of plasma. Indeed many plasma constituents (urea, amino acids, uric acid) are found in the CSF. The existence of these exceptions indicates that active metabolic processes are involved in the formation of this highly specialized fluid.

Most of the values listed in Table 8-1 are in terms of milliequivalents. This terminology is used because these substances are ionized in solution and thus carry an electrical charge: hence the term *electrolyte*. A *milliequivalent* is the atomic weight in milligrams divided by the valence; a *millimol (mmol)* is the molecular weight in milligrams; a *milliosmol (mOsmol)* is the weight of an osmotically active particle in milligrams. Hence 1 mmol NaCl contains 1 mEq Na^+ and 1 mEq Cl^-, and 2 mOsmol; 1 mM $CaCl_2$ contains 2 mEq Ca^{2+} and 2 mEq Cl^-, and 3 mOsmol; 1 mM glucose

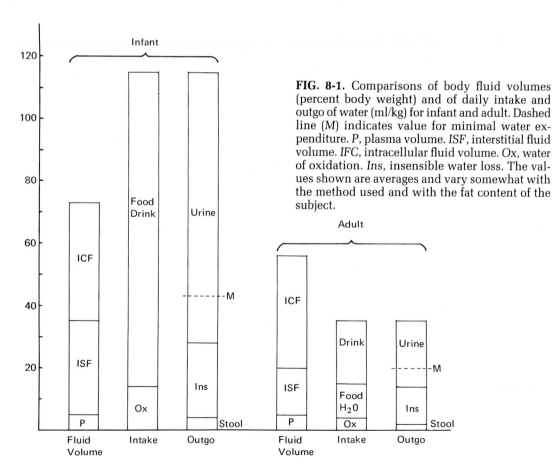

FIG. 8-1. Comparisons of body fluid volumes (percent body weight) and of daily intake and outgo of water (ml/kg) for infant and adult. Dashed line (M) indicates value for minimal water expenditure. P, plasma volume. ISF, interstitial fluid volume. IFC, intracellular fluid volume. Ox, water of oxidation. Ins, insensible water loss. The values shown are averages and vary somewhat with the method used and with the fat content of the subject.

TABLE 8-1. Body Fluid Constituents

	Blood Plasma (mEq/liter)		Cerebrospinal Fluid (mEq/liter)*	Intracellular Fluid (mEq/liter cell water)†
	Infant	Adult		
Cations				
Na$^+$	140	142	144	10
K$^+$	5	4	3	150
Ca^{2+}	5 (10 mg/dl)	5	2.5	2
Mg^{2+}	2 (2 mg/dl)	2	2.1	25
Anions				
Cl$^-$	103	100	123	
HCO$_3^-$	24	27	20	10
Phosphate	3 (5.5 mg/dl)	2 (3.5 mg/dl)	1	100
Sulfate	1	1	1	20
Organic acids	7	6	4	
Protein	14 (6 g/dl)	16 (7 g/dl)	20 mg/dl	60
Nonelectrolytes				
Glucose (fasting)	75 mg/dl	90 mg/dl	⅔ blood value	

*There is disagreement on precise values for CSF ion concentrations; the values here represent averages of those reported in the literature.

†Intracellular ion concentrations ae calculated from the Cl$^-$ space.

represents 1 mOsmol. The osmotic equivalents of the various ions in body fluids are actually slightly less than this owing to the fact that ionic activity is somewhat below that observed in dilute aqueous solutions. Thus the predicted osmolality of blood plasma,

$$(Na^+ + K^+) \times 2 + \frac{glucose\ mg/dl}{18}$$

$$+ \frac{Blood\ urea\ nitrogen\ (BUN)\ mg/dl}{2.8}$$

$$= 296\text{--}305$$

is greater than the measured value of 285 mOsmols/liter.

The composition of intracellular fluid differs markedly from that of extracellular fluid: K$^+$, Mg^{2+}, and P are much higher in the former as is protein, and Na$^+$ is much lower. In muscle cells Cl$^-$ content is very low (many investigators consider it to be zero), whereas brain and nerve are said to contain 10 mEq Cl$^-$/kg to 50 mEq Cl$^-$/kg. The sum total of all cations is somewhat greater in intracellular fluid owing to a certain amount of ion binding, particularly in brain, by protein and phospholipid. In the young animal, brain and muscle have a somewhat higher total content of water, Na$^+$, and Cl$^-$, and a lower content of K$^+$.[5]

However, careful studies have shown that the total concentration of osmotically active materials in interstitial and intracellular fluids is equal. This state of osmotic equality is maintained principally by the free diffusion of water across cell walls. Decreases in extracellular osmolality thus lead to cellular overhydration, and increases to cellular dehydration. This is the basis for the use of hyperosmolar solutions in the treatment of cerebral edema.

FUNCTIONAL ASPECTS

Not only is water continually diffusing across capillary walls and entering and leaving cells, but isotope studies have shown that the same is also true of all electrolytes. The older idea that compositional differences were maintained by virtue of the selective permeability of cell membranes has given way to the modern view that such differences are the result of metabolic processes, the so-called active transport. Sodium, for example, diffuses readily into cells and out again. It does not accumulate in cells because it is being continuously pumped out of the cell at a rapid rate; hence the low concentration of Na^+ in the cell in the face of a high external concentration. The exact nature of the Na^+ pump is not certain, but it is known to be linked to certain metabolic processes within the cell and to be adenosine triphosphate (ATP)-dependent. Application of certain cell poisons causes the pump to fail, whereupon Na^+ accumulates within the cell. An inability to generate sufficient ATP, either due to decreased substrate delivery or inefficient (anerobic) metabolism, is one of the characteristic features of cell injury, whether due to heat, anoxia, physical trauma, cardiac failure, or metabolic inhibitors. Under normal circumstances an appreciable fraction of the total energy expended by the cell is used to drive the Na^+ pump.

The situation presented by the CSF has some unique features. In addition to certain concentration differences (Table 8-1), the entry of many substances (deuterium, bromide, radiosodium, radiopotassium, radiophosphorus) into CSF from blood is 3 times to 30 times slower than that into the interstitial fluid of other soft tissues. This phenomenon, noted many years ago for certain vital dyes, has been ascribed to the existence of a "blood–brain barrier." The anatomic basis for such a barrier may well consist of the continuous, rather thick, basement membrane that surrounds the capillary endothelium and that is in turn closely invested by sheaths of neuroglial processes. The brain's endothelial cells are densely packed with mitochondria, thereby providing the enormous amounts of ATP that are required for the maintenance of the organic and ionic pumps. Brain extracellular ionic composition is regulated by these cells, whose enzymatic activity of Na^+, K^+-activated ATPase is even greater than that of the cells of the choroid plexus.[10]

Thus the nerve cell body does not share the same intimacy with interstitial fluid as do the cells of other soft tissues; hence the central nervous system is afforded a certain degree of protection against sudden perturbations in extracellular fluid volume and composition. Cerebral blood flow is maintained nearly invariant of changes in systemic blood pressure and plasma volume over a wide range by the vascular tone (autoregulation); this protection may not be fully developed in the newborn. Fortunate it is that such protection does exist because the brain, encased in its rigid calvarium that precludes changes in tissue volume, would otherwise suffer violent and symptomatic changes in pressure. Were it not for a "barrier" of some type the very existence of the CSF reservoir would be in jeopardy because the oncotic pressure exerted by the plasma proteins together with high CSF pressure would drain it away.

There is some evidence to show that the blood–brain barrier is not as efficient in young infants. Perhaps the open cranial fontanels that permit a certain degree of volume change constitute a safety factor in this age group. It is of interest that the blood–brain barrier is either absent or nonfunctional in certain regions: the pineal body, pituitary, endocrine areas of the hypothalamus, and the area postrema. The barrier is rendered less efficient by anoxia, inflammation, physical trauma, or convulsions, and is largely lacking in tumor tissue. The latter is the basis for iostopic localization of brain tumors.*

The hydraulic function of the CSF is easily appreciated: the effective weight of the brain is reduced to a thirtieth of its actual weight and its inertia is increased in the face of external acceleration. It has also been suggested that the CSF constitutes a large reservoir for the dilution of materials discharged from nerve cells during cell activity, thus avoiding local disturbances. On the other hand, it may also hold nearby the substances that are lost during neuronal discharge and that must be replaced rapidly during recovery, substances that might otherwise be swept away by the bloodstream. It may be more than fortuitous therefore that the most active part of the brain (gray matter) is turned toward the subarachnoid and ventricular surfaces.[17]

Earlier, note was taken of the fact that the ECF volume of brain is lower than that of muscle. Of the total brain water, about

---

*Invertebrate species do not possess CSF, and it is only the higher mammals that have a fully formed subarachnoid space with cisternal expansions.

half is in neurons, a fourth is in glia, and the remainder is equally divided between the interstitial space and the CSF. Hence cerebral edema is primarily intracellular in location, rather than interstitial as in muscle, and the volume of CSF may not be altered significantly. This is why a spinal tap is hazardous in such patients.

Cerebrospinal fluid composition (see Table 8-1), differing in certain respects from that of blood plasma, tends to resist change.[7] Potassium concentration in CSF varies but little in response to changes in plasma K^+, and CSF pH (normally about 0.1 unit below that of the blood) is more stable than blood pH, as is CSF HCO_3^- concentration.[9,24] Since CO_2 equilibration between plasma and CSF is more rapid than that of hydrogen ions, it follows that respiratory alkalosis influences acid–base balance within the CNS (and hence electrical excitability) to a greater extent than metabolic alkalosis does.[26] This accounts for the well known response to hyperventilation in children with petit mal epilepsy.

Body fluid electrolytes serve a number of important functions in addition to osmoregulation. They act as buffers, helping to preserve acid–base equilibrium, as colloid stabilizers, as enzyme activators, and as facilitators of synaptic transmission. Ca^{2+} and Mg^{2+} are required for the synthesis of an important compound, adenosine 3′:5′-cyclic phosphate (cyclic AMP), from ATP and for its conversion to 5′-adenosine monophosphate (5′-AMP). Another regulator of cellular metabolism is the recently identified Ca^{2+}-binding protein, calmodulin.[4]

The action of many hormones and some drugs is mediated through the formation of cyclic AMP, which is now known as the "second messenger." There is an optimal ionic environment for efficient tissue function. Major alterations in pH, ionic concentration, or osmolality cannot be tolerated.[11]

DISTURBANCES OF WATER AND SODIUM

The resting electrical potential of cells (about −70 mV) is primarily due to the separation of Na^+ and K^+ across the cell wall; during excitation the potential becomes positive, a process known as *depolarization*. The upstroke of the action potential is associated with a sudden influx of Na^+, followed by an efflux of K^+. The nerve impulse is propagated by means of a wave of positive charges traveling down the axon, the so-called electrotonic current.[28]

The height of the action potential is directly proportional to the external Na^+ concentration and the concentration of other ions (Ca^{2+}, Mg^{2+}, H^+) affects the threshold for excitability. Changes in plasma pH or Ca^{2+} can therefore produce marked alterations in the electroencephalogram (EEG). At least two drugs used in the treatment of epilepsy (phenytoin and acetazolamide) are known to affect ionic transport, the former by stimulating the Na^+ pump, the latter by reducing Na^+ influx and K^+ exchange.[29] Barbiturates and chlorpromazine act to increase the threshold for neuronal excitability.

Although lithium (Li^+) can substitute for Na^+ to a certain extent in *in-vitro* tissue systems, high concentrations are toxic, especially when the ECF Na^+ level is low. Once accumulated by cells, the Na^+ pump cannot remove Li^+, K^+ reentry during repolarization is impeded, resting potential falls, and nerve conduction is impaired. This element inhibits adenylcyclase, and therapeutic levels induce changes in the human EEG.[25] The basis for using Li^+ in certain psychiatric states is not known, but various theories suggest that it may alter cyclic AMP-mediated processes in the central nervous system (CNS) and other organs, prevent supersensitivity of dopamine receptors, and interfere with the active membrane transport of catecholamines.[3] Lithium also antagonizes the action of (antidiuretic hormone) ADH on the renal tubule, thereby accounting for the occurrence of diabetes insipidus in some patients treated with this element, and for the salutary effects of the ion in situations involving inappropriate ADH secretion.

The regulation of body fluid volume and its Na^+ content is achieved through the interaction of a number of organ systems including kidney, adrenal, skin, central nervous system, and lung. Carotid and hypothalamic osmoreceptors have been identified, and volume receptors located in the left atrium, carotid sinus, and pulmonary veins. Posterior pituitary hormone influences water reabsorption by the renal tubule. Thirst is a function of central nervous system activity. The question of whether the CNS has a direct effect on Na^+ metabolism is still an open one.[6]

Etiology.   Dehydration results from excessive losses of water and electrolyte by way of the gastrointestinal tract (diarrhea or vomiting), the kidney (polyuria of renal failure, diabetes insipidus, or diabetes mellitus), or the skin (excessive sweating). Since water is being continuously lost through skin and lung (insensible perspiration) and since there is a certain obligatory renal water loss (Fig. 8-1), thirsting alone eventually leads to dehydration. The rapidity with which a state of dehydration develops and its extent depend on the magnitude of the negative water balance (intake minus output).

Usually some loss of Na^+ also occurs. If the negative balance of Na^+ relative to that of water is equivalent to the Na^+ concentration in body fluids (140 mEq/liter), the resulting state of dehydration is spoken of as *isotonic*. If the negative balance of Na^+ relative to that of water exceeds this value then serum Na^+ falls, a condition designated as *hypotonic dehydration*. The hypertonic variety can be similarly visualized.

Note that the term *negative balance* is used in this context. It is not only the actual loss of water and salt from the body that is important, but also the net loss (intake minus output) that determines the degree and type of dehydration that ensues. Thus the clinical evaluation of the dehydrated patient must include the volume of intake and its composition (rich or poor in salt) as well as the nature and volume of fluid lost from the body.[18]

Water retention can also occur in the face of Na^+ loss, as for example when water is freely consumed in the face of pitressin administration. Certain nervous system lesions and pulmonary disorders apparently cause excess ADH release and a similar train of circumstances. Such patients have been described as suffering from the cerebral salt-wasting syndrome or the syndrome of inappropriate ADH release.[23] The manifold disturbances seen in neurosurgical patients are the result of a train of complicated circumstances: respiratory embarrassment, disturbed thirst, coma, damage to endocrine areas of the hypothalamus, inappropriate fluid and electrolyte administration, and so on.

Overhydration results whenever intake of water exceeds the capacity of the body to excrete it. Some patients have a pathologic desire (*psychogenic polydypsia*) to drink water. Included in this group are those who have been severely burned. More frequently, the excess water loads are given parenterally in a mistaken impression of actual need. Although overhydration is in actuality rather difficult to achieve in the normal individual, it can readily occur in persons whose ability to excrete water loads is, for one reason or another, impaired. These include the newborn, patients with certain types of renal, cardiac, or hepatic failure, and those who have been subjected to surgical procedures. Excess water retention results in an increase in body fluid volume, a fall in serum Na^+, and, if carried far enough, to actual water intoxication. On the other hand, if the net increase in body water content is accompanied by an equivalent amount of salt so that serum Na^+ and osmolality remain normal, edema is the principal consequence.[8]

Pathology.   Hypotonic states may result in swelling and edema of the brain and obliteration of the perivascular spaces, shrunken ventricles, and flattened gyri. Hypertonic states produce shrinkage of brain cells and retraction of the brain with congestion of the meninges and vascular stasis. The brain, unlike most tissues, can in such situations generate intracellular "idiogenic osmols" in order to preserve cell volume. As a consequence, too vigorous therapy with hypotonic fluids can result in massive cerebral edema because the removal or inactivation of these intracellular osmols may take several hours. Hemorrhagic encephalopathy has been described in hypertonic dehydration, as have pyknosis of microglial nuclei and loss of staining in the outer cortical layers.[13,14]

Since dehydration is usually accompanied by circulatory insufficiency and hypoxia, some of the pathologic changes may be a consequence of these. Occasionally thrombosis of one of the large cerebral veins or dural sinuses occurs. Perivascular and focal necrosis have been described in uremic states.

Symptoms and Signs. The clinical manifestations of dehydration are dependent to a certain extent on the concomitant status of Na^+ balance. In the hypotonic or isotonic form, the earliest symptoms are weight loss, fatigue, and weakness. Later drowsiness, alternating irritability and stupor, delirium, decreased visual acuity, dysconjugate eye movements and nystagmus, cutaneous anesthesia, suppression of the deep tendon reflexes, and muscle hypotonia occur. Anorexia and vomiting are common complaints. Coma may develop in the final stages.

Other signs include dryness of the mucous membranes, diminished subcutaneous tissue turgor, enophthalmus, and in infants depression of the cranial fontanels. Eventually signs of circulatory insufficiency ensue including tachycardia, hypotension, peripheral cyanosis, and coolness. Body temperature may fall, in contrast to the fever that is so characteristic of the earlier stages. The end result is a state of shock that can progress to irreversibility and death. These above-mentioned physical signs reflect primarily the depletion of ECF volume.

Certain variations are seen in the hypertonic form of dehydration, in which a considerable share of the fluid loss represents intracellular fluid (ICF) volume. Thirst is avid, vomiting less common. Irritability, restlessness, and occasionally convulsions are characteristic, in addition to confusion and stupor. The deep tendon reflexes are hyperactive, and increased muscle tone and even opisthotonus may occur. Peripheral signs of dehydration are less profound because the increased osmolality of extracellular fluid causes water to shift from cells to this compartment, thus preserving to a certain degree its volume.

In infants with nephrogenic diabetes insipidus the clinical picture may be dominated by persistent fever, mental apathy, growth failure, irritability, and recurrent convulsions. Many of these abnormalities disappear when there is adequate water intake and dietary solute reduction.

Overhydration with water intoxication leads to headache, vomiting, confusion, muscle pain and spasm, and occasionally coma and convulsions. Signs of increased intracranial pressure may be present together with hypertension. If the retention of water is accompanied by an equivalent amount of Na^+, there are usually no signs referable to the CNS and peripheral edema (which usually spares the CNS) is the principal manifestation.

Note should be taken here of the entity known as *asymptomatic hyponatremia*. Certain patients with cardiac or hepatic failure, tuberculosis (particularly tuberculous meningitis), pyogenic meningitis, pneumonia, and starvation have a consistently reduced serum Na^+ concentration. Serum Cl^- is also reduced, and it is this that accounts for the characteristically lowered Cl^- content of the CSF in tuberculous meningitis. Some of these patients undoubtedly have inappropriate ADH release. The lack of symptoms from the hyponatremia is due to the fact that ECF volume is maintained.

Laboratory Examination. In most situations the serum Na^+ value is a reliable index of serum osmolality. Hyperglycemic, lipemic, and azotemic states are exceptions to this rule. Furthermore, a large disparity between measured and calculated serum osmolality may be seen with the ingestion of certain low molecular weight toxins, such as ethylene glycol: a useful clue in the diagnosis of the comatose patient who has consumed an unknown poison. The total CO_2 content of the serum is an index of acid–base status unless respiratory abnormalities exist. In such instances determination of blood pH is necessary. Evidence for a fall in intravascular fluid volume can be sought in a rising hematocrit or plasma protein content. Diminution in renal function is reflected in an elevated BUN and creatinine. Oliguria is common in dehydrated patients, as is the presence of albumin, casts, and leukocytes in the urine. Theoretically it should be possible to document changes in body fluid volume by use of the various dilution techniques described above, but these are difficult to apply to the bedside situation. The clinical history and appraisal of the patient (history of fluid intake and losses, signs of dehydration or overhydration, changes in body weight, and so on) are of the utmost importance here.

In infants with hypertonic dehydration the protein content of the CSF is often increased and the pressure may be low. Pressure may be elevated in water intoxication, and the EEG reveals a reduction in amplitude and wave frequency.

Differential Diagnosis. It is evident that disturbances in water and Na^+ metabolism can mimic certain types of primary CNS diseases such as those associated with confusion, delirium, convulsions, and coma, or those resulting in increased intracranial pressure. It is helpful that water and electrolyte disturbances are usually acute in onset and that peripheral manifestations of fluid imbalance are usually evident. When such disturbances occur in a patient with preexisting CNS disease, the differential diagnosis may be most difficult and may be made with certainty only after the water and electrolyte abnormalities have been corrected.[20]

Treatment. As a rule, treatment involves parenteral administration of fluids (the intravenous route is preferred). In dehydration, water and salt must be given and often potassium as well (the latter only after it has been established that renal function is reasonably adequate). Sodium bicarbonate should be used when acidosis is severe. Whole blood, plasma, or serum albumin is indicated in situations complicated by malnutrition or blood loss.

Two phases in treatment of dehydration can be recognized. The first involves restoration of the plasma and interstitial fluid volume in order to reestablish, to a certain extent, circulatory and renal function. This can be accomplished by the relatively rapid intravenous infusion, in amounts of 10 ml/kg body weight to 30 ml/kg body weight of normal saline or, if acidosis is severe, a mixture of 1 part normal saline and 1 part Molar/6 $NaHCO_3$, with or without added dextrose.

The isotonic solutions are indicated in isotonic or hypotonic states, particularly when shock is present, and the more dilute solutions when dehydration is of the hypertonic variety. The aim of this phase is not to repair completely the postulated deficit of body fluids but rather to effect a sufficient degree of repair so that shock and acidosis are alleviated and renal function restored to the point where selective renal processes can once again aid the body in its adjustment of the underlying disturbance.

The second phase of treatment involves completion of the reparative process plus giving sufficient fluid and electrolyte to allow for maintenance of body needs during the period when oral feedings may be proscribed. Ordinarily, this phase lasts 2 days to 5 days. Since extrarenal losses of water are high in infants, hypotonic fluids must be used for this phase. Potassium should always be given (unless the serum K^+ is high or renal function seriously compromised) because K^+ losses are usually appreciable in states of underhydration. An appropriate solution is one that provides 40 mEq Na^+ to 50 mEq Na^+, 20 mEq K^+ to 30 mEq K^+, 30 mEq Cl^- to 40 mEq Cl^-, 10 mEq phosphate, 20 mEq HCO_3 or lactate, and 50 g dextrose per liter. If neither acidosis nor K^+ deficiency is present or anticipated, a mixture of 1 part normal saline and 2 parts 5% dextrose in water (50 mM NaCl) is satisfactory. The proportions can be varied to suit the particular circumstances. The amounts given depend on the age of the patient, the presence or absence of fever, the degree of dehydration, and whether abnormal fluid and electrolyte losses continue to occur. Ordinarily the amounts are 70 ml/kg per day to 100 ml/kg per day in the newborn, 100 ml/kg per day to 150 ml/kg per day in infants, and 50 ml/kg per day to 80 ml/kg per day in children. Maintenance needs for Na^+ and K^+ are 2 mEq to 3 mEq of each per kilogram per day.

It is important to remember that no scheme of fluid therapy yet devised is foolproof. One must make an estimate of fluid needs and then carefully observe the course of the patient during therapy, being prepared to change the character or amount of fluid if need be. Repeated determinations of serum Na^+, K^+, total CO_2, BUN, and on occasion pH and PCO_2 are of great help in evaluating the progress of therapy.

Infants suffering from hypertonic dehydration present special problems in therapy because the rapid alleviation of hypernatremia is often followed by convulsions. Since hypocalcemia may occur during treatment, the addition of 20 ml 10% calcium gluconate per liter of infusate is desirable. The rate of fluid administration should be relatively slow, the aim being to repair the fluid deficit over a 48-hour period; and the Na^+ concentration should be at least 40 mEq/liter to 60 mEq/liter so that the serum Na^+ level falls slowly to normal.

Water intoxication is treated with hypertonic saline (2.5% or 427 mEq Na^+/liter) given intravenously in sufficient quantity to alleviate symptoms; 5 ml/kg to 10 ml/kg (about 2 mEq Na^+/kg–4 mEq Na^+/kg) given over a period of an hour or so is usually sufficient. There is no need to raise the serum Na^+ concentration to normal because symptoms usually disappear long before this point is reached and the potential hazard of giving too much salt is thereby avoided. Water must be withheld. Other osmotically active substances, for example, mannitol (1 g/kg in 15% solution), have proved effective in experimental water intoxication. When hyponatremia is due to psychogenic polydypsia or inappropriate ADH release, restriction of total water intake (food plus drink) to a level below that of obligatory urine and insensible losses corrects the situation.

An important phase of therapy is that directed at the underlying cause of the disturbed water and sodium metabolism. Such treatment (e.g., antibiotics for infectious diarrhea) can often proceed simultaneously with that aimed at the disturbance itself. Pitressin therapy is indicated in diabetes insipidus.

Prognosis. Under ordinary circumstances prognosis is good. Infants and children recover from the effects of fluid and electrolyte imbalance with amazing rapidity, and ordinarily within a few days there is no evidence of abnormal CNS function.

Thrombosis of one of the cerebral veins or dural sinuses can occur in severe cases of dehydration. In the hypertonic form particularly, the associated encephalopathy can lead to permanent brain damage.

DISTURBANCES OF CALCIUM

In contrast to Na^+ only a minute fraction (less than 1%) of the total body Ca^{2+} is found in body fluids, the remainder being an integral part of bone mineral. The concentration of Ca^{2+} in serum is maintained by the action of a number of factors: parathyroid activity, vitamin D, thyrocalcitonin, renal and gastrointestinal processes, and bone itself because a small portion of this vast reservoir of mineral readily exchanges with ECF. Only a fraction (55%) of the total serum Ca^{2+} is in ionic form under normal conditions, 12% being present as diffusible undissociated complexes, and the remainder (33%) bound to protein. Since it is the total serum Ca^{2+} that is determined in the clinical laboratory, it follows that the low levels encountered in hypoproteinemic states do not always result in symptoms.

Calcium is firmly bound to cell membranes, and the ion has a prominent role in tissue excitability. It modulates the excitatory threshold and Na^+ permeability of cells, and it is required for acetylcholine release at the nerve terminal and for formation of cyclic AMP. A fall in the level of ionized Ca^{2+} leads to depolarization of the cell membrane, increased permeability to Na^+ and K^+, and increased cell irritability. This is manifested by spasm of skeletal, smooth, and cardiac muscle as a result of enhanced excitability of the peripheral myoneural apparatus and autonomic ganglia. Full expression of these effects is dependent on the integrity of the spinal reflex arc.[2]

Paradoxical effects are observed at high levels of serum Ca^{2+}. Permeability to Na^+ and K^+ is decreased; acetylcholine release at the myoneural junction is increased; ventricular fibrillation occurs; and yet synaptic transmission is blocked.

Etiology. Hypocalcemia is seen in a number of situations: vitamin D deficiency, hypoparathyroidism, malabsorption syndromes, Mg^{2+} deficiency, certain types of renal failure, pseudohypoparathyroidism, acute pancreatitis, and during the neonatal period. Temporary hypocalcemia may be encountered in infants receiving parenteral fluids for the treatment of severe dehydration.

The etiology of neonatal hypocalcemia is not known. The fact that it rarely occurs in breast-fed babies suggests that the excessive load of phosphorus provided by cows' milk is a factor. The existence of a state of temporary "functional hypoparathyroidism" has also been postulated and excessive release of thyrocalcitonin has been incriminated. The incidence is increased in babies with intercurrent illness and in those whose mothers have hyperparathyroidism.

Recently it was reported that anticonvulsant medication is associated with an appreciable incidence of mild hypocalcemia, and a few subjects who sustained clinical rickets and osteomalacia have been found.[1] The current hypothesis is that these drugs (particularly phenytoin and phenobarbital) induce hepatic enzyme activity leading to altered metabolism of vitamin D.

A reduction in ionized Ca^{2+} results from the intravenous infusion of large quantities of citrate as in massive transfusions of whole blood. It is common practice to give Ca^{2+} salts periodically during the course of an exchange transfusion. Hypocalcemia can also follow the use of chelating agents such as ethylenediaminetetraacetic acid (EDTA) and pediatric hypertonic phosphate enemas.

Hypercalcemia occurs in hyperparathyroidism, vitamin D intoxication, and in immobilized patients who have poor renal function. It is also associated with sarcoidosis, milk-alkali syndrome, thyrotoxicosis, chronic thiazide usage, and extensive malignancy, particularly when skeletal metastases are present. In recent years the syndrome of "hypercalcemia of infancy with failure to thrive" has been described as occurring in association with generous intakes of vitamin D and Ca^{2+}.[19] Although the cause is not known, these patients lack the ability to handle oral or intravenous Ca^{2+} loads in an efficient manner.[16]

Pathology.   No specific changes are seen in the brain as a result of acute hypocalcemia. In hypoparathyroidism intracranial calcification may be noted, involving principally the basal ganglia. Microscopically the Ca^{2+} deposits are located within and about the walls of the finer blood vessels and are associated with colloid deposits of an unknown type.

Symptoms and Signs.   Muscle pain and stiffness, spontaneous tremor, fibrillary twitching, awkward movements, facial grimacing, laryngospasm, and the peculiar posturing of the hands and feet known as *carpopedal spasm* are the characteristic symptoms of hypocalcemic tetany. Carpopedal spasm consists of flexion of the wrist, abduction of the hands, flexion of the metacarpophalangeal joints with extension of the phalanges, and adduction of the thumb; the feet are in equinovarus with the toes flexed and the plantar surfaces arched. Both sides of the body are usually involved, and the spasm is of variable duration. Laryngospasm manifests as hoarseness, lowering of voice pitch, and stridor; if severe, a pertussislike whoop may occur and on rare occasions complete respiratory obstruction may ensue. In certain patients the clinical picture is dominated by generalized tonic–clonic seizures with loss of consciousness. This is particularly true in young infants.

Symptoms and signs of acute hypocalcemia are intensified by febrile states, excitement, physical activity, hyperkalemia, and elevation of blood pH. Conversely, symptoms of tetany improve in the face of acidosis or hypokalemia.

A number of characteristic signs may be elicited. Chvostek's sign consists of contraction of facial muscles on tapping over the facial nerve trunk. The ophthalmic division is most easily provoked, and sometimes the three major divisions of the nerve can be delineated. Trousseau's sign consists of carpal spasm in response to circumferential pressure applied to the upper arm. The peroneal sign consists of dorsiflexion and abduction of the foot in response to tapping over the peroneal nerve trunk. In addition, attacks of tetany may be accompanied by muscle rigidity, adduction of the extremities, and mild opisthotonus. The deep tendon reflexes are hyperactive.

The term *latent tetany* is used to describe hypocalcemic states in which there are no spontaneous manifestations but in which signs of increased neuromuscular irritability can be elicited by appropriate mechanical or electrical stimulation. A certain amount of tolerance may develop during the course of chronic hypocalcemia so that tetany is not always manifest at serum levels that would regularly lead to symptoms in the acute state.

Chronic hypocalcemia, particularly that due to hypoparathyroidism, may result in a number of additional features.[15] Typical grand mal seizures are common. Symptoms of increased intracranial pressure with papilledema, congestive heart failure, mental dullness and confusion, and psychotic behavior have been described. Punctate lenticular cataracts are common, and some patients have photophobia. A number of other ectodermal defects may also occur: dental caries, enamel hypoplasia, dry skin, brittle nails, and loss of scalp and body hair. Occasional patients have chronic moniliasis and adrenocortical insufficiency. It is not certain whether these interesting abnormalities are due to hypocalcemia *per se*, or to the existence of autoimmune processes involving a number of organ systems.

Patients with pseudohypoparathyroidism are usually short of stature, mentally retarded, and exhibit shortening of one or more metacarpal bones. Siblings may be afflicted, and this is also true in occasional cases of idiopathic hypoparathyroidism.

Acute hypercalcemia, the result of intravenous administration of Ca^{2+} salts, may be associated with vasodilatation and bradycardia. In experimental animals death from cardiac failure occurs at serum Ca^+ levels of about 60 mg/dl.

The infantile hypercalcemic syndrome is manifested by growth failure, muscle weakness, and hypotonia. Some patients have mental retardation, cardiac murmurs, and hypertension, and exhibit a peculiar elfinlike facies. Additional features seen in chronic hypercalcemia of various causes include headache, constipation (due to gastrointestinal atony), listlessness, changes in sensorium, pruritus, neuromuscular symptoms, paresthesias, anorexia, and vomiting. Secondary renal damage and stone formation may occur. Uremic encephalopathy may complicate the picture in extreme cases. Certain patients show minute crystalline deposits in cornea and conjunctiva, and a whitish lesion of the cornea known as *band keratitis*.

Laboratory Examination. Symptoms and signs of hypocalcemia are usually evident at serum Ca^{2+} levels below 7 mg/dl, providing serum protein concentration is normal. Associated abnormalities of serum phosphorus and alkaline phosphatase are often present, depending on the underlying disease (Table 8-2). Prolongation of the Q–T interval of the electrocardiogram is characteristic, and in chronic hypocalcemia the EEG usually reveals slowing of wave frequencies and paroxysmal dysrhythmia.

In chronic hypocalcemia calcification of the basal ganglia may be detected roentgenographically (Fig. 8-2). Cerebrospinal fluid pressure may be elevated.

Hypercalcemic states are associated with shortening of the Q–T interval of the electrocardiogram. Skull roentgenograms may show osteosclerosis in the infantile hypercalcemic syndrome (Fig. 8-3) and osteitis fibrosa in hyperparathyroidism. Cal-

TABLE 8-2. Values for Serum Calcium, Inorganic Phosphorous, and Alkaline Phosphatase in Normal Subjects and Those with Certain Diseases

	Serum Calcium (mg/dl)	Serum Phosphorus (mg/dl)	Serum Alkaline Phosphatase (International Units per liter)
Normal infant	10	6–7	15–275
Normal child	10	4–5	15–295
Normal adult	10	3–4	20–90
Nutritional rickets	N or ↓	↓	↑
Resistant rickets	N or ↓	↓	↑
Hypoparathyroidism	↓	↑	N
Pseudohypoparathyroidism	↓	↑	N
Hyperparathyroidism	↑	↓	N or ↑
Infantile hypercalcemia	↑	N	N
Hypoproteinemia	↓	N	N
Neonatal tetany	↓	↑	N

N, normal; ↓ decrease; ↑ increase

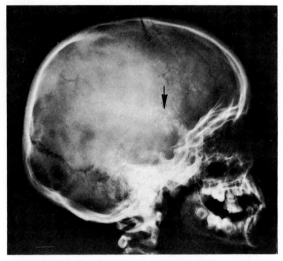

FIG. 8-2. Skull roentgenogram of child with idiopathic hypoparathyroidism, showing calcification in region of basal ganglia (retouched). (From Forbes GB: Ann NY Acad Sci 64:437, 1956)

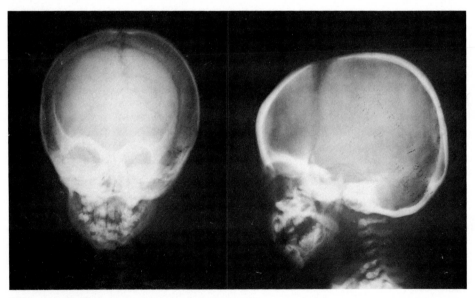

FIG. 8-3. Skull roentgenogram of 21.5-month-old infant with the infantile hypercalcemic syndrome, showing marked osteosclerosis.

cification in basal ganglia or choroid plexus may be seen in the latter. In experimental hypercalcemia a progression of cardiac effects has been described: vagal bradycardia occurs at serum Ca^{2+} levels of 13 mg/dl to 35 mg/dl; tachycardia, ectopic beats, and ventricular fibrillation at 30 mg/dl to 60 mg/dl; and arrest at higher levels. Temporary (nonfatal) arrest and syncope have been observed in man following rapid intravenous administration of Ca^{2+} salts.

Differential Diagnosis. Hypocalcemic states must be differentiated from conditions associated with increased neuromuscular irritability and convulsions such as tetanus, phenothiazine poisoning, and certain acute encephalopathies. Although in rare cases carpopedal spasm does occur in toxic encephalopathy, tetany in all of its various manifestations is the distinguishing and diagnostic feature of hypocalcemia. The presence of some underlying disease, such as rickets or a history of neck surgery, helps to orient the thinking of the physician. In chronic hypocalcemia the greatest difficulty comes in excluding idiopathic epilepsy, acute psychosis, and diseases causing increased intracranial pressure. The difficulties in clinical diagnosis can be appreciated from the fact that many patients with hypoparathyroidism have masqueraded as epileptics for months or years.

The tetany of hypocalcemia must be differentiated from that due to hyperventilation or metabolic alkalosis. Tetany also occurs in hyperaldosteronism, and a positive Chvostek's sign can occur in hyperkalemic periodic paralysis. Hypercalcemic states must be distinguished from the various myopathies because weakness, hypotonia, and decreased tendon reflexes are common to both. In the last analysis, it is the assay of serum for its Ca content that must provide the definitive diagnosis of both hypo- and hypercalcemic states.

Treatment. Calcium salts* may be given orally or intravenously, *never subcutaneously or intramuscularly* because they are sufficiently irritating to cause extensive tissue necrosis, especially in infants. Immediate control of tetany follows the intravenous use of calcium gluconate, given slowly in doses of 5 ml to 10 ml of the 10% solution; the effect is temporary. Oral calcium chloride, 0.5 g every 6 hours to 8 hours, usually suffices to maintain the serum Ca^{2+} at a level high enough to avoid symptoms. It is best given as a 10% solution in milk in order to obviate gastric irritation. For patients requiring protracted therapy, as for hypoparathyroidism, calcium lactate or gluconate (3 g–10 g of the salt daily) is commonly used.

Vitamin D should be given to those patients suffering from deficient intake or malabsorption. In the former condition, doses of 5000 units daily should be sufficient. Theoretically, ordinary rickets should respond to exposure of the skin to ultraviolet light. Calcium should always be given at the same time. Since one of the first actions of vitamin D is to raise the level of serum phosphorus, there may be a concomitant fall in serum Ca^{2+} with resurgence of tetany if Ca^{2+} is not given. In resistant rickets doses of vitamin D ranging from 10,000 units to 500,000 units daily are required. For hypoparathyroidism the usual doses are in the range of 50,000 units to 200,000 units daily.

Dihydrotachysterol (A.T.10), a nonantirachitic sterol, is effective in the treatment of hypoparathyroidism. The dose range is 0.625 mg to 2.5 mg of the pure sterol daily. With this drug, as with vitamin D, overdosage leading to hypercalcemia can occur; hence dosage must be individualized and monitored by frequent determinations of serum Ca^{2+}.

The dose of vitamin D required to treat hypocalcemia and rickets caused by anticonvulsant drugs has not been established, although various reports place it at 1000 units to 50,000 units daily. In view of the frequency of hypocalcemia (as high as 30% in some series) it would seem prudent to ensure an intake of 800 units daily (or twice the normal requirement) in all children being treated with such drugs.

Two metabolic conversion products of vitamin D, 25-hydroxycholecalciferol and the 1,25-dihydroxy compound, are known to be effective in the treatment of the hypocalcemia of renal and hepatic disease and of some forms of resistant rickets.

Parathyroid hormone in doses of 50 units to 250 units intravenously causes an immediate rise in urinary phosphorus excretion and an increase in urinary cyclic AMP. Repeated intramuscular doses at 6-hour intervals for several days cause the serum phosphorus to fall and Ca^{2+} to rise. (Pseudohypoparathyroidism is distinguished from true hyposecretion in that this characteristic response is lacking.) The hormone is not suitable for long-term therapy because refractoriness develops in time. For patients with phosphate retention, oral aluminum hydroxide may be of help by virtue of its effect on intestinal absorption of phosphate.

Symptoms of tetany may be relieved temporarily by acidosis, and herein lies one of the reasons why $CaCl_2$ is preferred over

---

*$CaCl_2 \cdot 2H_2O$ contains 27% calcium, $CaCl_2$ 36% calcium, calcium lactate 13% calcium, calcium gluconate 9% calcium, and calcium gluceptate 8% calcium.

neutral Ca^{2+} salts for therapy. Sedatives and anticonvulsants are of help in controlling tetanic and epileptiform seizures.

Hypercalcemic states present a more formidable therapeutic problem as far as the serum Ca^{2+} per se is concerned. Chelating agents such as EDTA offer the only available means of direct attack. Administration of large volumes of isotonic saline (200 ml/kg per day) together with intravenous (IV) furosemide will augment urinary Ca^{2+} excretion. In the idiopathic hypercalcemic syndrome and in vitamin D intoxication, treatment consists of a diet low in both Ca^{2+} and vitamin D.*

Cortisone or sodium sulfate may help by virtue of their ability to increase fecal Ca^{2+} excretion. Immobilized or paralyzed patients may be helped by the rocking bed and passive exercises. The use of methramycin and thyrocalcitonin remains experimental. The treatment of hyperparathyroidism is surgical.

Prognosis. Rarely hypocalcemia leads to fatality through laryngospasm or cardiac failure. In fact, very few postmortem examinations have been reported in patients with hypoparathyroidism. Even in patients with long, continued hypocalcemic seizures, recovery of adequate mental function is expected under adequate therapy.

The principal hazard from hypercalcemia is renal damage. In infants with the mild form of infantile hypercalcemic syndrome, recovery of normal physical and mental growth is the rule. In those infants with the severe form, some features of the disease may be ameliorated by treatment, although complete recovery is not to be expected.

DISTURBANCES OF MAGNESIUM

Magnesium is found in all body tissues. This ion serves to activate a large number of enzymes, including those involved with phosphorylation reactions, such as hexokinase or phosphofructokinase, adenyl cyclase, and those for which thiamine pyrophosphate is a cofactor. Oxidative phosphorylation is greatly reduced in the absence of Mg^{2+} Excessive quantities inhibit ATPase in brain and muscle, and interfere with acetylcholine release at neuromuscular junctions and sympathetic ganglia.

Little is known of the factors regulating Mg^{2+} metabolism. The possible influence of the parathyroid and adrenal is suggested by reports of low serum levels and negative balance of Mg^{2+} in some hyperparathyroid and hyperadrenal patients, but the role played by hormonal factors is speculative at best. It is known that intestinal absorption is enhanced by acidic solutions and that the kidney is the main avenue of excretion. Vitamin D is not involved.

Magnesium sulfate was commonly employed at one time as a sedative and anticonvulsant, and as an antihypertensive, especially for eclampsia and the hypertensive encephalopathy of acute nephritis. Magnesium is the only metallic electrolyte capable of producing anesthesia.

Etiology. Hypomagnesemia readily occurs in growing animals fed a Mg^{2+} deficient diet. With the exception of grass tetany in cattle, adult animals and man are more tolerant of deficient diets. Deficiency develops more quickly on high intakes of protein and Ca^{2+}.

In man, low serum levels of Mg^{2+} have been encountered in diabetic acidosis, acute pancreatitis, hyperaldosteronism, malabsorption syndromes, and congestive heart failure when mercurial diuretics are used. Symptomatic deficits have occurred in patients receiving Mg^{2+} free parenteral fluids for long periods, especially when gastric suction was used. There are descriptions in the literature of infants who have a congenital defect in gastrointestinal absorption of Mg^{2+} and others who have a defect in renal tubular reabsorption of Mg^{2+}. Of interest is the observation that such patients also have hypocalcemia, and that serum Ca^{2+} returns to normal when Mg^{2+} is administered.[21] Reduced secretion of parathormone (PTH) and end organ unresponsiveness may be involved in the pathogenesis of hypocalcemia associated with hypomagnesemia.

Hypermagnesiemia is encountered in

---

*It should be remembered that many drinking waters contain appreciable amounts of Ca^{2+} and that milk is usually fortified with vitamin D.

uremic patients, in adrenocortical insufficiency, and following parenteral administration of Mg^{2+} salts. Poisoning has been reported from the use of enemas in children with megacolon. Oral administration may be hazardous in patients who have reduced renal function.

Of interest is the common occurrence of elevated serum levels of Mg^{2+} in hibernating animals. Marine invertebrates normally carry a serum level high enough to be fatal to mammals.

Pathology. Magnesium deficiency results in widespread perivascular necrosis (though the brain is spared) and Ca^{2+} deposits in renal tubules. Some observers report degeneration of Purkinje cells, whereas others find no evidence of CNS damage.

Symptoms and Signs. Magnesium deficiency, in both animals and man, results in tetany, choreiform movements, irritability, awkward gait, disorientation, and generalized convulsions. Fibrillary twitching and gross tremor may occur. On examination, increased muscle tone, carpopedal spasm, and positive Chvostek's and Trousseau's signs can be elicited. The clinical picture closely resembles that seen in hypocalcemic tetany.[27]

That Mg has a toxic effect on brain and nerve can be appreciated from the fact that Mg^{2+} salts have been used to effect both local and general anesthesia. This ion thus acts to depress the activity of the peripheral and central nervous systems, competing with Ca^{2+} ions for specific sites on the presynaptic membrane. The clinical result is that of a curarelike peripheral neuromuscular paralysis with loss of the tendon reflexes. At the central level effects include somnolence, lethargy, coma, loss of all reflexes, and respiratory failure. Vasodilation, at both the arteriolar and venous levels, leads to flushing of the skin and a fall in blood pressure. Cardiac arrhythmias occur, and at very high serum levels cardiac arrest occurs in diastole. Since respiratory failure occurs at lower serum levels, the latter phenomenon is not ordinarily seen unless artificial respiration is being used.[12]

Laboratory Examination. The normal concentration of Mg^{2+} in serum is 2 mg/dl (range 1.4 mg/dl to 2.5 mg/dl). Symptoms and signs of deficiency may be manifest at levels below 1 mg/dl and those of toxicity at levels of 4 mg/dl to 5 mg/dl and above. Hypotension, prolongation of P–R and QRS intervals of the electrocardiogram, and evidence of sedation appear at concentrations of 4 mg/dl to 10 mg/dl; disappearance of tendon reflexes, respiratory depression, and slowing of the EEG at 6 mg/dl to 20 mg/dl; and cardiac arrest and loss of corneal reflexes at 25 mg/dl to 44 mg/dl. Magnesium deficiency is associated with hypocalcemia in several species including man; the rat differs in that serum Ca^{2+} is elevated.

Differential Diagnosis. Magnesium deficiency can be differentiated from hypocalcemic states only on the basis of the history and analysis of blood serum because the clinical picture is so similar. Magnesium toxicity must be differentiated from the host of conditions that cause peripheral paralysis and central depression. These include uremia and the various encephalopathies, including those due to depressant drugs and lead. The occurrence of concomitant hypotension and electrocardiographic abnormalities may provide a clue to the possibility of Mg^{2+} toxicity.

Treatment. Magnesium deficiency responds promptly to oral administration of Mg^{2+} salts. Experience has shown that a daily dose of Mg^{2+} in the range of 6 mg/kg to 30 mg/kg given in divided doses is sufficient. A convenient solution for oral use is a mixture of 4% sexhydrated magnesium chloride and 6% magnesium citrate, which provides 10 mg/ml.[21]

Immediate relief of symptoms can be obtained by the intramuscular injection of 0.1 ml/kg body weight to 0.2 ml/kg body weight of a 25% solution of $MgSO_4$ (equivalent to 5 mg–10 mg Mg^{2+}). This is the usual dose (repeated every 8 hours) employed in normomagnesemic patients for the treatment of convulsions.

Treatment of Mg^{2+} toxicity is more difficult. Peripheral paralysis may respond to administration of Ca^{2+} salts because this ion facilitates release of acetylcholine at the myoneural junction. Neostigmine, particularly when used in combination with an analeptic such as metrazol, is an effective antagonist of Mg^{2+} action. High fluid intake combined with ethacrynic diuretics are beneficial because the kidney is the main avenue of excretion. Failing this, peritoneal dialysis or the artificial kidney may have to be used. In extreme cases artificial respiration and measures to alleviate hypotension may be necessary.

Prognosis. No sequelae are anticipated from mild to moderate states of either Mg^{2+} deficiency or excess. Death occurs in experimental animals from protracted and severe deficiency. Magnesium intoxication can also be lethal because of the severe cardiac and medullary effects of this ion.

REFERENCES

1. **Borgstedt A, Bryson MF, Young L et al:** Long term administration of antiepileptic drugs and the development of rickets. J Pediatr 81:9, 1972

2. **Brink F:** The role of calcium ions in neural processes. Pharmacol Rev 6:243, 1954

3. **Bunney WE, Pert A, Rosenblatt J et al:** Mode of action of lithium. Arch Gen Psychiatry 36:898, 1979

4. **Cheung WY:** Calmodulin plays a pivotal role in cellular regulation. Science 207:19, 1980

5. **Comar C, Bronner F (eds):** Mineral Metabolism: Advanced Treatise, Vols 1 and 2. New York, Academic Press, 1961–1962.

6. **Cooke RE, Ottenheimer EJ:** Clinical and experimental interrelations of sodium and the central nervous system. Adv Pediatr 11:81, 1960

7. **Davson H:** Physiology of the Ocular and Cerebrospinal Fluids. Boston, Little, Brown & Co, 1956

8. **Dodge PR, Crawford JD, Probst JH:** Studies in experimental water intoxication. Arch Neurol 3:513, 1960

9. **Downman CBB (ed):** Modern Trends in Physiology. New York, D Appleton, 1972

10. **Eisenberg HM, Suddith RL:** Cerebral vessels have the capacity to transport sodium and potassium. Science 206:1083, 1979

11. **Elkinton JR, Danowski TS:** The Body Fluids. Baltimore, Williams & Wilkins, 1955

12. **Engbaek L:** The pharmacologic actions of magnesium ions with particular reference to the neuromuscular and the cardiovascular system. Pharmacol Rev 4:396, 1952

13. **Finberg L:** Pathogenesis of lesions in the nervous system in hypernatremic states. Part I. Clinical observations of infants. Pediatrics 23:40, 1959

14. **Finberg L, Luttrell C, Reed H:** Pathogenesis of lesions in the nervous system in hypernatremic states. Part II. Experimental studies of gross anatomic changes and alterations of chemical composition of the tissues. Pediatrics 23:46, 1959

15. **Forbes GB:** Clinical features of idiopathic hypoparathyroidism in children. Ann NY Acad Sci 64:432, 1956

16. **Forbes GB, Bryson MF, Manning JA et al:** Impaired calcium homeostasis in the infantile hypercalcemia syndrome. Acta Paediatr Scand 61:305, 1972

17. **Javid M, Settlage P:** Effect of urea on cerebrospinal fluid pressure in human subjects. JAMA 160:943, 1956

18. **Kerpel-Fronius E, Varga F, Kun K:** Cerebral anoxia in infantile dehydration. Arch Dis Child 25:156, 1950

19. **Lowe KG, Henderson JL, Park WW et al:** The idiopathic hypercalcemic syndromes of infancy. Lancet 2:101, 1954

20. **Lyon G, Dodge PR, Adams RD:** The acute encephalopathies of obscure origin in infants and children. Brain 84:680, 1961

21. **Paunier L, Radde IC, Kooh SW et al:** Primary hypomagnesemia with secondary hypocalcemia in an infant. Pediatrics 41:385, 1968

22. **Ruch TC, Fulton JF (eds):** Medical Physiology and Biophysics. Philadelphia, WB Saunders, 1960

23. **Schwartz WB, Tassel D, Bartter FC:** Further observations on hyponatremia and renal sodium loss probably resulting from inappropriate secretion of antidiuretic hormone. N Engl J Med 262:743, 1960

24. **Siesjö BK, Sørensen SC (eds):** Ion Homeostasis of the Brain. New York Academic Press, 1971

25. **Singer I, Rotenberg D:** Mechanisms of lithium action. N Engl J Med 289:254, 1973

26. **Tschirgi RD:** Blood-brain barrier: fact or fancy? Fed Proc 21:665, 1962

27. **Vallee BL, Wacker WEC, Ulmer DD:** The magnesium-deficiency tetany syndrome in man. N Engl J Med 262:155, 1960

28. **Welt, LG:** Clinical Disorders of Hydration and Acid-Base Equilibrium, 2nd ed. Boston, Little, Brown & Co, 1960

29. **Wyke BD:** Principles of General Neurology. New York, Elsevier, 1969

Inherited Metabolic Diseases 9

Robert S. Greenwood
Stephen G. Kahler
Arthur S. Aylsworth

In this chapter we will describe the inherited metabolic diseases that affect the nervous system. The number of recognized diseases has increased dramatically in the recent past as a result of both advances in our understanding of metabolic pathways and improved analytic techniques. This increase in the number of metabolic diseases and their complexity make it more difficult for the physician to correctly identify children with these neurologic disorders. Correct and early identification of children with metabolic disorders is essential because the ill effects may become irreversible over time. In addition, correct diagnosis is important for genetic counseling.

PRINCIPLES OF GENETICS

It is beyond the scope of this book to provide more than the barest outline of genetic principles. Full discussion can be found in several textbooks, ranging from introductory to advanced.[223,389,428,531,667,843]

The genetic material deoxyribonucleic acid (DNA) is present in the nucleus of each cell in long strands, the chromosomes. Regions of the chromosome that code for peptide chains are *genes*. A single or haploid set of chromosomes (23 in man) is inherited from each parent, to create a diploid zygote at conception. The 22 autosomes are identical in the two sexes. The sex chromosomes are different, in that males have one X chromosome and one Y, whereas females have two X chromosomes. The X chromosome of males is inherited from the mother.

Genes at the same locus on a pair of chromosomes may be identical or may be different; if different they are called *alleles*. An individual with identical genes at the same locus is said to be *homozygous*, whereas an individual with two different alleles is *heterozygous*. Males are *hemizygous* for genes on the X chromosome.

By definition, autosomal dominant genes are detectable when present in a single dose, regardless of the allele present on the homologous chromosome. Detectability is usually defined at the level of the organism, which is called the *phenotype*. Autosomal recessive genes are usually evident only in the homozygote, but often the heterozygote (or carrier) may have some subtle manifestations, such as a modest but clinically unimportant depression of enzyme activity. One X chromosome in each cell of females is inactive from early in development, so recessive genes on the active chromosome will be expressed in some cells. The pattern of inactivation is usually random, so women heterozygous for X-linked recessive disorders are usually clinically normal, but in some cases may be identified through special testing.

A given gene in one parent has a 50% (½) chance of being inherited by a child. Thus, there is a 50% chance that a child of a parent with a dominant disorder will inherit it. If both parents are heterozygous for a recessive gene each child has a 25% (½ × ½) chance of being homozygous. Each child of either sex has a 50% chance of inheriting X-linked genes from the mother. X-linked genes from the father are inherited by all of the daughters and none of the sons.

Genes that are unpredictable in their manifestations display *variable expression*.

Penetrance refers to the proportion of gene carriers who express a particular trait. Penetrance may be complete or incomplete, and may be expressed as a percentage.

The incidence of autosomal recessive disease is the square of the gene frequency. The carrier rate is approximately twice the gene frequency. If a disorder is present in one of 40,000 individuals, the gene frequency is $\frac{1}{200}$ and the carrier rate is 1%. It is thought that all individuals are carriers of four to six genes for severe autosomal recessive disorders. For autosomal dominant disorders the incidence is approximately twice the gene frequency.

For X-linked recessive disorders, the incidence in men is equal to the gene frequency (half the carrier rate) in women. For lethal X-linked recessive disorders, loss of genes by death of affected males is probably balanced by mutation of normal to abnormal genes. Whether this happens equally in oocytes and spermatocytes, or mainly in the latter (yielding daughters who are carriers), is not settled at present. This is an important point because the prior probability that the mother of an isolated case of an X-linked disorder is a carrier influences the estimate of recurrence risk, in the absence of effective carrier testing.

A recent summary of genetic disorders in man lists 736 proven autosomal dominant traits and disorders and a further 753 for which the evidence is suggestive.[533] Relatively few biochemical defects are known for dominant disorders. The 521 proven autosomal recessive disorders (and another possible 596) include nearly all the disorders discussed in this chapter. A few metabolic disorders are X-linked, including Fabry's disease, adrenoleukodystrophy, Hunter's syndrome, Lesch-Nyhan syndrome, and ornithine transcarbamylase deficiency. Unless otherwise specified, disorders discussed in this chapter are inherited in an autosomal recessive manner.

The family history may prove quite helpful when evaluating a child with an unknown disorder. A history of affected males related through females suggests an X-linked disorder. A history of unaffected parents and affected siblings, particularly if girls are affected, suggests autosomal recessive inheritance, as does finding parental consanguinity or the same surname on both sides of the family. Even for the rarest of disorders, however, consanguinity is not present in all cases.

GENETIC COUNSELING

The patient and his family should be given genetic counseling after a genetic disease has been diagnosed. Genetic counseling by trained personnel is available at many medical centers. It is often wise to postpone formal counseling for a few weeks, until the family has adjusted to the impact of the diagnosis. Counseling should be done under unhurried circumstances, so the family can understand and respond to the information presented.

Issues to be addressed include the family's understanding of the disorder and its adjustment to it; assessing the impact of the disorder on family life; relieving guilt over having a child with genetic disease; understanding genetic principles including the risks of having affected children in the future; and understanding the risks (usually low) to their relatives.

Directive counseling, in which the family is told what to do about future children, should be avoided. Decisions about family planning are based on the parents' desire for children, perception of risk as high or low, perception of the child's disorder as a burden, and religious and ethical beliefs. The counselor cannot substitute his or her judgment for the family's.

The availability of heterozygote testing, prenatal diagnosis if possible, and selective abortion of affected fetuses must be mentioned. In the case of autosomal recessive disorders, artificial insemination by an unrelated donor may provide the family with children who are at very low risk of having genetic disease.

A follow-up visit solely for the purpose of genetic counseling is often useful.[131,428] A letter of summary should be sent to the family after diagnosis and counseling are completed.

INCIDENCE

The incidence of many of the metabolic diseases is not known, but these are rare disorders. Most of the incidence figures have come from large newborn screening programs. In using these estimates of incidence it is important to know the population from which they were obtained and the age group that was screened. For example, the Tay-Sachs disease carrier frequency is approximately ten times greater in Jews in the United States who have descended from northeastern European ancestors than in other groups. Incidence figures, then, are most applicable to the population from which they have been derived and in some instances may not be applicable at all to other populations. It should also be remembered that the incidences are estimates that are usually based upon incomplete samples. Assumptions have to be made about the unsampled portion of the population.

Some of the metabolic diseases affecting the nervous system, their incidence, and the population from which the incidence was derived are listed below. When possible we have listed the incidence in the United States and the highest and lowest frequency for all populations that have been screened.

DIAGNOSIS OF METABOLIC DISEASES OF THE NERVOUS SYSTEM

The biochemical basis of neurological function and disease is beginning to be understood.[737] Conclusive diagnosis of metabolic diseases affecting the nervous system requires that the enzymatic defect or excessive storage or excretion product(s) be defined. It is impractical, however, to study all patients with neurologic diseases for all metabolic disorders affecting the nervous system. A clinical approach to the diagnosis of metabolic disorders and sensitive and practical laboratory screening methods must

Incidence of Inherited Metabolic Diseases Affecting the Nervous System

Disease	Population	Frequency per 100,000 live births
Phenylketonuria[721]	United States	7.1
	Ireland	20.0
	Israel	5.5
Hyperphenylalaninemia[721]	Worldwide mean	3.3
	Poland	0.5
	Switzerland	3.7
Histidinemia[448,487]	Massachusetts	2.0
	England	4.5
Homocystinuria[448,487]	Massachusetts	2.0
	England	0.5
Maple syrup urine disease[149,482]	Massachusetts	0.6
	Europe	0.8
Methylmalonic aciduria[154]	Massachusetts	2.1
Nonketotic hyperglycinemia[482]	Massachusetts	0.6
Argininosuccinic acidemia[482]	Massachusetts	1.4
Hartnup disease[482]	Massachusetts	5.6
Galactosemia[482]	Massachusetts	0.9
Hurler's syndrome[502]	British Columbia	1.0
Hunter's syndrome[502]	British Columbia	0.7
Abetalipoproteinemia[230]	United States	2.5
Tay-Sachs disease[598]	United States, Non-Jewish	0.2
	United States, Jewish	17.0
Gaucher's disease type I[321]	Ashkenazic Jews	40.0
Globoid cell leukodystrophy[337]	Sweden	1.9
Metachromatic leukodystrophy[330]	Sweden	2.5
Acute intermittent porphyria[235,850]	Ireland	1.2
	Lapland	100.0

be employed to evaluate patients with neurologic disorders.

The inherited disorders of metabolism affecting the nervous system generally occur early in life and are progressive. Exceptions to this rule, however, are frequent enough that metabolic disorders must be considered in nonprogressive neurologic disturbances beyond infancy. Infants and children with an idiopathic loss of milestones or a plateau in development after normal development should be evaluated for disorders of metabolism. Metabolic disorders in these circumstances are particularly likely when a sibling or close relative has a neurodegenerative disease or expires early in life. Cerebellar disturbances, peripheral or cranial neuropathies, vomiting, alterations in consciousness, and seizures during infancy are some of the most frequent neurologic manifestations of metabolic disorders.

In the following lists and tables 9-1 through 9-4, we have listed the inherited metabolic disorders that produce various clinical features. We have chosen signs and symptoms that are most likely to limit the number of possible diagnoses and that commonly occur in disorders other than inherited metabolic diseases. Where it is relevant, the disorders in each table or list are grouped according to age at onset of the symptom or sign: infancy (birth–1 yr), late infancy (1 yr–2 yr), childhood (2 yr–10 yr), adolescence (10 yr–20 yr), and adult (20 yr and older). These tables and lists are intended to supplement the text and guide the reader to a specific reference or to the appropriate subsection where the disease is discussed. The symptoms in these tables and lists are presenting or prominent symptoms of the diseases listed.

A clinical approach to the diagnosis of metabolic diseases affecting the nervous system is most applicable to the lysosomal storage diseases. Physical signs and symptoms can be quite distinctive, for example, the appearance of a child with Hurler's syndrome. Disorders of amino acid and organic acid metabolism generally do not produce

Behavioral and Psychiatric Disturbances

Disorder (Reference)	Onset
Phenylketonuria[614]	Infancy
Blue diaper syndrome[206]	Infancy
Lowe's syndrome[501]	Infancy to childhood
Maple syrup urine disease, variant[169]	Childhood
Methylmalonic aciduria and homocystinuria[311]	Childhood
Hartnup disease[50]	Childhood
Hunter's syndrome[535]	Childhood
Sanfilippo's syndrome (MPS III)[174]	Childhood
Aspartylglycosaminuria[30]	Childhood
Metachromatic leukodystrophy, juvenile[75]	Childhood
Neuronal ceroid-lipofuscinosis, juvenile[907]	Childhood
Cerebrotendinous xanthomatosis[833]	Childhood to adolescence
Neuronal ceroid-lipofuscinosis, adult (Kufs' disease)[319]	Childhood to adulthood
Wilson's disease[855]	Childhood to adulthood
Methylene-tetrahydrofolate reductase deficiency[253]	Adolescence
Acute intermittent porphyria[670]	Adolescence
Homocystinuria[214]	Adulthood
Gamma-glutamylcysteine synthetase deficiency[668,669]	Adulthood
Fabry's disease[193,688]	Adulthood
Metachromatic leukodystrophy[638,639]	Adulthood
Taurine deficiency[629]	Adulthood

Recurrent Vomiting

Disorder (Reference)	Onset
Propionic acidemia[142]	Newborn to childhood
Phenylketonuria[616]	Infancy
Isovaleric acidemia[483]	Infancy
Beta-ketothiolase deficiency[178]	Infancy
Hypervalinemia[167]	Infancy
3-Methylcrotonyl-glycinuria[804]	Infancy
3-Hydroxy-3-methylglutaryl CoA-lyase deficiency[898]	Infancy
Glutaric aciduria-type II[309]	Infancy
Pyruvate decarboxylase deficiency[76]	Infancy
Pyruvate carboxylase deficiency[21]	Infancy
Globoid cell leukodystrophy[334]	Infancy
Wolman's disease[1]	Infancy
Lipogranulomatosis[229]	Infancy
Galactosemia[572]	Infancy
Menkes' kinky hair syndrome[256]	Infancy
Maple syrup urine disease[544]	Infancy to childhood
Methylmalonic aciduria[880]	Infancy to childhood
Carbamoyl phosphate synthetase deficiency[730]	Infancy to childhood
Citrullinemia[730]	Infancy to childhood
Subacute neurotizing encephalomyelopathy[642]	Infancy to childhood
Lysinuric dibasic aminoaciduria[426]	Childhood
Argininemia[759]	Childhood
Fabry's disease[686]	Childhood to adulthood

distinctive physical symptoms or signs. Developmental regression, cessation of development, or a reduced rate of development may in certain cases be the only abnormality. Laboratory tests, therefore, are very important in guiding the physician toward a diagnosis of these disorders. In the section that follows we will describe the laboratory tests used in the diagnosis of the disorders of amino and organic acid metabolism. After this we describe a clinical and laboratory approach to the diagnosis of patients with suspected lysosomal storage diseases.

LABORATORY DIAGNOSIS OF DISORDERS OF AMINO AND ORGANIC ACID METABOLISM

The anion gap is readily calculated from the serum electrolyte concentrations. It is the sum of chloride plus bicarbonate subtracted from the sodium concentration. The normal value for adults is $+12$ mEq/dl or less; in children, it may be as high as $+15$.[605] A persistently elevated anion gap, particularly due to low HCO_3^- and accompanied by tachypnea, indicates the presence of an unidentified anion. The urine pH will often be inappropriately low. The serum pH is of less use because respiratory compensatory mechanisms will lower the pCO_2 in proportion to the lowering of HCO_3^-, so the

Acute Encephalopathy and Hepatic Dysfunction (Reyelike Syndrome)

Disorder (Reference)
Ornithine transcarbamylase deficiency[456]
Propionic acidemia[351]
Isovaleric acidemia[615]
Glutaric aciduria[309]
Systemic carnitine deficiency[858]
Carnitine acetyltransferase deficiency[196]
Methylmalonyl-CoA apomutase deficiency[880]
Hydroxymethylglutaryl-CoA lyase deficiency[673]

Bulbar Abnormalities (Dysphagia, Dysarthria, Hoarseness)

Disorder (Reference)	Onset
Pyruvate decarboxylase deficiency[411]	Infancy
Gaucher's disease, infantile[251]	Infancy
Lipogranulomatosis[229]	Infancy
Subacute necrotizing encephalomyelopathy[642]	Infancy to childhood
G_{M1} gangliosidosis, juvenile[601]	Infancy to childhood
Gaucher's disease, juvenile[251]	Infancy to childhood
Salla disease[24]	Infancy to childhood
Sandhoff's disease, infantile[233]	Late infancy
Wilson's disease[190]	Childhood to adulthood
Glutamate dehydrogenase deficiency[645]	Adolescence to adulthood
Taurine deficiency[629]	Adulthood

pH may be essentially normal unless the patient is overwhelmingly ill. Dehydration, lactic acidosis due to seizures or other hypermetabolic states, and ketoacidosis due to fasting will cause an increased anion gap. Low serum HCO_3^- without an anion gap suggests renal tubular acidosis (as might be seen in tyrosinemia type I, galactosemia, Wilson's disease, Lowe's syndrome, and so on) or other cause for bicarbonate loss.

Identification of a missing anion can be done indirectly or directly. Indirect tests include the ferric chloride test (for aromatic compounds), the dinitrophenylhydrazine (DNPH) reaction for alpha-keto acids, and amino acid analysis, which seeks elevation of amino acid precursors of organic acids. Direct measurements of blood lactate, pyruvate, and other organic acids can also be performed. Blood lactate level is often secondarily elevated in many of the organic acidurias.

The ferric chloride test is performed by gradually adding 10% ferric chloride to urine. A positive reaction indicates the need for further investigation. Common positive reactions may be due to the presence of salicylate (purple) and phenylpyruvic acid (green). The DNPH reagent will cause alpha-ketoacids (including acetoacetate during ketosis) to precipitate. Tentative identification of some substances can be made by testing the precipitate. The sodium nitroprusside test is for sulfur-containing compounds. Patients with homocystinuria will have a strongly positive test, but the

TABLE 9-1. Psychomotor Regression and Visceromegaly

Disorder (Reference)	Onset
With Coarse Facies	
Hurler's Syndrome[532]	Infancy
Beta-glucuronidase deficiency[62]	Infancy
Sialidosis type 2[500]	Infancy
I-cell disease[775]	Infancy
Mannosidosis[439]	Infancy
G_{M1}-gangliosidosis, infantile[36]	Infancy
Hunter's syndrome[532]	Late infancy
Hurler-Scheie compound[404]	Late infancy
Fucosidosis-Type 2[453]	Late infancy
Multiple sulfatase deficiency[26]	Late infancy
Sanfilippo's syndrome[173]	Late infancy–childhood
Without Coarse Facies	
Argininosuccinic aciduria[296]	Infancy
Sandhoff's disease[698]	Infancy
Gaucher's disease, infantile[252]	Infancy
Niemann-Pick disease-type A[252]	Infancy
Wolman's disease[1]	Infancy
Gaucher's disease, juvenile[252]	Infancy–adulthood
G_{M1} gangliosidosis, juvenile[601]	Late infancy
Niemann-Pick disease-type C[252]	Late infancy–adulthood
Juvenile dystonic lipidosis[218]	Childhood
Wilson's disease[789]	Childhood

(Text continues on p. 290)

TABLE 9-2.   Abnormalities of Posture and Movement

ATAXIA

Intermittent Ataxia

Disorder (Reference)	Onset
Isovaleric acidemia[483]	Infancy
Multiple carboxylase deficiency[694]	Infancy
Citrullinemia[730]	Infancy
Hyperornithinemia and homocitrullinuria[732]	Infancy
Pyruvate dehydrogenase defects[77]	Infancy
Subacute necrotizing encephalomyelopathy[642]	Infancy
Maple syrup urine disease[168]	Infancy–childhood
Ornithine transcarbamylase deficiency[691]	Infancy–childhood
Argininosuccinic acidemia[559]	Infancy–childhood
Hartnup disease[393]	Infancy–adolescence

Ataxia and Spasticity

Disorder (Reference)	Onset
Pyruglutamic aciduria[862]	Infancy
G_{M1} gangliosidosis, late infantile[598]	Late infancy
Niemann-Pick disease-type C[252]	Late infancy–childhood
Salla disease[24]	Late infancy–childhood
Methylmalonic acidemia and homocystinuria[311]	Childhood
Nonketotic hyperglycinemia[777]	Childhood
G_{M2} gangliosidosis, juvenile[796]	Childhood
G_{M1} gangliosidosis, juvenile[865]	Childhood
Gaucher's disease, juvenile[325]	Childhood
Globoid cell leukodystrophy, late onset[160]	Childhood
Sialidosis-type 2[500]	Childhood–adolescence
Metachromatic leukodystrophy (MLD)[569,333]	
Late infantile	Late infancy
Juvenile	Childhood
Adult	Young adulthood
Cerebrotendinous xanthomatosis[833]	Adolescence–adulthood
Gaucher's disease, adult[550]	Adulthood

Chronic Progressive Ataxia

Disorder (Reference)	Onset
Beta-ketothiolase deficiency[184]	Infancy
Sanfilippo's syndrome[174]	Childhood
Aspartylglycosaminuria[30]	Childhood
G_{M2}-gangliosidosis, juvenile[398]	Childhood
Metachromatic leukodystrophy[569,333]	Childhood–young adulthood
Cerebrotendinous xanthomatosis[772]	Adolescence–young adulthood

Spinocerebellar Syndrome*

Disorder (Reference)	Onset
Abetalipoproteinemia[54]	Childhood
Nonketotic hyperglycinemia[777]	Childhood
Glutamate dehydrogenase deficiency[646]	Childhood
G_{M2} gangliosidosis, adult[662]	Childhood–adulthood
Refsum's disease[663]	Childhood–adulthood
Hyperuricemia[681]	Adolescence to adulthood
Gamma-glutamyl cysteine synthetase[668]	Young adulthood
Sandhoff's disease, adult[610]	Young adulthood

*Ataxia, peripheral neuropathy and upper motor neuron disease

(Continued)

TABLE 9-2.   Abnormalities of Posture and Movement (*Continued*)

Myoclonus and Myoclonic Seizures

Disorder (Reference)	Onset
Dihydrobiopterin reductase deficiency[423]	Infancy
Sulfite oxidase deficiency[731]	Infancy
Multiple carboxylase deficiency[694]	Infancy
Nonketotic hyperglycinemia[60]	Infancy
Hyperornithinemia and homocitrullinuria[732]	Infancy
Carnosinemia[819]	Infancy
Globoid cell leukodystrophy[335]	Infancy
G_{M1} and G_{M2} gangliosidoses[598]	Infancy to childhood
Gaucher's disease, juvenile[325]	Infancy to childhood
Menkes' kinky hair syndrome[256]	Infancy to childhood
Niemann-Pick disease-type C[91]	Late infancy to childhood
Neuronal ceroid lipofuscinosis, late infantile[907]	Late infancy to childhood
Wilson's disease[190]	Childhood
Sialidosis-type 1[500]	Childhood to adolescence

Choreoathetosis

Disorder (Reference)	Onset
Dihydrobiopterin reductase deficiency[422]	Infancy
Propionic acidemia[49]	Infancy
3-Methylglutaconic acidemia[338]	Infancy
Pyruvate decarboxylase deficiency[79]	Infancy
Beta-ketothiolase deficiency[309]	Infancy
Glutaric aciduria[309]	Infancy–childhood
Lesch-Nyhan syndrome[593]	Infancy–childhood
Tyrosine aminotransferase deficiency[300]	Childhood
Sulfite oxidase deficiency[731]	Childhood
Hartnup disease[880]	Childhood
Sialidosis[768]	Childhood
G_{M2}-gangliosidosis, juvenile[798]	Childhood
G_{M1} gangliosidosis, juvenile[866]	Childhood
Dystonic lipidosis[218]	Childhood
Wilson's disease[190]	Childhood
Niemann-Pick disease-type C[579]	Childhood–adulthood
Fabry's disease[193]	Childhood–adulthood
Metachromatic leukodystrophy[338]	Childhood–adulthood

Rigidity, Tremor, Bradykinesa or Dystonia

Disorder (Reference)	Onset
Isovaleric acidemia[483]	Childhood
Neuronal ceroid-lipofuscinosis, juvenile[748]	Childhood
Neuronal ceroid-lipofuscinosis, adult[319]	Childhood–adulthood
Wilson's disease[190]	Childhood–adulthood
Homocystinuria[334]	Adolescence
Taurine deficiency[629]	Adulthood
Metachromatic leukodystrophy[333]	Adulthood

TABLE 9-3. Ophthalmologic Abnormalities

Corneal Clouding

Disorder (Reference)	Onset
Lowe's syndrome[501]	Infancy
Hurler's syndrome[536]	Infancy
G_{M1} gangliosidosis,[536] infantile[36]	Infancy
Fabry's disease[762]	Infancy–adulthood
Hurler-Scheie compound[404]	Childhood
Scheie's syndrome[708]	Childhood
I-cell disease[478]	Childhood
Mucolipidoses III & IV[30,39]	Childhood
Aspartylglycosaminuria[30]	Childhood

Cataracts

Disorder (Reference)	Onset
Systemic carnitine deficiency[196]	Infancy
Lowe's syndrome[501]	Infancy
Galactosemia[572]	Infancy
Mannosidosis[439]	Childhood
Wilson's disease[877]	Childhood
Cerebrotendinous xanthomatosis[833]	Adolescence–adulthood

Ophthalmoplegia

Disorder (Reference)	Onset
Maple syrup urine disease[509]	Infancy–childhood
Hartnup disease[50]	Infancy–childhood
Subacute necrotizing encephalomyelopathy[642]	Infancy–childhood
Pyruvate decarboxylase deficiency[78]	Infancy–adolescence
G_{M1} gangliosidosis, juvenile[866]	Late infancy–childhood
Niemann-Pick disease-type C[251]	Childhood
Gaucher's disease, juvenile[251]	Childhood
Juvenile dystonic lipidosis[218]	Childhood
Abetalipoproteinemia[451]	Childhood
Tangier disease[225]	Adolescence

Retinal Abnormalities

Disorder (References)	Onset
Cherry-red macula	
Tay-Sachs disease[598]	Infancy
Sandhoff's disease[598]	Infancy
Niemann-Pick disease-type A[92]	Infancy
Lipogranulomatosis[146]	Infancy
Metachromatic leukodystrophy, early onset[335]	Late infancy
G_{M2} gangliosidosis, juvenile[398]	Childhood
Sialidosis[500]	Childhood–adolescence

(Continued)

TABLE 9-3.   Ophthalmologic Abnormalities (*Continued*)

Retinal Abnormalities

Disorder (References)	Onset
Retinitis Pigmentosa	
Pipecolatemia[272]	Infancy
Hunter's syndrome[283]	Infancy
Niemann-Pick disease-type C[252]	Late infancy
Neuronal ceroid lipofuscinosis, late infantile and juvenile[906]	Late infancy–childhood
Hyperornithinemia[808]	Childhood
Hurler's syndrome[152]	Childhood
Hurler-Sheie syndrome[536]	Childhood
Mucolipidosis IV[580]	Childhood
G_{M2} gangliosidosis, juvenile[598]	Childhood
Abetalipoproteinemia[894]	Childhood–adulthood
Hypobetalipoproteinemia[894]	Childhood
Refsum's disease[663]	Childhood–adulthood
Optic Atrophy	
Subacute necrotizing encephalomyelopathy[642]	Infancy
Multiple sulfatase deficiency[26]	Infancy
Sandhoff's disease[233]	Infancy
Niemann-Pick disease-type A[252]	Infancy
Neuronal ceroid-lipofuscinosis, infantile[699]	Infancy
Menkes' kinky hair syndrome[897]	Infancy
Metachromatic leukodystrophy[335]	Late infancy
Niemann-Pick disease-type C[252]	Infancy–childhood
Globoid cell leukodystrophy[335]	Infancy–adulthood
Homocystinuria[231]	Childhood
Nonketotic hyperglycinemia[777]	Childhood
G_{M2} gangliosidosis, juvenile[601]	Childhood

most common reason for a positive test is the heterozygous state of cystinuria. A positive nitroprusside test must be followed by identification of the sulfur compound(s) in the sample. These and other helpful tests are discussed by Thomas and Howell[822] and Schmidt.[712]

Most hospital laboratories can measure lactate and NH_3 levels, but arrangements for these tests may need to be made in advance. Amino acids can be quickly analyzed using one-dimensional high-voltage thin-layer electrophoresis (HVTLE). Further information can be obtained by using ascending paper chromatography in the second dimension, or by doing two-dimensional thin-layer chromatography (TLC).[712] Accurate quantification can be achieved using ion-exchange column chromatography, high-performance liquid chromatography (HPLC), or gas-liquid chromatography (GLC).[104]

Many techniques will separate or-ganic acids. Current practice centers around liquid partition, high-performance liquid, and gas chromatography.[803] All of these analytic techniques provide useful preliminary information. Most of the large number of organic acids in body fluids are subject to great variation owing to diet, drugs, and intestinal flora. Positive identification of abnormal organic acids is essential. A mass spectrometer coupled to the outlet of a chromatograph will provide rapid results.[306] These instruments are located in relatively few university medical centers, so samples must be collected and transported for analysis.

For amino acid and organic acid disorders, a single untimed sample is usually adequate. If symptoms are episodic, the samples should be obtained during the acute episode. Urine samples should be frozen quickly, and blood should be separated and the serum or plasma frozen. Diagnostic enzyme assays are usually performed on

TABLE 9-4   General Physical Signs of Disorders

Macrocephaly

Disorder (References)

Glutaric aciduria[460]
MPS I, II, III, VI, VII
Glycoproteinoses[194]
Gangliosidoses, infantile types[598]
Globoid cell leukodystrophy[903]
Menkes' kinky hair syndrome[256]

Cutaneous Manifestations

Disorder	Sign
Phenylketonuria	Eczema
Tyrosine aminotransferase deficiency	Palmar keratosis
Argininosuccinic aciduria	Trichorrhexis nodosa
Hartnup disease	Pellagralike eruption
Hurler's syndrome	Thickened skin
Hunter's syndrome	Nodular thick skin
Sanfilippo syndrome	Thickened skin
I-cell disease	Thickened skin
Fucosidosis	Angiokeratomas
Multiple sulfatase deficiency	Ichthiotic skin
Fabry's disease	Angiokeratomas
Refsum's disease	Ichthiosis
Cerebrotendinous xanthomatosis	Xanthomas
Lipogranulomatosis	Subcutaneous and periarticular nodules
Menkes' kinky hair syndrome	Pili torti

Unusual Odor

Disorder	Odor
PKU	Musty or mousy
Tyrosinosis	Rancid butter
Maple syrup urine disease	Maple syrup or burnt sugar
Isovalanic acidemia	Sweaty-feet
Glutaric aciduria	Sweaty-feet
Methionine malabsorption	Dried celery or yeastlike
Hydromethylglutaryl-CoA lyase deficiency	Cat's urine

serum, leukocytes, fibroblasts, or tissue obtained at biopsy. Procuring and handling such samples must be discussed with the laboratory involved.

If a patient is dying of a suspected metabolic disorder, a small piece of skin can be obtained up to several hours after death using a sterile technique but avoiding iodinated antiseptics (povidone and others) that interfere with cell growth. The sample should be placed in tissue culture medium, isotonic saline, or Ringer's lactate and refrigerated (not frozen) for transport to the laboratory. Other postmortem tissue samples should also be obtained as quickly as possible. Even a needle liver biopsy may provide some information, if permission for more extensive investigation cannot be obtained. Tissue should be procured as soon as possible after death and frozen quickly in liquid nitrogen to preserve enzyme activity. Routine pathologic examination, special stains, and electron microscopy are also helpful.

APPROACH TO THE PATIENT WITH A POSSIBLE LYSOSOMAL STORAGE DISEASE

The following discussion is meant to suggest a directed approach to follow in working up a patient for a lysosomal storage disease. We will cover individual areas of importance to the clinical diagnostician such as history, physical examination, and diagnostic studies, and then summarize with an approach combining these modalities. Features peculiar to specific conditions will be covered in the discussion of these diseases.

History and Physical Examination

Children with inborn errors of metabolism are typically normal at birth and subsequently develop postnatal changes typical of their particular disease. Patients with lysosomal storage disease generally follow this pattern. Various aspects of development such as linear growth and central nervous system maturation begin normally and then plateau. In general (there are a few exceptions) one can distinguish between an inborn error of metabolism and a static encephalopathy by paying attention to this point when beginning to take the medical history. The child with an inborn error that causes mental retardation typically will start with a normal passage of developmental milestones, then slow down in rate of progression, plateau with no gain or loss of skills, and finally regress and lose previously gained milestones. Notable exceptions to this rule include some patients with multiple sulfatase deficiency, mucolipidosis II, and G_{M1} gangliosidosis who may be affected clinically in the newborn period.

Linear growth may also follow the same pattern. Some children with certain mucopolysaccharidoses and glycoproteinoses may be relatively large for their ages during the early period of normal growth, subsequently crossing percentiles downward from the 97th to the third and ending up significantly dwarfed. The somatic dysmorphism discussed below, including skeletal radiographic features, follows the same progressive pattern. One exception to this is the macrocephaly and hydrocephalus seen in many patients with storage of mucopolysaccharides and glycoproteins; these may be present shortly after birth and continue throughout life. Also, many parents notice that affected children seem to have chronic upper respiratory congestion with rhinitis right from the newborn period. This rhinitis appears to be significant compared to normal sibs and other unaffected children.

Gradual coarsening of the facial features occurs after an initial period of normal appearance in most of the mucopolysaccharidoses and glycoprotein storage diseases. Physicians may find it difficult to state specifically what they mean when they use the term "coarse facies," but one should try to pay close attention to the specific features seen in the face of a patient. After all, many or perhaps most of the patients seen in any institution for the retarded might be considered to have a coarse face, characterized by a dull, expressionless affect, an open mouth with orthodontic abnormalities resulting from hypotonic musculature, and broad alveolar ridges due to poor oral–motor coordination resulting in a palate with a very narrow central arch that is frequently referred to as a "highly arched palate." Instead, the facial dysmorphia that is associated with mucopolysaccharide and glycoprotein storage disease and that we refer to in this chapter as coarse facies is characterized by frontal bossing, puffiness around the eyes, a flat, depressed nasal bridge with anteverted nose and flared nostrils, enlarged tongue and thick, pouting lips. The alveolar ridges are also broad and hyperplastic due to infiltration of storage material and may resemble the appearance of a child who chronically takes phenytoin anticonvulsants.

The hair may feel coarse (thick and wiry) and may extend down over the forehead and be confluent with the eyebrows. Generalized hirsutism may be present with hair most prominent over the back, shoulders, and arms. The skin feels thick, puffy, and firm. Angiokeratoma corporis diffusum is common in Fabry's disease and in milder forms of fucosidosis, and is reported in sialidosis.

Hepatomegaly or hepatosplenomegaly gradually progresses and frequently is not present at birth. Even though enlargement may be great, there is usually not any associated hepatic dysfunction. Children with storage diseases who are referred for evaluation of hepatomegaly may have unnecessary liver biopsies. Instead, one should realize that lysosomal storage diseases can usually be diagnosed without resorting to such invasive techniques. Liver biopsies are usually only necessary after other diagnostic procedures have not revealed any abnormality, or if glycogen storage disease or another cause of hepatomegaly is suspected. The abdomen becomes protuberant, and inguinal and umbilical hernias may be present.

The eyes should be checked for corneal clouding, which suggests a mucopolysaccharidosis, cataracts as found, for example, in mannosidosis, and for the cherry-red spots found in some of the sphingolipidoses and sialidoses.

Storage material may involve the vasculature, myocardium, and valves resulting in aortic and mitral regurgitation, myocardiopathy, and occlusive disease. This acquired heart disease, combined with frequent respiratory infections and compromised pulmonary function, leads to a cardiorespiratory death in many patients.

As infants with mucopolysaccharidoses and glycoproteinoses start to sit up, they sometimes develop a characteristic protrusion or prominence of the lumbar spine called a *gibbus*. This seems to be caused by hypotonia, muscle weakness, and dysplasia of the vertebral bodies resulting in anterior wedging and posterior displacement, usually of L1 or L2. Other progressive skeletal manifestations include limitation of extension of the elbows and fingers and decreased growth of both the long and short tubular bones resulting in dwarfism and short, broad hands and feet. Restriction of joint motion is progressive and may be severe. Typical patients with Hurler's and Hunter's syndromes, for example, develop extreme joint stiffness resulting in a crouched stance and a clawhand deformity.

This joint stiffness is a limitation of both extension and flexion, and it usually can be differentiated from the joint contractures that other children may develop in association with severe central nervous system dysfunction.

Hearing loss occurs commonly in the mucopolysaccharide and glycoprotein storage diseases and may be sensorineural, conductive, or mixed. This is a feature that requires aggressive attention in those conditions with the potential for normal or near normal intelligence, such as the milder forms of Hunter's syndrome, to prevent unnecessary retardation of development.

Grouping the lipidoses and related disorders according to whether early symptoms and signs are predominantly "gray matter" or "white matter" is a traditional approach to the clinical diagnosis of these disorders. The gray matter symptoms include dementia, seizures, and retinal changes such as the cherry-red macula. White matter symptoms are spasticity, ataxia, and peripheral neuropathy. This division of the lipidoses is most applicable to the diagnosis of those forms occurring in infancy. The implication in this approach is that the pathology of the disease occurs predominantly in either gray matter or white matter, which is usually an oversimplification of the actual pathology. The gray matter degenerations include the gangliosidoses, Neimann-Pick disease, Gaucher's disease, and neuronal ceroid lipofuscinosis. The white matter degenerations are globoid cell leukodystrophy, metachromatic leukodystrophy, and adrenoleukodystrophy.

A thorough family history must always be part of the workup. A three- or four-generation pedigree should be taken and medical records, radiographs, and autopsy summaries obtained on any relatives with similar problems. One should also probe carefully for consanguinity.

The clinical phenotype must be carefully documented. If the patient dies before studies are completed, a complete postmortem examination should be obtained including light and electron microscopic studies with special attention to brain, spleen, and liver; skeletal radiographs; photographs; sterile biopsies of skin or tendon for fibroblast culture; and fresh pieces of tissues, such as liver, brain, and spleen, that are taken as soon as possible after death, cut in thin slices, and frozen quickly in order to be available for future enzyme assay or extraction of storage material.

Diagnostic Studies

The typical radiographic features of lysosomal storage diseases are referred to as *dysostosis multiplex*. These changes include thickening of the calvaria and anterior extension of the sella sometimes referred to as a "shoe-shaped" or "boot-shaped" sella. The clavicles are widened. The ribs are irregular and broadened to the extent that the width exceeds that of the intercostal space. They also are narrower in the area next to the spine, giving rise to a spatulate or "oar-shaped" appearance. The vertebral bodies are more ovoid than usual and in MPS IV have generalized flattening called *platyspondyly*. Vertebral abnormalities are best appreciated in lateral projection. There are ossification defects of the anterior portions of the upper lumbar vertebral bodies, commonly an anterosuperior defect. This appearance is referred to as "hooking" or "beaking" (see Fig. 9-10). The pelvis has characteristic changes including shallow acetabulae and very narrow basal portions of the ilia. In the extreme, the normal shape of the ilium has disappeared; the body flares out in the upper portion and narrows down to a point at the base. One of the most characteristic features of dysostosis multiplex is a valgus deformity of the femoral necks. This finding is an important diagnostic sign that helps to differentiate between a lysosomal storage disease and one of the many osteochondrodysplasias (bone dysplasias such as spondyloepiphyseal dysplasia congenita) that have coxa vara as a prominent feature. In dysostosis multiplex both the long bones and the short tubular bones are broad and thick and there is coarsening of the trabecular pattern. These changes are usually much more prominent in the upper extremities than in the lower extremities. The diaphyses of the long bones are widened and there is poor modeling at the metaphyses. There is sometimes a varus deformity at the proximal humerus. The metacarpals and phalanges are broad in their midportions and taper at the ends, resulting in "bullet-shaped phalanges" and proximal pointing of the metacarpals. A notch in the lateral portion of the proximal fifth metacarpal may be a significant early diagnostic finding. Finally, the distal radius and ulna may be irregular and slanted toward each other (For further discussion the reader is referred to the discussion by Grossman and Dorst.[322])

Laboratory studies include biochemical assessment of urine or tissues for the characteristic storage material that can give a clue about what enzyme may be deficient; histologic studies of cells from peripheral blood, bone marrow, or other body tissues to look for the characteristic storage cells with vacuoles where material is stored; and biochemical studies of enzyme activity or substrate turnover in peripheral leukocytes or cultured fibroblasts.

The urine can be screened for the presence of abnormally large amounts of glycosaminoglycans (GAG; formerly called *mucopolysaccharides*) and other oligosaccharides derived from glycoproteins. The toluidine blue spot test and its modification by McKusick are qualitative tests to detect the presence of GAG by reaction with the metachromatic dye, toluidine blue.[66,532] Urine is dropped onto filter paper that is then dipped in the dye. A positive result is a purple spot. Other similar tests have been devised with azure A, which is used in commercially available test strips.

Turbidity tests seem to be more sensitive and specific and can be designed as semiquantitative assays. In these tests, the reagent is added to an acidified urine specimen and the mixture is observed for the development of turbidity. Reagents used include acidified albumin, cetyltrimethylammonium bromide (CTAB), and cetylpyridinium chloride (CPC). These assays may be made semiquantitative by measuring the optical density of the solution and comparing it to that developed by a standard solution (e.g., chondroitin sulfate). A good method using CPC was described by Pennock.[621] The measurement of urinary GAG is normalized for creatinine so that the test can be done on single spot urines rather than requiring the sometimes cumbersome collection of a 24-hour urine specimen. The normal GAG excretion is relatively higher at birth and in early infancy than in later childhood and adult life.[623]

There are other urine tests that have been used, but for practical purposes, the main one to be aware of is thin layer chromatography (TLC) for urinary oligosaccharides. This analysis is usually done in research laboratories when initial attempts at a specific diagnosis have been unsuccessful and one needs to get a better idea of what compounds are not being metabolized correctly. Thin layer chromatography is an essential part of the study of a newly discovered storage disease because biochemical characterization of the excretion products can sometimes point fairly clearly to the kind of enzyme activity that is deficient. Thin layer chromatography may also be an important part of the workup of a patient who may have aspartylglycosaminuria because the excretion product produces a clearly detectable spot after special development. All urine studies should be done on very fresh specimens or those that have been frozen immediately after collection.

Microscopic study of cells from blood, bone marrow, and other tissues may be valuable in detecting the presence of the key feature of all of these diseases, that is, abnormal storage of material within lysosomes. In the sphingolipidoses, large lipid-containing cells found throughout the body are called *foam cells* because of the bubbly appearance of the cytoplasm. The electron microscopic picture may be relatively specific for various disorders or at least should give a clue to the general type of diagnostic category. In the mucopolysaccharidoses and glycoproteinoses, histologic evidence for storage is usually more subtle than in the sphingolipidoses but, nonetheless, is present and detectable in most. A simple screening test is to look for abnormal vacuolization in peripheral lymphocytes and bone marrow cells. A stain such as toluidine blue may allow one to see metachromatic inclusions.[568]

A histologic picture of lysosomal storage may be present in numerous tissues throughout the body but is most consistently found in cells of the reticuloendothelial system. As mentioned above, one usually does not need to resort to a liver biopsy to diagnose one of these conditions, but if one has been done, all cell types should be examined carefully for signs of lysosomal storage. It has been suggested that ultra-structural examination of a skin biopsy specimen may be a convenient noninvasive technique and this has been used extensively enough now so that pitfalls, sources of error, and guidelines for interpretation have been elucidated.[599,747] Conjunctival biopsy has also proved to be a convenient way to obtain tissue that has histologic features of storage.[654]

Finally, perhaps the most important diagnostic step is as complete a delineation of the biochemical defect as possible. This is usually a deficiency in the activity of a lysosomal acid hydrolase due to a single gene mutation. It is not sufficient to make only a clinical diagnosis, even though supported by urinary and histologic studies, without documenting the specific enzyme deficiency in cultured skin fibroblasts, peripheral leukocytes, or other biopsy or postmortem tissue such as liver. In the past, many patients have been labeled with uncertain diagnoses based on physical, radiographic, and urinary findings but such an evaluation should no longer be considered complete, now that specific enzyme deficiencies can be accurately detected.

Abnormal ^{35}S incorporation into sulfated GAG in cultured fibroblasts may be helpful in discriminating between a mucopolysaccharidosis and other lysosomal storage disorders that have normal ^{35}S accumulation. This test is also used in cross-correction studies to determine whether cells from two patients have the same or allelic mutations (no correction of abnormal sulfate kinetics) or mutations at different loci.[879]

It is important to note that enzyme assays in the laboratory can be misleading. Synthetic substrates with properties different from naturally occurring substrates are used in relatively high concentrations. Preparation of lysed cells for enzyme assay may lead to loss of an enzyme's regulators, and other substances with which the enzyme may interact. In addition, many lysosomal disorders are characterized by secondary depression or augmentation of various enzyme activities. Misleading results may be obtained by the unwary, and some older case reports have been revised as newer diagnostic techniques have more correctly identified the primary defect.

For true enzyme deficiencies, confirming evidence may be found in the form of half-normal enzyme activity in obligate carriers. However, some obligate heterozygotes may be chemically indistinguishable from normal. Ideally, enzyme studies should be done on cultured fibroblasts so that several aliquots of growing cells can be saved by being frozen in liquid nitrogen in case other biochemical tests become available in the future. This is very important, not only for advancing knowledge about this group of crippling diseases, but also for purposes of counseling the families of affected patients.

Summary of Approach to the Patient

How does the busy physician efficiently evaluate children for lysosomal storage diseases? Clearly, one can not do skin biopsies on every child who presents with mental retardation, short stature, and slightly coarse facial features. These enzyme assays are usually done in research laboratories so one must have reasonably good evidence that such a disorder exists before asking the enzyme laboratory to become involved. Also, various laboratories may have different interests and areas of expertise so that before deciding to do a skin biopsy for enzyme studies, one should have in mind whether the condition is a mucopolysaccharidosis, a glycoproteinosis, or a sphingolipidosis.

As mentioned above, many mentally retarded children may have nonspecific features such as joint contractures, a somewhat coarse face, short stature, broad alveolar ridges, and hirsutism, especially if treated with hydantoins for seizures. If the patient who presents with neurologic symptoms has any one of the following major diagnostic criteria, then the likelihood of a lysosomal storage disease is great enough that one may proceed directly to enzyme studies: macular cherry-red spot; radiographic features of dysostosis multiplex; abnormal mucopolysacchariduria; or histologic evidence of lysosomal storage, for example, foam cells in the bone marrow or liver.

If the patient has any two of the following second level diagnostic criteria a lysosomal storage disease should be strongly suspected: corneal clouding; hepatomegaly or hepatosplenomegaly; stiff joints or thick-feeling skin; valvular heart disease, especially aortic or mitral regurgitation; the growth pattern of normal or above average early growth with subsequent crossing of percentiles downward resulting in dwarfism; and the characteristic type of facial coarsening consisting of frontal bossing, depressed nasal bridge, periorbital fullness, and thick, pouting lips. If two or more of these features are seen one should try to establish the presence of one or more of the major criteria above. Therefore, if the patient is dysmorphic, a urine specimen should be obtained for TLC or a semiquantitative GAG test and complete skeletal radiographs should be obtained to look for dysostosis multiplex. If the patient is not dysmorphic but developmentally retarded with hepatomegaly or hepatosplenomegaly, then a very careful ophthalmologic examination should be obtained. Cherry-red spots are found in some of the sphingolipidoses and sialidoses, whereas dysostosis multiplex is a feature of the mucopolysaccharidoses, glycoproteinoses, multiple enzyme deficiencies, and G_{M1} gangliosidosis.

The third level diagnostic criteria include the features we have listed above as "nonspecific" (coarse face, joint contractures, short stature, broad alveolar ridges, and hirsutism) plus the following: hernias, macrocephaly, coarse hair, and hearing loss. When three or four of these findings are present in a child referred with neurologic abnormalities, a storage disease should be considered. A careful examination should be done to look for gross corneal clouding, cherry-red spot, heart murmur, abdominal organomegaly, joint stiffness, and thick skin, and a urine screening test should be obtained. If the patient is found to have any other suggestive features, skeletal radiographs should be done.

In the list of second level diagnostic criteria the most important are corneal clouding and organomegaly. The skin and joint findings are also fairly specific. In the group of third level criteria, macrocephaly, hearing loss, and hernias (especially if both umbilical and inguinal are present) are of the greatest significance.

Because these enzymes are present in cultured skin fibroblasts and cells from the amniotic fluid, carrier detection and prenatal diagnosis should be at least theoretically feasible for most of the storage diseases owing to a deficiency of lysosomal hydrolase activity. In practice, the difficulty of doing such studies varies among the different conditions but has been accomplished for many of them.

After the diagnostic studies are completed, the immediate family must receive thorough counseling about the natural history and etiology of the disorder, and questions should be addressed about recurrence risks and options for those of childbearing age. Then a letter should be sent to the family summarizing the counseling session and including information about the specific enzyme deficiency, where the biochemical studies were done, and whom they should contact if anyone has further questions or needs information about prenatal diagnosis.

DEFECTS IN AMINO ACID METABOLISM AND TRANSPORT

PHENYLKETONURIA

Phenylketonuria (PKU) is a model metabolic disorder that illustrates the stages of understanding such diseases. The first stage occurred when Følling called attention to a group of mentally retarded children who excreted large amounts of phenylpyruvic acid.[244] Since then a succession of advances have led to the description of the basic biochemical defect in PKU, development of a dietary treatment for PKU, introduction of an effective and practical screening test, and delineation of PKU variants and normal variation.[73,331,395] PKU appears to be among the most common metabolic diseases. Incidence estimates vary from 1:4500 in Ireland to 1:19,000 in Israel[721]

Phenylalanine Metabolism

Phenylalanine is an essential amino acid in man. High quality protein contains 5% to 7% phenylalanine. Phenylalanine can be hydroxylated to tyrosine, which can be incorporated into protein, or further metabolized to dopamine, catecholamines, thyroid hormones, and melanin, or degraded (Fig. 9-1). Phenylalanine hydroxylase catalyses the conversion of phenylalanine to tyrosine.

This enzyme requires elemental oxygen and a cofactor, tetrahydrobiopterin (BH_4), which is regenerated through dihydrobiopterin reductase. The BH_4 is originally formed from dihydropteridine through the action of dihydrofolate reductase. These pterin cofactors are not derived from dietary folate. Dihydrobiopterin is formed at a step requiring dihydrobiopterin synthetase (Fig. 9-1). Tetrahydrobiopterin is also required by tyrosine and tryptophan hydroxylases, which form 3,4-dihydroxyphenylalanine (dopa) and 5-hydroxytryptophan, respectively. The latter is the immediate precursor of serotonin. Therefore, a deficiency of BH_4 interferes with the formation of two neurotransmitters.

Initially, during rapid growth as much as 50% of dietary phenylalanine is incorporated into protein. Later this fraction becomes 10% or less.[721] Consequently, defective phenylalanine hydroxylase activity would be expected to raise the serum phenylalanine level significantly. Phenylalanine by-products normally found in very small amounts would also be increased.

Isozymes of phenylalanine hydroxylase have been identified in rats by immunologic techniques and by isoelectric focussing. If isozymes exist in man, they are probably due to post-translational modifications.[823]

Classical PKU, an autosomal recessive disorder, is associated with virtually complete enzymatic and immunologic absence of phenylalanine hydroxylase. This implies a defective structural gene or the absence of an activator. In the presence of normal dietary phenylalanine intake, the blood phenylalanine level will be substantially elevated, and the metabolites phenylpyruvic, phenylactic, phenylacetic, and o-hydroxyphenylacetic acids, and phenylacetylglutamine will be present.[104] Infants with classical PKU never develop enzyme activity, and the blood phenylalanine level will be elevated whenever the diet contains more phenylalanine than is needed for growth.

Transient mild neonatal hyperphenylalaninemia is associated with low phenylalanine hydroxylase activity and absent immunologically cross-reacting material.[255] These findings suggest that this disorder is due to a structural alternation in phenylalanine hydroxylase. The inheritance of this

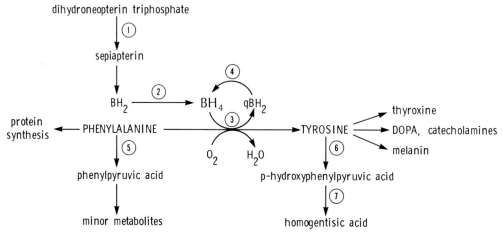

FIG. 9-1. Phenylalanine and tyrosine metabolism. Tyrosine also participates in protein synthesis. Tetrahydrobiopterin (BH_4) is a cofactor for dihydroxyphenylalanine (DOPA) synthesis. Enzymes indicated are: (1) dihydrobiopterin synthetase; (2) dihydrofolate reductase; (3) phenylalanine hydroxylase; (4) dihydropteridine reductase; (5) phenylalanine transaminase; (6) tyrosine-α-ketoglutarate transaminase; and (7) p-hydroxyphenylpyruvic acid oxidase. Other abbreviations used are BH_2 for dihydrobiopterin and qBH_2 for quinonoid-dihydrobiopterin.

disorder is probably also autosomal recessive because probands have had affected sibs.

The mechanism of brain damage in PKU is uncertain, but there are at least three possibilities: direct phenylalanine toxicity, toxicity due to phenylalanine metabolites, and a relative deficiency of tyrosine. Intestinal transport of L-tryptophan and tyrosine is diminished in untreated PKU. Phenylalanine may be incorporated into brain protein in place of tyrosine, and in untreated PKU, tryptophan and tyrosine metabolism is disrupted. The level of serotonin (5-hydroxytryptamine) in serum and its metabolite in urine, 5-hydroxyindolylacetic acid, are decreased, whereas derivatives of their precursors including indolyl-3-pyruvic acid, indolyl-3-lactic acid, indolyl-3-acetic acid, and indican are present in excess. These abnormalities may reflect interference with serotonin synthesis at several sites.[540] Altered activity of tyrosine hydroxylase may account for decreased melanin production in untreated PKU.[553]

Hyperphenylalaninemic Conditions

Table 9-5 shows the large number of conditions associated with hyperphenylalaninemia. Three of the conditions listed in the table, namely, persistent phenylketonuria, transient phenylketonuria, and transaminase deficiency, are generally considered to be benign. There are insufficient data to confirm the impression that mild hyperphenylalaninemia is benign and some indirect evidence indicates that elevated phenylalanine levels even those less than 20 mg/dl, may be harmful.[71] At most centers treating infants with hyperphenylalaninemia these children have been managed during the first few months of life in the same manner as infants with classical PKU. It is likely that these patients, especially those with persistent phenylketonuria, are heterogenous. Liver biopsy data in patients with moderate hyperphenylalaninemia (less than 20 mg/dl) revealed at least two groups of patients with low but detectable phenylalanine hydroxylase activity.[51] Those with enzyme activities of 6 μmol or less of tyrosine formed per gram protein-hour were more likely to be retarded than those with higher activities. The number of patients in each group was relatively small, however, and further study of this point is needed.

Patients with defects in tyrosine metabolism are also included in Table 9-5 because they also commonly have hyperphenylalaninemia. The distinction between these patients and patients with defects in

TABLE 9-5 Conditions Associated with Hyperphenylalaninemia

Disorder (Reference)	Defect	Blood Phenylalanine*	Blood Tyrosine	Clinical Features
Phenylketonuria[395]	Complete phenylalanine hydroxylase deficiency	>20 mg/dl	Low to normal	Psychomotor delay apparent by 4 mo–9 mo of age. Seizures, dry skin, and hypopigmentation.
Persistent phenylketonuria[407]	Partial phenylalanine hydroxylase deficiency	As above then 4 mg/dl–20 mg/dl	Low to normal	Normal
Transient phenylketonuria[444]	Transient phenylalanine hydroxylase deficiency	As above early, then normal	Low to normal	Normal
Dihydropteridine reductase deficiency[423]	Dihydropteridine reductase deficiency	>20 mg/dl	Normal	Marked psychomotor delay, seizures, feeding difficulties, and no clinical response to low phenylalanine diet.
Tetrahydrobiopterin deficiency[422]	7,8-dihydrobiopterin synthetase deficiency (presumed)	>20 mg/dl	Normal	Psychomotor delay, and hypotonia followed later by spasticity, dystonia, and hyperthermia despite low phenylalanine diet.
Transaminase defect[23]	Transaminase deficiency	Normal to >20 mg/dl	Normal	Normal
Transient neonatal tyrosinemia[488,525]	p-hydroxyphenylpyruvate hydroxylase inhibition	<12 mg/dl	Elevated	Commonly preterm infants. No definite adverse affect.
Tyrosinemia-type I[346]	p-hydroxyphenylpyruvate hydroxylase deficiency	<10 mg/dl	Elevated	Hepatic disease and renal tubule dysfunction.
Tyrosinemia-type II[431]	Cytosolic tyrosine aminotransferase deficiency	<10 mg/dl	Elevated	Mental retardation and skin and eye lesions.

*Normal blood phenylalanine level <4 mg/dl. Phenylalanine levels are those that occur with regular diet.

phenylalanine metabolism is discussed in the tyrosine metabolic defects section.

Classical Phenylketonuria

The natural evolution of classical PKU ideally should not be encountered by physicians in countries with PKU screening programs. However, screening programs may occasionally fail to detect every infant with PKU. It is important, therefore, that physicians seeing children be familiar with the clinical features of classical PKU.

On the average, affected children have lower birth weights than control infants or unaffected siblings.[702] This may in part be a consequence of the heterozygous state of the mothers of homozygous PKU infants. Phenylalanine levels of heterozygous women during pregnancy rise to approximately one and one-half times their previous level, but abnormalities at birth have not been observed in children born to mothers heterozygous for PKU.[408] Infants with PKU do seem to experience more perinatal difficulties than normal infants, are often irritable, and may vomit intermittently during infancy.[616,652] Other than these rather subtle clues little seems abnormal about the PKU infant until intellectual delay becomes apparent between 4 and 9 months.[616] The intellectual delay is progressive, so that the majority of untreated patients become severely retarded. The rate of deterioration is greatest in infants and is approximately linear for the first 10 months.[443] The untreated child with PKU continues to deteriorate more slowly until at least 3 years of age. Whether deterioration continues beyond early childhood is uncertain but is a question of importance because this could influence the duration of dietary treatment (see below). Only approximately 4% of untreated PKU patients escape with intelligence quotient (IQ) values greater than 60.[484]

The appearance of PKU patients is not distinctive. They appear to have less skin, hair, and eye pigment than their parents and 25% of patients have dry and eczematous skin. The perspiration and urine of PKU patients may have a musty or mousy odor because these excretions often contain excessive phenylacetic acid. This odor is not present in hyperphenylalaninemic patients with transaminase deficiency.

Seizures, usually generalized, are one of the frequent neurologic symptoms, occurring in approximately 25% of PKU patients.[614] In infancy, PKU patients may have infantile spasms and manifest the typical hypsarrhythmic electroencephalogram (EEG) pattern.[860] In as many as 80% of PKU patients the EEG is abnormal.[860] Diffuse or multifocal spikes or polyspikes are the most common abnormalities. Phenylketonuria patients also commonly have a photoconvulsive response to flashing light.[860] Other neurologic abnormalities include microcephaly, hypotonia, tremor, and pathologic reflexes.[614] Obviously, these are not distinctive features and do not convey the impression of a localized abnormality. Older PKU children behave in a manner not unlike autistic children. They are quite hyperkinetic and difficult to manage. Speech delay generally exceeds motor delay.

Compared to the general population untreated PKU patients have a shorter lifespan, an average of 30 years. Treatment does seem to reverse most of the abnormalities of classic PKU including the seizures, skin and hair changes, and behavioral abnormalities.[109] Retardation, however, does not improve. Treatment early in infancy is the only means of avoiding intellectual regression.

Atypical Phenylketonuria

Early in the treatment of PKU a group of patients was recognized who regressed mentally despite treatment; indeed, these children often developed treatment complications such as hypoglycemia or protein deficiency. As the details of phenylalanine metabolism were delineated, it was proposed that defects in other components of the phenylalanine hydroxylase system would be found.[419,421] Two such defects, dihydropteridine reductase deficiency and BH_4 deficiency, have now been discovered in atypical PKU patients.

Patients with dihydropteridine reductase deficiency account for perhaps 3% of PKU patients. Some of these patients have had hyperbilirubinemia in the newborn period; however, most of them are asymptomatic and without identifying features at this time.[423] The most distinguishing feature is the obvious progression of neurologic symptoms despite well-controlled serum phenylalanine levels. Psychomotor delay may become apparent at 3 months of age, but usually is detected at around 6 months of age.[106,172] Other common features include feeding difficulties, apparently on the basis of abnormal deglutition; increased muscle tone, at times taking the form of marked dystonia; and seizures.[106,172] Seizures in patients with dihydropteridine reductase deficiency are a particularly helpful symptom because they may help to distinguish these patients from those with BH_4 deficiency.[422] The EEG becomes progressively more abnormal as the disease progresses. By 2 years of age most of these patients are in a vegetative state. Death prior to 6 years of age usually follows.

Only a few patients with BH_4 deficiency have been reported.[163,422,666,704] The clinical features, therefore, are rather uncertain. In most respects the patients with BH_4 deficiency are clinically similar to those with dihydropteridine reductase deficiency. As noted above, these patients have not had seizures although one patient had continuous myoclonus with "diffuse dysrhythmia" on EEG. Hyperthermia has been a feature in at least two of the reported cases.[422] Hypotonia is the earliest neurologic abnormality; later, dystonia and increased and pathologic reflexes become apparent. The reason for BH_4 deficiency is not clear at present but it may be due to impaired BH_4 synthesis.

Diagnosis

Although diagnosis of PKU is considerably easier and more reliable once the child is clinically affected, diagnosis must be made within the first few weeks of life for maximal intellectual preservation. This can only be done by mass neonatal screening. Diagnosis in the symptomatic infant can be strongly suggested by the appearance of a forest green color when 10% ferric chloride is added to 1 ml of freshly voided urine. This test has been used in mass screening of infants; however, a considerable number of affected infants will be missed using this screening method. False negatives occur because the substance detected, phenylpyruvic acid, is unstable or may be absent from the urine of many infants owing to tran-

sient phenylalanine aminotransferase deficiency. Older, institutionalized patients with PKU may voluntarily restrict their protein intake, so that the urine ferric chloride reaction is negative. Under these circumstances, PKU may remain undiagnosed unless the blood phenylalanine level is measured.

Currently, the screening of newborns for PKU is done by way of blood phenylalanine measurements. This is required by law in most states within 3 days of birth because infants are generally discharged from the hospital after this time. Although phenylalanine levels may be elevated at birth, protein feeding leads to even higher blood levels. Screening, therefore, should be done after at least 24 hours of protein feedings. Questions have been raised about the adequacy of this timing because some feel that false negatives are too frequent. Follow-up testing at 2 weeks to 6 weeks after birth, in states with good early screening programs, however, does not appear to be very productive.[724]

Several screening tests can be used to test blood specimens collected on filter paper. The most common screening test for PKU is the Guthrie test, a test measuring the extent to which the blood in the filter paper allows bacteria to overcome growth inhibition by beta-2-thienylalanine, a competitive inhibitor of phenylalanine.[331] Fluorimetric methods and partition chromatographic methods have also been used. These screening tests currently come closest to fulfilling the criteria for a good screening test: they allow access to a whole target population (newborn infants); they have a near unity true positive rate; they have an acceptable false positive rate (1:15, false positives:true positives) they allow adequate followup of positive tests; and they have a favorable cost-benefit ratio.[368,521]

When a screening test reveals an elevated phenylalanine blood level (above about 4 mg/dl), the test should be repeated. If repeat testing reveals an increased phenylalanine level the child should be referred to a facility experienced in dealing with children with PKU. If the ferric chloride test is negative, quantitative serum amino acid determinations are run before and after 3 days of a dietary challenge, usually 200 mg of phenylalanine/kg each day. If phenylalanine levels exceed 20 mg/100 ml and the urine contains phenylpyruvic acid as evidenced by positive ferric chloride and dinitrophenylhydrazine (DNPH) tests, then the diagnosis of classical or atypical PKU is likely. Patients with transaminase deficiency will show elevations of phenylalanine above 20 mg/100 ml but will have negative urine ferric chloride and DNPH tests because they are unable to form phenylpyruvic acid. (Infants with PKU may have a temporary transaminase deficiency.) Infants with benign forms of hyperphenylalaninemia usually have phenylalanine levels below 20 mg/dl. Elevated blood tyrosine levels will identify infants with hereditary or transient defects in tyrosine metabolism (see Table 9-5).

The procedure for identification of infants with atypical PKU is as yet unsettled. Administration of BH_4 (2.0 mg/kg orally) to all patients with moderate to marked elevations of phenylalanine has been advocated.[176] Infants with a deficiency of BH_4, either on the basis of a defect in synthesis or secondary to a dihydropteridine reductase deficiency, should respond with a drop in serum phenylalanine. Unfortunately, BH_4 is not commercially available. Other means for diagnosis of PKU variants have been recently reviewed. Currently the American Academy of Pediatrics Task Force on Biopterin has recommended against routine screening for biopterin metabolic defects. Rather, they suggest that only infants with hyperphenylalaninemia who show neurologic deterioration despite an adequate dietary regimen be studied for biopterin metabolic defects.[595] To distinguish infants with biopterin metabolic defects, this committee recommends measuring 5-hydroxyindoleacetic acid, homovanillic acid, and vanillylmandelic acid in the urine. These metabolites are low in the urine of infants with biopterin metabolic defects and phenylalanine is not likely to be elevated in any other condition associated with low levels of these metabolites.[420,595] The most promising technique, high pressure liquid chromatography, can not only distinguish biopterin metabolic defects from classical PKU but also can determine whether the defect is due to dihydrobiopterin reductase deficiency or to BH_4 deficiency.[420,595] In dihydrobiopterin reductase deficiency, no BH_4

is in the urine, whereas in BH_4 deficiency, the ratio of urinary neopterin to biopterin is high.[420,552] Unfortunately, there are only a few research laboratories able to do this procedure. Ultimately, confirmation of the diagnosis requires measuring enzyme levels or biopterin in leukocytes or liver samples obtained by biopsy.

Efforts to detect heterozygotes for classical PKU have been moderately successful and are summarized elsewhere.[824] Prenatal diagnosis of classical PKU is not presently possible. The diagnosis of dihydropteridine reductase deficiency should be possible because dihydropteridine reductase can be measured in amniotic fluid cells.[551]

Maternal Phenylketonuria

The high blood phenylalanine levels in mothers with PKU not on a restricted diet apparently have a deleterious effect on the developing fetus. Growth and mental retardation, microcephaly, and heart defects are common among infants born to mothers with PKU.[117,507] Women with PKU should be on dietary restriction of phenylalanine from before they become pregnant. Studies are currently in progress to find ways to minimize the risk of fetal damage.[476]

Treatment

The treatment of PKU is based on providing adequate protein for growth while restricting phenylalanine intake. This is done by limiting the intake of regular formula and other dietary protein and using a special low-phenylalanine formula as the major protein source.

As the child gets older the diet is essentially vegetarian, with most protein still being given in a low-phenylalanine form. Tables of phenylalanine content of various foods allow the diet to be individualized to the child's tastes. The blood phenylalanine level should be kept between 3 and 10 mg/dl. The level should be checked twice a week at first, eventually tapering to once every 2 weeks.[445] Dietary restriction of phenylalanine in infancy and childhood has dramatically improved the outlook for intelligence in PKU patients. Some reports have suggested that the diet could be discontinued safely at school age.[370,446] Recent reports have suggested that there may be a loss of IQ points even after the age of 5 or 6 years if the diet is discontinued.[121,753] Further studies to test these observations are in progress. Dietary restriction of phenylalanine may be helpful in ameliorating hyperkinesis or seizures in those patients who were not treated in infancy.[729]

The need for treating benign hyperphenylalaninemia is not so clear. Most centers follow these children using dietary restrictions, if necessary, to keep the blood phenylalanine level less than 10 mg/dl. Treatment of BH_4-deficient states including dihydropterinine reductase deficiency is uncertain at present, but deterioration has lessened and biochemical markers have become more normal when L-dopa, 5-hydroxytryptophan, and a peripheral dopa decarboxylase inhibitor were used, along with BH_4. Since BH_4 cannot enter the brain, it is necessary to provide related substances that can.[177,422,583,665]

TYROSINEMIA AND TYROSINOSIS

Tyrosine is a nonessential amino acid that can be synthesized from phenylalanine except by patients with PKU. Catabolism occurs similarly to phenylalanine, with transamination to p-hydroxyphenylpyruvate and thence to homogentisate, and ultimately to acetoacetate and fumarate (Fig. 9-1). Excessive excretion of tyrosine derivatives called tyrosyluria is detectable by the ferric chloride reaction, and implies impaired tyrosine catabolism. In this situation conjugates of tyrosine derivatives may also be found, as well as secondary elevation of the blood phenylalanine level. One enzyme involved in tyrosine catabolism, p-hydroxyphenylpyruvic acid oxidase, catalyses the formation of homogentisate, and requires ascorbic acid (vitamin C) or another reducing substance as a cofactor.[313]

The most common cause of hypertyrosinemia is transient neonatal hypertyrosinemia. The blood tyrosine level is elevated, twofold to 20-fold, and the phenylalanine level is normal or only slightly elevated. The ferric chloride reaction may be positive. Prematurity, high protein intake, and vitamin C deficiency may all play a role. Most infants with this dis-

order are premature, and many of them have been receiving a high protein formula derived from whole or evaporated cow's milk. Restriction of protein to 3 gm/kg per day, and vitamin C supplementation (at least 60 mg/day) will rapidly return the blood tyrosine level to normal in most cases. Ascorbic acid, in addition to serving as a reducing agent for the enzyme, may also protect the enzyme against degradation.[42] Transient neonatal tyrosinemia may not be a completely benign condition because lethargy and delayed development have been reported in some of these infants.[32,542,617] Transient neonatal tyrosinemia has been reported to affect as many as 30% of premature and 10% of term infants.[488,525] The medical significance of this condition is not clear, and if damage occurs it may well be due to factors other than the high tyrosine level, factors such as prematurity or unsuspected mild hyperammonemia due to high protein intake, for example.

Other disorders of tyrosine metabolism are much less common. Tyrosinemia type I is an autosomal recessive disorder with progressive liver damage leading to cirrhosis, and renal damage leading to Fanconi's syndrome. Other findings include mental retardation, cataracts, and hyperpigmentation. Mental retardation occurs occasionally. A deficiency of p-hydroxyphenylpyruvate hydroxylase activity has been found, but this deficiency may be only a secondary phenomenon.[278,809] However, a dramatic improvement is seen following institution of a diet providing only minimal amounts of the aromatic amino acids.[350] Neonatal hepatitis in premature infants may simulate this disorder.[901] This disorder is occasionally referred to as tyrosinosis in the literature.

Tyrosinemia type II is characterized by high blood tyrosine levels, mental retardation, microcephaly, corneal ulcers, photophobia, and erythematous papular and pustular lesions on the palms and soles. A dramatic response to a low tyrosine diet occurs. A deficiency of the cytosolic tyrosine aminotransferase has been demonstrated.[300,431]

Tyrosinosis traditionally has referred to a condition reported by Grace Medes in a patient with myasthenia gravis.[538] The association of myasthenia with increased p-hydroxyphenylpyruvic acid was apparently a chance association. There were no other neurologic symptoms. The defect responsible for tyrosinosis is unknown, but a lack of p-hydroxyphenylpyruvic acid oxidase activity was proposed.[538] A defect in tyrosine transaminase is more likely. No other patients have been reported.

It should also be noted that hypertyrosinemia, often in association with hypermethioninemia, is a common but nonspecific feature of primary liver disease.

HISTIDINEMIA

Histidinemia is among the most common aminoacidurias. Histidinemia results from a deficiency in histidase, the enzyme necessary for histidine deamination and formation of urocanic acid.[464] Histidase is absent or low in skin and liver, although in one variant, skin histidase levels were normal.[464,897] Among reported cases speech abnormalities and mental retardation have been quite common.[463] Infants with histidinemia who have been identified by newborn screening, however, have often developed normally.[487] It is uncertain, therefore, whether mental retardation and speech abnormalities are, in fact, more common in histidinemia because the method of case selection may have biased the results.

The ill effect of histidinemia may be time-dependent. Histidinemic mice are normal, but the offspring of histidase-deficient mothers show a defect in balance due to vestibular damage.[118] Similarly, in one family five children of a histidinemic mother were found to have a mean IQ approximately 20 points less than the midparent value.[505]

Reduction of the elevated plasma histidine is possible by dietary therapy, but the importance of treatment remains in question.[271]

DEFECTS IN SULFUR AMINO ACID METABOLISM

The sulfur-containing amino acids and related compounds figure prominently in the nervous system. Some of the major reactions involving sulfur amino acids are shown in Fig. 9-2. Methionine is a direct precursor of S-adenosyl methionine (SAM), a methyl donor in over a hundred reactions including the formation of choline and epinephrine, the inactivation of serotonin and the catecholamines, and the modification of nucleotides and proteins. Loss of a methyl group from methionine results in homocysteine, which can be conjugated with serine to form cystathionine, a compound of unknown function abundant in the brain. Cystathionine can be cleaved to form alpha-ketobutyrate and cysteine, which can then be incorporated into protein or glutathione, or further metabolized to taurine. Methionine can be regenerated from homocysteine by way of a methyl donation from methyl tetrahydrofolate and a cofactor derived from vitamin B_{12}, methylcobalamin (Fig. 9-3). Methyl tetrahydrofolate (MethylTHF) is readily synthesized from methylene-THF, which can be derived from glycine cleavage.

Defects in sulfur amino acid metabolism include homocystinuria, cystathioninuria, hypermethioninemia, sulfite oxidase deficiency, and beta-mercaptolactate-cysteine-disulfiduria. Several of these defects have been associated with mental retardation because they were discovered in mentally retarded patients. It is now recognized, however, that the association of some of these defects with mental retardation is simply a reflection of case selection and that these metabolic variations are not necessarily harmful. Cystathioninuria described in 1959 in a mentally retarded patient with pituitary atrophy and orthopaedic deformities is one of the defects now considered to be a benign variant. The abnormalities in patients with cystathioninuria have been quite variable and some patients have had none.[631] The defect in cystathioninuria appears to be a deficiency in cystathionase, an enzyme responsible for cleaving cystathionine into cysteine and alpha-ketobutyric acid.[258]

Hypermethioninemia also is not presently recognized as a cause of neurologic dysfunction. Transient hypermethioninemia has been observed in the neonatal period, particularly in the premature infants fed a high protein diet.[792] In tyrosinemia Type I, hypermethioninemia may result from

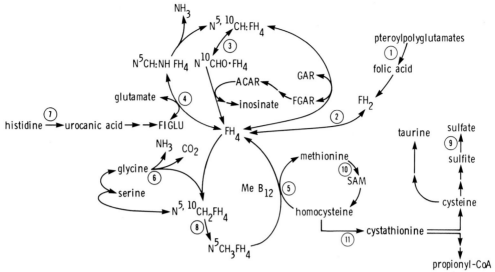

FIG. 9-2. Folate and sulfur amino acid metabolism. The role of folate in histidine, glycine, and homocysteine metabolism is shown. GAR → inosinate is the purine synthetic pathway. Enzymes indicated are: (1) folate absorption; (2) dihydrofolate reductase; (3) cyclohydrolase; (4) formiminotransferase; (5 homocysteine-methionine methyltransferase; (6) glycine cleavage system; (7) histidase; (8) $N^{5,10}$ methylene-FH_4 reductase; (9) sulfite oxidase; (10) S-adenosylmethionine synthetase; and (11) cystathionine beta-synthase. Abbreviations used are: ACAR for 5-aminoimidazole-4-carboxyamide ribonucleotide; FGAR for N-formylglycinamide ribonucleotide; FH_2 for dihydrofolate; FH_4 for tetrahydrofolate; FIGLU for formiminoglutamate; GAR for glycinamide ribonucleotide; MeB_{12} for methylcobalamin; N^5CH_3 for N^5methyl; $N^5CH:NH$ for N^5 formimino; $N^{5,10}$ CH: for $N^{5,10}$methenyl; $N^{5,10}CH_2$ for $N^{5,10}$ methylene; $N^{10}CHO·$ for N^{10}formyl; and PP for pyridoxal phosphate.

the liver dysfunction found in this condition because hypermethioninemia is a common feature of severe liver disease.[292,384,493] Hypermethioninemia may also accompany classical homocystinuria and could facilitate simple screening for homocystinuria if it were not for the fact that it may occur only with high protein intake.[332,449,875] Hypermethioninemia may also occur in association with a deficiency of hepatic S-adenosylmethionine synthetase activity.[276]

Homocystinuria

As the list, Incidence of Inherited Metabolic Diseases Affecting the Nervous System, shows, homocystinuria is one of the most common aminoacidurias. Homocystinuria frequently causes neurologic symptoms. Homocystinuria, however, is not one disease clinically or biochemically. Two types of inborn errors of metabolism may lead to increased homocystine in plasma and urine—a defect in cystathionine beta-synthase, or a defect in homocysteine remethylation. The defects in homocysteine remethylation are discussed with the defects in vitamin B_{12} (B_{12}) and folate.

Cystathionine Beta-Synthase Deficiency. *Pathology.* The dominant pathology involves vessels. Thrombosis is a common finding at autopsy and may involve arteries or veins in any region of the body. The wall of the vessels have marked intimal thickening. Muscle fibers are deranged and fragmented as are the elastic fibers. This process involves large or moderate sized arteries anywhere in the body. In the brain the principal neuropathology is arterial or venous infarction. Neuronal loss in the cerebral cortex and hippocampus has been reported even in the absence of infarction.[275]

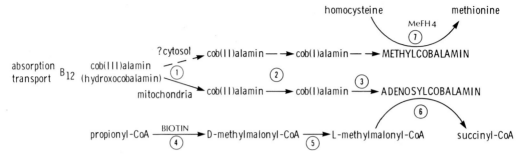

FIG. 9-3. B_{12} and methylmalonate metabolism. Methylcobalamin, found in the cytosol, is presumably formed there. Adenosylcobalamin is in the 5'-deoxy form. Succinyl-CoA is a member of the Krebs cycle. Enzymes indicated are: (1) cob(III)alamin reductase; (2) cob(II)alamin reductase; (3) adenosyl transferase; (4) propionyl-CoA carboxylase; (5) methylmalonyl-CoA racemase; (6) methylmalonyl-CoA mutase; and (7) homocysteine-methionine methyltransferase. Vitamin B_{12} is abbreviated B_{12}; Methyltetrahydrofolate is abbreviated $MeFH_4$. Cofactors are in bold type.

Biochemistry. The condensation of homocysteine with serine is catalyzed by cystathionine-beta-synthase. The enzyme purified from rat liver has two pairs of non-identical peptide chains, namely, $\alpha_2\ \beta_2$ structure.[416] Pyridoxal phosphate bound to the enzyme is necessary to activity.[434] The biochemical defect in some cases may be due to homozygosity for a mutant gene (i.e., $\alpha'_2\beta_2$ or $\alpha_2\ \beta'_2$), whereas in others it may be due to a compound heterozygous state ($\alpha\alpha'\beta_2$ or $\alpha_2\beta\beta'$). This enzyme can be measured in cultured skin fibroblasts, lymphocytes stimulated with phytohemagglutinin, liver, and amniotic fluid cells.[301,563,564,828]

The enzyme deficiency results in elevation of plasma homocysteine and its dimer homocystine–the mixed disulfide homocysteine–cysteine; methionine; and methionine sulfoxide. These substances and several others are present in abnormal amounts in urine.[104,630]

Clinical Features. The eye, the central nervous system, the vascular system, and the skeletal system are affected in homocystinuria. Patients have physical features similar to those found in Marfan's syndrome. Ectopia lentis, vascular accidents, and mental retardation are the other principal features.

Ectopia lentis, or lens dislocation, is the most common clinical manifestation. Lens dislocation, typically downward, appears to be a consequence of disruption of zonular fibers of the ciliary body. Lens dislocation occurs between the ages of 3 and 10 years in more than 90% of patients.[250] Other ocular manifestations may occur including acute glaucoma, iridodynesis (wavering of the iris when not stabilized by the lens), myopia, and optic atrophy.

Nervous system abnormalities may be either localized or nonlocalized. The localized abnormalities are the result of the vascular accidents that occur in this disease. Thromboembolism of cerebral vessels may occur even in infancy.[873] Acute hemiplegia is the most common localized neurologic abnormality. Mental retardation is the most common nonlocalized abnormality. The reported incidence of this complication is quite variable not only because of the disease variability, but also because of variable ascertainment. Various estimates have placed the risk of retardation at between 50% to 80%.[566] Retardation may be evident early in the first year but typically is detected at around 1 year of age, not as regression but as failure to progress. Retardation is apparently progressive because older patients with homocystinuria have lower IQs than younger patients. The degree of retardation varies from mild to marked. Homocystinuric patients are, however, generally less retarded than patients with PKU. Retardation may result from multiple small strokes, but there is little evidence to document this pathogenesis other than plausibility and the absence of a more tenable hypothesis. Mental retardation, moreover, is not invariably seen in patients with strokes. Seizures may also occur in homocystinuric patients. These can be focal or generalized. Since many of these seizures accompany the onset of focal neurologic deficits, they may be another manifestation of vascular accidents.[214,374] The gait of homocystinuric patients may be quite unusual and can be a mode of disease presentation. This gait abnormality has been termed the "Charlie Chaplin" gait.[269,450] Psychiatric disturbances may also be more common among patients with homocystinuria and their relatives.[214]

The skeletal manifestations are among the most common manifestations of homocystinuria. Many of the abnormalities are obvious on gross inspection of the patients, including the Marfanoid habitus, arachnodactyly, genu valgum, cubitus valgum, pectus carinatum or excavatum, high-arched palate, pes cavus, and kyphoscoliosis. Radiographically, osteoporosis, especially of the spine, is extremely common and along with lens dislocation, may be the only abnormality in mild cases. Osteoporosis is usually not evident until late childhood.

Other systems may also be involved. Cutaneous manifestations include livido reticularis, malar flush, and friable, light hair. Hepatomegaly is also quite common and results from fatty infiltration of the liver.

Homocystinuria is inherited in an autosomal recessive manner.[238,565] The expression of the disease is variable among sibships. This fact along with several other observations suggests that there is considerable genetic heterogeneity in cystathionine beta-synthase deficiency. Genetic heterogeneity probably also accounts for the considerable biochemical variation found in these patients (see above).

Diagnosis. The nitroprusside reaction in urine of patients with homocystinuria is almost always strongly positive. Excessive homocysteine and methionine in plasma and urine reflect the metabolic block, as do unusual conjugates of those compounds. Likewise, diminished synthesis and excretion of products distal to the block is the rule, including cystine, inorganic sulfate, and perhaps taurine.[630] The enzyme defect can be demonstrated in cultured skin fibroblasts, lymphocytes, and liver.[238,301,564,828] Prenatal diagnosis is probably possible using cultured amniotic fluid cells.[243] At least three distinct subgroups of patients with homocystinuria are distinguishable, based on laboratory studies of enzyme activity and pyridoxal phosphate binding.[247] Pyridoxine responsiveness should, however, be tested *in vivo* as well.

Heterozygotes detection is possible in many cases, particularly using methionine loading.[566,695] Newborn screening has been attempted using urine (measuring homocystine) or blood (measuring methionine).[482,485,827] Mudd and Levy discuss the pitfalls of newborn screening.[566]

Treatment. About one half of patients with this disorder show significant improvement in the biochemical abnormalities when treated with large doses of vitamin B_6, usually taken orally as pyridoxine hydrochloride.[46,47] The response may be proportional to the dose. A patient should receive 500 mg to 1000 mg each day without effect for several weeks before being considered a nonresponder.[627] Dietary methionine restriction with cystine supplementation may also be helpful clinically. It certainly can diminish or eliminate the biochemical abnormalities.[566]

Sulfite Oxidase Deficiency

This rare defect has been reported in only 3 patients. The clinical features have been similar to some extent. The first patient was abnormal at birth with severe mental retardation, seizures, opisthotonus, and later, bilateral dislocated lenses.[565] Another child developed seizures at 17 months of age followed by hemiparesis.[731] This child later developed progressive choreoathetosis and lens dislocation. Sulfur-containing metabolites were increased in the urine of these patients and sulfite oxidase activity was decreased. A single case of what appears to be a combined xanthine oxidase and sulfite oxidase deficiency has been reported.[215,397] This patient presented in the neonatal period with dysmorphic facial features, enophthalmus, nystagmus, and bilateral superiorly dislocated lens. The child also had generalized seizures. Later the child was found to have renal xanthine stones. Development and growth were extremely poor and hypertonicity had become prominent. Xanthine oxidase deficiency was demonstrated in a jejunal biopsy. Sulfite oxidase was implied from the increased urinary S-sulfocysteine and taurine and the decreased sulfate in the urine. Since molybdenum is a cofactor for xanthine oxidase and sulfite oxidase, a defect in molybdenum metabolism could explain this combination of deficiencies.

BRANCHED-CHAIN AMINO ACID AND VITAMIN B₁₂ METABOLIC DEFECTS, AND RELATED ORGANIC ACIDEMIAS

Biochemistry

The branched-chain amino acids, leucine, isoleucine, and valine, are essential in man. They are used in protein synthesis and as an energy source. Branched-chain amino acids in excess of protein synthesis requirements can be catabolized (Fig. 9-4). The initial step in these similar metabolic pathways is deamination. In this step, leucine and isoleucine appear to share a common enzyme, whereas valine has another.[847] Decarboxylation and formation of coenzyme

A (CoA) derivatives occur through a common branched-chain ketoacid dehydrogenase. This is a multienzyme complex similar to pyruvate dehydrogenase (see Fig. 9-8). The sequence of decarboxylation, transfer to a lipoic acid derivative, and transfer to CoA occurs in both complexes. Dihydrolipoyl dehydrogenase, an enzyme apparently identical with the enzyme found in pyruvate dehydrogenase, regenerates the lipoic acid derivative. After formation of the CoA derivatives, further oxidation of the branched-chain ketoacids occurs (Fig. 9-4). Leucine is catabolized to acetyl-CoA and acetoacetate; isoleucine yields acetyl-CoA and propionyl-CoA, and valine yields propionyl-CoA (Fig 9-4). Propionyl-CoA is carboxylated by an enzyme requiring biotin as a cofactor (propionyl-CoA carboxylase), yielding L-methylmalonyl-CoA. L-methylmalonyl CoA is racemized to D-methylmalonyl-CoA and the second carboxyl group

FIG. 9-4. Branched-chain amino acid metabolism. Enzymes that are indicated have been associated with clinical deficiency states. Vitamin cofactors are shown in bold type. Enzymes indicated are: (1) valine transaminase; (2) branched-chain ketoacid dehydrogenase complex; (3) isovaleryl-CoA dehydrogenase; (4) beta-methylcrotonyl-CoA carboxylase; and (5) acetoacetyl-CoA thiolase (beta-ketothiolase); (6) beta-hydroxy beta-methylglutaryl CoA lyase. Abbreviations used are: PP for pyridoxal phosphate and TTP for thiamine pyrophosphate.

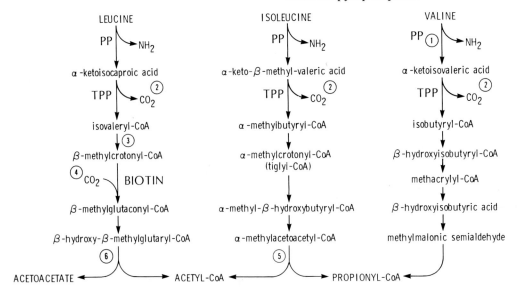

is then shifted to the terminal carbon yielding succinyl-CoA, a member of the Krebs cycle. This last step requires a vitamin B_{12} cofactor, 5'-deoxyadenosyl cobalamin (see Fig. 9-3). Propionyl-CoA is also derived from threonine and methionine.

Inborn errors of metabolism of these amino acids occur at many of the metabolic steps. Symptoms may be produced directly through accumulation of substrates or by interference with other metabolic pathways. The syndrome of ketotic hyperglycinemia was originally observed in a patient who was eventually found to have propionic acidemia. Other disorders that can present this way include methylmalonic aciduria, isovaleric acidemia, and beta-methyl-crotonyl-CoA carboxylase deficiency. These four disorders are clinically almost indistinguishable and constitute one category of the organic acidemias.

Maple Syrup Urine Disease

Maple syrup urine disease (MSUD) or branched-chain ketoaciduria was first observed in 1954 in a newborn infant who was normal at birth but who developed lethargy, vomiting, hypertonicity, seizures, and finally coma and death within the first week of life.[544] The incidence of this disorder, estimated from routine newborn screening by means of a bacterial inhibition assay is approximately 1 in 22,400 newborns worldwide and in the United States.[576] Cases have been reported in blacks, Japanese, Samoans, and Caucasians. Maple syrup urine disease is not unusually prevalent in any particular ethnic group.

Pathology. The pathologic changes in the brain of MSUD patients are dependent upon the stage of the disease during which the patient dies. Patients with classic MSUD dying during the acute illness in the newborn period may have spongy white matter and neuronal migration defects such as heterotopic gray matter and abnormal cortical lamination.[544] The patients who have survived the acute episodes and are mentally retarded have additional abnormalities including the absence of myelination of pathways known to become myelinated after birth, and status spongiosus of white matter.[160,738] Biochemically, total lipid, proteo-

lipid, and cerebroside content are markedly reduced in untreated patients.[649,650] Dietary treatment of MSUD prevents these lipid changes.[546,649]

Biochemistry. Maple syrup urine disease is due to a defect in branched-chain ketoacid decarboxylase, a multienzyme complex. Earlier suggestions that there were separate decarboxylases for each of the three branched-chain ketoacids have not been borne out.[169] A defect in the decarboxylase subunit itself has been suggested in two cases of MSUD.[221,689]

The block in branched-chain ketoacid metabolism results in excretion of large amounts of these substances and a rise in the plasma and urine levels of branched-chain amino acids. Leucine is always more strikingly elevated than the other two branched-chain amino acids. There have been repeated suggestions that elevation of the serum concentration of any one of these amino acids impairs the metabolism of the other two.[757]

Clinical Features. Although the newborn infant with classical MSUD appears normal at birth, the child becomes symptomatic by one week after birth. The first symptoms are poor feeding and vomiting. Subsequently, hypertonicity and a strained cry develop. If the infant thus affected remains untreated, coma, seizures, and apnea appear. Death may even occur within the first week of life. Patients with classical MSUD rarely survive beyond 2 years of age. Those patients who survive the initial episode generally have been severely retarded. The only characteristic feature is the odor of the urine, which has been likened to the odor of maple syrup, or, for those unfamiliar with this odor, to the odor of burnt sugar. This odor may be present in the urine by 5 days of age. Patients with classical MSUD may have a family history of mentally retarded siblings or siblings expiring in infancy.

Four variants of MSUD have been described: mild branched-chain ketoaciduria, intermittent branched-chain ketoaciduria, thiamine-responsive branched-chain ketoaciduria, and valine-sensitive intermittent MSUD. In mild branched-chain ketoaciduria, branched-chain amino acids are continuously elevated as are the urinary keto acids. Branched-chain amino acid decarboxylase activity is reduced but is greater than 8% of normal activity in skin fibroblasts. Such patients are generally mildly to moderately retarded and may suffer an acute attack when infected or when similarly stressed.[774,717] During these attacks personality changes and ataxia often appear.[717] The urine, at such times, may have the characteristic maple syrup odor even though at other times this odor will be absent. Coma and death may occur during these attacks.

In intermittent branched-chain ketoaciduria, branched-chain amino acid decarboxylase activity is in the range of 2% to 8% of normal in cultured fibroblasts.[168] These patients frequently do not tolerate high protein diets and often avoid them. Children with this form of MSUD are often diagnosed in late infancy or childhood when they deteriorate during an intercurrent illness. During these periods there may be variable alterations of consciousness and ataxia. Death may occur during such episodes of deterioration.

Thiamine administration produced a reduction in levels of blood branched-chain amino acids and an amelioration of symptoms in one moderately retarded infant 11 months of age who had a mild elevation of these acids.[719] Activity of branched-chain ketoacid decarboxylase was 20% of normal in cultured leukocytes and fibroblasts. Thiamine administration *in vitro* did not improve this activity.

The fourth variant was recently described. All branched-chain amino acid challenges except valine were tolerated by this 18-month-old child with an intermittent form of MSUD. Fibroblasts from this child had 5% to 10% of normal activity when valine was the substrate in the decarboxylase assay. When leucine was the substrate in this same assay, activity was 30% of normal.[908] In the other forms of MSUD defective leucine metabolism accounts for most of the neurologic symptoms.

Genetics.   Classical MSUD is inherited as an autosomal recessive disorder. Several families with multiple affected siblings have been reported. Males and females are equally affected. The parents of patients with MSUD are not affected. Carrier detection has not been perfected although, in general, leukocytes from obligate carriers have reduced branched-chain keto acid decarboxylase activity. The variants of MSUD are presumed to be autosomal recessive.

Laboratory Features.   In addition to the elevation of branched-chain amino acids in the blood and branched-chain keto acids in the urine, several other laboratory abnormalities occur. One of the most common abnormalities in MSUD is metabolic acidosis. This may be reflected by an increased anion gap. Hypoglycemia may also occur episodically.[510] The hypoglycemia is secondary to defective gluconeogenesis.[358]

Diagnosis.   The diagnosis of classical MSUD can be suspected in the sick infant with hypertonicity, vomiting, and the characteristic maple syrup urine or body odor. A simple screening test can be performed on the urine, 2,4-DNPH when added to urine of a patient with MSUD will produce a yellow precipitate. Identification of the specific branched-chain amino acid elevations in plasma and the excretion pattern of branched-chain keto acids in the urine can be accomplished by the various chromatographic techniques. Paper chromatography of plasma from patients suspected of having classic MSUD on the basis of family history has revealed elevated branched-chain amino acids on the third day of life.[868]

Enzymatic studies are necessary to define the type of MSUD. The most rapid method uses leukocytes incubated with 1-^{14}C-leucine.[165] Greater accuracy and precision in defining the decarboxylase activity can be achieved by use of cultured skin fibroblasts, but this is a more time-consuming method.[168]

Treatment.   During the acute episode, acidosis, dehydration, and hypoglycemia must be corrected. If neurologic signs are present peritoneal dialysis or exchange transfusion should be performed because brain damage apparently occurs rather quickly during these episodes.[274] Leucine may be the most significant toxic metabolite.[757,758] Long-term management centers around providing only enough of the branched-chain amino acids for growth, while providing adequate amounts of other essential amino acids and calories. Frequent monitoring of the plasma amino acid pattern is essential.[758] Commercially prepared infant formulas without the branched-chain amino acids are available so that the harmful amino acids can be regulated tightly without jeopardizing overall nutrition.[756,757] The treatment probably must be continued for life.

Methylmalonic Acidemia and Defects of Vitamin B_{12} Metabolism

Methylmalonic acidemia refers to a group of diseases that have in common excessive blood and urine methylmalonic acid. These are rare conditions with perhaps no more than 20 patients with this condition recorded in the literature.[682] Defects in B_{12} metabolism and primary defects in methylmalonic acid catabolic enzymes have been associated with methylmalonic acidemia.

Biochemistry of Cobalamin and Methylmalonic Aciduria. Two cofactors are derived from vitamin B_{12}-adenosylcobalamin, which is necessary for the action of methylmalonyl-CoA mutase, and methylcobalamin, which is a cofactor for homocysteine-methionine methyl transferase. No other functions for vitamin B_{12} in human metabolism are known. Dietary vitamin B_{12} is in the hydroxocobalamin (cob[III]alamin) form, a form in which the cobalt atom is trivalent. Hydroxocobalamin must be reduced to the cob[I]alamin form before the adenosyl or methyl group can be transferred to it (see Fig. 9-3). Methylmalonyl-CoA mutase is a mitochondrial enzyme. The reduction and final synthesis of its cofactor, adenosylcobalamin, take place in the mitochondrion. Reduction of cob[III]alamin for methylcobalamin synthesis probably takes place in the cytosol.[682]

Errors in vitamin B_{12} metabolism that lead to deficient formation of only adenosylcobalamin are discussed below. Two forms of methylmalonic acidemia, separable by complementation, are accompanied by impaired homocysteine methylation.[317,494] In these disorders the activity of both adenosylcobalamin and methylcobalamin are deficient, possibly due to defective retention or accumulation of hydroxocobalamin.[682]

Methylmalonic aciduria is due to deficient conversion of D-methylmalonyl-CoA to succinyl-CoA. Two enzymes are involved sequentially, methylmalonyl-CoA

racemase and carbonylmutase. Adenosylcobalamin is a cofactor in the second reaction, converting L-methylmalonyl-CoA to succinyl-CoA (see Fig. 9-4). Defects in the mutase enzyme activity are more common than defects in the racemase enzyme activity.[409,557] Four groups of patients (A–D) with defects in cobalamin metabolism have been identified by complementation studies.[317,882] The enzyme defect in the cobalamin B group affects the last step of adenosylcobalamin synthesis, the adenosyltransferase reaction.[512] The defect in the other groups is not known. Many of the patients with defects in synthesis of adenosylcobalamin will respond to pharmacologic doses of vitamin B_{12} with a decrease in methylmalonic acid excretion.[683]

The metabolic block leads to excretion of methylmalonic acid in large quantities during times of illness, and lesser amounts at other times. Secondary elevations of glycine, propionic acid, and its excretion products (3-hydroxypropionate, propionylglycine, tiglylglycine, and methylcitrate), and NH_3 may also be seen.[682,726]

Clinical Features. Methylmalonic acidemia due to deficient methylmalonyl-CoA mutase activity usually presents clinically as severe ketoacidosis in infancy. Later presentation and less severe illness than infantile ketoacidosis has also been reported occasionally.

Infants with methylmalonic acidemia presenting as infantile ketoacidosis are usually detected quite early in life, usually within the first year.[682] These infants have no clinically distinctive feature.

Other patients with much less severe illness than infantile ketoacidosis have had reduced methylmalonyl-CoA mutase activity.[286,880] Two of these patients were brothers 62 and 70 years of age who were completely asymptomatic.[286] The other two patients presented in late infancy with acute onset of metabolic acidosis manifested clinically by symptoms resembling those occurring in Reye's Syndrome. The growth and development of these children were otherwise normal.

At least five cases of the combined deficiency of adenosylcobalamin and methylcobalamin activity have been reported. No uniform clinical picture emerges from these cases. Even in the same family the manifestations of the disorder have been variable.[311] In one instance, in a 2½-year-old-child, this disorder was completely asymptomatic. In other patients the symptom complex has included organic psychosis, Marfanoid habitus, feeding difficulties, seizures, ataxia, and growth failure often associated with psychomotor delay.[61,486] Several of these patients have had anemia with evidence of megaloblastic changes in the bone marrow. Pathologically, these patients often show prominent vascular lesions quite similar to those seen in homocystinuria, thus suggesting that the elevation in homocystine may be responsible for the vascular lesions seen in these two diseases, which otherwise are quite different.[61]

The defects leading to methylmalonic acidemia are inherited in an autosomal recessive fashion. Siblings have been affected, but in no instance has a parent of a child with methylmalonic acidemia been affected.

Diagnosis. Methylmalonic acidemia should be considered in any case of infantile ketoacidosis or ketotic hyperglycinemia. A colorometric test is available. Filter paper saturated with urine, when exposed to diazotized p-nitroaniline, develops a green color if the urine contains methylmalonic acid.[822] Patients with combined defective synthesis of adenosylcobalamin and methylcobalamin will also excrete excessive amounts of homocystine in the urine. Gas liquid chromatography, TLC, or HPLC may also be used and are more specific and sensitive. Vitamin B_{12} deficiency, leading to mild methylmalonic aciduria, can usually be excluded by the absence of megaloblastic anemia and normal vitamin B_{12} levels. Confirmation of the diagnosis and delineation of the defect usually require leukocyte or fibroblast assays. The diagnosis can be made in an affected fetus by demonstrating elevated methylmalonic acid levels in amniotic fluid and maternal urine or by assaying for methylmalonyl-CoA mutase activity in cultured amniotic cells.[513,558]

Treatment. Acute episodes of ketoacidosis are treated in a manner similar to that described under MSUD. All patients with methylmalonic acidemia should be treated with vitamin B_{12} supplements at least until it is known that the patient does not respond to vitamin B_{12}.[377] Oral doses of 1 mg to 2 mg of cyanocobalamin or hydroxocobalamin should be administered. A fetus with a B_{12}-responsive form of methylmalonic acidemia treated continuously from the prenatal period did well.[8] Restriction of protein intake to the minimum needed for growth will minimize the methylmalonic aciduria and episodes of ketoacidosis.

Vitamin B_{12} Absorption and Transport Defects

Malabsorption of vitamin B_{12} may occur in two inherited disorders, intrinsic factor deficiency and absence of the ileal receptor for the B_{12}-intrinsic factor complex.[353,467,530] Patients with these disorders develop megaloblastic anemia and increased excretion of methylmalonic acid and homocystine in late infancy to childhood. Serum levels of vitamin B_{12} are low. A minority of these children develop neurologic manifestations. The onset of the neurologic complications occurs later than the hematologic signs. The signs and symptoms are those of subacute combined degeneration.[467] These are discussed in the chapter on nutritional deficiencies.

A hereditary deficiency of transcobalamin II that results in abnormal transport of vitamin B_{12} has also been reported.[340] Infants with this disorder develop frequent infections, growth failure, lethargy, vomiting, diarrhea, and megaloblastic anemia. Methylmalonic acid excretion is not increased.

Organic Acidurias

Isovaleric Acidemia or Sweaty Feet Syndrome. Approximately 25 patients with this disorder have been reported. This defect in leucine metabolism may present as an acute organic acidosis in the first week of life and may, therefore, be confused with MSUD.[483] A characteristic feature of these patients is their offensive odor, an odor likened to that of "sweaty feet." One patient has been reported who did not have this odor.[11]

Other patients with isovaleric acidemia are unaffected until late in the first year of life, at which time they begin having repeated episodes of metabolic acidosis of gradually decreasing frequency.[115,810] During these episodes they manifest symptoms of vomiting, lethargy, ataxia, tremulousness, and, if the acidosis is severe, coma. Patients with isovaleric acidemia are generally mildly retarded but may be normal between attacks.

Associated features include depressed white blood cell counts and thrombocytopenia. The defect in isovaleric acidemia is in the catabolic pathway of leucine at the isovaleryl-CoA dehydrogenase step (Fig. 9-4). This results in elevated serum isovaleric acid that is usually conjugated with glycine to form isovalerylglycine which is present in the urine.[811] Particularly during periods of illness, there is an elevation of serum and urine isovaleric acid, the substance responsible for the odor of sweaty feet. The metabolite, beta-hydroxyisovaleric acid, is also elevated when urine is analyzed by TLC, liquid partition chromatography, or gas chromatography. Beta-methylcrotonic acid levels are not elevated because the defect appears to be in the enzyme responsible for its formation, isovaleryl-CoA dehydrogenase. This defect can be demonstrated by measuring enzyme activity in leukocytes or cultured fibroblasts.[734,810]

Treatment consists of a dietary regimen similar to that described for MSUD with the exception that only one of the branched-chain amino acids, leucine, must be restricted.[483] Another treatment that shows great promise is the administration of glycine.[148,457] Administration of glycine to an infant with isovaleric acidemia and severe ketoacidosis rapidly reduced the serum isovalerate level and led to clinical improvement within a few weeks.[148] Continuous administration of glycine after resolution of the acute acidosis prevented recurrence of acidosis and development proceeded normally. This beneficial effect of glycine is probably due to enhanced elimination of free isovaleric acid through conjugation to form isovalerylglycine, which is rapidly excreted in the urine.[148]

Propionic Acidemia or Ketotic Hyperglycinemia. Propionic acidemia was first recognized in an infant with recurrent, severe metabolic ketoacidosis.[142] Since then at least 60 other cases of propionic acide-

mia have been reported. The general picture is that of overwhelming ketoacidosis, usually accompanied by significant dehydration.

Pathology. In an infant dying in the newborn period during an episode of ketoacidosis, the only changes were those of a fatty liver and nonspecific alterations in the cerebellum.[372] Children surviving longer have had defective myelinization and status spongiosus of the white matter.

Biochemistry. Propionic acidemia is caused by deficient activity of the enzyme propionyl-CoA carboxylase (Fig. 9-4).[303,379] This enzyme is probably a tetramer, containing two pairs of identical amino acid chains. Biotin, essential for enzyme function, is incorporated into the apoenzyme. Cell fusion experiments using Sendai virus have demonstrated production of functioning enzyme from fused cells derived from different patients with propionic acidemia. Successful pairings have determined complementation groups, whose members are thought to have similar defects. (Cells from the same group cannot complement each other.) There is no good correlation between a complementation group and symptoms or severity of disease.[316,891] Even within the same family the variability of propionic acidemia can be impressive.[432]

Some of the metabolic derangements that are present in untreated propionic acidemia are easily explained. Propionic acid, normally present in serum at 5 μM or less, may be elevated tenfold to 1000-fold in a very sick patient. Propionic acid will be present in the urine, as will metabolic by-products of excess propionyl-CoA including 3-hydroxypropionate, propionylglycine, tiglylglycine, and methylcitrate. The last compound is a highly specific marker for propionic and methylmalonic acidemias. It apparently is formed by condensation of propionyl-CoA with oxaloacetate, analogous to acetyl-CoA condensing with oxaloacetate to form citrate as it enters the Krebs cycle.[14] Methylcitrate is usually identified using mass spectroscopy, which precludes its identification in most laboratories.

Other findings are more difficult to explain, although they may be more conspicuous. These include ketonuria, elevated glycine and NH_3, and bone marrow depression. The principal ketones excreted are the usual, acetone, acetoacetate, and beta-hydroxybutyric acid, but lesser amounts of butanone, pentanone, and hexanone are also excreted.[539] Hyperglycinemia has been thought to be due to impaired function of the glycine cleavage system.[12,447,725] The hyperammonemia may be due to low activity of carbamoyl-phosphate synthetase, which is due to deficiency of its activator, N-acetylglutamate. The hyperammonemia correlates with the elevation of propionate. (Fig. 9-5)[153,889]

Clinical Manifestations. Most patients with this disorder present in the newborn period with severe metabolic ketoacidosis that may be fatal.[372] Survivors may have episodic attacks of ketoacidosis, generally associated with infections or protein ingestion. During such attacks, patients are often quite ill with hyperventilation, vomiting, and varying degrees of alteration of consciousness. Areflexia has been noted during the attacks of metabolic acidosis in some patients.[373] Between attacks of ketoacidosis, children with propionic acidemia are often developmentally retarded and may have evidence of spastic-

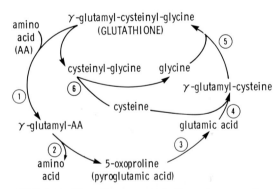

FIG. 9-5. Glutathione metabolism. 5-oxoprolinuria (pyroglutamic aciduria) results from cleavage of gamma-glutamyl glycine by enzymes (1) and (2), when glutathione synthetase (enzyme 5) is deficient. Enzymes indicated are: (1) gamma-glutamyl transpeptidase; (2) gamma-glutamyl cyclotransferase; (3) 5-oxoprolinase; (4) gamma-glutamylcysteine synthetase; (5) glutathione synthetase; and (6) peptidase. Amino acid is abbreviated AA.

ity and extrapyramidal disturbances. In some children, attacks of ketoacidosis do not occur and the disease presents as developmental retardation.[378,379] Even normal growth and development have been reported in propionic acidemia.[99,890] In one Mennonite family, a male child was affected by multiple episodes of ketoacidosis, hyperglycinemia, and hyperammonemia. This child was mentally retarded and had seizures. His sister, however, who was also deficient in enzyme activity, suffered no episodes of ketoacidosis and developed entirely normally.[890] Episodic or persistent neutropenia or thrombocytopenia are also common. Autonomic dysfunction has been reported in one infant with this disorder.[351] This infant did not have abnormal fungiform tongue papillae, a constant feature of familial dysautonomia.

This disorder is inherited in an autosomal recessive fashion.[682] Genetic complementation cited above has demonstrated at least three major and two minor complementation groups.[316] This suggests that even among propionic acidemia patients with the same clinical features genetic and biochemical variation is likely.

Laboratory Abnormalities. Most often the predominant laboratory abnormality is the ketoacidosis. In addition to serum and urine elevations of propionic acid, other propionate derivatives accumulate including methylcitrate, propionylglycine, beta-hydroxypropionate, and tiglic acid. Hyperglycinemia has been a regular feature. Hyperammonemia is frequently present and may be marked.[725] Long bone films have revealed osteoporosis in some cases.[141]

Diagnosis. The diagnosis of propionic acidemia should be considered in infants with unexplained ketoacidosis and in children with psychomotor delay, seizures, and nonlocalizing neurologic abnormalities. Since ketoacidosis is not specific for propionic acidemia, and may even be absent, it is necessary to determine serum or urine concentrations of propionic acid and its metabolites.[849] The determination should not be performed after a prolonged period of starvation because metabolite levels may not be elevated.[848] Methylmalonic acidemia may also produce secondary propionic acidemia. Definite diagnosis is possible by demonstrating reduced levels of propionyl CoA carboxylase activity in white blood cells, liver, cultured fibroblasts, or cultured amniotic fluid cells. Prenatal diagnosis has also been achieved by demonstrating increased methylcitrate in amniotic fluid and maternal urine.[806]

Treatment. Treatment consists of protein restriction, vigorous treatment of any acute infection, and treatment of the acute episodes of ketoacidosis. Administration of $NaHCO_3$ and peritoneal dialysis may be effective during the bouts of ketoacidosis. In one patient with propionic acidemia, administration of biotin (10 mg daily) was effective in reducing the ketoacidosis.[49]

Multiple Carboxylase Deficiency. Several patients initially suspected of having propionic acidemia have been found to have deficiencies of three carboxylases that require biotin as a cofactor. In addition to propionyl-CoA carboxylase, pyruvate carboxylase and beta-methylcrotonyl-CoA carboxylase are deficient. All patients reported to date with this autosomal recessive disorder have responded to oral biotin.

Patients present in infancy with intermittent ataxia and myoclonus. In addition to the neurologic symptoms, immunologic defects suggestive of combined immunodeficiency have been seen in some patients.[155] These symptoms include *Candida* dermatitis, keratoconjunctivitis, and alopecia. All symptoms resolved after a few days of biotin treatment. Defects in transport or incorporation of biotin into the apoenzyme are a likely explanation.[703]

Beta-Ketothiolase Deficiency. Beta-ketothiolase (acetoacetyl-CoA thiolase) deficiency is a recently described cause of protein intolerance and infantile ketoacidosis. The defect in this condition involves the deficiency of beta-ketothiolase, an enzyme in the isoleucine catabolic pathway that is responsible for the conversion of alpha-methylacetoacetyl-CoA to acetyl-CoA and propionyl-CoA (Fig. 9-4).

At least eight patients in five families have been reported to have this recessively inherited defect.[178,179,305,362,425,675] In all cases these patients have had acute episodes of ketoacidosis, often at the time of febrile illnesses, manifested by a reduced level of consciousness, vomiting, hyperventilation, and seizures. Some patients, although suffering episodic ketoacidosis, have developed normally, whereas others, including siblings of children with normal psychomotor development, have been retarded.

In addition to ketoacidosis, neutropenia, thrombocytopenia, hyperglycinemia, hyperglycinuria, and hyperammonemia can be found during attacks. Urinary alpha-methylhydroxybutyrate, alpha-methylacetoacetate, and butanone are increased. This pattern of urinary organic acids, the excretion of tiglylglycine, normal levels of propionate and methylmalonic acid, and reduced ^{14}C-isoleucine metabolism by fibroblasts from these patients imply a defect in beta-ketothiolase deficiency. This deficiency, however, has not been directly demonstrated because the substrate for beta-ketothiolase is not available for direct assays.

The diagnosis of beta-ketothiolase deficiency depends upon demonstration of the abnormal urinary organic acids by gas-liquid chromatography during attacks of ketoacidosis or after an isoleucine challenge. This condition can be easily confused with salicylism, which may also result in ketoacidosis. Indeed, one child with this disorder had a falsely elevated salicylate level, apparently a consequence of elevated levels of acetoacetate.[675] Treatment, as in other organic acidurias, consists of restriction of protein intake to the minimum required for growth.

FOLATE METABOLIC DEFECTS

The folates are a large group of compounds involved in one-carbon transfers. They are derived from a common precursor, folic acid. At least 144 different forms are possible, based on the known one-carbon substitutes, the state of reduction of the pteridine rings, and the number of glutamate residues present.[687] Some of the important aspects of folate metabolism are drawn in Figure 9-2. The interrelationship between disorders of folate and disorders of B_{12} metabolism is due to the central nature of THF, as an intermediate for the synthesis of 5-methylTHF polyglutamates, the predominant folate derivative in erythrocytes. 5-Methyl tetrahydrofolate is the form of folate that is carried across cell membranes. Impaired synthesis of THF (due to methylcobalamin deficiency, for example) would lead to accumulation of 5-methylTHF and diminished intracellular transport of this compound, which would be overcome either by B_{12} or by pharmacologic doses of folate.[687]

The inborn defects of folate metabolism are generally so rare that a description of a typical patient with one of these defects is not possible. At least five defects have been described: a folate absorption defect, dihydrofolate reductase deficiency, formiminotransferase deficiency, methylene-THF reductase deficiency, and THF-methyltransferase deficiency. In dihydrofolate reductase deficiency, megaloblastic anemia is the principal clinical feature; neurologic symptoms are not a constant feature. Among the patients with folate malabsorption there has been considerable clinical variation. In two patients neurologic features were prominent. These patients were retarded and had movement disorders and seizures.[470,503] The features of the patients with THFmethyltransferase deficiency are given in Table 9-6.

Formiminotransferase Deficiency

This defect in folate metabolism results in a deficiency in the formation of 5-formiminotetrahydrofolate from THF. In addition, there is an abnormally large amount of formiminoglutamic acid (FIGLU) excreted in the urine. The defect is thought to be a deficiency in formiminotransferase.[16] The patients described by Arakawa presented in infancy and were physically and mentally retarded.[16] Pneumoencephalography showed cortical atrophy and the EEG was abnormal in all of these patients.[16] Megaloblastosis was not observed in these patients. Elevated serum folate was another prominent feature. Other patients, presumably having this same deficiency, have not been as severely affected and have had variable neurologic abnormalities.[584,628]

Methylenetetrahydrofolate Reductase Deficiency

Approximately 12 patients with this disorder have been described.[349] The defective conversion of 5,10-methylene-THF to 5-methyl-THF, a cofactor required for methylation of homocysteine (see Fig. 9-2), leads to moderate homocystinemia and homocystinuria accompanied by normal or low plasma methionine. Serum folate levels are low.

All patients with methylenetetrahydrofolate reductase deficiency have been affected neurologically, but there is striking variation in symptoms. The disorder presents either in late childhood and adolescence or in infancy. Presentation in infancy is characterized by seizures, apnea, and death.[349,574] One patient with this disorder responded dramatically to treatment with methionine, folinic acid, pyridoxine, and vitamin B_{12}.[349]

Patients presenting later in life have more variable symptoms. Most have been retarded. One patient had schizophrenic-like behavior, whereas another had proximal muscle weakness, a waddling gait and a paroxysmal, proximal upper extremity movement disorder.[253,567] Vascular lesions, less severe than in cystathionine beta-synthase deficiency, have been described.[410]

NONKETOTIC HYPERGLYCINEMIA

Biochemistry

Glycine, the simplest amino acid, participates in at least twenty major pathways, including the synthesis of heme, creatine, glutathione, ethanolamine, choline and sarcosine.[280] The major catabolic mechanism is cleavage into NH_3, CO_2, and methylene-THF (see Fig. 9-2). This occurs through the action of an enzyme complex, the glycine cleavage system. This system is defective in nonketotic hyperglycinemia, and glycine then accumulates in the brain, liver, plasma, urine, and cerebrospinal fluid.[12,13,632] The plasma glycine level is markedly increased. Urinary glycine excretion is significantly elevated, but excretion of other amino acids is normal. The cerebrospinal fluid (CSF): plasma glycine ratio is elevated. Normally this ratio is .02 to .03, but it may be ten times higher in nonketotic hyperglycinemia.[632]

Glycine is a presumed neurotransmitter, so some of the symptoms from this disorder may be due to glycine excess. However, normalizing the serum glycine level does not improve the patients with the classical form of this disease (see below). One possibility is that the serum glycine level does not reflect the concentration of glycine in the synapses.

Hyperglycinemia may be seen in association with sodium valproate administration.[390]

Hyperglycinemia also occurs in a number of other metabolic defects, especially in the ketotic hyperglycinemia syndromes (see above). In most instances hyperglycinemia is accompanied by ketoacidosis and appears to be an indirect effect of the primary enzymatic defect. Causes of ketotic hyperglycinemia include isovaleric acidemia, propionic acidemia, methylmalonic acidemia, and type I glutaric acidemia. Nonketotic hyperglycinemia should be distinguished from ketotic hyperglycinemia because the latter is treatable whereas the former has generally not been treatable. These disorders can generally be distinguished clinically and biochemically.

Clinical and Laboratory Features

As in ketotic hyperglycinemia, symptoms of nonketotic hyperglycinemia usually appear in the newborn period. In some cases these infants have been severely affected with seizures and inability to maintain respiration.[60,607] Movement is often conspicuously absent except for seizures and myoclonus, including hiccups.[60,279] If the infant survives, increased muscle tone gradually appears so that the patient may become opisthotonic. Development is often severely delayed, although less severe retardation has also been reported.[607] Failure to thrive often accompanies this profound delay.

Typically, patients with nonketotic hyperglycinemia have generalized seizures. These have most often been myoclonic seizures, although tonic or clonic seizures may also occur. The EEG often reveals a hypsarrhythmic pattern.[289,857]

Neutropenia, although much less common in nonketotic hyperglycinemia than in ketotic hyperglycinemia, does occasionally occur.[60]

Glycine is elevated in blood, urine, and CSF and may reach a level as high as 12 mg/dl.[60] Unless respiratory complications occur, acidosis and ketosis are absent, unlike the acidosis and ketosis in ketotic hyperglycinemia.

Some patients have not followed the clinical course described above. One child had slowly progressive optic atrophy and spinocerebellar degeneration beginning at 4 years of age.[777] This child's defect was thought to be an intestinal and renal tubular glycine transport defect. This patient and three brothers with progressive spastic paraparesis and nonketotic hyperglycinemia most likely do represent a different metabolic defect than that causing infantile nonketotic hyperglycinemia.[44]

Prenatal diagnosis of non-ketotic hyperglycinemia is likely to be available in the future.

Treatment

No treatment has been consistently effective. Exchange transfusion can temporarily produce clinical improvement but this is not a practical long-term method of treatment.[60] Sodium benzoate and protein restriction reduce the hyperglycinemia but this has not changed the neurologic outcome. Recently strychnine has been used, based on the theory that since glycine is an inhibitory neurotransmitter in the central nervous system, then a direct receptor antagonist, strychnine, might effectively reverse the neurologic symptoms. Unfortunately, although some patients have responded transiently to strychnine, most have not had a significant alteration in the usual course of the disease. Moreover, in one instance the strychnine may have exacerbated a status epilepticus that was fatal.[20,290,508,858,864]

UREA CYCLE DEFECTS

Hyperammonemia

Disposition and detoxification of NH_3 is largely dependent upon urea production by way of the Krebs-Henseleit urea cycle. Defects in this cycle are chiefly manifested by hyperammonemia. Hyperammonemia is not specific for urea cycle defects because it occurs in many other conditions (see list, Disorders Associated with Hyperammonemia).

(Text continues on p. 320)

TABLE 9-6 Very Rare Aminoacidopathies with Neurologic Dysfunction

Disorder (Reference)	Enzyme or Transport Defect	Onset	Clinical Features	Laboratory Features
Taurine deficiency[629]	Unknown	Adulthood	Psychiatric disturbances, bulbar symptoms, dyspnea, and faulty depth perception. Later Parkinsonism and respiratory failure	Low taurine in plasma and CSF
Molybdenum cofactor deficiency[397]	Combined sulfite oxidase and xanthine oxidase[2]	Infancy	Bilateral dislocated lens, enophthalmus, nystagmus, Brushfield spots, tonic–clonic seizures, and severe psychomotor retardation	Increased urine sulfite, S-sulfocysteine, taurine, xanthine, hypoxanthine, and uric acid. Xanthine stones
Hypervalinemia[847]	Reduced transamination of valine[4]	Newborn	Poor feeding and vomiting followed by psychomotor retardation, nystagmus, and failure to thrive	Elevated serum valine
3-Methylcrotonyl-glycinuria[302,304,786,804]	Biotin-responsive 3-methylcrotonyl-CoA-carboxylase and propionyl-CoA carboxylase[4]	Infancy	Variable but includes spinal muscular atrophy, mental retardation and vomiting, and reduced level of consciousness; cat urine odor	Ketoacidosis, increased urine 3-methylcrotonylglycinuria, 3-hydroxyisovaleric acid, tiglylglycine, methylcitric acid, and 3-hydroxypropionic acid
Tetrahydrofolate methyltransferase deficiency[15]	Tetrahydrofolate methyltransferase[2]	Infancy	Growth failure, psychomotor delay, hepatosplenomegaly, and infantile spasms	Megaloblastic acemia, cerebral atrophy, elevated serum folate
Pipecolatemia[272]	Unknown	Infancy	Hepatomegaly and hypotonia then tremor, ataxia, horizontal nystagmus and retinitis pigmentosa. Several patients with the cerebrohepatorenal syndrome	Generalized aminoaciduria, high plasma pipecolic acid levels
3-Hydroxy-3-methyl-glutaryl CoA lyase deficiency[898,216,232]	3-Hydroxy-3-methylglutaryl CoA lyase[4]	Infancy	Newborn or episodic hypotonia, vomiting and symptoms of acidosis	Acidosis; hypoglycemia; increased urine 3-hydroxy-3-methylglutaric acid
Hyperornithinemia[72]	Ornithine ketoacid transaminase	Childhood	Retardation	Hyperornithinemia, renal tubular abnormalities, liver dysfunction
Saccharopinuria[740,741,133]	Saccharopine-dehydrogenase[6]	Childhood	Mental retardation and spastic diplegia	Elevated urine and plasma lysine, citrulline, and homocitrulline. Increased CSF saccharopine
Glutathionemia[307]	Glutathione transpeptidase[5]	Adulthood	Mental retardation	Elevated serum glutathione

Disorder	Enzyme defect	Age of onset	Clinical features	Laboratory findings
Gamma-glutamylcysteine synthetase deficiency[668]	Gamma-glutamylcysteine synthetase[5]	Young adulthood	Spinocerebellar degeneration, peripheral neuropathy and in one patient, psychotic behavior	Hemolytic anemia; generalized aminoaciduria
Pyroglutamic aciduria[862]	Glutathione synthetase[5]	Infancy	Spastic quadriparesis, cerebellar ataxia, and tremor in one older, untreated patient; some mentally retarded	5-Oxoprolinuria and 5-Oxoprolinemia; hemolytic anemia; acidosis in infancy
Glutamate dehydrogenase deficiency[645]	Glutamate dehydrogenase[8]	Childhood Adulthood	Slowly progressive spinocerebellar ataxia, lower cranial nerve palsies and dyskinesias and tremors	Glutamic dehydrogenase deficiency in cultured fibroblasts and leukocytes
Hyperbeta-alaninemia[720]	Beta-alanine-alpha-ketoglutarate transaminase	Newborn	Lethargy and intractable seizures	Elevated serum and urine beta-alanine, beta-aminoisobutyric acid, and GABA
Carnosinemia[819]	Carnosinase	Infancy	Psychomotor regression, spasticity, and tonic-clonic and myoclonic seizures	Elevated serum and urine carnosine
Homocarnosinosis	Unknown	Adulthood	Psychomotor retardation and spastic tetraparesis	Elevated CSF homocarnosine
Carnitine acetyltransferase deficiency[196]	Carnitine acetyl transferase	Childhood	Episodes of disturbed consciousness. Later episodes of ataxia, hypotonia, hyporeflexia, and ophthalmoplegia, then coma, spasticity, and liver dysfunction	Moderately elevated lactate and pyruvate
Tryptophanemia[807]	Possible tryptophan pyrolase or kynurenine formylase[7]	Childhood	Cerebellar ataxia, photosensitive dermatitis, mental retardation, and growth failure	Elevated urine and plasma tryptophan without indicanuria or indolacetic aciduria
Methionine malabsorption (oasthouse urine disease)[394]	Intestinal and renal methionine, aromatic, and branched-chain amino acid malabsorption	Infancy	Episodic hypertonus, seizures, fever and respiratory disturbances. Psychomotor retardation. Unusual odor	Elevated fecal methionine; increased β-hydroxybutyric acid, branched-chain amino acids, phenylalanine, and tyrosine in urine
Blue diaper syndrome[206]	Intestinal tryptophan transport defect	Adulthood	Irritability	Elevated tryptophan in urine, hypercalcemia
Hyperornithinemia and homocitrullinemia[732]	Ornithine decarboxylase deficiency or mitochondrial transport defect	Infancy	Variable retardation, seizures, and ataxia. Episodic stupor	Hyperammonemia, ornithinemia, and homocitrullinemia

*Figure number for relevant metabolic pathway

Disorders Associated with Hyperammonemia

Urea cycle defects
Carbamyl phosphate synthetase deficiency (CPS 1)
Ornithine transcarbamylase deficiency (OTC)
Citrullinemia
Argininosuccinic aciduria
Arginase deficiency

Other metabolic defects
Propionic acidemia
Methylmalonic acidemia
Alpha-methylacetoacetic aciduria
Nonketotic hyperglycinemia
Hyperlysinemia
Familial lysinuric protein intolerance with dibasic
    aminoaciduria
Hyperornithinemia
Hyperornithinemia and homocitrullinemia
Hyperlysinuria
N-Acetylglutamate synthase deficiency[40]
Systemic carnitine deficiency
Transient hyperammonemia of the newborn

Miscellaneous disorders
Excessive protein intake
Stress/hypoxia
Prematurity
Reye's syndrome
Toxins
Biliary obstruction
Infections, infestations

These conditions can be divided into those that are familial and those that represent acquired hepatic insults. It is usually possible to separate these two groups on the basis of clinical features, family history, and laboratory evidence of hepatic dysfunction in acquired hepatic disease. In some instances, however, this distinction is not easy. Most notable among the acquired diseases that can be confused with the inherited deficiencies of the urea cycle enzymes is Reye's syndrome. Reye's syndrome is an illness characterized by a combination of encephalopathy and liver disease. During the active phase of Reye's syndrome, decreased activity of the mitochondrial enzymes, ornithine transcarbamylase and carbamyl phosphate synthetase, may occur.[108,741] Conversely, the clinical and biochemical features of late onset congenital ornithine transcarbamylase deficiency are easily confused with those in the Reye's syndrome.[266,381] Liver pathology, however, will distinguish these two conditions because in Reye's syndrome there is microvesicular fatty infiltration and mitochondrial changes that are not found in ornithine transcarbamylase deficiency.[462]

Another transient cause of hyperammonemia that can easily be confused with an inherited defect in the urea cycle occasionally occurs in the newborn preterm infant.[43,298] Although in some of these infants there is obvious severe perinatal asphyxia and evidence of liver dysfunction, others may have only mild respiratory distress and no hepatic dysfunction.[43] These patients are distinguished from neonates with defects in the urea cycle enzymes by the former's normal levels of these enzymes in liver tissue and by their normal levels of urea cycle metabolites. This is an important distinction because the hyperammonemia in these infants is often transient and responds well to prompt and aggressive treatment.

Other familial conditions may also be associated with hyperammonemia. As noted previously, the organic acidemias that produce the ketotic hyperglycinemia syndrome that is, beta-ketothiolase deficiency, propionic acidemia, methylmalonic acidemia, and isovaleric acidemia, may be associated with hyperammonemia. The origin of the hyperammonemia in these disorders is uncertain. Proposed mechanisms of hyperammonemia include inhibition of the transport of aspartic acid into mitochondria, secondary inhibition of hepatic urea cycle enzyme activity, deficiency of N-acetylglutamate, (an activator of carbamyl phosphate synthetase I) and diversion of ornithine from the urea cycle by the energy-generating arginine to alpha-ketoglutarate pathway.[327,341,791,891]

Hyperammonemia may also be seen in at least two other familial disorders. In congenital lysine intolerance a defect in transport of basic amino acids results in protein intolerance.[426,739] Symptoms of this disorder include feeding difficulties, vomiting, diarrhea, and aversion to protein. These patients often grow poorly and some are mentally retarded.[739] Hyperammonemia in this condition is intermittent and is associated with increased urinary excretion of lysine. Most of these patients have been Finnish. Citrulline supplement corrects the deficiency of urea cycle intermediates.[658] Hyperammonemia may also be associated with hyperornithinemia and homocitrul-linuria syndrome. In this syndrome there is often intermittent symptomatology including changes in mental status, ataxia, and seizures.[732] The defect in this disorder is not known.

Biochemistry

There are five enzymes involved in the elimination of free NH_3 derived from various deaminations (Fig. 9-6). Carbamyl phosphate synthetase (CPS) forms carbamyl phosphate from NH_3, adenosine triphosphate (ATP), and CO_2. CPS has two forms: the mitochondrial isozyme CPS I, which is involved in urea synthesis, and the cytosol form CPS II, which is active in pyrimidine synthesis.[815] The mitochondrial enzyme CPS I requires N-acetylglutamate as an activator.

Ornithine transcarbamylase (OTC) or ornithine carbamyl transferase (OCT) catalyzes the condensation of ornithine with carbamyl phosphate to form citrulline. The gene controlling OTC is located on the X chromosome. Symptoms of deficient activity are, therefore, much more severe in affected males (hemizygotes) than in heterozygous females. Carbamyl phosphate synthetized in mitochrondria, if not metabolized further, will accumulate in the cytosol, where it will enter the pyrimidine synthetic pathway and be excreted as orotic acid.[64]

Citrulline formed by the action of OTC is transported into the cytoplasm where it condenses with aspartate to form argininosuccinic acid (ASA) through the action of ASA synthetase. This compound is cleaved to arginine and fumarate by ASA lyase. Arginine is then cleaved to urea and ornithine, which can be transported back into the mitochondria to begin the cycle again.[267]

The urea cycle enzymes are present mainly in liver and to a much lesser extent in leukocytes.[656] These enzymes undergo great changes in activity depending on intercurrent illness and protein intake. For this reason as well as because of the considerable biochemical heterogeneity of these enzymes, measurement of their activity is difficult.[134,656] Tissue samples need to be processed rapidly for enzyme assay, which should be performed by an established laboratory familiar with the pitfalls of diagnosing urea cycle disorders.

Carbamyl Phosphate Synthetase Deficiency

This condition was first described in 1964 in a newborn infant who developed vomiting, lethargy, and hypertonia in response

FIG. 9-6. Urea cycle, ammonia metabolism, and relationships to the Krebs cycle. Reactions 1, 2, and the Krebs cycle take place in mitochondria. Enzymes indicated are: (1) carbamyl phosphate synthetase; (2) ornithine transcarbamylase; (3) argininosuccinic acid synthetase; (4) argininosuccinic acid lyase; and (5) arginase. Abbreviations used are: ADP for adenosine diphosphate; ARG for arginine; ASA for argininosuccinic acid; ASP for aspartate; ATP for adenosine triphosphate; αKG for alpha-ketoglutarate; OAA for oxaloacetate; ORN for ornithine; and Pi for inorganic phosphate.

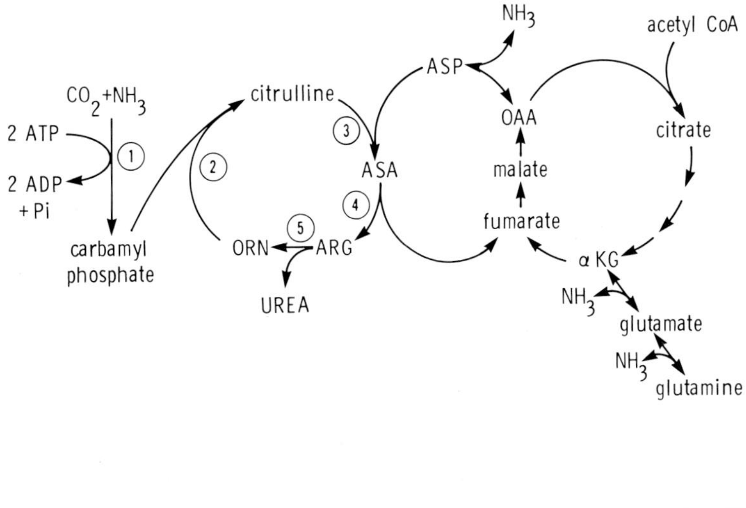

to protein feedings.[254] The child also had a mild metabolic acidosis, hyperglycinemia, and cyclic neutropenia. In fact, this infant may have had one of the ketotic hyperglycinemias. At least a dozen additional cases have been described since the original case. In each case, hyperammonemia and related symptoms have been the predominant features. Neurologically, these children are often hypotonic, although in at least one infant hypertonicity was noted. The natural course of the disease is poorly defined. One 13-year-old child with this disorder was retarded and had spastic quadriparesis and hemiparesis.[56] In contrast, two children with this disorder who had been treated developed normally during the first 18 months of life.

Hyperammonemia may be the only laboratory abnormality, although mild changes in blood amino acids may occur. Urine orotic acid is either normal or low, a feature useful in differentiating CPS deficiency from OTC deficiency. A family history of other affected children is often obtained. The mode of inheritance is uncertain but may be autosomal recessive.

The pathologic changes in CPS deficiency have not been defined. In one autopsied case reported as a case of CPS deficiency, the patient was deficient in glycolytic enzymes as well as urea cycle enzymes and hyperammonemia was not documented.[371] The diagnosis in this patient, therefore, is somewhat questionable.[730]

Ornithine Transcarbamylase Deficiency

Ornithine transcarbamylase deficiency is one of the most instructive inherited metabolic diseases. Initially, it appeared that OTC deficiency predominantly affected females.[735] We now know that males are also affected; however, males affected by this X-linked disorder were severely affected and died shortly after birth before a diagnosis could be made.[127,735]

Clinical Features and Diagnosis. The clinical features in males and females with OTC deficiency differ considerably. As noted above, this results from the more complete deficiency of OTC in males. A few examples of partial OTC deficiency in males have been associated with normal development or delayed onset of symptoms.[456,902]

The disease in males is generally fatal. The onset of the symptoms occurs very soon after birth, usually within the first day of life. The symptoms are those of extreme hyperammonemia, including vomiting, a gradual reduction in level of consciousness ultimately reaching coma, rapid respirations, hypotonia, hypothermia, and convulsions. Death often occurs within the first week of life. Infants surviving this initial illness are usually left profoundly retarded. Several males with partial OTC deficiency have been reported.[730] These patients often have had normal development until a sudden attack of hyperammonemia. These attacks occurred at variable ages ranging from 4 weeks to 10 years of age.

Heterozygous females have a partial OTC deficiency. The clinical symptomatology in females has been quite variable. The disease is occasionally fatal but more often results in episodic symptoms, commonly including vomiting and variable disturbances of consciousness and motor function. Headache often accompanies these symptoms and may be misdiagnosed as migraine headaches, especially complicated migraine headache.[691] This error is understandable because the symptomatology in the heterozygous female may be quite similar to that encountered in so-called acute confusional migraine. A family history of similar headaches in female relatives may even be elicited. Other symptoms in the heterozygous female include failure to thrive and mental retardation. Even among supposedly asymptomatic carriers of OTC deficiency, cerebral dysfunction may be much more common than previously suspected. Performance on intelligence tests has been reported to be below that of their protein-tolerant siblings.[56]

Laboratory features of OTC deficiency are principally hyperammonemia associated with increased urinary excretion of orotic acid. This increased orotate excretion, especially after a protein load, is a sensitive indicator of the OTC heterozygous state.[58] Other laboratory abnormalities that are inconsistently reported include elevated plasma glutamine, lysine, and alanine, subnormal plasma alpha-ketoglutarate, and increased urinary excretion of N-carbamylaspartate and N-carbamyl-beta-alanine.[594]

The enzyme defect cannot be diagnosed in leukocytes, so liver must be used for enzyme assays.[656,754] Measurements of orotic acid in amniotic fluid have failed to detect an affected fetus.[537]

Pathologically, the changes in the brain seem to be rather nonspecific. Alzheimer type II astrocytic changes have been noted, a result of the marked hyperammonemia. Loss of cerebral white matter has also been reported.[113]

Citrullinemia

Citrullinemia is a defect in the third step of the urea cycle. Citrulline accumulates in the urine and plasma. Argininosuccinic acid synthetase activity is reduced or undetectable in the liver but may be normal in other organs.[678,840] The enzyme defect is variable and may be found in liver, brain, cultured fibroblasts, and leukocytes.[870] Prenatal diagnosis is possible using cultured amniotic fluid cells.[278] Several clinical syndromes have occurred in association with citrullinemia. The disorder may present in the newborn period in a manner quite similar to that described above for OTC deficiency. Associated with the neonatal form, one may also find hypocalcemia, hypoglycemia or elevations in liver enzymes. Other infants with citrullinemia have a more gradual onset of symptoms manifested by episodes of vomiting and feeding problems. These episodes may be associated with alterations of consciousness and other neurologic abnormalities such as ataxia, tremor, and seizures. These patients may also have signs of hepatic dysfunction in the form of hepatomegaly and elevated liver transaminases. Mental retardation may accompany this disorder. At least one asymptomatic patient has been reported.[875] One patient with onset at 21 years of age had episodic disturbances of consciousness and later developed a myelopathy.[554]

Citrullinuria has also been encountered in a patient with cystinuria. Citrulline, in this case, was not elevated in the plasma, and other basic amino acids, (cystine, lysine, arginine, and ornithine) were also elevated in the urine.[842]

Argininosuccinic Aciduria

Argininosuccinic aciduria is caused by the deficiency of the enzyme L-argininosuccinic acid lyase. It is probably the most common defect in the urea acid cycle. The incidence of argininosuccinic acid lyase deficiency is variously estimated to be between 1 in 70,000 to 1 in 250,000 live births.[721] Hyperammonemia in this condition is a variable finding.

Clinical Features. As in the case of the other defects in urea cycle metabolism, the clinical features of argininosuccinic aciduria are variable. The most severe form of this disease begins in the neonatal period and is characterized by prominent hyperammonemia that produces lethargy, feeding problems, seizures, and ultimately coma.[296] Death usually follows within a few weeks.

In other infants the disease runs a much more protracted course but is also characterized by feeding difficulties and vomiting. These children grow and develop poorly. Hepatomegaly has generally been a prominent feature. Trichorrhexis nodosa (friable hair with a characteristic microscopic appearance) is a typical feature of this disorder. In some children the psychomotor delay and feeding disturbances are not recognized until late infancy or early childhood.[559] These patients often manifest intermittent ataxia. Seizures occur frequently. Patients with normal or borderline normal intelligence have also been described in argininosuccinic aciduria.[559,730] A mild form responsive to protein restriction has been described recently.

Laboratory Abnormalities. The markedly increased ASA is readily detectable in the urine of these patients. Citrulline and orotic acid may also be increased in the urine. Ammonia levels may be normal, particularly in the late onset varieties of argininosuccinic aciduria. A protein load usually causes a protracted rise in blood NH_3.[355] The enzyme defect can be detected in red blood cells, cultured fibroblasts, and amniotic fluid cells. Prenatal diagnosis is possible by this means or by measurement of ASA in amniotic fluid.[308]

Argininemia

At least 10 cases of argininemia, a defect in urea cycle metabolism due to arginase deficiency, have been reported.[759] Symptoms of hyperammonemia usually begin in infancy. These bouts of hyperammonemia usually occur episodically and are manifested by vomiting followed by irritability, drowsiness, seizures, and coma. Mental retardation is a common sequela of this defect. Marked spastic diplegia has also been noted in all of the reported cases.

Urine chromatography reveals elevated arginine unless the patient is on a low protein diet. The urinary amino acid pattern may resemble that in cystinuria but the elevated blood NH_3 level, along with the clinical history, should allow argininemia to be distinguished from cystinuria. Absence of arginase activity in red blood cells confirms the diagnosis of argininemia.[136]

General Treatment of Hyperammonemia

The acute management of hyperammonemia is directed toward correcting the functional derangements and lowering the NH_3 level. Shock, acidosis, increased intracranial pressure, and respiratory failure should be treated with the usual supportive measures. All exogenous protein intake should be stopped. Blood products should be used only as needed because of the nitrogen load. Production of NH_3 in the gut can be diminished with oral neomycin or lactulose.

Specific treatment to lower the NH_3 level centers around direct removal and enhanced excretion. Exchange transfusion and peritoneal dialysis are both effective, but the latter may be preferable because of the enhanced removal of the NH_3 precursors alanine, glutamine, and glutamate. Arginine (4 mmol/kg per day) should be provided to ensure that a deficiency of ornithine does not limit NH_3 detoxification.[55,111] Sodium benzoate (250 mg/kg per day) can enhance NH_3 excretion by conjugation with glycine to form hippurate.[55,112]

Chronic treatment of urea cycle disorders is imperfect at present. Protein restriction, perhaps with essential amino acids added in an amount necessary for growth, is important.[759] The carbon skeletons of five essential amino acids given as their alpha-keto analogs can cut nitrogen intake further in CPS deficiency, citrullinemia, and presumably other disorders.[56,820] Enhancing the excretion of nitrogen as citrulline by providing arginine supplementation daily has been useful in citrullinemia and OTC deficiency.[57] It appears that arginine supplementation will be useful except in arginase deficiency and benzoate therapy may be generally useful. The long-term prognosis is guarded for patients with severe deficiencies of urea cycle enzymes, but with vigorous emergency treatment and careful nutritional management satisfactory growth and development appear possible.

DEFECTS IN LYSINE METABOLISM

Defects in lysine metabolism include persistent and intermittent hyperlysinemia, saccharopinuria, hyperpipecolatemia, and glutaric aciduria.

Most of the defects in lysine metabolism are very rare. These rare defects in lysine metabolism are shown in Table 9-6. Only glutaric aciduria has been described in a sufficient number of patients to have established a clinical picture.

BIOCHEMISTRY

Lysine is an essential amino acid. Like ornithine, it has a terminal amino group. Lysine can be incorporated into protein, hydroxylated, or decarboxylated to cadaverine. Like ornithine in the urea cycle it can accept a carbamyl group to become homocitrulline and be metabolized analogously to homoarginine. The catabolism of lysine proceeds by two pathways (Fig. 9-7). The major pathway is through conjugation with alpha-ketoglutarate to form saccharopine, then alpha-aminoadipate, then alpha-ketoadipate, and finally glutaryl-CoA.[361] An alternate pathway through epsilon-N-acetyllysine and pipecolate to alpha-aminoadipate also exists.[685] Glutaryl-CoA undergoes oxidation by its dehydrogenase to glutaconyl-CoA. The end-product of lysine catabolism is acetoacetyl-CoA.

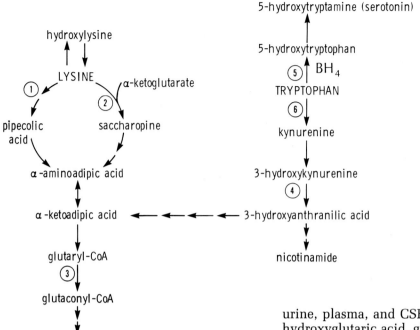

FIG. 9-7. Lysine and tryptophan metabolism. BH_4 is a cofactor for tryptophan hydroxylase. Enzymes indicated are: (1) lysine dehydrogenase; (2) lysine alpha-ketoglutarate reductase; (3) glutaryl-CoA dehydrogenase; (4) kynureninase; (5) tryptophan hydroxylase; and (6) tryptophan pyrrolase. Tetrahydrobiopterin is abbreviated BH_4.

Glutaric Aciduria

There are at least two disorders associated with massive increases in glutaric acid in the urine. These two conditions have been labeled type I and type II and are associated with rather distinctive clinical pictures.

Type I glutaric aciduria typically has its onset at several months of age, but may go undetected until several years of age. Although infants may present with ketoacidosis, more commonly the condition has been detected in childhood. In childhood, the disorder presents a striking neurologic picture of mental retardation, choreoathetosis, dystonia, facial grimacing, spastic quadriparesis, and occasional seizures.[101,309,460,871] These patients may also have hypoglycemia or ketoacidosis.[871]

Patients with type I glutaric aciduria have markedly increased glutaric acid in the urine, plasma, and CSF. In addition, beta-hydroxyglutaric acid, glutaconic acid, aminoadipic acid, and saccharopine have also been elevated in the urine. This pattern of elevated organic acids is consistent with the demonstrated defect in glutaryl-CoA dehydrogenase (Fig. 9-7). This enzyme has been absent or inactive in patients with type I glutaric aciduria, whereas the parents of these children have had intermediate enzyme activity.[871]

Pathologic studies of the brain of one child with type I glutaric aciduria revealed gliosis and neuronal loss in the putamen and caudate, histologic changes resembling those in Huntington's chorea.[309]

Type II glutaric aciduria is associated with a considerably different clinical picture from that seen in type I. These patients generally present in the neonatal period or in early infancy with ketoacidosis and are acutely ill.[310,651,805] As in isovaleric aciduria, these patients may have a sweaty-feet odor. In addition mild dysmorphic features, especially of dermatoglyphics, are sometimes noted. In at least one instance, an infant presented in a fashion similar to that seen in Reye's syndrome.[309]

Unlike type I glutaric aciduria, in type II glutaric aciduria ketoacidosis has been a constant finding. In addition, hyperammonemia and hypoglycemia are regular features. Elevated lactic acid, glutaric acid, and other dicarboxylic acids are found in the urine. The enzymatic defect appears to affect several metabolic pathways at steps involving acyl-CoA dehydrogenases.

Treatment of type I glutaric aciduria has included dietary restriction, riboflavin, and a gamma-amino butyric acid (GABA) analogue, 4-amino-3-(chlorophenyl)butyric acid. Dietary treatment has consisted of a low protein diet or a diet low in lysine and tryptophan; the former has resulted in no or slight improvement, whereas the latter was associated with moderate improvement.[102,312] The GABA analogue was associated with marked improvement.[102] No effective treatment for the severe infantile form of glutaric aciduria type II has been found.

DEFECTS IN AMINO ACID TRANSPORT

Transport of amino acids is a property of most mammalian cell membranes. Much has been learned about amino acid transport from the study of amino acid transport disorders. A large number of these defects has been described. Some of these defects are now considered benign, normal variations (see list, Aminoacidurias of Questionable Neurologic Significance), others do not produce significant neurologic symptoms (cystinuria), and some of those amino acid transport disorders that produce neurologic symptoms are extremely rare (Table 9-6). In this section we will discuss only Hartnup disease and Lowe's syndrome. Both of these disorders affect renal and intestinal amino acid transport. Other transport disorders, such as tryptophan malabsorption, affect amino acid transport in only one organ.

Hartnup Disease

Hartnup disease is a defect in neutral (monoamino-monocarboxylic) amino acid transport that in its classical form produces a pellagralike skin eruption, intermittent cerebellar ataxia, mental retardation, and psychosis. The disorder is named for the original family in which this condition was described.[50] As the list of the incidence of inherited metabolic diseases affecting the nervous system shows, Hartnup disease is one of the more common aminoacidurias; the incidence is approximately 1:26,000 live births.[481,482]

Biochemistry.   There are three major renal transport systems for monocarboxylic alpha-amino acids. One transports glycine, proline, and hydroxyproline. A defect in this system results in iminoglycinuria, which is probably of no clinical significance. A second system is for cystine, arginine, lysine, and ornithine. A defect in this system results in cystinuria, a disorder of questionable neurologic significance. If cystine is transported but arginine, lysine and ornithine are not, hyperdibasicaminoaciduria (asymptomatic) or lysinuric protein intolerance (discussed with hyperammonemia and the urea cycle defects) occurs.

The third system transports a group of thirteen monoamine-monocarboxylic acids. This transport system is defective in the kidney and intestine in Hartnup disease. The intestinal absorption of most amino acids in Hartnup disease is variable, but tryptophan is always affected. Bacterial metabolism of unabsorbed tryptophan results in the production of metabolites (indoles) that may be absorbed and then appear in the urine.

Symptoms in Hartnup disease are apparently due to a deficiency of nicotinamide and its precursor, tryptophan (Fig. 9-7). The diagnosis depends more on the pattern of aminoaciduria than on the quantity.[104,393]

Clinical and Laboratory Features.   The clinical features of Hartnup disease are quite variable. It seems likely that genetic and environmental factors can influence the manifestations of Hartnup disease. It even appears that a nutritious diet may protect the patient with Hartnup disease from developing symptoms.[881] Ataxia is the most common neurologic symptom. This ataxia generally begins acutely often in infancy or early childhood but can also begin as late as 18 years of age.[393] The onset of the ataxia often corresponds to periods of stress, poor nutrition, or intercurrent illness. The ataxia is appendicular, involves both upper and lower extremities, and is often accompanied by nystagmus. Recovery from ataxia usually occurs over a period of days to weeks. A skin eruption often accompanies these attacks but may occur alone. This eruption, quite similar to that seen in pellagra, is a dry, scaly eruption occurring on exposed body parts. During severe skin eruptions, vesicular and bullous skin lesions may occur.

Other neurologic symptoms that may occur intermittently include vascular headaches, myalgia, syncope, and personality changes. Mild mental retardation has been a common, but by no means constant, feature in Hartnup disease. Indeed, some patients may have superior intelligence even though other neurologic symptoms may be prominent.[895] In general, all symptoms tend to improve as the patient grows older.

Hartnup disease appears to be transmitted as an autosomal recessive trait. It seems likely, however, that multiple alleles are involved. Individuals heterozygous for Hartnup disease may have photosensitive skin eruptions.[345]

Diagnosis. Hartnup disease should be suspected in patients with intermittent ataxia, especially if the ataxia is accompanied by a pellagralike skin eruption. The differential diagnosis for intermittent ataxia is given in Table 9-2. Hartnup disease can be differentiated from the other conditions producing intermittent ataxia and from pellagra on the basis of the urinary amino acid excretion pattern. In Hartnup disease neutral amino acids are increased in the urine; these include tryptophan, alanine, asparagine, citrulline, glutamine, histidine, valine, isoleucine, leucine, phenylalanine, serine, threonine, and tyrosine. In addition, urinary indicans are excreted in large amounts. Hartnup disease can be distinguished from tryptophanemia on the basis that serum tryptophan is normal in Hartnup disease (Table 9-6).

Treatment. Treatment of Hartnup disease consists of administration of nicotinic acid and supplemental protein. The response to this therapy, however, has been hard to evaluate because the disease is variable and tends to remit spontaneously.

Lowe's Syndrome

Lowe's syndrome is another disorder in which there appears to be a defect in amino acid transport. This X-linked syndrome, described in 1952, consists of dysmorphic facial features, psychomotor retardation, growth failure, and renal rickets. The renal rickets appears to be due to a renal tubular transport defect that leads to hypercalcuria, renal tubular acidosis, and generalized aminoaciduria. The renal tubular defect does not appear to be distinctive. Transport defects involving other organs have not been described in Lowe's syndrome.[501]

The neurologic signs and symptoms in this disorder are nonlocalizing. Infants with Lowe's syndrome may present as floppy infants. Deep tendon reflexes may be absent or reduced. Blindness is a common feature and seems to be a result of the congenital cataracts seen in this condition.

The neuropathologic features have been variable but have included hypoplastic cerebellum, hydrocephalus, multiple cyst formation, and evidence of abnormal neuronal migration.[669] Lowe's syndrome is treated symptomatically. Patients with this disorder expire early in life even though the metabolic abnormalities do tend to improve as the child grows older.

VERY RARE AMINOACIDOPATHIES WITH NEUROLOGIC DYSFUNCTION AND AMINOACIDURIAS OF QUESTIONABLE NEUROLOGIC SIGNIFICANCE

In Table 9-6 we have listed aminoacidopathies which have been reported in only a few families (usually less than three). The

Aminoacidurias of Questionable Neurologic Significance

Histidinemia
Methioninemia
Cystathioninemia
Beta-mercaptolactate-cystine disulfiduria
Persistent hyperlysinemia
Alpha-ketoadipic aciduria
Xanthurenic aciduria
Hyperprolinemia types 1 and 2
Hydroxyprolinemia[471]
Alpha-aminoadipic acidemia
Sarcosinemia
Dicarboxylic aciduria
Cystinuria
Cystine-lysinuria
Glycinuria
Beta-aminoisobutyric aciduria

clinical features and to some extent the enzyme defects of these disorders should be viewed as tentative. In addition, we have listed below the aminoacidurias which are of questionable neurologic significance either because these are viewed as benign variants or because there are no definite neurologic signs and symptoms.

DISORDERS OF PYRUVATE METABOLISM AND SUBACUTE NECROTIZING ENCEPHALOMYELOPATHY

BIOCHEMISTRY

Pyruvate occupies a pivotal position in several metabolic pathways. In particular, pyruvate is important in energy metabolism. It is not surprising, therefore, that pyruvate metabolism is under very tight control and even minor alterations in the metabolism of pyruvate produce substantial metabolic consequences. Several inborn errors of pyruvate metabolism have been described.[76] Those entities with neurologic consequences include hereditary pyruvate dehydrogenase deficiency, pyruvate carboxylase deficiency, and defects in pyruvate dehydrogenase activity resulting from deficient cofactors or abnormal modulation.

Pyruvate dehydrogenase (PDH) complex (Fig. 9-8) is a prototype enzyme complex, with three separable components present together in the mitochondria. The complex catalyzes the conversion of pyruvate to acetyl-CoA. In the nervous system, most of the product enters the Krebs cycle, but small amounts are necessary for acetylcholine synthesis.

The first catalytic step involves PDH itself, also called *pyruvate decarboxylase*, or E_1. Thiamine pyrophosphate is a cofactor in this reaction, in which CO_2 is released. Pyruvate decarboxylase is the regulated step of the PDH complex. Regulation is accomplished by an activator, PDH kinase, and an inactivator, PDH phosphorylase. They in turn are governed by the concentration of substrates (pyruvate, reduced CoA and the oxidized form of nicotinamide-adenine dinucleotide [NAD^+]), products (acetyl-CoA and the reduced form of NAD.

[NADH]),[582,613,773] and insulin to adjust the rate of acetyl-CoA synthesis to fluctuating needs.

After E_1, the resulting hydroxyethyl moiety is transferred to E_2, dihydrolipoate transacetylase. In this step, the disulfide bond of the lipoate arm is broken, and the acetyl group is transferred to CoA to form acetyl-CoA. The disulfide bond of E_2 is reformed through the action of E_3, dihydrolipoate dehydrogenase. This enzyme uses a flavoprotein electron acceptor, which itself is regenerated by transfer of electrons to NAD^+.

Disorders in PDH have been difficult to identify. The clinical severity usually reflects the degree of enzyme impairment *in vitro*. Pyruvate dehydrogenase disorders may be suspected by an increased anion gap, lactic acidosis, and elevated alanine in the blood and urine (reflecting the elevation in pyruvate, its alpha-keto acid analog). Elevated pyruvate is more difficult to demonstrate than lactic acidosis because the equilibrium between the two is heavily toward lactate. Disturbances of PDH complex may lead to abnormal sensitivity to fats or carbohydrates.

Pyruvate may also enter the Krebs cycle as oxaloacetate. Pyruvate carboxylase catalyzes this reaction, which requires biotin as a cofactor. Deficiency of pyruvate carboxylase may result in lactic acidosis and impaired gluconeogenesis from alanine.

Cautious dietary challenges with glucose, galactose, fructose, glycerol, and alanine can help to define the origin of lactic acidosis. Fasting hypoglycemia, often accompanied by ketosis, suggests impaired gluconeogenesis, with excess production of hexose or triose intermediates and diversion to pyruvate and lactate. (The phosphorylated intermediates are unable to leave the cell.) Such disorders include glucose-6-phosphatase deficiency (von Gierke's disease) fructose 1,6-diphosphatase deficiency, and phosphoenolpyruvate carboxykinase (PEPCK) deficiency. These disorders may produce acute and recurrent symptoms, but usually do not result in neurologic deterioration. Defects in PDH may result in fasting acidosis, carbohydrate dependence, and fat intolerance, and less commonly, carbohydrate intolerance. Stepwise or progressive disease is more likely a

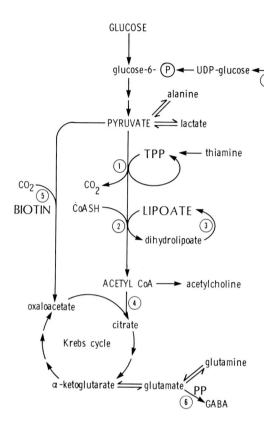

FIG. 9-8. Galactose and pyruvate metabolism. Enzymes *1*, *2*, and *3* comprise the pyruvate dehydrogenase (PDH) complex. Vitamin-derived cofactors are shown in bold type. Synthesis of the neurotransmitters acetylcholine and GABA is indicated. Enzymes indicated are: *(1)* pyruvate decarboxylase (E_1); *(2)* dihydrolipoyl transacetylase (E_2); *(3)* dihydrolipoyl dehydrogenase (E_3); *(4)* citrate synthetase; *(5)* pyruvate carboxylase; *(6)* glutamate decarboxylase; *(7)* galactokinase; *(8)* galactose-1-phosphate uridyl transferase; and *(9)* UDP-galactose-4-epimerase. Abbreviations used are: GABA for gamma-aminobutyric acid; (P) for phosphate; PP for pyridoxal phosphate; TPP for thiamine pyrophosphate; and UDP for uridine diphosphate.

result of impairment within the PDH complex, perhaps as a result of inadequate production of energy or acetylcholine.

PYRUVATE DEHYDROGENASE ENZYME COMPLEX ABNORMALITIES

Although deficiency of PDH complex activity may be a consequence of deficient activity of any of the component enzymes of the PDH complex, the clinical symptoms seem more dependent upon the degree of deficiency.[76] Based upon 50 reported cases Blass has identified three groups of patients with PDH deficiency.[76,411,876] In the first group, enzyme activity is generally less than 15% of control activity. The onset of the illness in this group occurs in infancy or early childhood and is characterized by severe psychomotor delay, growth failure, absent subcutaneous fat, and neurologic signs including spasticity, hypotonia, muscle wasting, and optic atrophy. The second group of patients have intermediate PDH enzyme activity generally ranging from 20% to 35% of normal activity. In these children, the disease usually begins in late infancy or early childhood. The onset of the disease and exacerbations of the disease usually correspond to periods of infections, commonly respiratory. Frequent symptoms include lethargy, ataxia, bulbar and oculomotor paresis, and motor regression. During these exacerbations, which generally last 2 weeks or more, the patient may be areflexic. In periods between these exacerbations the patient may have few neurologic signs but often has growth failure and is intellectually delayed. The third group of patients may be clinically indistinguishable from patients with Friedreich's ataxia, and have a disorder characterized by progressive posterior column signs, absent deep tendon reflexes in the lower extremities, gait ataxia, kyphoscoliosis, pes cavus, positive Babinsky responses, and cardiomyopathy. The activity of the PDH complex in this group of patients has been found to be only mildly reduced, 35% to 50% of control activity. Although some investigators find that patients with PDH complex deficiency constitute a significant percentage of patients with Friedreich's ataxia, others have been unable to demonstrate an enzymatic abnormality in these patients. One other clinical group of patients, those with "ragged-red ataxia," may also have reduced PDH complex activity.[411]

Whether any of these defects in PDH complex activity are primary deficiencies of the component enzymes or simply reductions in activity secondary to perturbations in regulatory factors remains unclear. The purified PDH complex proteins have not been studied in any of these disorders.

PYRUVATE CARBOXYLASE DEFICIENCY

Approximately 12 patients have been described with pyruvate carboxylase deficiency.[195] The onset of this disorder generally tends to occur within the first six months of life. Metabolic acidosis and seizures are the most common mode of presentation. Other common features include psychomotor regression, hypotonia, which may later be replaced by spasticity, and failure to thrive. This disorder is reported to imitate subacute necrotizing encephalomyelopathy, but this contention has been challenged on the basis that little pathologic confirmation of subacute necrotizing encephalomyelopathy or confirmation of pyruvate carboxylase deficiency has been given.[21]

Lactate and pyruvate levels in pyruvate carboxylase deficiency tend to be moderately to markedly elevated.[110] In addition, serum alanine may also be increased because pyruvate carboxylase is an important enzyme in the gluconeogenic pathway leading from alanine. Mild elevation in serum NH_3 is occasionally noted.[701] In one patient renal tubular acidosis was also encountered.[21]

The pathologic changes in pyruvate carboxylase deficiency have been studied in only a few infants. Degenerative changes and changes consistent with developmental arrests have been described. The degenerative changes appear to involve chiefly white matter where there is evidence of white matter destruction. In addition, subependymal gliosis and protoplasmic astrocytic hyperplasia has been observed.[21] The sibling of one child with pyruvate carboxylase deficiency had pathologic features of subacute necrotizing encephalomyelopathy.[373]

SECONDARY DEFECTS OF PYRUVATE METABOLISM

Several disorders are known to alter pyruvate metabolism by altering the activities of regulated enzymes involved in pyruvate metabolism. These disorders include carnitine acetyltransferase deficiency and disorders of branched-chain amino acid metabolism.

TREATMENT OF PYRUVATE METABOLIC DISORDERS

Treatment of these disorders must be individualized because patients with apparently similar enzyme defects may require different treatments. The first priority is preventing the episodes of acidosis. Some patients may require a high fat, ketogenic, diet that generates acetyl-CoA from lipid and minimizes the use of carbohydrates as an energy source. Other patients may do better on a high carbohydrate diet, with frequent feedings.

Patients with PDH complex disorders have responded favorably to both high protein[80] and high carbohydrate diets;[676] or they have worsened on a high carbohydrate diet.[135] One patient with PDH phosphatase deficiency required a high carbohydrate diet, which apparently kept the PDH complex fully activated at all times.[674]

Patients with pyruvate carboxylase deficiency have responded to a low carbohydrate diet or a special diet with amino acid supplements of glutamine or aspartate to provide 4-carbon substrates for the Krebs cycle.[110,183,812]

The vitamin cofactors should certainly be given as well, even if the enzyme defect does not seem to warrant it. The patients of Lonsdale and associates and of Wick responded to thiamine.[497,876] In one case the response to thiamine was perhaps due to stabilization of the enzyme complex, which increased overall activity.[459,497,876]

Some patients have responded favorably for reasons that were not clear. The patients of Brunette with pyruvate carboxylase (PC) deficiency were improved on thiamine, a cofactor for pyruvate decarboxylase (PDC).[110] A patient of Maesaka and associates with PC deficiency required both thiamine and lipoic acid for improvement.[511] All patients so far described with PC deficiency due to multiple carboxylase deficiency (q.v.) have responded well to biotin.

SUBACUTE NECROTIZING ENCEPHALOMYELOPATHY

This disorder is a clinical syndrome that was first described by Denis Leigh in 1951.[474] Although a biochemical abnormality has been associated with subacute necrotizing encephalomyelopathy (SNE), the diagnosis ultimately requires pathologic confirmation.

Pathology

The brain of patients with SNE typically appears grossly normal. Microscopically, bilateral, often symmetric lesions occur in the periventricular regions, periaqueductal region, brain stem tegmentum, cerebellum, substantia nigra, optic nerves, and spinal cord. These lesions are characterized by loss of myelin, and by gliosis, tissue rarefaction, capillary proliferation, and relative sparing of neurons and axons. These lesions are similar to those in Wernicke's encephalopathy but the distribution of the lesions is different in the two conditions. In contrast to Wernicke's encephalopathy, in SNE the brain stem, basal ganglia, and optic nerves are commonly affected but the thalamus and mamillary bodies are usually unaffected.

Biochemistry

SNE in different patients has been associated with a defect in PDH activity; deficient cytochrome oxidase activity; a urinary inhibitor of thiamine diphosphate phosphoryl transferase; and elevated CSF and brain beta-endorphin levels.[21,100,151,883] The most commonly reported abnormality has been the urinary inhibitor of thiamine diphosphate phosphoryl transferase. Although there is a 20% false negative rate and false positives can accompany other neurologic diseases, neurologic abnormalities in the large pedigree cited above did correlate well with the presence of the urinary inhibitor.[646] Thiamine triphosphate (TTP), the end product of the reaction catalyzed by the transferase enzyme, has been found to be decreased in brains of patients with SNE.[644] The function of TTP in brain is not clear, and the significance of the inhibitor is controversial.

Clinical and Laboratory Features

The clinical features are extremely variable.[642] In one well-studied family in which one member died with pathologically proven SNE seven of the 68 family members examined had neurologic abnormalities.[646] Mental retardation was the most common abnormality, but the severity of clinical abnormality was quite variable. The age of onset of neurologic abnormalities varied from infancy to early childhood and these abnormalities began insidiously or abruptly. Partial or complete neurologic remissions usually occured in this family. Exacerbation of neurologic symptoms is common in SNE and has been observed in half of the reported cases.[642] Clinical features reported in more than half of the cases include hypotonia, weakness, dysphagia, psychomotor retardation, and episodes of vomiting.[642] Other frequent signs are spasticity (at times superimposed on lower motor neuron signs, e.g., absent reflexes), ataxia, seizures, and blindness due to optic atrophy.[642] The most diagnostically helpful signs in SNE are the frequent disturbances of ocular movement and of respiration. Nystagmus, strabismus, oculomotor apraxia, and even pupillary abnormalities may occur. Respiratory disturbances include sighing respiration, hyperventilation, and apnea.

Most laboratory tests are normal in SNE patients. Lactic acidosis and hyperalanemia have been described.[67,143,323,373] One patient with pathologically proven SNE had a unique cerebral angiogram that revealed prominent, small, perforating vessels supplying the diencephalon and mesencephalon, the sites of greatest involvement as demonstrated pathologically.[318]

Genetics

Most forms of SNE are transmitted in an autosomal recessive manner. Males and females are affected. No vertical transmission occurs but siblings are commonly affected.[646] The expression of this condition is quite variable. Two families have been reported in which spinocerebellar degeneration and SNE occurred in successive generations suggesting an autosomal dominant mode of transmission.[318,328]

Treatment

Effective treatment of SNE is not well documented. Thiamine in high doses was administered but did not produce sustained improvement.[643] Other therapeutic attempts have been aimed at supplying Krebs cycle intermediates, the assumption being that there was decreased pyruvate carboxylase activity.[143] The patients with elevated beta-endorphin levels were given naloxone.[100] There was an initial response to the naloxone but repeated doses were ineffective.

MITOCHONDRIAL METABOLIC DISEASE

Numerous reports of patients with presumed mitochondrial defects associated with encephalopathy, myopathy, or both have appeared in the recent literature. In most of these patients the nature of the mitochondrial defect has not been directly demonstrated; rather, the defect has been inferred from the histochemical abnormality, the so-called ragged red appearance of muscle fibers stained with the Gomori trichrome stain, or ultrastructural mitochondrial abnormalities. Many of these patients have had lactic acidemia. Clinically, the symptoms have been quite variable. In some patients a proximal myopathy predominates.[354,517] Several of these patients have also had growth failure. In other patients an encephalopathy predominates.[354] The features of the encephalopathy have been quite inconsistent. In general, psychomotor retardation has been common. Some of the clinical syndromes in which mitochondrial abnormalites have been found include SNE, cerebral poliodystrophy, and acute focal or hemispheric syndromes.[107,161,354,728,749,883] A variety of mitochondrial defects have been found in patients including loose coupling of oxidative phosphorylation, cytochrome c oxidase deficiency, deficient reduceable cytochrome b, and both cytochrome aa_3 and cytochrome b deficiencies.[556,832,839,883]

THE LYSOSOMAL STORAGE DISEASES

The lysosomal storage diseases are characterized by storage within lysosomes of excessive amounts of various complex cellular or extracellular substances, usually because their degradation is impaired. In many cases, the nature of the stored substance has provided a clue to the deficient enzyme. The relevant enzymes are usually expressed in readily available tissue, such as fibroblasts or leukocytes.

The lysosomes are single-membrane-bound intracellular structures in which degradative enzymes act upon their substrates, particularly membranes and extracellular substances. The substrate must be taken into the lysosome. There is evidence that enzymes must be taken up as well. An enzyme probably has sites necessary for recognition by and uptake into the lysosome and may undergo modification or activation once it is internalized. Lysosomal enzymes characteristically are most active at a pH of 4 to 5, which is much more acidic than the milieu in the surrounding cytoplasm. Modern concepts of lysosomes and lysosomal storage diseases are discussed in a recent text.[124]

Classification of the lysosomal storage diseases is somewhat arbitrary and may undergo further revision in the future. We find it helpful to think in terms of mucopolysaccharidoses, glycoproteinoses, sphingolipidoses, multiple enzyme deficiencies, lipidoses, and then a miscellaneous group (see list, Lysosomal Storage Diseases). An example of the lack of precision of this classification scheme is multiple sulfatase deficiency, which could be classified as a sphingolipidosis, a mucopolysaccharidosis, or as we have done, as one of a special group of disorders characterized by multiple enzyme deficiencies. Therefore, it should be emphasized that one should not be too inflexible in thinking about categorization of these diseases.

Lysosomal Storage Diseases

Clinical Conditions	Enzyme Defect
Mucopolysaccharidoses (MPS)	
MPS I H (Hurler's syndrome)	α-L-Iduronidase
MPS I S (Scheie's syndrome)	α-L-Iduronidase
MPS I Intermediate types (including Hurler/Scheie compound)	α-L-Iduronidase
MPS II (Hunter's syndrome)	
Severe, mild, and intermediate forms	Iduronate sulfatase
MPS III (Sanfilippo's syndrome)	
Type A	Heparan N-sulfate sulfatase
Type B	N-Acetyl-α-glucosaminidase
Type C	Acetyl CoA: α-glucosaminide N-acetyltransferase
Type D	Heparan sulfate-specific N-acetylglucosamine-6-sulfate sulfatase
MPS IV (Morquio's syndrome)	
Classic severe forms and milder variants	N-Acetylgalactosamine-6-sulfate sulfatase
Milder variants	β-Galactosidase
MPS V Vacant (formerly Scheie's syndrome)	
MPS VI (Maroteaux-Lamy syndrome)	
Severe, mild, and intermediate forms	N-Acetylgalactosamine-4-sulfate sulfatase
MPS VII	
Severe, mild and intermediate forms	β-Glucuronidase
Glycoproteinoses	
Mannosidosis	
Severe and mild forms	α-Mannosidase
Fucosidosis	
Severe and milder forms	α-Fucosidase
Aspartylglycosaminuria	Amidase
Sialidosis	
Severe, mild, and intermediate forms (includes ML I)	Neuraminidase
Multiple Enzyme Deficiencies	
Multiple sulfatase deficiency	Multiple sulfatases
ML II	Recognition site phosphorylation defect
ML III	Recognition site phosphorylation defect
Sphingolipidoses	
G_{M1} gangliosidosis	
Type 1 (Landing)	β-Galactosidase A,B, and C
Type 2 (juvenile)	β-Galactosidase B and C
G_{M2} gangliosidoses	
Tay-Sachs	β-Hexosaminidase A
Sandhoff's	β-Hexosaminidase A and B
Juvenile	β-Hexosaminidase A (partial)
AB Variant	Enzyme normal (activator protein deficiency)
Metachromatic leukodystrophy (MLD)	
Late infantile, juvenile, and adult forms	Arylsulfatase A
Gaucher's disease	
Infantile, juvenile, and adult forms	Glucocerebroside β-glucosidase
Krabbe's disease	Galactosylceramide α-galactosidase
Fabry's disease	α-Galactosidase A
Farber's disease	Ceramidase
Niemann-Pick disease	
Type A and B	Sphingomyelinase
Type C	Sphingomyelinase (partial)
Type D	Unknown
Other	
ML IV	Unknown
Glycogen storage disease II (Pompe's disease)	
Severe and milder forms	α-Glucosidase
Wolman's disease (Infantile cholesterol ester storage disease)	Acid lipase
Adult cholesterol ester storage disease	Acid lipase (partial)
Acid phosphatase deficiency	Acid phosphatase
Cystinosis	Unknown
Salla disease	Unknown
Neuronal ceroid-lipofuscinoses	Unknown

THE MUCOPOLYSACCHARIDOSES

The mucopolysaccharidoses are a group of conditions caused by lysosomal enzyme defects that result in accumulation of GAG (formerly referred to as mucopolysaccharides) and excessive excretion of partially degraded GAG. Clinically these conditions are manifested by variable coarsening of the facies, skeletal abnormalities, hepatosplenomegaly, thick-feeling skin, heart disease, ocular defects, and neurologic abnormalities. The classification of these disorders is shown in the list of lysosomal storage diseases. A classification was originally established by McKusick on the basis of the clinical features, mode of inheritance, and the mucopolysaccharide excreted in the urine.[535] This classification has undergone revision as the enzyme defects have been delineated and new disorders described.

Hurler's syndrome has been estimated to have an incidence of 1:100,000, Scheie's syndrome 1:500,000, Hurler-Scheie compound 1:112,000, Hunter's syndrome 1:150,000, and Morquio's syndrome 1:300,000.[502,536] No estimates of incidence for the other disorders are available but most appear to be less common than Hurler's syndrome.

All of the mucopolysaccharidoses are inherited as autosomal recessive disorders, except Hunter's syndrome, which is usually inherited in an X-linked recessive fashion.

There are several general reviews of the mucopolysaccharidoses (MPS) diseases that we recommended for further reading.[128,204,532,536,578,622,727]

Mucopolysaccharidosis Type I

This category includes several conditions associated with a deficiency of lysosomal alpha-L-iduronidase. The three clinical syndromes are Hurler's syndrome, Scheie's syndrome, and an intermediate phenotype usually referred to as Hurler/Scheie compound. Hurler's syndrome and Scheie's syndrome are quite different clinically, although the enzyme defect appears to be the same in both disorders.[38,879] With the development of newer substrates for assaying iduronidase activity, Hopwood and Muller have been able to detect residual enzyme activity in both Hurler's and Scheie's syndromes and have found apparent differences between the two by enzyme kinetic studies.[375] McKusick and associates have proposed that the genes that cause Hurler's and Scheie's syndromes are allelic, that is, they are the result of two different mutations at a single locus.[534] This hypothesis predicts that patients who carry both of the mutant alleles would have a disorder with severity intermediate between Hurler's and Scheie's syndromes and such patients have been described.[784] Note that this hypothesis also implies that the genetic compound mucopolysaccharidosis Type I Hurler/Scheie compound (MPS I H/S) will have an incidence that is at least as great as the least common homozygous condition (in this case, Scheie's syndrome). As noted above, the estimated incidence of MPS I H/S is 1:112,000, which would make it approximately as common as the Hurler's syndrome. By using the Hardy-Weinberg formula and assumptions, it can be shown that the genetic compound will be more common than either of the homozygous conditions if the ratio between the incidences of the two homozygous conditions is less than four to one.

It should also be noted that although we expect an increase in consanguinity among parents of children homozygous for rare autosomal recessive traits, one would not expect to see any increase in consanguinity among parents of children with a condition such as the Hurler/Scheie compound because one parent must carry the Hurler gene and the other parent must carry the Scheie gene. This point will become important in the discussion of MPS I intermediate phenotypes.

Somatic cell genetic studies support the hypothesis that the Hurler and Scheie mutations are allelic. Fusing fibroblasts from patients with Hurler's syndrome, Scheie's syndrome, and Hurler/Scheie compound resulted in no correction of the iduronidase deficiency.[246] Correction of the enzyme deficiency in fused cells would be expected if the mutations occurred at different genetic loci.

Mucopolysaccharidosis Type I H or Hurler's Syndrome

Hurler's syndrome is considered to be the archetypal lysosomal storage disease, not only because it was probably the first to be described, but also because it is characterized by storage in tissue throughout the body, including the nervous system, the skeleton, and the viscera. Patients with Hurler's syndrome are not obviously affected at birth. Symptoms generally become obvious during the second half of the first year. Although dwarfism becomes apparent after infancy in Hurler's syndrome, these patients may actually grow more rapidly than average during the first year.[477] Macrocephaly with scaphocephaly is a regular feature. Patients typically present at about 6 months to 12 months of age with slow development. Other features that gradually develop include hepatomegaly, stiff joints, kyphosis with a gibbus deformity, chest deformity, chronic nasal congestion and rhinorrhea, and umbilical and inguinal hernias. By 2 or 3 years of age, the child has developed the typical coarse facies characterized by prominent forehead (frontal bossing), hirsutism with heavy eyebrows and hair extending down over the forehead, flat nasal bridge, broad nose, periorbital fullness, thick lips, gingival hypertrophy, and large tongue (Fig. 9-9). Progressive corneal clouding, thickened skin, hepatosplenomegaly, abdominal protuberance, and short, broad stiff hands also appear. Death usually occurs before the age of 10 years, a consequence of respiratory or cardiac complications that result from cardiac valvular involvment, myocardial disease, and chronic airway obstruction.[458,477]

Mental retardation is a prominent and often presenting feature. Development appears to cease in the second year of life. The disposition of these children is sometimes notably agreeable. Funduscopic changes are common and include retinitis pigmentosa and, late in the course of the disease, optic atrophy.[152] Deafness occurs in most patients. Other neurologic signs may include weakness and hypotonia or spasticity. Communicating hydrocephalus is quite common but only infrequently is it massive hydrocephalus. It is probably due to storage material in the leptomeninges that interferes with absorption of CSF.

Radiographically, the typical changes of dysostosis multiplex are invariably present and severe (Fig. 9-10). Although these changes are not present at birth or in early infancy, they usually become apparent during the first year of life as other dysmorphic features develop. Abnormal mu-

copolysacchariduria is present and should be detectable by the methods discussed elsewhere in this chapter.

Pathology. The clinical features of Hurler's syndrome reflect multisystem storage of the compounds dermatan sulfate and heparan sulfate. Histologic and biochemical studies of skin, cartilage, periosteum, blood vessels, fascia, liver, spleen, lymph nodes, lymphocytes, leukocytes, glomeruli, heart, and brain reveal excessive mucopolysaccharide storage. Van Hoof and Hers correctly suggested that the vacuoles in hepatic cells from a patient were mucopolysaccharide-filled lysosomes.[834] In the brain the mucopolysaccharide appears to accumulate in glial cells and perithelial cells surrounding capillaries. Neurons also reveal lysosomal storage material. This material, however, is thought to be lipid. By electron microscopy this storage material appears as parallel membranes oriented perpendicularly to the long axis of the cytosome, the so-called zebra body.[5] Similar storage material has been observed in neurons in Hunter's syndrome (MPS II) and Sanfilippo's syndrome (MPS III) as well as in Tay-Sachs disease.[573,852] Biochemically, an increase in brain mucopolysaccharide content above normal and elevated gangliosides, G_{M2} and G_{M3}, have been found.[794] Abnormal neuronal cytosomes are not observed in those patients with a mucopolysaccharidosis who are mentally normal or mildly affected.[893] The origin of the elevation in gangliosides is uncertain because the deficient enzymes degrade mucopolysaccarides. Kint and his associates have demonstrated that mucopolysaccharides inhibit beta-galactosidase activity in fibroblasts.[437] Avila and Convit have extended this observation to show that GAG may inhibit many acid hydrolases.[33] The ganglioside accumulation then may be a secondary effect of the excessive GAG accumulation.

Mucopolysaccharidosis Type I S or Scheie's Syndrome

The fact that this disorder was first reported in the ophthalmologic literature illustrates the importance of corneal clouding as one of the most troublesome symptoms of this mucopolysaccharidosis.[708] Joint limitations leading to hand deformities and aortic

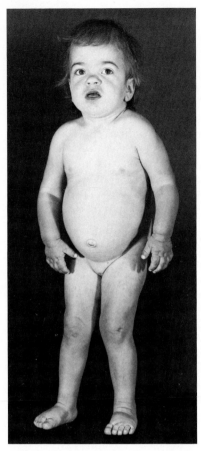

FIG. 9-9. Twenty-two-month old patient with the Hurler syndrome (mucopolysaccharidosis IH). Note coarsening facies, crouched stance, claw hands, and abdominal protuberance.

years of age, the majority of these patients are diagnosed as adults.[784] This condition is compatible with a normal life span.

Mucopolysaccharidosis Type I, Intermediate Forms

As mentioned above, a number of patients have been observed with iduronidase deficiency but with clinical phenotypes intermediate between the syndromes of Hurler (severe) and Scheie (mild). For representative cases, the reader is referred to reports by Kajii and associates, Stevenson and associates, Danes, Leisti and associates, Winters and associates, Jensen and associates, and Kaibara and associates.[170,391, 392,403,404,475,886]

These patients with intermediate phenotypes display considerable variability of phenotypic expression. Craniofacial dysmorphism may be mild to severe whereas skeletal changes are usually of moderate severity. The patients usually have short stat-

FIG. 9-10. Hurler's syndrome. Hook-shaped deformity of bodies of the second and third lumbar vertebrae are present.

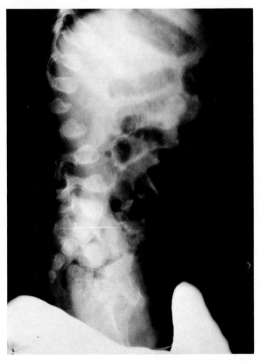

valve dysfunction are the other prominent features of this disorder. Stature and intelligence are normal. Complications that may bring these patients to the attention of the neurologist are retinitis pigmentosa, carpal tunnel syndrome, pes cavus deformity, and deafness. Bone cysts may be associated with pathologic fractures and degenerative arthritis.[466] Radiographic changes of dysostosis multiplex may not be present or, if present, are very mild. As in Hurler's syndrome, abnormal mucopolysacchariduria consisting of heparan sulfate and dermatan sulfate should be detectable by the usual screening tests for urinary GAG. Although the corneal clouding, joint stiffness, and mild facial dysmorphia appear between 7 and 10

ure and either normal intelligence or mild mental retardation. Hepatosplenomegaly, thickened skin, hernias, and cardiac valve abnormalities are also found. Symptoms may begin as early as the second year of life and survival into adulthood is common. Arachnoid cysts can occur in the parasella region and act as mass lesions, thus leading in one instance to CSF rhinorrhea and optic atrophy.[532]

It seems appropriate to think of this group of patients with conditions of intermediate severity as being genetically heterogeneous. Clearly, if the Hurler and Scheie genes are truly allelic, as the somatic cell complementation studies suggest, the existence of a true Hurler/Scheie compound is a necessary consequence of that fact and the incidence of the compound should be close to that seen for Hurler's syndrome.[246] However, the marked clinical variability of this group of patients suggests heterogeneity, that is, that there may be more mutations at the hypothesized Hurler/Scheie locus, and possibly at other loci necessary for normal intracellular expression of alpha-L-iduronidase. In fact, evidence for the existence of other mutations resulting in iduronidase deficiency and an intermediate phenotype in the homozygote has been presented by Jensen and associates and Kaibara and associates, who have observed affected sibs who were the offspring of consanguineous matings.[391,392,403] The presence of consanguineous parents suggests that the affected children are homozygous for a gene inherited from a common ancestor through both parents. This would seem to be a more likely explanation than to suppose that both parents are, by chance, heterozygous for two different rare mutations (i.e., the Hurler gene and the Scheie gene). Note that a third mutant allele at the Hurler/Scheie locus would necessarily imply the existence of three different genetic compounds in addition to the three homozygous conditions. Therefore, this mechanism could easily result in an almost continuous spectrum of clinical phenotypes expressed as manifestations of what would appear to be the same enzyme deficiency. On the other hand, single mutations at other loci involved in the expression of iduronidase would be expressed only in the homozygous state and the nonallelic mutations would not be expected to interact, that is, one would not expect the compound heterozygote to be clinically affected.

It seems likely that the above discussion applies to many if not most of the inborn errors of metabolism covered in this chapter. Future studies of patients can be expected to delineate the clinical and molecular complexity of these conditions, for which the iduronidase-deficient mucopolysaccharidoses serve as an interesting example.

Mucoplysaccharidosis Type II or Hunter's Syndrome

Hunter's syndrome (MPS II) is caused by a deficiency of lysosomal iduronate sulfatase, and both dermatan sulfate and heparan sulfate are stored in tissues throughout the body. Most cases have been male and family studies clearly indicate X-linked inheritance. However, genetic heterogeneity may also exist in Hunter's syndrome.

There is great variability of severity seem among patients with MPS II. Severity tends to "breed true" in families but this is not invariable, suggesting the need for caution in counseling.[226] Some of the observed variability may be due to genetic heterogeneity, that is different genetic mutations (genes) resulting in iduronate sulfatase deficiency and "Hunter's syndrome."

At the present time, MPS II patients are divided into a severe group (MPS IIA) and a mild group (MPS IIB), based on the degree of physical impairment and the presence or absence of mental retardation. However, it is clear that variability still remains in each of these two categories. Some "severe" Hunter patients are much more severely affected than others, although all are significantly retarded, whereas some "mild" Hunter patients are much less severely physically handicapped than others, even though all have intelligence in the normal range.

All patients with MPS II have short stature, coarse facial features, visceromegaly, and joint stiffness. Macrocephaly and hydrocephalus may also occur. Affected babies are normal at birth and show normal or accelerated linear and head growth in early infancy, followed by plateauing of linear growth with subsequent dwarfism.

The severe form is similar in most respects to Hurler's syndrome but progression is slightly slower so that death, usually from cardiac failure, occurs before 15 years of age. Corneal clouding is usually absent, although it has been observed in both severe and mild forms.[767] The degree of nervous system involvement is also less. Compared to Hurler patients, patients with Hunter's syndrome are less severely retarded and are more active. They are not docile like Hurler patients; rather, aggressive behavior as in Sanfilippo's syndrome is common. A nodular skin eruption over the shoulders may offer an additional clue to the diagnosis. Radiographic changes of dysostosis multiplex are present but they may be somewhat milder than in Hurler's syndrome. Abnormal urinary excretion of dermatan sulfate and heparan sulfate results in a positive screening test for urinary GAG.

These patients may present with neurologic symptoms of speech retardation, deafness, or behavioral disturbances.[473] Other neurologic symptoms and signs include convulsions, retinitis pigmentosa, and papilledema in patients with hydrocephalus.

In the mild form of the disease, patients survive into adulthood and intellect is relatively intact. As adults these patients may develop entrapment of peripheral nerves and joint stiffness may lead to severe limitation of motion, pain, and disability.[412] Degenerative arthritis, especially of the hips, may also occur.

Hearing loss probably occurs in most, if not all, patients with MPS II, and may, if undiagnosed and untreated, lead to unnecessary learning difficulties for school-age children with milder forms of Hunter's syndrome. For this reason, it is recommended that neurologists, pediatricians, and other physicians who follow children with MPS IIB and potentially normal intelligence, be aware of the almost certain problem of hearing loss and be aggressive in treatment. Hearing loss may be conductive, sensorineural, or mixed. Many patients with MPS II have chronic serous otitis that should receive prompt attention. However, one should not be lulled into complacency by the fact that the serous otitis is being treated medically or surgically. If a significant hearing loss is present, amplification should be considered in order to allow normal development to proceed. Perhaps undiagnosed and untreated hearing loss is the reason for the observation that in patients with MPS II B mathematical ability is better than verbal ability.[532] Laryngeal edema and tracheal narrowing are also significant problems as patients grow older and probably contribute to already compromised cardiorespiratory function.[900] Cardiac involvement occurs in MPS II and usually contributes to morbidity and mortality.

As predicted by the Lyon principle, fibroblasts from female carriers of Hunter's syndrome are of two types depending on which X chromosome is active. Fibroblasts from female carriers may or may not show metachromasia or excessive ^{35}S-mucopolysaccharide accumulation.[130,171,549] Carrier detection is hazardous because the mutant phenotype may be masked by normal cells in the same culture. Extensive cloning of cells, a complicated and time-consuming process, is necessary for heterozygote detection to be at all reliable but, even then, a normal result does not rule out carrier status. An abnormal result would clearly indicate heterozygosity, but, for the purposes of genetic counseling, one needs to be able to test potential carriers and tell them if they are not carriers. Tests have been devised to improve carrier testing but so far no test has been reliable for ruling out carrier status.[84,203,904] For this reason, it has been suggested that all close female relatives of Hunter patients, namely, mothers, sisters, maternal aunts, cousins, and nieces consider themselves carriers.[226] This means that they should all be counseled about the availability of prenatal diagnosis. The use of Bayes' theorem may allow one to calculate a risk figure for counseling purposes.[257,506,570] However, one must be very careful when interpreting such calculations because they are usually done assuming equal mutation rates in the sperm and the egg. If mutations turn out to be more common during spermatogenesis than oogenesis, then one will calculate too low a risk if the usual methods are used. One way of compensating for this in the calculations is to assume that all mothers of affected boys are carriers. One should make sure that the potential carrier sees an experienced genetic counselor who can explain the risks and options to her.

In addition, two females with iduronate sulfatase deficiency and features consistent with Hunter's syndrome have been described.[577] However, subsequent studies have revealed that the first patient also has deficiencies in the activities of other sulfatases, suggesting that she should be thought of as having a type of multiple sulfatase deficiency.* In the case of the second patient, an autosomal recessive etiology seems more likely than extreme Lyonization in a heterozygous carrier for X-linked iduronate sulfatase deficiency because her parents were second cousins. We know that at least one autosomal locus affects iduronate sulfatase expression (see below, section on multiple sulfatase deficiency). There is still a great deal to be learned about the spectrum of clinical and biochemical phenotypes determined by alleles at autosomal loci that affect the expression of iduronate sulfatase and other sulfatases.

Mucopolysaccharidosis Type III or Sanfilippo's Syndrome

Four different enzyme defects involving heparan sulfate degradation have been reported in patients with the Sanfilippo's syndrome (see list, Lysosomal Storage Diseases). Unlike the other mucopolysaccharidoses, differentiation between the types of MPS III is not based on clinical findings. Patients of all four types have the same phenotype so that classification is not possible on clinical grounds. Rather, each of the types (MPS III, A,B,C, and D; see list, Lysosomal Storage Diseases) is due to a different enzyme deficiency and all appear to be inherited in an autosmal recessive manner. Heparan sulfate is the material stored.

Sanfilippo's syndrome is characterized by central nervous system involvement manifested eventually as severe mental retardation, but only mild skeletal and visceral involvement. Early development is normal. In some patients psychomotor delay becomes apparent in the second year of life whereas others appear to function fairly normally until the first or second grade in school. Somatic features such as coarse facies may be very mild in the first decade of life so that an abnormality is not suspected until learning problems manifest themselves in the first grade. On the other hand, some patients do have mild but definite phenotypic features such as coarse facies, thick skin, and coarse hair by the second or third year of life. A typical history is that the child is thought to be normal until the age of 3 or 4 years when parents complain of hyperactivity and behavioral problems. By the age of 5 years developmental plateauing is evident.[173] Regression occurs but the child continues to have normal growth. Parents and other caretakers are then faced with a large, strong, retarded, hyperactive, and frequently destructive child who gradually becomes more dysmorphic and retarded through the teenage years. The hyperactive, aggressive, and destructive behavior is a very real problem for families who have children with Sanfilippo's syndrome and special attention, help, and support must be given by professionals involved in their care.

Physical signs in Sanfilippo's syndrome are mild and, in addition to the features noted above, include joint contractures of fingers and knees, hepatomegaly, hirsutism, and valvular heart disease. Symptoms and signs that are usually absent in Sanfilippo's syndrome include corneal opacity, dwarfism, and splenomegaly.

Mild changes of dysostosis multiplex may be present. Although usually positive, the usual urine screening tests for the mucopolysaccharidoses can be negative in Sanfilippo's syndrome, necessitating studies of cultured fibroblasts in order to confirm the diagnosis.

A coarse tremor and ataxia in these children manifesting psychomotor regression have also been noted. As adolescents, some Sanfilippo patients develop bulbar palsy, which may account for the fact that pneumonia is a frequent cause of death in the second decade of life.[173] Taori and his coworkers have reported fibrillation in electromyograms (EMGs), reduced nerve conduction velocity, and grouped muscle fiber atrophy consistent with involvement of anterior horn cells.[813]

The basic defect in Sanfilippo type A is a deficiency of Heparan N-sulfatase ac-

---

*Neufeld, E. F. and Thomas, G. H.: Personal communication, 1982

tivity, and in Sanfilippo type B it is a deficiency in the activity of N-acetyl-alpha-glucosaminidase (for a more detailed discussion and original references, see the general review references given above). Sanfilippo type C has been defined as a deficiency in the activity of acetyl-CoA: alpha-glucosaminide N-acetyl transferase and several patients with this defect have been reported.[52,440] More recently, two patients with Sanfilippo's syndrome were found to be deficient in the activity of N-acetylglucosamine-6-sulfate sulfatase directed specifically at heparan sulfate, resulting in the classification of this condition as Sanfilippo type D.[455] The patients' cells had normal N-acetylglucosamine-6-sulfate sulfatase activity as measured with a substrate derived from keratan sulfate, suggesting that two different enzymes may exist, one of which is specific for only heparan sulfate.

Mucopolysaccharidosis Type IV or Morquio's Syndrome

Morquio's syndrome is characterized by marked skeletal involvement, normal intelligence, and urinary excretion of keratan sulfate. Patients usually present with a chief complaint of dwarfism with orthopaedic and neurologic problems, especially involving the spine, spinal cord, and legs, and a diagnosis of one of the osteochondrodysplasias may be entertained. (See Rimoin and associates for a classification of constitutional diseases of bone that includes the lysosomal storage diseases and the osteochondrodysplasias, as well as others.[671]) Indeed, the diagnosis of a spondyloepiphyseal dysplasia may be mistakenly made on the basis of clinical and radiographic findings if one is not aware of the unique features such as dysostosis multiplex, corneal clouding and heart involvement, which should immediately suggest that one is dealing with a lysosomal storage disease. Conversely, one should be very careful in reading the older literature because a number of different types of short-trunk dwarfism have been erroneously reported as examples of "Morquio's syndrome" between the 1930s and 1960s. Even today, it is not uncommon for practicing physicians to lump all short-trunk dwarfism under the term Morquio's syndrome. This practice should be strongly discouraged and the term should be used only to refer to patients with one of the types of MPS IV, characterized by the reasonably specific although somewhat variable clinical phenotype described in this section.

Patients with Morquio's syndrome present with a short trunk form of dwarfism and frequently with genu valgum (knock knee deformity), after relatively normal growth and development over the first year of life. Growth plateaus as spine and joint deformities progress throughout childhood. Radiographically, signs of dysostosis multiplex may be present in the first year and then progress to a pattern that includes universal platyspondyly and is fairly specific for MPS IV.[469]

The odontoid is hypoplastic and ligamentous laxity contributes to the frequent complication of cervical spinal cord compression due to subluxation of C_1 on C_2. Weakness and long tract signs should warn one of the presence of cervical compression that may lead to paraplegia and even respiratory paralysis. Patients with MPS IV should be followed carefully for this complication, which may be acute. Although MPS IV patients typically are intellectually normal, neuronal inclusions have been found in cerebral cortex, Ammon's horn, basal ganglia, and thalamic nuclei.[284,452]

Classic Morquio's syndrome is an autosomal recessive condition due to a deficiency of lysosomal N-acetylgalactosamine-6-sulfate sulfatase.[522,744] Milder expression of the Morquio phenotype has been recognized in many patients over the years and in some of these beta-galactosidase activity is reduced.[17,320,600,825] Further heterogeneity is illustrated by the patient described by Fujimoto and Horwitz who also had a mild expression of the Morquio phenotype but complete absence of N-acetylgalactosamine-6-sulfate sulfatase, the enzyme absent in classic Morquio's syndrome.[261] Thus, heterogeneity in the MPS IV diseases may be analogous to that seen in both MPS I, where different mutations affecting the expression of a single enzyme may produce a spectrum of clinical severity, and in MPS III, where different mutations affecting different enzymes may result in the same phenotype. The relative consistency of the different clinical syndromes associated with deficiencies in beta-galactosidase activity seems to be reasonable evidence in support of the hypothesis that these are truly different mutations rather than simply variable expression of a single gene.[765] (See also the section on G_{M1} gangliosidosis).

Mucopolysaccharidosis Type V

This category is now vacant because Scheie's syndrome, which was formerly classified as MPS V, has been reclassified as MPS type I S.

Mucopolysaccharidosis Type VI or Maroteaux-Lamy Syndrome

The Maroteaux-Lamy syndrome is typically characterized by marked involvement of the skeleton and viscera but with normal intelligence. It is autosomal recessive and is caused by a deficiency of lysosomal N-acetylgalactosamine-4-sulfatase (arylsulfatase B) that results in massive excretion of GAG, predominantly dermatan sulfate. Dysostosis multiplex, dwarfism, corneal opacities, hepatosplenomegaly, cardiac involvement, and facial dysmorphia may be almost as severe as is seen in Hurler's syndrome. A mild form of the syndrome has been described that has the same enzymatic defect as the severe form and other patients with intermediate severity have also been described.[641,655]

Neurologic problems in Maroteaux-Lamy syndrome include communicating hydrocephalus, peripheral nerve entrapment, and myelopathy. Myelopathy can result from either odontoid hypoplasia with atlantoaxial dislocation or cervical pachymeningitis.[37,634,641] Hydrocephalus may be more severe in MPS VI than in the other MPS conditions and some patients have required shunting procedures.

Mucopolysaccharidosis Type VII

This rare disorder of mucopolysaccharide metabolism, beta-glucuronidase deficiency, has been described in a few patients with variable clinical manifestations. The first patient described had dysostosis multiplex, short stature, dysmorphic facies, umbilical hernia, frequent infections, and hepatosplenomegaly in infancy with subsequent slow mental and physical development.[751] Other patients have been reported with only very mild features, including normal intelligence and deficiency of beta-glucuronidase.[62,291,329]

MPS VII appears to be inherited in an autosomal recessive fashion. Evidence for this includes observation of half-normal enzyme levels in parents of affected children as well as studies that conclude that the structural gene for human beta-glucuronidase is on chromosome 7.[140,248]

Mucopolysaccharidosis Type VIII

Two patients have been reported with phenotypes that appeared to be combinations of Morquio's syndrome and Sanfilippo's syndrome.[285,523] However, the hypothesized deficiency of N-acetylglucosamine-6-sulfate sulfatase has not been confirmed, and the reader should be aware of the questionable status of this condition.[197]

THE GLYCOPROTEINOSES

These disorders are often confused with the mucopolysaccharidoses. In most of them there is storage of mucopolysaccharides and lipids.[766] The disorders of glycoprotein metabolism include mannosidosis, fucosidosis, aspartylglycosaminuria, and the sialidoses. So far, all appear to be autosomal recessive.

Mannosidosis

Mannosidosis is characterized by most of the somatic features found in the mucopolysaccharidoses including coarse facies, hepatosplenomegaly, dwarfism, dysostosis multiplex, macrocephaly, and joint stiffness. Patients also have mental retardation, hearing loss, hypotonia, frequent respiratory infections, cataracts, and vacuolization of peripheral lymphocytes and bone marrow cells.[34,194,604,841] They store and excrete mannose-rich oligosaccharides as a result of a deficiency in the lysosomal component of alpha-mannosidase.[604,817] A wide spectrum of clinical severity has been reported; some patients have rapid progression over the first several years and die during the first decade of life, whereas others have been identified as teenagers and adults.[83,841] Significant mental retardation seems to be present in all patients, even those with milder somatic manifestations. Hearing loss appears to be a relatively common finding in mannosidosis.

Fucosidosis

A deficiency of lysosomal alpha-fucosidase results in storage throughout the body of fucose-containing oligosaccharides and glycosphingolipids.[835] As with most lysosomal enzyme deficiencies, the clinical phenotypes found in fucosidosis have been variable.[87,217,453,496,618] Various authors have suggested a division into types I (severe) and II (mild) whereas others advocate three clinical subtypes. Some patients who are severely affected have the onset of hypotonia in the first year of life with progression to hypertonicity and eventual decerebrate rigidity. They may have coarse facies, dysostosis multiplex, organomegaly, thick skin, corneal opacities, hypohidrosis, recurrent respiratory infections, seizures, and vacuolization of peripheral lymphocytes. Some patients may have the onset in the second year and some even later with a much slower progression of symptoms. Those with early onset and rapid progression usually die by the age of 5 or 6 years. Those with later onset and more gradual progression may survive into the third decade. A very interesting feature of the "milder" types is the presence of angiokeratoma corporis diffusum, which is consistently seen in Fabry's disease and has also been reported in one case of sialidosis. Angiokeratomas are not seen in the severe, early onset, rapidly progressive type of fucosidosis. They are frequently but not always seen in the less severe forms.[717] Lysosomal alpha-galactosidase activity has been normal in all patients tested. Diagnosis is made by enzyme assay on cultured skin fibroblasts or leukocytes. Serum or plasma is not adequate for enzymatic diagnosis because of the existence of a polymorphism in the normal population; some normal individuals have very low serum or plasma fucosidase activity but normal leukocyte enzyme activity. Ng and associates suggest that this low level variant is a heritable trait.[581]

Aspartylglycosaminuria

This condition has been diagnosed in over 130 patients, most of whom are Finnish. The incidence in Finland has been estimated at 1:26,000 making it one of the more common inborn errors of metabolism in that country. It is the result of a deficiency of lysosomal 1-aspartamido-beta-N-acetylglucosamine amidohydrolase (amidase or AADGase), which causes storage of N-acetylglucosamine-asparagine in tissues throughout the body.[526]

Affected patients have normal growth and development in early infancy. Recurrent respiratory infections, diarrhea, and delayed speech development may be the first symptoms between the ages of 1 and 4 years. Speech abnormalities including very indistinct articulation and occasional stammering continue to be a prominent part of the neurologic picture through adult life. A thick tongue may contribute to the indistinct speech. Slightly coarse facial features and motor incoordination may appear prior to 4 years of age and progress during the early school-age years. Patients develop coarse facies including a depressed nasal bridge, anteverted nostrils, and thick lips. A unique but consistent feature of aspartylglycosaminuria (AGU) is increased skin laxity resulting in a wrinkled face with sagging skin. Other features may include kyphosis and scoliosis, protuberant abdomen, joint laxity, hernias, heart disease, poor secondary sexual development, cataracts, vacuolized lymphocytes in peripheral blood and bone marrow, dysostosis multiplex with anterosuperior ossification defects and anterior wedging of vertebral bodies, a thickened calvaria, thinned cortex of the long bones with broadening of short tubular bones, occasional small bone cysts, and spontaneous fractures. There is progressive mental retardation to a severe degree by adult life. Hypotonia is present in childhood; later mild spasticity may develop. Seizures are rare. Brain atrophy has been found with pneumoencephalography.[30,31,387]

If this condition is suspected, urine TLC can be used to identify the characteristic excretion product, 2-acetamido-1-[beta-L-aspartamido]-1,2-dideoxy-beta-D-glucose (AADG).[382,387] The diagnosis should then be confirmed by enzyme assay using either leukocytes or cultured skin fibroblasts.

The Sialidoses

A wide spectrum of clinical manifestations has been described for patients with primary deficiencies of lysosomal neuraminidase who accumulate and excrete increased amounts of sialic acid bound to various oligosaccharides. Lowden and O'Brien have divided patients into those with normal physical appearance and body proportions (normosomatic, type 1) and those who are dysmorphic (type 2).[500] All of the clinical syndromes described so far appear to be autosomal recessive. These include the cherry-red spot-myoclonus syndrome, the Goldberg syndrome, mucolipidosis I, and nephrosialidosis.

The cherry-red spot-myoclonus syndrome (Lowden and O'Brien normosomatic type 1) is the mildest clinical subtype associated with neuraminidase deficiency. It is characterized by macular cherry-red spots, occasional corneal punctate opacities, slowly progressive myoclonus, gradually decreasing visual activity, normal appearance, normal growth, and relatively normal intelligence. The age of onset of visual loss or myoclonus is usually between 8 and 15 years but there may be significant intrafamilial variability as illustrated by a family in which the proband had the onset of neurologic symptoms at 29 years whereas his brother developed weakness prior to the age of 10 years. The myoclonus is stimulated by movement, touch, sound, or emotion, decreases during sleep, is gradually progressive, may initiate grand mal seizures, and appears to be refractory to treatment.[347,661] A patient of Rapin and associates also developed severe intermittent pain in the hands, legs, and feet during hot weather, symptoms similar to those seen in patients with Fabry's disease.[661] Electroencephalogram abnormalities have also been found. Other features include vacuolization of peripheral leukocytes and bone marrow cells. Nephrotic syndrome also occurred in a patient reported by Rapin and associates.[661]

The Goldberg syndrome (Lowden and O'Brien type 2, dysmorphic with juvenile onset) is characterized by mental retardation, ataxia, corneal clouding, hearing loss, coarse facies, and short stature with skeletal dysplasia in addition to cherry-red spots with progressive visual impairment, myo-clonus with occasional seizures and EEG abnormalities, and vacuolization of bone marrow cells. Hepatosplenomegaly does not appear to occur. Many of these patients were originally reported as having primary deficiencies of beta-galactosidase, but it is now clear that deficiency of this enzyme is secondary.

Mucolipidosis I is more severe than either of the other two types previously discussed. In addition to macular cherry-red spots, myoclonus, dwarfism with skeletal dysplasia, coarse facial features, mental retardation and other features of the Goldberg syndrome, they may also have hepatomegaly.[429,768] Some survive into the second decade of life.

In addition, a more severe clinical phenotype has been described characterized by nephrosis, congenital ascites, pericardial effusion, and death usually before 5 years of age and sometimes before the age of 2 years.[35,519] It is not clear whether these patients represent one or more distinct clinical subtypes or whether they simply represent the severe end of the mucolipidosis I spectrum. Several patients with ascities, nephrosis, and a severe clinical course have now been observed, and the name "nephrosialidosis" has been suggested for this group.

The diagnosis of a sialidosis is made by demonstrating a deficiency of lysosomal neuraminidase in cultured skin fibroblasts. Quantitative measurement of urinary sialic acid will aid in the diagnosis; there should be a significantly increased excretion of bound sialic acid. Free urinary sialic acid excretion is normal.[34,129]

MULTIPLE ENZYME DEFICIENCIES

Multiple Sulfatase Deficiency

This is a rare autosomal recessive disorder caused by deficiency of multiple sulfatases including glycosaminoglycan sulfatases, cerebroside sulfatases, and steroid sulfatase.[53,212] Therefore patients can be thought of as having a combination of several different diseases, each of which is due to deficiency of a single enzyme, including Hunter's, Sanfilippo's, Morquio's, and Maroteaux-Lamy syndromes, as well as metachromatic leukodystrophy and steroid sulfatase deficiency ichthyosis. Onset is in the first 2 years of life. Retardation is progressive and severe and the neurologic manifestations are those of the late infantile type of metachromatic leukodystrophy. There are also features of the mucopolysaccharidoses such as mild facial coarsening, hepatomegaly, and dysostosis multiplex. In addition, ichthyosis may be present.

Mucolipidosis Types II and III

Mucolipidosis II (ML II; I-cell disease) is one of the most severe of the lysosomal storage diseases with clinical manifestations present at birth, whereas ML III (pseudo-Hurler polydystrophy) has a much milder phenotype. Both are autosomal recessive conditions due to defective intracellular localization of lysosomal enzymes. Mucolipidosis II is characterized by severe growth and developmental retardation, coarse facies, thick, firm skin, gingival hypertrophy, stiff joints, dysostosis multiplex, and early death.[769] However, even in these patients, variability of expression has been observed.[282] The name is derived from characteristic refractile inclusions that are seen in cells (I-cells)

The clinical features of ML III are much milder than those of ML II. The diagnostic criteria for ML III outlined by Kelly and associates are onset after 2 years of age, short stature, progressive joint stiffness, mild mental retardation, fine corneal opacities, dysostosis multiplex with severe pelvic and peculiar vertebral changes, valvular heart disease, normal mucopolysacchariduria, and cytoplasmic inclusions in cultured fibroblasts.[430]

Activities of a number of lysosomal hydrolases are intracellularly decreased whereas levels of enzyme activity are markedly increased extracellularly, for example, in the serum or in the medium from a culture of growing cells. These biochemical features are similar in both ML II and III. Initially this observation suggested that the lysosomal enzymes were leaking from the cells.[878] Hickman and Neufeld, however, have proposed that normal enzymes are released by cells and then must be taken up and internalized.[360] Studies of ML II and ML III cells in tissue culture have been very

productive of new knowledge about the normal cycle of lysosomal enzyme synthesis within the cytoplasm, transfer of the enzyme molecules out of the cell, and then uptake and internalization of the enzymes.[357] Mucolipidosis II and ML III appear to be caused by a defect in the process necessary for normal uptake of the enzymes by cells, which may involve specific recognition markers with phosphorylated mannose residues. There is also some recent evidence suggesting that ML II and ML III are due to allelic mutations but one should keep in mind the possibility of further heterogeneity within this group of conditions.

THE SPHINGOLIPIDOSES

The sphingolipidoses are characterized by accumulation of glycolipids within the nervous system and other organs. The classical descriptions of these disorders on clinical and morphologic grounds have been augmented by enzymatic analysis. A large number of phenotypes resulting from defects in a small number of enzymes has resulted. In most cases the degree of impairment of enzyme activity bears a rough resemblance to the severity of symptoms and rapidity of progression.

Sphingolipids are derivatives of sphinogosine, an amino alcohol with a terminal unsaturated fatty acid. Ceramide, or N-acyl sphingosine, is formed by condensing sphingosine with a fatty acid to form an amide-ester link on the second carbon (Fig. 9-11). The various sphingolipids are formed by adding phosphatidylcholine, glucose, or galactose to the first carbon, followed by other hexoses, hexosamines or a sialic acid, usually N-acetylneuraminic acid (NANA). Because chain elongation is an enzymatic process, there are probably inherited defects in these enzymes. These defects have not been recognized, so it is possible that they are lethal during development. This would be in keeping with the proposed function of sphinoglipids as membrane constituents such as receptors, binding sites, and so on. All known defects of sphingolipid metabolism are disorders of breakdown, or catabolism and result in lysosomal storage (Fig. 9-12). (A reported defect in the synthesis of G_{M3} ganglioside has recently become less certain.[91])

The neutral sphingolipids have one or more simple sugars linked to ceramide. The acid sphingolipids include sulfatide and the gangliosides, which are sphingolipids that contain sialic acid. Sphingomyelin, in which phosphorylcholine is linked to ceramide, is a phosphosphingolipid. The enzymatic breakdown of these substances proceeds toward the ceramide from the distal molecule. Extensive reviews of the sphingolipidoses have recently been published.[124,295,625,697]

The Gangliosidoses

The gangliosidoses are defects in lipid metabolism characterized by excessive accumulation of ganglioside, a sphingolipid composed of ceramide and an oligosaccharide chain to which one or more N-acetylneuraminic acid (sialic acid) molecules are attached. The term *gangliosidosis* was coined by Klenk who noted that lipid storage in these disorders tended to occur in ganglion cells.

The gangliosidoses are one subgroup of the sphingolipidoses. There are two main forms of gangliosidosis based upon the ganglioside stored, G_{M1} and G_{M2} ganglioside. Both G_{M1} and G_{M2} gangliosidoses occur in different clinical and biochemical forms.

Generalized Gangliosidosis. Generalized gangliosidosis (G_{M1} gangliosidosis) was first described by Norman and coworkers in 1959.[592] This recessively inherited disorder is characterized by neonatal or infantile onset of coarse facial features, visceromegaly, dysostosis multiplex, and psychomotor regression.

PATHOLOGY. The chief pathologic features in generalized gangliosidosis are visceral histiocytosis, vacuolation of renal glomerular epithelial cells, and neuronal lipidosis. The visceral histiocytes occur in liver, bone marrow, spleen, and lymph nodes. Vacuolization occurs not only in glomerular epithelial cells but may also be seen in epithelial cells in skin biopsies.

The neuronal lipid inclusions are found throughout the brain in infantile G_{M1} gangliosidosis. By electron microscopy the inclusions appear as concentric laminated membranes, so-called membranous cytoplasmic bodies. These same inclusions are found in Tay-Sachs disease and other G_{M2} gangliosidoses. The neuronal inclusions are also found in type 2 or juvenile G_{M1} gangliosidosis. The visceral histiocytosis in juvenile G_{M1} gangliosidosis, however, is much less severe than that which occurs in infantile G_{M1} gangliosidosis.

BIOCHEMISTRY. G_{M1} gangliosidosis is due to a deficiency of G_{M1} ganglioside beta-galactosidase[196] (Fig. 9-12). The disorder is extremely heterogeneous, and the enzymology is not at all certain, owing to problems mentioned in the section on the approach to the patient. Beta-galactosidase is found in acid forms with pH optima of 4 to 5, and neutral forms, which are also less heat-labile.[364] The acid forms are a monomer, a dimer, and a polymeric arrangement of the same protein.[260,589] The purified enzyme is active against water-soluble artificial substrates, but bile salts must be added to detect activity against G_{M1} ganglioside and other amphophilic substances.[589] A naturally occurring activator protein serving as a detergent has been described for this system.[490,491] Another beta-galactosidase is deficient in Krabbe's disease (q.v.). This enzyme and the neutral beta-

FIG. 9-11. Sphingosine and ceramide. The breakdown reaction of ceramide to sphingosine is shown. Synthesis of ceramide is from sphingosine and fatty acid acyl-CoA. Enzyme (1) is ceramidase. Fatty acid is abbreviated FA.

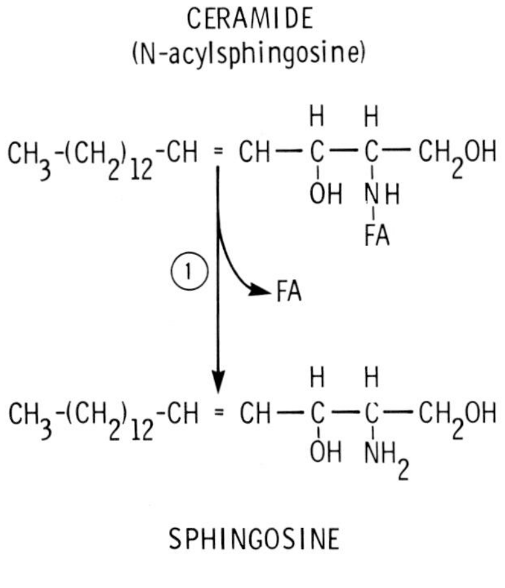

CERAMIDE
(N-acylsphingosine)

$$CH_3\text{-}(CH_2)_{12}\text{-}CH = CH - \underset{\underset{OH}{|}}{\overset{\overset{H}{|}}{C}} - \underset{\underset{\underset{FA}{|}}{\overset{H}{|}}}{\overset{\overset{H}{|}}{C}} - CH_2OH$$

(1) ↘ FA

$$CH_3\text{-}(CH_2)_{12}\text{-}CH = CH - \underset{\underset{OH}{|}}{\overset{\overset{H}{|}}{C}} - \underset{\underset{NH_2}{|}}{\overset{\overset{H}{|}}{C}} - CH_2OH$$

SPHINGOSINE

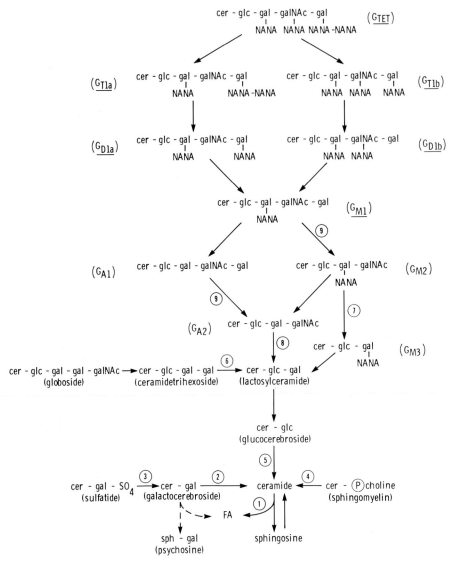

FIG. 9-12. Sphingolipid catabolism and enzyme deficiencies. The gangliosides are named according to the number of sialic acid (NANA) residues present, eg., M for mono, D for di, T for tri, and TET for tetra. G_A gangliosides are asialogangliosides. Sialidase activity in catabolism is not specifically labeled. The major brain gangliosides are underlined. *Globoside* is the major neutral glycosphingolipid of erythrocyte stroma and is not present in large quantities in the brain. Psychosine is formed only when reaction (2) is blocked. Enzymes indicated are: (1) ceramidase (Farber disease); (2) galactocerebroside beta-galactosidase (globoid-cell leukodystrophy); (3) arylsulfatase A (metachromatic leukodystrophy); (4) sphingomyelinase (Niemann-Pick disease); (5) glucocerebroside beta-glucosidase (Gaucher disease); (6) alpha-galactosidase A (Fabry disease); (7) hexosaminidase A (G_{M2}-gangliosidosis); (8) hexosaminidase A and B (Sandhoff disease); (9) G_{M1}-beta-galactosidase (G_{M1}-generalized gangliosidosis). Abbreviations used are: cer for ceramide; FA for fatty acid; gal for galactose; galNAc for N-acetylgalactosamine; glc for glucose; NANA for N-acetylneuraminic acid (a sialic acid); ℗ for phosphoryl; and sph for sphingosine.

galactosidases are not allelic with the acidic enzyme.

The great range of phenotypic variability may be due to the presence of several mutant genes in the population, so that many patients are heterozygous for two mutant alleles, rather than homozygous for one.[597,602] In addition, complementation (cell fusion) has suggested the necessity of post-translational modification of the primary gene product to generate functional enzymes.[85]

CLINICAL FEATURES. Two major clinical forms of generalized gangliosidosis have been delineated, type 1 or infantile and type 2 or juvenile G_{M1} gangliosidosis. Several other patients have had features atypical for either type 1 or type 2 generalized gangliosidosis. Some of these atypical patients probably have had beta-galactosidase deficiency that was secondary to another enzyme defect such as sialidase deficiency (q.v.).

Infantile Generalized Gangliosidosis. Development is slow from birth in infantile generalized gangliosidosis (type 1 G_{M1} gangliosidosis). The infant with generalized gangliosidosis has dysmorphic facies: frontal bossing, depressed nasal bridge, large low-set ears, elongated philtrum, gingival hypertrophy, and hirsutism.[596] Facial and peripheral edema occur. A cherry-red macula is present in approximately half the infants.[596] In contrast to the mucopolysaccharidoses corneal clouding is generally absent although it has been noted in one patient.[36]

Affected infants have a poor appetite and poor sucking ability and perhaps for these reasons grow poorly. Developmentally, these infants usually do not become able to sit alone or walk. Fine hand and finger movements are never well developed. Tonic–clonic seizures frequently occur. These infants may have macrocephaly, although it is less frequent and not usually as massive as in Tay-Sachs disease. Hepatomegaly is present after 6 months of age. Splenomegaly is not usually prominent. Lymph node enlargement is usually minor. Dorsolumbar kyphoscoliosis often is present in infancy. Joint stiffness and contractures occur in the hands, elbows, and knees.

Neurologic signs include hyperactive deep tendon reflexes, hypotonia, poor muscle strength, strabismus, and nystagmus. An exaggerated acoustic motor or startle response may sometimes be demonstrable. If survival is prolonged, decerebrate rigidity, blindness, and deafness appear and the patient loses all contact with the environment.

The radiographic abnormalities of the spine and upper extremity can be helpful diagnostically, although these are by no means specific for generalized gangliosidosis. Vertebral bodies are hypoplastic and beaked, and long bones often show cortical rarefaction and periosteal cloaking.

Juvenile Generalized Gangliosidosis. Juvenile generalized gangliosidosis (type 2 G_{M1} gangliosidosis) begins later (6 mo–20 mo of age) than infantile generalized gangliosidosis.[598,601] Coarse facial features, hepatosplenomegaly, and skeletal deformities are not present. Development is usually normal until the second year of life when psychomotor regression appears. Neurologic signs and symptoms include hyperacusis, seizures, ataxia, strabismus, and progressive spasticity. These children often expire as a result of infections between the ages of 3 and 10 years. Radiographic changes are mild. Vacuoles in lymphocytes and foamy histiocytes in bone marrow may be found.

DIAGNOSIS. Infantile generalized gangliosidosis is most often confused with mucopolysaccharidosis I H (Hurler's syndrome), Niemann-Pick disease and Tay-Sachs disease. In generalized gangliosidosis the absence of corneal clouding, normal urinary mucopolysaccharides, and rapid neurologic deterioration helps exclude mucopolysaccharidosis I. The facial dysmorphic features and bony abnormalities in generalized gangliosidosis are not seen in Tay-Sachs disease or Niemann-Pick disease.

The diagnosis of generalized gangliosidosis can be confirmed by demonstrating deficient activity of the enzyme beta-galactosidase in white blood cells or cultured skin fibroblasts.[742,750] A partial deficiency of beta-galactosidase occurs in heterozygotes.[742] In utero diagnosis is possible using cultured amniotic fluid cells.[716,750]

The G_{M2} Gangliosidoses. At least four clinical disorders are currently designated G_{M2} gangliosidoses: Tay-Sachs disease (G_{M2} gangliosidosis type 1), Sandhoff's disease (G_{M2} gangliosidosis type 2), juvenile G_{M2} gangliosidosis (G_{M2} gangliosidosis type 3), and adult G_{M2} gangliosidosis. These disorders are all characterized by excessive accumulation of G_{M2} gangliosides.

BIOCHEMISTRY. Tay-Sachs disease is the best understood of the sphingolipidoses. Accumulation of G_{M2} ganglioside was shown over a decade ago to be due to deficiency of hexosaminidase A (Hex A; Fig. 9-12).[606,696] This enzyme is thought to be a tetramer made up of 2 pairs of identical subunits, $\alpha_2 \beta_2$, in a manner analogous to globin. Hexosaminidase B (Hex B) is the homopolymer $\beta_2 \beta_2$. Mild treatment of the purified enzyme has resulted in interconversion of Hex A to Hex B presumably due to dissociation and reassociation.[697] Reversal of this process using Hex B and hexosaminidase S (Hex S; a rare form $\alpha_2 \alpha_2$) has produced Hex A.[70] The α and β subunits are similar in size and composition, perhaps reflecting common genetic ancestry.[277] The genes for the two subunits are located on different chromosomes.[465]

Hex A and Hex B when purified are active against water-soluble artificial substrates, but not against G_{M2} ganglioside. An activator specific to Hex A has been described.[150]

Three biochemical forms of infantile G_{M2} gangliosidosis are distinguishable: Tay-Sachs disease, Sandhoff's disease and the AB variant. In classical Tay-Sachs disease (variant B) Hex A is absent by biochemical and immunologic assays, probably reflecting defective α-chain synthesis.

In Sandhoff's disease (variant O), both Hex A and Hex B are deficient, presumably reflecting abnormal β-chain structure or synthesis. Immunologic studies have shown cross-reacting material present in at least one patient.[771] Genetic compounds (heterozygotes) for two different mutant genes may have atypical disease and enzyme properties.[468,499] Juvenile and adult types of G_{M2} gangliosidosis due to partial deficiency of Hex A or Hex A and Hex B have been described. Residual activity of enzyme against synthetic substrate in serum and tissues may be quite variable and correlates poorly with clinical severity.

Enzyme activity of patients with the AB variant of infantile G_{M2} gangliosidosis is diminished when tested against natural substrate in the absence of detergent; when tested against synthetic substrate, enzyme activity is normal. This disorder is, therefore, thought to be due to a deficiency of the activator substance.[150]

Tay-Sachs Disease or Type 1 G_{M2} gangliosidosis. In 1881 Warren Tay reported an infant with a cherry-red macula and delayed development.[816] In 1887 Sachs further defined the clinical condition that now bears Tay's and his name.[692] This disorder is the most common disorder of lipid metabolism affecting the nervous system.

PATHOLOGY. Lipid storage in visceral organs is observable only at the ultrastructural level; the nervous system bears the brunt of this disease. The gross appearance of the brain is usually normal during the first few months of life. Later the brain may become larger than normal. Microscopically, neurons at all levels of the neuraxis are ballooned by stored lipid material. Lipid inclusions displace the nucleus towards the margin of the neuron. Gangliosides constitute the majority of the lipid in these inclusions. By electron microscopy, the neuronal cytosomes consist of laminated circular membranes and membranous cytoplasmic bodies. As the disease progresses neuronal depopulation occurs accompanied by cortical gliosis and demyelination of white matter.

CLINICAL FEATURES. Excessive accumulation of G_{M2} ganglioside occurs before birth, but symptoms do not become apparent until after the first 3 months of life.[603] Onset of symptoms after 6 months of life is unusual. Developmental arrest or regression, irritability, lethargy, and hyperacusis are common early symptoms. Hyperacusis represents an exaggerated startle or Moro response to abrupt sounds. Initially, affected infants are hypotonic but deep tendon reflexes are preserved. Late in the course of the disease the infant reaches a vegetative state characterized by spasticity and opisthotonus. Simple partial, complex partial, and generalized seizures almost invariably occur after 1 year of age. Macrocephaly is generally present in Tay-Sachs patients after 18 months of age.

An extremely useful diagnostic feature is the cherry-red macula. This ophthalmologic feature, although present in a subtle form even before obvious clinical onset of the disease, is present in virtually all patients with Tay-Sachs disease after 1 year of age. The cherry-red macula, which is not specific for Tay-Sachs disease (Table 9-3), results from the loss of cells from the macula region of the retina, thereby exposing the vasculature of the choroid. Blindness and, later, optic atrophy occur after 1 year of age. Pupillary reflexes may be preserved even when the infant is blind.

Death usually occurs at 2 years to 5 years. Hepatosplenomegaly, coarse facial features, and bony involvement do not occur in Tay-Sachs disease.

DIAGNOSIS AND GENETICS. The diagnosis is made by measuring total and heat-stable hexosaminidase activity in serum using an artificial substrate that yields the fluorogenic substance methylumbelliferone upon cleavage. Severe deficiency of the heat-labile form (Hex A) is found in Tay-Sachs disease. The enzyme can also be measured in leukocytes, tears, fibroblasts, and cultured amniotic fluid cells.[770]

The gene for Tay-Sachs disease is found in all peoples, but is most common among East European (Ashkenazic) Jews and their descendants, among whom roughly one in 30 individuals is a carrier, or heterozygote. This is about ten times the incidence in other groups. The reason for this discrepancy is not known at present. Evidence for heterozygote advantage, versus founder effect and genetic drift, has been cited by various authors.[139,571] In most instances there is no family history of the disease.

Tay-Sachs disease is the object of the first major effort at heterozygote screening and counseling in this country. It was a logical choice because most cases of Tay-Sachs disease occur in a well-defined population, the carrier test is inexpensive and reliable, and accurate prenatal diagnosis is available if both parents are found to be carriers.[400,401]

Carrier detection programs have al-lowed couples at 25% risk to discover this fact before having a child with Tay-Sachs disease. If the couple desires, amniocentesis can be performed at about the 16th gestational week to determine if the fetus has the disease. The assay is performed on cultured amniocytes.

If the fetus is affected, the parents may elect to terminate the pregnancy. Other reproductive options include artificial insemination (a donor in this situation should be screened for Tay-Sachs disease), and adoption.

Carrier detection using the serum assay is quite reliable. "False positive" results may occur due to chronic disease (especially diabetes), oral contraceptives, and pregnancy. If a woman is pregnant, the father should be tested first. If the serum assay shows him to be in the inconclusive or carrier range, the hexosaminidase assay must then be done on the mother's leukocytes instead of serum. For this reason women desiring testing should be screened before becoming pregnant.[598,770]

Sandhoff's Disease or type 2 G_{M2} gangliosidosis. The clinical and pathologic features of Sandhoff's disease are very similar to Tay-Sachs disease. Visceral storage of gangliosides is evident in histiocytes.[698] Clinically, this may be detectable as mild hepatosplenomegaly. The onset of the disease is earlier and the progression is more rapid than in Tay-Sachs disease.

Juvenile and Adult G_{M2} Gangliosidoses or type 3 G_{M2} gangliosidosis. As noted at the introduction to the G_{M2} gangliosidoses, partial deficiency of Hex A or Hex A and B have been reported.[398,610,764,798] The juvenile variants have usually had a disease onset in early childhood. Frequent signs and symptoms have included dementia, seizures (including myoclonic seizures), spasticity, ataxia, tremor, and choreoathetosis. The macula is usually normal although in one patient a cherry-red macula was observed.[105] Retinitis pigmentosa and optic atrophy have been noted in a few patients.[105] The usual absence of retinitis pigmentosa and the late onset of visual loss helps exclude late infantile neuronal ceroid lipofuscinosis.

Adult onset of G_{M2} gangliosidosis, whether due to partial Hex A deficiency or partial Hex A and B deficiency, has presented clinically as a spinocerebellar degeneration.[610,661] Ataxia, pyramidal tract involvement, peripheral neuropathy, and absence of dementia are the usual signs and symptoms.

G_{M3} Gangliosidosis.   Three patients with excessive accumulation of G_{M3} ganglioside have been reported.[527,639,680] No consistent clinical picture emerges from these cases. Onset of symptoms has been in infancy and all patients have been severely affected. Visceral storage and seizures were noted in two cases. The defect in these patients is no longer believed to be an abnormality in biosynthesis of higher gangliosides.[91]

Metachromatic Leukodystrophy

The phenomenon of metachromasia in a patient with the pathologic changes of a leukodystrophy was first described in 1910 by Alzheimer.[6] Scholz in 1925 described the clinical features of this familial leukodystrophy.[715] Since that description three other conditions have been added so that four forms of metachromatic leukodystrophy (MLD) are recognized, namely late infantile MLD, juvenile MLD, adult MLD, and multiple sulfatase deficiency. The late infantile, juvenile, and adult forms of MLD probably represent distinct entities because the age of onset tends to be constant in families with adult and juvenile MLD. Moreover, studies indicate differences both in the quantities of stored material and in the nature of the enzyme defect.[211,231]

Pathology.   The characteristic feature of MLD is the storage of metachromatic lipid material in cells. *Metachromasia* refers to the color change of a dye induced by substances with particular anionic groups, for example, the usual purple color of acidic cresyl violet is changed to brown by the sulfatide in MLD. Metachromatic storage material in MLD occurs in cells of the peripheral and central nervous system, in epithelial cells of the renal tubules, gall bladder, liver, pituitary, pancreas, and adrenal gland.[893]

At autopsy the brain usually reveals an obvious, widespread loss of white matter. The white matter is firm, has a gray discoloration, and may even be cavitated in the areas of the brain in which the white matter is severely involved. The U-fibers in the cerebral cortical white matter are usually spared. Microscopically, demyelination is apparent and the number of oligodendroglia is decreased. Metachromatic lipid storage material in the central nervous system is found in macrophages, in oligodendroglia, and outside of cells in the tissue. The lipid storage material may also be found in neurons in the dentate nucleus, cranial nerve nuclei, the hypothalamus, the thalamus, the basal ganglia, the pons, the anterior horn cells, the dorsal root ganglia, and Betz cells. In peripheral nerves segmental demyelination can usually be found in teased nerve fiber preparations. Metachromatic granules are usually found in Schwann cells and phagocytes. In adult MLD the changes may be absent until late in the course of the disease. The ultrastructure of the lipid storage material has a characteristic appearance that resembles a herring bone pattern. The lipid inclusions in Schwann cells, oligodendroglia, and cultured fibroblasts grown in a medium high in sulfatide may display this typical ultrastructural pattern.

Biochemistry.   In this disorder galactosyl sulfatide, also known as *galactosyl-3-sulfate ceramide*, accumulates in the central and peripheral nervous system, as well as in the kidney, liver and other organs. This substance is ordinarily cleaved to galactosyl ceramide and phosphoadenosine phosphosulfate (Fig. 9-12). The enzyme responsible for this reaction is generally called *arylsulfatase A*.[199,200,688] The term arylsulfatase refers to enzymes with activity against synthetic sulfate esters of phenols. The insoluble fraction is microsomal arylsulfatase C. The soluble lysosomal fraction is comprised of arylsulfatases A and B. These last two enzymes are clearly distinguished by their chemical and physical properties. Nevertheless, care must be taken because they may both contribute to an enzyme assay.[211] Several forms of arylsulfatase A can be found in various fluids and tissues. These probably represent post-translational modifications of the same protein rather than separate enzymes.[782,783] In MLD an antigenically active protein can be found by immunologic techniques, but it has low or no activity.[790] Patients with atypical forms of

MLD may have enzyme activity demonstrable on gel electrophoresis but with atypical properties or altered behavior with respect to substrate or detergent interaction.[207]

Arylsulfatase A can be studied using urine, serum, and amniotic fluid.[64,86,745,821,822] The activity in urine is considerably higher than in the other fluids. Nevertheless, for definitive diagnosis, a tissue sample should be used. Leukocytes and cultured skin and amniotic fluid fibroblasts are satisfactory. Assay of other enzymes can be used as controls.[211] Obligate heterozygotes often are distinguishable from patients and normal controls but there is some overlap so that carrier detection is not completely certain.[433]

Arylsulfatase A deficiency is also part of the disorder of multiple sulfatase deficiency, in which at least five enzymes can be demonstrated to be deficient. This disorder is discussed in a separate section.

Clinical Features. All forms of MLD have a recessive mode of inheritance. The most common form of arylsulfatase A deficiency is late-infantile MLD. It is approximately four times as common as juvenile MLD.[330] Adult MLD is rare; no more than 50 cases have been reported.

The onset of late infantile MLD may occur between 1 year and 4 years, and occurs typically near the end of the second year.[212] The onset occurs after apparently normal early development so that the child is usually ambulatory before disease onset. Difficulty in walking is a common early symptom. The child is often weak, hypotonic, and hyporeflexic early in the disease. Evidence of upper motor neuron involvement may be relatively inconspicuous, perhaps consisting of no more than an extensor plantar response. As the disease progresses, ataxia becomes more obvious, muscle tone increases, and the child clearly begins to deteriorate mentally. After 18 months to 2 years the patient becomes bedridden, loses contact with the environment, and displays decorticate or decerebrate posturing in response to stimuli. The child usually dies at 3 years to 6 years of age.

Ocular symptoms and signs include strabismus, optic atrophy, and a red macula that, unlike Tay-Sachs disease, is surrounded by a grayish discoloration of the retina.[14] These changes usually appear late in the course.

Juvenile MLD begins between 4 and 21 years of age.[342] This form of MLD is only one fourth as common as late infantile MLD.[330] Some patients have developmental delay preceding the presumed onset but most have developed normally until the onset of the disease. Common first symptoms are clumsiness and weakness, school failure, and behavioral disturbances. Other early symptoms are speech disturbances, hand tremor, and seizures. At the time of examination the patient usually has signs of mental retardation, spastic quadriplegia, pseudobulbar paresis, ataxia of upper and lower extremities, strabismus, nystagmus, optic atrophy, and macular changes similar to those seen in late infantile MLD. The rate of progression of the disease is quite variable, but usually patients survive for several years.

Adult MLD begins after 21 years in the third and fourth decades of life. The onset is so subtle as to make the diagnosis difficult during life. Commonly the disorder presents as a slowly progressive dementia or organic psychosis. Peripheral neuropathy and ataxia occur much later in adult MLD than in late infantile or juvenile MLD. Nerve conduction velocity, cerebrospinal fluid protein and the EEG are usually normal until late in the disease. The EEG is often abnormal in the earlier stages of the other forms of MLD. Background activity is slow and paroxysmal epileptiform activity may occur, especially in late infantile MLD.

Diagnosis. The diagnosis of late infantile MLD is often suggested by the typical clinical features of late infantile onset of spastic ataxia associated with lower motor neuron signs and elevated cerebrospinal fluid (CSF) protein. Elevated CSF protein and slow nerve conduction velocities are present in most patients with late infantile and adult MLD. It should be noted that in juvenile MLD, CSF protein and nerve conduction velocity may be normal.[342] A nonfunctioning gall bladder may also help confirm the diagnosis but the availability of other tests has largely supplanted this procedure. Recently cranial computed tomography has shown abnormalities in MLD.[119,672] In late infantile and juvenile MLD computerized tomograms reveal low-density lesions involving the entire centrum ovale. The low density is bilateral, symmetric, and homogeneous. The margins of the low-density lesion are scalloped and do not enhance with contrast. These features serve to differentiate the low-density lesions of MLD from those of other leukodystrophies and multiple sclerosis. Another means of confirming the diagnosis of MLD is a sural nerve biopsy demonstrating stored metachromatic lipid material that has the characteristic ultrastructure.[608]

Assays of arylsulfatase A activity are necessary to establish the diagnosis conclusively. The activity of this enzyme may be measured in urine, serum, leukocytes, cultured fibroblasts, and cultured amniotic fluid cells.[27,211,624] The last two assays allow detection of heterozygotes, in most cases, and intrauterine diagnosis of MLD.

Globoid Cell Leukodystrophy or Krabbe's Disease

The first complete clinical and pathologic description of globoid cell leukodystrophy was by Krabbe in 1916.[454] He described the globoid cell that is the characteristic pathologic feature of this disease. In 1970 a deficiency of galactosylcerebroside beta-galactosidase was described in the brain, liver, spleen, and kidney of a patient with globoid cell leukodystrophy.[796] Although this biochemical defect presently confirms the diagnosis of the disorder, in most of the reported cases the diagnosis was based upon finding globoid cells in the brain at autopsy. The clinical disorder described below, therefore, is best termed *globoid cell leukodystrophy*.

Pathology.   The nervous system is the only system that shows pathologic changes that are of any clinical significance. Renal tubule cell lipid inclusions were noted in one patient but this finding was without clinical consequence.[25]

The changes in the brain are largely restricted to the white matter. That these changes begin quite early is demonstrated by white matter involvement in a fetus with globoid cell leukodystrophy.[220] In infants dying of this disorder the brain is usually atrophic. The white matter has a darker appearance and is firmer than usual. The cerebral white matter with the exception of the subcortical arcuate fibers, the cerebellar white matter, the corticospinal and corticobulbar tracts, and the spinal cord are the most involved areas in the brain. Microscopically, demyelination and gliosis are noted.[591] Oligodendroglial cells are diminished or absent. Axon sheaths and axons alike are destroyed.

The most characteristic pathologic feature is the globoid cell. These cells are moderate to large (up to 50 μm) and may contain multiple nuclei. They are periodic acid-Schiff (PAS)-positive and stain with lipid stains. Globoid cells are similar to Gaucher's cells but unlike Gaucher's cells they do not occur outside the central nervous system. Globoid cells tend to be found in perivascular clusters in the most recent lesions.

The origin of globoid cells is uncertain. Although the origin was originally thought to be glial, presently a mesodermal origin is favored. This view is supported by observations made in an experimental model in which galactocerebroside is injected intracerebrally into rats.[25,29] At the site of injection globoid cells appeared, but only after galactocerebroside injection. No other material is capable of inducing their formation. The lipid material in the large, multinucleated globoid cells is galactocerebroside. This material has a tubular or crystalline ultrastructure.

The peripheral nervous system is also involved.[213,366] Loss of myelin sheaths and axons occurs. Inclusions with an ultrastructure similar to that of the lipid inclusions in globoid cells are found in histiocytes. Globoid cells, however, are not found in peripheral nerves.

Biochemistry.   The primary defect in this disorder is a deficiency of a beta-galactosidase, galactosylceramidase.[796] Enzyme deficiency can be shown in serum, leukocytes, and cultured fibroblasts as well as in kidney, brain, spleen, and liver.[795,797] The deficiency in cerebroside sulfotransferase also reported in brains of patients with globoid cell leukodystrophy is probably a secondary deficiency.[28]

As shown in Figure 9-12, galactosylceramide (galactocerebroside) is degraded to sphingosine by removal of the galactose and a fatty acid. Removal of the fatty acid first will create galactosyl sphingosine or psychosine, an extremely toxic compound. Psychosine is present in the brain of patients with globoid cell leukodystrophy at ten times to one hundred times the normal concentration.[836,837] Psychosine accumulation could account for the drastic loss of myelin in Krabbe's disease, and the absence of a discrete storage compound.

Galactosylceramidase can be measured using a radioactively labeled natural substrate.[795] An assay using artificial substrate is also available.[264]

Clinical Features. Globoid cell leukodystrophy is inherited as an autosomal recessive trait. More than one affected sibling and parental consanguinity have been noted.

Globoid cell leukodystrophy may be divided into infantile-onset and late-onset forms according to the age of onset of symptoms. Infantile-onset globoid cell leukodystrophy begins between 3 and 6 months after birth.[334] Rarely, onset may even be as early as the neonatal period. Hagberg has identified three stages of the disease.[324] In the first stage the child is irritable and may have feeding difficulties and vomiting, seizures, episodic fever, or psychomotor retardation. In the second stage marked psychomotor regression becomes apparent. Spasticity increases and intermittent decerebrate or decorticate posturing may occur. Deep tendon reflexes are usually increased. Evidence of visual failure and optic atrophy appear in this stage. In the third stage the patient reaches a state of decorticate or decerebrate posturing with little or no response to sensory stimuli. Deep tendon reflexes are often absent in this stage of the disease.[213] Terminally the infants develop dysphagia, bulbar paralysis, and hypotonia. Death usually occurs before the end of the first year.

At least 14 cases of late-onset globoid cell leukodystrophy have been reported.[160] The age of onset has been quite variable, ranging from 2 years to 35 years. Commonly these patients have gait disturbances, failing vision, or psychomotor regression as their earliest symptoms. Hemiplegia, progressing to spastic quadriplegia, is common. Vision is usually impaired but optic atrophy is much less common than in the infantile-onset form of globoid cell leu-

kodystrophy. Seizures are unusual and deep tendon reflexes are usually normal or increased. The course of the disease is surprisingly short considering the late onset; death usually occurs within less than 2 years after onset.

At autopsy all patients with the late-onset disease have had globoid cells and demyelination in the brain. Rarely, have patients not had the elevated cerebroside:sulfatide ratio in cortical white matter, a typical biochemical abnormality in infantile globoid cell leukodystrophy. Galactosylceramide beta-galactosidase activity has been deficient in several patients.[899]

Niemann-Pick Disease or Sphingomyelin Lipidosis

This sphingolipidosis is clinically and biochemically heterogeneous. The infantile form was described in 1914 and since then several other forms have been described.[158,251,585] The disorder has been reported in many races and ethnic groups but most of the infantile cases have been children of Jewish parents. Inheritance is autosomal recessive.

Pathology. Storage of sphingomyelin occurs in cells in lymphoreticular tissue, kidney, intestine, and endocrine organs. Histiocytes (20 mm–90 μm in diameter) in these tissues may be filled with clear lipid droplets that give them a foamy appearance. The brain is firm and atrophic, and upon microscopic examination neurons are seen to be moderately distended with lipid. The cytosomes in these neurons appear intrastructurally as concentric laminated membranes.[405] The cerebral and cerebellar cortex, basal ganglia, brain stem, spinal cord, peripheral ganglia, meninges, blood vessel endothelium, and choroid plexus are involved. Only slight demyelination is found in the cerebral white matter.

Biochemistry. In these disorders the problems mentioned earlier of correlating stored material with an enzyme defect are especially obvious. By definition, these disorders are characterized by an increase in intracellular sphingomyelin.[441] This highly polar compound is found in almost all mammalian membranes and is composed of ceramide and phosphorylcholine. It makes up about 20% of liver and plasma membrane phospholipids, and a slightly smaller proportion of human myelin phospholipids.[864] Specific enzymes in the cystosol and lysosomes that cleave sphingomyelin into phosphorylcholine and ceramide (see Fig. 9-12) have been described. The cytosolic form has optimal activity at a neutral pH, whereas another form, presumably lysosomal, has optimal activity at around pH 5.[660] The lysosomal enzyme when partially purified requires added detergent for activity to be significant.[359] The sphingomyelinase enzymes have been noted generally to have high specificity and have little or no activity against other phospholipids. These enzymes have been found in leukocytes, cultured skin fibroblasts, liver, spleen, and brain. Enzyme activity has been assessed using radioactive substrate, and a synthetic substrate has also been developed.[263,600,714,785]

Advances in biochemistry have added confusion to the original five categories of Crocker and Mayes.[158] Two of the categories have remained somewhat homogeneous. Type A, the acute neuropathic form, is characterized by a severe deficiency of sphingomyelinase activity as measured at pH 5.0 Heterozygotes for this form may have an intermediate level of sphingomyelinase in cultured skin fibroblasts.[864] Sphingomyelinase activity in spleens from patients with Neimann-Pick disease type B is also quite low, and was low in one patient whose liver sphingomyelinase activity was measured.[89,714]

The other forms of sphingomyelin lipidosis are not as clear-cut. They fall into two groups, the juvenile forms, with nervous system involvement, and a smaller group of adults who have an asymptomatic increase of sphingomelin in liver and spleen.[92,637] The Nova Scotian variant, called type D by Crocker and Mayes, is best considered a genetically distinct form of juvenile sphingomyelin lipidosis.[158] In these disorders, sphingomyelinase activity has ranged from moderately depressed to normal in early reports. Close examination of sphingomyelinase has disclosed at least two isozymes separable by isoelectric focusing, with a demonstrable defect in one of these isozymes in some patients.[123] In another

family, sphingomyelinase activity was not lower than normal but it was distinctly difficult to extract from brain, liver, and spleen, perhaps reflecting poor bioavailability.[356] In summary, intracellular accumulation of sphingomyelin does not correlate well with the degree of gross sphingomyelinase activity measured by most techniques. Further characterization of normal and abnormal enzymes and the stored material is needed.

Clinical Features. Five clinical types of Niemann-Pick disease have been delineated, Types A, B, C, D, and E.[157,158] The most common form is the acute infantile form, Type A. In this form the infant begins to feed poorly and loses weight, usually within the first 6 months of life. Development lags and the abdomen becomes distended as the liver and spleen enlarge. Occasionally jaundice is present. Lymph node enlargement occurs in approximately one-half of patients. About one-third of the patients show cutaneous abnormalities consisting of a brownish-yellow pigmentation, which may be diffuse or confined to extensor surfaces of the limbs. Xanthomatous eruptions may occur. Emaciation rapidly develops and there may be irregular fever, sweating, and salivation. Concomitantly motor development fails and gross mental deficit appears. The infant does not sit and loses strength in his limbs. Some patients develop brisk reflexes and generalized rigidity. About one-half of the patients have a cherry-red macula indistinguishable from that found in Tay-Sachs disease, and pale optic disks. Blindness, however, appears late in the disease. In contrast to Tay-Sachs disease, the head does not enlarge, there is no abnormal reponse to auditory stimuli, and seizures rarely occur. Death usually occurs before 3 years of age.

Type B Niemann-Pick disease also begins in infancy but is characterized by visceral involvement, especially hepatosplenomegaly, without nervous system involvement. Type C has been extremely variable.[252,356] The onset of the disease in this form occurs between 2 and 5 years of age. Neurologic symptoms are the most prominent symptoms. Psychomotor retardation, spasticity and seizures, often myoclonic, frequently occur. Hepatosplenomegaly is less prominent than in the infantile form. Visceromegaly may even decrease during the course of the illness.[356] A macular cherry-red spot may also occur in this form. One group of patients often considered to have Type C Niemann-Pick disease have vertical supranuclear ophthalmoplegia and ataxia.[414,579,590] These patients have been felt by some to have a special form of sphingomyelin lipidosis.[579] One recent report of a patient with features of Type C Niemann-Pick disease but with vertical supranuclear ophthalmoplegia was found to have both normal sphingomyelin levels and sphingomyelinase activity.[336] Lactose levels were increased in the spleen and beta-galactosidase activity was deficient. The proposed defect was in lysosomal beta-galactosidase with a substrate specificity for lactose and other oligosaccharides with a terminal beta-galactoside.

Type D Niemann-Pick disease is the variant that occurs only in patients with a Nova Scotian ancestry. The age of onset is quite variable but symptoms usually begin in childhood. Hepatosplenomegaly, slowly progressive psychomotor retardation, ataxia, and pyramidal and extrapyramidal signs characterize the disease. Death occurs 12 years to 20 years after onset of the disease.

Type E Niemann-Pick disease is characterized by the adult onset of hepatosplenomegaly without neurologic involvement.

Diagnosis. The diagnosis of the infantile form of Niemann-Pick disease is suggested by the clinical picture of psychomotor regression and visceromegaly. The presence in the bone marrow of foam cells can help confirm the diagnosis in this form and in the B and C Types. The diagnosis must be confirmed by enzyme assay. The assay may be performed on leukocytes or skin fibroblasts.[263,406] Heterozygotes for type A may also be detected in this manner. *In utero* diagnosis of type A Niemann-Pick disease is possible using cultured amniotic cells.[864]

Treatment. No effective treatment is currently available for patients with Niemann-Pick disease. Enzyme replacement is being intensively investigated as a treatment. Splenectomy in patients with the visceral forms may be of value when thrombocytopenia becomes severe.

Gaucher's Disease or Glucocerebroside Lipidosis

Gaucher's disease is one of the earliest of the sphingolipidoses described.[273] It was also the first lipidosis in which the storage material was identified and the first lipidosis in which the enzymatic defect was delineated. It is the most common sphingolipidosis but usually presents in the adult form (Type I) that affects the nervous system only minimally. Type I Gaucher's disease is 30 times more common in Ashkenazic Jews than in other groups, but the infantile form (Type II) and juvenile form (Type III) are not. Type II Gaucher's disease usually presents in infancy with hepatosplenomegaly, anemia, developmental regression, spasticity, retroflexion of the neck, and bulbar paralysis.

Pathology. The distinctive pathologic abnormality in Gaucher's disease is the Gaucher's cell. This is a ballooned cell, 20 μm to 100 μm in size, that can be found in reticuloendothelial cells and other organs including the brain. The cell's nucleus is displaced toward the cell wall and the cytoplasm has an unusual reticulated or wrinkled appearance when viewed after a trichrome stain or observed under a phase contrast microscope. Neuronal loss and neuronophagia is prominent in brain stem nuclei (especially the bulbar nuclei), the dentate nucleus, the basal ganglia, and the middle layers of the cerebral cortex. The changes in the cortex are most prominent in the calcarine cortex.

Biochemistry. The accumulation of glucocerebroside (glucosylceramide) in this disorder is due to a deficiency of glucocerebrosidase, which hydrolyses its substrate to glucose and ceramide (Fig. 9-12). The enzyme can be found in liver, spleen, intestinal mucosa, brain, fibroblasts, and leukocytes. The last are a convenient source of enzymes for diagnostic assay.[755] Using labeled glucocerebroside as substrate avoids the problems encountered with nonspecific beta-glucosidase activity associated with synthetic substrate. The contribution of other glucosidases can be minimized by using an acid *p*H or detergent for the assay.[68,633] In general, the severity of the enzyme defect is proportional to the clinical severity.[90] The major source of glucocerebroside is probably leukocytes, with a smaller contribution from erythrocytes and brain gangliosides.[417] In view of the neurologic progression of types II and III Gaucher's disease, and the perivascular location of Gaucher's cells, it is possible that the material stored in the nervous system is derived from plasma.[181]

Clinical Features.   Type II Gaucher's disease begins before 6 months to 7 months of age. Rarely the disease may be recognized in the neonatal period. Hepatosplenomegaly and enlargement of lymph nodes are early features. In unusual cases, the disease appears to begin later and may lack clinically apparent hepatosplenomegaly.[325] The infant usually has undergone psychomotor regression by the time medical help is sought. A consistent early sign of the neurologic disease is a powerful but intermittent retraction of the head that may antedate any disturbance of posture and tone in the rest of the body. Symptoms and signs of bulbar paresis are often prominent. The cry is feeble. Feeding is difficult because it is difficult to swallow and material accumulates in the pharynx. Extraocular muscle paresis is often noted, usually taking the form of convergent strabismus. An initial trismus may later be replaced by a sagging jaw. Laryngeal stridor occurs as the disease progresses. Seizures occur in some patients. A cherry-red macula has rarely been reported in Gaucher's disease but this observation has been questioned recently.[145] As the disease progresses spasticity increases so that a state of decerebration is reached. Death usually occurs before the infant reaches 2 years of age, often as a result of respiratory complications.

Type III Gaucher's disease is much less common than Type II and is less clearly defined as well. The onset is in childhood. Splenomegaly, anemia, and seizures are the most common manifestations. In some Type III patients dementia, spasticity, strabismus, and ataxia also occur.

Type I or adult Gaucher's disease is principally manifested by hepatosplenomegaly without significant neurologic dysfunction. Other frequent features are bony abnormalities, thrombocytopenia, pulmonary symptoms related to Gaucher's cell infiltration of the lungs, and a bleeding diathesis. Some adult patients with Gaucher's disease have both clinical and pathologic nervous system involvement.[586,760] It is not clear if these patients should be separated from Type I patients and included with Type III patients or whether they represent one end of the clinical spectrum seen in Type I Gaucher's disease. The most common neurologic symptoms are dementia and seizures, often myoclonic.[586] Patients may also have spasticity, ataxia, strabismus, and dysphagia. An adult variant of Gaucher's disease that is found in Sweden also includes dementia as a symptom.[205]

Laboratory Findings.   Anemia is quite common in all forms of Gaucher's disease and is often associated with thrombocytopenia. Acid phosphatase, also a lysosomal hydrolase, is increased in the serum and spleen. The isozyme profile of this increase in Type I Gaucher's disease has been shown to be distinguishable from that in prostatic carcinoma.[547] The EEG is frequently abnormal in Types II and III but in a nonspecific way.[587]

Diagnosis.   Gaucher's disease Types II and III should be suspected in an infant or child with hepatosplenomegaly and psychomotor regression or arrest. Other metabolic diseases producing psychomotor regression and visceromegaly without coarse facies are listed in Table 9-1. Gaucher's cells may be identified in bone marrow aspirates. Glucocerebrosidase deficiency can be demonstrated in leukocytes, and cultured fibroblasts.[365,406] Carrier detection using leukocytes and prenatal diagnosis using cultured amniotic cells are also possible.[95,713]

Treatment.   No treatment is currently available for Type II and III forms of Gaucher's disease. Genetic counseling and intrauterine diagnosis currently offer the best approach to prevention of the recurrence of this disase. A promising approach to the treatment of the lipid storage disorders has been pioneered in Gaucher's disease. This approach, enzyme replacement, involves the administration of exogenous enzyme.[97] Enzyme replacement is particularly applicable to Type I Gaucher's disease because the lipid storage predominantly occurs outside of the nervous system, so one can avoid the problem of getting enzyme across the blood–brain barrier. Administration of glucocerebrosidase isolated from human placental tissue has produced a 26% reduction in the quantity of accumulated glucocerebroside in erythrocytes.[97] This reduction persists in some patients years after the infusions. Evidence for reduction in liver size and improved reticuloendothelial function during enzyme infusion has also been presented.[93]

Fabry's Disease

This disorder was first described in 1898 by Anderson and Fabry who were struck by the cutaneous lesions leading Fabry to label this condition *angiokeratoma corporis diffusum universalis*.[10,228] In addition to the angiokeratoma, this X-linked disease is characterized by corneal opacities, pain crises, acroparesthesias, and renal and cardiovascular disease.

Pathology. Storage of neutral glycolipids occurs in many tissues, especially in endothelial cells, epithelial cells, muscle cells and neurons. Cells of the perineural sheaths of peripheral nerves may contain lipid material in excess. Often there is a predominant loss of small axons from the peripheral nerves. Neuronal storage of neutral glycospingolipids occurs in dorsal root ganglia, the intermediolateral cell column, the vagus nucleus, the reticular formations of the pons and medulla, the accessory nucleus, the amygdala, and the presubiculum.[657] Ultrastructural studies of intraneuronal inclusions reveal several types including zebra bodies and granulomembranous bodies similar to those in Hurler's syndrome.[326]

Biochemistry. Globotriosylceramide (ceramide trihexoside), galabiosylceramide, and hexaglycosylceramide are the major lipids stored in the lysosomes of cells of patients with Fabry's disease.[802,872] These neutral glycosphingolipids with alpha-galactosyl moieties accumulate as a result of deficient alpha-galactosidase A deficiency (ceramide trihexosidase) (Fig. 9-12)[94,436] The gene controlling this enzyme is apparently on the X chromosome. Fabry's disease is the only known sphingolipidosis transmitted as an X-linked recessive trait. Two forms (A and B) of alpha-galactosidase have been characterized.[69] Males with the defective gene have absent alpha-galactosidase A activity, although total alpha-galactosidase activity is 10% to 25% of that of normal controls. Heterozygous females have intermediate alpha-galactosidase A activity. Plasma globotriosylceramide levels are 3 times to 10 times that of normal. The predominance of storage in cells lining blood-containing structures perhaps occurs because of the absence of necessary catabolic mechanisms in plasma. Red cell membranes are the principal source of globoside, the precursor of the neutral glycosphingolipids. Excess neutral glycosphingolipids ultimately appear in the urine in Fabry's disease.

Clinical Features. Fabry's disease usually begins in childhood or adolescence but may not begin until adulthood. Early symptoms include angiokeratomas, corneal dystrophy and consequent visual loss, pain in extremities, and hypohydrosis.[887] The angiokeratomas occur in the skin between the umbilicus and the knees. These lesions appear as macular or papular, dark red to blue, punctate lesions.[838] The pain is usually most intense in the hands and feet but may extend into the proximal portions of the extremities. Fever often accompanies the pain. Thus Fabry's disease may imitate an arthritis.[887] Other non-specific symptoms and signs include vomiting, diarrhea, growth failure, and maturational delay.

With increasing age the vascular and lympathic complications begin to dominate the clinical condition. Cardiovascular symptoms, renal failure, lymphedema, and cerebrovascular accidents occur. The cerebrovascular accidents may be either hemorrhagic or ischemic. These generally occur in the third or fourth decade. As a consequence of these strokes, personality changes, seizures, and focal neurologic symptoms appear.

Corneal opacification, called cornea verticillata, can be detected in males with the disease as early as 6 months of age.[62] The corneal lesions, however, are not unique to Fabry's disease and may be seen after chloroquin administration.

Females heterozygous for Fabry's disease are commonly affected. The severity of the disease in the heterozygote is quite variable. Often corneal dystrophy and sparse angiokeratoma occur. Rarely the heterozygote may have manifestations as severe as the male with Fabry's disease. Renal failure is rare. Young adult heterozygote females have been described with cerebrovascular symptoms, which may be intermittent.[75]

Diagnosis. The diagnosis of Fabry's disease is usually suggested by the angiokeratoma. These cutaneous lesions may be limited in distribution so that careful examination, particularly of the scrotum, may be necessary to find them. Patients with fever and pain may be particularly difficult to diagnose and laboratory tests may be necessary.

Screening laboratory tests for Fabry's disease include ophthalmologic examination for corneal dystrophy and examination of urine sediment for birefringent lipid globules that appear similar to a "Maltese cross."

Confirmation of the diagnosis requires demonstration of reduced alpha-galactosidase A activity in tears, urine, plasma, leukocytes, or cultured fibroblasts, or increased plasma or urinary levels of ceramide trihexoside.[188,192]

Prenatal diagnosis is possible by amniocentesis.[98] Alpha-galactosidase activity is measured in amniotic fluid. Cultured amniotic cells are used to establish male sex (XY karyotype), and alpha-galactosidase A and B activity are then measured. Reduced alpha-galactosidase A activity but normal alpha-galactosidase B activity would confirm the diagnosis of Fabry's disease. A rapid prenatal diagnostic test has also been developed.[265]

Treatment. Although enzyme replacement is theoretically possible, attempts have not been successful, in part because the enzyme is rapidly destroyed.[182,514] The efficacy of renal transplantation, an alternate means of enzyme replacement, is presently controversial but may be effective.[635] Relief of the excruciating pain that occurs in Fabry's disease frequently may be achieved

by chronic administration of the anticonvulsants phenytoin or carbamazepine.[22,495] Corticosteroids may also be helpful.[849]

Lipogranulomatosis or Farber's Disease

Lipogranulomatosis is a disorder characterized by subcutaneous nodules, joint contractures, hoarseness, failure to thrive, irritability, mental retardation, and intermittent fever. This is a rare condition; only 13 patients have been reported since the description of the condition in 1957.[229,620] The disease usually begins before 4 months of age, often with the appearance of painful, swollen joints. As the disease progresses subcutaneous nodules appear around joints, over the occiput, over the spine, and in other areas subjected to trauma. The diagnosis can usually be made from the clinical features because they are unique. Death, usually due to the severe pulmonary involvement, generally occurs before 2 years of age.

Neurologic symptoms include mental retardation, which is usually severe. A few patients have been reported with mild retardation or normal intellect and long survival.[620] Involvement of the peripheral nervous system is suggested by the frequent finding of areflexia. Seizures and more localized neurologic symptoms and signs have not been reported.

Pathology. This disorder is characterized by granulomatous changes in the subcutaneous nodules. Macrophages and foam cells found in these lesions contain PAS-positive material that is extractable in lipid solvents. In the nervous system the neurons of the anterior horn of the spinal cord, the brain stem nuclei, cerebellum, peripheral ganglia, dorsal root ganglia, and retinal ganglion cells are swollen with similar material.

The material stored in the inflammatory cells of the granulomatous lesions and in the other tissues affected in this disorder is in large part ceramide, an important component of the sphingolipids. Glycolipids and, at times, polysaccharides also occur in excess. The accumulation of ceramide appears to be a consequence of a deficiency in acid ceramidase.[793]

Biochemistry. The main storage substance, ceramide, is found in the subcutaneous nodules, kidney, liver, spleen, lung, and brain.[562,693] Activity of ceramidase, which cleaves ceramide into sphingosine and a fatty acid (Fig. 9-11), is severely deficient when measured at an acid pH using natural substrate, radioactively labeled.[210]

Diagnosis and Treatment. The diagnosis of lipogranulomatosis is suggested by the clinical features. Confirmation of the diagnosis depends upon demonstrating a deficiency in acid ceramidase activity in cultured fibroblasts, leukocytes, or autopsy material.[210,793] Prenatal diagnosis has been possible using cells cultured from amniotic fluid.[237]

No specific treatment is currently available for this disorder, therefore, treatment has consisted of supportive care.

OTHER LYSOSOMAL STORAGE DISEASES

Salla Disease

This is a condition recently described by Aula and associates in four adults.[24] It has now been recognized in other patients in Finland and is characterized by severe mental retardation and somewhat coarse facial features resembling those of patients with AGU. The first signs of retardation occur between 6 and 24 months. Other neurologic manifestations include ataxia, spasticity, spastic tetraplegia, athetosis, and severe dysarthria. There is vacuolization of peripheral lymphocytes but no organomegaly. Except for thickening of the calvaria and curving of the tibia, changes of dysostosis multiplex have not been present. Skin and nerve biopsies have revealed cytoplasmic storage vacuoles typical of a lysosomal storage disease. The urinary excretion of free sialic acid is increased tenfold compared to normal (as opposed to the increased excretion of bound sialic acid in the sialidoses). All lysosomal enzymes assayed so far have been normal. The basic defect is unknown. Autosomal recessive inheritance is suggested by the occurrence in sibs of both sexes, parental consanguinity, and the fact that most cases so far have come from a small area in northeastern Lapland.

Recently, increased tissue storage and increased urinary excretion of free sialic acid have been found in two severely affected infants. One infant with fetal hydrops had persistent ascites and hepatosplenomegaly until his death at 5 months of age.[376] The other had hepatosplenomegaly at 6 weeks, severe mental retardation, and coarse facies by 16 months of age.* Both children have histologic evidence of lysosomal storage. All lysosomal enzyme activities assayed so far have been normal. These patients clearly have a more severe condition than the Finnish patients with Salla disease. However, experience with heterogeneity in other storage diseases suggests that the causes and pathogeneses of these conditions may be related.

Mucolipidosis IV

Mucolipidosis IV (ML IV) is an autosomal recessive disease described so far only in Ashkenazi Jews. It is characterized by mental retardation, corneal clouding, and storage of both gangliosides and GAG. There has been no specific enzyme deficiency detected and diagnosis is based on clinical findings plus the microscopic demonstration of lysosomal storage bodies containing both lamellar inclusions and amorphous granular material. A partial deficiency of ganglioside sialidase has been described but additional studies are needed.[39]

Neuronal Ceroid-Lipofucinoses

Early in this century Batten described a familial progressive neurologic deterioration beginning in late infancy.[59] He recognized that this disorder, which he called *familial cerebral degeneration with macular changes,* was not the same as Tay-Sachs disease. Vogt, however, classified similar patients as *juvenile amaurotic idiocy.*[844] Age of onset was the only distinguishing feature among the familial amaurotic idiocies. The disorders that have been included among the familial amaurotic idiocies are all characterized by neuronal storage of excessive lipid material. Some of the patients of all ages have been found to have enzymatic defects in

---

*Stevenson, RE: Personal communication, 1981.

sphingolipid metabolism. These cases are now classified according to the enzyme defect. Other patients have excessive neuronal lipid storage but no enzymatic defect has been found to account for this accumulation. The stored material in some of these patients shares some of the characteristics of ceroid and lipofuscin, substances that accumulate in neurons during aging as well as in other conditions. Zeman and Dyken therefore, have labeled these diseases the *neuronal ceroid-lipofuscinoses*.[907] The lipid material that accumulates in neurons and other cells in neuronal ceroid-lipofuscinosis is PAS-positive, is insoluble in polar and nonpolar solvents, and is autofluorescent in ultraviolet light.

All of the conditions grouped under the term neuronal ceroid-lipofuscinoses (NCL) are characterized clinically by progressive neurologic deterioration without clinical evidence of involvement outside of the nervous system. Inheritance of these disorders is autosomal recessive. The only exceptions are several rare cases of adult NCL in which a dominant mode of transmission appeared to occur.[82] Several clinical and pathologic subtypes have been delineated: infantile NCL, late infantile NCL (Bielschowsky-Jansky syndrome), juvenile NCL (Spielmeyer-Sjögren syndrome), and adult NCL (Kufs' disease).

Pathology. All forms of NCL are to some extent characterized by neuronal lipid storage, neuronal loss, and gliosis. The distribution of neuronal involvement and the ultrastructure of cytosomes varies with the clinical subtypes. The brain is severely involved in infantile NCL. Severe neuronal loss and gliosis occur throughout the cerebral and cerebellar cortex, resulting in marked atrophy.[343,344] In late infantile NCL ballooned neurons are found in most gray matter and in all cortical laminae.[187,907] The brain in juvenile NCL is less severely involved than it is in the infantile and late infantile forms. Cortical layers one and five are less affected than layers two, four, and six.[187,907] In adult NCL the basal ganglia, thalamus, cerebellum and brain stem are more severely involved than is the cerebral cortex.[187]

The ultrastructure of the neuronal cytosomes also varies to some extent with the clinical disorder. The ultrastructure of the inclusions does not correlate as consistently with the clinical condition as the type of inclusion in the gangliosidoses correlates with the enzymatic defect. The neurons and the phagocytes in the cerebral cortex of infants with infantile NCL contain inclusions with a homogeneous, granular ultrastructure.[343] The most typical cytosome in late infantile NCL is characterized by convoluted membranes, sometimes called *curvilinear bodies*.[187,209] In other patients with late infantile NCL the inclusions are more pleomorphic and may appear similar to the concentric circular membranes (membranous cytoplasmic bodies) found in Tay-Sachs disease or to the arrays of parallel membranes (zebra bodies) seen in Hurler's syndrome. The typical inclusions in juvenile NCL are characterized by short, linear membrane segments that may be arranged in a so-called finger print pattern.[187,824,907] Inclusions in adult NCL resemble lipofuscin granules.

Biochemistry. The storage material in NCL resembles so-called aging pigments seen in older individuals, but the chemical identity of the material is unknown. The terms *ceroid* and *lipofuscin* sometimes have been used interchangeably for the stored lipopigments, but some investigators refer to two different substances when using the terms.[736] These authors distinguish ceroid from lipofuscin on the basis of different lipid content, density, metal content, and fluorescence excitation and emission spectra.[736,814] Both substances contain lysosomal enzymes and, therefore, probably are lysosomal material. The autofluorescence of the storage material may be due to a condensation product of malonaldehyde. Since this substance is a product of lipid peroxidation, a defect in peroxidation has been cited as a possible cause of NCL.[906] A deficiency in leukocyte peroxidase has been described but this finding has been quite inconsistent.[19,640] It is doubtful, therefore, that this observation is directly related to the pathogenesis or that it will prove diagnostically useful. No definite abnormality in sphingolipids has been detected.[906] In infantile NCL an abnormal serum lecithin fatty acid pattern and a marked reduction of brain lipids have been found.[799] The ethanolamine phosphoglycerides of the gray matter of these patients have higher proportions of oleic acid and arachidonic acid and much lower proportions of dodecosatetraenoic (C_{24}) acid and dodecosahexaenoic (C_{26}) acid.[799] Svennerholm has proposed that these alterations are manifestations of a generalized defect in metabolism of arachidonic acid.[800]

Infantile Neuronal Ceroid-Lipofuscinosis. This disorder is a form of NCL recently described in Finnish infants.[339,343,344,699] The disease begins between the ages of 8 and 18 months with rapid psychomotor regression, ataxia, and hypotonia. Infants with this disorder usually have begun speaking single words and may have begun to walk. Seizures usually do not occur and, if they are part of the illness, are infrequent. Myoclonus is common. Retinal blindness usually occurs before 2 years of age and is accompanied by optic atrophy and macular degeneration without a cherry-red spot like that seen in Tay-Sachs disease. Retinal pigmentary degeneration does not occur as it does in late infantile NCL. In marked contrast to the gangliosidoses, microcephaly is prominent. Deep tendon reflexes are hyperactive even though hypotonia is prominent. Death has occurred before the age of 6 years.

Late Infantile Neuronal Ceroid-Lipofuscinosis or Bielschowsky-Jansky Syndrome. Typically this disorder begins in early childhood, but the clinical and pathologic features of this type of NCL can occur in older children.[187,807,906] The onset of the disease is usually marked by seizures. These are often minor motor seizures, but a mixture of other types of seizures may occur as well. Myoclonic seizures are the most typical seizure type. The seizures are usually resistant to anticonvulsant treatment. Subsequently, ataxia appears and there is rapid mental, motor, and visual deterioration. Retinal pigmentary degeneration is a characteristic feature, but may be absent early in the course of the illness. Death usually occurs within 5 years of disease onset.

Juvenile Neuronal Ceroid-Lipofuscinosis or Spielmeyer-Sjögren Syndrome. The onset of juvenile NCL usually occurs between the ages of 3 and 10 years. Early symptoms include psychomotor regression, school failure, behavioral changes, and visual symptoms. In contrast to the late infantile form, seizures are usually a late symptom and when seizures occur early, they are not as frequent or as difficult to control. The clinical features of this disorder have been well delineated in several old and recent series of patients.[222,748,763,906] Visual symptoms are the most common symptom, but mental impairment often accompanies and occasionally precedes the visual symptoms.[222,748,763] The visual failure is often first recognized as night blindness or central visual field defects. The retina may appear normal or may show only slight abnormality, even when vision is markedly affected. The opposite circumstance may also occur, atrophic retinal changes may be present when visual acuity is normal. The most common funduscopic abnormalities are the bull's-eye macular dystrophy (pigmentary or tapetoretinal degeneration) and retinal vessel attenuation. These abnormalities are often subtle and may only be appreciated in a careful examination of the retina through dilated pupils. Other funduscopic abnormalities include optic atrophy, which may be mild, and peripheral pigmentary retinal changes.

The intelligence of chidlren with juvenile NCL is usually borderline or lower. Poor impulse control, fluctuations in mood, poor frustration tolerance, and self-mutilation are the typical behavioral disturbances. Motor disturbances are not the initial manifestations very often, but are usually detected early in the disease. Extrapyramidal dysfunction is particularly common and is manifested by bradykinesia, dystonia, loss of associated movements, and gait disturbances.[748] Cerebellar signs occur later in the course of the illness. Pyramidal tract symptoms and signs may be present but are usually overshadowed by the extrapyramidal and cerebellar disturbances.[907] Pseudobulbar palsy often develops late in the illness. Strabismus commonly appears when vision is severely affected. The motor signs and symptoms are slowly progressive. Death usually occurs in the third decade of life.

Adult Neuronal Ceroid-Lipofuscinosis or Kufs' Disease. The adult form of NCL usually begins in late adolescence or young adulthood. The range of age at onset, however, is quite broad, 5 years old to 40 years old.[319] The clinical syndrome, nevertheless, is quite similar in children and adults. The initial symptoms are usually dementia or psychiatric disturbances, although seizures and movement disorders are occasionally the first manifestation. The course of the disease may be remarkably protracted. This fact in part accounts for the difficulty in diagnosing this disease before death. The typical duration of the illness is 7 years to 10 years but the range of duration is 4 years to 53 years. Dementia is an invariable symptom. In order of frequency, extrapyramidal, pyramidal, and cerebellar dysfunctions are commonly observed. Extrapyramidal signs include choreoathetosis and tremors. Seizures and myoclonus may also occur.

Laboratory Features and Diagnosis. The most important progress in our understanding of NCL in the last decade has been the recognition of the involvement of cells outside of the nervous system. This observation has also facilitated diagnosis. Two tissues, blood lymphocytes and skin, are particularly accessible tissues with abnormalities that facilitate diagnosis.[201,518,588,888] Lymphocyte vacuolization is the most frequent and diagnostically useful abnormality. These vacuoles are found in 10% to 20% of lymphocytes.[222] Lymphocyte vacuoles are found in other conditions, most notably in the lipidoses and mucopolysaccharidoses, as well as occasionally in normal individuals. In these patients the percentage of lymphocytes with vacuoles is generally much lower than in patients with NCL. By electron microscopy the vacuoles have revealed lamellar and tubular cytosomes, curvilinear bodies, and fingerprint bodies.[201,518,588,888] These may be present even in the absence of lymphocyte vacuoles by light microscopy.[518] Cells in the bone marrow may contain autofluorescent material and when stained with the Wright stain may be sea blue.[262] This observation suggests that the family reported by Swaiman and associates with sea blue histiocytes in the bone marrow and posterior column dysfunction may have a form of NCL.[801]

Many other biopsy sites have been used to establish the diagnosis of NCL. Until recently, the procedure most widely used was the rectal biopsy. Skin and muscle biopsy, however, have largely supplanted this procedure.

The electroretinogram (ERG) and visual evoked potential (VEP) are other tests that may be diagnostically helpful. The ERG may be quite abnormal at a time when the VEP is normal.[348] This combination helps to distinguish NCL from the gangliosidoses because in the gangliosidoses the ERG is normal even when the patient is blind and the VEP is abnormal. In addition, the ERG may help assess visual function in patients incapable of cooperating in subjective tests of vision. The ERG abnormality may be present even when the retina is normal. The EEG is frequently abnormal but the abnormalities are nonspecific. The electroencephalographic abnormalities and clinical deterioration proceed together, so that the EEG may help to confirm a clinical impression of disease progression.[219] Mildly slowed motor and sensory nerve conduction velocities have been observed.

Wolman's Disease

The disorder was described in 1956 and since then only a few additional cases have been described.[1] In this disorder cholesteryl esters and triglycerides accumulate in many different tissues. This accumulation appears to be the consequence of a deficiency in acid hydrolase activity that facilitates hydrolysis of cholesteryl esters and triglycerides.[619]

The disorder consistently begins in the first few weeks of life. The first symptoms are usually abdominal distention and vomiting, although diarrhea or fever may also be the initial symptoms. The abdominal distention probably results from ileus and hepatosplenomegaly. The hepatosplenomegaly is usually detectable at the initial visit and becomes more prominent with increasing age. Anemia appears by the second month of life. Malnutrition becomes increasingly apparent and death occurs before 6 months of age.

Neurologically, patients with Wolman's disease appear normal at birth, but as the symptoms appear, development begins to wane. Hypotonia gradually predominates. Neurologic signs are nonlocalizing and funduscopic abnormalities and seizures do not occur.

The most characteristic feature of this disorder is adrenal gland calcification that may be seen on a plain film of the abdomen.

Other clues to the diagnosis include vacu-olization of peripheral lymphocytes and histiocytes and foam cells in the bone mar-row. The deficiency in acid hydrolase ac-tivity may be demonstrated in skin fibro-blasts, leukocytes, or hepatic tissue.[461,619]

Treatment consists in supportive management because no specific treatment is available.

OTHER DEFECTS IN LIPID METABOLISM

REFSUM'S DISEASE OR PHYTANIC ACID STORAGE DISEASE

This disorder was first clearly defined in 1946 by Refsum under the title of *heredo-pathia atactica polyneuritiformis*.[663] The usual components of this disease include retinitis pigmentosa, peripheral polyneu-ropathy, cerebellar ataxia, and CSF cytoal-bumin dissociation.

The disease usually begins before 20 years of age. Children often present with symptoms related to the peripheral poly-neuropathy seen in this disorder. Dimin-ished vision may also be a presenting symptom. Typically, this visual loss is worse at night or in the dark. Other features in-clude nystagmus, deafness, anosmia, pu-pilary abnormalities, ichthyotic skin changes, cataracts, and orthopaedic de-formities of the feet including pes cavus and hammer toes. The course of the disease is one of gradual deterioration often inter-rupted by abrupt worsening of the symp-toms followed by partial recovery.[664]

Laboratory features of the disorder in-clude an elevation of CSF protein up to 500 mg/dl without pleocytosis. Electrocardio-graphic changes are also common. Cardiac arrhythmias may account for the high in-cidence of sudden death among patients with Refsum's disease.

The disease appears to be inherited in an autosomal recessive fashion. Many of the reported cases have been in patients of Scandinavian origin.

Autopsy study of patients with Ref-sum's disease reveals extensive involve-ment of the brain and most other organs of the body. There is loss of myelin in the brain stem and posterior columns of the spinal cord, atrophy of the inferior olivary nuclei, and loss of neurons in the sympathetic gan-glia.[125,126] The peripheral neuropathy is an interstitial hypertrophic polyneuropathy. Other organs have substantial neutral fat storage.

Most organs contain excessive amounts of lipid. A major and unusual component of the lipid is accounted for by a fatty acid, phytanic acid. This same branched-chain lipid is found in excess in the plasma as well.[442] The most likely source of this lipid is exogenous dietary sources that supply phytanic acid, phytol, and phylloquinone. Phytanic acid appears to be supplied chiefly from dairy products and ruminant fats. Phytol is provided by green vegetables.

The defect accounting for the accu-mulation of the phytanic acid is a reduced phytanic acid hydroxylase activity. This enzyme is responsible for the conversion of phytanic acid to alpha-hydroxyphytanic acid.[555,776]

Treatment of Refsum's disease con-sists of eliminating phytanic acid and its precursors from the diet. This maneuver appears to reduce the plasma phytanic acid and also results in stabilization or improve-ment in the neurologic symptoms and signs.[504] This diet must be maintained for long periods of time before plasma phy-tanic acid begins to fall. Dietary manage-ment, however, must be done cautiously so as to avoid rapid weight loss because this has been associated with neurologic dete-rioration.[504] Plasma exchange is also a promising new approach to the treatment of Refsum's disease.[504]

LIPOPROTEIN DEFICIENCY

The lipoprotein deficiencies are abetali-poproteinemia, hypolipoproteinemia, and an-alphalipoproteinemia (Tangier disease). Analphalipoproteinemia is considered elsewhere.

Abetalipoproteinemia is a disorder of lipoprotein metabolism characterized by ataxia, loss of proprioception, retinitis pig-mentosa, acanthocytosis, and fat mal-absorption. This rare disorder was first described in 1950.[54] The absence of apolipoprotein B in the plasma is the only unique biochemical abnormality. Other lipids are absent including very low density lipoproteins, low density lipoproteins, and chylomicrons.

Pathology.   The involvement of the nervous system is characterized by involvement of large axon pathways including the spinocerebellar tracts and the posterior columns. Cerebellar involvement in the form of loss of neurons in the molecular layer and Purkinje cell layer has been described.[761] Anterior horn cell loss of a mild degree has also been noted.[761] Peripheral nerves may be normal or show mild segmental demyelination. Neurons in the cerebellum and brain stem may contain ceroid-lipofuscin in excessive amounts.

Biochemistry.   The pathogenesis of this disorder is unclear. The lipid abnormalities found in this condition may interfere with normal membrane function of cells. Alternatively the deficiency of fat-soluble vitamins may be important in the pathogenesis of the nervous system abnormalities. A deficiency of vitamin E may lead to increased lipid peroxidation and secondary neuronal degeneration. Other conditions in which there is chronic vitamin E deficiency such as biliary atresia have now been associated with a neurologic deterioration similar to that in abetalipoproteinemia.[684] Vitamin A deficiency may also account for some of the ocular manifestations of this disorder. Electroretinographic improvement has been reported in two patients treated with pharmacologic doses of vitamin A.[314]

Clinical Features.   In infancy abetalipoproteinemia may be manifested by failure to thrive, anorexia, vomiting, and loose bulky stools. As the affected child grows older he may learn to avoid fat in his diet and, as a result, will no longer have prominent gastrointestinal symptoms. Growth is generally poor so that many of these children are below the normal range for height and weight.

Neurologic symptoms invariably appear by the third decade. The earliest sign is deep tendon reflex loss, which may begin as early as 17 months of age. Usually, the first neurologic symptom is gait ataxia. This appears sometime after infancy but before 20 years of age. The gait ataxia appears to result from the involvement of both the spinocerebellar tracts as well as the posterior columns. As the disease progresses other features of spinocerebellar involvement appear including scanning speech, hypotonia, and dysmetria. Ocular signs include nystagmus, color blindness, scotoma, and ophthalmoplegia. Visual actuity may begin to fail as early as 7 years or as late as 30 years of age.[718,761] Retinal pigmentary degeneration appears sometime between the ages of 2½ years and 20 years.[63,743] Although corticospinal tract involvement is not a typical feature several patients have had extensor plantar reflexes. The skeletal abnormalities in this disorder are similar to those in other spinocerebellar degenerations and include equinovarus deformity of the feet, and curvature of the spine.

Involvement of other organs outside of the central nervous system also occurs in abetalipoproteinemia. Electrocardiographic changes, arrhythmias, and cardiac enlargement may appear.

In the context of the typical clinical features the diagnosis of abetalipoproteinemia is quite likely when acanthocytes (spiny red blood cells) and a low serum cholestrol are present. Confirmation of the diagnosis depends upon the demonstration of the absence of apolipoprotein B in the plasma. In order to distinguish this condition from hypobetaliproteinemia in which apolipoprotein B is also absent from the plasma, low density lipids must be measured in all obligate heterozygotes. In abetalipoproteinemia the levels of these lipids are normal but in hypobetalipoproteinemia the heterozygote has reduced levels.

Treatment.   Treatment of this disorder consists in restricting dietary fat to between 8% and 12% of the diet, by calories. Fat-soluble vitamins should be administered if possible in a water-soluble form as follows: vitamin A (Aquasol A), 200 international units (IU)/kg per day to 400 IU/kg per day, vitamin K_1 (Mephyton), 5 mg every 2 weeks, and vitamin E, 200 to 300 IU/day.[386] The use of medium-chain triglycerides as a source of fat may not be desirable because this may hasten the development of hepatic abnormalities.[386]

ADRENOLEUKODYSTROPHY

Adrenoleukodystrophy is an X-linked disorder characterized by demyelination in the nervous system and adrenal cortical insufficiency. The disorder was first described in 1923 by Siemerling and Creutzfeld. Until recently this disease might have been placed among the familial degenerative diseases and would have been considered a form of Schilder's disease.[489] Adrenoleukodystrophy is now viewed as a lipidosis because excessive amounts of unbranched saturated or monounsaturated fatty acids with a carbon chain length of 24 to 30 are found in the nervous system.[385,543,659] The disorder has been grouped among the sudanophilic leukodystrophies because the lipid that accumulates in the demyelinated areas stains with Sudan black stain.

Pathology. The main pathologic changes occur predominantly in the white matter of the occipital and parietal regions of the cerebral cortex. In the affected regions the arcuate fibers are spared but otherwise there is extensive demyelination and gliosis. Macrophages in the area of demyelination are filled with material that stains with PAS stain and oil-red O stains.[707] Lipid inclusions are also found in cells in the zona reticularis and zona fasciculata of the adrenal gland, and the testes.[560]

Biochemistry. Unbranched saturated or monounsaturated fatty acids accumulate in the white matter. Fatty acids 24 to 30 carbons long constitute up to 40% of the fatty acids of the cholesteryl esters and gangliosides, a unique biochemical feature not found in other demyelinating conditions.[385,543,659] This accumulation of long-chain fatty acids appears to be of exogenous or dietary origin, at least in part, because deuterated hexocosanoic acid administered orally accumulates in the white matter lesions. Similar accumulation of fatty acids have been found in cultured skin fibroblasts, muscle cells, and in the plasma.[560,561,609] Clones of fibroblasts from females who are obligate heterozygotes for adrenoleukodystrophy reveal two populations, one with excessive long-chain fatty acid accumulation and the other with normal amounts of fatty acid.

Clinical Features. Several clinical forms of this disorder are recognized including: the classical childhood adrenoleukodystrophy, adrenomyeloneuropathy, and neonatal adrenoleukodystrophy. All patients are male. In childhood adrenoleukodystrophy the disease usually appears between 4 and 8 years of age.[81,705] Behavioral and intellectual disturbances are the most common presenting complaints. These may include temper outbursts and irritability, school failure, and memory changes. Other frequent signs include dysarthria, dysphagia, spasticity (especially in the lower extremities), hemiparesis, ataxia, and visual disturbances. The visual disturbances include visual field defects, optic atrophy, and visual agnosia. Seizures are uncommon. The pace of the disease is rapid after onset and within several months to several years the patient reaches a state of decortication in which there is little response to the environment. Improvement after clinical deterioration has rarely been noted.[561] Even a relapsing and remitting course has been observed.[853]

A brown skin pigmentation may be clinically evident when the patient presents. The skin pigmentation occurs even in areas that are not sun-exposed, for example, the buccal mucosa and skin folds. The pigmentation is the most common manifestation of the adrenal insufficiency in this disorder and is also, perhaps the most diagnostically helpful clinical feature. Clinical evidence for adrenal insufficiency, however, may be completely absent. Rarely, overt adrenal insufficiency may precede the onset of neurologic symptoms.[705]

Uncommon variants of adrenoleukodystrophy have been noted in recent years. The neonatal form begins in the first few days of life.[560,829] The infants are hypotonic and suck poorly.[560,829] Thereafter, seizures, severe phychomotor delay, blindness and deafness and spasticity may occur. The clinical course has been quite variable; one patient expired at 20 months whereas another lived until 6½ years of age. The demyelination in infantile adrenoleukodystrophy is not predominantly in the parietal and occipital lobes but rather occurs either in the brain stem and cerebellum or the frontal and temporal lobes.

Adrenomyeloneuropathy begins in the

third decade and is manifested as progressive spastic paraparesis, bowel and bladder disturbances, and peripheral neuropathy.[180,706] Dementia and ataxia are not present until late in the course of the disease. Adrenal insufficiency may be severe and hypogonadism may occur. A close association between adrenomyeloneuropathy and childhood adrenoleukodystrophy is suggested by the occurrence of the disorders in brothers.[180]

Laboratory Features. The laboratory tests most helpful in the diagnosis of adrenoleukodystrophy are tests of adrenal function, the radionuclide brain scan, and the cranial computerized tomogram. The urinary excretion of adrenal corticosteroids and plasma cortisol may be decreased and adrenocorticotropic hormone (ACTH) stimulation does not produce a rise in 17-hydroxycorticosteroid excretion.[245] Radionuclide brain scans and computerized tomograms in childhood adrenoleukodystrophy reveal bilateral symmetric parieto-occipital lesions. These are seen as areas of increased uptake on the brain scan and as low density lesions that enhance with contrast on the cranial computerized tomogram.[208,861] Forward migration of radionuclide uptake as the disease progresses is also characteristic.[861]

Cerebrospinal fluid abnormalities are frequently noted late in the disease. These include elevation of CSF protein, mild lymphocytic pleocytosis, and a first zone elevation in the colloid gold curve.

SYSTEMIC CARNITINE DEFICIENCY

Carnitine (gamma-trimethylamino-beta-hydroxybutyrate) is necessary for the transport of fatty acids into mitochondria. Palmitoyl carnitine is synthesized on the outer mitochondrial membrane by carnitine palmitoyl transferase I (CPT I), translocated across the membrane, and palmitoyl-CoA and carnitine are regenerated by CPT II. Carnitine is synthesized from lysine and is present in the diet. The origin of systemic carnitine deficiency is not known. Diminished synthesis or absorption, abnormal distribution in the tissues, defective uptake into various organs, or excessive turnover

are all possible. Systemic deficiency of carnitine would be expected to lead to impaired energy production in liver and muscle. The consequences might be inadequate gluconeogenesis without ketosis, generalized mitochondrial dysfunction similar to Reye's syndrome, weakness, cardiomyopathy, and lipid storage. Serum, liver, and muscle carnitine assays are necessary to demonstrate systemic carnitine deficiency.

Patients with this disorder usually present in childhood with chronic progressive proximal weakness interrupted by episodes of alteration of consciousness and hepatic disease.[88,138,224,413,858] Patients with systemic carnitine deficiency may present during an episode of acute deterioration in consciousness and closely resemble patients with Reye's syndrome.[138] During these acute episodes weakness may be obscured by coma. Hepatomegaly, hypoglycemia, elevated liver enzymes, and hyperammonemia may occcur. Cardiac involvement as evidenced by cardiac enlargement and electrocardiographic changes has also occurred.[858] Between the acute episodes the patients have a clinically apparent proximal weakness and delayed development but normal physical growth.

This disorder should be considered in patients with progressive proximal myopathies or in patients with Reyelike presentations. Muscle and liver biopsies reveal fatty changes at the light level. Electron microscopy of liver reveals abnormal mitochondria and electron-dense material in hepatocytes. Verification of the diagnosis depends upon finding low plasma and tissue carnitine levels.

CEREBROTENDINOUS XANTHOMATOSIS

This rare disorder of lipid metabolism was first described by van Bogaert and his associates in 1937.[833] Since this original report, fewer than 30 reported cases have been added. The disorder is characterized biochemically by an accumulation of cholestanol in the tissues of the body, especially the brain and tendons.[545] The metabolic defect accounting for this accumulation is unknown, although a defect in cholestanol removal secondary to a membrane transport abnormality has been suggested.[545]

Pathology. The disease is characterized by xanthomas in tendons, bone, and in various white matter structures of the brain.[636,711,833] In the brain, the xanthomas can be found in the cerebellum, basal ganglia, cerebral peduncles, and brain stem.[711,833] Demyelination is prominent in many areas of the brain and spinal cord. Often cystic necrosis with perivascular mononuclear cellular infiltrates and giant cells is present in the regions of demyelination. Gliosis may also become prominent in the affected areas.

Clinical Features. The cardinal features are a progressive cerebellar ataxia, dementia, cataracts, and tendon xanthomas beginning in childhood.[545,833] The disease is often insidious in onset and slowly progressive. Cerebrotendinous xanthomatosis may be extremely difficult to diagnose because some of the typical symptoms and signs may be absent initially. In a few cases, one or more of the typical features, ataxia, dementia, and cataracts, never appeared. Tendon xanthomas are most commonly found in the Achilles tendon. Tendons of the elbow, fingers, and knee may also contain xanthomas. Death in this disorder usually occurs before 60 years of age. Cerebrotendinous xanthomatosis is probably transmitted in an autosomal recessive fashion. Diagnosis of cerebrotendinous xanthomatosis depends upon finding elevated cholestanol in plasma or tissue, especially from xanthomas.

Currently, there is no effective treatment for this disorder, although dietary elimination of cholesterol and choletanol and the use of cholesterol-lowering drugs have been tried.

GALACTOSEMIA

The term *galactosemia* has generally referred to the classical form of the disorders of galactose metabolism. However, several enzyme defects result in elevations of serum galactose. The clinical features of these defects are quite different. Three enzyme deficiencies have been described including galactose-1-phosphate uridyl transferase deficiency, galactokinase deficiency, and uridine diphosphate galactose-4-epimerase deficiency.[287,288,388] The classical form or galactose-1-phosphate uridyltransferase deficiency consists, clinically, of four main features: hepatosplenomegaly, cataracts, mental retardation, and failure to thrive.[520,846] Inheritance is autosomal recessive. The incidence of classical galactosemia has been estimated to range from 1:40,000 live births in Australia to 1:170,000 live births in Massachusetts.[733] The estimated frequency of galactokinase deficiency is 1:40,000 live births, with a frequency of 1:107 for the heterozygote carrier state.[67,528]

Biochemistry. Galactose is metabolized to glucose-6-phosphate through four steps (Fig. 9-8). Galactose is first phosphorylated through galactokinase. The resulting phosphate reacts with uridine-diphosphate-glucose (UDP-glucose) to create UDP-galactose and glucose-1-phosphate. This is catalyzed by galactose-1-phosphate uridyltransferase. Uridine-diphosphate galactose is epimerized to UDP-glucose, which is then converted to glucose-1-phosphate, the first compound in the Embden-Myerhoff glycolytic pathway. All the steps of galactose metabolism are reversible. Galactose is a part of membrane glycolipids, and it can be synthesized from glucose if not present in the diet.

Isozymes of galactokinase are known, and severely deficient activity can cause cataracts.[818] The accumulated galactose is reduced to its alcohol, galactitol, in the lens. Galactitol is osmotically active and will cause water accumulation and cataracts.[435]

Classical galactosemia is caused by severe deficiency of the transferase enzyme. Homozygotes for the classical form have no measurable activity. Homozygotes for the form generally termed the Negro variant may have some residual activity, and, therefore, have symptoms only in infancy, when galactose intake is at its peak.[41] Other alleles of the transferase are relatively common, but in the homozygous state, or even in combination with a severely deficient allele, do not cause symptoms.

The origin of cataracts can be related to galactose excess and galactitol formation. The reasons for liver and kidney toxicity, pseudotumor cerebri, and mental retardation in transferase deficiency are not clear.[723]

Clinical Features. Infants with classical galactosemia are generally normal at birth. Cataracts have been observed as early as 7 days after birth in infants with classical galactosemia.[380] Symptoms usually begin a few days after the initiation of milk containing lactose. Poor feeding, vomiting, diarrhea, and failure to thrive are the initial symptoms.[572] With continued milk ingestion, jaundice, hepatosplenomegaly, and cataracts appear. The jaundice may not only be due to hepatic dysfunction but also to hemolysis that can occur as a consequence of this disorder. The bilirubin is mainly conjugated, reflecting cholestasis. Sepsis with gram-negative organisms, particularly *Escherichia coli*, is common. The underlying metabolic defect is often overlooked when treating the infection.

Because the cataracts in galactosemia occur in the neonatal period, they appear as ring opacities, then become capsular. Hypoglycemia may occur and appears to be a consequence of the hepatic dysfunction produced by galactosemia. Neurologic symptoms and signs are prominent in galactosemia. Initially, the severely affected infant is hypotonic and if the disease remains untreated, development becomes obviously delayed by a few months of age. Psychomotor retardation, however, is usually not severe even in those infants treated late.[202] Pseudotumor cerebri has also been reported to occur in galactosemia.[383]

If infants with classical galactosemia remain untreated, many will ultimately expire, some as a consequence of the complications of their hepatic disease but most from infection. Occasionally, patients with classical galactosemia will present at several months of age with mental retardation and growth failure without a history of neonatal problems. In some cases this can be attributed to a partial restriction of galactose intake, often by using a soy formula. Some infants never develop cataracts.[380]

Laboratory Features and Diagnosis. Laboratory features of classical galactosemia include evidence of hepatic dysfunction, aminoaciduria, hypochloremic acidosis, and evidence of erythroblastosis. The aminoaciduria is a sign of renal toxicity and resolves when galactosemia is treated. Reducing substances will be found in the urine only after intake of milk containing galactose. Dependence upon this finding as a means of screening or diagnosing galactosemia, however, is hazardous because several cases without galactosuria have been reported.[352,396] In addition, conditions other than galactosemia can result in nonglucose-reducing substances in the urine, including severe hepatic disease, fructose intolerance, and intestinal lactase deficiency.[492] When galactosemia is suspected, all galactose should be withdrawn from the diet immediately. This usually happens if the infant is septic and placed on intravenous feeding. The infant should *never* be challenged with galactose. The diagnosis can be made easily and safely by other means. Reducing substances in the urine are identified using Benedict's reagent or reagent tablets containing copper sulfate (Clinitest [Ames] tablets.) Glucose, which will also make this test positive, will be identified using a specific glucose oxidase test strip. To confirm that a reducing substance found in the urine is galactose, chromatography can be performed. The diagnosis of classical galactosemia can be confirmed by demonstrating a deficiency of galactose-1-phosphate uridyl transferase. This enzyme is generally assayed in a hemolysate of the patient's red cells.[9] Erythrocyte galactose-1-phosphate can be measured as well.[241,438]

Treatment. Since enzyme replacement is not feasible, the principal mode of treatment consists in restricting dietary intake of galactose. In infants this is done by providing a formula that does not contain galactose in an absorbable form. Soybean milks (e.g., Nutramigen and Neomullsoy) have been used quite successfully for this purpose. Milk is added to many of the foods ordinarily used in this country, so labels must be read carefully when infants start to eat solid foods. Treatment with a low-galactose diet results in rapid resolution of diarrhea, vomiting, hepatic dysfunction, and renal tubular dysfunction. Cataracts also appear to regress but this may be a consequence of continued lens growth.[144] Hepatic cirrhosis and mental retardation are not reversed by dietary management; these effects of galactosemia must be prevented by early institution of dietary treatment. Patients with galactosemia who receive dietary treatment from birth exhibit better intellectual progress than those treated later.[241] However, even in these patients there may be perceptual problems and, when compared to siblings, patients treated from birth may still have lower IQs.[241,572] This difference between siblings may be due to prenatal exposure of galactosemic infant to galactose and has led some to restrict lactose intake in pregnant females with previous galactosemic children.[240] Adherence to the low-galactose diet has been determined by measurements of galactose-1-phosphate in red cells.[241] A procedure to measure red cell galactose-1-phosphate on filter paper samples mailed to a laboratory allows dietary compliance to be monitored.[438] It appears unlikely that galactose metabolism improves with age, so relaxation of dietary restrictions should be done cautiously. Social factors will probably necessitate some dietary relaxation at school age but regular milk ingestion is best avoided.

The pathologic alterations in the nervous system are nonspecific. The changes in the liver, however, are more specific and may be helpful in establishing the diagnosis.[752] In the early stages of the disease, the hepatic cells are filled with large fat vacuoles.

Other Forms of Galactosemia. Galactokinase deficiency results in elevated blood and urine galactose levels. This rare disorder results in the appearance of cataracts at a young age. No definite neurologic abnormalities have been associated with this defect in galactose metabolism.

Uridine diphosphate galactose-4-epimerase deficiency is an apparently benign abnormality that has been reported in only one patient.[288] The blood galactose level was not elevated in this disorder but red blood cell galactose-1-phosphate was elevated.

Newborn Screening and Diagnosis. The diagnosis of classical galactosemia should be made as early as possible in order to limit the permanent effects of galactosemia. *In utero* diagnosis is possible and could be used to determine the need for a galactose-free diet in a mother heterozygous for classical galactosemia.[236] A simpler approach is to restrict galactose intake during pregnancy and feed the newborn galactose-free milk

for a day or two until the enzyme can be tested.[202]

The rapidity of onset of symptoms has generally precluded effective newborn screening, but better follow-up and faster testing have allowed some states to use the PKU filter paper sample to screen for galactosemia as well. All infants with congenital cataracts, protracted jaundice, or failure to thrive should have their urine tested for reducing substances or for galactose by galactose oxidase test.[164] Sources of false negatives should be kept in mind. In particular, the test may be negative if the infant has not received milk containing galactose just before the test is run. A challenge of milk may be fatal (see above). Care should be taken to see that the urine is not extremely dilute. False positives are often seen with these tests and are due to the presence of reducing substances other than galactose in the urine, the normal galactosuria seen in normal prematures, and galactosuria that can occur with ingestion of large amounts of milk.

LESCH-NYHAN SYNDROME

Lesch-Nyhan syndrome is a disorder of purine metabolism first definitively described in 1964.[479] This disorder affects males and is characterized by mental retardation, spasticity, choreoathetosis, and self-mutilation in association with hyperuricemia.

Pathology. Although neurologic symptoms and signs are quite prominent in Lesch-Nyhan syndrome, no consistent pathologic changes have been found in the central nervous system. Those changes that have been found appear to be related to renal failure or other complications of the disease.

Biochemistry. Synthesis of purines proceeds from ribose-5-phosphate to 5-phosphoribosyl-1-phosphate (PRPP or PP-ribose-P), eventually to inosine-5-phosphate (IMP or inosinic acid), and then to the nucleotides adenosine-5-phosphate (AMP) and guanosine-5-phosphate (GMP). Purine synthesis occurs mainly in liver and placenta. Purines, mainly ATP, are transported to the peripheral tissues by erythrocytes. The peripheral tissues depend on recycling purines from DNA, RNA and nucleotides such as ATP and adenosine $3':5'$-cyclic phosphate (cyclic AMP) to ensure an adequate supply. Bases can be recycled in two steps by first condensing with ribose (forming nucleosides), then being phosphorylated (to nucleotides); or in one step through a phosphoribosyl transferase (PRT) reaction. Adenine has its own enzyme, adenine PRT (APRT). Hypoxanthine (the base analog of IMP) and guanine share an enzyme, hypoxanthine-guanine PRT, or HGPRT. The PRT reactions require PRPP as a second substrate.

Impaired HGPRT activity leads to diminished purine salvage and overproduction of the purine excretion product uric acid. There is also a secondary increase in PRPP synthesis, resulting in a further acceleration of purine synthesis.

Moderate impairment of HGPRT leads to gout. Severe impairment leads to the Lesch-Nyhan syndrome. It is unclear whether other factors besides HGPRT deficiency may influence the nervous system disease.[427] HGPRT activity in the Lesch-Nyhan syndrome is often undetectable but may be as high as 30% of normal. Enzyme activity in erythrocytes or fibroblasts does not correlate well with activity in brain and liver. In most patients there is a diminished amount of immunologically cross-reacting material, suggesting absence of the structural gene, increased turnover of the enzyme, or a mutation affecting both the antigenic and catalytic sites.[281,830]

Heterozygotes for severe HGPRT deficiency are generally asymptomatic, but some have an elevated serum uric acid concentration and urinary excretion of uric acid, and a few have had recurrent monarticular arthritis.[427] Heterozygote detection is best done by assay of HGPRT in hair roots. Each follicle starts from a few cells, and therefore may be a clone, expressing only one of the female's two X chromosomes in all cells of the follicle.[270] Fibroblasts cultured in medium that is lethal to normal cells but allows Lesch-Nyhan cells to proliferate can also detect heterozygotes.[234,548]

A recent report suggests that nearly all mothers of patients with Lesch-Nyhan syndrome are carriers.[249] Classical genetic theory predicts that one-third of the cases of a lethal X-linked disorder represent new mutations. It is suggested, therefore, that perhaps there is a greater mutation rate in sperm cells producing carrier females than in oocytes producing affected sons or carrier daughters. This difference could be due to differences in sperm and egg production. This possibility is being investigated for other lethal X-linked diseases because the genetic counseling with respect to recurrence risk for an isolated case, in the absence of definitive carrier testing, depends on the relative likelihood of where the mutation occurred.

Clinical Features.   Infants with Lesch-Nyhan syndrome are usually normal at birth. In the first few months of life there are few manifestations of this disorder although irritability and feeding problems have been infrequently described.[479] Developmental delay becomes increasingly apparent during the first year. Psychomotor retardation is generally in the mild to moderate range. A patient with Lesch-Nyhan syndrome and normal intelligence despite communication difficulties has been reported.[710]

The extrapyramidal disturbances generally appear during the second year of life and are characterized by choreoathetosis and dystonia. Spasticity, too, becomes obvious after the first year of life and ultimately becomes so severe that it obliterates the choreoathetosis. Dysarthria similar to that found in other patients with athetosis appears later in life. Seizures occur in a substantial percentage of patients but may be unrelated to the disease itself.

The most characteristic feature of this syndrome is self-destruction. This self-destructive behavior can appear as early as 2 years of age or as late as 16 years of age.[427,593] Although these children experience pain during this self-destructive behavior, they are somehow unable to prevent it. As a consequence of this self-destructive behavior, mutilation of the lips and fingers then occurs. Although self-destructive behavior is also common in mentally retarded patients, tissue loss is not common except in the Lesch-Nyhan syndrome. Physical restraint to prevent self-mutilation seems to relieve these children greatly. Children with Lesch-Nyhan syndrome are not only aggressive toward themselves but may be physically and verbally aggressive toward others as well.

Problems related to the hyperuricemia are encountered frequently. Included among the problems are hematuria, crystalluria, gouty tophi, arthritis, and renal failure.

Laboratory Features and Diagnosis. All patients with Lesch-Nyhan syndrome excrete excessive quantities of uric acid. This may be manifested in infancy by orange discoloration of the diaper or by crystalluria in a urine specimen. The best screening test appears to be measurement of the uric acid-to-creatinine concentration ratio in urine. This ratio is usually above two in Lesch-Nyhan syndrome.[418] The enzyme defect can be demonstrated in cultured skin fibroblasts, amniotic fluid cells, and blood cells.[65,189,722]

The diagnosis should be considered in males with extrapyramidal disturbances and self-mutilation. In this context, the laboratory abnormalities are diagnostic.

Treatment. Patients with Lesch-Nyhan syndrome should be treated with allopurinol. This xanthine oxidase inhibitor inhibits the formation of uric acid and reduces the complications of gout and urate nephropathy. Unfortunately, allopurinol does not influence the appearance of the neurologic abnormalities. During treatment with allopurinol urine output must be maintained in order to prevent formation of xanthine stones. Since this treatment does not alleviate the neurologic symptoms, addition therapies have been attempted. Most of these therapies have not had any obvious beneficial effect.[427] 5-Hydroxytryptophan, a precursor of serotonin (Fig. 9-7), has been shown in a double-blind study to produce both a significant reduction of athetoid movements and a sedative effect but did not reduce the aggressive or self-mutilating behavior.[239] Physical restraints are not only an effective means of preventing self-mutilation, but also seem to reduce the anxiety accompanying this behavior.

DISORDERS OF COPPER METABOLISM

Copper is an essential but potentially toxic trace element in the human diet. Copper is an important element in such molecules as cytochrome oxidase, tyrosinase, and superoxide dismutase. Abnormally low levels of copper can occur in malnutrition, malabsorption, renal disease, and specific inborn errors of metabolism. Abnormally high levels occur in accidental intoxication and in Wilson's disease. In conditions in which copper is abnormally low the copper-containing enzymes are deficient whereas in those conditions in which copper is excessive other enzymes such as microsomal ATPase and glycolytic pathway enzymes are inhibited.

Considering requirements, the copper in a balanced diet (2 mg/day–5 mg/day) is more than adequate. Absorption of this amount of copper is incomplete and is probably dependent on an energy-requiring transport mechanism.[156] Copper is absorbed in a nonionic form. In contrast to iron, the absorption is not known to be controlled according to body needs. After an oral load of copper, serum copper reaches an early peak, falls, then rises again reaching a second peak 4 hours to 6 hours after ingestion.

Copper is transported by attachment to albumin and amino acids and by incorporation in ceruloplasmin. Very little ionic copper is found in tissue; most of the copper is bound to protein or incorporated in enzymes. Copper in the liver may account for as much as 15% of the total body copper content. In the liver and in other tissues the copper is bound to metallothionein and related proteins.[116,227,402] Lysosomal methionine may also be important in copper binding.[648] Copper-containing enzymes account for 1% to 2% of total body copper. Ceruloplasmin is the principal copper-containing enzyme. Ceruloplasmin is formed in the liver, its amount depending on age. Ceruloplasmin is elevated in a variety of conditions such as hyperthyroidism, infection, pregnancy, and liver disease. Ceruloplasmin can be low in children with chronic active hepatitis, nephrotic syndrome, malabsorption syndromes, protein-losing enteropathy, protein-caloric malnutrition, small bowel scleroderma, Menkes' kinky hair syndrome, and Wilson's disease.[626] The function of this enzyme is uncertain. Ceruloplasmin has oxidase activity and may function as a catalyst in a reaction converting the ferrous form of iron to the ferric form and as a copper donor in cytochrome c oxidase synthesis.[515,516,679] Other copper-containing proteins have been identified in various tissues. These proteins are structurally similar to each other and have been labeled *cytocupreins*.[132] At least one of these cytocupreins has been shown to have the same activity as superoxide dismutase.[529]

Under normal circumstances the vast majority of copper lost from the body is excreted by the liver in bile in a variety of bound forms, some of which prevent subsequent reabsorption from the bowel.[120,259] The nature of the substances binding copper in bile is uncertain but it is doubtful if ceruloplasmin plays a significant role.

WILSON'S DISEASE

Although scattered reports of a progressive neurologic disease associated with liver disease appeared in the medical literature of the late 19th and early 20th centuries, the delineation of Wilson's disease did not begin until Kayser and, later, Fleischer described the pathognomonic corneal ring.[242,424] The clinical and pathologic delineation of Wilson's disease by Kinnier Wilson completed the first phase in our understanding of this disease.[885] A year after Wilson's description, an increased hepatic copper content was noted in patients with Wilson's disease.[690] Unfortunately, 20 years passed before the excessive tissue copper in Wilson's disease was rediscovered.[294]

In its classical form, Wilson's disease, or hepatolenticular degeneration, is clinically a combination of liver disease, progressive pyramidal and extrapyramidal dysfunction and Kayser-Fleischer corneal rings presenting in the second or third decade. The disease, however, is quite variable in its clinical manifestations. In general, in Wilson's disease the earlier the onset the less likely are neurologic symptoms and the more likely is hepatic disease. It has been observed that there is a progression of symptoms that allow the division of Wilson's disease into four stages.[186] In stage one, although there is laboratory evidence of abnormal copper metabolism, the patients are asymptomatic. Stage two begins after the liver is saturated with copper and is characterized by hemolytic anemia and liver failure. A minority of patients present in

this stage. Most proceed to stage three in which there is extrahepatic copper accumulation. Kayser-Fleischer rings appear and renal abnormalities are present although rarely symptomatic. Stage four is characterized by the appearance of neurologic symptoms.

Some patients with Wilson's disease develop neurologic symptoms in childhood (7 yr–15 yr of age), whereas others do not develop them until adulthood (19 yr–35 yr of age).[190] These two groups of patients differ in their symptoms and prognosis. The juvenile form is characterized by frequent associated hepatic disease. The first neurologic signs are limb dystonia. Other prominent signs include a characteristic, fixed, open-mouth grin and a movement disorder that progresses from an early tremor to a "flapping" tremor and finally to an athetotic or myoclonic movement disorder. The terminal neurologic picture is fixed rigidity in flexion. This form of Wilson's disease was termed *progressive lenticular degeneration*.[190] Other prominent features in the juvenile form include dysarthria, drooling, gait disturbances, difficulty in writing, and school failure.[18,190] Death often occurs within 4 years of onset. Acute exacerbations of symptoms or partial remission can occur. In contrast to the juvenile form, the adult form of Wilson's disease, the pseudosclerosis form, is characterized by tremor and dysarthria. Progression in pseudosclerosis is much slower than in the juvenile form. Characteristically, the tremor in pseudosclerosis has a flapping or wing-beating quality. Dysphagia is common in Wilson's disease and seems to be oropharyngeal because patients have difficulty initiating deglutition.[789]

The variations in presenting symptoms and severity of various components of Wilson's disease among patients have not been explained. As noted above, this variation may in part reflect disease stage.[186,789,855] Familial factors are also important because similar symptoms and age of onset are found in members of the same family.[790] The poor prognosis in progressive lenticular degeneration compared to the pseudosclerosis form may, in part, be a consequence of the associated hepatic disease in the progressive lenticular degeneration form.[18,190]

Other neurologic and psychiatric symptoms may occur in Wilson's disease. These include psychiatric symptoms ranging from frequent mild behavioral and personality changes to severe psychosis. Clinical symptoms resembling those of parkinsonism or a progressive choreoathetosis have also been reported. Seizures, usually myoclonic or partial, occur occasionally. In general, Wilson's disease should be considered in any patient with extrapyramidal symptoms or organic brain syndromes no matter how bizarre they appear because diagnosis may be delayed beyond a point at which symptoms are reversible.[854]

Patients with neurologic symptoms invariably have a golden-brown, brownish-green, greenish-yellow, bronze, or tannish-green bilateral corneal discoloration at the limbus of the cornea.[242,424,877] Pathologically, the pigment represents copper granules located in Descemet's membrane.[831] The pigment can often be seen with the unaided eye, especially in blue-eyed patients. It is advisable, however, to perform a slit lamp exam on any patient with neurologic symptoms suspected of having Wilson's disease whether or not a pigmented corneal ring is found on initial examination. The pigmentation of the Kayser-Fleischer ring is most intense in the peripheral cornea.[877] It must be differentiated from pigmented corneal rings seen in other conditions including cirrhosis, carotenemia, arcus senilis, multiple myeloma, trypanosomiasis, topical copper use for eye conditions, and intraocular foreign bodies containing copper alloys.[877] The superior cornea may be the first part of the cornea pigmented during copper deposition and is the last part to lose pigment during penicillamine treatment.[877] Asymptomatic, "sunflower" cataracts may also occur in patients with Wilson disease.

Other systems are commonly involved in Wilson's disease. Hepatic disease is quite common and often the presenting complaint in childhood.[867] Wilson's disease patients with hepatic involvement may present as young as 4 years of age.[18] The usual progression of the hepatic disease is from asymptomatic liver enlargement to a picture of hepatitis and finally to nodular cirrhosis. Although the hepatic disease usually runs a chronic course, it may be fulminant.[472,779,780,789] The laboratory abnormalities of liver dysfunction and the liver histology at the light microscopic level are not distinctive. Ultrastructural changes in the mitochondria of hepatocytes, however, may be specific for Wilson's disease.[778]

Renal tubular dysfunction is quite common but rarely symptomatic. Bone lesions in Wilson's disease probably are a consequence of renal tubular dysfunction and secondary hyperparathyroidism.[789] Hemolytic anemia occasionally is the first sign of Wilson's disease and may be the consequence of increased oxidative stress produced by copper accumulation in erythrocytes.[185,867]

Pathophysiology. The principal cause for the dysfunction and the lesions in Wilson disease appears to be excessive copper deposition in various tissues. Although ceruloplasmin concentration is reduced in this disorder it is unlikely that this is the basic defect. The reduced ceruloplasmin is a consequence of decreased production. Apoceruloplasmin, a ceruloplasmin precursor, is found in normal amounts, suggesting that failure of copper incorporation is the defective step in ceruloplasmin synthesis.[369,524] Failure of ceruloplasmin synthesis is also not likely to be the basic defect because occasional Wilson's disease patients have normal ceruloplasmin, and raising ceruloplasmin levels with estrogen has no beneficial effect. Alternatively, it has been suggested that ceruloplasmin in Wilson's disease is defective; studies, however, have failed to support this contention.[369] Total serum copper is low in Wilson's disease but is higher than expected considering ceruloplasmin concentration. Increased copper binding to amino acids and proteins other than ceruloplasmin appears to account for this excess copper. This increased binding may be an important factor influencing copper deposition. Tissue copper content and urinary copper excretion are increased. The liver is affected earliest by this increased copper accumulation. The predominant site of the copper accumulation is in lysosomes of the hepatocytes.[299] Lysosomal copper storage may protect the hepatocyte. Ultimately, however, this lysosomal copper accumulation may result in destruction of the lysosomal membrane with consequent release of copper into the cell. Excessive copper also accumulates in the brain, especially in the basal ganglia. This increased body burden of copper appeared at first to be a consequence of increased absorption but now seems more likely to represent defective biliary excretion.[611,709,787] In Wilson's disease the appearance of copper in the blood after an oral copper load is diagnostic. The initial rise in copper concentration reaches higher levels in Wilson's disease patients than in normal persons. The subsequent fall is slower and the second rise in copper concentration normally seen at 4 hours to 6 hours fails to appear.[700] This latter abnormality is highly characteristic of Wilson's disease and is found in presymptomatic patients. The abnormal copper kinetics are the consequence of defective copper incorporation in ceruloplasmin. It now seems likely that a defect in copper metabolism is present even in cultured fibroblasts from patients with Wilson's disease because they have elevated intracellular copper concentration.[137]

Gross and microscopic tissue changes follow the copper accumulation. In the brain the basal ganglia are the structures most severely affected. At the gross level cavitation of the putamen and globus pallidus and red discoloration of the basal ganglia are seen; this abnormality is especially common in the juvenile or progressive lenticular degeneration form.[190,885] Microscopically one finds neuronal loss even though copper accumulates predominantly in glial cells. Gliosis is prominent. These degenerative changes predominantly involve the pallidum, putamen, frontal lobe, dentate nucleus, and brain stem.

Laboratory Abnormalities. The patient with Wilson's disease who presents with overt neurologic symptoms is not usually difficult to diagnose. The essential features, progressive extrapyramidal symptoms, hepatic disease, and a Kayser-Fleischer ring, are often present in the child with Wilson's disease presenting with neurologic symptoms. A family history of affected siblings is commonly elicited. The Kayser-Fleischer ring should be seen on slit lamp exam of the eye. It is present in virtually all Wilson's disease patients with neurologic symptoms.

Laboratory tests are useful in confirming the diagnosis of Wilson's disease. Serum ceruloplasmin is low in the majority of patients with symptomatic or presymptomatic Wilson's disease. In comparison to adults ceruloplasmin levels generally are higher in children beyond infancy, therefore, appropriate standards must be used. Urinary copper excretion and hepatic copper concentration are increased whereas serum copper is low.[789,867] In some patients, particularly those being screened for presymptomatic Wilson's disease radioactive copper uptake tests can be performed. This test may also be used to exclude the heterozygous carrier state (see above).[781] As noted above, cultured fibroblasts from patients with Wilson's disease have elevated intracellular copper concentration and may, therefore, serve as a noninvasive method for early diagnosis.[137]

Treatment. Untreated Wilson's disease progresses to death; treated late, many of the symptoms are irreversible. Timely treatment, therefore, is essential. Treatment consists of oral administration of penicillamine.[854] In children less than 10 years of age, penicillamine is given at an initial dose of 0.5 g to 0.75 g daily; over 10 years of age the adult dose, 1 g daily, may be given. The daily dose is administered in two divided doses and adjusted according to patient response. Patients with Wilson's disease usually have a marked cupresis after the start of penicillamine therapy.[826] In adults with Wilson's disease, the daily copper excretion may reach 4 mg daily. With continued treatment daily urine copper excretion, serum copper, and ceruloplasmin levels fall. These tests and hepatic copper content can be used to monitor response to treatment.

Adverse reactions to penicillamine are common. These include nephrotic syndrome; hypersensitivity reactions, including cutaneous eruptions, fever, lymphadenopathy, thrombocytopenia, and leukopenia; and optic neuritis. The hypersensitivity reactions occur in 20% to 30% of patients at 5 days to 10 days after initiating treatment. Penicillamine should be stopped and the hypersensitive reaction allowed to resolve. The penicillamine should then be reinstituted at a low dose and gradually increased. Corticosteroids and antihistamines can be used if necessary to treat hypersensitivity reactions or the nephrotic syndrome occurring with penicillamine. Pyridoxine administration for prophylaxis against optic neuritis and the use of D-penicillamine rather than the racemic form also help reduce adverse reactions. If penicillamine cannot be tolerated other chelating agents may be used including 2,3-dimercaptopropanol (BAL) and triethylene tetramine. These drugs are effective but not as effective as penicillamine.[162,191,198,856]

Patients should also be placed on a diet eliminating chocolate, nuts, mushrooms, liver, shellfish, and other foods containing high quantities of copper. Oral administration of potassium disulfide (30 mg/day–50 mg/day) has been advocated to reduce copper absorption.

As a general rule, the earlier the diagnosis and initiation of treatment the better the prognosis.[18] Asymptomatic children with Wilson's disease treated prophylactically with penicillamine do not develop symptoms.[18,480,788] Children with progressive lenticular degeneration respond less well to chelation than those with the pseudosclerotic form of the disease.[18,190,789] In those that have residual extrapyramidal dysfunction L-dopa and surgical ablative treatment have been helpful.[45,190]

MENKES' KINKY HAIR SYNDROME

Menkes' kinky hair syndrome (Menkes' syndrome, X-linked copper malabsorption) is an X-linked defect in copper metabolism that presents in infancy as a neurodegenerative disease associated with stubby, friable scalp hair.[174,541] This is a rare disease with less than 50 cases reported in the world's literature, although in Australia the frequency has been estimated to be one in 35,000 live births.[174]

Pathology. On gross examination of the brain of patients with Menkes syndrome, the most striking features are decreased brain weight and volume. Ventricular size is usually increased. Commonly, evidence of meningoencephalitis or subdural hematoma or hygromas is found.[2,48,541] Microscopically, the most prominent abnormality is cortical, basal ganglia, and thalamic

neuronal loss and gliosis.[48,884] The neuronal loss particularly affects the granular cells in the neocortex and cerebellum.[48,884] Calcification and ferrugination may accompany this neuronal loss.[48] White matter involvement in the form of myelin loss and gliosis is also a constant feature.[48] Golgi impregnation and ultrastructural studies have shown that the Purkinje cell soma contains an excessive number of primary dendrites and that the dendritic arborization of the Purkinje cell is less elaborate than normal.[363,653,884] These neuronal aberrations along with other pathologic features such as neuronal heterotopia and microgyria noted in one case of Menkes' syndrome, are consistent with an antenatal disturbance in brain development.

Biochemistry. As noted above, serum copper and ceruloplasmin are low in Menkes' syndrome. Copper levels are reduced in brain and liver but not in erythrocytes.[114,174] Orally administered ^{64}Cu is not absorbed normally.[114,498] Copper content of the intestinal wall, however, is increased.[114,175] These observations have been interpreted as indicating a defect in intestinal copper transport. Some observations, however, cannot be explained in this way. Copper content in erythrocytes is normal or slightly elevated despite low serum Cu levels. In addition, although serum ceruloplasmin rises after copper is administered by parenteral injection, a similar rise is not observed when serum copper is raised to comparable levels by high oral dose of Cu.[498] Finally, fibroblast cultures from patients with Menkes syndrome exhibit elevated copper concentration, a defect that appears to be due to reduced Cu efflux.[268,297] Thus, it would appear that the basic defect remains to be defined. The most plausible explanation to date suggests that there is an abnormality in the Cu transport protein(s) or a Cu-transport protein complex.[367]

The reduced Cu levels in Menkes syndrome probably results in deficient activity of enzymes that require Cu.[367] The deficient enzymes that might account for the observed clinical symptoms include ceruloplasmin, connective tissue amine oxidases, cytochrome oxidase, dopamine-beta-hydroxylase, superoxide dismutase, and tyrosinase.

Clinical Features. Typically the disease is recognized at 2 months to 3 months of age after a relatively normal early development. Menkes' syndrome, however, has been detected in a 3-day-old infant.[324] The most common presenting symptom is seizures, usually generalized or focal, but also myoclonic. All patients with Menkes' syndrome ultimately develop seizures.[256] Other presenting symptoms include gastrointestinal symptoms (vomiting, diarrhea), failure to thrive, psychomotor delay or regression, and autonomic disturbances (hypotension or hypothermia).

At the time of presentation patients with Menkes' syndrome often have other features that may suggest the diagnosis. Typical facial features include micrognathia, prominent forehead, and a full or coarse facial appearance. With one exception, the scalp hair has been sparse, coarse, friable, or light in color at some time during the course of the disease.[612] "Kinky hair" is not visible to the unaided eye. Microscopically, one typically finds pili torti (twisted hair shaft) alone or in combination with monilethrix or trichorrhexis nodosa. Pili torti is not pathognomic for Menkes' syndrome.[122,647,677] Microcephaly and growth failure are common and early features. Macrocephaly, often a consequence of subdural hematoma or hydroma, or normal head circumference may be seen.[103,541]

Congenital anomalies consistent with a developmental defect are frequent in Menkes' syndrome. Included among these anomalies are high-arched palate, pectus excavatum, club feet, undescended testes, and inguinal or hiatal hernias.[74,114,541,746]

Neurologic signs suggest diffuse brain involvement. Abnormalities of muscle tone (hypotonia or hypertonia), are present in the majority of cases. Signs of spasticity, such as hyperactive deep tendon reflexes, are commonly present. Ocular signs include nystagmus, blindness, and optic atrophy or optic disc pallor.[897] Developmental delay and persistent primitive reflexes are present in the majority of patients at the time of the initial examination. Unless obscured by a neonatal onset, the progressive nature of the disease usually becomes apparent as the child gets older.[114,174,541]

Menkes' syndrome is an invariably fatal disease. Most patients expire before 2 years of age. The longest known surviving patient expired at 3.5 years. Sudden death is not unusual.[174] Death frequently is a result of the common complications. Neonatal jaundice, spontaneous subdural hematoma and subdural hygroma formation, frequent infections, and autonomic disturbances, hypotension and hypothermia, are the most common complications seen in Menkes syndrome.[256]

Laboratory Features. Diagnostically, the most important laboratory abnormalities are low serum Cu and ceruloplasmin levels. Few conditions are associated with low serum Cu and ceruloplasmin levels. Malnutrition in infants, hyperalimentation in prematures, and one case of idiopathic Cu deficiency in a 3-month-old infant are the only other conditions in children in which Cu deficiency has been described.[4,315,415]

Radiographic abnormalities are also helpful in making a diagnosis of Menkes' syndrome. Bone films reveal wormian bones of the skull, flaring of the rib cage, diaphyseal periosteal reaction, and metaphyseal spurring or cupping in the majority of patients with Menkes' syndrome.[2] Skull films may rarely reveal craniosynostosis.[541] Angiographic abnormalities are quite distinctive and perhaps pathognomic of Menkes' syndrome.[3] Pneumoencephalography or computerized tomography may demonstrate unsuspected subdural fluid collections, and more or less pronounced internal hydrocephalus and atrophy.[3] Abnormalities of the urinary tract, hydronephrosis, hydroureter, and bladder diverticuli, have also been demonstrated radiographically.[869]

Electroencephalographic abnormalities have been found in all cases except one.[324] A variety of abnormalities have been described, most commonly multifocal epileptiform activity initially restricted to one hemisphere then later involving both hemispheres. Other frequent patterns include slowing and hypsarrhythmia. Electroretinograms and VERs are often abnormal.

Other laboratory tests are less helpful in diagnosing Menkes' syndrome. Hypochromic anemia and thrombocytopenia have been reported.[256] Aminoaciduria and increases in various serum amino acids are occasionally observed. Elevated alkaline phosphatase and low serum albumin have also been observed. Normal laboratory tests, which are helpful because they distinguish Menkes' syndrome from other infantile neurodegenerative diseases, include nerve conduction velocity and CSF.

Genetics. Menkes' syndrome cases have been reported from at least six countries, and in Caucasians, blacks, and orientals. Only males have been reported to be affected by Menkes' syndrome. In the original report five males in one pedigree were affected and in several other reported families males on the maternal side but not on the paternal side have been affected in generations preceding the proband. These observations suggest an X-linked pattern of inheritance. Suspected female carriers can manifest kinky hair (pili torti) or cutaneous abnormalities.[174,845,851]

Treatment. If the pathologic abnormalities are an indirect consequence of Cu deficiency, the Cu replacement should be effective when administered prior to irreversible change. This may be a difficult goal to achieve because some of the defects appear to occur *in utero*. Nevertheless, in at least one infant receiving Cu infusions from 28 days of age, developmental progress continued and electroencephalographic abnormalities did not occur.[324] Others have failed to demonstrate a beneficial effect of Cu infusion.

REFERENCES

1. **Abramov A, Schorrs S, Wolman M:** Generalized xanthomatosis with calcified adrenals. Am J Dis Child 91:282, 1956

2. **Aguilar MJ, Chadwick DK, Okuyama K et al:** Kinky hair disease: Part I, clinical and pathological features. J Neuropathol Exp Neurol 25:507, 1966

3. **Ahlgren P, Vester M:** Menkes' kinky hair disease. Neuroradiol 13:159, 1977

4. **Al Rashid RA, Spangler J:** Neonatal copper deficiency. N Engl J Med 285:841, 1971

5. **Aleu FP, Terry RD, Zellweger H:** Electron microscopy of two cerebral biopsies in gargoylism. J Neuropathol Exp Neurol 24:306, 1965

6. **Alzheimer A:** Beitrage zur Kenntnis der patho-logischen Neuroglia und ihrer Beziehung zu den Abbauvorgange in Nervengewebe Nissl Alzheimer's Histol Histopathol Arb 3:493, 1910

7. **Ampola MG, Efron ML, Bixby EM et al:** Mental deficiency in a new aminoaciduria. Amer J Dis Childhood 117:66, 1969

8. **Ampola MG, Mahoney MJ, Nakamura E et al:** Prenatal therapy of a patient with vitamin B_{12}-responsive methylmalonic aciduria. N Engl J Med 293:313, 1975

9. **Anderson EP, Kalckar HM, Isselbacher KJ:** Defect in the uptake of galactose-1-phosphate into liver nucleotides in congenital galactosemia. Science 125:113, 1957

10. **Anderson W:** A case of angiokeratoma. Br J Dermatol 10:113, 1898

11. **Ando T, Lingburg WG, Ward AN et al:** Isovaleric acidemia presenting with altered metabolism of glycine. Pediatr Res 5:478, 1971

12. **Ando T, Nyhan WL, Connor JD et al:** The oxidation of glycine and propionic acid in propionic acidemia with ketotic hyperglycinemia. Pediatr Res 6:576, 1972

13. **Ando T, Nyhan WL, Gerritsen T et al:** Metabolism of glycine in the nonketotic form of hyperglycinemia. Pediatr Res 2:254, 1968

14. **Ando T, Rasmussen K, Wright JM et al:** Isolation and identification of methylcitrate, a major metabolic production of propionate in patients with propionic acidemia. J Biol Chem 247:2200, 1972

15. **Arakawa T:** Congenital defects in folate utilization. Am J Med 48:594, 1970

16. **Arakawa T, Narisawa K, Tanno K et al:** Megaloblastic anemia and mental retardation associated with hyperfolicacidaemia. Probably due to N^5-methyltetrahydrofolate transferase deficiency. Tohoku J Exp Med 93:1, 1967

17. **Arbisser AI, Donnelly KA, Scott CI Jr et al:** Morquio-like syndrome with beta-galactosidase deficiency and normal hexosamine sulfatase activity: mucopolysaccharidosis IVB. Am J Med Genet 1:195, 1977

18. **Arima M, Takeshita K, Yoshino K et al:** Prognosis of Wilson's disease in childhood. Eur J Pediatr 126:147, 1977

19. **Armstrong D, Dimmit S, van Wormer DE:** Studies in Batten disease: Part I. Peroxidase deficiency in granulocytes. Arch Neurol 30:114, 1974

20. **Arneson D, Ch'ien LT, Chance P et al:** Strychnine therapy in nonketotic hyperglycinemia. Pediatr 63:369, 1979

21. **Atkin BM, Buist NRM, Utter MF et al:** Pyruvate carboxylase deficiency and lactic acidosis in a retarded child without Leigh's disease. Pediatr Res 13:109, 1979

22. **Atzopodien W, Kremer GJ, Schnellbacher E et al:** Angiokeratoma corporis diffusum (Morbus Fabry): Biochemische diagnostik im Blutplasma. Dtsch Med Wochenschr 100:423, 1975

23. **Auerbach VH, DiGeorge AM, Brigham MP et al:** Delayed maturation tyrosine metabolism in a full-term sibling of a child with phenylketonuria. J Pediatr 62:938, 1963

24. **Aula P, Autio S, Raivio KO et al:** Salla disease: a new lysosomal storage disorder. Arch Neurol 36:88, 1979

25. **Austin J:** Recent studies in the metachromatic and globoid forms of sclerosis. Res Publ Assoc Res Nerv Ment Dis 40:189, 1962

26. **Austin J:** Studies in metachromatic leukodystrophy. Part XII. Multiple sulfatase deficiency. Arch Neurol 28:258, 1973

27. **Austin J, Armstrong D, Shearer L et al:** Metachromatic form of diffuse cerebral sclerosis. Part VI. A rapid test for the sulfatase A deficiency in metachromatic leukodystrophy (MLD) urine. Arch Neurol 14:259, 1966

28. **Austin J, Armstrong D, Stumpf D et al:** Defective sulfatide synthesis in Krabbe's disease (globoid leukodystrophy). Trans Am Neurol Assoc 175:179, 1967

29. **Austin J, Lehfeldt D, Maxwell W:** Experimental "globoid bodies" in white matter and chemical analysis in Krabbe's disease. J Neuropathol Exp Neurol 20:284, 1961

30. **Autio S:** Aspartylglucosaminuria. Analysis of thirty-four patients. J Ment Def Res Monogr Ser 1:1, 1972

31. **Autio S, Palo J, Perheentupa J:** Aspartylglucosaminuria: a gargoyle-like syndrome with autosomal recessive inheritance. Birth Defects: Original Article Series, 10, no 4:193, 1974

32. **Avery ME, Clow CL, Menkes JH et al:** Transient tyrosinemia of the newborn: dietary and clinical aspects. Pediatr 39:378, 1967

33. **Avila JL, Convit J:** Inhibition of leukocytic lysosomal enzymes by glycosaminoglycans in vitro. Biochem J 152:57, 1975

34. **Aylsworth AS, Taylor HA, Stuart CM et al:** Mannosidosis: Phenotype of a severely affected child and characterization of alpha-mannosidase activity in cultured fibroblasts from the patient and his parents. J Pediatr 99:814, 1976

35. **Aylsworth AS, Thomas GH, Hood JL et al.** A severe infantile sialidosis: clinical biochemical, and microscopic features. J Pediatr 96:662, 1980

36. **Babrik A, Benson PF, Fensom AH et al:** Corneal clouding in G_{M1}-generalized gangliosidosis. Brit J Ophthalmol 60:565, 1976

37. **Bacchus H, Peterson DI:** Pregnancy complicated by myelopathy due to Maroteaux-Lamy syndrome. Am J Obstet Gynecol 136:259, 1980

38. **Bach G, Friedman R, Weissman B et al:** The defect in the Hurler and Scheie Syndromes: deficiency of alpha-L-iduronidase. Proc Natl Acad Sci USA 69:2048, 1972

39. **Bach G, Zeigler M, Kohn G:** Biochemical investigations of cultured amniotic fluid cells in mucolipidosis type IV. Clin Chim Acta 106:121, 1980

40. **Bachmann C, Krahenbuhl S, Colombo JP et al:** Letter: N-acetyl-glutamate synthetase deficiency: a disorder of ammonia detoxification. N Engl J Med 304:543, 1981

41. **Baker L, Mellman WJ, Tedesco TA et al:** Galactosemia: symptomatic and asymptomatic homozygotes in one Negro sibling. J Pediatr 68:551, 1966

42. **Bakker HD, Wadman SK, van Sprang FJ et al:** Tyrosinemia and tyrosyluria in healthy prematures: time courses not vitamin C-dependent. Clin Chim Acta 61:73, 1975

43. **Ballard RA, Vinocour B, Reynolds JW et al:** Transient hyperammonemia of the preterm infant. New Engl J Med 299:920, 1978

44. **Bank WJ, Morrow G:** A familial spinal cord disorder with hyperglycinemia. Arch Neurol 27:136, 1972

45. **Barbeau A, Frieseu H:** Treatment of Wilson's disease with L-dopa after failure with pencillamine. Lancet 1:1180, 1970

46. **Barber GW, Spaeth GL:** Pyridoxine therapy in homocytinuria. Lancet 1:337, 1967

47. **Barber GW, Spaeth GL:** The successful treatment of homocystinuria with pyridoxine. J Pediatr 75:463, 1969

48. **Barnard RO, Best PV, Erdohazi M:** Neuropathology of Menkes' disease. Dev Med Child Neurol 20:586, 1978

49. **Barnes ND, Hull D, Balgobin L et al:** Biotin-responsive propionic acidaemia. Lancet 2:244, 1970

50. **Baron DN, Dent CE, Harris H et al:** Hereditary pellagra-like skin rash with temporary cerebellar ataxia, constant renal aminoaciduria, and other bizarre biochemical features. Lancet 2:421, 1956

51. **Bartholome K, Lutz P, Bickel H:** Determination of phenylalanine hydroxylase activity in patients with phenylketonuria and hyperphenylalaninemia. Pediatr Res 9:899, 1975

52. **Bartsocas C, Grobe H, van de Kamp JJP et al:** Sanfilippo type C disease: clinical findings in four patients with a new variant of mucopolysaccharidosis III. Eur J Pediatr 130:251, 1979

53. **Basner R, von Figura K, Glossl J et al:** Multiple deficiency of mucopolysaccharide sulfatase in mucosulfatidosis. Pediatr Res 13:1316, 1979

54. **Bassen F, Kornzweig A:** Malformation of the erythrocytes in a case of atypical retinitis pigmentosa. Blood 5:381, 1950

55. **Batshaw M, Brusilow S:** Treatment of hyperammonemic coma caused by inborn errors of the urea synthesis. J Pediatr 97:893, 1980

56. **Batshaw M, Brusilow S, Walser M:** Treatment of carbamyl phosphate synthetase deficiency with keto-analogues of essential amino acids. New Engl J Med 292:1085, 1975

57. **Batshaw ML, Painter MJ, Sproul GT et al:** Therapy of urea cycle enzymopathies: three case studies. Johns Hopkins Med J 148:34, 1981

58. **Batshaw ML, Roan Y, Jun AL et al:** Cerebral dysfunction in asymptomatic carriers of ornithine transcarbamylase deficiency. New Engl J Med 302:482, 1980

59. **Batten FE:** Cerebral degeneration with symmetrical changes in the maculae in two members of a family. Trans Ophthalmol Soc U K 23:386, 1903

60. **Baumgartner RE, Nyhan WL:** Nonketotic hyperglycinemia. J Pediatr 75:1022, 1969

61. **Baumgartner RE, Wick H, Maurer R et al:** Congenital defect in intracellular cobalamin metabolism resulting in homocystinuria and methylmalonic aciduria. Helv Paediat Acta 34:465, 1979

62. **Beaudet AL, DiFerrante NM, Ferry GD et al:** Variation in the phenotypic expression of beta-glucuronidase deficiency. J Pediatr 86:388, 1975

63. **Belanger M, Tremblay M, Lapointe JR:** Absence congenitale des beta-lipoproteines; syndrome rare et bizzare. Nouvelle observation. Laval Med 42:332, 1971

64. **Beratis NG, Aron AM, Hirschhorn K:** Metachromatic leukodystrophy: detection in serum. J Pediatr 83:824, 1973

65. **Berman PH, Balis ME, Dancis J:** Congenital hyperuricemia, an inborn error of purine metabolism associated with psychomotor retardation, athetosis, and self-mutilation. Arch Neurol 20:44, 1969

66. **Berry HK, Spinanger J:** A paper spot test useful in the study of Hurler's syndrome. J Lab Clin Med 55:136, 1960

67. **Beutler E, Baluda MC, Sturgeon P et al:** The genetics of galactose-1-phosphate uridyl transferase deficiency. J Lab Clin Med 68:646, 1966

68. **Beutler E, Kuhl W:** Diagnosis of the adult type of Gaucher's disease and its carrier state by demonstration of a deficiency of glucosidase activity in peripheral blood leukocytes. J Lab Clin Med 76:747, 1970

69. **Beutler E, Kuhl W:** Fabry's disease: structural or regulatory mutation. J Lab Clin Med 78:977, 1971

70. **Beutler E, Villacorte D, Kuhl W et al:** Nonenzymatic conversion of human hexosaminidase A. J Lab Clin Med 86:195, 1975

71. **Bickel H:** Phenylalaninemia or classical phenylketonuria. Neuropaediatrie 1:379, 1970.

72. **Bickel H, Feist D, Muller H et al:** Ornithinamie, eine weiter Aminosaurenstoff-wechselstorung mit Hirnschadijung. Dtsch Med Worchenschr 47:2247, 1968

73. **Bickel H, Gerrard J, Hickman EM:** Influence of phenylalanine intake on phenylketonurics. Lancet 2:812, 1953

74. **Billings DM, Degnan M:** Kinky hair syndrome. Amer J Dis Child 121:447, 1971

75. **Bird TD, Lagunoff D:** Neurological manifestations of Fabry disease in female carriers. Ann Neurol 4:537, 1978

76. **Blass JP:** Disorders of pyruvate metabolism. Neurology 29:280, 1979

77. **Blass JP, Avigan J, Uhlendorf BW:** A defect in pyruvate decarboxylase in a child with an intermittent movement disorder. J Clin Invest 49:423, 1970

78. **Blass JP, Cederbaum SD, Dunn HG:** Biochemical defect in Leigh's disease. Lancet 1:1237, 1976

79. **Blass JP, Kark RAP, Engel WK:** Clinical studies of a patient with pyruvate-decarboxylase deficiency. Arch Neurol 25:449, 1971

80. **Blass JP, Schulman JD, Young DS et al:** An inherited defect affecting the tricarboxylic acid cycle in a patient with congenital lactic acidosis. J Clin Invest 91:1845, 1972

81. **Blaw ME:** Melanodermic type leukodystrophy (adrenoleukodystrophy). In Vinken PJ, Bruyn GW (eds): Handbook of Clinical Neurology, pp 128–133. New York, Elsevier Publishing, 1970

82. **Boehme DH, Cottrell JC, Leonberg SC et al:** A dominant form of neuronal ceroid-lipofuscinosis. Brain 94:745, 1971

83. **Booth CW, Chen KK, Nadler HL:** Mannosidosis: clinical and biochemical studies in a family of affected adolescents and adults. J Pediatr 88:821, 1976

84. **Booth CW, Nadler HL:** Demonstration of the heterozygous state in Hunter's syndrome. Pediatr 53:396, 1974

85. **Bootsma D, Galjaard H:** Heterogeneity in genetic diseases studied in cultured cells. In Hommes FA (ed): Models for the Study of Inborn Errors of Metabolism, pp 241–256. Amsterdam, Elsevier Publishing, 1979

86. **Borreson AL, van der Hagen CB:** Metachromatic leukodystrophy. Part II. Direct determination of arylsulfatase A activity in amniotic fluid. Clin Genet 4:442, 1973

87. **Borrone C, Gatti R, Trias X et al:** Fucosidosis: clinical, biochemical, immunologic and genetic studies in two new cases. J Pediatr 84:727, 1974

88. **Boudin G, Mikol S, Guillard A et al:** Fatal systemic carnitine deficiency with lipid storage in skeletal muscle, heart, liver and kidney. J Neurol Sci 30:313, 1976

89. **Brady RO:** Cerebral lipidoses. Ann Rev Med 21:317, 1970

90. **Brady RO:** Glucosyl ceramide lipidosis: Gaucher's disease. In Stanbury JB, Wyngaarden JB, Fredrickson DS (eds): The Metabolic Basis of Inherited Disease, 4th ed, pp 731–746. New York, McGraw-Hill, 1978

91. **Brady RO:** Inherited metabolic diseases and pathogenesis of mental retardation. Ann Biol Clin 36:113, 1978

92. **Brady RO:** Sphingomyelin lipidosis: Niemann-Pick disease. In Stanbury JB, Wyngaarden JB, Fredrickson DS (eds): The Metabolic Basis of Inherited Disease, 4th ed, pp 718–730. New York, McGraw-Hill, 1978

93. **Brady RO, Barranger JA, Gal AE et al:** Treatment of lipidoses by enzyme infusion. In Callahan JW, Lowden JA (eds): Lysosomes and Lysosomal Storage Diseases, pp 373–379. New York, Raven Press, 1981

94. **Brady RO, Gal AE, Bradley RM et al:** Enzymatic defect in Fabry's disease: ceramide trihexosidase deficiency. N Engl J Med 276:1163, 1967

95. **Brady RO, Johnson WG, Uhlendorf BW:** Identification of heterozygous carriers of lipid storage diseases. Am J Med 51:423, 1971

96. **Brady RO, O'Brien JS, Bradley RM et al:** Sphingolipid hydrolases in brain tissue of patients with generalized gangliosidosis. Biochim Biophys Acta 210:193, 1970

97. **Brady RO, Pentchev PG, Gal AE:** Replacement therapy for inherited enzyme deficiency. Use of purified glucocerebrosidase in Gaucher's disease. N Engl J Med 291:989, 1974

98. **Brady RO, Uhlendorf BW, Jacobson CB:** Fabry's disease: antenatal diagnosis. Science, 172:172, 1971

99. **Brandt I, Hsia YE, Clement DH et al:** Propionic acidemia (ketotic hyperglycinemia) dietary treatment resulting in normal growth and development. Pediatr 53:391, 1974

100. **Brandt JB, Terenius L, Jacobesen BB et al:** Hyperendorphin syndrome in a child with necrotizing encephalomyelopathy. N Engl J Med 303:914, 1980

101. **Brandt NJ, Christensen E, Gregersen N et al:** Glutaric aciduria in progressive choreoathetosis. Clin Genet 13:77, 1978

102. **Brandt NJ, Gregorsen N, Christensen E et al:** Treatment of glutaryl-CoA dehydrogenase deficiency (glutaric aciduria). J Pediatr 94:669, 1979

103. **Bray PF:** Sex-linked neurodegenerative disease associated with monilethrix. Pediatr 36:417, 1965

104. **Bremer HJ, Duran M, Kamerling JP et al:** Disturbances of Amino Acid Metabolism: Clinical Chemistry and Diagnosis. Baltimore, Urban and Schwarzenberg, 1981

105. **Brett EM, Ellis RB, Haas L et al:** Late onset G_{M2}-gangliosidosis: clinical, pathological, and biochemical studies on eight patients. Arch Dis Child 48:775, 1973

106. **Brewster TG, Moskowitz MA, Kaufman S et al:** Dihydropteridine reductase deficiency associated with severe neurologic disease and mild hyperphenylalaninemia. Pediatr 63:94, 1979

107. **Britton DE, Pollock JM, Eiven RM:** Acute hemiplegia of childhood, lactate-pyruvate acidemia and mitochrondrial disorder. Ann Neurol 2:265, 1977

108. **Brown T, Hugg G, Lansky L et al:** Transiently reduced activity of carbamyl phosphate synthetase and ornithine transcarbamylase in the liver of children with Reye's syndrome. New Engl J Med 294:861, 1976

109. **Bruhl HH:** Dietary treatment in older PKU patients. In Proceedings of a Conference on Nutrition and the Inherited Diseases of Man as Related to Public Health, p 73. Minneapolis, 1966

110. **Brunette MG, Delvin E, Hazel B et al:** Thiamin-responsive lactic acidosis in a patient with a deficient low-Km pyruvate carboxylase activity in liver. Pediatr 50:702, 1972

111. **Brusilow S, Batshaw ML:** Arginine therapy of argininosuccinase deficiency. Lancet 1:124, 1979

112. **Brusilow SW, Valle DL, Batshaw ML:** New pathways of nitrogen excretion in inborn errors of urea synthesis. Lancet 2:452, 1979

113. **Bruton CJ, Corsellis JAN, Russell A:** Hereditary hyperammonemia. Brain 93:423, 1970

114. **Bucknall WE, Haslam RHA, Holtzman NA:** Kinky-hair syndrome: response to copper therapy. Pediatr 52:653, 1973

115. **Budd MA, Tanaka K, Holmes LB et al:** Isovaleric acidemia: clinical features of a new genetic defect of leucine metabolism. N Engl J Med 277:321, 1967

116. **Buhler RHO, Kagi JHR:** Human hepatic metallothioneins. FEBS Letter, 39:229, 1974

117. **Buist NRM, Lis EW, Tuerck JM et al:** Maternal phenylketonuria. Lancet II:589, 1979

118. **Bulfield G, Kacser H:** Histidinaemia in mouse and man. Arch Dis Child 49:545, 1974

119. **Buonanno FS, Ball MR, Laster DW et al:** Computed tomography in late-infantile metachromatic leukodystrophy. Ann Neurol 4:43, 1978

120. **Bush JA, Mahoney JP, Markowitz H et al:** Studies on copper metabolism. Radioactive copper studies in normal subjects and in patients with hepatolenticular degeneration. J Clin Invest, 34:1766, 1955

121. **Cabalska B, Duczyniska N, Borzymowska J et al:** Termination of dietary treatment in phenylketonuria. Eur J Pediatr 126:253, 1977

122. **Calderon R, Gonzales-Cantu N:** Kinky hair, photosensitivity, broken eyebrows and eyelashes, and nonprogressive mental retardation. J Pediatr 95:1007, 1979

123. **Callahan JW, Lassila EL, Phillippart M:** Phosphodiesterases in human tissues. II. Decreased hydrolysis of synthetic substrate by tissues from patients with the Niemann-Pick syndrome. Biochem Med 11:262, 1974

124. **Callahan JW, Lowden JA (eds):** Lysosomes and Lysosomal Storage Diseases. New York, Raven Press, 1981

125. **Cammermeyer J:** Neuropathological changes in hereditary neuropathies: manifestation of the syndrome heredopathia atactica polyneuritiformis in the presence of interstitial hypertrophic polyneuropathy. J Neuropathol Exp Neurol 15:340, 1956

126. **Cammermeyer J, Haymaker W, Refsum S:** Heredopathia atactica polyneuritiformis: the neuropathologic changes in three adults and one child. Am J Pathol, 30:643, 1954

127. **Campbell AGM, Rosenberg LE, Snodgrass PJ et al:** Ornithine transcarbamylase deficiency: a cause of lethal neonatal hyperammonemia in males. New Engl J Med 288:1, 1973

128. **Cantz M, Gehler J:** The mucopolysaccharidoses: inborn errors of glycosaminoglycan catabolism. Hum Genet 32:233, 1976

129. **Cantz M, Gehler J, Spranger J:** Mucolipidosis I: increased sialic acid content and deficiency of an alpha-N-acetylneuraminidase in cultured fibroblasts. Biochem Biophys Res Commun 74:732, 1977

130. **Capobianchi MR, Romeo G:** Mosaicism for sulfoiduronate sulfatase deficiency in carriers of Hunter's syndrome. Experientia. 32:459, 1976

131. **Capron AM, Lappe M, Murray RF et al:** Genetic counseling: facts, values, and norms. Birth Defects Original Article Series, 15, no 2, 1970

132. **Carrico RJ, Deutsch HF:** Isolation of human hepatocuprein and cerebrocuprein: their identity with erythrocuprein. J Bio Chem 244:6097, 1969

133. **Carson NA, Scally BG, Neill DW et al:** Saccharopinuria: a new inborn error of lysine metabolism. Nature (Lond) 218:679, 1968

134. **Cathelineau L, Saudubray J-M, Polonovski C:** Heterogenous mutations of the structural gene of human ornithine carbamyltransferase as observed in five personal cases. Enzyme 18:103, 1974

135. **Cederbaum SD, Blass JP, Minkoff N et al:** Sensitivity to carbohydrate in a patient with familial

intermittent lactic acidosis and pyruvate dehydrogenase deficiency. Pediatr Res 10:713, 1976

136. **Cederbaum SD, Shaw KN, Valente M:** Hyperargininemia. J Pediatr 90:569, 1977

137. **Chan W-Y, Cushing W, Coffman MA et al:** Genetic expression of Wilson's disease in cell culture: a diagnostic marker. Science 208:299, 1980

138. **Chapoy PR, Angelini C, Brown WJ et al:** Systemic carnitine deficiency—a treatable inherited lipid-storage disease presenting as Reye's syndrome. N Engl J Med 303:1389, 1980

139. **Chase GA:** The TSD gene among Askenazic Jews: founder effect and genetic drift. In Kaback MM, Rimoin DL, O'Brien JS (eds): Tay-Sachs Disease: Screening and Prevention, pp 109–110. New York, Alan R Liss, 1977

140. **Chern CJ, Croce CM:** Assignment of the structural gene for human beta-glucuronidase to chromosome 7 and tetrameric association of subunits in the enzyme molecule. Am J Hum Genet 28:350, 1976

141. **Childs B, Nyhan WL:** Further observations of a patient with hyperglycinemia. Pediatr 33:403, 1964

142. **Childs B, Nyhan WL, Borden M et al:** Idiopathic hyperglycinemia and hyperglycinuria: new disorder of amino acid metabolism. Part I. Pediatr 27:522, 1961

143. **Clayton BE, Dobbs RH, Patrick AD:** Leigh's subacute necrotizing encephalopathy: clinical and biochemical study, with special reference to therapy with lipoate. Arch Dis Child 42:467, 1967

144. **Cogan DG:** The lens, cataracts, and galactosemia. N Engl J Med 288:1239, 1973

145. **Cogan DG, Chu FC, Gittinger J et al:** Fundal abnormalities of Gaucher's disease. Arch Ophthalmol 98:2292, 1980

146. **Cogan DG, Kuwabara T, Moser H et al:** Retinopathy in a case of Farber's lipogranulomatosis. Arch Ophthalmol 75:752, 1966

147. **Cogan DG, Kuwabara T, Moser H:** Metachromatic leukodystrophy. Ophthalmology. 170:2, 1970

148. **Cohn RM, Yudkoff M, Rothman R et al:** Isovaleric acidemia: use of glycine therapy in neonates. N Engl J Med 299:996, 1978

149. Collective results of mass screening for inborn metabolic errors in eight European countries. Acta Paediatr Scand, 62:413, 1973

150. **Conzelmann E, Sandhoff K:** AB variant of infantile G_{M2}-gangliosidosis: Deficiency of a factor necessary for stimulation of hexosaminidase A-catalyzed degradation of ganglioside G_{M2} and glycolipid G_{M2}. Proc Natl Acad Sci (USA) 75:3979, 1978

151. **Cooper J, Itokawa Y, Pincus J:** Thiamine triphosphate deficiency in subacute necrotizing encephalomyelopathy. Science 164:75, 1969

152. **Cotlier E:** Corneal cloudiness and retinitis pigmentosa in the mucopolysaccharidoses. Lancet 1:993, 1973

153. **Coude FX, Sweetman L, Nyhan WL:** Inhibition by propionyl-coenzyme A of N-acetylglutamate synthetase in rat liver metochondria. J Clin Invest 64:1544, 1979

154. **Coulombe JT, Shih VE, Levy HL:** Massachusetts metabolic disorders screening program. Part II. Methylmalonic aciduria. Pediatr 76:26, 1981

155. **Cowan MJ, Packman S, Wara DW et al:** Multiple biotin-dependent carboxylase deficiencies associated with defects in T-cell and B-cell immunity. Lancet 2:115, 1979

156. **Crampton RF, Matthews DV, Poisner R:** Observations on the mechanism of absorption of copper by the small intestine. J Physiol (London) 178:11, 1965

157. **Crocker AC:** The cerebral defect in Tay-Sachs disease and Niemann-Pick disease. J Neurochem 7:69, 1961

158. **Crocker AC, Mays VA:** Sphingomyelin synthesis in Niemann-Pick disease. Am J Clin Nutr 9:63, 1961

159. **Crome L, Dutton G, Ross CF:** Maple syrup urine disease. J Pathol 81:379, 1961

160. **Crome L, Hanefeld F, Patrick D et al:** Late onset globoid cell leukodystrophy. Brain 96:84, 1973

161. **Crosby TW, Chou SM:** "Ragged-red" fibers in Leigh's disease. Neurol 24:49, 1974

162. **Cumings JN:** The copper and iron content of brain and liver in the normal and in hepato-lenticular degeneration. Brain 71:410, 1948

163. **Curtis H-Ch, Niederwieser A, Viscontini M et al:** Atypical phenylketonuria due to tetrahydrobiopterin deficiency: diagnosis and treatment with tetrahydrobiopterin, dihydrobiopterin and sepiapterin. Clin Chim Acta 93:251, 1979

164. **Dahlqvist A:** Test paper for galactose in urine. Scan J Clin Lab Invest 22:87, 1968

165. **Dancis J, Hutzler J, Levitz M:** The diagnosis of maple syrup urine disease (branched-chain ketoaciduria) by the in vitro study of the peripheral leucocyte. Pediatr 32:234, 1963

166. **Dancis J, Hutzler J, Rokkones T:** Intermittent branched-chain ketonuria. N Engl J Med 276:84, 1967

167. **Dancis J, Hutzler J, Tada K et al:** Hypervalinemia: a defect in valine transamination. Pediatr 39:813, 1967

168. **Dancis J, Hutzler J, Snyderman SE et al:** Enzyme activity in classical and variant forms of maple syrup urine disease. J Pediatr 81:312, 1972

169. **Dancis J, Levitz M:** Abnormalities of branched chain amino acid metabolism. In Stanbury JB, Wyngaarden JB, Fredrickson DS (eds): The Metabolic Basis of Inherited Disease, 4th ed, pp 397–410. New York, McGraw-Hill, 1978

170. **Danes BS:** Variant of iduronidase deficient mucopolysaccharidoses. Further evidence for genetic heterogeneity. J Med Genet 14:346, 1977

171. **Danes BS, Bearn AG:** Hurler's syndrome: a genetic study of clones in cell culture with particular reference to the Lyon hypothesis. J Exp Med 125:509, 1967

172. **Danks DM, Bartholome K, Clayton B et al:** Current status of malignant hyperphenylalanemia. J Inherited Metab Dis 1:49, 1978

173. **Danks DM, Campbell PE, Cartwright E et al:** The Sanfilippo syndrome: clinical, biochemical,

radiological, haematological and pathological features of nine cases. Aust Paediat J 8:174, 1972

174. **Danks DM, Campbell PE, Walker-Smith J et al:** Menkes' kinky hair syndrome. Lancet 1:1100, 1972

175. **Danks DM, Cartwright E, Stevens BJ et al:** Menkes' kinky hair disease: further definition of the defect in copper transport. Science 179:1140, 1973

176. **Danks DM, Cotton RGH:** Early diagnosis of hyperphenylalaninemia due to tetrahydrobiopterin deficiency (malignant hyperphenylalaninemia). J Pediatr 96:854, 1980

177. **Danks DM, Schlesinger R, Firgaira F et al:** Malignant hyperphenylalaninemia—clinical features, biochemical findings, and experience with administration of biopterins. Pediatr Res 13:1150, 1979

178. **Daum RS, Lamm PH, Mamer OA et al:** A "new" disorder of isoleucine catabolism. Lancet 2:1289, 1971

179. **Daum RS, Scriver CR, Mamer OA et al:** An inherited disorder of isoleucine catabolism causing accumulation of alpha-methylacetoacetate and alpha-methyl-beta-hydroxybutyrate, and intermittent metabolic acidosis. Pediatr Res 7:149, 1973

180. **David LE, Orth DN, Kornfeld M et al:** Adrenoleukodystrophy and adrenomyeloneuropathy associated with partial adrenal insufficiency in three generations of a kindred. Am J Med 66:342, 1979

181. **Dawson G, Sweeley CC:** In vivo studies on glucosphingolipid metabolism. J Biol Chem 245:410, 1970

182. **Dean KJ, Sweeley CC:** Fabry's disease. In Glew RH, Peters SP: Practical Enzymology of the Sphingolipidoses, pp 173–216. New York, Alan R Liss, 1977

183. **DeGroot CJ, Hommes FA:** Letter: Further speculation on the pathogenesis of Leigh's encephalopathy. J Pediatr 82:541, 1973

184. **DeGroot CJ, Luit-DeHaan G, Hulstaert CE et al:** A patient with severe neurologic symptoms and acetoacetyl-CoA thiolase deficiency. Pediatr Res 11:1112, 1977

185. **Deiss A, Lee GR, Cartwright GE:** Hemolytic anemia in Wilson's disease. Ann Intern Med 73:413, 1970

186. **Deiss A, Lynch RE, Lee GR et al:** Long-term therapy of Wilson's disease. Ann Intern Med 75:57, 1971

187. **Dekaban AS, Hermann MM:** Childhood, juvenile and adult cerebral lipidoses. Are these different nosological entities? Arch Pathol 97:65, 1974

188. **Del Monte MA, Johnson DL, Cotlier E et al:** Diagnosis of Fabry's disease by tear alpha-galactosidase A. N Engl J Med 290:57, 1974

189. **DeMars R, Sarto G, Felix JS et al:** Lesch-Nyhan mutation: prenatal detection with amniotic fluid cells. Science 164:1303, 1969

190. **Denny-Brown D:** Hepatolenticular degeneration (Wilson's disease): two different components. N Eng J Med 270:1149, 1964

191. **Denny-Brown D, Porter H:** The effect of BAL (2,3-dimercaptopropanol) on hepatolenticular degeneration (Wilson's disease). N Eng Med 245:917, 1951

192. **Desnick RJ, Allen KY, Desnick SJ et al:** Fabry's disease: enzymatic diagnosis of hemizygotes and heterozygotes. J Lab Clin Med 81:157, 1973

193. **Desnick RJ, Klionsky B, Sweeley CC:** Fabry's disease (alpha-galactosidase A deficiency). In Stanbury JB, Wyngaarden JB, Frederickson DS (eds): The Metabolic Basis of Inherited Disease, 4th ed, pp 810–840. New York, McGraw-Hill, 1978

194. **Desnick RL, Shart HL, Grabowski GA et al:** Mannosidosis: clinical, morphologic, immunologic, and biochemical studies. Pediatr Res 10:985, 1976

195. **DeVivo DC, Haymond MW, Leckie MP et al:** The clinical and biochemical implications of pyruvate carboxylase deficiency. J Clin Endocrinol Metab 45:281, 1977

196. **DiDonato S, Rimoldi M, Moise A et al:** Fatal ataxic encephalopathy and carnitine acetyltransferase deficiency: a functional defect of pyruvate oxidation? Neurol 29:1578, 1979

197. **DiFerrante N:** N-Acetylglucosamine-6-sulfate sulfatase deficiency reconsidered. Science 210:448, 1980

198. **Dixon HBF, Gibbs K, Walshe JM:** Preparation of triethylenetetramine dihydrochloride for the treatment of Wilson's disease. Lancet 1:853, 1972

199. **Dodgson KS, Spencer B:** Studies on sulphatases. Part I. The choice of substrate for the assay of rat-liver arylsulphatase. Biochem J 53:444, 1953

200. **Dodgson KS, Spencer B, Thomas J:** Studies on sulphatase. The arylsulphatases of mammalian livers. Biochem J 59:29, 1955

201. **Dolman CL, MacLeod PM, Chang E:** Skin punch biopsies and lymphocytes in diagnosis of lipidoses. Can J Neurol Sci 2:67, 1975

202. **Donnell GN, Koch R, Bergren WR:** Observations of results of management of galactosemic patients. In Hsia DYY (ed): Galactosemia, pp 247–268. Springfield, Ill., Charles C Thomas, 1969

203. **Donnelly PV, DiFerrante N:** Reliability of the Booth-Nadler technique for the detection of Hunter heterozygotes. Pediatr 56:429, 1975

204. **Dorfman A, Matalon R:** The mucopolysaccharidoses (a review). Proc Natl Acad Sci 73:630, 1976

205. **Dreberg S, Erikson A, Hugberg B:** Gaucher disease—Norrbottaian type. Eur J Pediatr 133:107, 1980

206. **Drummond KN, Michael AF, Ulstrom RA et al:** The blue diaper syndrome: familial hypercalcemia with nephrocalcinosis and indicanuria. Am J Med 37:928, 1964

207. **Dubois G, Turpin JC, Baumann N:** Arylsulfatase isoenzymes in metachromatic leucodystrophy. Detection of a new variant by electrophoresis. Improvement of quantitative assay. Biomedicine 23:116, 1975

208. **Duda EE, Huttenlocker PR:** Computed tomography in adrenoleukodystrophy: correlation of radiological and histological findings. Radiology 120:349, 1976

209. **Duffy PE, Kornfeld MD, Suzuki K:** Neurovisceral storage disease with curvilinear bodies. J Neuropathol Exp Neurol 27:351, 1968

210. **Dulaney JT, Milunsky A, Sidbury JB et al:** Diagnosis of lipogranulomatosis (Farber disease)

by use of cultured fibroblasts. J Pediatr 89:59, 1976

211. **Dulaney JT, Moser HW:** Metachromatic leukodystrophy. In Glew RH, Peters SP (eds): Practical Enzymology of the Sphingolipidoses, pp 137–171. New York, Alan R Liss 1977

212. **Dulaney JT, Moser HW:** Sulfatide Lipidosis: Metachromatic leukodystrophy. In Stanbury JB, Wyngaarden JB, Fredrickson DS (eds): The Metabolic Basis of Inherited Disease, 4th ed, pp 770–809. New York, McGraw-Hill, 1978

213. **Dunn HG, Lake BD, Dolman CL et al:** The neuropathy of Krabbe's infantile cerebral sclerosis (Globoid cell leucodystrophy). Brain 92: 329, 1969

214. **Dunn HG, Perry TL, Dolman CL:** Homocystinuria. Neurology 16:407, 1966

215. **Duran M, Beemer FA, Heiden CVD et al:** Combined deficiency of xanthine oxidase and sulphate oxidase: a defect of molybdenum metabolism or transport? J Inherited Metab Dis 1:175, 1978

216. **Duran M, Ketting D, Wadman SK et al:** Organic acid excretion in a patient with 3-hydroxy-3-methylglutaryl CoA lyase deficiency: facts and artefacts. Clin Chim Acta 90:187, 1978

217. **Durand P, Borrone C, Della Cella G:** Fucosidosis. J Pediatr 75:665, 1969

218. **Elfenbein IB:** Dystonic juvenile idiocy without amaurosis, a new syndrome: light and electron microscopic observations of cerebrum. Johns Hopkins Med J 123:205, 1968

219. **Ellingson RJ, Schain RJ:** EEG patterns in juvenile cerebral lipidosis. Electroenceph Clin Neurophysiol 27:191, 1969

220. **Ellis WG, Schneider EL, McCulloch JR et al:** Krabbe disease. Arch Neurol 29:253, 1973

221. **Elsas LJ, Priest JH, Wheeler FB et al:** Maple syrup urine disease: coenzyme function and prenatal monitoring. Metabolism 23:569, 1974

222. **Elze KL, Koepp P, Lagenstein I et al:** Juvenile type of generalized ceroid-lipofuscinosis (Spielmeyer-Sjogren syndrome). Clinical findings. Neuropaediatrie 9:3, 1978

223. **Emergy AEH:** Elements of Medical Genetics, 4th ed. Berkeley University of California Press, 1975

224. **Engel AG, Banker BQ, Eiben RW:** Carnitine deficiency: clinical morphological and biochemical observations in a fatal case. J Neurol Neurosurg Psychiatry, 40:313, 1977

225. **Engel WK, Dorman JD, Levy RI et al:** Neuropathy in Tangier disease: alpha-lipoprotein deficiency manifesting as familial recurrent neuropathy and intestinal lipid storage. Arch Neurol 17:1, 1967

226. **Epstein CJ, Yatziv S, Neufeld E et al:** Genetic counselling for Hunter syndrome. Lancet 2:737, 1976

227. **Evans GW, Hahn CJ:** Copper and zinc-binding components in rat intestine. Adv Exp Med Biol 48:285, 1974

228. **Fabry J:** Ein Beitrag zur Kenntnis der Purpura haemorrhagica nodularis (Purpura papulosa hemorrhagica Hebrae). Arch Dermatol Syphilol 43:187, 1898

229. **Farber S, Cohen J, Uzman L:** Lipogranulomatosis: a new lipoglycoprotein "storage" disease. J Mt Sinai Hosp 24:816, 1957

230. **Farquhar JW, Ways P:** Abetalipoproteinaemia. In Stanbury JB, Wyngaarden JB, Fredrickson DS (eds): The Metabolic Basis of Inherited Disease, 2nd ed, pp 509–522. New York, McGraw-Hill, 1960

231. **Farrell DF, MacMartin MP, Clark AF:** Multiple molecular forms of arylsulfatase A in different forms of metachromatic leukodystrophy (MLD). Neurology 29:16, 1979

232. **Faull K, Bolton P, Halpern B et al:** Patient with defect in leucine metabolism. N Engl J Med 294:1013, 1976

233. **Felding I, Hultbert O:** An atypical form of Sandhoff's disease. Case report and biochemical studies. Neuropaediatrie 9:74, 1978

234. **Felix JS, DeMars R:** Detection of females heterozygous for the Lesch-Nyhan mutation by alpha-arginine-resistant growth of cultured fibroblasts. J Lab Clin Med 77:596, 1971

235. **Fennelly JJ, Fitzgerald O, Hingert DJ:** Observations on porphyria with special reference to Ireland. Irish J Med Sci 411:130, 1960

236. **Fensom AH, Benson PF, Blunt S:** Prenatal diagnosis of galactosemia. Br Med J 4:386, 1974

237. **Fensom AH, Neville BRG, Moser AE et al:** Prenatal diagnosis of Farber's disease. Lancet 2:990, 1979

238. **Finkelstein JD, Mudd SH, Irreverre F et al:** Homocystinuria due to cystathionine synthetase deficiency: the mode of inheritance. Science 146:785, 1964

239. **Firth CD, Johnstone EC, Joseph MH et al:** Double-blind clinical trials of 5-hydroxytryptophan in a case of Lesch-Nyhan syndrome. J Neurol Neurosurg Psychiatry 39:656, 1976.

240. **Fishler K, Donnell GN, Bergren WR et al:** Intellectual and personality development in children with galactosemia. Pediatr 50:412, 1972

241. **Fishler K, Koch R, Donnell GN et al:** Developmental aspects of galactosemia from infancy to childhood. Clin Pediatr 19:38, 1980

242. **Fleischer B:** Zwei weitere Falle von grublicher Verfarbung der Kornea. Klin Monatsbl Augenheilds 41:489, 1903

243. **Fleisher LD, Longhi RC, Tallan HH et al:** Homocystinuria: investigations of cystathionine synthase in cultured fetal cells and the prenatal determination of genetic status. J Pediatr 85:677, 1974

244. **Følling A:** Uber Ausscheidung von Phenylbenztraubensaure in den Harn als Stoffwechselanomalie in Verbindung mit Imbezzillitat. Hoppe-Seyler's Z Physiol Chem 227:169, 1934

245. **Forsyth CC, Forbes M, Cumings JN:** Adrenocortical atrophy and diffuse cerebral sclerosis. Arch Dis Child 46:273, 1971

246. **Fortuin JJH, Kleijer WJ:** Hybridization studies of fibroblasts from Hurler, Scheie, and Hurler/Scheie compound patients: support for the hypothesis of allelic mutants. Hum Genet 53:155, 1980

247. **Fowler B, Kraus J, Packman S et al:** Homocystinuria. Evidence for three distinct classes of cystathionine beta-synthase mutants in cultured fibroblasts. J Clin Invest 6:645, 1978

248. **Francke U:** The human gene for beta glucuronidase is on chromosome 7. Am J Hum Genet 28:357, 1976

249. **Francke U, Felsenstein J, Gartler SM et al:** The occurrence of new mutants in the X-linked recessive Lesch-Nyhan disease. Am J Hum Genet 28:123, 1976

250. **Francois J:** Ocular manifestations in aminoacidopathies. Adv Ophthalmol 25:28, 1972

251. **Fredrickson DS, Sloan HR:** Glucosyl ceramide lipidosis: Gaucher's disease. In Stanbury JB, Wyngaarden JB, Fredrickson DS (eds): The Metabolic Basis of Inherited Disease, 3rd ed, pp 730–759. New York, McGraw-Hill, 1972

252. **Fredrickson DS, Sloan HR:** Sphingomyelin lipidosis. Niemann-Pick disease. In Stanbury JB, Wyngaarden JB, Fredrickson DS (eds): The Metabolic Basis of Inherited Disease, 3rd ed, pp 783–807. New York, McGraw-Hill, 1972

253. **Freeman JM, Finkelstein JD, Mudd SH:** Folate-responsive homocystinuria and "schizophrenia": a defect in methylation due to deficient 5,10 methylenetetrahydrofolate reductase activity. N Engl J Med 292:491, 1975

254. **Freeman JM, Nicholson JF, Maslind WS et al:** Ammonia intoxication due to a congenital defect in urea synthesis. J Pediatr 10:39, 1964

255. **Freidman PA, Kaufman S, Kang ES:** On the nature of the molecular defect in phenylketonuria and hyperphenylalaninemia. Nature 240:187, 1972

256. **French JH:** X-chromosome linked copper malabsorption. In Vinkin PJ, Bruyn GW (eds): Handbook of Neurology. Metabolic and Deficiency Diseases of the Nervous System pp 279–304. Amsterdam, Elsevier Publishing 1977

257. **Friedman JM, Fish RD:** The use of probability trees in genetic counselling. Clin Genet 18:408, 1980

258. **Frimpter GW:** Cystathioninuria: nature of the defect. Science 149:1095, 1965

259. **Frommer FJ:** Defective biliary excretion of copper in Wilson's disease. Gut 15:125, 1974

260. **Frost RG, Holmes EW, Norden AGW et al:** Characterization of purified human liver acid beta-D-galactosidases A$_2$ and A$_3$. Biochem J 175:181, 1978

261. **Fujimoto A, Horwitz A:** Mild form of Morquio disease, a new variant? Clin Res 28:98A, 1980

262. **Gadoth N, O'Croinin P, Butler IJ:** Bone marrow in the Batten-Vogt syndrome. J Neurol Sci 25:197, 1975

263. **Gal AE, Brady RO, Hibbert SR et al:** A practical chromogenic procedure for the detection of homozygotes and heterozygous carriers of Niemann-Pick disease. N Engl J Med 293:632, 1975

264. **Gal AE, Brady RO, Pentchev PG et al:** A practical chromogenic procedure for the diagnosis of Krabbe's disease. Clin Chim Acta 77:53, 1977

265. **Galjaard H, Niermyer MF, Hahnemann N et al:** An example of rapid prenatal diagnosis of Fabry's disease using microtechnique. Clin Genet 5:368, 1979

266. **Gall DG, Cutz E, McCling HJ et al:** Acute liver disease in encephalopathy mimicking Reye syndrome. J Pediatr 87:869, 1975

267. **Gamble JG, Lehninger AL:** Transport of ornithine and citrulline across the mitochondrial membrane. J Biol Chem 248:610, 1973

268. **Garnica AD, Chan WY, Rennert OM:** Role of metallothioneins in copper transport in patients with Menkes syndrome. Ann Clin Lab Sci 8:302, 1978

269. **Garston JB, Gordon RR, Hart CT et al:** An unusual case of homocystinuria. Br J Ophthalmol 54:248, 1970

270. **Gartler SM, Scott RC, Goldstein JL et al:** Lesch-Nyhan syndrome: rapid detection of heterozygotes by the use of hair follicles. Science 72:572, 1971

271. **Gatfield PD, Knights RM, Devereux M et al:** Histidinemia: report of four new cases in one family and the effect of low-histidine diets. Canad Med Assoc J 101:71, 1969

272. **Gatfield PD, Tallerd E, Hinton GG:** Hyperpipecolatemia, a new metabolic disorder associated with neuropathy and hepatomegaly. A case study. Canad Med Assoc J 99:1215, 1968

273. **Gaucher PCE:** De L' epitheliome primitif de la rate. These de Paris, 1882

274. **Gaull GE:** Pathogenesis of maple syrup urine disease: observations during dietary management and treatment of coma by peritoneal dialysis. Biochem Med 3:130, 1969

275. **Gaull GE, Carson NAJ, Dent CE et al:** Homocystinuria: clinical and pathological description of 10 cases. In Oster J (ed): Proceedings of the International Copenhagen Congress on the Scientific Study of Mental Retardation, Vol 1, pp 91–93. Denmark, Det Berlingke Bogtrykker 1964

276. **Gaut J-P, Serre J-C, Dieterlen M et al:** Une nouvelle cause d'hypermethionemie de l'enfant; le deficit en S-adenosylmethionine-synthase. Arch Fr Pediatr 34:416, 1977

277. **Geiger B, Aron R:** Chemical characterization and subunit structure of human N-acetylhexosaminidases A and B. Biochemistry 15, 3484, 1976

278. **Gentz J, Lindblad B:** p-Hydroxyphenylpyruvate hydroxylase activity in fine-needle aspiration liver biopsies in hereditary tyrosinemia. Scand J Clin and Lab Inves 29:115, 1972

279. **Gerritsen T, Kaveggie LS, Waismare HA:** A new type of idiopathic hyperglycinemia with hypooxaluria. Pediatr 36:883, 1965

280. **Gerritsen T, Waisman AJ:** Hypersarcosinemia. In Stanbury JB, Wyngaarden JB, Fredrickson DS (eds): The Metabolic Basis of Inherited Diseases, 4th ed, pp 514–517. New York, McGraw-Hill, 1978

281. **Ghargas GS, Milman G:** Radioimmune determination of hypoxanthine phosophoribosyl transferase cross-reacting material in erythrocytes of Lesch-Nyhan patients. Proc Natl Acad Sci USA 72:4147, 1975

282. **Gilbert E, Dawson G, Zu Rhein GM et al:** I-cell disease, mucolipidosis II. Pathological, histochemical, ultrastructural, and biochemical observations in four cases. Z. Kinderheilk 114:259, 1973

283. **Gill JP, Holson R, Hanley C:** Electroretinography and fundus oculi findings in Hurler's disease and allied mucopolysaccharidoses. Arch Ophthalmol 74:596, 1965

284. **Gilles FH, Deuel RM:** Neuronal cytoplasmic globules in the brain in Morquio's syndrome. Arch Neurol 25:393, 1971

285. **Ginsburg LC, Donnelly PV, DiFerrante DT et al:** N-acetylglucosamine-6-sulfate sulfatase in man: deficiency of the enzyme in a new mucopoly-saccaridosis. Pediatr Res 12:805, 1978

286. **Giorgio AJ, Trowbridge M, Boone AW et al:** Methylmalonic aciduria without vitamin B_{12} deficiency in an adult sibship. New Engl J Med 295:310, 1976

287. **Gitzelmann R:** Hereditary galactokinase deficiency, a newly recognized cause of juvenile cataracts. Pediatr Res 1:14, 1967

288. **Gitzelmann R:** Deficiency of uridine diphosphate galactose-4-epimerase in blood cells of an apparently healthy infant. Helv Paediatr Acta 27:125, 1972

289. **Gitzelmann R, Steinmann B, Cuenod M:** Strychnine for the treatment of nonketotic hyperglycinemia. New Engl J Med 298:1424, 1978

290. **Gitzelmann R, Steinmann B, Otten A et al:** Nonketotic hyperglycinemia treated with strychnine, a glycine receptor antagonist. Helv Paediat Acta 32:517, 1977

291. **Gitzelmann R, Wiesmann UN, Spycher MA et al:** Unusually mild course of beta-glucuronidase deficiency in two brothers (mucopolysaccharidosis VII). Helv Paediat Acta 33:413, 1978

292. **Gjessing LR, Halvorsen S:** Letter: Hypermethioninemia in acute tyrosinosis. Lancet 2:1132, 1965

293. **Gjessing LR, Sjaastad O:** Homocarnosinosis: a new metabolic disorder associated with spasticity and mental retardation. Lancet 2:1028, 1974

294. **Glazebrook AJ:** Wilson's disease. Edinburgh Med J 42:83, 1945

295. **Glew RH, Peters SP (eds):** Practical Enzymology of the Sphingolipidoses. New York, Alan R Liss, 1977

296. **Glick NR, Snodgrass PJ, Schafer IA:** Neonatal argininosuccinic aciduria with normal brain and kidney but absent liver argininosuccinate lysase activity. Am J Hum Genet 28:22, 1976

297. **Goka TJ, Stevenson RE, Hefferan PM et al:** Menkes disease: a biochemical abnormality in cultured human fibroblasts. Proc Natl Acad Sci USA 73:604, 1976

298. **Goldberg RN, Cagal LA, Sinatra FR et al:** Hyperammonemia associated with perinatal asphyxia. Pediatr 64:336, 1979

299. **Goldfischer S, Sternlieb I:** Changes in the distribution of hepatic copper in relation to the progression of Wilson's disease (hepatolenticular degeneration). Am J Pathol 53:883, 1968

300. **Goldsmith LA, Reed J:** Tyrosine-induced eye and skin lesions. JAMA 236:382, 1976

301. **Goldstein JL, Campbell BK, Gartler SM:** Homocystinuria: heterozygote detection using phytohemagglutinin-stimulated lymphocytes. J Clin Invest 52:28, 1973

302. **Gompertz D, Bartlett K, Blair D et al:** Child with a defect in leucine metabolism associated with beta-hydroxyisovaleric aciduria and beta-methylcrotonylglycinuria. Arch Dis Child 48:975, 1973

303. **Gompertz D, Bau DCK, Storrs CN et al:** Localization of enzyme defect in propionicacidemia. Lancet I:1140, 1970

304. **Gompertz D, Draffan GH, Watts JL et al:** Biotin-responsive beta-methylcrotonylglycinuria. Lancet 11:22, 1971

305. **Gompertz D, Saudubray J-M, Charpentier C et al:** A defect in isoleucine metabolism associated with alpha-methyl-beta-hydroxybutyric and alpha-methyl-acetoacetic aciduria: quantitative in vivo and in vitro studies. Clin Chim Acta 57:269, 1974

306. **Goodman SI:** An introduction to gas chromatography—mass spectrometry and the inherited organic acidemias. Am J Hum Genet 32:781, 1980

307. **Goodman SI, Mace JW, Pollak S:** Serum gamma-glutamyl transpeptidase deficiency. Lancet 1:234, 1971

308. **Goodman SI, Mace JW, Turner B et al:** Antenatal diagnosis of argininosuccinic aciduria. Clin Genet 4:236, 1973

309. **Goodman SI, Markey SP, Moe PG et al:** Glutaric aciduria; a "new" disorder of amino acid metabolism. Biochem Med 12:12, 1975

310. **Goodman SI, McCabe ERB, Fennesey PL et al:** Multiple acyl-CoA dehydrogenase deficiency (Glutaric aciduria type II) Pediatr Res 13:419, 1979

311. **Goodman SI, Moi PG, Hammond KB et al:** Homocystinuria with methylmalonic aciduria: two cases in a sibship. Biochem Med 4:500, 1970

312. **Goodman SI, Norenberg MD, Shikes RH et al:** Glutaric aciduria: biochemical and morphologic considerations. J Pediatr 90:746, 1977

313. **Goswami MND, Knox WE:** An evaluation of the role of ascorbic acid in regulation of tyrosine metabolism. J Chron Dis 16:363, 1963

314. **Gouras P, Carr RE, Gunkel RD:** Retinitis pigmentosa in abetalipoproteinemia: effects of vitamin A. Invest Ophthalmol 19:784, 1971

315. **Graham GE, Cordano A:** Copper depletion and deficiency in the malnourished infant. Johns Hopkins Med J 124:139, 1969

316. **Gravel RA, Lam K-F, Scully KJ et al:** Genetic complementation of propionyl-CoA carboxylase deficiency in cultured fibroblasts. Am J Hum Genet 29:378, 1977

317. **Gravel RA, Mahoney MJ, Ruddle FH et al:** Genetic complementation in heterokaryons of human fibroblasts defective in cobalamin metabolism. Proc Natl Acad Sci USA 72:3181, 1975

318. **Greenwood RS, DeVivo DC, Nelson JS et al:** An autosomal dominant form of necrotizing encephalomyelopathy resembling a spinocerebellar degeneration. Trans Am Neurol Assoc 100:47, 1975

319. **Greenwood RS, Nelson JS:** Atypical neuronal ceroid lipofuscinosis. Neurology 28:710, 1978

320. **Groebe H, Krins M, Schmidberger H et al:** Morquio Syndrome (mucopolysaccharidosis IV B) associated with beta-galactosidase deficiency. Report of two cases. Am J Hum Genet 32:258, 1980

321. **Groen JJ:** Gaucher's disease: Hereditary transmission and racial distribution. Arch Intern Med 113:543, 1964

322. **Grossman H, Dorst JP:** The mucopolysacchari-

doses and mucolipidoses. Prog Pediatr Radiol 4:495, 1973

323. **Grover W, Auerback V, Patel M:** Biochemical studies and therapy in subacute necrotizing encephalomyelopathy. J Pediatr 81:39, 1972

324. **Grover WD, Scrutton MC:** Copper infusion therapy in trichopoliostrophy. J Pediatr 86:216, 1975

325. **Grover WD, Tucker SH, Wenger DA:** Clinical variation in 2 related children with neuronopathic Gaucher disease. Ann Neurol 3:281, 1978

326. **Grunnet ML, Spilsbury PR:** The central nervous system in Fabry's disease. An ultrastructural study. Arch Neurol 2:231, 1973

327. **Gruscay JA, Rosenberg LE:** Inhibition of hepatic mitochondrial carbamyl phosphate synthetase (CPS I) by acyl CoA esters: possible mechanism of hyperammonemia in the organic acidemias. Pediatr Res 13:475, 1979

328. **Guggenheim MA, Stumpf DA:** Familial metabolic disease with clinicopathological findings of both Leigh's disease and adult type spinocerebellar degeneration. Ann Neurol 2:264, 1977

329. **Guibaud P, Maire I, Goddon R et al:** Mucopolysaccharidose type VII par deficit en beta-glucoronidase. Etude d'une famille. J Genet Hum 27:29, 1979

330. **Gustavson KH, Hagberg B:** The incidence and genetics of metachromatic leucodystrophy in northern Sweden. Acta Pediatr Scand 60:585, 1971

331. **Guthrie R:** Blood screening for phenylketonuria. JAMA 178:863, 1961

332. **Guthrie R:** Screening for inborn errors of metabolism of newborn infants: a multiple test program. Birth defects: Original Article Series 4:92, 1968

333. **Haberland C, Brunngraber E, Witting L et al:** Juvenile metachromatic leukodystrophy: case report with clinical, histopathological, ultrastructural and biochemical observations. Acta Neuropathol 26:93, 1973

334. **Hagberg B:** The clinical diagnosis of Krabbe's infantile leucodystrophy. Acta Pediatr Scand 52:213, 1963

335. **Hagberg B:** Clinical symptoms, signs and tests on metachromatic leucodystrophy. In Folch-Pi J, Bauer H (eds): Brain Lipids and Lipoproteins and the Leucodystrophies, pp 134–146. Amsterdam, Elsevier Publishing, 1963

336. **Hagberg B, Haltia M, Sourander P, et al:** Neurovisceral storage disorder simulation Niemann-Pick disease. A new form of oligosaccharidosis? Neuropaediatrie, 9:59, 1978

337. **Hagberg B, Kalberg H, Sourander P et al:** Infantile globoid cell leucodystrophy (Krabbe's disease): A clinical and genetic study of 32 Swedish cases 1953–1967. Neuropaediatrie, 1:74, 1970

338. **Hagberg B, Kyllerman M, Steen G:** Dyskinesia and dystonia in neuromuscular disorders. Neuropaediatrie 10:305, 1979

339. **Hagberg B, Sourander P, Svennerholm L:** Late infantile progressive encephalopathy with disturbed polyunsaturated fat metabolism. Acta Paediat Scand 57:495, 1968

340. **Hakami N, Neiman PE, Canellos GP et al:** Neonatal megaloblastic anemia due to inherited transcobalamin II deficiency in two siblings. N Engl J Med 285:1163, 1971

341. **Halperin ML, Schiller CM, Fritz IB:** The inhibition by methylmalonic acid of malate transport by the dicarboxylate carrier in rat liver mitochondria. A possible explanation for hypoglycemia in methylmalonic aciduria. J Clin Invest 50:276, 1971

342. **Haltia M, Rapola J, Haltia M et al:** Juvenile metachromatic leukodystrophy. Clinical, biochemical, and neuropathologic studies in nine new cases. Arch Neurol 37:42, 1980

343. **Haltia M, Rapola J, Santavuori P:** Infantile type so-called neuronal ceroid lipofuscinosis. Histological and electron microscopic studies. Acta Neuropathol 26:157, 1973

344. **Haltia M, Rapola J, Santavuori P et al:** Infantile type so-called neuronal ceroid-lipofuscinosis. Part 2. Morphological and biochemical studies. J Neurol Sci 18:269, 1973

345. **Halvorsen K, Halvorsen S:** Hartnup disease. Pediatr 31:29, 1963

346. **Halvorsen S, Pande H, Christie-Loken A et al:** Tyrosinosis. Arch Dis Child 41:238, 1966

347. **Hambert O, Peterson I:** Clinical, electroencephalographical and neuropharmacological studies in syndromes of progressive myoclonus epilepsy. Acta Neurol Scand 46:149, 1970

348. **Harden A, Pampiglione G, Picton-Robinson N:** Electroretinogram and visual evoked response in a form of 'neuronal lipidosis' with diagnostic EEG features. J Neurol Neurosurg Psychiatry 36:61, 1973

349. **Harpey J-P, Rosenblatt DS, Cooper BA et al:** Homocystinuria caused by 5,10-methylenetetrahydrofolate reductase deficiency: a case in an infant responding to methionine, folinic acid, pyridoxine, and vitamin B_{12} therapy. J Pediatr 98:275, 1981

350. **Harries JT, Seakins GWT, Ersser RS et al:** Recovery after dietary treatment of an infant with features of tyrosinosis. Arch Dis Child 44:258, 1969

351. **Harris DJ, Yang BI, Wolf B et al:** Dysautonomia in an infant with secondary hyperammonemia due to propionyl coenzyme A carboxylase deficiency. Pediatr 65:107, 1980

352. **Harris RC:** Negative urine sugars in galactosemia. Pediatr 53:768, 1974

353. **Harris-Jones JN, Swan HT, Tudhope GR:** Pernicious anemia without gastric atrophy and in the presence of free hydrochloric acid: report of a case. Blood 12:461, 1957

354. **Hart ZH, Chang C, Perrin EVD et al:** Familial poliodystrophy, mitochondrial myopathy and lactic acidemia. Arch Neurol 34:180, 1977

355. **Hartlage PL, Coryell ME, Hall WK et al:** Argininosuccinic aciduria: perinatal diagnosis and early dietary management. J Pediatr 85:86, 1974

356. **Harzer K, Schlote W, Peiffer J et al:** Neurovisceral lipidosis compatible with Niemann-Pick disease Type C: morphological and biochemical studies of a late infantile case and enzyme and

lipid assays in a prenatal case of the same family. Acta Neuropathol (Berl), 43:97, 1978

357. **Hasilik A, Neufeld EF:** Biosynthesis of lysosomal enzymes in fibroblasts. J Biol Chem 255:4937, 1980

358. **Haymond MW, Karl IE, Feigin RD et al:** Hypoglycemia and maple syrup urine disease-defective gluconeogenesis. Pediatr Res 7:500, 1973

359. **Heller M, Shapiro B:** Enzymatic hydrolysis of sphingomyelin by rat liver. Biochem J 98:76, 1966

360. **Hickman S, Neufeld EF:** A hypothesis for I-cell disease: defective hydrolases that do not enter lysosomes. Biochem Biophys Res Commun 49:992, 1972

361. **Higashimo K, Tsukada K, Lieberman I:** Saccharopine, a product of lysine breakdown by mammalian liver. Biochem Biophys Res Commun 20:285, 1965

362. **Hillman RE, Keating JP:** Beta-ketothiolase deficiency as a cause of the "ketotic hyperglycinemia syndrome." Pediatr 53:221, 1974

363. **Hirano A, Lena JF, French JH et al:** Fine structure of the cerebellar cortex in Menkes kinky-hair disease. Arch Neurol 34:52, 1977

364. **Ho MW, Norden AGW, Alhadeff JA et al:** Glycophingolipid hydrolases: properties and molecular genetics. Mol Cell Biochem 17:125, 1977

365. **Ho MW, Seck J, Schmidt D et al:** Adult Gaucher's disease: kindred studies and demonstration of a deficiency of acid beta-glucosidase in cultured fibroblasts. Am J Hum Genet, 24:37, 1972

366. **Hogan GR, Gutmann L, Chou SM:** The peripheral neuropathy of Krabbe's (globoid) leukodystrophy. Neurology 19:1093, 1969

367. **Holtzman NA:** Menkes' kinky hair syndrome: a genetic disease involving copper. Fed Proc 35:2276, 1976

368. **Holtzman NA:** Newborn screening for inborn errors of metabolism. Pediatr Clin N Amer 25:411, 1978

369. **Holtzman NA, Naughton MA, Iber FL et al:** Ceruloplasmin in Wilson's disease. J Clin Invest 46:993, 1967

370. **Holtzman NA, Welcher DW, Mellits ED:** Termination of restricted diet in children with phenylketonuria: a randomized controlled study. N Engl J Med 293:1121, 1975

371. **Hommes FA, DeGroot CJ, Wilmink CW et al:** Carbamyl phosphate synthetase deficiency in an infant with severe cerebral damage. Arch Dis Child 44:688, 1969

372. **Hommes FA, Kuipers JRG, Elema GD et al:** Propionicacidemia, a new inborn error of metabolism. Pediatr Res 2:519, 1968

373. **Hommes FA, Polman HA, Reerink JD:** Leigh's encephalomyelopathy: an inborn error of gluconeogenesis. Arch Dis Child 43:423, 1968

374. **Hopkins I, Townley RRW, Shipman RT:** Cerebral thrombosis in a patient with homocystinuria. J Pediatr 75:1082, 1969

375. **Hopwood JJ, Muller V:** Biochemical discrimination of Hurler and Scheie syndrome. Clin Sci 57:265, 1979

376. **Horwitz AL, Hancock L, Dawson G et al:** Generalized sialic acid storage disease (abstr). Pediatr Res 15:563, 1981

377. **Hsia YE, Scully K, Lilljeqvist A-C et al:** Vitamin B_{12} dependent methylmalonic aciduria. Pediatr 46:497, 1970

378. **Hsia YE, Scully KJ, Rosenberg LE:** Defective propionate carboxylation in ketotic hyperglycinaemia. Lancet 1:757, 1969

379. **Hsia YE, Scully KJ, Rosenberg LE:** Inherited propionyl-CoA carboxylase deficiency in "ketotic hyperglycinemia." J Clin Invest 50:127, 1971

380. **Hsia YE, Walker FA:** Variability in the clinical manifestations of galactosemia. J Pediatr 59:872, 1961

381. **Hug G, Lansky L, Bove K et al:** Human hepatocytes in acquired vs inheritable defects of urea cycle enzymes. J Cell Biol 70:157A, 1976

382. **Humbel R, Marchal C:** Screening test for aspartylglycosaminuria. J Pediatr 84:456, 1974

383. **Huttenlocher PR, Hillman RE, Hsia YE:** Pseudotumor cerebri in galactosemia. J Pediatr 76:902, 1970

384. **Iber SL, Rosen H, Levenson SM et al:** Plasma amino acids in patients with liver failure. J Lab Clin Med 50:417, 1957

385. **Igarashi M, Schaumburg HH, Powers J et al:** Fatty acid abnormality in adrenoleukodystrophy. J Neurochem 26:851, 1976

386. **Illingworth Dr, Connor WE, Miller RG:** Abetalipoproteinemia. Report of two cases and review of therapy. Arch Neurol 37:659, 1980

387. **Isenberg JN, Sharp HL:** Aspartylglucosaminuria: psychomotor retardation masquerading as a mucopolysaccharidosis. J Pediatr 86:713, 1975

388. **Isselbacher KJ:** Galactose metabolism and galactosemia. Am J Med 26:715, 1959

389. **Jackson LG, Schimke RN:** Clinical Genetics. New York, John Wiley & Sons, 1979

390. **Janken J, Corbeel L, Casaer P et al:** Dipropylacetate (valproate) and glycine metabolism. Lancet 2:617, 1977

391. **Jensen OA, Pedersen C, Schwartz M et al:** Hurler-Scheie phenotype-report of an inbred sibship with tapeto-retinal degeneration and electromicroscopic examination of the conjunctiva. Ophthalmologica, Basel 176:194, 1978

392. **Jensen OA, Pederson C, Vestermark S et al:** The Hurler-Scheie phenotype in children from a consanguineous marriage: case report with electronmicroscopy of the conjunctiva and ERG. Metab Pediatr Ophthalmol 4:133, 1980

393. **Jepson JB:** Hartnup disease. In Stanbury JB, Wyngaarden JB, Fredrickson DF (eds): The Metabolic Basis of Inherited Disease, 4th ed, pp 1563–1577. New York, McGraw-Hill, 1978

394. **Jepson JB, Smith AJ, Strang LB:** An inborn error of metabolism with urinary excretion of hydroxyacids, ketoacids, and aminoacids. Lancet 2:1334, 1958

395. **Jervis GA:** Phenylpyruvic oligophrenia: deficiency of phenylalanine oxidizing system. Proc Soc Exp Med 82:514, 1953

396. **Johnson JD:** Unconjugated hyperbilirubinemia in galactosemia. N Engl J Med 292:924, 1975

397. **Johnson JL, Wand WR, Rajagopalan KV et al:** Inborn errors of molybdenum metabolism: combined deficiencies of sulfite oxidase and xanthine dehydrogenase in a patient lacking the molybdenum cofactor. Proc Natl Acad Sci USA 77:3715, 1980

398. **Johnson WG, Chutorian A, Maranda A:** A new juvenile hexoaminidase deficiency disease presenting as cerebellar ataxia. Neurology 27:1012, 1977

399. **Johnston AW, Weller SD, Warland BJ:** Angiokeratoma corporis diffusum: some clinical aspects. Arch Dis Child 43:73, 1968

400. **Kaback MM, Nathan RJ, Greenwald S:** Tay-Sachs disease: heterozygote screening and prenatal diagnosis—US experience and world perspective. In Kaback MM, Rimoin DL, O'Brien JS, (eds): Tay-Sachs Disease: Screening and Prevention, pp 13–36. New York, Alan R Liss, 1977

401. **Kaback MM, Rimoin DL, O'Brien JS (eds):** Tay-Sachs Disease: Screening and Prevention. New York, Alan R Liss, 977

402. **Kagi JHR, Valle BL:** Metallothionein: a cadmium and zinc-containing protein from equine renal cortex, II. Physiochemical properties. J Biol Chem 236:2435, 1961

403. **Kaibara, N, Eguchi M, Shibata K et al:** Hurler-Scheie phenotype: a report of two pairs of inbred sibs. Hum Genet 53:37, 1979

404. **Kajii T, Matsuda I, Ohsawa T et al:** Hurler/Scheie genetic compound (mucopolysaccharidosis IH/IS) in Japanese brothers. Clin Genet 6:394, 1974

405. **Kamoshita S, Aron AM, Suzuki K et al:** Infantile Niemann-Pick disease: a chemical study with isolation and characterization of membranous cytoplasmic bodies and myelin. Am J Dis Child 117:379, 1969

406. **Kampine JP, Brady RO, Kanfer JN et al:** Diagnosis of Gaucher's disease and Niemann-Pick disease with small samples of venous blood. Science 155:86, 1967

407. **Kang ES, Kaufman S, Gerald PS:** Clinical and biochemical observations of patients with atypical phenylketonuria. Pediatr 45:83, 1970

408. **Kang ES, Paine RS:** Elevation of plasma phenylalanine during pregnancies of women heterozygous for phenylketonuria. J Pediatr 63:283, 1963

409. **Kang ES, Snodgrass PJ, Gerald PS:** Methylmalonyl coenzyme A racemase defect: another cause of methylamalonic aciduria. Pediatr Res 6:875, 1972

410. **Yanwar YS, Manaligod JR, Wong PWK:** Morphologic studies in a patient with homocystinuria due to 5, 10 methylenetetrahydrofolate reductase deficiency. Pediatr Res 10:598, 1976

411. **Kark RAP, Rodriquez-Budelli M, Blass JP:** Evidence for a primary defect of lipoamide dehydrogenase in Friedreich's ataxia. In Kark RAP, Rosenberg RN, Schut LJ (eds): The Inherited Ataxias: Biochemical, Viral and Pathological Studies, Adv Neurol, 21:163, New York, Raven Press, 1978

412. **Karpati G, Carpenter S, Eisan AA et al:** Multiple peripheral nerve entrapments: an unusual phenotypic variant of the Hunter syndrome (mucopolysaccharidosis II) in a family. Arch Neurol 31:418, 1974

413. **Karpati G, Carpenter S, Engel AG et al:** The syndrome of systemic carnitine deficiency: clinical, morphologic, biochemical, and pathophysiologic features. Neurology (Minneap) 25:16, 1975

414. **Karpati G, Carpenter S, Wolfe LS:** Juvenile dystonic lipidosis: an unusual form of neurovisceral storage disease. Neurology 27:32, 1977

415. **Karpel JT, Peden VH:** Copper deficiency in long term parenteral nutrition. J Pediatr 80:32, 1972

416. **Kashiwamata S, Greenberg DM:** Studies on cystathionine synthase of rat liver. Properties of the highly purified enzyme. Biochem Biophys Acta 212:488, 1970

417. **Kattlove ME, Williams JC, Graynor E et al:** Gaucher cells in chronic myelocytic leukemia: an acquired abnormality. Blood 33:379, 1969

418. **Kaufman JM, Greene ML, Seegmiller JE:** Urine uric acid to creatinine ratio—a screening test for inherited disorders of purine metabolism. J Pediatr 73:583, 1968

419. **Kaufman S:** Phenylalanine hydroxylation cofactor in phenylketonuria. Science 128:1506, 1958

420. **Kaufman S:** Differential diagnosis of variant forms of hyperphenylalaninemia. Pediatr 65:840, 1980

421. **Kaufman S:** Unanswered questions in the primary metabolic block in phenylketonuria. In Anderson JA, Swaiman KF (eds): Proceedings of the Conference on the Treatment of Phenylketonuria and Allied Diseases. DHEW [HEW68-2], pp 205–213. Washington, DC, Government Printing Office, 1967

422. **Kaufman S, Berlow S, Summer GK et al:** Hyperphenylalaninemia due to a deficiency of biopterin: a variant form of phenylketonuria. N Engl J Med 299:673, 1978

423. **Kaufman S, Holtzman NA, Milstein S, et al:** Phenylketonuria due to a deficiency of dihydropteridine reductase. N Engl J Med 293:785, 1975

424. **Kayser B:** Uber einen Fall von ageboerener grunlicher Verfarbung der Kornea. Dtsch Monatsbl Augenheilkd 40:22, 1902

425. **Keating JP, Feigin RD, Tennenbaum SM et al:** Hyperglycinemia with ketosis due to a defect in isoleucine metabolism: a preliminary report. Pediatr 50:890, 1972

426. **Kekomaki M, Visakorpi JK, Perahentupa J:** Familial protein intolerance with deficient transport of basic amino acids. An analysis of 10 patients. Acta Paediatr Scand 56:617, 1967

427. **Kelley WN, Wyngaarden JB:** The Lesch-Nyhan syndrome. In Stanbury JB, Wyngaarden JB, Fredrickson DS (eds): The Metabolic Basis of Inherited Disease, 4th ed, pp 1011–1036. New York, McGraw-Hill, 1978

428. **Kelly TE:** Clinical Genetics and Genetic Counseling. Chicago, Year Book Medical Publishers 1980

429. **Kelly TE, Graetz G:** Isolated acid neuraminidase

deficiency: a distinct lysosomal storage disease. Am J Med Genet 1:31, 1977

430. **Kelly TE, Thomas GH, Taylor HA et al:** Mucolipidosis III (Pseudo-Hurler polydystrophy). Clinical and laboratory studies in a series of 12 patients. Johns Hopkins Med J 137:156, 1975

431. **Kennaway NG, Buist NRM:** Metabolic studies in a patient with hepatic cytosol tyrosine aminotransferase deficiency. Pediatr Res 5:287, 1971

432. **Kidd JR, Wolf B, Hsia YE et al:** Genetics of propionic acidemia in a Mennonite-Amish kindred. Am J Hum Genet 32:236, 1980

433. **Kihara H, Porter MT, Fluharty AL et al:** Metachromatic leukodystrophy: ambiguity of heterozygote identification. Am J Ment Defic 77:389, 1973

434. **Kim YJ, Rosenberg LE:** On the mechanism of pyridoxine-responsive homocystinuria. Part II. Properties of normal and mutant cystathionine beta-synthase from cultured fibroblasts. Proc Natl Acad Sci USA 71:4821, 1974

435. **Kinoshita JH, Merola LU:** Hydration of the lens during the development of galactose cataract. Invest Ophthalmol 3:577, 1964

436. **Kint JA:** Fabry's disease, alpha-galactosidase deficiency. Science 167:1968, 1970

437. **Kint JAG, Dacremont G, Carton D et al:** Mucopolysaccharidosis: secondarily induced abnormal distribution of lysosomal isoenzymes. Science 181:352, 1973

438. **Kirkman HN, Lanier DC, Clemons EH et al:** Estimation of galactose-1-phosphate in blood spotted on filter paper. J Lab Clin Med 88:515, 1976

439. **Kjellman B, Ganstorp I, Brun A et al:** Mannosidosis: a clinical and histopathologic study. J Pediatr 75:366, 1969

440. **Klein U, Kresse H, von Figura K:** Sanfilippo syndrome type C: deficiency of acetyl-CoA: alpha-glucosaminide N-acetyl transferase in skin fibroblasts. Proc Natl Acad Sci USA 75:5185, 1978

441. **Klenk E:** Uber die Natur der Phosphatide der Milz bei der Nieman-Pickschen Krankheit. Z Physiol Chem 229:151, 1934

442. **Klenk E, Kahlke W:** Uber das Vorkommen der 3, 7, 11, 15-Tetra-methylehexadecansaure (Phytansaure) in den Cholesterinestern und anderen Lipoidfraktionen der Organe bei einem Krankheitsfall unbekannter Genese Verdacht auf Heredopathia atactica polyneuritiformis (Refsum's syndrome). Hoppe Seyler's Z Physiol Chem 333:133, 1963

443. **Knox WE:** Phenylketonuria. In Stanbury JB, Wyngaarden JB, Fredrickson DS (eds): The Metabolic Basis of Inherited Disease, pp 266–295. New York, McGraw-Hill, 1972

444. **Koch R, Blaskovics M, Wenz E et al:** Phenylalaninemia and phenylketonuria. In Nyhan WL (ed): Heritable Disorders of Amino Acid Metabolism, pp 109–140. New York, John Wiley & Sons 1974

445. **Koch R, Shaw KN, Acosta PB et al:** An approach to the management of phenylketonuria. J Pediatr 76:815, 1970

446. **Koff E, Kannerer B, Boyle P et al:** Intelligence and phenylketonuria: effects of diet termination. J Pediatr 94:534, 1979

447. **Kolvraa S:** Inhibition of the glycine cleavage system by branched-chain amino acid metabolites. Pediatr Res 13:889, 1979

448. **Komrower GM:** The philosophy and practice of screening for inherited diseases. Pediatr 53:182, 1974

449. **Komrower GM, Lambert AM, Cusworth BC et al:** Dietary treatment of homocystinuria. Arch Dis Childhood 41:666, 1966

450. **Komrower GM, Wilson VK:** Homocystinuria. Proc R Soc Med 56:996, 1961

451. **Kornzweig AL, Bassen FA:** Retinitis pigmentosa, acanthocytosis, and heredodegenerative neuromuscular disease. Arch Ophthalmol 58:183, 1957

452. **Koto A, Horwitz AL, Suzuki K et al:** The Morquio syndrome: neuropathology and biochemistry. Ann Neurol 4:26, 1978

453. **Kousseff BG, Beratis NG, Strauss L et al:** Fucosidosis type 2. Pediatr 57:205, 1976

454. **Krabbe K:** A new familial, infantile form of diffuse brain sclerosis. Brain 39:74, 1916

455. **Kresse H, Paschke E, von Figura K et al:** Sanfilippo disease type D: deficiency of N-acetylglucosamine-6-sulfate sulfatase required for heparan sulfate degradation. Proc Natl Acad Sci USA 77:6822, 1980

456. **Krieger I, Snodgrass PJ, Roskump J:** Atypical clinical course of ornithine transcarbamylase deficiency due to new mutant (comparison with Reye's disease). J Clin Endocrinol Metab 48:388, 1979

457. **Krieger I, Tanaka T:** Therapeutic effect of glycine in isovaleric acidemia. Pediatr Res 10:25, 1976

458. **Krovetz LJ, Schiebler GL:** Cardiovascular manifestations of the genetic mucopolysaccharidoses. In Bergsma D (ed): The Cardiovascular System Birth Defects—Original Article Series, Vol 8, No 5, pp 192–196. Baltimore, Williams & Wilkins, 1972

459. **Kuroda Y, Kline JJ, Sweetman L et al:** Abnormal pyruvate and alpha-ketoglutarate dehydrogenase complexes in a patient with lactic acidemia. Pediatr Res 13:928, 1979

460. **Kyllerman M, Stein G:** Intermittently progressive dyskinetic syndrome in glutaric aciduria. Neuropaediatrie 8:397, 1977

461. **Kyriakides EC, Paul B, Balint JA:** Lipid accumulation and acid lipase deficiency in fibroblasts from a family with Wolman's disease, and their apparent correction in vitro. J Lab Clin Med 80:810, 1972

462. **LaBrecque DR, Latham PS, Reily CA et al:** Heritable urea cycle enzyme deficiency-liver disease in 16 patients. J Pediatr 94:580, 1979

463. **La Du BN:** Histidinemia. In Stanbury JB, Wyngaarden BJ, Fredrickson DS (eds): The Metabolic Basis of Inherited Disease, 4th ed, pp 317–327. New York, McGraw-Hill, 1978

464. **La Du BN, Howell RR, Jacoby GA et al:** The enzymatic defect in histidinemia. Biochem Biophys Res Commun 7:398, 1962

465. **Lalley PA, Rattazzi MC, Shows TB:** Human beta-D-acetylhexosaminidases A and B: expression and linkage relationships in somatic cell hybrids. Proc Nat Acad Sci USA 71:569, 1975

466. **Lamon JM, Trojak JE, Abbott MH:** Bone cysts in mucopolysaccharidosis I S. (Scheie syndrome). Johns Hopkins Med J 146(2):73, 1980

467. **Lampkin BC, Schubert WK:** Pernicious anemia in the second decade of life. J Pediatr 72:387, 1968

468. **Lane AB, Jenkins T:** Two variant hexosaminidase beta-chain alleles segregating in a South African family. Clin Chim Acta 87:219, 1978

469. **Langer LO, Carely LS:** The roentgenographic features of the KS mucopolysaccharidosis of Morquio (Morquio-Brailsford's disease). Am J Roentgenol Rad Ther Nucl Med 97:1, 1966

470. **Lanzkowsky P:** Congenital malabsorption of folate. Am J Med 48:580, 1970

471. **Lapiere CHM, Nusgens B:** Plaies cutanees torpides et trouble du metabolisme bucollage no. Arch Belg Dermatol Syph 25:353, 1969

472. **Lawrie NR, Carter RA:** Acute case of Wilson's disease (hepatolenticular degeneration). Lancet 1:1309, 1958

473. **Legum CP, Schorr S, Berman ER:** The genetic mucopolysaccharidoses and mucolipidoses: review and comment. Adv Pediatr 22:305, 1976

474. **Leigh D:** Subacute necrotizing encephalomyelopathy in an infant. J Neurol Neurosurg Psychiatry 14:216, 1951

475. **Leisti J, Rimoin DL, Kaback M et al:** Allelic mutations in the mucopolysaccharidoses. Birth Defects—Original Article Series, 12, No 6:81, 1976

476. **Lenke RR, Levy HL:** Maternal phenylketonuria and hyperphenylalaninemia: an international survey of the outcome of untreated and treated pregnancies. N Engl J Med 303:12102, 1980

477. **Leroy JG, Crocker AC:** Clinical definition of the Hurler-Hunter phenotypes. Am J Dis Child 112:518, 1966

478. **Leroy JG, Spranger JW, Feingold M et al:** I-cell disease. A clinical picture. J Pediatr 79:360, 1971

479. **Lesch M, Nyhan WL:** A familial disorder of uric acid metabolism and central nervous system function. Am J Med 36:561, 1964

480. **Levi AJ, Sherlock S, Scheuer PJ et al:** Presymptomatic Wilson's disease. Lancet 2:575, 1967

481. **Levy HL:** Genetic Screening. In Harris H, Hirschhorn K, (eds): Advances in Human Genetics, Vol 4, pp 1–104. New York, Plenum Press, 1973

482. **Levy HL:** Newborn screening for metabolic disorders. N Engl J Med 288:1299, 1973

483. **Levy HL, Erickson AM, Lott IT et al:** Isovaleric acidemia: results of family study and dietary treatment. Pediatr 52:83, 1973

484. **Levy HL, Karolkewicz V, Houghton SA et al:** Screening the 'normal' population in Massachusetts for phenylketonuria. New Engl J Med 282:1455, 1970

485. **Levy HL, Madigan PM, Shih VE:** Massachusetts metabolic disorders screening program. Part I. Technics and results of urine screening. Pediatr 49:825, 1972

486. **Levy HL, Mudd SH, Schulman JD et al:** The derangement of B_{12} metabolism associated with homocystinemia, cystathioninemia, hypomethioninemia, and methylmalonic aciduria. Am J Med 48:390, 1970

487. **Levy HL, Shih VE, Madigan PM:** Routine newborn screening for histidinemia. Clinical biochemical results. New Engl J Med 291:1214, 1974

488. **Levy HL, Shih VE, Madigan PM et al:** Transient tyrosinemia in full-term infants. JAMA 209:249, 1969

489. **Lhermitte F:** Les Leuco-encephalites. Paris, Flammarion, 1950

490. **Li S-C, Wan CC, Mazzotta MY et al:** Requirement of an activator for the hydrolysis of sphingoglycolipids by glycosidases of human liver. Carbohydr Res 34:189, 1974

491. **Li Y-T, Mazzotta MY, Wan C-C et al:** Hydrolysis of Tay-Sachs ganglioside by beta-hexosaminidase A of human liver and urine. J Biol Chem 248:7512, 1973

492. **Lieberman E, Shaw KND, Donall GN:** Cystathioninuria and galactosemia in certain types of liver disease. Pediatr 40:828, 1967

493. **Linblad B, Linstadt S, Steen G:** On the enzymatic defects in hereditary tyrosinaemia. Proc Natl Acad Sci USA 74:4641, 1977

494. **Linnell JL, Mathews DM, Mudd SH et al:** Cobalamin in fibroblasts cultured from normal control subjects and patients with methylmalonic aciduria. Pediatr Res 10:179, 1976

495. **Lockman LA, Hunninghake DB, Krivit W et al:** Relief of the pain of Fabry's disease by diphenylhydantoin. Neurol 23:871, 1973

496. **Loeb H, Tondeur M, Jonniaux G et al:** Biochemical and ultrastructural studies in a case of mucopolysaccharidosis "F" (Fucosidosis). Helv Paediat Acta 24:519, 1969

497. **Lonsdale D, Faulkner WR, Price JW et al:** Intermittent cerebellar ataxia associated with hyperpyruvic acidemia, hyperalaninemia, and hyperalaninuria. Pediatr 43:1025, 1969

498. **Lott IT, DiPaolo R, Schwartz D et al:** Copper metabolism in the steely-hair syndrome. N Engl J Med 292:197, 1975

499. **Lowden JA:** Evidence for a hybrid hexosaminidase isoenzyme in heterozygotes for Sandhoff disease. Am J Hum Genet 31:281, 1979

500. **Lowden JA, O'Brien JS:** Sialidosis: a review of human neuraminidase deficiency. Am J Hum Genet 31:1, 1979

501. **Lowe CU, Terry M, MacLachlan EA:** Organic-aciduria, decreased renal ammonia production, hydroophthalmos, and mental retardation: a clinical entity. Am J Dis Child 83:164, 1952

502. **Lowry RB, Renwick HG:** Relative frequency of the Hurler and Hunter syndromes. N Engl J Med 284:221, 1971

503. **Luhby AL, Eagle FJ, Roth E et al:** Relapsing megaloblastic anemia in an infant due to a specific defect in gastrointestinal absorption of folic acid. Am J Dis Child 102:482, 1961

504. **Lundberg A, Lilja LG, Lundberg PO et al:** Heredopathia atactica polyneuritiformis (Refsum's

disease): experience of dietary treatment and plasmaphoresis. Eur Neurol 8:309, 1972

505. **Lyon ICT, Gardner RJM, Veale AMO:** Maternal histidinemia. Arch Dis Child 49:581, 1974

506. **Maag VR, Gold RJM:** A simple combinatorial method for calculating genetic risks. Clin Genet 7:361, 1975

507. **Mabry CC, Denniston JC, Coldwell JG:** Marked retardation in children of phenylketonuric mothers. N Engl J Med 275:1331, 1966

508. **MacDermot KD, Nelson W, Reichert CM, et al:** Attempts at use of strychnine sulfate in the treatment of nonketotic hyperglycinemia. Pediatr 65:61, 1980

509. **MacDonald JT, Sher PK:** Ophthalmoplegia as a sign of metabolic disease in the newborn. Neurology 27:971, 1977

510. **MacKenzie DY, Wolff LI:** Maple syrup urine disease: An inborn error of metabolism of valine leucine, and isoleucine associated with gross mental deficiency. Br Med J 1:90, 1959

511. **Maesaka H, Komiya K, Misugi K, et al:** Hyperalaninemia, hyperpyruvicemia, and lactic acidosis due to pyruvate carboxylase deficiency of the liver: Treatment with thiamine and lipoic acid. Eur J Pediatr 122:159, 1976

512. **Mahoney MJ, Hart AC, Steen VD, et al:** Methylmalonic acidemia: biochemical heterogeneity in defects of 5-deoxyadenosylcobalamin synthesis. Proc Natl Acad Sci USA 72:2799, 1975

513. **Mahoney MJ, Rosenberg LE, Lindblad D, et al:** Prenatal diagnosis of methylmalonic aciduria. Acta Paediatr Scand 64:44, 1975

514. **Mapes CA, Anderson RL, Sweeley CC et al:** Enzyme replacement in Fabry's disease, an inborn error of metabolism. Science 169:987, 1970

515. **Marceau N, Aspin N:** The intracellular distribution of the radiocopper derived from ceruloplasmin and from albumin. Biochim Biophys Acta, 329:33, 1973

516. **Marceau N, Aspin N:** The association of the copper derived from ceruloplasmin with cytocuprein. Biochim Biophys Acta 329:351, 1973

517. **Markesberry WR:** Lactic acidemia, mitochondrial myopathy and basal ganglia calcification. Neurology 29:1057, 1979

518. **Markesberry WR, Shield LK, Egel RT et al:** Late-infantile neuronal ceroid-lipofuscinosis. An ultrastructural study of lymphocyte inclusions. Arch Neurol 33:630, 1976

519. **Maroteaux P, Humbel R, Strecker et al:** A new type of sialidosis with renal impairment: nephrosialidosis. Arch Fr Pediatr 35:819, 1978

520. **Mason HH, Turner ME:** Chronic galactosemia. Am J Dis Child 50:359, 1935

521. **Massachusetts Department of Public Health:** Cost-benefit analysis of newborn screening for metabolic disorders. N Engl J Med 291:1414, 1974

522. **Matalon R, Arbogast B, Justice P et al:** Morquio's syndrome. Deficiency of a chondroitin sulfate N-acetylhexosamine sulfate sulfatase. Biochem Biophys Res Comm 61:709, 1974

523. **Matalon R, Horowitz A, Wappner R et al:** Kera-

tan and heparan sulfaturia—a new mucopolysaccharidosis with N-acetylglucosamine 6-sulfatase deficiency (abstr). Pediatr Res 12:453, 1978

524. **Matsuda I, Pearson T, Holtzman NA:** Determination of apoceruloplasmin by radioimmunoassay in nutritional copper deficiency. Menkes' kinky hair syndrome, Wilson's disease, and umbilical cord blood. Pediatr Res 8:821, 1974

525. **Matthews J, Partington MW:** The plasma tyrosine levels of premature babies. Arch Dis Child 39:371, 1964

526. **Maury CPJ, Palo J:** N-acetylglucosamine-asparagine levels in tissues of patients with aspartylglycosaminuria. Clin Chim Acta 108:293, 1980

527. **Max SR, Maclaren NK, Brady RO et al:** G_{M3} (hematoside) sphingolipodystrophy. N Engl J Med 291:929, 1974

528. **Mayes JS, Guthrie R:** Detection of heterozygotes for galactokinase deficiency in a human population. Biochem Genet 2:219, 1968

529. **McCord JM, Fridovich I:** Superoxide dismutase; an enzymic function for erythrocuprein (hemocuprein). J. Biol Chem 244:6049, 1969

530. **McIntyre OR, Sullivan LW, Jeffries GH et al:** Pernicious anemia in childhood. N Engl J Med 272:981, 1965

531. **McKusick VA:** Human Genetics, 2 ed. Englewood Cliffs, Prentice-Hall, 1969

532. **McKusick VA:** Heritable Disorders of Connective Tissue, 4th ed. St Louis, CV Mosby, 1972

533. **Mc Kusick VA:** Mendelian Inheritance in Man, 5th ed. Baltimore, Johns Hopkins University Press, 1978

534. **McKusick VA, Howell RR, Hussels IE et al:** Allelism, non-allelism and genetic compounds among the mucopolysaccharidoses: hypothesis. Lancet 1:993, 1972

535. **McKusick VA, Kaplan D, Wise D et al:** The genetic mucopolysaccharidoses. Medicine 44:445, 1965

536. **McKusick VA, Neufeld EF, Kelly TE:** The mucopolysaccharide storage diseases. In Stanbury JB, Wyngaarden JB, Fredrickson DS (eds): The Metabolic Basis of Inherited Disease. New York, McGraw-Hill, pp 1282–1307. 1978

537. **McReynolds JW, Montagos S. Brusilow S et al:** Treatment of complete ornithine transcarbamylase deficiency with nitrogen-free analogues of essential amino acids. J Pediatr 93:421, 1978

538. **Medes G, Berglund H, Lohmann A:** An unknown reducing urinary substance in myasthenia gravis. Proc Soc Exp Biol Med 25:210, 1927

539. **Menkes JH:** Idiopathic hyperglycinemia: isolation and identification of three previously undescribed urinary ketones. J Pediatr 69:413, 1966

540. **Menkes JH:** The pathogenesis of mental retardation in phenylketonuria and other inborn errors of metabolism. Pediatr 39:296, 1967

541. **Menkes JH, Alter M, Steigleder GK et al:** A sex-linked recessive disorder with retardation of growth, peculiar hair, and focal cerebral degeneration. Pediatr 29:764, 1962

542. **Menkes JH, Chernick V, Rengel B:** Effect of ele-

vated blood tyrosine on subsequent intellectual development of premature infants. J Pediatr 69:583, 1966

543. **Menkes JH, Corbo LM:** Adrenoleukodystrophy. Accumulation of cholesterol esters with long chain fatty acids. Neurology (Minneap) 27:928, 1977

544. **Menkes JH, Hurst PL, Craig JM:** A new syndrome: progressive familial infantile cerebral dysfunction associated with unusual urinary substance. Pediatr 14:462, 1954

545. **Menkes JH, Schimschock JR, Swanson PD:** Cerebrotendinous xanthomatosis: the storage of cholestanol within the nervous system. Arch Neurol 19:47, 1968

546. **Menkes JH, Solcher H:** Maple syrup urine disease: effects of diet therapy on cerebral lipids. Arch Neurol 16:486, 1967

547. **Mercer DW, Peters SP, Glew RH et al:** Acid phosphatase isoenzymes in Gaucher's disease. Clin Chem 23:631, 1977

548. **Migeon BR:** X-linked hypoxanthine-guanine phosphoribosyl-transferase deficiency: detection of heterozygotes by selective medium. Biochem Genet 4:377, 1970

549. **Migeon BR, Sprenkle JA, Liebaers I et al:** X-linked Hunter syndrome: the heterozygous phenotype in cell culture. Am J Hum Genet 29:448, 1977

550. **Miller JD, McCluer R, Tanfer JN:** Gaucher's disease: neurologic disorder in adult siblings. Ann Intern Med 78:833, 1973

551. **Milstein S, Holtzman NA, O'Flynn ME et al:** Hyperphenylalaninemia due to dihydropteridine reductase deficiency: assay of the enzyme in fibroblasts from affected infants, heterozygotes, and in normal amniotic fluid cells. J Pediatr 89:763, 1967

552. **Milstein S, Kaufman S, Summer GK:** Hyperphenylalaninemia due to dihydropteridine reductase deficiency: diagnosis by measurement of oxidized and reduced pterins in urine. Pediatr 65:806, 1980

553. **Miyamoto M, Fitzpatrick TB:** Competitive inhibition of mammalian tyrosinase by phenylalanine and its relationship to hair pigmentation in phenylketonuria. Nature 179:199, 1957

554. **Miyazaki M, Fukuda S, Aki M et al:** A case of hepatic encephalomyelopathy associated with citrullinemia. Brain and Nerve (Tokyo) 23:19, 1971

555. **Mize CE, Herndon JH Jr, Blass JP et al:** Localization of the oxidative defect in phytanic acid degradation in patients with Refsum's disease. J Clin Invest 48:1033, 1969

556. **Morgan-Hughes JA, Darveniza SN, Kahn DN et al:** A mitochondrial myopathy characterized by a deficiency in reducible cytochrome-b. Brain 100:617, 1977

557. **Morrow G, Barnes LA, Cardinale GJ et al:** Congenital methylmalonic acidemia: enzymatic evidence for two forms of the disease. Proc Natl Acad USA 63:191, 1969

558. **Morrow G. Schwartz RH, Hallock JA et al:** Prenatal detection of methylmalonic acidemia. J Pediatr 77:120, 1970

559. **Moser HW, Efron ML, Brown H et al:** Arginino-succinicaciduria: report of two new cases and demonstration of intermittent elevation of blood ammonia. Am J Med 42:9, 1967

560. **Moser HW, Moser AB, Kawamura N et al:** Adrenoleukodystrophy: studies of the phenotype, genetics, and biochemistry. Johns Hopkins Med J 147:217, 1980

561. **Moser HW, Moser AB, Kawamura N et al:** Adrenoleukodystrophy: elevated C_{26} fatty acid in cultured skin fibroblasts. Ann Neurol 7:542, 1980

562. **Moser HW, Prensky AL, Wolfe HJ et al:** Farber's lipogranulomatosis: report of a case and demonstration of excess of free ceramide and ganglioside. Am J Med 47:869, 1969

563. **Mudd SH: Discussion. In Carson NAJ, Raine DN (eds):** Inherited Disorders of Sulphur Metabolism, p 311. Edinburgh, Churchill Livingstone, 1971

564. **Mudd SH, Finkelstein JD, Irreverre F et al:** Homocystinuria: an enzyme defect. Science 148:1443, 1964

565. **Mudd SH, Irreverre F, Laster L:** Sulfite oxidase deficiency in man: demonstration of the enzymatic defect. Science 156:1599, 1967

566. **Mudd SH, Levy HL:** Disorders of transulfuration. In Stanbury JD, Wyngaarden JB, Fredrickson DS (eds): The Metabolic Basis of Inherited Disease, 4th ed, pp 458–503. New York, McGraw-Hill, 1978

567. **Mudd SH, Uhlendorf BW, Freeman JM et al:** Homocystinuria associated with decreased methylenetetrahydrofolate reductase activity. Biochem Biophys Res Commun 46:905, 1972

568. **Muir H, Mittwoch V, Bitter T:** The diagnostic value of isolated urinary mucopolysaccharides and of lymphocytic inclusions in gargoylism. Arch Dis Child 38:358, 1963

569. **Muller D, Pilz H, Muden VT:** Studies on adult metachromatic leukodystrophy. Part 1, clinical, morphological and histochemical observations in two cases. J Neurol Sci 9:567, 1969

570. **Murphy EA, Chase GA:** Principles of Genetic Counseling, Chicago, Year Book Medical Publishers, Chicago, 1975

571. **Myrianthopoulos NC, Melnick MM:** Tay-Sachs disease: a genetic-historical view of selective advantage. In Kaback MM, Rimoin DL, O'Brien JS: Tay-Sachs Disease: Heterozygote Screening and Prevention, pp 95–106. New York, Alan R Liss, 1977

572. **Nadler HL, Inouye T, Hsia DYY:** Clinical galactosemia: a study of fifty-five cases. In Hsia DYY (ed): Galactosemia, pp 127–162. Springfield, Ill. Charles C Thomas, 1969

573. **Nagashima K, Endo H, Sakakibara K et al:** Morphological and biochemical studies of a case of mucopolysaccharidosis II (Hunter's syndrome). Acta Pathol Jpn 26:115, 1976

574. **Narisawa K, Wada Y, Saito T et al:** Infantile type homocystinuria with $N^{5,10}$-methylenetetrahydrofolate reductase deficiency. Tohoku J Exp Med 121:185, 1977

575. **Natale PJ, Tremblay GL:** On the availability of intramitochondrial carbamylphosphate for the

extramitochondrial biosynthesis of pyrimidines. Biochem Biophys Res Commun 37:512, 1969

576. **Naylor EW, Guthrie R:** Newborn screening for maple syrup urine disease (Branched-chain ketoaciduria). Pediatr 61:262, 1978

577. **Neufeld EF, Liebaers I, Epstein CJ et al:** The Hunter syndrome in females: is there an autosomal recessive form of iduronate sulfatase deficiency? Amer J Hum Genet 29:455, 1977

578. **Neufeld EF, Lim TW, Shapiro LJ:** Inherited disorders of lysosomal metabolism. Ann Rev Biochem 44 357, 1975

579. **Neville BGR, Lake BD, Stephens R et al:** A neurovisceral storage disease with vertical supranuclear ophthalmoplegia, and its relationship to Niemann-Pick disease. A report of nine patients. Brain 96:97, 1973

580. **Newell FW, Matalon R, Meyer S:** A new mucolipidosis with psychomotor retardation, corneal clouding and retinal degeneration. Am J Ophthalmol 80:440, 1975

581. **Ng WG, Donnell GN, Koch R et al:** Biochemical and genetic studies of plasma and leukocyte alpha-L-fucosidase. Am J. Hum Genet 28:42, 1976

582. **Ngo TT, Barbeau A:** Regulation of brain pyruvate dehydrogenase multienzyme complex. Canad J Neurol Sci 8:231, 1978

583. **Niederwieser A, Curtius H-C, Bettoni O et al:** Atypical phenylketonuria caused by 7,8-dihydrobiopterin synthetase deficiency. Lancet I:131, 1979

584. **Niederwieser A, Giliberti P, Matosovic A et al:** Folic acid non-dependent formiminoglutamicaciduria in two siblings. Clin Chim Acta 54:293, 1974

585. **Niemann A:** Ein unbekanntes Krankheitsbild. Jahrb Kinderheilkd, 79:1, 1914

586. **Nishimura RN, Barranger JA:** Neurologic complications of Gaucher's disease, Type 3. Arch Neurol 37:92, 1980

587. **Nishimura R, Omos-Lau N, Ajmone Marsan C et al:** Electroencephalographic findings in Gaucher disease. Neurol 30:152, 1980

588. **Noonan SM, Desousa J, Riddle JM:** Lymphocyte ultrastructure in two cases of neuronal ceroid-lipofuscinosis. Neurol 28:472, 1978

589. **Norden AGW, Tennant LL, O'Brien JS:** G$_{M1}$ ganglioside β-galactosidase A. Purification and studies of the enzyme from human liver. J Biol Chem 249:167, 1974

590. **Norman RM, Forrester RM, Tingey AH:** The juvenile form of Niemann-Pick disease. Arch Dis Child 42:91, 1967

591. **Norman RM, Oppeheimer DR, Tingey AH:** Histological and chemical findings in Krabbe's leukodystrophy. J Neurol Neurosurg Psychiatry 24:223, 1961

592. **Norman RM, Urich H., Tingey AH et al:** Tay-Sachs disease with visceral involvement and its relationship to Niemann-Pick's disese. J Pathol 72:409, 1959

593. **Nyhan WL:** Clinical features of the Lesch-Nyhan syndrome. Arch Intern Med 130:186, 1972

594. **Oberholzer VG, Palmer T:** Increased excretion of N-carbamyl compounds in patients with urea cycle defects. Clin Chim Acta 68:73, 1976

595. **O'Brien D, Berlow S. Donnell G et al:** New developments in hyperphenylalaninemia. Pediatr 65:844, 1980

596. **O'Brien JS:** Generalized gangliosidosis. J Pediatr 75:167, 1969

597. **O'Brien JS:** Molecular genetics of G$_{M1}$ Beta-galactosidase. Clin Genet 8:303, 1975

598. **O'Brien JS:** The gangliosidoses. In Stanbury JB, Wyngaarden JB, Fredrickson DS (eds): The Metabolic Basis of Inherited Disease, 4th pp 841–915. New York, McGraw-Hill, 1978

599. **O'Brien JS, Bernett J, Veath MC et al:** Lysosomal storage disorder. Diagnosis by ultrastructual examination of skin biopsy specimens. Arch Neurol 32:592, 1975

600. **O'Brien JS, Gugler E, Giedion A et al:** Spondyloepiphyseal dysplasia, corneal clouding, normal intelligence, and acid beta-galactosidase deficiency. Clin Genet 9:495, 1976

601. **O'Brien JS, Ho MW, Veath ML et al:** Juvenile G$_{m1}$ gangliosidosis: clinical, pathological, chemical and enzymatic studies. Clin Genet 3:411, 1972

602. **O'Brien JS, Norden AGW:** Nature of the mutation in adult beta-galactosidase deficient patients. Am J Hum Genet 29:184, 1977

603. **O'Brien JS, Okada S. Fillerup DL et al:** Tay-Sachs disease: prenatal diagnosis. Science 172:61, 1971

604. **Ockerman PA:** Manosidosis. In Hers HG, Van Hoof F (eds): Lysosomes and Storage Disease, pp 291–304. New York, Academic Press, 1973

605. **Oh MS, Carroll HJ:** The anion gap. N Engl J Med 297:814, 1977

606. **Okada S, O'Brien JS:** Tay-Sachs disease: generalized absence of a beta-D-N-acetylhexosaminidase component. Science 165, 698, 1969

607. **Okken A, DeGroot CJ, Hommes FA:** Nonketotic hyperglycinemia. J. Pediatr 75:1022, 1969

608. **Olsson Y, Sourander P:** The reliability of the diagnosis of metachromatic leukodystrophy by peripheral nerve biopsy. Acta Paediatr Scand, 48:15, 1969

609. **O'Neill BP, Moser HW, Marmion LC:** The adrenoleukomyeloneuropathy (ALMN) complex: elevated C$_{26}$ fatty acid in cultured skin fibroblasts and correlations with disease expression in three generations of kindred. Neurology (Minneap) 30:353, 1980

610. **Oonk JGW, van der Helm HJ, Martin JJ:** Spinocerebellar degeneration: hexosaminidase A and B deficiency in two adult sisters. Neurology 29:380, 1979

611. **O'Reilly A, Pollycove M, Bank WT:** Iron metabolism in Wilson's disease. Neurology 18:634, 1968

612. **Osaka K, Sato N, Matsumoto S et al:** Congenital hypocupraemia syndrome with and without steely hair. Report of two Japanese infants. Dev Med Child Neurol 19:62, 1977

613. **Paetzke-Brunner I, Schon H, Wieland OM:** Insulin activates pyruvate dehydrogenase by lowering the mitochondrial acetyl-CoA/CoA ratio as

evidenced by digitonin fractionation of isolated fat cells, FEBS letters 93:307, 1978

614. **Paine RS:** The variability in manifestations of untreated patients with phenylketonuria (phenylpyruvic aciduria). Pediatr 20:290, 1957

615. **Partin JC:** Hepatic encephalopathy and Reye's syndrome. Pediatr Ann May 101, 1977

616. **Partington MW:** The early symptoms of phenylketonuria. Pediatr 27:465, 1961

617. **Partington MW, Delahaye DJ, Masotti RE et al:** Neonatal tyrosinaemia: a follow-up study. Arch Dis Child 43:195, 1968

618. **Patel V, Watanabe I, Zeman W:** Deficiency of alpha-1-fucosidase. Science 176:426, 1972

619. **Patrick AD, Lake BD:** An acid lipase deficiency in Wolman's disease. Biochem J 112:29P, 1969

620. **Pavone L, Moser HW, Mollica F et al:** Farber's lipogranulomatosis: ceramidase deficiency and prolonged survival in three relatives. Johns Hopkins Med J 147:193, 1980

621. **Pennock CA:** A modified screening test for glycosaminoglycan excretion. J Clin Path 22:379, 1969

622. **Pennock CA, Barnes IC:** The mucopolysaccharidoses. J. Med Genet 13:169, 1976

623. **Pennock CA, White F, Murphy D et al:** Excess glycosaminoglycan excretion in infancy and childhood. Acta Paediat Scand 62:481, 1973

624. **Percy AK, Brady RO:** Metachromatic leukodystrophy: diagnosis with samples of venous blood. Science 161:594, 1968

625. **Percy AK, Shapiro LJ, Kaback MM:** Inherited lipid storage diseases of the central nervous system. Curr Prob Pediatr 9:1, 1979

626. **Perman JA, Werlin S, Grand FJ et al:** Laboratory measures of copper metabolism in the differentiation of chronic active hepatitis and Wilson disease in children. J Pediatr 94:564, 1979

627. **Perry TL:** Homocystinuria. In Nyhan WL (ed): Heritable Disorders of Amino Acids Metabolism, pp 395–428. New York, John Wiley & Sons, 1974

628. **Perry TL, Applegarth DE, Evans ME et al:** Metabolic studies of a family with massive formiminoglutamicaciduria. Pediatr Res 9:117, 1975

629. **Perry TL, Bratly PJA, Hansen S et al:** Hereditary mental depression and parkinsonism with taurine deficiency. Arch Neurol 32:108, 1975

630. **Perry TL, Hansen S. MacDougall L et al:** Sulfur-containing amino acids in the plasma and urine of homocystinurics. Clin Chim Acta 15:409. 1967

631. **Perry TL, Hardwick DF, Hansen S et al:** Israel's cystathioninuria in two healthy siblings. N Engl J Med 278:590, 1968

632. **Perry TL, Urgulent N, MacLean J et al:** Non-ketotic hyperglycinemia. Glycine accumulation due to absence of glycine cleavage in brain. N Engl J Med 292:1269, 1975

633. **Peters S, Lee RE, Glew RH:** Microassay for Gaucher's Disease. Clin Chim Acta 60:391, 1975

634. **Peterson DI, Bacchus A, Seaich L et al:** Myelopathy associated with Maroteaux-Lamy syndrome. Arch Neurol 32:127, 1975

635. **Philippart M, Franklin SS, Gordon A:** Reversal of an inborn sphingolipidosis (Fabry's disease) by kidney transplantation. Ann Int Med 77:195, 1972

636. **Philippart M, van Bogaert L:** Cholestanolosis (cerebrotendinous xanthomatosis): A follow-up study on the original family. Arch Neurol 21:603, 1969

637. **Pilz H:** Niemann-Picksche Krankheit in Erwachsenenalter. Dtsche Med Wochenschr, 38:1905, 1970

638. **Pilz H, Duensing I, Heipertz R et al:** Adult metachromatic leukodystrophy. Part I. Clinical manifestation in a female 44 years, previously diagnosed in the preclinical state. Eur Neurol 15:301, 1977

639. **Pilz H, Sandhoff K, Jatzkewitz H:** Eine Gangliosidstoffwechselstorung mit Anhaufung von Ceramidlactosid, Monosialoceramidlactosid und Tay-Sachs-Gangliosid im Gehirn. J Neurochem 13:1273, 1966

640. **Pilz H, Schwendemann G, Goebel HH:** Diagnostic significance of myeloperoxidase assay in neuronal ceroid-lipofuscinoses (Batten-Vogt syndrome). Neurology 28:924, 1978

641. **Pilz H, von Figura K, Goebel HH:** Deficiency of arylsulfatase B in two brothers aged 40 and 38 years (Maroteaux-Lamy syndrome, type B). Ann Neurol 6:315, 1979

642. **Pincus J:** Subacute necrotizing encephalomyelopathy (Leigh's disease): a consideration of clinical features and etiology. Dev Med Child Neurol 14:87, 1972

643. **Pincus J, Cooper J, Itokawa Y et al:** Subacute necrotizing encephalomyelopathy: Effects of thiamine and thiamine propyl disulfide. Arch Neurol 24:511, 1971

644. **Pincus JH, Solitare GB, Cooper JR:** Thiamine triphosphate levels and histopathology. Correlation in Leigh's disease. Arch Neurol 33:759, 1976

645. **Plaitakis A, Nicklas WJ, Desnick RJ:** Glutamate dehydrogenase deficiency in three patients with spinocerebellar syndrome. Ann Neurol 7:297, 1980

646. **Plaitakis A, Whetsell WO Jr, Cooper JR et al:** Chronic Leigh disease: a genetic and biochemical study. Ann Neurol 7:304, 1980

647. **Pollitt RJ, Jennor FA, Davies M:** Sibs with mental and physical retardation and trichorrhexis nodosa with abnormal amino acid composition of the hair. Arch Dis Child 43:211, 1968

648. **Porter H:** The particulate half-cystine-rich copper protein of newborn liver. Relationship to metallothionein and subcellular localization in nonmitochondrial particles possibly representing heavy lysomes. Biochem Biophys Res Commun 56:661, 1974

649. **Prensky AL, Carr S, Moser HW:** Development of myelin in inherited disorders of amino acid metabolism. Arch Neurol 19:552, 1968

650. **Prensky AL, Moser HW:** Brain lipids, proteolipids, and free amino acids in maple syrup urine disease. J Neurochem 13:863, 1966

651. **Pryzrembel H, Wendel U, Becker K et al:** Glutaric aciduria type II: report on a previously undescribed metabolic disorder. Clin Chim Acta 66:227, 1976

652. **Pueschel SM, Rotteman KJ:** Birth weight analysis of children with phenylketonuria. Pediatr Res 10:419, 1976

653. **Purpura DP, Hirano A, French JH:** Polydendritic Purkinje cells in X-chromosome linked copper malabsorption: a Golgi-study. Brain Res 117:125, 1976

654. **Quigley HA, Goldberg MF:** Conjunctival ultrastructure in mucolipidosis III. Invest Ophthalmol 10:568, 1971

655. **Quigley HA, Kenyon KR:** Ultrastructural and histochemical studies of a newly recognized form of systemic mucopolysaccharidosis (Maroteaux-Lamy syndrome, mild phenotype). Am J Ophthalmol 77:809, 1974

656. **Rabir D, Cathelineau L, Kamouu P:** Lack of mitochondrial enzymes of the urea cycle in human white blood cells. Pediatr Res 13:207, 1979

657. **Rahman AN, Lindenberg R:** The neuropathology of hereditary dystopic lipidosis. Arch Neurol 9:373, 1963

658. **Rajantie J, Simmell O, Rapola J et al:** Lysinuric protein intolerance: a two year trial of dietary supplementation with citrulline and lysine. J Pediatr 97:927, 1980

659. **Ramsey RB, Banik NL, Davison AN:** Adrenoleukodystrophy: brain cholesterol esters and other neutral lipids. J Neurol Sci 40:189, 1979

660. **Rao BG, Spence MW:** Sphingomyelinase activity at pH 7.4 in human brain and a comparison to activity at pH 5.0. J Lipid Res 17:506, 1976

661. **Rapin I, Goldfischer S, Katzman R et al:** The cherry-red spot-myoclonus syndrome. Ann Neurol 3:234, 1978

662. **Rapin I, Suzuki K, Valsamis MP:** Adult (chronic) GM_2 gangliosidosis. Arch Neurol 33:120, 1976

663. **Refsum S:** Heredopathia atactia polyneuritiformis. Acta Psychiatr Scand (Suppl)38:9, 1946

664. **Refsum S:** Heredopathia atactia polyneuritiformis reconsideration. World Neurol 1:334, 1960

665. **Rembold H:** Metabolism and metabolic roles of 6-polyhydroxyalkylpterins. J Inherited Metab Dis 1:61, 1978

666. **Rey F, Harpey JP, Leeming RJ et al:** Les hyperphenylalanenemies area avitivite normale de al phenylalanine hydroxylase: le deficit en tetrahydrobiopterin et le deficit en dihydropterdine reductase. Arch Fre Pediatr (Suppl)34:109, 1977

667. **Riccardi VM:** The Genetic Approach to Human Disease. New York, Oxford University Press, 1977

668. **Richards F II, Cooper MR, Pearce LA et al:** Familial spinocerebellar degeneration, hemolytic anemia, and glutathione deficiency. Arch Intern Med 134:534, 1974

669. **Richards W, Donnell GN, Wilson WA:** The oculocerebro-renal syndrome of Lowe. Am J Dis Child 109:185, 1965

670. **Ridley A:** The neuropathy of acute intermittent porphyria. Am J Med 38:307, 1969

671. **Rimoin DL, Hall J, Maroteaux P:** International nomenclature of constitutional diseases of bone with bibliography. Birth Defects Original Article Series, vol 15, No 10, 1979

672. **Robertson WC, Gomez MR, Reese DF et al:** Computerized tomography in demyelinating disease of the young. Neurology (Minneap) 27:838, 1977

673. **Robinson BH, Oci J, Sherwood WG et al:** Hydroxymethylglutaryl CoA lyase deficiency: features resembling Reye Syndrome. Neurology 30:714, 1980

674. **Robinson BH, Sherwood WG:** Pyruvate dehydrogenase phosphatase deficiency: a cause of congenital chronic lactic acidosis in infancy. Pediatr Res 9:935, 1975

675. **Robinson BH, Sherwood WG, Taylor J et al:** Acetoacetyl CoA thiolase deficiency: a cause of severe ketoacidosis in infancy simulating salicylism. J Pediatr 95(2):228, 1979

676. **Robinson BH, Taylor J, Kahler SG et al:** Lactic acidemia, neurologic deterioration and carbohydrate dependence in a girl with dihydrolipoyl dehydrogenase deficiency. Eur J Pediatr 136:35, 1981

677. **Robinson GC, Johnston MM:** Pili torti and sensory neural hearing loss. J Pediatr 70:621, 1967

678. **Roerdink FH, Gouw WLM, Okken A et al:** Citrullinemia, report of a case, with the studies of antenatal diagnosis. Pediatr Res 7:863, 1973

679. **Roeser HP, Lee GR, Nacht S et al:** The role of ceruloplasmin in iron metabolism. J Clin Invest 49:2408, 1970

680. **Rose AL, Pullarkat RK, Farmer PM et al:** A new gangliosidosis with accumulation of G_{M3} ganglioside. Ann Neurol 2:266, 1977

681. **Rosenberg AL, Bergstrom L, Troost T et al:** Hyperuricemia and neurologic deficits: a family study. N Engl J Med 282:992, 1970

682. **Rosenberg LE:** Disorders of propionate, methylmalonate, and cobalamin metabolism. In Stanbury JB, Wyngaarden JB, Fredrickson DS (eds): The Metabolic Basis of Inherited Diseases, 4th ed, pp 411–429. New York, McGraw-Hill, 1978

683. **Rosenberg LE, Lilljeqvist AC, Hsia YE et al:** Vitamin B_{12} dependent methylmalonicaciduria: defective B_{12} metabolism in cultured fibroblasts. Biochem Biophys Res Commun 37:607, 1969

684. **Rosenblum JL, Keating JP, Prensky AL et al:** A progressive neurologic syndrome in children with chronic liver disease. N Engl J Med 304:503, 1981

685. **Rothstein M, Miller LL:** The conversion of lysine to pipecolic acid in the rat. J Biol Chem 211:851, 1954

686. **Rowe JW, Gilliam JI, Warthin TA:** Intestinal manifestations of Fabry's disease. Ann Intern Med 81:628, 1974

687. **Rowe PB:** Inherited Disorders of folate metabolism. In Stanbury JB, Wyngaarden JB, Fredrickson BS (eds): The Metabolic Basis of Inherited Disease, 4th ed, pp 430–457. New York, McGraw-Hill, 1978

688. **Roy AB:** The sulphatase of ox liver. I. The complex nature of the enzymes. Biochem J 53:12, 1953

689. **Rudiger HW, Langenbeck U, Schulze-Schencking M et al:** Defective decarboxylase in branched chain ketoacid oxidase multienzyme complex in classic type of maple syrup urine disease. Humangenetik 14:257, 1972

690. **Rumpel A:** Uber Das Wesen und die Bedeutung der Leberverandorung en und der Pigmentierungen bei den damit verbundensen Fallen von Pseudosklerose, zugleich ein Beitrag zur Lehre von der Pseudosklerose (Westphal-Strumpell). Dtsch Z Nervenheilkd 49:54, 1913

691. **Russell A, Levin B, Oberholzer BG et al:** Hyperammonemia, a new instance of an inborn enzymatic defect of biosynthesis of urea. Lancet 2:699, 1962

692. **Sachs B:** On arrested cerebral development with special reference to its pathology. J Nerv Ment Dis 14:541, 1887

693. **Samuelsson E, Zetterstom R:** Ceramide in a patient with lipogranulomatosis (Farber's disease) with chronic course. Scan J Clin Lab Invest 27:393, 1971

694. **Sander JE, Malamud N, Cowan MJ et al:** Intermittent ataxia and immunodeficiency with multiple carboxylase deficiencies: a biotin-responsive disorder. Ann Neurol 8:544, 1980

695. **Sandharwaller JB, Fowler B, Robins AJ et al:** Detection of heterozygotes for homocystinuria. Study of sulphur-containing amino acids in plasma and urine after L-methionine loading. Arch Dis Child 49:553, 1974

696. **Sandhoff K:** Variation of β-N-acetylhexosaminidase-pattern in Tay-Sachs disease. FEBS Letter 4:351, 1969

697. **Sandhoff K, Christomanou H:** Biochemistry and genetics of gangliosidoses. Hum Genet 50:107, 1979

698. **Sandhoff K, Harzer K, Wassle W et al:** Enzyme alterations in lipid storage in three variants of Tay-Sachs disease. J Neurochem 18:2469, 1971

699. **Santavuori P, Haltia M, Rapola J et al:** Infantile type of so-called neuronal ceroid-lipofuscinosis. Part 1. A clinical study of 15 patients. J Neurol Sci 18:257, 1973

700. **Sass-Kortask A, Bearn AG:** Hereditary disorders of copper metabolism. In Stanbury JB, Wyngaarden JB, Fredrickson DS (eds): The Metabolic Basic of Inherited Disease, 4th ed, pp 1098–1126. New York, McGraw-Hill, 1978

701. **Saudebray JM, Marsac C, Charpentier C et al:** Neonatal congenital lactic acidosis with pyruvate carboxylase deficiency in two siblings. Acta Pediatr Scand 65:717, 1976

702. **Saugstad LF:** Birthweights in children with phenylketonuria and in their siblings. Lancet I:809, 1972

703. **Saunders M, Sweetman L, Robinson B et al:** Biotin-responsive organicaciduria. J Clin Invest 64:1695, 1979

704. **Schaub J, Daumling S, Curtius HC et al:** Tetrahydrobiopterin therapy of atypical phenylketonuria due to defective dihydrobiopterin biosynthesis. Arch Dis Child 53:674, 1978

705. **Schaumburg HH, Powers JM, Raine CS et al:** Adrenoleukodystrophy: a clinical and pathological study of 17 cases. Arch Neurol 32:577, 1975

706. **Schaumburg HH, Powers JM, Raine CS:** Adrenomyeloneuropathy: a probable variant of adrenoleukodystrophy: Part II. General pathological, neuropathologic and biochemical aspects. Neurology (Minneap) 27:1114, 1977

707. **Schaumburg HH, Powers JM, Suzuki K et al:** Adrenoleukodystrophy (sex-linked Schilder disease): ultrastructural demonstration of specific cytoplasmic inclusions in the central nervous system. Arch Neurol 31:210, 1974

708. **Scheie HG, Hambrick GW Jr, Barness LA:** A newly recognized forme fruste of Hurler's disease (gargoylism). Am J Ophthalmol 53:753, 1962

709. **Scheinberg IH, Sternlieb I:** Wilson's disease. Ann Rev Med 16:119, 1965

710. **Scherzer Al, Ilson JB:** Normal intelligence in the Lesch-Nyhan syndrome. Pediatr 44:116, 1969

711. **Schimshock JR, Alvord EC, Swanson PD:** Cerebrotendinous xanthomatosis: clinical and pathological studies. Arch Neurol 18:688, 1968

712. **Schmidt L:** The biochemical detection of metabolic disease: screening tests and a systematic approach to screening. In Nyhan WL (ed): Heritable Disorders of Amino Acid Metabolism: Patterns of Clinical Expression and Genetic Variation, pp 675–697. New York, John Wiley & Sons, 1974

713. **Schneider EL, Ellis WG, Brady RO et al:** Infantile (type II) Gaucher's disease: in utero diagnosis and fetal pathology. J Pediatr 81:1134, 1972

714. **Schneider PB, Kennedy EP,** Sphingomyelinase in normal human spleens and in spleens from subjects with Niemann-Pick disease. J Lipid Res 8:202, 1967

715. **Scholz W:** Klinische pathologisch-anatomische und erbbiologische Untersuchungen bei familiarer, diffuser Hirnsklerose in Kindesalter. Z Gesamte Neurol Psychiatr 99:42, 1925

716. **Schoonderwaldt AC, Lamers KJB, Kleijnen FM et al:** Two patients with an unusual form of type II fucosidosis. Clin Genet 18:348, 1980

717. **Schulman JD, Lustberg TJ, Kennedy JL et al:** A new variant of maple syrup urine disease (branched chain ketoaciduria). Clinical and biochemical evaluation. Am J Med 49:118, 1970

718. **Schwartz JF, Rowland LP, Eder H et al:** Bassen-Kornzweig syndrome: deficiency of serum beta-lipoprotein. Arch Neurol 8:438, 1963

719. **Scriver CR, MacKenzie S, Clow CL et al:** Thiamine responsive maple syrup urine disease. Lancet 1:310, 1971

720. **Scriver CR, Pueschel S, Davies E:** Hyperbeta-alaninemia associated with beta-aminoaciduria and gamma-aminobutyric-aciduria, somnolence and seizures. N Engl J Med 179:636, 1966

721. **Scriver CR, Rosenberg LE:** Amino Acid Metabolism and Its Disorders. Philadelphia, WB Saunders, 1973

722. **Seegmiller JE, Rosenbloom FM, Kelley WN:** An enzyme defect associated with a sex-linked human neurological disorder and excessive purine synthesis. Science 155:1682, 1967

723. **Segal S:** Disorders of galactose metabolism. In Stanbury JB, Wyngaarden JB, Fredrickson DL (eds): The Metabolic Basis of Inherited Disease, 4th ed, pp 160–181. New York, McGraw-Hill, 1978

724. **Sepe SJ, Levy HL, Mount FW:** An evaluation of routine follow-up blood screening of infants for phenylketonuria. N Engl J Med 300:606, 1979

725. **Shafai T, Sweetman L, Weyler W et al:** Propionic acidemia with severe hyperammonemia and defective glycine metabolism. J Pediatr 92:84, 1978

726. **Shapiro LJ, Bocian ME, Reijman L et al:** Methylmalonyl CoA mutase deficiency associated with severe neonatal hyperammonemia: activity in the urea cycle enzymes. J Pediatr 93:986, 1978

727. **Shapiro LJ, Neufeld EF:** Genetic Mucopolysaccharidoses and Mucolipidoses. In Siegel GJ, Albers RW, Katzman R (eds): Basic Neurochemistry, pp 569–580. Little, Brown & Co, 1976

728. **Shapiro Y, Cedarbaum SD, Cancilla PA et al:** Familial poliodystrophy, mitochondrial myopathy and lactate acidemia. Neurology 25:614, 1975

729. **Shear CS, Wellman NS, Nyhan WL:** Phenylketonuria: experience with diagnosis and management. In Nyhan WL (ed): Heritable Disorders of Amino Acid Metabolism, pp 141–159. New York, John Wiley & Sons, 1974

730. **Shih VE:** Urea cycle disorders and other congenital hyperammonemic syndromes. In Stanbury JB, Wyngaarden JB, Fredrickson DS (eds): The Metabolic Basis of Inherited Disease, 4th ed, pp 362–386. New York, McGraw-Hill, 1978

731. **Shih VE, Abroms IF, Johnson JL et al:** Sulfite oxidase deficiency: biochemical and clinical investigations of a hereditary disorder in sulfur metabolism. New Engl J Med 297:1022, 1977

732. **Shih VE, Efron ML, Moser HW:** Hyperornithinemia, hyperammonemia, and homocitrullinemia. A new disorder of amino acid metabolism associated with myoclonic seizures and mental retardation. Am J Dis Child 117:83, 1969

733. **Shih VE, Levy HL, Karolkewicz V et al:** Galactosemia screening of newborns in Massachusetts. N Engl J Med 284:753, 1971

734. **Shih VE, Mandell R, Tanaka K:** Diagnosis of isovaleric acidemia in cultured fibroblasts. Clin Chim Acta 48:437, 1973

735. **Short EM, Conn HO, Snodgrass PJ et al:** Evidence for X-linked dominant inheritance of ornithine transcarbamylase deficiency. N Engl J Med 288:7 1973

736. **Siakotos AM, Watanabe I, Saito A et al:** The isolation of two distinct lipopigments from human brain: lipofuscin and ceroid. Biochem Med 4:361, 1970

737. **Siegel GJ, Albers RW, Katzmann R et al (eds):** Basic Neurochemistry, 2nd ed. Boston, Little, Brown & Co, 1976

738. **Silberman J, Dancis J, Feigin IH:** Neuropathological observations in maple syrup urine disease: branched chain ketoaciduria. Arch Neurol 5:351, 1961

739. **Simell O, Perahentupa J, Rapola J et al:** Lysinuric protein intolerance. Am J Med 59:229, 1975

740. **Simell O, Visakorpi JK, Donner M:** Saccharopinuria. Arch Dis Child 47:52, 1972

741. **Sinatra F, Yoshida T, Applebaum M et al:** Abnormalities of carbamyl phosphate synthetase and ornithine transcarbamylase in liver of patients with Reyes syndrome. Pediatr Res 9:829, 1975

742. **Singer HS, Schafer IA:** White cell B-galactosidase activity. N Engl J Med, 232:571, 1970

743. **Singer K, Fisher B, Perlstein MA:** Acanthocytosis: a genetic erythrocyte malformation. Blood 7:577, 1952

744. **Singh J, DiFerrante N, Niebes P et al:** N-acetylgalactosamine 6-sulfate sulfatase in man. Absence of the enzyme in Morquio disease. J Clin Invest 57:1036, 1976

745. **Singh J, Tavella D, DiFerrante N:** Measurements of arylsulfatases A and B in human serum. J Pediatr 86:574, 1975

746. **Singh S, Bresnan MJ:** Menkes kinky-hair syndrome (trichopoliodystrophy). Am J Dis Child 125:572, 1973

747. **Sipe JC, O'Brien JS:** Ultrastructure of skin biopsy specimens in lysosomal storage diseases: common source of error in diagnosis. Clin Genet 15:118, 1979

748. **Sjögren T:** Die juvenile amaurotische Idiotie. Klinische und erblichkeitsmedizinische Untersuchungen. Hereditas (Lund) 14:197, 1931

749. **Skoglund RR:** Reversible alexia, mitochondrial myopathy, and lactic acidemia. Neurology 29:717, 1979

750. **Sloan HR, Uhlendorf BW, Jacobson CB et al:** Beta-Galactosidase in tissue culture derived from human skin and bone marrow: enzyme defect in G_{M1} gangliosidosis. Pediatr Res. 3:532, 1969

751. **Sly WS, Quinton BA, McAlister WH et al:** Beta-Glucuronidase deficiency: report of clinical, radiological, and biochemical features of a new mucopolysaccharidosis. J Pediatr 82:249, 1973

752. **Smetana HF, Olen F:** Hereditary galactose disease. Am J Clin Pathol 38:3, 1962

753. **Smith I, Lobascher ME, Stevenson JE et al:** Effect of stopping low-phenylalanine diet on intellectual progress of children with phenylketonuria. Brit Med J 2:723, 1978

754. **Snodgrass PJ, Wappner RS, Brandt IK:** Letter to the Editor: White cell ornithine transcarbamylase activity cannot detect the liver enzyme deficiency. Pediatr Res 12:873, 1978

755. **Snyder RA, Brady RO:** The use of white cells as a source of diagnostic material for lipid storage diseases. Clin Chim Acta, 25:331, 1969

756. **Snyderman SE:** Maple syrup urine disease. In Nyhan WL (ed): Heritable Disorders of Amino Acid Metabolism, pp 17–31. New York, John Wiley & Sons, 1974

757. **Snyderman SE:** Medical and nutritional aspects of maple syrup urine disease. In Koch RF, Shaw KNF, Durkin F (eds): Maple Syrup Urine Disease Symposium. DHEW (HSA) 79–5294, Washington DC, Government Printing Office, 1979

758. **Snyderman SE, Norton PM, Roitman E et al:** Maple syrup urine disease with particular reference to diet therapy. Pediatr 34:454, 1964

759. **Snyderman SE, Sansarcq C, Norton PM et al :** Argininemia treated from birth. J Pediatr 75:61, 1979

760. **Soffer D, Yamanaka T, Wenger DA et al:** Central nervous system involvement in adult-onset Gaucher's disease. Acta Neuropathol (Berl) 49:1, 1980

761. **Sorbrevilla LA, Goodman ML, Kane CA:** Demyelinating central nervous system disease, macular atrophy and acanthocytosis (Bassen-Kornzweig syndrome). Am J Med 37:821, 1964

762. **Spaeth GL, Frost P:** Fabry disease: its ocular manifestations. Arch Ophthalmol 74:760, 1965

763. **Spalton DJ, Taylor DSI, Sanders MD:** Juvenile Batten's disease: an ophthalmological assessment of 25 patients. Br J Ophthalmol 64:726, 1980

764. **Spence MW, Ripley BA, Embil JA et al:** A new variant of Sandhoff's disease. Pediatr Res 8:628, 1974

765. **Spranger JW:** Beta galactosidase and the Morquio syndrome. Am J Med Genet 1:207, 1977

766. **Spranger JW:** Catabolic disorders of complex carbohydrates. Postgrad Med J 53:441, 1977

767. **Spranger JW, Cantz M, Gehler J et al:** Mucopolysaccharidosis II (Hunter disease) with corneal opacities. Report on two patients at the extremes of a wide clinical spectrum. Eur J Pediatr 129:11, 1978

768. **Spranger JW, Gehler J, Cantz M:** Mucolipidosis I—A sialidosis. Am J Med Genet 1:21, 1977

769. **Spritz RA, Doughty RA, Spackman TJ et al:** Neonatal presentation of I-cell disease. J Pediatr 93:945, 1978

770. **Srivastava SK:** Tay-Sachs and Sandhoff diseases. In Glew RH, Peters SP (eds): Practical Enzymology of the Sphingolipidoses, pp 217–2460. New York, Alan R Liss, 1977

771. **Srivastava SK, Beutler E:** Hexosaminidase A and hexosaminidase B: studies in Tay-Sachs' and Sandhoff's disease. Nature 241:463, 1973

772. **Stahl WL, Sumi SM, Swanson PD:** Cerebrotendinous xanthomatosis. J Neurochem 18:403, 1971

773. **Stansbie D:** Regulation of the human pyruvate dehydrogenase complex. Clin Sci Mol Med 51:445, 1976

774. **Steen-Johnson J, Vellan EJ, Gjessing LR:** Maple syrup-urine disease variant—amino acid pattern and problems of treatment during acute attacks. Acta Paediatr Scand (Suppl) 206:71, 1970

775. **Steinbach HL, Preger L, Williams HE et al:** The Hurler syndrome without abnormal mucopolysacchariduria. Radiol 90:472, 1968

776. **Steinberg D, Herndon JG Jr, Uhlendorf BW et al:** Refsum's disease. Nature of the enzyme defect. Science 156:1740, 1967

777. **Steinmann GS, Yudkoff M, Berman PH et al:** Late-onset nonketotic hyperglycinemia and spinocerebellar degeneration. J Pediatr 94:907, 1979

778. **Sternlieb I:** Mitochondrial and fatty changes in hepatocytes of patients with Wilson's disease. Gastroenterol 55:354, 1968

779. **Sternlieb I:** Evolution of the hepatic lesion in Wilson's disease (Hepatolenticular degeneration). Prog Liver Dis 4:511, 1972

780. **Sternlieb I:** The development of cirrhosis in Wilson's disease. Clin Gastroenterol 4:367, 1975

781. **Sternlieb I, Scheinberg IH:** Chronic hepatitis as a first manifestation of Wilson's disease. Ann Intern Med 76:59, 1972

782. **Stevens RL, Fluharty AL, Killgrove AR, et al:** Microheterogeneity of human arylsulfatase A on isoelectric focusing. Fed Proc 35:1726, 1976

783. **Stevens RL, Fluharty AL, Skokut MH et al:** Purification and properties of cortical arylsulfatase A from human urine. J Biol Chem 250:2495, 1975

784. **Stevenson RE, Howell RR, McKusick VA et al:** The iduronidase-deficient mucopolysaccharidoses: clinical and roentgenographic features. Pediatr 57:11, 1976

785. **Stoffel W, LeKim D, Tschung TS:** A simple chemical method for labeling phosphatidylcholine and sphingomyelin in the choline moiety. Hoppe-Seyler's Z Physiol Chem 352:1058, 1971

786. **Stokke O, Eldjarn L, Jellum E et al:** Beta-methylcrotonyl-CoA carboxylase deficiency: a new metabolic error in leucine degradation. Pediatr 49:726, 1972

787. **Strickland GT, Beckner WM, Leu ML:** Absorption of copper in homozygotes for Wilson's disease and controls: isotope tracer studies with ^{67}Cu and ^{64}Cu. Clin Sci 43:617, 1972

788. **Strickland GT, Frommer D, Leu M-L et al:** Wilson's disease in the United Kingdom and Taiwan. Part I. General characteristics of 142 cases and prognosis. Part II. A genetic analysis of 88 cases. Q J Med 42:619, 1973

789. **Strickland GT, Leu M-L:** Wilson's disease: clinical and laboratory manifestations in 40 patients. Med (Baltimore) 54:113, 1975

790. **Stumpf D, Neuwelt E, Austin J et al:** Metachromatic leukodystrophy (MLD) X. Immunological studies of the abnormal sulfatase A. Arch Neurol 25:427, 1971

791. **Stumpf DA, Parks JK:** Urea cycle regulation: I. Coupling of ornithine metabolism to mitochondrial oxidative phosphorylation. Neurology 30:178, 1980

792. **Sturman JA, Gaull G, Raiha NC:** Absence of cystathionase in human fetal liver: is cystine essential? Science 169:74, 1970

793. **Sugita M, Dulaney J, Moser HW:** Ceramidase deficiency in Farber's disease. Science 178:1100, 1972

794. **Suzuki K:** Neurochemical aspects of mucopolysaccharidoses. In Lajtha A (ed): Handbook of Neurochemistry, Vol VII, pp 17–32. New York, Plenum Press, 1972

795. **Suzuki K:** Globoid leukodystrophy (Krabbe's disease) and G_{M1}-gangliosidosis. In Glew RH, Peters SP: Practical Enzymology of the Sphingolipidoses, pp 101–136. New York, Alan R Liss, 1977

796. **Suzuki K, Suzuki Y:** Globoid cell leukodystrophy (Krabbe's disease): deficiency of galactocerebroside B-galactosidase. Proc Natl Acad Sci USA 66:304, 1970

797. **Suzuki Y, Suzuki K:** Krabbe's globoid cell leukodystrophy: deficiency of galactocerebrosidase in serum, leukocytes and fibroblasts. Sci 171:73, 1971

798. **Suzuki Y, Suzuki K, Rapin I et al:** Juvenile GM_2-

gangliosidosis. Clinical variant of Tay-Sachs disease or a new disease. Neurology 20:190, 1970

799. **Svennerholm L:** Polyunsaturated fatty acid lipidosis: a new nosological entity. In Volk BW, Schneck L (eds): Current Trends in Sphingolipidosis and Allied Disorders, pp 389–402. New York, Plenum Press, 1976

800. **Svennerholm L, Hagberg B, Haltia M et al:** Polyunsaturated fatty acid lipidosis. Part II. Lipid biochemical aspects. Acta Paediatr Scand 64:489, 1975

801. **Swaiman KF, Garg BP, Lockman LA:** Sea-blue histiocytes and posterior column dysfunction: a familial disorder. Neurology 25:1084, 1975

802. **Sweeley CC, Klionsky B:** Fabry's Disease: classification as a sphingolipidosis and partial characterization of a novel glycolipid. J Biol Chem 238:3148, 1963

803. **Sweetman L:** Liquid partition chromatography and gas chromatography—mass spectroscopy in identification of acid metabolites of amino acids. In Nyhan WL (ed): Heritable Disorders of Amino Acid Metabolism: Patterns of Clinical Expression and Genetic Variation, pp 730–751. New York, John Wiley & Sons, 1974

804. **Sweetman L, Bates SP, Hull D et al:** Propionyl-CoA carboxylase deficiency in a patient with biotin responsive 3-methylcrotonylglycinuria. Pediatr Res 11:1144, 1977

805. **Sweetman L, Nyhan WL, Trauner DA et al:** Glutaric aciduria type II. J Pediatr 96:1020, 1980

806. **Sweetman L, Weyler W, Shafai T et al:** Prenatal diagnosis of propionic acidemia by organic acid analysis. Clin Res 24:295A, 1976

807. **Tada K, Ito H, Wada Y et al:** Congenital tryptophanuria with dwarfism ("A disease-like clinical feature without indicanuria and generalized aminoaciduria"): a probable new inborn error of tryptophan metabolism. Tohoku J Exp Med 80:118, 1963

808. **Takki K:** Gyrate atrophy of the choroid and retina associated with hyperornithinemia. Br J Ophthalmol 58:3, 1974

809. **Tanaguchi K, Gjessing LI:** Studies on tyrosinosis: 2. Activity of the transaminase, p-hydroxyphenylpyruvate oxidase and homogentisic acid oxidase. Brit Med J 1:968, 1965

810. **Tanaka K, Budd MA, Efron ML et al:** Isovaleric acidemia: a new genetic defect of leucine metabolism. Proc Natl Acad Sci USA 56:236, 1966

811. **Tanaka K, Isselbacher KJ:** The isolation and identification of N-isovalerylglycine from urine of patients with isovaleric acidemia. J Biol Chem 242:2966, 1967

812. **Tang T, Good T, Dyken P et al:** Pathogenesis of Leigh's encephalomyelopathy. J Pediatr 81:189, 1972

813. **Taori GM, Iyer GV, Mokashi S et al:** Sanfilippo syndrome (mucopolysaccharidosis III). J Neurol Sci 17:323, 1972

814. **Tappel AL:** Vitamin E and free radical peroxidation of lipids. Ann NY Acad Sci 293:12, 1972

815. **Tatibana M, Shigisada K:** Two carbamyl phosphate synthetases of mammals: specified roles in control of pyrimidine and urea biosynthesis. Adv Enz Regul 10:249, 1972

816. **Tay W:** Symmetrical changes in the region of the yellow spot in each eye of an infant. Trans Ophthalmol Soc UK, 1:1155, 1881

817. **Taylor HA, Thomas GH, Aylsworth A et al:** Mannosidosis: deficiency of a specific alpha-mannosidase component in cultured fibroblasts. Clin Chim Acta 59:93, 1975

818. **Tedesco TA, Borrow R, Miller K et al:** Galactokinase: evidence for a new racial polymorphism. Science 178:176, 1972

819. **Terplan KL, Caves HL:** Histopathology of the nervous system in carnosinase enzyme deficiency with mental retardation. Neurology (Minneap) 22:644, 1972

820. **Thoene J, Batshaw M, Spector E et al:** Neonatal citrullinemia: treatment with keto-analogues of essential amino acids. J Pediatr 90:218, 1977

821. **Thomas GH, Howell RR:** Arylsulfatase A activity in human urine: quantitative studies on patients with lysosomal disorders including metachromatic leukodystrophy. Clin Chim Acta 36:99, 1972

822. **Thomas GH, Howell RR (eds):** Selected Screening Tests for Genetic Metabolic Diseases, pp 67–72. Chicago, Year Book Medical Publishers, 1973

823. **Tourian AY, Sidbury JB:** Phenylketonuria. In Stanbury JB, Wyngaarden JB, Fredrickson DS (eds): The Metabolic Basis of Inherited Disease, 4th ed. pp 240–255. New York, McGraw-Hill, 1978

824. **Towfighi J, Baird HW, Gambetti P et al:** The significance of cytoplasmic inclusions in late infantile and juvenile amaurotic idiocy. An ultrastructural study. Acta Neuropath 23:32, 1973

825. **Trojak JE, Ho C, Roesel RA et al:** Morquio-like syndrome (MPS IV B) associated with deficiency of a Beta-galactosidase. Johns Hopkins Med J 146:75, 1980

826. **Tu JB, Blackwell RQ:** Studies on levels of penicillamine-induced cupriuresis in heterozygotes of Wilson's disease. Metabolism 16:507, 1967

827. **Turner B, Brown DA:** Amino acid excretion in infancy and early childhood. Med J Aust 1:62, 1962

828. **Uhlendorf BW, Mudd SH:** Cystathionine synthase in tissue culture derived from human skin: enzyme defect in homocystinuria. Science 160:1007, 1968

829. **Ulrich J, Herschkowitz N, Heitz P et al:** Adrenoleukodystrophy. Preliminary report of a connatal case. Light and electron microscopical, immunohistochemical and biochemical findings. Acta Neuropathol (Berl) 43:77, 1978

830. **Upchurch KS, Leyva A, Arnold WF et al:** Hypoxanthine-guanine phosphoribosyl transferase deficiency: association of reduced catalytic activity with reduced levels of immunologically detectable enzyme protein. Proc Natl Acad Sci USA 72:4147, 1975

831. **Uzman LL, Jakus MA:** The Kayser-Fleisher ring. Neurology 7:341, 1957

832. **van Biervliet JPGM, Bruinvis D, Ketting PK et al:** Hereditary mitochondrial myopathy with lactic acidemia, a DeToni-Fanconi-Debre syndrome, and

a defective respiratory chain in voluntary striated muscles. Pediatr Res 11:1088, 1977

833. **van Bogaert L, Scherer HJ, Epstein E:** Une Forme Cerebrale de la Cholesterinose Generalisee. Paris, Masson et Cie, 1937

834. **Van Hoof F, Hers HG:** The ultrastructure of hepatic cells in Hunter's disease (gargoylism). C R Acad Sci (Paris) 259:1281, 1964

835. **Van Hoof F, Hers HG:** Mucopolysaccharidosis by absence of alpha-fucosidase. Lancet 1:1198, 1968

836. **Vanier M-T, Svennerholm L:** Chemical pathology of Krabbe's disease. Part III. Ceramide-hexosides and gangliosides of brain. Acta Paediatr Scand 64:641, 1975

837. **Vanier M-T, Svennerholm L:** Chemical pathology of Krabbe disease: the occurrence of psychosine and other neutral sphingolipids. In Volk BW, Schneck L (eds): Current Trends in Sphingolipidoses and Allied Disorders, p. 115. New York, Plenum Press, 1976

838. **Van Roey A, Wellens W:** Angiokeratoma corporis diffusum van Fabry. Arch Belg Dermatol Syphilig 17:325, 1961

839. **Van Wijngaarden GK, Bethlem J, Meijer AEFH et al:** Skeletal muscle disease with abnormal mitochondria. Brain 90:577, 1967

840. **Vidailhet M, Levin B, Dautravaux M et al:** Citrullinemia. Arch Fr Pediatr 28:521, 1971

841. **Vidgoff J, Lovrien EW, Beals RK et al:** Mannosidosis in three brothers—A review of the literature. Medicine 56:335, 1977

842. **Visakorpi JK:** Citrullinuria. Lancet 1:1357, 1962

843. **Vogel F, Motulsky AG:** Human Genetics. New York, Springer-Verlag, 1979

844. **Vogt H:** Uber familiare amaurotische Idiotie und verwandte Krankheitsbilder. Mschr Psychiat Neurol 18:161, 1905

845. **Volpintesta EJ:** Menkes kinky hair syndrome in a Black infant. Am J Dis Child 128:244, 1974

846. **Von Reuss A:** Zuckerausscheidung im Sauglingsalter. Wien Med Wochenschr 58:799, 1980

847. **Wada Y, Taka K, Minagawa A et al:** Idiopathic hypervalinemia: probably a new entity of inborn error of valine metabolism. Tokohu J Exp Med 81:46, 1963

848. **Wadlington WB, Kilroy A, Ando T et al:** Hyperglycinemia and propionyl CoA carboxylase deficiency and episodic severe illness without consistent ketosis. J Pediatr 86:707, 1975

849. **Wadskov S, Anderson V, Kobayasi T et al:** On the diagnosis of Fabry's disease. Acta Derm Venereol (Stockholm) 55:363, 1975

850. **Waldenstrom J:** The porphyrias as inborn errors of metabolism. Am J Med 22:758, 1957

851. **Walker-Smith JA, Turner B, Blomfield J et al:** Therapeutic implications of copper deficiency in Menkes' steely-hair syndrome. Arch Dis Child 48:958, 1973

852. **Wallace BJ, Kaplan K, Adachi M et al:** Mucopolysaccharidosis type III. Arch Pathol 82:462, 1966

853. **Walsh PJ:** Adrenoleukodystrophy. Report of two cases with relapsing and remitting courses. Arch Neurol 37:448, 1980

854. **Walshe JM:** Wilson's disease: new oral therapy. Lancet 25, 1956

855. **Walshe JM:** Wilson's disease: the presenting symptoms. Arch Dis Child 37:253, 1962

856. **Walshe JM:** Copper chelation in patients with Wilson's disease: a comparison of penicillamine and triethylene tetramine dihydrochloride. Q J Med NS 42:441, 1973

857. **Warburton D, Boyle RJ, Keats JP et al:** Nonketotic hyperglycinemia: effects of therapy with strychnine. Am J Dis Child 134:273, 1980

858. **Ware AJ, Burton WC, McGarry JD et al:** Systemic carnitine deficiency: report of a fatal case with multisystemic manifestations. J Pediatr 93:959, 1978

859. **Warner JO:** Juvenile onset metachromatic leukodystrophy. Failure of response on a low vitamin A diet. Arch Dis Child 50:735, 1975

860. **Watson CW, Nigam MP, Paine RS:** Electroencephalographic abnormalities in phenylpyruvic oligophrenia. Neurology 18:203, 1968

861. **Weisbaum SD, Garnett ES:** Brain scan in Schilder's disease. J Nucl Med 14:291, 1973

862. **Wellner VP, Sekura R, Meister A et al:** Glutathione synthetase deficiency, an inborn error of metabolism involving the gamma-glutamyl cycle in patients with 5-oxoprolinuria (pyroglutamic aciduria). Proc Natl Acad Sci USA 71:2505, 1974

863. **Wendt LV, Simila S, Saukkoren A-L et al:** Failure of strychnine treatment during the neonatal period in three Finnish children with nonketotic hyperglycinemia: effects of therapy with strychnine. Am J Dis Child 134:273, 1980

864. **Wenger DA:** Niemann-Pick Disease. In Glew RH, Peters SP (eds): Practical Enzymology of the Sphingolipidoses, pp 39–70. Alan R Liss, New York, 1977

865. **Wenger DA, Goodman SI, Myers GG:** Beta-galactosidase deficiency in young adults. Lancet 2:1319, 1974

866. **Wenger DA, Sattler M, Mueller OT et al:** Adult G_{M1} gangliosidosis: clinical and biochemical studies on two patients and comparison to other patients called variant or adult G_{M1} gangliosidosis. Clin Genet 17:323, 1980

867. **Werlin SL, Grand RJ, Perman JA et al:** Diagnostic dilemmas of Wilson's disease: diagnosis and treatment. Pediatr 62:47, 1978

868. **Westall RG:** Dietary treatment of a child with maple syrup urine disease (branched-chain ketoaciduria). Arch Dis Child 38:485, 1963

869. **Wheeler EM, Roberts PF:** Menkes's steely hair syndrome. Arch Dis Child 51:269, 1976

870. **Whelan DT, Brusso T, Spate M:** Citrullinemia: phenotypic variants. Pediatr 56:935, 1976

871. **Whelan DT, Hill R, Ryan ED et al:** L-glutaric acidemia: investigation of a patient and his family. Pediatr 63:88, 1979

872. **Wherret JR, Hakomore S-J:** Characterization of a blood group B glycolipid accumulating in the

pancreas of a patient with Fabry's disease. J Biol Chem 248:304 b, 1973

873. **White HH, Rowland LP, Araki S et al:** Homocystinuria. Arch Neurol 13:455, 1966

874. **Whiteman PD, Clayton BE, Ersser RS et al:** Changing incidences of neonatal hypermethionemia: implications for the detection of homocystinuria. Arch Dis Child 54:593, 1979

875. **Wick H, Bachmann C, Baumgartner RL:** Variants of citrullinaemia. Arch Dis Child 48:636, 1973

876. **Wick H, Schweizer K, Baumgartner R:** Thiamine dependency, a patient with congenital lactic acidemia due to pyruvate dehydrogenase deficiency. Agents in Action 7:405, 1977

877. **Wiebers DO, Hollenhorst RW, Goldstein NP:** The ophthalmologic manifestations of Wilson's disease. Mayo Clin Proc 52:409, 1977

878. **Wiesman UN, Lightbody J, Vassella F et al:** Multiple lysosomal enzyme deficiency due to enzyme leakage? N Engl J Med 284:109, 1971

879. **Wiesmann U, Neufeld EF:** Scheie and Hurler Syndromes: apparent identity of the biochemical defect. Science 169:72, 1970

880. **Wilcken B, Kilham HA, Faulk K:** Methylmalonic aciduria: a variant form of methylmalonyl CoA apomutase deficiency. J Pediatr 91:428, 1977

881. **Wilcken B, Yu JS, Brown DA:** Natural history of Hartnup disease. Arch Dis Child 52:38, 1977

882. **Willard HF, Mellman I, Rosenberg LE:** Genetic complementation among inherited deficiencies of methylmalonyl—CoA mutase activity: evidence for a new class of human cobalamin mutant. Amer J Hum Genet 30:1, 1978

883. **Willems JL, Monnens LAH, Trijbels JMF et al:** Leigh's encephalomyelopathy in a patient with cytochrome c oxidase deficiency in muscle tissue. Pediatr 60:850, 1977

884. **Williams RS, Marshall PC, Lott IT et al:** The cellular pathology of Menkes steely hair syndrome. Neurol 28:575, 1978

885. **Wilson SAK:** Progressive lenticular degeneration: a familial nervous disease associated with cirrhosis of the liver. Brain 34:295, 1912

886. **Winters PR, Harrod MJ, Molenich-Heefred SA et al:** alpha-L-Iduronidase deficiency and possible Hurler-Scheie genetic compound. Clinical, pathologic, and biochemical findings. Neurol 26:1003, 1976

887. **Wise D, Wallace HJ, Jellinck EH:** Angiokeratoma corporis diffusium: a clinical study of eight affected families. Am J Med 31:177, 1962

888. **Witzleben CL:** Lymphocyte inclusions in late-onset amaurotic idiocy. Value as a diagnostic test and genetic marker. Neurol 22:1075, 1972

889. **Wolf B, Hsia YE, Tanaka K et al:** Correlation between serum propionate and blood ammonia concentrations in propionic acidemia. J Pediatr 93:471, 1978

890. **Wolf B, Paulsen EP, Hsia YE:** Asymptomatic propionyl-CoA carboxylase deficiency in a 13-year-old girl. J Pediatr 95:563, 1979

891. **Wolf B, Rosenberg LE:** Heterozygote expression in propionyl coenzyme A carboxylase deficiency. J Clin Invest 62:931, 1978

892. **Wolfe HJ, Blennerhasset JB, Young GF et al:** Hurler's syndrome: a histochemical study. New techniques for localization of very water-soluble mucopolysaccharides. Amer J Path 45:1007, 1964

893. **Wolfe HJ, Pietra GG:** The visceral lesions of metachromatic leukodystrophy. Am J Pathol 44:921, 1962

894. **Wolfe OH, Lloyd JK, Tonks EL:** A-beta-lipoproteinaemia with special reference to the visual defect. Exp Eye Res 3:439, 1964

895. **Wong PWK, Pillai PM:** Clinical and biochemical observations in 2 cases of Hartnup disease. Arch Dis Child 41:383, 1966

896. **Woody NC, Snyder CH, Harris JA:** Histidinemia. Am J Dis Child 110:606, 1965

897. **Wray SH, Kuwabara T, Sanderson P:** Menkes' kinky hair disease: a light and electron microscopic study of the eye. Invest Ophthalmol 15:128, 1976

898. **Wysocki SJ, Wilkinson SP, Hahnel R et al:** 3-Hydroxy-3-methylglutaric aciduria, combined with 3-methylglutaconic aciduria. Clin Chim Acta 70:399, 1976

899. **Young E, Wilson J, Patrick AD et al:** Galactocerebrosidase. A deficiency in globoid cell leukodystrophy of late-onset. Arch Dis Child 47:449, 1972

900. **Young ID, Harper PS:** Long-term complications in Hunter's syndrome. Clin Genet 16:125, 1979

901. **Yu JS, Walker-Smith JA, Barnard EB:** Neonatal hepatitis in premature infants simulating hereditary tyrosinosis. Arch Dis Child 46:306, 1971

902. **Yudkoff M, Yang W, Snodgrass PJ et al:** Ornithine transcarbamylase deficiency in a boy with normal development. J Pediatr 96:441, 1980

903. **Yunis EJ, Lee RE:** The ultrastructure of globoid (Krabbe) leukodystrophy. Lab Invest 21:425, 1969

904. **Yutaka T, Fluharty AL, Stevens RL et al:** Iduronate sulfatase analysis of hair roots for identification of Hunter Syndrome heterozygotes. Am J Hum Genet 30:575, 1978

905. **Zeman W:** Presidential address. Studies in the neuronal ceroid-lipofuscinoses. J Neuropathol Exp Neurol 33:1, 1974

906. **Zeman W, Donahue S, Dyken P et al:** The neuronal ceroid-lipofuscinoses (Batten-Vogt syndrome). In Vinken PJ, Bruyn GW (eds): Handbook of Clinical Neurology, Vol 10, pp 588–679. New York, Elsevier Publishing, 1970

907. **Zeman W, Dyken P:** Neuronal ceroid-lipofuscinosis (Batten's disease). Relationship to amaurotic familial idiocy? Pediatr 44:570, 1969

908. **Zipf WB, Hieber V, Allen RJ:** Valine-toxic intermittent maple syrup urine disease: a previously unrecognized variant. Pediatr 63:286, 1979

Nutritional, Vitamin, and Endocrine Disorders

10

Michael J. Bresnan
E. M. Hicks

NUTRITIONAL DISORDERS

MALNUTRITION

The lack of adequate amounts of food, although no longer a significant problem in the United States of America, still accounts for much morbidity and mortality worldwide. Malnutrition is classified according to degree and type.[51] *Kwashiorkor* is the term used for the child who is subject to inadequacy of protein intake but who receives enough calories, and *marasmus* the term for the condition in which the reverse is true. Intermediate states are referred to as *protein-calorie malnutrition*. The neuromuscular system usually shows abnormalities in the acute state, namely, apathy, muscle-wasting and weakness, hypotonia, decreased to absent deep tendon reflexes, and pallor of the disks. General signs include loss or lack of gain in weight, stunted growth, edema, dermatitis, lowered serum proteins, and infection.[15] It is now clear that many of these effects may be severe enough to be permanent despite appropriate refeeding, and this is true for the neurologic aspects as well as the systemic effects. Studies of malnutrition in infancy have to begin with those of pregnant women because the fetus is particularly prone to the effects of malnutrition and its diet is the mother's diet. Malnutrition during the first trimester may cause malformations such as hydrocephalus, anencephaly, and myelomeningocoele. These may be related to specific deficiencies of vitamins or trace elements such as copper, zinc, and manganese. Malnutrition during early brain development has been shown to curtail both protein synthesis and deoxyribonucleic acid (DNA) synthesis, resulting in a permanently stunted brain containing fewer cells of normal size. Later, malnutrition causes a decrease in cell size. Myelination is also impaired by malnutrition occurring during the time that this process is most active. The mechanisms for these changes, as well as their functional significance, is, as yet, unknown. Long-lasting effects on behavior in children suffering from severe malnutrition have also been noted, although it is difficult to separate the many factors operative in these children, such as poor housing, lack of opportunity in education, and so on, which in themselves cause behavioral problems.[17] It seems clear that the earlier the malnutrition occurs, the less likely it is that there will be a full recovery with treatment, and the converse also seems true.

The emergence of various unorthodox diets has made a small but important impact on nutrition. In particular, infants of parents who follow strict vegetarian regimes may be at risk of developing deficiency disorders if their diet is not supplemented.[31] It may be difficult to ensure adequate intake of protein, calories, and especially of some vitamins if a very restricted program is maintained. Vitamins B_{12} and D are of particular concern.[54]

Failure to thrive in infancy and childhood, despite adequate diet, is a common clinical problem in pediatrics, and the underlying causes are many. Of particular interest to the neurologist are those that result from disorders of the brain and neuromuscular system.

Neurologic Causes of Failure to Thrive

Central
  Malformations
  Cerebral palsy
  Mental retardation
  Degenerative disorders
  Toxins, for example, lead
Peripheral
  Decreased intake
    Neuromuscular disorders
    Cerebral palsy
    Mental retardation
    Dementia
    Psychiatric disorders
  Increased loss
    Vomiting (Increased intracranial pressure
      [ICP], tumors, infections)
  Inappropriate use
    Tumors, for example, diencephalic
    Infections
    Inborn errors of metabolism

VITAMINS

Vitamin deficiencies like malnutrition are no longer a major problem in the developed world. This chapter is intended to serve as an outline of neurologic features of vitamin-related disorders. For a full discussion of all aspects of these problems, the reader is referred to a more comprehensive text.[3]

Vitamins are substances present in foods that, in small amounts, are necessary for normal metabolic processes. Three main types of disease are associated with abnormalities of vitamins, namely, deficiency, toxicity, and dependency states. Specific deficiency states have helped identify each vitamin, and characteristic toxicity states exist particularly for the fat-soluble vitamins A and D. Several conditions involving defects in vitamin metabolism have been described. They usually have an autosomal recessive mode of inheritance, and are often serious, sometimes lethal, disorders that may respond to large doses of vitamin.[41] Among these so-called vitamin-dependency states are several with neurologic implications involving deficits in the metabolism of vitamins B_1, B_6, B_{12}, folate, biotin, and niacin.

Vitamin A

Vitamin A is a fat-soluble vitamin, wholly of animal origin, and found in milk, eggs, and animal fats, especially fish liver oils. It is essential for maintenance of normal growth and integrity of epithelial tissues, and for normal retinal function. Daily requirement is 1500 international units IU during the first year of life increasing to 5000 IU during adolescence. Deficiency of vitamin A is manifested early by night blindness (nyctalopia), then by squamous metaplasia and keratinization of epithelium and endothelium throughout the body, causing xerophthalmia and keratomalacia of the cornea. Bitot's spots appear on the bulbar conjunctiva, and the skin shows follicular hyperkeratosis. In infants, mental and physical retardation may occur, as well as anemia, hepatosplenomegaly, cranial nerve palsies, neck and back stiffness, and raised intracranial pressure probably related to changes in arachnoid villi.

Toxicity due to excessive ingestion may be acute or chronic. Acute hypervitaminosis A may occur in infants following ingestion of 300,000 IU or more, and presents with an acute encephalopathic picture of pseudotumor cerebri. The symptoms and

Disease	Untreated Clinical State	Vitamin
Maple syrup urine disease	Hypotonia, ataxia, seizures, death	B_1
Hyperpyruvic acidaemia	Ataxia, retardation	B_1
Homocystinuria	Marfanoid habitus, retardation, thrombosis, ectopia lentis	B_6, folate
Pyridoxine dependency	Intractible neonatal seizures	B_6
Xanthenuric aciduria	Retardation	B_6
Formiminotransferase	Retardation	Folate
Methylmalonic aciduria	Retardation	B_{12}
β-Methylcrotonyl glycinuria	Lethargy, coma	Biotin
Hartnup Disease	Pellagralike rash, ataxia, retardation	Niacin

signs include nausea, vomiting, drowsiness, bulging fontanelle, papilledema, diplopia, and strabismus. These findings may suggest intracranial tumor. Venous occlusion and arachnoid villi changes are likely causes. The latter syndrome also occurs in chronic, excessive vitamin A ingestion, resulting from doses such as 20,000 to 50,000 IU daily for several weeks or months. Other features include skin-itching and desquamation, hair loss, hepatomegaly, and subperiosteal hyperostosis.

Vitamin B-complex

The B-complex vitamins are water-soluble substances that are chemically unrelated, but are often found together in foodstuffs. Those of neurologic significance are thiamine or B_1, pyridoxine or B_6, B_{12}, niacin, and folate.

Vitamin B_1 or Thiamine

Thiamine deficiency causes beri-beri, a disease now rare in the United States and Europe except in alcoholics. It is seen where polished rice is a staple of the diet, and therefore, could occur as part of a food faddism. Beri-beri occurs in three forms: wet, dry, and mixed. Wet beri-beri is so-called because of the predominant features that are secondary to cardiac failure of high-output type. Symptoms and signs of neuropathy may also be present, but are less common in children than adults. These include paresthesias, hyperesthesias with pain and burning of the feet, muscle atrophy, ataxia and loss of deep sensation, followed by signs of increased intracranial pressure, meningismus, and finally coma. Dry beri-beri is an ascending, bilateral, usually symmetric polyneuropathy with tenderness of muscles, anesthesia, and loss of vibratory sense. The patellar and Achilles tendon jerks, initially hyperactive, become hypoactive, and footdrop occurs causing a "steppage" gait. There may be painful burning of the soles of the feet, nystagmus, ptosis, optic atrophy, and laryngeal nerve paresis causing hoarseness. In the infant anorexia, hypotonia, and retarded growth are frequent features.

Wernicke's encephalopathy, found particularly in alcoholics, may occur in infants in whom it takes a pseudoencephalitic form with ataxia, various ophthalmoplegias, and peripheral neuropathy. Pathologically, the brain shows changes in small vessels, swollen and pyknotic nerve cells, and occasional petechial hemorrhages in the walls of the third and fourth ventricles, periaqueductal gray matter (especially the nuclei of the third, fourth, and other cranial nerves), and the corpora quadrigemina, dentate, and olivary nuclei. The mamillary bodies are characteristically spared in children.

Leigh's Disease, a subacute necrotizing encephalomyelopathy, is an inborn error of thiamine metabolism inherited as an autosomal recessive trait, which shows pathologic changes similar to Wernicke's encephalopathy. The clinical syndrome is variable, but most affected children manifest as progressive neurologic disorders with seizures, impairment of intellect, and signs of brain stem dysfunction, including ophthalmoplegias and cardiorespiratory irregularities.[37] Alterations in muscle tone and tendon reflexes, and extrapyramidal movement disorders may be prominent. Diagnosis rests on demonstration of abnormalities of thiamine metabolism, that is, increased pyruvate and lactate in blood and the presence of a thiamine triphosphate (TTP) inhibitor in urine.[38] Treatment is rarely successful in preventing deterioration, although large doses of thiamine may benefit some patients. Since the disease often shows a spontaneously remitting–relapsing course, the effects of therapy are difficult to evaluate.

Niacin

Deficiency of niacin causes pellagra, which as recently as 1930 was still common in some of the southern states, especially where corn or maize formed the dietary staple. The disease manifests as a classic triad of dermatitis, diarrhea, and dementia. The dermatitis is a photosensitive, itching, vesicular eruption that causes desquamation and healing with dyspigmentation. Almost all patients have foul-smelling, watery diarrhea, and in children with concurrent parasitic infestations, the disease is particularly severe. Nervous system manifestations include insomnia, irritability progressing to tremor, jerky movements, and rigidity. Numbness of the extremities is followed by paralysis with apparent insanity. Pathologically, changes in the nervous system occur late in the disease, and consist of patchy areas of demyelination and degeneration of the ganglion cells, including those of the spinal cord. Diagnosis is made by obtaining an appropriate dietary history, and by rapid clinical response to niacin administration.

Vitamin B₆ or Pyridoxine

Deficiency of pyridoxine is very rare owing to its widespread presence in many foodstuffs, but has been described in several clinical situations. Of relevance to this chapter is the occurrence of infantile convulsions when a vitamin B_6-deficient formula is fed.[33] Infants develop irritability, generalized seizures, intestinal colic, and an increased startle response. The symptoms respond to the addition of physiological doses of B_6 to the formula.

Peripheral neuropathy occurs in B_6-deficient states, the most common situation being individuals treated for tuberculosis with isonicotinic acid hydrazide (INH), a B_6 antagonist that binds pyridoxal-5-phosphate. The neuropathy is less common in children so treated than in adults and can be prevented by prophylactic administration of pyridoxine. A similar problem can occur in children taking penicillamine, for example, for Wilson's disease.

A vitamin B_6-dependency state exists that causes severe seizures in the neonate (first month of life). This is considered to be an autosomal recessive condition in which the exact biochemical abnormality is still uncertain.[23] The seizures respond to maintenance pharmocologic doses of pyridoxine (10 mg–25 mg par os (po) daily). The mechanism of seizure production is thought to be due to decreased synthesis of gamma-amino butyric acid (GABA) because B_6 is necessary for its manufacture.[33] Gamma-aminobutyric acid is a central synaptic inhibitor that acts on post-synaptic transmission, and decreased GABA availability leads to seizures. Infants with B_6-dependency seizures usually have refractive generalized and myoclonic convulsions from early in life, and the electro-

encephalogram is generally markedly abnormal, occasionally hypsarrhythmic. Diagnosis may be made by seeing a normalization of the electroencephalogram (EEG) tracing when pyridoxine is given intravenously in large doses (50 mg).

Folic Acid

Folic acid deficiency is not associated with neurologic disorders, but some children with inborn errors of folate metabolism show mental retardation as part of the dependency state. Folate may be necessary for brain myelinization. Serum and cerebrospinal fluid folate levels are approximately 50% of normal in patients on phenytoin and other related anticonvulsants.[26] This may be related to the increased incidence of birth defects in the offspring of pregnant epileptics (fetal hydantoin syndrome). For this reason very early treatment with folate is suggested in pregnancy complicated by epilepsy and anticonvulsants.

Vitamin B₁₂

Clinically, two features of vitamin B_{12}-deficiency are important, namely, pernicious anemia and combined system disease. The latter is a B_{12}-deficient neuropathy that, in childhood, occurs only in the presence of megaloblastic anemia. Pernicious anemia is uncommon in childhood, but neurologic abnormalities occur in approximately one-third of these children, taking the form of numbness and weakness of the extremities, loss of vibration sense, reflex changes, and ataxia.[36] Secondary B_{12} deficiency occurs in disorders of the terminal ileum including operative resection, in children with blind-loop syndromes, and in cases of infestation with the fish tapeworm *Diphyllobothrium latum*. Neurologic involvement is less common in these secondary B_{12}-deficiency states.

Vitamin D

This fat-soluble vitamin is essential for normal calcium and phosphorus metabolism.[12] It is derived from two main sources, ingested ergocalciferol (D2) and cholecalciferol (D3) produced in the skin by ultraviolet irradiation and converted to 7-dehydrocholesterol. Both forms undergo transformation in the liver to 25-hydroxy forms, and further alteration takes place in the kidney to the active form of the vitamin, 1,25-dihydroxycholecalciferol. Vitamin D deficiency in childhood is called *rickets*, and may be dietary in origin or secondary to other disease states. In infancy the disorder in calcium metabolism causes softening in many bones; in the skull this is called *craniotabes*. Such a finding can be physiologic in the first 3 months, and can also occur in hydrocephalus and osteogenesis imperfecta. Muscle weakness and hypotonia occur, and are the likely cause of the delay in standing and walking seen in these children, and also of the abdominal distension frequently seen. The serum calcium is maintained at normal levels until late in the disease, but when it falls to 7.5 mg/dl or less, muscular irritability increases and tetany may occur. Trousseau's and Chvostek's signs may be elicitable, and carpopedal spasm, laryngospasm, and seizures may be evident.

Metabolic bone disease may be associated with long-term anticonvulsant usage, phenytoin, phenobarbital, and primidone being the main drugs implicated.[26] Radiograms may show bony changes of rickets, a lowered (5%–10%) serum level of calcium, and marked elevation of alkaline phosphatase. The changes are considered to be due to anticonvulsant drug induction of hepatic enzymes involved in vitamin D metabolism with accelerated turnover to inactive products. Treatment is to administer vitamin D, usually in higher doses than for dietary deficiency. It has been suggested that all epileptic children requiring chronic anticonvulsant medication should receive vitamin D supplementation, but this does not seem necessary. Most likely to be affected are those who are black, retarded, institutionalized, have poor diets, or little exposure to sunlight.

Excessive ingestion of vitamin D causes signs and symptoms of hypercalcemia, namely, hypotonia, anorexia, irritability, poor concentrating power, constipation, polydipsia, and polyuria. Pallor, vomiting, hypertension, retinopathy, clouding of the cornea and conjunctiva, and metastatic calcification in the kidneysa and other organs may develop. Treatment is by withdrawal of the vitamin, and in severe cases, corticosteroids may be used.[7]

Pseudotumor Cerebri or Benign Intracranial Hypertension

Pseudotumor cerebri is characterized by signs of ICP, typically headache and papilledema, but without focal neurologic signs.[4,21] A sixth nerve palsy is common and causes diplopia, but is a non-localizing sign due to the diffusely raised pressure, and its effect on the path of exit of that cranial nerve. In all cases, pseudotumor is a diagnosis of exclusion.[52] A true intracranial tumor, often in the midline, either supra- or infratentorial, can easily produce these signs by blocking cerebrospinal fluid (CSF) circulation. Similarly, other causes of CSF obstruction must be ruled out, for example, aqueductal stenosis. A low-grade meningeal infection with blockage, or a brain abscess in a clinically silent area, for example, the frontal lobe, might have similar symptoms and signs without focality.

Careful initial and serial visual examinations are important. Typically, there is enlargement of the blind spot that may merge into a scotoma with decreased visual acuity and ultimately blindness if untreated.

Computed tomography scanning has dramatically changed the workup in this syndrome and has obviated the necessity for other radiological studies, for example, arteriography or air studies.[50] The skull x-ray film may show signs of pressure such as split sutures and an enlarged, thinned sella. In the face of a normal CT scan, the diagnosis is confirmed by the presence of increased pressure with normal CSF composition.

Once the diagnosis has been established, a search should be made for known causes[4,21]

Venous sinus occlusion; Otitis–Mastoiditis; trauma to head or neck

Endocrine: Addison's disease, steroid withdrawal; hypoparathyroidism; obesity and menstrual irregularities (empty-sella syndrome; pregnancy, contraceptives)

Drugs: Vitamin A, hyper- and hypovitaminosis; tetracycline; nalidixic acid

Hematologic: Anemia, infectious mononucleosis; Wiskott-Aldrich syndrome

Idiopathic: In infancy a period of rapid growth after deprivation and malnutrition

Occasionally a child presenting with headache, papilledema, and no signs will be suspected to have pseudotumor, but will have normal pressure at lumbar puncture. Such children may have instead pseudo-papilledema, which is usually caused by a drusen in the optic nerve. Drusens are not as obvious on funduscopic examination in childhood as they are in adulthood. Examination of the parents' and siblings' fundi can be very revealing and reassuring because drusen are often familial. In cases with residual concern, true papilledema can be distinguished from pseudopapilledema by the presence of leakage of dye about the disk with fluoroscein angiography.

Cases related to venous sinus obstruction are particularly common in childhood and used to be called "otitic hydrocephalus." Sinus obstruction in cases not related to ear and mastoid infections will be missed by all studies short of angiography with delayed venous pictures or direct jugular venography. In most other cases, the block is postulated to be at the arachnoid villae, for example, vitamin A.[43]

In cases without specific etiologies, and, therefore, without specific treatments, serial lumbar punctures are necessary to lower the pressure and preserve vision, the one system subject to damage in this syndrome. In childhood, the pressure usually drops after two or three taps. Rarely does the increased pressure persist. In such cases, acetazolamide, or subsequently furosemide can be used to decrease CSF production. If these drugs fail, dexamethasone can be used, often successfully.[52] In the rarest of cases, a lumboperitoneal shunt will have to be placed as a sight-saving procedure.[50]

NEUROENDOCRINOLOGY

It is no longer possible to discuss the hypophysis (pituitary) in isolation. Although previously thought to be the conductor of the endocrine orchestra, it is now clear that the hypothalamus is the primary site of neuroendocrine control and that it is more appropriate to talk of the hypothalamic–hypophysial system. Embryologically the neurohypophysis (posterior pituitary) develops as an outpouching of the floor of the third ventricle, the future hypothalamus.

The supraoptic, paraventricular, and tuberal nuclei of the hypothalamus are connected by their nerve fibers to the neurohypophysis. The adenohypophysis (anterior pituitary) originates in the ectoderm of the roof of the mouth as Rathke's pouch and migrates upward to envelope the neurohypophysis anteriorly. There it becomes related to the hypothalamus by a vascular portal system. The combined gland, the pituitary or hypophysis, is anatomically situated in the sella turcica. These close anatomical quarters and the intimate relationships of the hypothalamus, hypophysis, optic nerves, third ventricle, cavernous sinus, and oculomotor nerves (third, fourth, sixth) explain the plethora of clinical signs associated with relatively small lesions in this area.[22,32]

ADENOHYPOPHYSIS OR ANTERIOR PITUITARY

The adenohypophysial system consists of neurons in the ventral hypothalamus that produce the various hypophysiotropic (releasing) factors, the portal system that carries them through the pituitary stalk, and the adenohypophysial parenchymal cells that synthesize and store the hormones that on release control the growth and activity of the endocrine glands. The eosinophilic (acidophilic) cells contain growth hormone (GH) and prolactin. The basophilic cells contain adrenocorticotrophic hormone (ACTH), melanocyte-stimulating hormone (MSH), beta-lipotropin, thyroid-stimulating hormone (TSH), luteinizing hormone (LH), and follicle-stimulating hormone (FSH). Chromophobe cells are thought of as inactive but do secrete, especially prolactin, but also GH, ACTH, TSH, FSH when tumorous. The complex interactions between neurologic input, serum levels, and releasing factors in the hypothalamus and the release of hormones in the pituitary have been well reviewed.[35] Figure 10-1 is a simplified schematic representation of the hypothalamic–hypophysial system and some of its controls.

Diseases affecting the anterior pituitary in childhood almost invariably affect the hypothalamus; therefore they are best thought of as hypothalamic–anterior pituitary diseases.[9] Many also involve the posterior pituitary (*vide infra*).

Clinical Hypothalamic—Anterior Pituitary Disorders in Childhood

I. **Developmental**
   A. Congenital
      Aplasia, anencephaly
      Holoprosencephaly
      Cleft lip and palate
      Septo-optic dysplasia (deMorsier's syndrome)
      Kallmann's syndrome (probable X-linkage with anosmia, hypogonadism)
      Aicardi's syndrome (affects females, agenesis of corpus collosum with retinal colobomas)
   B. Idiopathic
      Isolated specific pituitary hormone deficiencies

II. **Acquired**
   A. Primary Brain Tumors
      Craniopharyngioma
      Astrocytomas of third ventricle (diencephalic syndrome)
      Optic chiasm gliomas (neurofibromatosis)
      Pinealomas, ectopic pineolomas, dysgerminomas
      Hamartomas (neurofibromatosis)
      Pituitary adenomas (very rare under 10 years of age), usually eosinophilic, with gigantism, acromegaly
   B. Infiltrative
      Histiocytosis X, leukemia, granulomatous
   C. Vascular
      Carotid aneurysm, hemorrhage
   D. Trauma
      Birth trauma (breech), head trauma
   E. Iatrogenic
      Surgical, irradiation

III. **Miscellaneous**
   A. Empty sella syndrome, benign intracranial hypertension pseudotumor
   B. Laurence-Moon-Bardet-Biedl syndrome, associated with retinitis pigmentosa and mental retardation
   C. Polyostotic fibrous dysplasia (Albright's syndrome)
   D. Familial dysautonomia (Riley-Day syndrome)
   E. Cerebral gigantism (Sotos syndrome)
   F. Ataxia telangiectasia
   G. Prader-Willi syndrome (hypogonadism, hypomentia, hypotonia, obesity)

The clinical signs of these diseases may involve abnormalities of the optic chiasm and nerves with visual field defects and also oculomotor palsies. With greater extension signs of third ventricular blockage and intracranial pressure may result. Their workup requires a combination of endocrine tests and careful ophthalmologic and visual field examination. X-ray studies including tomography, CT scanning with intravenous contrast and CSF contrast injection, angiography, and pneumoencephalography should be performed, as indicated.

Treatment of these conditions includes hormone replacement and specific treatment of the underlying cause, especially with tumors. The surgical approach can be either intracranial or transsphenoidal. Unfortunately such approaches almost invariably increase the endocrine deficit. X-irradiation can be used as a primary therapy in some tumors and as an adjunct to surgery in others.[48] Irradiation is less likely to increase endocrine deficits and may indeed restore normal function in hypersecretion states.

NEUROHYPOPHYSIS OR POSTERIOR PITUITARY

Antidiuretic Hormone or Vasopressin

The neurohypophyseal system consists of hypothalamic magnocellular neurosecretory neurons situated in the supraoptic and paraventricular nuclei that are responsible for the production, storage, and release of antidiuretic hormone (ADH), and their axons that terminate in the posterior pituitary (neurohypophysis.)[53] The hormones (neurosecretory granules) produced in the hypothalamus are carried down the axons to their terminal storage sites in the pituitary. The release of ADH is mainly controlled by osmoreceptors in the anterior hypothalamus and preoptic area. But nonosmotic stimuli including hypotension, pain, psychosis, temperature, drugs, hypoxia–hypercapnea (chemoreceptors), and blood volume (cardiovascular baroreceptors, renin-angiotensin systems) are also involved. Hormone release is the result of the sum of competing stimulatory and inhibitory impulses. The actual stored hormone is released into the systemic venous system by exocytosis.

Diabetes Insipidus

Diabetes insipidus (DI) is due to a deficiency of ADH which results in the failure of renal conservation of free water. Simple damage of the posterior pituitary alone will not produce permanent DI. Such DI, which

Causes of Diabetes Insipidus

1. Idiopathic, congenital, familial (both autosomal dominant and X-linked recessive)
2. Tumors, supra- and intrasellar, the latter involving the hypothalamus, craniopharyngioma, pinealoma, astrocytoma of third ventricle, leukemia
3. Post-hypophysectomy (iatrogenic), by surgery or irradiation
4. Basal skull fractures
5. Histiocytosis X
6. Granulomatous diseases
7. Vascular malformation or aneurysm
8. Acute infection, for example, meningitis, encephalitis
9. Hemorrhage, pituitary apoplexy, intraventricular hemorrhage

is neurogenic, is ADH-sensitive as opposed to nephrogenic DI, which is the result of end-organ unresponsiveness. Acquired neurogenic DI, for example, neurosurgical DI, may have a triphasic pattern of onset with an initial polyuric polydipsic syndrome, as if there is hypothalamic shock, then a period of return toward normal urinary volumes and concentrations that can still, however, be offset by a water load resulting in water intoxication and hyponatremia. Assumedly this phase is the result of the release of whatever stored ADH remains. Thereafter DI reappears that may be temporary or permanent, partial or complete, depending on the extent of damage to the hypothalamus.

Diagnosis and Treatment. Polyuria, especially nocturnal, polydipsia, normal blood chemistries, mild plasma hyperosmolality, and low urine specific gravity are the typical clinical findings. The diagnosis is confirmed by the lack of antidiuresis in response to extremely carefully controlled water restriction in older children, by the failure of antidiuresis to develop during the infusion of hypertonic saline solution and by the response to exogenous ADH (vasopressin).

Treatment is by replacement of ADH most commonly by the synthetic analogue 1, desamino, 8-D-arginine vasopressin (d DAVP) administered transnasally.

Syndrome of Inappropriate Secretion of Antidiuretic Hormone

A syndrome of inappropriate secretion of ADH (SIADH) is a common complication of a number of pediatric illnesses and surgical procedures. Neurologic conditions causing the syndrome include meningitis, encephalitis, polyneuritis (Guillain-Barré), brain tumors, brain abscesses, subdural hematomas, and seizures in which it may be related to barbiturates and carbamazepine (Tegretol). Headache, lethargy, confusion, stupor, coma, and seizures, focal or generalized, result, and the serum sodium is usually less than 120 mEq/liter. It is corrected by water restriction occasionally supplemented by hypertonic saline or mannitol depending on the severity of symptoms and signs.

Oxytocin, which has a similar neuroregulatory system to ADH, has no clinical relevance in childhood.

ENDORPHINS

Currently there is great interest in several polypeptide hormones found in brains and pituitary glands. They are called *endorphins* and have effects similar to opiate alkaloids, the effects being rapidly reversible by opiate antagonists such as naloxone. They also modify mood and behavior. They have in common the protein β-lipotropin and are synthesized in conjunction with ACTH. Although the endorphins are an exciting development, their place in clinical neuroendocrinology and disease is undetermined.[22,25]

PINEAL GLAND

Although the pineal gland has no currently recognized normal function in man it is likely to have some neuroendocrine function.[32] In childhood it can be the site of tumors that cause endocrine malfunction. The cells of the pineal, pinealocytes and glia, can cause primary tumors that may stay

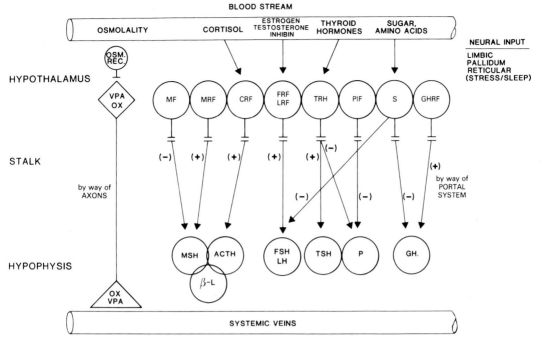

FIG. 10-1. A schematic representation of the hypothalamic–hypophyseal system, and some of its controls.

localized and by exerting pressure on the collicular area, cause Parinaud's syndrome, that is, difficulty with upward gaze, unreactive pupils, and hydrocephalus secondary to aqueductal blockage. If the tumor invades, or originates in the third ventricular area it may interfere with hormonal regulation centers in the hypothalmus and lead to precocious puberty. These tumors are rarely removable neurosurgically and are treated by shunting and irradiation.

The pineal gland, and the paraventricular area, as well as the testis and anterior chest, are occasionally the sites of embryonic rests, which contain undifferentiated germ cells, and which develop into tumors called *dysgerminomas*. These produce all the signs of a pineal tumor. In addition they produce DI, hypogonadism, and ocular abnormalities because of hypothalamic invasion and blockage of the posterior third ventricle. They may also secrete human chorionic gonadotropin (HCG), which can mimic puberty, and occasionally alpha-fetoprotein (AFP). They have a tendency to seed by way of the CSF throughout the neuraxis. Surgical approaches should be avoided in favor of irradiation, to which they are quite sensitive.

Key: Osm. = Osmoreceptors
Rec.

VPA = Vasopressin (ADH)

OX = Oxytocin

MIF = Melanophoretic Inhibiting Factor

MRF = Melanophoretic Releasing Factor

MSH = Melanocyte Stimulating Hormone

CRF = Corticotropin Releasing Factor

ACTH = Adrenocirticotrophic Hormone

β-L = β-Lipotropin

FRF, = Follicle Releasing Factor and
LRF   Luteinizing Hormone Releasing Factor

FSH, LH = Follicle Stimulating Hormone and Luteinizing Hormone

TRH = Thyrotropin Releasing Hormone

TSH = Thyroid Stimulating Hormone

PIF = Prolactin Inhibiting Factor

P = Prolactin

S = Somatostatin

GHRF = Growth Hormone (Somatotropin) Releasing Factor

GH = Growth Hormone

ENDOCRINE DISORDERS

This section is intended as a review of the neurologic problems encountered in patients with endocrinological diseases, and not as an exhaustive review of endocrinology. For further details, the reader is referred to more comprehensive texts.[5,13]

ADRENAL

The adrenal cortex is divided into three zones of cells: the outer zona glomerulosa, the middle zona fasciculata, and the inner zona reticularis, which lies closest to the medulla. Aldosterone is secreted by the zona glomerulosa, the inner two layers producing glucocorticoids and adrenal androgens.

Glucocorticoid excess results in Cushing's syndrome, a disorder that is rare in children, the most common variant being secondary to steroid therapy, iatrogenic Cushing's syndrome.[24] The most common primary cause in children under the age of 7 years is adrenal tumor (65%), rather than bilateral hyperplasia, which is the most common cause in adults and older children. The hyperplasia can be autonomous, but often will be secondary to increased hypothalamic secretion (70%). The clinical features include obesity with growth retardation (as opposed to dietary obesity in which linear growth is typically accelerated), muscular weakness, thinning of the skin causing purple striae, osteoporosis and delayed epiphyseal maturation, impaired carbohydrate intolerance, hypertension, and headaches. Many children with Cushing's syndrome also exhibit virilization, hirsutism, and acne. Laboratory tests show hypokalemic metabolism alkalosis. Plasma cortisol levels are usually high with loss of diurnal variation, and absence of suppression on dexamethasone administration.

Identification of the source of the hypersecretion may be possible with plain tomography and computerized tomography, both of the sella turcica and the adrenals, thus eliminating the necessity in many cases for more invasive radiologic techniques.[10]

The weakness in Cushing's syndrome has been shown to be due to a true myopathy, which is characteristically of proximal predominance with the lower limbs especially affected.[39] Atrophy of skeletal muscles may be apparent on limb radiographs.[11] Myopathy secondary to ingested glucocorticoids has been demonstrated in children taking steroids for dermatomyositis.[14]

Treatment of Cushing's syndrome depends on the underlying cause. Surgery may be undertaken for pituitary or adrenal tumor, and for bilateral adrenal hyperplasia. In the latter instance, there is a significant incidence of postoperative emergence of a pituitary microadenoma that manifests as hyperpigmentation (Nelson's syndrome). Chemicals such as aminoglutethimide and mitotane may be indicated in some instances to suppress hypercortisolism.

Adrenal Cortical Insufficiency

Acute adrenocortical failure may be due to a number of causes including hemorrhage and fulminating septicemia, and presents as a shocklike state that is rapidly fatal unless promptly treated. Chronic adrenocortical insufficiency of Addison's disease may be due to tuberculosis, autoimmune destruction of the glands, or in a significant number of affected males, to an association with a demyelinating disorder of the nervous system, adrenoleukodystrophy (ALD). Adrenal failure may also be secondary to hypopituitarism.[24]

Addison's Disease

In the original description of this disorder, the patients had tuberculous destruction of the adrenal glands, an uncommon cause of Addison's disease in the United States today. An autoimmune phenomenon is now the most frequent underlying disease. In some cases, there may be a familial incidence, and it can occur in association with other autoimmune endocrinopathies producing multiple endocrine deficiency. The outstanding features of this disorder are progressive weakness and hyperpigmentation, and despite the former feature, no pathologic abnormality of muscle has been described. Laboratory diagnosis rests on demonstration of hyponatremia, hyperkalemia, and often, a low blood glucose. Adrenocorticotropic hormone levels are high, unless hypopituitarism is the underlying cause.

Therapy consists of treatment of the underlying cause if it is tuberculosis (TB) and replacement of glucocorticoids and mineralocorticoids.

Adrenoleukodystrophy (ALD) is a familial condition that is inherited in a sex-linked recessive manner. The onset is usually in the first two decades of life, and the disease is relentless to death. Early features are neurologic, and include behavioral changes, school difficulties, abnormalities of gait, dysphasia, visual disorders, and seizures.[6,44] There is often an asymmetry of onset suggesting tumor, which may be misleading. Ultimately all patients develop a progressive spastic quadriparesis with decorticate posturing, visual field defects, optic atrophy, nystagmus, and occasionally deafness. The CT scan is particularly useful in delineating the demyelination.[34] Characteristic signs of adrenocortical insufficiency may be lacking, but in a few cases, they antedate the neurologic illness. Biochemical evidence of glucocorticoid deficiency can occasionally be demonstrated, that is, hyponatremia, hyperkalemia, and metabolic acidosis with low serum cortisol in the face of high ACTH levels. A lack of adrenal response to injected ACTH can be demonstrated, and is a useful confirmatory test. The best single test in ALD is skin biopsy with demonstration of elevated C_{26} fatty acids in fibroblasts.[34] Cerebral biopsy from an affected region shows demyelination. Characteristically, the brain at autopsy shows loss of white matter (which spreads in a typical caudal–rostral direction) with sparing of the subcortical regions. Ultrastructural cytoplasmic inclusions similar to those seen in the adrenal gland may be present, suggesting a common metabolic disorder.

Conn's Syndrome

Conn's syndrome of mineralocorticoid excess, or hyperaldosteronism, is rare in childhood. In the original description episodes of muscular weakness were noted, presumably due to hypokalemia, although the low potassium persists between attacks. Other symptoms and signs include headache, hypertension, polyuria, paresthesias, and alkalosis. Affected children often have severe hypertension and retinopathy, but less marked muscle weakness than adults.

The usual etiology in childhood is idiopathic benign hyperplasia, although secondary hyperaldosteronism may occur more often. Aldosterone-producing adenomas are very rare in childhood.

Pheochromocytoma

This neoplasm of chromaffin tissue is uncommon in childhood. Its association with neurofibromatosis is well recognized as is its association with other autosomal dominant syndromes, for example, multiple endocrine adenomatosis (MEA), Type II (Sipple's syndrome), and Type III (mucosal neuromas syndrome).[28] (See list, Multiple Endocrine Adenomatosis Syndromes.) In such cases, the tumor may be bilateral. Another phakomatosis, von Hippel-Lindau disease (retinal cerebellar hemangioblastoma), also has an increased incidence of pheochromocytoma. The most common presenting features are headaches and hypertension, visual blurring, and sweating.[46] Diagnosis is made by finding both raised urinary vanillylmandelic acid (VMA) and catecholamines. Intravenous pyelography with tomography and angiography may be superceded by computerized tomography as an aid to tumor localization. Careful preoperative preparation with alpha-sympathetic blockade and stabilization of circu-

Multiple Endocrine Adenomatosis Syndromes

Type I, Wermer
Autosomal dominant
Anterior pituitary tumors
Hyperparathyroidism
Pancreatic islet cell tumors
  Insulinoma
  Glucogonoma
Zollinger-Ellison syndrome (peptic ulcers)

Type II, Sipple
Autosomal dominant
Medullary thyroid carcinoma
Hyperparathyroidism
Pheochromocytoma (bilateral)

Type III, Multiple Mucosal Neuroma Syndrome
Autosomal dominant/sporadic
medullary thyroid carcinoma (CA)
Pheochromocytoma (bilateral)
Marfanoid habitus
Mucosal neuromas
Dysmorphic face, lips, and eyes
Neuromas of tongue, buccal muscosa, eyes, and
  gastrointestinal tract

lating blood volume is necessary, and controlled anesthesia is essential for low morbidity and mortality. Tumor may occur anywhere along the sympathetic chain, although in childhood the great majority arise from the adrenal medulla, and may be multiple. They are usually benign in childhood, but prolonged follow-up is essential.

THYROID GLAND

Disorders of thyroid function, both hypo- and hyperthyroidism, are common pediatric problems, and because the actions of thyroid hormones are ubiquitous, neurologic symptoms may be the mode of presentation in each.[18,20,27]

Thyroid Development

The fetus is free of maternal influence, that is, maternal thyroid hormones do not cross the placental barrier. The hypothalamic regulatory system (thyrotropin releasing hormone [TRH], thyroid stimulating hormone [TSH]) develops independently of the thyroid gland. When pituitary portal vascular connections are established, the thyroid then comes under pituitary control. By understanding this sequence, it is possible to divide the congenital–neonatal dysfunctions according to ontogenesis.

Phase I: Embryogenesis
             (a) Thyroid
                 Agenesis, hypoplasia, ectopy, dishormonogenesis
             (b) Pituitary
                 Aplasia, hypoplasia, decreased TSH
Phase II: Hypothalamic maturation
             Dysplasia, decreased TRH
             May be associated with midline defects, cleft lip–palate, septo-optic dysplasia
Phase III: Thyroid system malfunctions
             Transient hypothyroidism in prematures (decreased thyroxine T_4, increased TSH)
             Transient hypothyroxinemia in prematures (de-

creased T_4, normal TSH)
             Antithyroid compounds
             Iodine abnormalities (deficiency, excess)
             Thyroxine–binding globulin (TBG) abnormalities
             Peripheral thyroid hormone unresponsiveness

Neonatal screening programs indicate an incidence of hypothyroidism of approximately 1 in 4000 live births, which makes it a very common problem, more common than many other diseases included in neonatal screening programs. Only 5% of such affected infants have been clinically suspect. With the strong evidence that early treatment is important, the value of such screening can not be overemphasized.

Because the fetus is dependent on its own thyroid production, the extent of the intrauterine deficiency state in hypothyroidism plays some part in prognosis. Neuropathologic studies have shown a decrease in all cellular elements without gliosis. In the experimental animal, there is a reduction in the number and size of neurons in the cerebral cortex and cerebellum, decreased axonal and dendritic arborizations and connections in addition to delayed myelination.[2,42]

Hypothyroidism

The hypothyroid neonate looks normal. There is a tendency to postmaturity, high birth weight, and prolonged jaundice. Later, hypotonia, umbilical hernia, large anterior and posterior fontanelles, macroglossia, and slowed deep tendon reflexes should make one suspicious. Considering the incidence of hypothyroidism, a thyroid screen is probably more important than an amino acid screen in the infant and child presenting with developmental delay, especially when early treatment is so important.

Hypothyroidism developing in childhood and adolescence is most frequently from thyroiditis and is usually insidious in onset. In early childhood, there may be delayed development and a slowing growth rate. Such children (1 year–3 years of age) may represent patients with congenital illness who are outgrowing their hypoplastic thyroid gland production. In later childhood school problems, cold intolerance, and later, in both ages, the obvious signs of myxedema with puffiness, pallor, dry, carotinemic skin, and thin hair become evident. A short, stocky habitus with apparent muscle hypertrophy may be seen ("infant Hercules"), and is called the *Kocher-Debré, Sémélaigne syndrome.* Muscle biopsy can show Type I fiber atrophy, abnormal glycogen collections, and distention of the sarcoplasmic reticulum.[45] The condition is reversible by treatment. In the adolescent hypothyroidism may cause a myotonialike phenomenon with difficulty in contraction and relaxation. True myotonia cannot be demonstrated electromyographically. Muscle biopsy is usually unrevealing.[42]

In areas where goiters are endemic, there may be severe associated central nervous system (CNS) abnormalities including spasticity, choreoathetosis, and deafmutism; this is sometimes called *neurologic cretinism.* It is likely that the neurologic damage is caused by iodine deficiency in the first trimester.[42]

Laboratory. The pathognomic blood abnormalities are a low T_4, normal or low triiodothyronine (T_3) resin uptake, and an elevated TSH. Ancillary neurologic tests may show abnormalities; for example, an EEG may be slow, a CSF examination may show an increased protein.

Treatment. Synthetic L-T_4 is now the accepted treatment of choice. The serum T_4, T_3 resin uptake, and TSH should be monitored; the latter is the best indication of adequacy of treatment. In severe cases or cases with definite heart disease, gradual introduction of L-T_4 is advised because of rare sudden deaths. Craniosynostosis can be a complication of treatment.[27]

Prognosis. The prognosis is related to the age of diagnosis and also to etiology. If hypothyroidism develops after age 2 years of age, all neurologic and muscular abnormalities should resolve with treatment.

In patients with congenital illness, earlier treatment generally leads to a better outlook, with those patients treated before 3 months of age having a normal intelligence. However, many such children have minor neurologic disabilities including clumsiness, behavioral disturbances, speech disorders, learning disorders, and strabismus. Athyreosis and dyshormonogenesis seem to carry a poorer prognosis.[30]

Hyperthyroidism

Hyperthyroidism increases cerebral blood flow and oxygen use. There is an increase in alpha-rhythm frequency. The hypermetabolic state produces a plethora of neurologic and muscular syndromes.[1,42]

Neurologic syndromes
 Tremor, chorea
 Seizures
 Irritability, nervousness, psychosis
 Delirium, stupor, coma
 Thyroid storm, fever, tachycardia, hyper- or hypotension, diarrhea, vomiting, weakness, tremor, and altered mental state
Muscle syndromes
 Myopathy
  Acute: Bulbar musculature is affected with dysarthria and dysphagia. It may be associated with mental changes (encephalopathy).
  Chronic: Virtually all patients with hyperthyroidism will complain of muscle weakness and fatigability, especially of the proximal muscles. Deep tendon reflexes remain brisk. Electromyography shows mild myopathic features. Rarely a more chronic insidious weakness and atrophy will occur to such an extent as to suggest a primary spinal muscular atrophy or limb girdle dystrophy. Extraocular and bulbar musculature are not affected as they are in the myasthenic syndrome and in acute myopathy. Muscle biopsy is in general unrevealing.
 Exophthalmic ophthalmoplegia: Whereas eye prominence and exophthalmos are common in hyperthyroid children and adolescents, they are usually mild, and impairment of ocular motility is minimal.
 Hyperthyroidism with myasthenia gravis: This rare combination does occur in childhood, and the distribution of weakness is similar to that in classical myasthenia, that is, ocular, facial, bulbar, and generalized. The conditions can occur simultaneously or one can

precede the other. Treatment of the hyperthyroidism improves the myasthenia.

Hyperthyroidism with periodic paralysis: This combination is seen virtually exclusively in Japanese persons, and rarely in the first two decades of life.

Because of the influence of the thyroid hormones on muscle, it is important to check thyroid function in virtually all cases of muscle weakness.

Neonatal Hyperthyroidism or Graves' Disease

Infants of mothers with hyperthyroidism, even those under treatment, may be born hyperthyroid secondary to transplacental transfer of thyroid-stimulating immunoglobulins in a clinical situation very similar to that of the infant of the myasthenic mother. The former infants are frequently premature, and show a hypermetabolic state. This may be suppressed during the first week by maternal antithyroid medication. It is possible for permanent neurologic sequelae to result, and the course may be complicated by premature closure of the sutures.[29]

Laboratory.   The diagnosis is confirmed by the presence of an elevated T_3 and T_4.

Treatment.   Antithyroid drugs (either propylthiouracil or methimazole) are indicated in the medical treatment of hyperthyroidism. In resistant cases, radioactive iodine or surgery may be considered. Thyroid storm constitutes a medical emergency requiring life supports, corticosteroids, and propanolol.[19]

PARATHYROID GLAND

The parathyroid glands are of central importance in calcium homeostatis. Neurologic manifestations of their dysfunction therefore relate to abnormal calcium levels.

Hypoparathyroidism

Two forms of deficient parathyroid function occur in childhood: the first, idiopathic hypoparathyroidism, the second, pseudohypoparathyroidism.[49]

In the former, secretion of parathryoid hormone (PTH) is deficient; there are no dysmorphic features; cutaneous moniliasis is common; and there may be headaches and papilledema caused by pseudotumor cerebri. The serum shows low calcium, high phosphate, and low PTH levels.

In pseudohypoparathyroidism, the child is of short stature with a round face, short metacarpals, and stubby fingers. There is often subcutaneous calcification, and many affected children are mentally retarded. A few have papilledema. The serum calcium is low, and phosphate high, but the PTH is high, this disorder being one of target-organ unresponsiveness. Radiographs show subcutaneous bone formation and shortened metacarpal and metatarsal bones. Symmetric punctate calcification of the basal ganglia may be present in either disorder, and is best seen on CT scan.

Seizures, tetany, muscle cramps, and twitching may occur in either type due to the hypocalcemia, and the EEG may show high voltage slow wave abnormalities.[47]

Diagnosis rests on demonstration of the abnormalities as mentioned above, and treatment consists of calcium supplements and vitamin D. Prognosis in idiopathic hypoparathyroidism is good, and the outlook for intellectual function may be improved by early diagnosis and treatment. Hypocalcemic seizures mandate treatment with intravenous calcium.

Neonatal hypoparathyroidism can occur secondary to maternal hyperparathyroidism, and may uncover the asymptomatic condition in the mother. However, in the neonate, the disorder is usually a transient phenomenon related to prematurity, maternal diabetes, and neonatal asphyxia, and may coexist with hypoglycemia and hypomagnesemia. Rarely neonatal hypocalcemia will be the first sign of DiGeorge's syndrome (III and IV branchial arch anomaly) with its parathyroid and thymic aplasia, associated immunologic deficits, midline defects, and mental retardation.

Hyperparathyroidism

This is a rare occurrence in childhood. A few cases in the neonatal period have been described, and many cases in later childhood are secondary to disorders causing hypocalcemia, for example, renal disease.[40,49]

Neurologic problems result from hypercalcemia, namely, confusion, memory impairment, depression, decreased level of consciousness, weakness, easy fatigability, and muscular atrophy. The neonatal cases present with hypotonia, poor feeding, weight loss, dehydration, and respiratory disorders due to rib fractures. Fractures also occur in the long bones.

Diagnosis is made by demonstration of both raised serum calcium and PTH. Treatment is by subtotal parathyroidectomy. Emergency treatment of hypercalcemia may be necessary in severe cases and consists of high fluid intake, and administration of furosemide, calcitonin and corticosteroids.[16]

Idiopathic hypercalcemia of infancy occurs as part of a syndrome that also includes "elfin" facies, rarely noticeable before the age of 1 year to 3 years, mental retardation, and supravalvular aortic stenosis. The hypercalcemia is temporary, resolving spontaneously during the first few months of life. The current popular thesis suggests that the basic defect is hypersensitivity to vitamin D.

Treatment involves high fluid intake with both a low calcium and vitamin D diet.

DIABETES MELLITUS

Neurologic complications of diabetes in childhood are less prominent than in adults, but retinopathy and neuropathy are present in a significant number of teenagers whose diabetes had its onset in early infancy. Neuropathy is usually asymptomatic, but careful examination may reveal minimal peripheral weakness and diminished deep tendon reflexes.

Neurologic impairment occurs in diabetic coma, presumably due to a number of causes, including decreased cerebral blood flow, and possibly accumulation of abnormal metabolites. Diabetic ketoacidosis may be associated with more serious effects such as acute cerebral edema, and nonketotic coma may be responsible for focal neurologic disorders secondary to hyperosmolarity with intracellular dehydration. Diabetic coma may be complicated by acute pressure neuropathies affecting especially the sciatic nerve and most particularly its lateral division (peroneal).

HYPOGLYCEMIA

A low blood sugar is a relatively common occurrence in childhood from birth to adolescence, with many different causes resulting either from inadequate availability of substrate (glycogen, amino acids, glycerol, pyruvate, and lactate), deficiency of glycogenolytic or gluconeogenic enzyme systems in the liver, or disorders of the endocrine system responsible for maintaining glucose homeostasis.[8]

The normal neonate or child under 5 years of age possesses less reserve (liver and muscle) for maintenance of glucose during fasting than the normal adult, and this may be exaggerated by disease states.

Causes of Hypoglycemia

Neonatal
Low birth weight
Intrauterine growth retardation
Maternal diabetes, especially treated with oral drugs
Rhesus hemolytic disease
Birth asphyxia
Multiple pregnancy
Late feeding
Sepsis
Chronic Undernutrition
Inadequate food
Chronic disease
Malabsorption, for example, celiac disease
Pancreatic (Hyperinsulinism)
Islet cell tumors (nesidioblastoma)
Islet cell hyperplasia
Functional hyperinsulinism
Prediabetes
Hepatic
Toxic, for example, alcohol, aspirin, carbon tetrachloride
Infection, viral or bacterial
Cirrhosis
Glycogen storage diseases, Types I and 3
Neoplastic infiltration
Galactosemia, fructose intolerance
Pituitary
Panhypopituitarism
Adrenal
Addison's disease, primary or secondary
Others
Ketotic hypoglycemia (fasting/illness)
Leucine-sensitivity
Maple syrup urine disease
Beckwith-Wiedemann's syndrome (fetal gigantism, macroglossia, abdominal wall defects)

Children usually become symptomatic when blood glucose concentrations fall to 50 mg/100 ml or less. For full-term newborns, levels of 30 mg/100 ml are considered abnormally low, whereas levels of 20 mg/100 ml are considered abnormally low for prematures.

Since the brain stores no glucose, it needs a constant supply, and in hypoglycemia the symptoms and signs reflect that dependency. A blood sugar determination at the time of symptom presentation is important in any complaint of prolonged behavior change or seizure.

Clinical symptoms and signs of hypoglycemia include pallor, sweating, weakness, tachycardia, nervousness, hunger, headache, confusion, combativeness, decreased level of consciousness, seizures, and prolonged coma. Permanent deficit may result from prolonged or repeated episodes. In the neonatal period, the symptoms may be absent or subtle, such as respiratory irregularity including apnea, jitteriness, irritability, lethargy, hypotonia, seizure, poor sucking ability, and tachycardia.

Diagnosis depends on demonstration of a low blood glucose and then further investigation as indicated by the clinical situation.

Treatment in acute symptomatic hypoglycemia is urgent. Glucose should be administered intravenously at once. Care should be taken to avoid reactive hypoglycemia that may follow treatment with hypertonic glucose solution. Further management will depend upon the underlying cause.

REFERENCES

1. **Adams RD, Rosman NP:** Hyperthyroidism, neuromuscular system. In Werner SC, Ingbar SH (eds): The Thyroid, a Fundamental and Clinical Text, 4th ed, pp 742–752. Hagerstown, Harper & Row, 1978

2. **Adams RD, Rosman NP:** Hypothyroidism, neuromuscular system. In Werner SC, Ingbar SH (eds): The Thyroid, a fundamental and Clinical Text, 4th ed, pp 901–910. Hagerstown, Harper & Row, 1978

3. **Barness LA:** Vitamins in nutrition. In Kelley VC (ed): Practice of Pediatrics, pp. 1–36. Hagerstown, Harper & Row, 1980

4. **Bell WE, McCormick WF:** Increased Intracranial Pressure in Children, 2nd ed. Philadelphia, WB Sauders, 1978

5. **Bondy PK, Rosenberg LE (eds):** Metabolic Control and Disease, 8th ed. Philadelphia, WB Saunders, 1980

6. Case records of the Massachusetts General Hospital, Case No. 18–1979. N Engl J Med 300:1037, 1979

7. Clinical nutrition cases, vitamin D intoxication treated with glucocorticoids. Nutr Rev 37:323, 1979

8. **Cornblath M, Schwartz R:** Disorders of Carbohydrate Metabolism in Infancy, 2nd ed. Philadelphia, WB Saunders, 1976

9. **Costin G:** Endocrine disorders associated with tumors of the pituitary and hypothalamus. Ped Clin North Amer 26:15, 1979.

10. **Curtis JA, Brennan RE, Kurtz AB:** Evaluation of adrenal disease by computed tomography. Comput Tomogr 4:165, 1980

11. **Darling DB, Loridan L, Senior B:** The roentgenographic manifestations of Cushing's syndrome in infancy. Radiology 96:503, 1970

12. **DeLuca HF:** Some new concepts emanating from a study of the metabolism and function of vitamin D. Nutr Rev 38:1969, 1980

13. **Dillon RS:** Handbook of Endocrinology, 2nd ed. Philadelphia, Lea & Febiger, 1980

14. **Dubowitz V:** Treatment of dermatomyositis in childhood. Arch Dis Child 51:494, 1976.

15. **Duckett S, Winick M:** Malnutrition and brain dysfunction. In Black P (ed): Brain Dysfunction in Children: Etiology, Diagnosis and Management. New York, Raven Press, 1981

16. Editorial, Management of severe hypercalcemia. Br Med J 280:204, 1980

17. **Evans D, Bowie M, Hansen JDL et al:** Intellectual development and nutrition. J Pediat 97:358, 1980

18. **Fisher D:** Pediatric aspects. In Werner SC, Ingbar SH (eds): The Thyroid, a Fundamental and Clinical Text, 4th ed, Hagerstown, Harper & Row, 1978

19. **Fisher DA:** Thyroid Disease. In Gellis, SS, Kagan BM (eds): Current Pediatric Therapy, 9th ed, pp 302–307. Philadelphia, WB Saunders, 1980

20. **Fisher DA, Klein AH:** Thyroid development and disorders of thyroid function in the newborn. N Engl J Med 304:702, 1981

21. **Fishman RA:** Cerebrospinal Fluid in Diseases of the Nervous System. Philadelphia, WB Saunders, 1980

22. **Guillemin R:** Neuroendocrine interrelations. In Bondy PK, Rosenberg LE (eds): Metabolic Control and Disease 8th ed, pp 1155–1164. Philadelphia, WB Saunders, 1980

23. **Heeley A, Pugh RJP, Clayton BE et al:** Pyridoxal metabolism in vitamin B6-responsive convulsions of early infancy. Arch Dis Child 53:794, 1978

24. **Kaplan SA:** Disorders of the adrenal cortex. Pediatr Clin North Amer 26:65, 1979

25. **Krieger DT, Martin JB:** Brain peptides Parts 1 and 2. New Engl J Med 304, p. 876, 1981

26. **Kutt H, Solomon GE:** Phenytoin relevant side effects. In Glaser GH, Penry JK, Woodbury DM (eds): Antiepileptic Drugs: Mechanisms of Action, Advances in Neurology Series No 27, 1st ed, pp 435–445. New York, Raven Press, 1980

27. **LaFranchi SH:** Hypothyroidism. Pediatr Clin North Am 26:33, 1979

28. **Landsberg L, Young JB:** Catecholamines and the adrenal medulla. In Bondy PK, Rosenberg LE (eds): Metabolic Control and Disease, 8th ed, pp 1621–1693. Philadelphia, WB Saunders, 1980

29. **Lee WNP:** Thyroiditis, hyperthyroidism, and tumors. Pediatr Clin North Am 26:53, 1979

30. **MacFaul R, Dorner S, Brett EM et al:** Neurological abnormalities in patients treated for hypothyroidism from Early Life. Arch of Dis Child 53:611, 1978

31. **MacLean W, Graham GG:** Vegetarianism in children. Am J Dis Child 134:513, 1980

32. **Martin JB, Reichlin S, Brown GM:** Clinical Neuroendocrinology. Philadelphia, FA Davis, 1977

33. **Minns R:** Vitamin B_6 deficiency and dependency. Dev Med Child Neurol, 22:795, 1980

34. **O'Neill BP, Forbes GS:** Computerized tomography and adrenoleukomyeloneuropathy. Arch Neurol 38:293, 1981

35. **Ontjes DA, Walton J, Ney RL:** The anterior pituitary gland. In Bondy PK, Rosenberg LE (eds): Metabolic Control and Disease, 8th ed, pp 1165–1239. Philadelphia, WB Saunders, 1980

36. **Pearson HA, Vinson R, Smith RT:** Pernicious anemia with neurologic involvement in childhood. J Pediatr. 65:334, 1964

37. **Pincus JH:** Subacute necrotising encephalomyelopathy (Leigh's disease), consideration of clinical features and etiology. Dev Med Child Neurol 14:87, 1972

38. **Pincus JH:** Letter: Urine Test in SNE. Neurology 29:424, 1979

39. **Pleasure DE, Walsh GO, Engel WK:** Atrophy of skeletal muscle in patients with Cushing's syndrome. Arch Neurol 22:118, 1970

40. **Rhone DP:** Primary neonatal hyperparathyroidism, report of a case and review of the literature. Am J Clin Path, 64:488, 1975

41. **Rosenberg LE, Scriver CR:** Disorders of amino acid metabolism. In Bondy PK, Rosenberg LE (eds): Metabolic Control and Disease, 8th ed, pp 583–776. Philadelphia, WB Saunders, 1980

42. **Rosman NP:** Neurological and muscular aspects of thyroid dysfunction in childhood. Pediatr Clin North Am 23:575, 1977

43. **Rottenberg DA, Foley KM, Posner JB:** Hypothesis: the pathogenesis of pseudotumor cerebri. Med Hypothesis 6:913, 1980

44. **Schaumberg HH, Powers JM, Raine CS et al:** Adrenoleukodystrophy: a clinical and pathological study of 17 cases. Arch Neurol 32:577, 1975

45. **Spiro AJ, Hirano A, Bellin RL et al:** Cretinism with muscular hypertrophy (Kocher-Debre-Semelaigne Syndrome). Arch Neurol 23:340, 1970

46. **Stringel G, Ein SH, Creighton R et al:** Pheochromocytoma in children—an update. J Pediatr Surg 15:496, 1980

47. **Sugar O:** Central neurological complications of hypoparathyroidism, AMA Arch Neurol Psychiatry 70:86, 1953

48. **Thomsett MJ, Conte FA, Kaplan SL et al:** Endocrine and neurologic outcome in childhood craniopharyngioma: review of effect of treatment in 42 patients. J Ped 97:728, 1980

49. **Tsang R, Noguchi A, Steichen JJ:** Pediatric parathyroid disorders, Pediatr Clin North Am 26:223, 1979

50. **Vassilouthis J, Utley D:** Benign intracranial hypertension: clinical features and diagnosis using computed tomography and treatment. Surg Neurol 12:389, 1979

51. **Waterlow JC:** Classification and definition of protein-calorie malnutrition. Br Med J 3:566, 1972

52. **Weisberg LA, Chutorian AM:** Pseudotumor cerebri of childhood. Am J Dis Child 131:2343, 1977

53. **Weitzman R, Kleeman CR, Vorherr H:** Water metabolism and the neurohypophyseal hormones. In Bondy PK, Rosenberg LE (eds): Metabolic Control and Disease, 8th ed, pp 1241–1323. Philadelphia, WB Saunders, 1980

54. **Zmora E, Gordischer R, Bar-Ziv J:** Multiple nutritional deficiencies in infants from a strict vegetarian community. Am J Dis Child 133:141, 1979

Intoxications of the Nervous System

11

Lorcan A. O'Tuama
Chung S. Kim

LEAD POISONING

ETIOLOGY

Lead is a cumulative protoplasmic poison that may enter the body by ingestion, inhalation, or rarely by absorption through the skin. The pharmacology and systemic effects of lead are much influenced by whether the metal is ingested as inorganic lead or inhaled as organic lead. The former is a greater clinical problem and this discussion will refer to inorganic lead, unless otherwise indicated. Children are universally exposed to lead at low levels in food, water, air, dust, and soil. This level is commonly accepted as safe, although this assumption has recently been questioned. In addition, sporadic ingestions of lead result in clinically manifest neurotoxicity. Paint-chewing is the classical cause of this exposure. More than half such cases occur at teething time, namely, during the second year, and this presentation is rare under the age of 12 months or over the age of 5 years in the child of normal intelligence. Paint exposure as a cause of lead poisoning is now rivaled by many additional modes of exposure that are being reported. These include ingestion of lead from parental work clothing and lead acquisition through living near smelters.[35]

PATHOGENESIS

Central Nervous System Effects

The well established toxicity of large amounts of lead is assumed to involve direct effects (irreversible binding to carboxyl- and sulfhydryl-containing active sites in nerve cells), as well as indirect effects attendant to vasculopathy, hypoxia, and cerebral edema.[30] A myriad of theories have been advanced to explain the mechanisms of low-level lead neurotoxicity. Postulated mechanisms include a lead-induced imbalance of neurotransmitters, competitive displacement by lead of calcium at the nerve cell ending or other organelle, and effects of lead on transport of nutrients and neurotransmitters into brain.[54]

Peripheral Nervous System

The effects of lead are most likely felt at the dorsal root ganglion.

PATHOLOGY

The gastrointestinal tract appears normal in chronic cases. Intranuclear acidophilic inclusion bodies may be found in the liver and kidneys. When death is due to lead encephalopathy, the changes in the nervous system consist of an acute encephalopathy with acute neuronal degeneration and swelling of the vascular epithelium. Edema of diffuse and perivascular distribution may be seen, as may fibroblastic proliferation of the leptomeninges. In cases with peripheral neuropathy, the brunt of the damage is borne by motor nerve fibers, particularly those supplying muscles that have undergone the greatest fatigue. The principal change consists of intermittent or segmental myelin degeneration with varying amounts of axonal damage.[113]

CLINICAL FEATURES

Three clearly distinctive syndromes can be recognized, depending mainly on the level of exposure.

1. Acute lead encephalopathy follows exposure to moderate or massive amounts of metal. Its incidence has steadily decreased pari passu with urban renewal programs and environmental deleading. This syndrome is rare in adults. The reasons for its childhood predilection are unknown but may be related to the decreased absorption and retention of inorganic lead by adults compared to children. Alternatively or as an additional factor, alterations in transport and metabolism of lead by the immature brain as compared to the adult brain may play a role. This important aspect of lead metabolism has as yet been only partly investigated.[89] Symptoms of systemic plumbism may precede the encephalopathy. These features are nonspecific and hence their diagnostic significance may be overlooked. The symptoms are irritability, fretfulness, gastrointestinal upsets with anorexia and failure to gain weight, constipation, and occasional vomiting. Secondary anemia is classically described but may be absent. Lead lines are rarely found in the gums of children. The onset of encephalopathy is dramatic; the tempo and neurologic findings may mimic a brain mass lesion. The picture of raised intracranial pressure becomes manifest over several days. Persistent vomiting is common, and the clouded mental state deepens to stupor, sometimes alternating with lucid intervals, and eventual coma with convulsions. Papilledema may occur and the risks of lumbar puncture in this situation have been emphasized.

2. A syndrome of chronic lead encephalopathy is shown by survivors of acute intoxication and by children exposed to lower doses of the metal over a longer period. The standard description of this syndrome was provided by Byers and Lord, and includes motor regression with loss of skillful movements as well as ataxia, muscular weakness, or paralysis.[15] Changes in personality, confusion, or delirium may appear.

3. In addition to the above syndromes that reflect central neural effects, lead may cause a peripheral neuropathy. This is an extremely rare manifestation of lead poisoning in children with the recently described exception of children suffering from sickle cell disease.[58] The reasons for this association are unknown. Chisolm has suggested a role for the zinc deficiency that is associated with sickle cell disease and notes experimental evidence that zinc protects against lead. Also, altered intravascular binding of lead to the mutant hemoglobin may change its tissue availability.

LABORATORY EXAMINATION

Most diagnostic methods come under two main headings. The first group consists of tests that establish evidence of biochemical dysfunction compatible with, but not pathognomonic of, lead intoxication. Secondly, lead measurements in body fluids can be used to detect the metal directly. In the first category, measurement of serum erythrocyte-free protoporphyrin (FEP) now plays a key part.[47] Abnormal elevations of this compound reflect a disturbance in porphyrin metabolism that is extremely typical of lead exposure. The test has the great advantages of being a relatively simple chemical procedure, and yielding speedy results. The interlaboratory variability of this test is also very low. A disadvantage lies in its relative nonspecificity because abnormal values can also be obtained in some anemias. However, this situation does not usually pose a serious problem given the other clinical features suggesting neurotoxicity.

Additional laboratory findings compatible with, but not diagnostic of, lead poisoning include elevations in urinary coproporphyrin III and delta-aminolevulinic acid, proteinuria, a generalized aminoacidruia, glycousuria, and increased urinary urobilinogen. X-ray films of the bones give useful information in children. Lines of increased density appear at the growing ends and are left in the shafts as growth proceeds. In cases of multiple exposure several of these "lead lines" might be apparent. (Fig 11-1) A plain x-ray film of the abdomen might reveal shadows caused by ingested lead-containing material (Fig 11-2).

Direct estimation of whole blood lead by atomic absorption spectrometry offers the

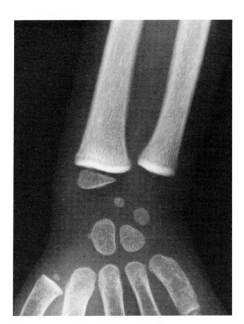

FIG. 11-1. "Lead lines" in bones.

most specific confirmation of an increased body lead burden. Correlations of subtle biochemical evidence of lead toxicity in the human with whole blood levels have resulted in a downward revision of the acceptable whole blood lead in children to 20 μg/dl.[86] It is less clear what level of blood lead corresponds with clinically detectable lead toxicity and in particular there is no clear relationship between moderate elevation of whole blood lead and neurologic symptoms. In resolving these questions, the overall clinical status of the patient has to be considered and tests such as the ethylenediaminetetraacetic acid (EDTA) mobilization test, discussed below, may be useful.

Assay of urinary lead levels offers an additional estimation of increased lead exposure. Urinary excretions greater than 80 μg/24 hours are considered excessive. Typically, a delay of several days is required for processing this assay, and this factor limits its effectiveness as a screening device. The major usefulness of urinary lead estimation lies in its employment as part of the calcium disodium edetate mobilization test in borderline cases of lead intoxication. This test is considered positive if Ca EDTA (50 mg/kg intramuscularly [IM]) leads to a urinary excretion of greater than 500 μg lead in 24 hours or if a greater than 20% increase over preinjection values occurs.

TREATMENT

Presymptomatic

Due to improved detection techniques and the increased prevalence of early detection programs, an increasing number of children are now being seen who have biochemical evidence of lead exposure without definite associated neurologic or other symptoms. Some patients of this type may be detected by the neurologist in the course of screening studies done as part of the workup of children with unexplained seizures or encephalopathy. The neurologist can make an important contribution to ensuring early detection of these patients and should actively initiate prophylactic treatment or refer them to an appropriate resource for this purpose. Further decisions about the management of these patients depend on assessing the type and source of lead exposure, the age of the child, and his or her neurologic and developmental status. In borderline cases, a diagnostic che-

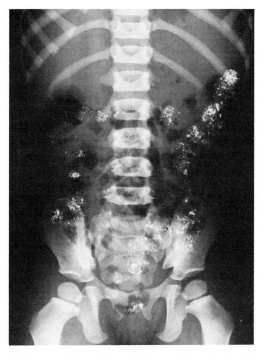

FIG. 11-2. X-ray film shadow of lead paint in bowel.

lation test with EDTA may be needed. Where pharmacologic treatment is felt to be needed, penicillamine is generally adequate. If it is indicated, EDTA is given as injections in a dose of 12.5 mg/kg IM every 4 hours as a 20% solution for 3 to 5 days. The injection is painful and the sites should be rotated and 0.5% procaine added to the injectate. Courses of EDTA should not exceed 500 mg/kg in children and an interval of 2 weeks should elapse between courses. When the overall evidence for lead neurotoxicity is mild or marginal, a more appropriate approach to treatment would involve oral penicillamine, 30 mg/kg daily for up to 6 months and a maximal daily dose of 500 mg. The exact duration of the course of treatment will depend on the clinical response and on the reduction of blood lead to a value of 40 μg/dl.

Acute Lead Encephalopathy and Established Neurotoxicity

This subject is reviewed comprehensively by Chisolm and Barltrop (1979).[22] Supportive measures are important. Intravenous fluid replacement should err slightly on the side of underhydration, and should comprise dextrose in hypotonic saline (rather than water) to avoid exacerbating cerebral edema. Acidosis should be corrected if present. Seizures and hyperthermia should be controlled. Acute lead encephalopathy has been traditionally regarded, together with brain abscess, as one of the pediatric conditions most likely to predispose to herniation after lumbar puncture, which should therefore be stringently avoided. Standard measures for combating cerebral edema should be used as indicated. In refractory cases, surgical decompression may be used. Pharmacologic treatment involves a combination of EDTA and dimercaprol (BAL), 4 mg/kg IM every 4 hours for 30 doses. Complications of treatment with EDTA include proximal tubular necrosis that may be first shown by aminoaciduria. Hypersensitivity reactions that may mimic systemic lupus may also occur. A clinical complication that follows from the basic properties of the chelating agents is their tendency to remove additional ions. By this mechanism, deficiencies of essential metals such as calcium and iron may occur and the pa-

tient should be screened periodically to detect this event. Dimercaprol has a similar toxicity to EDTA. In addition, it acts more powerfully on the erythrocyte to remove lead. It therefore has a greater tendency to promote internal redistribution of the metal. In the early stages of treatment, this effect can sometimes lead to a transfer of newly mobilized lead from bone into brain and other soft tissues. This factor is thought to underlie the transient worsening of lead encephalopathy sometimes observed early in treatment with BAL.

DIFFERENTIAL DIAGNOSIS

In mild cases this embraces all the causes of failure to thrive, including insufficient caloric intake, vitamin deficiency disease, congenital heart disease, chronic respiratory and other infections, malabsorption syndromes, and chronic renal disease. Cases with encephalopathy must be distinguished from other forms of encephalopathy, as well as from brain abscess, tumor, and meningitis (especially tuberculosus meningitis).

Lead lines in the bones must be differentiated from similar opacities resulting from bismuth, phosphorus, and strontium poisoning, cretinism, and the early stages of osteopetrosis.

A causal association between low-level lead exposure and mild, unexplained encephalopathies of childhood has not been proven.[32] There is, however, substantial evidence suggesting at least a contributory role for low-level lead exposure in certain cases of learning disability and "attention deficit syndrome." In these patients the physician should bear in mind the possibility of lead exposure and include a measurement of free erythrocyte porphyrin in his investigation.

PROGNOSIS

The prognosis of acute lead encephalopathy is poor. Not only is the mortality high, but in those children who recover, some impairment of mental development is the rule. Recurrent epileptic convulsions, permanent motor disabilities, and behavioral disorders are common.

The prognosis of low-level lead exposure is uncertain. This problem should be clarified when one can assess the performance in lower school grades of children documented earlier to have minor degrees of exposure to the metal.

ORGANIC LEAD NEUROTOXICITY

The organic lead compounds tetraethyl- and tetramethyllead are lipid-soluble compounds used as "anti-knock" additives in gasoline and are occasionally neurotoxic following inhalation. Their lipophilicity promotes central nervous system entry and they tend to cause a marked encephalopathy. Early mild symptoms are nonspecific and include insomnia and headache. Delusions, ataxia, and a state of mania ensue at higher doses. Diagnosis is heavily dependent on clinical suspicion. Urinary lead levels may be markedly increased but blood lead levels tend to remain normal and porphyrin metabolism is unchanged. In nonfatal cases, residual neurologic damage may occur.

ARSENIC POISONING

Arsenic, an amphoteric element of ubiquitous distribution, is a general tissue poison. Its toxic effects may involve the gastrointestinal tract, liver, kidneys, heart, skin and mucous membranes, hematopoietic system, and central and peripheral nervous systems.

ETIOLOGY

Although arsenic exists as a trace element in food, glass, and metal, toxicity in children results usually from accidental ingestion. Administration with homicidal intent also occurs. Most cases of poisoning are due to arsenical insecticides and weed killers, which, despite the advent of newer synthetic insecticides, continue to be used in large quantities. The main arsenic salts encountered are lead arsenate, calcium triarsenate, and cupric acetoarsenite (Paris green).

PATHOGENESIS

Arsenic occurs in the elemental form (As^0) or as trivalent (As^{3+}) or pentavalent (As^{5+}) oxidation states. The As^{3+} or As^{5+} forms are linked covalently to carbon in the organic arsenicals. Toxicity depends in part on the physicochemical properties of the As ion. For example, As^{5+} has a much lower affinity for thiol groups and consequently less toxicity than As^{3+} forms, such as occur in potassium arsenite ($KAsO_2$) and salts of arsenious acids ($H_2S_2O_3$).

A well-known mechanism of arsenic toxicity involves uncoupling of oxidative phosphorylation through competitive substitution of arsenate for inorganic phosphate. Arsenic has a marked tendency to attach itself to sulfhydryl and hydroxyl groups of enzymes. This tendency leads to the element becoming fixed in keratin-containing tissues such as skin, hair, and nails; and also explains arsenic-induced poisoning of several enzymes involved in the tricarboxylic acid cycle and elsewhere. These enzymatic interactions of arsenic mimic those produced by thiamine deficiency. This fact is reflected in the similar clinical features of the neuropathy produced by thiamine deficiency and arsenical exposure.

PATHOLOGY

Fatal cases of encephalopathy usually follow trivalent organic arsenical exposure and may show the features of an acute hemorrhagic encephalopathy with scattered "ring hemorrhages" due to capillary extravasation. These changes are nonspecific and indistinguishable from the picture produced by numerous other toxins. They probably represent a direct toxic effect upon the capillary walls rather than an anaphylactic effect.

Pathologic data on patients with arsenical polyneuropathy are sparse. Changes have been described both in the spinal cord (anterior horn cell loss) as well as in peripheral nerves (abnormalities of the myelinated nerves).[38]

CLINICAL FEATURES

Acute ingestion of inorganic arsenic is usually painless, but solutions of it may produce severe burning pain in the mouth and esophagus followed by abdominal pain, nausea, and vomiting, which may be bloody. A profuse diarrhea frequently occurs, which also may be bloody. Conjunctival suffusion and rhinorrhea are common, and a number of patients have epistaxis. There may be mild transitory jaundice. Rarely, ingestion of a massive dose of a soluble form of arsenic can cause severe cardiomyopathy, heart failure, and death. Polyneuropathy may appear in 10 days to 14 days, but it occurs less frequently in children than in adults following chronic industrial exposure.[59] The CSF is acellular and typically shows a normal protein concentration. Electromyographic studies show a mild to moderate delay in motor nerve conduction with marked slowing of sensory action potentials.

Arsenic encephalopathy or myelopathy is usually a complication of organic arsenic intoxication and follows within a day or so of intravenous or oral administration. The encephalopathy is characterized by headache, irritability and fretfulness, confusion, convulsions, and coma. Arsenical aphonia has been described, but cranial nerve involvement is otherwise uncommon.

In chronic cases a history of one or more acute gastrointestinal illnesses is frequently obtained, and in others it is surmised that the ingestion was of smaller doses over a prolonged period. The presence of transverse striate leukonychia (Aldrich-Mees lines; see Fig. 18-9) is highly significant if other features of arsenic poisoning are present.[60] The child may be anemic. Arsenites are well known to have a granulocytopenic effect. Aplastic anemia may follow administration of organic arsenicals. Nephropathy with albuminuria, cardiomyopathy, and hepatotoxic effects occur.

LABORATORY EXAMINATION

Following acute ingestion abnormally large quantities of arsenic are excreted in the urine (upper limit of normal is 0.1 mg/24 hr), but this drops within a few weeks as the arsenic becomes fixed to the tissues. After some weeks arsenic is found in the hair. Because of its slower growth, lesser bulk, and protection from external contamination, such as arsenic-containing cosmetics, pubic hair is more suitable than head hair for analytic purposes and should be used if present. If head hair is used, it might be advisable to test a separate sample cut from the portion nearest the scalp; 0.1 mg arsenic/100 g of hair is regarded as the upper limit of normal. Arsenic may also be found in the nails once they have grown out.

TREATMENT

Profuse emesis usually follows ingestion of arsenic by children, and in this case, gastric lavage may safely be omitted. Dimercaprol should be given in a dose of 3 mg/kg every 4 hours on the first and second days, every 6 hours on the third day, every 12 hours on the fourth and fifth days, and once a day thereafter until completion of a 10-day course. On no account should BAL treatment be withheld in order to obtain a 24-hour urine specimen when a clear history of acute ingestion has been obtained. An alternative approach involves chelation with DL-penicillamine. In severe acute cases, dehydration and shock should be treated by the usual methods. The residual effects from polyneuropathy are treated with physical therapy and suitable prostheses such as below-knee braces with toe-raising springs.

DIFFERENTIAL DIAGNOSIS

This includes gastroenteritis from various causes and other forms of encephalopathy and polyneuropathy.

PROGNOSIS

The prognosis for life and for preventing the appearance of polyneuropathy is good in children. If the neuropathy is confined to sensory symptoms or if the motor disability is relatively minor and of distal distribution, prognosis for complete recovery is excellent. On the other hand, once profound muscular wasting and weakness appear and are present for any length of time, the prognosis for complete recovery becomes correspondingly less favorable. Furthermore, recent studies suggest that neurotoxicity due to arsenic may occasionally progress. This event may be explained by the strong binding of arsenic to the brain and raises the question of whether presently available chelating agents can act on such a bound fraction. Clinical observations such as these illustrate the lack of fundamental knowledge about certain aspects of the basic neuropharmacology of toxic metals, in particular the factors regulating their transport into and compartmentation in the brain.

THALLIUM POISONING

ETIOLOGY

The principal source of this substance is thallous sulfate, a tasteless, odorless compound found in rodenticides and insecticides, especially ant and roach powder. Thallium poisoning is more common in the south than in the other parts of the United States and particularly affects children in the lowest socioeconomic strata because of the practice of making the poison attractive to pests by mixing it with stale, crumbled cake, cookie, or other palatable foodstuffs.[85]

PATHOGENESIS

Thallium-induced depletion of succinic dehydrogenase and other striatal enzymes occurs in rat brain and may be part of the mechanism of neurotoxicity.[49] The tissue compartmentation of thallium in the brain has not been directly studied. Avid binding of the metal to soft tissues is suggested by the typically high urinary and fecal levels associated with low plasma levels.

PATHOLOGY

Necropsy may reveal hyperemia and petechiae in the upper gastrointestinal tract, fatty infiltration of the liver and kidneys, small medullary hemorrhages, and cortical de-

generation of the adrenal glands. The central nervous system shows engorgement of cortical blood vessels with swelling and varying degrees of chromatolysis of the neurons, affecting especially those of the pyramidal tracts, globus pallidus, and substantia nigra. Pathologic studies in the peripheral neuropathies show distal axonal degeneration of a "dying back" type.[16]

CLINICAL FEATURES

Following ingestion of large doses the patient is stricken with abdominal pain, vomiting, diarrhea, and hemorrhage, accompanied by severe headache and tachycardia. Neurologic symptoms follow 2 days to 5 days later and take the form of confusion, delirium, convulsions, and coma. Death may follow from respiratory paralysis during the next week. Ataxia and paresthesia are the main manifestations of ingestion of smaller doses. This may progress to a frank, predominantly motor polyneuropathy with muscular wasting and only minimal objective sensory loss. Tremor, chorea, athetosis, myoclonus, encephalopathy, and retrobulbar neuritis also occur.[98] Black pigment may appear at the bases of hairs a few days after ingestion; almost invariably alopecia starts about the tenth day and becomes complete within a month. Transverse striate leukonychia appears about 4 weeks after ingestion (see Fig. 18-9).

LABORATORY EXAMINATION

Diagnosis may be confirmed by finding thallium sulfate in the urine, using a spectroscopic screening test.[134] Its presence, even in small concentrations, is evidence of thallium intoxication. In cases with encephalopathy, the electroencephalogram shows diffuse continuous high-voltage slow activity that predominates frontally.

DIFFERENTIAL DIAGNOSIS

Initially the illness may resemble arsenic and other forms of poisoning or gastroenteritis. Other forms of predominantly motor polyneuropathy are discussed in Chapter 18.

TREATMENT

Results of treatment with chelating agents such as BAL, penicillamine, EDTA, or dithiocarbamate are difficult to assess, but a regimen of dithizone 20 mg/kg per day in four divided oral doses plus KCl and charcoal has been recommended. Hemodialysis may be used in patients with renal failure. Supportive therapy should be given, as outlined by Chamberlin.[18] Treatment with KCl and chelators such as dithiocarbamate may also help.[90]

PROGNOSIS

Reed described an overall mortality of 13% of 72 cases.[98] Moreover, 54% of 48 survivors showed residual abnormalities of which mental retardation and psychosis were the most common. Abnormal reflexes, tremor, ataxia, and residual muscular weakness were also seen.

MERCURY POISONING

ETIOLOGY

Mercury is capable of being absorbed through the alimentary tract, lungs, or skin. Inorganic mercury occurs either as the elemental vapor (Hg^0 valency), mercuric (Hg^{2+}), or mercurous (Hg^+) salts, whereas in organic mercury compounds, aliphatic or aromatic radicles are attached to the metal. Mercuric chloride is about the most common mercury salt to be ingested accidentally, but consumption of seed wheat and other cereals treated with organic mercurial compounds (e.g., fungicides) have produced epidemics of poisoning. Toxicity can result from mercury vapor inhalation, although this is rare in children. Calomel, usually as an ingredient of teething powder, can produce toxic effects, as can ammoniated mercury ointment. Inhalation of mercury vapor particularly affects the nervous system.

PATHOGENESIS

Organic mercurials show major physicochemical differences from inorganic mercury compounds. In particular, their greater lipophilicity promotes easier passage across biologic membranes with enhanced tissue uptake. Experimental studies show that gastrointestinal absorption of methylmercury exceeds by more than 40-fold that of mercuric chloride.[11,24] Similarly, transport of methylmercury across the blood–brain barrier exceeds that of inorganic mercury.[123] These pharmacokinetic properties may, in part, explain the somewhat different patterns of neurotoxicity produced by inorganic and organic mercurials. Mercury is toxic because of its property of forming highly stable linkages with sulfhydryl and other groups, which causes it to inhibit a variety of enzyme systems. The immediate factors determining mercury neurotoxicity are still undefined. The effects of the metal on blood to brain transport of nutrients may perturb neural metabolism of mercury.[120] Direct effects of mercury on brain metabolic systems such as sulfhydryl enzymes may further contribute to its toxicity.[136]

PATHOLOGY

Detailed descriptions of human neuropathologic changes exist only for organic mercurials.

Nervous system lesions consist of cortical and subcortical atrophic areas involving particularly the striate area, the pre- and postcentral gyri, the left central temporal gyrus, and the calcarine cortex. There is also cerebellar atrophy, tending particularly to select the granular cell layer.[126]

In the peripheral nerve, evidence of both myelinopathy and axonopathy is found.

CLINICAL FEATURES

Inorganic Mercury Exposure, Acute Poisoning

Most cases result from adult industrial exposure and this event is rare in children and occurs mostly by accidental ingestion.[112] The clinical picture is dominated by acute gastrointestinal disturbance and neurologic dysfunction is not marked.

Organic Mercury Exposure

Most human cases are acute and due to methylmercury. Modern recognition of the potential health risk of methylmercury exposure dates from the massive outbreak at

Minamata City in Southern Japan during the 1950s, which was due to consumption of mercury-contaminated fish and which was traced to a seed grain treated with a fungicide containing methylmercury.[88] The United States has been spared outbreaks on this scale but a need for constant vigilance was shown by an outbreak of methylmercury toxicity documented in New Mexico.[118]

Chronic mercury poisoning is manifested by malaise, anorexia, dyspepsia, loss of weight, anemia, increased salivation, gingivitis with a possible blue mercury line in the gums, stomatitis, and colitis. Mercury is said to be capable of absorption across the cornea causing the appearance of mercuria lentis, a brown band in the front of the lens. There may be proteinuria. Nervous system symptoms comprise a coarse "shaking" tremor possibly superimposed on a background finer tremor, cerebellar ataxia, and a curious shyness, timidity, and diffidence known as mercurial erethism. Gross constriction of the visual fields has been described.

A syndrome of combined upper and lower motor neuron degeneration resembling amyotrophic lateral sclerosis has appeared in adults who had consumed flour made from seed wheat treated with an organic mercurial preservative. Four siblings were poisoned by eating pork from a hog fed mercury-treated seed grain. In one of the children the mercury was transferred transplacentally. Symptoms included tremor, ataxia, choreoathetosis, myoclonus, and blindness. In the Minamata City outbreak the encephalopathy affected all ages but mostly children under 10 years of age, and also infants born to apparently healthy mothers. Its chief manifestations were numbness of the limbs and lips, concentric constriction of visual fields, dysarthria, hearing defects, truncal and limb ataxia, and intention and resting tremor with slight mental disturbance. Excessive sweating and salivation were noted in some cases. Domestic animals and seabirds were similarly affected with ataxia and inability to stand. The victims were found to be excreting mercury in the urine; the cause was traced to the consumption of fish and shellfish whose tissues contained mercury derived from factory effluent discharged into Minamata Bay.

Fetal and Infantile Effects

The enhanced sensitivity of the fetus to methylmercury exposure was dramatically shown in the Minamata epidemic by the occurrence of encephalopathic neonates in infants born to clinically asymptomatic but exposed mothers. A comparison of maternal and neonatal mercury concentrations show clearly that methylmercury is transferred transplacentally from the mother's blood to the fetus. The Iraqui epidemic also showed that mercury is transferred to milk, where it achieves about 3% of the blood concentration, thus providing another source of mercury for infants born after the start of the epidemic.[69,70] The clinical neurologic features of methylmercury encephalopathy were studied intensively in 29 infants–mother pairs and included overall developmental retardation with or without focal neurologic symptoms such as microcephaly, extensor plantar responses, and a motor picture resembling cerebral palsy. This study also established a relationship between maximal maternal hair mercury levels and the severity of neurologic involvement.[80]

LABORATORY FINDINGS

The diagnosis of mercury poisoning is confirmed by determining the mercury level in the whole blood; 0.2 $\mu g/g$ is considered excessive; 0.1 $\mu g/g$ is considered the maximum allowable for individuals occupationally exposed. Methylmercury concentrates in the red blood cell so that erythrocyte mercury levels give a better indication of the body's methylmercury burden than is provided by whole blood alone.

TREATMENT

General supportive care is important with acute mercury exposure. Rehydration with control of fluid and electrolytes is undertaken if required. The care of renal shutdown may be necessary. In chronic cases the outlook is variable. Stomatitis, gingivitis, and loosening of the teeth are treated appropriately with mouthwashes, oral hygiene, and dental care. It can be anticipated that the colitis will heal. Many patients require special nursing care and rehabilitation consisting of coordination exercises, speech therapy, and possibly various limb prostheses.[31]

The objective of pharmacologic treatment is to enhance mercury excretion and hopefully prevent further neurologic worsening and hasten improvement.[23] In an attempt to achieve these aims, chelation treatment has been attempted in many patients with methylmercury poisoning although its effectiveness is limited by the poor dissociation of organic mercury compounds to yield available chelatable ions in tissues. Of the chelating agents, BAL has been used both for acute and chronic mercury poisoning in doses comparable to those described for lead toxicity. In acute cases, this approach has been accompanied by gastric lavage. Some authorities have advocated abandoning BAL treatment because of reports of its limited usefulness in clinical trials, and also because of experimental evidence that it increases brain mercury levels in animals treated with methylmercury.[10] The chelators N-acetyl-DL-penicillamine or D-penicillamine are also effective in the clearance of methylmercury from blood.

An alternative approach to chelation is offered by thiol resins that trap methylmercury secreted in the bile and so prevent its reabsorption from the intestine and thereby enhance fecal excretion of the metal.[6] These agents are theoretically preferable to chelators for two reasons. First, they do not enter the systemic circulation and hence do not result in redistribution of body mercury. Secondly, they are not prone to cause the toxicity associated with blood dissemination of agents that act as ligands to free sulfhydryls. These compounds were first used in humans during the Iraqi epidemic.

Experimentally, an interaction between selenium and inorganic mercury has been described such that dietary supplementation with selenium considerably lessens the chronic toxicity of methylmercury.[40] Addition of selenium to human diets might therefore help in reducing some of the clinical features of mercury neurotoxicity. This potentially useful new therapeutic approach has apparently not yet been exploited.

PESTICIDE POISONING

Thanks to the efforts of the chemical industry, large and growing numbers of chemicals are in use as insecticides. With the exception of arsenic and the organic phosphates, they have proved remarkably safe in practice; accidental poisoning is rare, and noxious effects due to ingestion of fruits and vegetables sprayed with the agents are as yet undocumented despite the known propensity of some to accumulate in body fat. Three major classes of pesticides are recognized: (1) inorganic arsenicals; (2) botanical, naturally occurring compounds such as the pyrethrins, which cause clinical neurotoxicity only rarely; and (3) synthetic insecticides. Three subgroups of these compounds exist, namely, organochlorines, organophosphates, and carbamates.

ORGANOCHLORINES

The pathogenesis of neurologic effects from organochlorines is unknown but may involve central acetylcholine release or uncoupling of oxidative phosphorylation.[114] Chlorophenothane (DDT) is generally viewed as the prototype of the organochlorines. However, DDT is one of the least toxic of the group and may owe at least some of its toxicity to coadministered solvents.

Pathology

The few neuropathologic studies of fatal DDT exposure have reported unimpressive and nonspecific changes, for example brain congestion and edema.[121]

Clinical Features

The neurologic features of toxicity due to organochlorines are somewhat variable and are not highly specific for individual compounds. Tremors and seizures are frequent and are not produced by synthetic insecticides other than the organochlorine group. Retrobulbar neuritis and a predominantly motor polyneuropathy have been recorded less commonly.[60,61] A recent epidemiologic study suggests that prior exposure to organochlorines may play a role in predisposing to Reye's syndrome in some children, but this connection is unproven.[119] In young children, accidental ingestion of DDT has been reported both individually and as part of a familial ingestion. Childhood poisoning by skin exposure is also possible. A further concern about DDT relates to possible chronic effects of this compound, which is still found in detectable amounts in most people despite the restrictions on its widespread use that were introduced in 1972. It is noteworthy that levels on the order of 300 parts per billion (ppb) have been found in pregnant mothers and that there are detectable levels in all newborns. Of further pediatric interest are the detection of residues of DDT and of polychlorinated biphenyls (PCBs) in human breast milk and the possible deleterious consequences of this exposure on the breast-fed baby and its developing nervous system.[103] Significant developmental delay was found at a 9-year follow-up of Japanese children exposed to PCBs by way of breast milk.

Several pediatric cases of hexachlorocyclohexane (benzene hexachlorine) poisoning have been described. Myoclonic seizures are typical. Recovery is the rule, presumably because of the relatively rapid metabolism of this compound. Childhood poisoning has also been reported with chlordane, one of the cyclodiene group of organochlorine pesticides, and its clinical expression ranged from seizures to mild ataxia. An outbreak of intoxication among factory workers due to chlordecone (Kepone), a product of myrex degradation, was intensively studied when expanding contamination resulted from its manufacture at the Hopewell Plant in Virginia.[125] Neurologic symptoms unique to this compound included opsoclonus and the occasional occurrence of a pseudotumorlike syndrome. In contrast to other organochlorines, seizures were not found. Of family members, 94% have detectable blood levels of the compound. Chlordecone is stored in human fat and is secreted in milk. The intake of this compound by breast-fed infants whose mothers consumed contaminated seafood is comparable to that of their parents. Chronic effects observed in laboratory animals at levels of exposure similar to those at Hopewell include neuromuscular and reproductive disorders. These observations indicate that delayed neurotoxicity may become manifest in children of the Hopewell families as well as in children reported as exposed to chlordecone through contact with insect traps. Chlordecone crosses the placenta of mice and accumulates in fetuses.[20] It has caused fetal mortality and congenital malformations, including enlargement of the cerebral ventricles in rodents. The molecular size and lipophilicity of chlordecone suggests that it could cross the human placenta. Although no data on human placental effects or newborn human toxicity are available, a potential hazard must be assumed.

Treatment

General supportive measures include gastric lavage, artificial respiration, and other intensive care measures. The nonabsorbable resin cholestyramine, which binds chlordecone *in vitro,* hastens the excretion of this pesticide when given in doses of 16g/day orally and continued over a period of several weeks.

ORGANOPHOSPHATE AND CARBAMATE INSECTICIDES

Etiology

The organophosphate and carbamate insecticides share the properties of acting as both true and pseudocholinesterase inhibitors.

Pathogenesis

Some agents are active *in vivo* whereas others are activated in the body to substances that inhibit cholinsterase, for example, paraoxon, the metabolite of parathion. The mechanism of organophosphate neurotoxicity depends on actions at three levels of the central nervous system: (1) muscarinic effects involving peripheral autonomic cholinergic overactivity; (2) nicotinic effects operating at the neuromuscular junction and consisting of initial stimulation followed by an increase in amplitude and number of miniature end-plate potentials leading to eventual blockade; and (3) diffuse central neural overactivity due to activation of cortical, subcortical, and spinal cholinergic terminals.

Pathology

Pathologic studies are limited and the findings have included generalized edema of most body organs, including the brain.

Clinical Symptoms

Symptoms of organophosphate neural toxicity reflect the different levels of action of the toxins described and fall into three corresponding groups: (1) muscarinic effects including anorexia, nausea, vomiting, abdominal cramps, diarrhea, sweating, salivation, lacrimation, shortness of breath, pallor, miosis, and urinary and fecal incontinence; (2) nicotinic effects, principally early stimulation soon followed by generalized muscular weakness and paralysis; and (3) central nervous system effects including headaches, dizziness, ataxia, tremor, drowsiness, convulsions, and coma, as well as psychic symptoms that vary from excitation to depression.

Treatment

Supportive measures are indicated as described for the organochlorines. Patients with organophosphate poisoning are remarkably tolerant to atropine and as much as 2 to 4 mg is given intramuscularly every hour to adults to counter the muscarinic effects of acetylcholine. Administration is continued until signs of atropinization (mydriasis, tachycardia, dry, flushed skin, mental excitement, and so on) appear. Various oximes, particularly pralidoxime, can produce dramatic improvement because of their ability to reactivate phosphate-bound cholinesterase. Pralidoxime (pyridine-2-aldoxime methochloride, 2-PAM), 20 to 40 mg/kg, is given intravenously (IV), slowly in aqueous solution. A second injection may be given in 30 minutes if necessary. This dosage may be repeated twice within a 24-hour period. It is important to note that pralidoxime is *not* suitable for carbamate pesticide toxicity. A pressor agent such as metaraminol is a useful adjuvant.

CARBAMATE INSECTICIDES

This group of insecticides is exemplified by carbaryl (1-naphthyl-N-methyl carbamate). In contrast to the organophosphates, carbamates combine reversibly with cholinesterase. As a consequence, clinical symptoms of carbamate neurotoxicity tend to clear after 8 hours and there is no cumulative effect of repeated daily exposure. In further contrast to organophosphates, pralidoxime is not indicated for carbaryl poisoning and actually tends to increase the hazard from this pesticide.

BARBITURATE POISONING

ETIOLOGY

Simple overdosage with barbiturate in a child may occur during treatment of epilepsy and is dealt with by temporary withdrawal of the drug or diminution of the dose. Occasionally hypersomnolence due to overdosage by a parent with psychiatric problems presents diagnostic difficulties. More often ingestion is accidental owing to the child's attaining access to brightly colored or pleasantly flavored medicine. In adolescents, deliberate ingestion of barbiturates is encountered during suicidal behavior.

PATHOGENESIS

The neurologic features of barbiturate poisoning are heavily dependent on certain aspects of their physical chemistry and physiology. Approximately 50% of plasma barbiturate is nonprotein-bound and is therefore available to equilibrate with tissues. The ability of the nonbound fraction to cross cell membranes is inversely correlated with its degree of ionization. Thus phenobarbital ($pK_a = 7.3$) can be made substantially more ionizable by raising the pH: hence urinary alkalinization promotes enhanced excretion of phenobarbital and is a useful therapeutic modality in treatment of barbiturate poisoning. This approach is much less effective with a short-acting barbiturate such as pentobarbital ($pK_a = 8.0$), which therefore has a greater tendency to be reabsorbed across the renal tubule and to cross other tissue membranes. This tendency is accentuated by the greater lipophilicity of the short-acting barbiturates. Barbiturates in maternal plasma cross the placenta freely and equilibrate with fetal blood within 1 or 2 hours, thus providing a pharmacokinetic basis for neonatal withdrawal seizures.

CLINICAL FEATURES

The child's clinical state when seen by his physician depends upon the amount and type of drug consumed and the time elapsed since its ingestion. In general, the shorter-acting barbiturates not only take effect more rapidly but the patient also achieves faster recovery from them than from the longer-acting ones such as phenobarbital and barbital. Coma may also occur sooner when the drug is contained in a liquid vehicle than when it is in capsules or sugar-coated tablets.

In the early stages of intoxication the child is sleepy, ataxic, dysarthric, and shows nystagmus. The respirations are slow but adequate, and the blood pressure is normal. He is easily aroused by noise, passive movement of the limbs, or painful stimuli. The corneal reflexes are present, and the pupils react briskly to light. The superficial reflexes tend to disappear fairly early. Later the limbs become flaccid and the deep tendon reflexes disappear. The plantar reflexes may be extensor or become areflexic. The eyes become still and the pupils constricted although they continue to respond to light unless they are pinpoint in size. Peripheral vasodilatation does not occur, and the skin appears pale. Sometimes bullous eruptions appear. In the terminal phases respiration becomes shallow and periodic, the blood pressure falls, and the patient enters a state of shock.

LABORATORY EXAMINATION

Stomach washings and blood can be tested for the presence of barbiturate. The electroencephalogram demonstrates fast activity and slows progressively with deepening unconsciousness. In patients in deep coma the record may be isoelectric but gradually reverts to normal as the patient recovers.

TREATMENT

Many of the principles of the treatment for severe barbiturate neurotoxicity provide a model for the treatment of encephalopathies due to central nervous system depressants as a group.[101] All patients with barbiturate-induced encephalopathy should be treated in an intensive care setting. The keystone of treatment involves careful support with emphasis on maintenance of the airway, optimizing ventilation ($PO_2 = -70$ torr–100 torr; $PCO_2 = 20$ torr–40 torr), and control of hypotension. Initial laboratory tests should include estimation of plasma electrolytes and arterial blood gases. Serial estimations of blood barbiturate levels may also be helpful. A blood level of 3.5 mg/dl may be lethal with short-acting barbiturates, whereas a level of 8.0 mg/dl may be reached before death is seen with longer-acting compounds. Careful nursing care with frequent turning of the patient is important. Head elevation of 15 degrees may help to reduce cerebral venous pressure and the possibility of cerebral edema. Oxygen, 40% to 50%, by way of oronasal airway may be necessary for depressed respiration and an endotracheal airway or tracheostomy may be needed for respiratory obstruction. Hypotension may often be controlled by adjusting fluid balance with electrolyte administration. Plasma administration may be required in order to keep central venous pressure at 5 cm of water to 8 cm of water. In severe cases, pressor agents such as metaraminol, 50 mg in 500 ml of 5% dextrose by intravenous infusion may be needed. Gastric lavage, repeated if necessary, is useful in removing the as yet unabsorbed drug from the gastrointestinal tract. A wide bore tube, which can be used in quite young children, is recommended, especially if tablets or capsules have been eaten. Forced alkaline diuresis is useful in phenobarbital poisoning. This is usually given as an undiluted 7.5% solution of sodium bicarbonate directly into a vein. Alkalinization is maintained by adding a sufficient amount of this solution to an intravenous drip to keep the urine at a pH of 7.5 to 8.0. This should be checked regularly by means of pH papers, which is easy to do in the catheterized patient. If the patient continues to deteriorate after forced alkaline diuresis, dialysis or hemoperfusion may help, especially in patients with encephalopathy due to long-acting agents. These measures are generally indicated with a blood phenobarbital level of 15 mg/dl and are much less effective with short-acting barbiturates that are highly bound to protein. Analeptic agents produce only transient improvement and their use is often followed by worsening of the encephalopathy.

PROGNOSIS

The prognosis is now very good, the danger of death occurring virtually only in cases with severe coma. Complications are aspiration of vomitus, pulmonary atelectasis, pneumonitis, respiratory failure, and vasomotor collapse.

TRANQUILIZERS AND ANALEPTICS

The tranquilizers or ataractic (from the Greek word *ataraktos* meaning peace of mind) drugs may be classified into two groups: the first contains those that are primarily sedative in action, and the second those possessing the more specific capability of calming mentally disturbed, agitated, and anxious patients without causing somnolence or confusion. Examples of the first group are phenobarbital and meprobamate, and of the second the phenothiazines, *Rauwolfia*, and benzodiazepine derivatives.

In children these drugs may be prescribed for their tranquilizing properties, but more toxic effects also commonly follow their use as hypnotic, antiemetic, antihistaminic, and hypotensive agents. Children appear to be more susceptible to the side-effects of phenothiazine drugs, on a weight-to-weight basis, than are adults; furthermore, certain individuals show a lower tolerance than their fellows.

MEPROBAMATE

This general depressant muscle relaxant is a substituted propanediol that is absorbed rapidly but has a relatively prolonged plasma half-life (up to 11 hr). This property may account for described symptoms of meprobamate habituation and withdrawal. Inactivation of meprobamate depends partly on acetylation in liver and brain. Genetic variations in the rate of acetylation contribute substantially to the individual clinical picture seen with encephalopathy associated with meprobamate toxicity. Serum levels of 10 mg/dl to 20 mg/dl are usually associated with severe toxicity. Dependency, drowsiness, ataxia, paradoxical excitement, and extraocular palsies have been described, as have allergic skin rashes, which may be pruritic, erythematous, purpuric, urticarial, or take the form of angioneurotic edema. Bronchospasm or hypotension appears in some patients, and massive overdosage may result in coma and vasomotor and respiratory collapse. The concentration of drug in breast milk may be several times greater than that in the mother's plasma.

Treatment in mild cases is supportive. Dialysis or forced diuresis may be needed for severe cases.[111]

PHENOTHIAZINES

Chlorpromazine and related synthetic chemicals are generally derived from phenothiazine. They are used as antiemetics, as tranquilizers, and as potentiators of analgesics and sedatives. Acute fatal doses are in the range of 50 mg/kg to 150 mg/kg. Depending on the subgroup attached to the phenothiazine nucleus, three types of derivative are recognized. The aliphatic derivatives include chlorpromazine (Thorazine), promazine (Sparine), trifupromazine (Vesprin), and methoxpromazine (Tentone). The piperidine derivatives include mepazine (Pacatal) and thioridazine (Mellaril). The piperazine derivatives include prochlorperazine (Compazine), trifluoperazine (Stelazine), perphenazine (Trilafon), fluphenazine (Permitil and Prolixin), and Thiopropazate (Dartal).

Mental effects include excitement and restlessness, the piperazine derivatives being more prone to produce this than the others. Occasional patients become depressed and deluded and may experience hallucinations. A catatonic state has followed the use of some of these drugs.

Side-effects on the central nervous system include a Parkinsonlike syndrome with rigidity, bradykinesia for initiation as well as performance of movements, mask-like facies, loss of associated movements, resting tremor, salivation, and seborrhea. Other complaints include a state of uncontrollable restlessness (akathisia) and various dystonic and dyskinetic symptoms. The latter may take the form of oculogyric crises or spasms of the neck or limbs, sometimes accompanied by loud involuntary shrieks and involuntary orofacial grimaces and tongue movements (tardive dyskinesia). These crises are aggrivated by dehydration and occur mostly in children receiving prochlorperazine (Compazine). The symptoms may be misdiagnosed as hysteria. Other patients exhibit myoclonic twitchings or hiccups. Grand mal convulsions may occur and generalized dysrhythmias or focal slowing appear on the electroencephalogram. Phenothiazines may interfere with temperature regulation, and the danger of heat stroke exists when the environmental temperature is high.

Autonomic symptoms include dry mouth, pallor, tachycardia, blurred vision, paralytic ileus, and bladder paralysis. Toxic effects on other systems include leukopenia, jaundice, skin rashes, weight gain, and breast enlargement. Pigmentary retinopathy has followed large doses of thioridazine.

Toxic effects may appear within a day or two of starting treatment, especially if the drugs were given parenterally; tardive dyskinesias are commonly associated with chronic administration. Helpful laboratory findings in phenothiazine toxicity include characteristic abnormalities in liver function tests (elevated serum and urine bilirubin with high serum alkaline phosphatase). A few drops of ferric chloride solution added to urine acdified with diluted nitric acid yield a violet color, providing a simple and reliable screening test. Treatment of toxicity involves intensive support of autonomic functions. Diphenhydramine (Benadryl), 1 mg/kg to 5 mg/kg IV, given over several minutes provides a dramatically effective antidote for acute extrapyramidal crises.[8] Rauwolfia derivatives are used only rarely as tranquilizers in children. The drug causes depletion of the chemical transmitter dopamine in the brain. Adverse symptoms include depressed mental state, extrapyramidal rigidity or involuntary movements, epileptiform convulsions, optic atrophy, autonomic manifestations, hypotension, and syncope. Allergic symptoms such as perennial rhinitis or bronchospasm may be exacerbated. A case of true thrombocytopenia has been described.

CHLORDIAZEPOXIDE AND DIAZEPAM

These drugs are of low toxicity, although occasionally skin rash, dependency, drowsiness, ataxia, or withdrawal symptoms can occur. Paradoxical rage has been described in psychotic patients and hyperactive children. This is possibly a release phenomenon brought about by the alleviation of anxiety. Diazepam is sometimes used as an anticonvulsant, particularly to treat status epilepticus; seizures may follow its abrupt withdrawal. Respiratory arrest has followed its intravenous use.

DIFFERENTIAL DIAGNOSIS

In the case of the phenothiazines, and to a lesser degree with diazepam, differential diagnosis includes hysteria, pseudotetanus with trismus and muscle spasms, epilepsy, encephalitis, lesions of the extrapyramidal system, and bulbar poliomyelitis.

TREATMENT

Gastric lavage and supportive measures are undertaken when accidental ingestion has occurred. In those common cases where the side-effects are secondary to administration of doses within the therapeutic range, withdrawal of the drug and sedation with a barbiturate or paraldehyde, if indicated, may suffice. Dystonic spasms respond to intravenous or intramuscular benztropine methanesulfonate (Cogentin).

BROMISM

Bromides are usually ingested in sedatives containing potassium, sodium, or ammonium bromide. They are used occasionally to treat intractable epilepsy in children. Signs of acute poisoning are nausea, vomiting, metal changes, and various paralyses. Chronic poisoning may lead to mental dullness, confusion or frank psychosis, weakness, tremors, or pyramidal signs. A small proportion of patients show acneform rashes, blisters, ulceration of the mucous membranes, or lacrimation. Ordinarily blood levels above 75 mg/dl are considered excessive, but a blood level of 100 mg/dl to 125 mg/dl may be therapeutic for the control of seizures. Chronic poisoning is treated by withdrawing the drug and giving chloride supplements by mouth; acute poisoning is treated with intravenous 2N saline with or without chloruretic agents.

AMPHETAMINE AND METHYLPHENIDATE POISONING

Amphetamines and methylphenidate are often used to modify behavior and increase performance in children with hyperactivity, distractibility, low frustration tolerance, impulsiveness, and other symptoms comprised in the term *minimal brain dysfunction*. Overdosage may occur from accidental ingestion. Adolescents may ingest amphetamines ("speed") for thrills and may also be exposed to the drug in the form of diet pills.[26] Loss of appetite, loss of weight, and insomnia are the most common side-effects, and the growth of children taking these drugs may be retarded. Other side-effects include irritability, headache, depression, abdominal pains, involuntary facial and other dyskinesias, and hallucinations. Intravenous injection of methamphetamine by young drug users has resulted in cerebrovascular occlusions due to emboli, vasculitis, or spasm. The skin may be pale and sweating. Coma and convulsions may be terminal events. Treatment consists of withdrawal of the drug, gastric lavage if indicated, and sedation, especially with chlorpromazine 0.5 mg/kg to 1 mg/kg every 30 minutes as needed. The use of hypotensive agents may sometimes be indicated.

SALICYLATE POISONING

ETIOLOGY

Many different salicylates are used therapeutically, including salicylic acid, sodium salicylate, para-aminosalicylic acid, acetylsalicylic acid, and methyl salicylate (oil of wintergreen). Most cases of poisoning in children are due to the latter two, which account for approximately 15% of reported

fatal accidental poisoning in children under five years of age. Infants account for about 40% of all cases. Oil of wintergreen is a particularly dangerous substance because of its high salicylate content: one teaspoonful contains the equivalent of 14 adult-size aspirin tablets. Tolerance for acetylsalicylic acid varies widely, and death has been reported following dosage within the normal therapeutic range for the age of the child. The average fatal dose ranges from 0.2 g/kg to 0.5 g/kg.[25,66]

PATHOGENESIS

Toxic amounts of salicylate stimulate the central nervous system directly to cause hyperpnea; they also produce a metabolic derangement with accumulation of organic acids. The resulting metabolic acidosis is aggravated by urinary losses of sodium and potassium as well as by ketosis and starvation. These changes are especially pronounced in the child under four years of age. The accompanying hyperpnea may later lead to respiratory alkalosis. In addition to the initial acidosis acidemia decreases the ionization of salicylic acid ($pK_a = 3.6$) and therefore enhances its entry into the brain.

PATHOLOGY

Severe salicylcate poisoning leads to irreversible toxic effects on the nervous system. Improvements in intensive care and the consequent reduction in mortality have reduced the incidence of fatal salicylate encephalopathy. At necropsy massive hyperemia is seen in the brain, and numerous scattered petechiae are seen in the peritoneum, pleura, pericardium, and lungs. In the central nervous system petechiae are found in the cerebrum, basal ganglia, thalamus, brain stem, cerebellum, and spinal cord. Subdural hematomas have been described.

CLINICAL FEATURES

Salicylates first stimulate then depress the central nervous system. The patient may appear deceptively well when first seen because the drug has not yet been absorbed.

When symptoms appear they consist of deafness, tinnitus, dizziness, nausea, and vomiting. Diaphoresis may occur. In severe cases vomiting is violent and protracted, especially following ingestion of oil of wintergreen, and marked dehydration is common. The patient usually hyperventilates. Kussmaul breathing is seen and is due to a direct stimulatory effect of salicylate on the respiratory center. The patient may manifest spontaneous tetany. Fever commonly occurs despite the antipyretic properties of salicylates in therapeutic dosages. States of mental confusion, excitement, disorientation, and delirium may progress to convulsions and coma. Myoclonic twitches may be seen. Respiratory failure is the common terminal event.

LABORATORY EXAMINATION

Blood salicylate levels are essential to adequate management of salicylate encephalopathy. In the first 6 hours after exposure, blood salicylate levels usually exceed 45 mg/dl in intoxicated patients. Levels over 90 mg/dl generally accompany moderately severe poisoning, whereas levels above 120 mg/dl are usually fatal. The level may drop sharply with dehydration. Determinations of blood glucose and electrolytes and arterial pH and blood gases are also essential to the management of the patient with toxic doses of salicylate. Blood gas and pH values reflect the acid–base disturbances outlined in section on pathogenesis. Older children at first develop respiratory alkalosis, which is followed by metabolic acidosis due to bicarbonate deficit caused by the appearance of excessive pyruvic and lactic acids. The venous serum electrolyte pictures of respiratory alkalosis and metabolic acidosis may be confusingly similar, and in order to assess the true state of affairs a pH determination of arterial blood is required. A complicating feature in the young child is his proneness to develop ketosis. Before 3 years of age this is almost invariable and of rapid onset, so that the stage of initial respiratory alkalosis might not be found. Hypokalemia may be a feature and is exacerbated by treatment with alkali. Characteristic abnormalities appear in the electrocardiogram.

The urine is at first alkaline owing to loss of base but later it becomes acidic. It may contain protein. A useful screening test for salicylate in urine is the addition of a few drops of ferric chloride to 5 ml of acidified urine. A violet color indicates the presence of salicylate and the color persists after boiling of the urine, in contrast to the positive reaction seen with ketones. In the presence of ketosis the nitroprusside test is also positive.

DIFFERENTIAL DIAGNOSIS

This includes diabetic and other forms of ketosis, ingestion of various toxic substances, meningitis, encephalitis and toxic encephalopathies including Reye's syndrome. Salicylate therapy may be a factor in the pathogenesis of Reye's syndrome.

TREATMENT

In mild cases discontinuance of the drug or decrease of the dosage and the provision of ample fluids is all that is necessary.

Emergency treatment of the severe case may need to deal with several grave complications. Serious hypotension is best treated by whole blood (10 ml/kg–15 ml/kg) and ventilatory depression may require artificial breathing and oxygenation. Repeated generalized motor seizures are best treated by early recourse to paralysis with pancuronium combined with ventilatory support and optimization of arterial blood gases and pH. The seizures generally reflect a transient metabolic encephalopathy and therefore usually do not require maintenance anticonvulsants. The latter may also increase the patient's respiratory difficulties. Because salicylates may continue to be absorbed for up to 12 hours after ingestion, gastric lavage should constitute part of the emergency treatment.[65]

Maintenance treatment of the seriously intoxicated child requires close attention to ventilatory status and adequate cardiovascular function along lines similar to those outlined for barbiturate poisoning. Monitoring of blood chemistry allows the physician to adjust the volume and composition of parenteral fluids in accordance with the evolution of the acid–base disturbance described under pathogenesis and clinical features. Fluid volume is adjusted according to renal function and blood chemistry and can approximate 2 liters per 24 hours with adequate renal function. Inappropriate antidiuretic hormone secretion may complicate treatment by promoting fluid retention and contributing to cerebral edema. This tendency may be aggravated by injudicious administration of dilute dextrose solutions. Hypokalemia may be produced or exacerbated by administration of sodium bicarbonate, but it can be controlled by adding potassium to the infusion. Dextrose is used to combat ketosis. Intravenous sodium bicarbonate is effective in increasing the urinary output of salicylate. Potassium deficit should be corrected. In cases of massive poisoning with severe acidosis the urine cannot be alkalinized with bicarbonate and it may be safer to treat the patient expectantly. Vitamin K and ascorbic acid are given, and blood transfusion or human albumin may be required to treat shock. Extracorporeal dialysis is highly effective in removing salicylate and may be indicated in the most severe cases.

The situation is more difficult in infants with whom closer metabolic control is required. In particular, maintenance of alkaline urine is difficult in this age group. Heel capillary blood gives results comparable to arterial blood for determination of pH.

PROGNOSIS

The outlook is good in the majority of poisoning cases for which oil of wintergreen is not responsible. Until recently, poisoning from this substance had a mortality of approximately 60% in all age groups and it was greater than this in infants.

CARBON MONOXIDE POISONING

Carbon monoxide is a colorless, odorless gas formed by incomplete combustion of carbon. Common sources are car exhaust, coal gas, water gas, and incomplete combustion of wood, coal, and charcoal.

PATHOGENESIS

Carbon monoxide has an affinity for hemoglobin that is several hundred times greater than that of oxygen. Furthermore, the presence of carboxyhemoglobin inhibits the release of oxygen by the remaining oxyhemoglobin, leading to tissue anoxia that is in excess of the degree of anoxemia. The proportion of carboxyhemoglobin in the blood depends on the proportion of carbon monoxide in the inspired air and on the length of time the person was exposed to it. Maternal carbon monoxide exposure indirectly causes fetal hypoxemia and possible long-term cognitive deficits have been seen in offspring of smoking mothers.[9]

PATHOLOGY

The brains of patients who die of acute carbon monoxide poisoning may be grossly edematous and show petechial hemorrhages in the white matter and corpus callosum. The long-term effect in patients who fail to recover completely is laminar degeneration of the third layer of the cerebral cortex, particularly of the junctional zones. Bilateral globus pallidus necrosis has been thought to be especially typical of carbon monoxide poisoning.[73]

CLINICAL FEATURES

The first symptoms may consist of impaired judgment, clumsiness, headache, confusion, and dyspnea on exertion. A cherry-red color may appear in the nail beds and elsewhere but is often not present. When the patient is exposed to high concentrations of carbon monoxide (blood saturation equal to or exceeding 50%) loss of consciousness may occur rapidly with respiratory failure, convulsions, and death. Rarely, a delayed encephalopathy develops and may involve combinations of neuropsychiatric dysfunction, diffuse hypertonicity, and a Parkinsonian picture.

Approximately 40 cases of maternal–fetal coexposure to carbon monoxide have been noted. Surviving babies have shown neonatal bulbar dysfunction, hypotonia, and seizures. Persistent encephalopathy with microcephaly was seen at later ages.[76] The blood carbon monoxide level is elevated.

TREATMENT

Pure oxygen is administered. This not only aids in the transformation of carboxy- to oxyhemoglobin but also increases the quantity of oxygen dissolved in the patient's plasma. Hyperbaric oxygen has been used. Hypothermia may help protect cerebral neurons from the effects of hypoxemia and cerebral edema.

MISCELLANEOUS NEUROTOXINS

ACETAMINOPHEN

This para-aminophenol derivative is an analgesic and antipyretic contained in numerous preparations often prescribed for younger children. Recently several case reports have appeared about toxic encephalopathy due to overdosage with this agent, especially in children under five years of age. Acetaminophen is normally metabolized by conjugation with glutathione. This mechanism is exhausted at high dosages, leading to an accumulation of toxic oxidation products.[95] Treatment involves general support along the lines described for depressants. In addition, specific treatment should be given using the surrogate glutathione acetylcysteine (Mucomyst), 140 mg/kg orally followed by one-half of this dose every 4 hours for 3 days. The patient should be watched carefully for signs of hepatic encephalopathy.

ALCOHOL

Although more commonly seen as a cause of adult-onset encephalopathy, the possibility of accidental ethyl alcohol ingestion should not be overlooked in younger children with unexplained encephalopathy. Childhood exposure to the toxin can occur through ingestion of beverages or cosmetic or pharmaceutical preparations containing alcohol. Symptoms in the younger child may include ataxia and, in the more severe cases, frank encephalopathy. The degree of the latter may vary from merely a subtle change in the child's usual behavior to frank coma. Treatment should include general supportive intensive care. Hypoglycemia and acidosis are disproportionately prominent features of alcoholic encephalopathy in younger children and need early and vigorous treatment. Specific treatments for cerebral edema may also be required.

Fetal Alcohol Syndrome

Heavy maternal alcohol use both before and during pregnancy is associated with the development of this syndrome. Multiple somatic malformations are seen and those involving the brain include microcephaly and callosal agenesis. These malformations express themselves clinically as an encephalopathy whose severity may range from an attention deficit disorder to severe mental retardation.[48]

ANTIHISTAMINES

Many forms of antihistaminic compounds are available both over the counter and by prescription as antiallergic or anticoryzal preparations. Diphenhydramine (Benadryl), chlorpheniramine (Chlor-trimeton), and hydroxyzine (Atarax) are examples of commonly prescribed antihistaminics. Toxic encephalopathy from overdosage with these agents is occasionally seen in younger children. Treatment involves general supportive measures as already discussed and may also require the use of physostigime (0.5 mg/kg IV) for anticholinergic neural symptoms.[74]

ATROPINE AND RELATED ALKALOIDS

Sources of exposure include ingestion of atropine-containing proprietary preparations. Younger children in particular may also be exposed through atropine-containing plants such as *Atropa belladonna* (deadly nightshade) and *Datura stramonium* (jimson weed). Rare but well documented cases of toxicity resulting from systemic absorption of atropine after its topical administration in the form of eye drops have been described. Symptoms of atropine exposure include classical features of cholinergic antagonism (such as dry mouth, fever resulting from hypohidrosis, and tachycardia). Treatment involves general support and the administration of physostigmine as needed. Lomotil, a commonly prescribed antidiarrheal agent, combines the synthetic narcotic diphenoxylate with atropine. Symptoms of neurotoxicity from this agent in part reflect its atropine content and may also involve seizures. Treatment is similar to that for other atropine alkaloids.

GLUTETHIMIDE

This sedative agent (Doriden) is an occasional source of toxic encephalopathy following accidental ingestion by children. The general clinical picture produced and the clinical management is similar to that described for barbiturates. A distinctive and noteworthy clinical feature of glutethimide encephalopathy is the frequent finding of mydriasis even in the absence of focal mesencephalic injury.

MUSHROOMS

Ingestion of toxic mushrooms is an important differential to remember as an occasional cause of acute encephalopathy in younger children. Neurologic symptoms reflect cholinergic (muscarinic) involvement as described under organophosphate insecticides. In addition to general supportive measures, treatment may include atropine (0.02 mg/kg–0.05 mg/kg, depending on age) for muscarinic symptoms. Hypoglycemia may also be a particular problem.

TRICYCLIC ANTIDEPRESSANTS

This chemically homogeneous group of psychotropic agents includes such commonly prescribed preparations as amitriptyline (Elavil), imipramine (Tofranil), and nortriptyline (Aventyl). These agents are commonly used as antidepressants in adolescents and somewhat less commonly as adjuvants in the treatment of refractory vascular headaches in older children. Imipramine is also used in the treatment of enuresis in the younger child. Toxic exposure can result from accidental ingestion in the younger child or deliberate intake by the adolescent in a suicidal gesture or serious attempt. Anticholinergic properties of this group of compounds strongly influence their clinical neurologic effects, which can include seizures and hallucinations. Alterations in blood pressure and cardiac arrhythmias may also occur. In addition to general supportive measures already described for depressants, specific treatment with physostigmine has been advocated to reverse the anticholinergic component of the patient's symptoms.[52] Guidelines for dosage have suggested that the child under 12 years of age receive 0.5 mg IV over a 60-second interval. This dose can be repeated up to a maximum of 2 mg or until the onset of clinical cholinergic symptoms. In older children an initial dosage of 2 mg IV repeated up to a maximum of 4 mg has been suggested. Initial enthusiasm for the use of physostigmine in the treatment of overdosage from tricyclic antidepressants and other agents with an anticholinergic component of action has been tempered by reports of seizures following even careful, slow administration of physostigmine. Current opinion favors its use in cases refractory to conventional treatment, especially for the symptoms of seizures, prolonged coma, or supraventricular tachyarrhythmias. Tricyclic-induced cardiac arrhythmias seem to result from an accumulation of catecholamines, reflecting a secondary consequence of cholinergic blockage. This symptom is not helped by physostigmine but may be aided by the use of sodium bicarbonate.

HEPATIC COMA

Hepatic coma (hepatic encephalopathy, portal systemic encephalopathy) and precoma are states characterized by alterations in the patient's mental processes or level of consciousness. They are usually associated with disturbances of motor function, which are due to disease of the liver.

ETIOLOGY

The causes of hepatic failure during infancy and childhood are numerous and include acute viral hepatitis; ascending cholangitis; ingestion of hepatotoxic substances such as phosphorus or carbon tetrachloride; Reye's syndrome; congenital hyperammonemia; α_1-antitrypsin deficiency; juvenile cirrhosis from such varying causes as infectious hepatitis, chronic active hepatitis, syphilis, Wilson's disease, and chronic heart failure; metabolic disorders such as galactosemia; arginosuccinic aciduria; hepatic venous obstruction (Budd-Chiari syndrome); and congenital atresia of the bile ducts.[96] The Crigler-Najjar syndrome is a form of congenital nonhemolytic jaundice in which, due to reduction in glucuronyl transferase activity, large quantities of unconjugated bilirubin are found in the plasma. Toxic effects occur in the central nervous system, and the typical changes of kernicterus are found in fatal cases. Patients who survive show a combination of mental retardation with pyramidal and extrapyramidal signs. Hepatic coma may be precipitated in these patients by intercurrent infection.

PATHOGENESIS AND PATHOLOGY

The appearance of hepatic coma is associated particularly with the development of internal or external shunts in the portal circulation. The brain of a patient with liver failure appears to be particularly sensitive to metabolic insults, so that when the liver fails to protect the systemic circulation by its detoxifying actions on the products of protein metabolism certain nitrogenous substances are free to exert their harmful effects upon it. Chief among these is ammonia produced in the gut, kidneys, and other tissues including the brain itself. Such patients' intolerance of high protein intake of certain amino acids and ammonium salts, as well as the proclivity of gastrointestinal hemorrhage to precipitate them into coma, is well known. Hypokalemia and alkalosis are common in hepatic coma; these factors favor conversion of the ammonium ion to ammonia, which diffuses more readily across cell membranes. Magnesium deficiency, accumulation of short- and medium-chain fatty acids, retention of porphyrin, failure of the liver to synthesize substances essential to the brain, and deficiency of serotonin precursors possibly play a part. Ammonia within brain cells may combine with α-ketoglutaric acid to form glutamic acid, which in turn combines with more ammonia to form glutamine. Coma may be due to this removal of α-ketoglutaric acid, which reduces the activity of the tricarboxylic acid cycle (of which it is a part). Diminished ATP and deranged dopaminergic mechanisms may also be invoked.[53,91]

The main histologic abnormality found in the brain is an increase in the number of protoplasmic astrocytes, many of which are increased in size and contain enlarged, pale nuclei with prominent nucleoli (Alzheimer type II cells). They occur in all parts of the cerebral cortex, especially layers 5 and 6, as well as in the immediately subjacent white matter. Changes in the neurons are less prominent and more difficult to evaluate because many patients pass through a phase of terminal circulatory collapse before death.

CLINICAL FEATURES

During the stage of precoma the level of consciousness usually falls insidiously, although occasionally it does so abruptly. The child may be apathetic and confused, and show impairment of intellectual abilities. Excessive somnolence alternating with wakefulness, as well as reversal of the sleep cycle, may be prominent features. Terrifying dreams and visual hallucinations sometimes occur, and some patients become hyperexcitable with episodes of screaming. Older patients can become frankly maniacal before the stage of coma is reached.

The hallmark of the motor dysfunction is the so-called liver flap, or asterixis, which consists of a coarse, flapping tremor due to intermittent loss of the sustained muscular contraction necessary for the maintenance of postural fixation. It may be seen in the hands when the patient holds them outstretched before him but is best demonstrated in a confused or stuporous patient by the examiner holding the patient's forearm up in the air with the hand extended at the wrist. The abnormality may also be found in the lower limbs, trunk, and face. Some patients show marked restlessness, and in others repeated grimacings and jerkings occur. Convulsions are not uncommon. Speech often shows a slurring dysarthria with dysphasia in the more advanced stages. Changes in the deep tendon reflexes are inconstant, although they are frequently hyperactive or asymmetrical. Babinski responses are frequently elicitable when the level of consciousness is at a deeply depressed stage but are sometimes found when consciousness is relatively intact. Grasp and sucking reflexes may be obtained in a large proportion of patients. Reversible decerebate posture may be seen, and some patients develop subdural hematomas because of a bleeding diathesis.[63] Hepatic fetor of the breath is almost invariably present. Diuretics, especially chlorothiazide and its analogues, are dangerous in these patients both because of increased production of ammonia by the kidneys and because of the brain's enhanced sensitivity to potassium depletion.[13]

LABORATORY EXAMINATION

Many or all of the liver function tests are abnormal, and the arterial blood ammonia level is usually elevated. The patient frequently shows a moderate to severe anemia, and a bleeding diathesis may be demonstrated. The spinal fluid is clear and under normal pressure, but a yellow tinge due to bilirubin may be apparent. Spinal fluid glutamine correlates closely with the severity of encephalopathy.[53] Cells and protein are normal. The electroencephalogram typically shows increased slowing with theta waves appearing at random in the early stages of coma. As obtundation increases, delta waves make their appearance. At first these tend to occur in short symmetrical runs most evident in the anterior leads. Later they become more widespread and of diminished amplitude. Some cases show a different form of abnormality, that is, triphasic waves that are most prominent in the frontal and sylvian leads, occurring during the phase of stupor rather than full coma. The normal slow activity seen in the records of young children makes these ab-normalities more difficult to interpret. The blood sugar is usually normal but can fall to hypoglycemic levels. Esophageal and gastric varices are sought by barium swallow or by splenography.

DIFFERENTIAL DIAGNOSIS

Deterioration of the level of consciousness in patients with known liver disease may be attributable directly to hepatic insufficiency, but other causes should also be considered, including bleeding into the gastrointestinal tract from varices or ulcerations producing shock and cerebral anoxia; cerebral hemorrhage or subdural hematoma due to the defects in the clotting mechanism; and hepatogenic hypoglycemia, which may masquerade under the diagnosis of hepatic coma. The involuntary twitchings, flaps, and grimacings may be mistaken for Sydenham's chorea. Various psychiatric syndromes may be mimicked. Asterixis is not pathognomonic of liver disease, occurring also in such states as uremia, heart failure, hypercapnia, and magnesium deficiency.

TREATMENT

In the acute phase precipitating factors should be sought and treated. The arrest of gastroesophageal bleeding may require administration of vitamin K and various mechanical measures such as introduction of a Sengstaken balloon. All diuretics should be withdrawn; intercurrent infection, uremia if present, and myocardial insufficiency must be treated. Oxygen should be administered if necessary and fluid and electrolyte balance restored to normal. Fresh rather than stored blood should be used for transfusion. Efforts are made to reduce the amount of ammonia produced in the gut, by such measures as giving magnesium sulfate by mouth, enemas to evacuate nitrogenous material, and administration of nonabsorbable broad-spectrum antibiotics such as neomycin or kanamycin to reduce bowel flora. Prednisone or other steroids and the administration of levodopa by stomach tube may be useful.[91] High titer antiserum to Australia antigen may be given to patients with fulminating acute hepatitis attributable to virus B.[44] Calories are given in the form of glucose, and vitamin supplements are added. No protein is given in the acute phase. Intravenous sodium glutamate may be given to fix serum ammonia by forming glutamine. Colectomy and ileosigmoid anastomosis are sometimes used in chronic cases, but mortality is high.

Regular electroencephalograms are a very useful monitor of the effect of treatment. If abdominal paracentesis is undertaken for the relief of ascites it is advisable to withdraw only part of the fluid at one time.

PROGNOSIS

This is dependent upon the nature of the underlying liver disease, the adequacy of liver cell function, and on the presence or absence of precipitating factors. The prognosis is worst in patients with fulminating hepatitis and in those with cirrhosis accompanied by ascites, jaundice, and low serum albumin. It is best in patients with well compensated liver disease in whom treatable precipitating factors are present.[28,107]

REYE'S SYNDROME

Reye and associates described in 1963 a rapidly progressive and often fatal encephalopathy seen in young children following a characteristic prodrome of varicella or upper respiratory infection.[99] Extended experience with the variable clinical expression indicates that Reye's syndrome must be considered in the differential diagnosis of any unexplained encephalopathy of childhood. Despite improvements in prognosis associated with intensive treatment by tertiary care medical centers, a 10% mortality is still encountered.[78] An additional level of interest has recently been added to these efforts by the findings of clinical and biochemical abnormalities shown in Reye's syndrome that seem common to other metabolic diseases. A better understanding of basic pathogenetic mechanisms in Reye's syndrome, and particularly of the events that

initiate encephalopathy, may have important implications for a wide variety of other childhood metabolic and toxic disorders. The treatment of the patient with severe Reye's syndrome requires an extensive knowledge of acute neurologic care.

ETIOLOGY AND PATHOGENESIS

A clear-cut temporal association of the occurrence of Reye's syndrome with the prevalence of specific infections has been repeatedly noted. The most systematic knowledge of this phenomenon derives from data compiled by the United States Center for Disease Control (CDC).[71] Using a combination of epidemiologic and viral isolation approaches, the CDC has produced evidence for temporal and geographical association of Reye's syndrome with influenza B (1973–1974) and influenza A (1978–1979) viruses. These cases have mainly occurred in persons 10 years of age to 14 years of age, whereas varicella-associated Reye's syndrome has especially affected 5-year-old to 9-year-old children. The role of associated viral infection in the causation of Reye's encephalopathy is unclear and several observations raise the possibility of additional pathogenetic factors. These include the findings of low attack rates of Reye's syndrome concurrently with high prevalence of influenza in some geographic areas, absence of histologic evidence of tissue inflammatory response, and the very limited success in recovery of virus from organs of patients with Reye's syndrome.

The possibility that environmental factors contribute to the etiology of Reye's syndrome was suggested by the studies of Crocker and his colleagues.[29] Their work was prompted by the observance of a striking areal correlation between the practice of intensive insecticide spraying and the occurrence of Reye's syndrome in the province of New Brunswick. Spray components have produced enhanced replication of encephalomyocarditis virus in animal models, thereby suggesting a mechanism whereby specific toxic chemical exposure might potentiate viral effects. Similar results were obtained from an epidemiologic survey in Northeast Thailand, where a correlation was noted between geographical use of pesticides (mainly parathion, but also carbamates and organochlorines) and the occurrence of a disease resembling Reye's syndrome.[34] Attention was also focused on the possible role of the fungal metabolite aflatoxin as a factor contributing to the onset of some cases of Reye's syndrome. Recent studies failed to find a significant difference in plasma and urinary levels of aflatoxin in Reye's syndrome patients compared to controls.[87] These results do not rule out a causal role in Reye's syndrome of more remotely acquired aflatoxin that would be stored in extravascular sites.

Recent thinking has attempted a partial unification of the differing theories of pathogenesis of Reye's syndrome by proposing the concept of toxin–virus or chemical–virus interaction. Muller has outlined a detailed scheme for this hypothetical sequence involving initial toxic chemical exposure that produces biochemical abnormalities with impairment of immune responses to viral infection.[84] Later, acute viral illness supervenes and induces further biochemical abnormalities that lead to liver failure and encephalopathy. This hypothesis remains unproven but derives some support from recent recognition of biochemical changes that appear common to the majority of children with Reye's syndrome. These abnormalities pertain especially to lipid metabolism and essentially comprise evidence of excessive beta-oxidation with accumulation of medium-chain fatty acids (C_6, C_8 and C_{10}) and their omega-oxidation dicarboxylic homologues.[79] A serum factor has been isolated from some patients that affects oxygen consumption by rat mitochondria at the cytochrome c level, but the specificity of this factor to Reye's syndrome is not yet established.[2,3] A further recent epidemiologic observation that may be of major importance in advancing our understanding of pathogenesis relates to the finding that high salicylate use in Reye's syndrome correlates with poor outcome.[119] If confirmed, these findings have obvious implications for the prescribing of antipyretics for children. In addition, they suggest a further line of potentially useful investigation, namely, whether salicylates or their metabolites may play an important part in the postulated chemical–viral interaction that may be involved in the initiation of Reye's syndrome.

It is gradually becoming apparent that a variety of metabolic disorders can clinically masquerade as Reye's syndrome. Such disorders include hydroxymethylglutaryl CoA lyase deficiency, β-hydroxy-β-methylglutaricaciduria, ethylmalonic-adipic aciduria, and "Jamaican vomiting sickness."[17,41,75,83,100,122,124] The recognition of disorders mimicking Reye's syndrome adds to the complexity of clinical diagnosis. However, this situation also provides an opportunity to study in detail metabolic pathways whose elucidation may eventually lead to a fundamental understanding of the pathogenesis of Reye's syndrome.

Trauner and colleagues have developed an animal model of Reye's syndrome based on sodium octanoate infusion and have demonstrated dose-dependent increases in intracranial pressure following exposure to this medium-chain fatty acid that is often elevated in Reye's syndrome serum.[130] It remains to be established how such intracranial changes are linked with the systemic metabolic defect in Reye's syndrome. The finding of a specific transport system in choroid plexus for organochlorine pesticides and organic acids may be important in this regard.[67] The operation of such systems in vivo would be critical in effecting rapid clearance from brain of toxic metabolites structurally akin to medium-chain fatty acids of the type elevated in Reye's syndrome serum. Impairment of the clearance systems by competing substrates would tend to cause prolonged elevations in the brain levels and may explain, at least, in part, the protracted encephalopathy in Reye's syndrome.

PATHOLOGY

Characteristic changes in liver at the ultrastructural level have been described particularly by Partin who has summarized criteria for the pathologic diagnosis of Reye's syndrome.[92] (Fig. 11-3) The criteria include mitochondrial matrix expansion and disorganization, cytoplasmic glycogen depletion and smooth endoplasmic increase, microvillar alterations, and nuclear swelling.[56,82,92] Less attention has been paid to the neuropathology of Reye's syndrome but ultrastructural changes have been reported

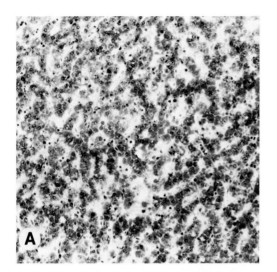

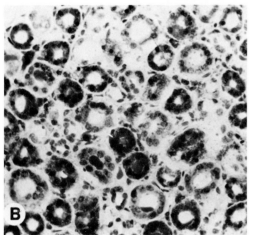

FIG. 11-3. *A*. Fat-laden liver cells in Reye's syndrome. *B*. Fatty infiltration of renal tubules. (Sudan black stain)

that resemble these found in liver and also bear some resemblance to the neuropathology of triethyltin intoxication.[93,135]

CLINICAL FEATURES

In the most classic presentation, the child with Reye's syndrome is first affected with a picture of upper respiratory infection or varicella that develops in a typical manner. Characteristically there ensues a period of 2 days to 3 days of clinical improvement following which profuse vomiting appears and heralds the first symptoms of encephalopathy. Sufficient variations in this clinical sequence have been encountered that

Reye's syndrome needs to be considered in the differential diagnosis of any otherwise unexplained childhood encephalopathy. Adult-onset cases are rarely seen.[5]

The initial symptoms of encephalopathy are subtle and may consist of merely a personality change detectable only to parents such as loss of interest in television. A phase of delirium, with increased psychomotor activity and agitated behavior, is followed by the development of obtundation. In severe cases, this stage rapidly merges into coma. The later stages of evolution are marked by the appearance of classical signs of progressive rostrocaudal deterioration, that is, decorticate and later decerebrate rigidity, with progressive loss of pupillomotor and oculocephalic reflexes. Staging criteria are a useful aid in evaluating the progress of the patient as well as in providing assessment of treatment response both for the individual patient and in clinical trials. A widely used classification is that of Lovejoy, which defines five stages in the clinical evolution of neurologic signs.[77] An additional level of classification involves electrocephalographic criteria that has also been proposed to be of prognostic value.[1,13] Increasingly frequent use of curarization engenders loss of clinical assessment criteria. Most patients in this category have on-line monitoring of intracranial pressure and their management may be aided by a recently proposed staging scheme based on the extent of intracranial pressure elevation.[14]

LABORATORY FINDINGS

An initial hyperammonemia (arterial blood ammonia greater than 80 μg/dl), first described in 1969 remains the most useful simple biochemical marker of Reye's syndrome.[51,55] Blood ammonia tends to normalize within 48 hours to 72 hours, irrespective of the clinical outcome, and at these later stages elevated serum transaminases are helpful diagnostically. Mild to moderate prolongation of prothrombin time is a common initial but transient abnormality. Evidence of cholestasis is also mild and persistent hyperbilirubinemia would strongly question the diagnosis of Reye's syndrome. Serum electrolyte and pH studies reveal a complex acid–base disturbance, initially involving metabolic acidosis with respiratory alkalosis and a relatively normal pH. Hypoglycemia is a particular problem in patients under 5 years of age, and is often associated with varicella. Short to medium–chain fatty acids are elevated, but their determination requires gas chromatography and mass spectroscopy. Abnormal plasma amino acids (especially alanine, glutamine, lysine, and alpha-aminon-butyrate) have been claimed to be characteristic. Elevations of plasma cortisol, glucagon, growth hormone and epinephrine are less consistently reported chemical disturbances that may be related to stress. Elevated muscle enzymes (serum creatine kinase and lactate dehydrogenase) have been reported to serve as a prognostic marker.[103]

The indications for liver biopsy remain a matter of contention and as yet no universally acceptable position has evolved. The spectrum of opinion ranges from advocacy of biopsy as a diagnostic requisite to an acceptance of clinical–biochemical criteria (e.g., hyperammonemia, elevated serum transaminases, and encephalopathy without other identifiable cause) as sufficient.[43,110] Recent experience suggests that nonhistologic criteria are inadequate since they may fail to distinguish a metabolic encephalopathy of known etiology, such as carnitine deficiency, from Reye's syndrome. This suggests an increasing breadth of indication for performance of liver biopsy, particularly in neonates and infants in whom the frequency of conditions potentially masquerading as Reye's syndrome (such as organic acidurias and other congenital metabolic errors) appears to be the highest. Cerebrospinal fluid examination by lumbar puncture is of importance primarily to exclude viral encephalitis, which can mimic many clinical features of Reye's syndrome. This can be accomplished by lumbar puncture early in the course of illness. Complications of this procedure such as cerebral herniation are extremely low, perhaps because of the symmetrical nature of the brain-swelling.

TREATMENT

The optimal treatment setting involves an intensive care unit located in a tertiary medical center with patient care delivered by pediatricians, neurologists, and neurosurgeons all of whom have had previous experience in Reye's syndrome.

The two major and critical aspects of treatment involve (1) meticulous supportive care and (2) particular attention to the assessment and management of intracranial hypertension.[128]

The principles of supportive care in the management of acute Reye's syndrome are similar to those outlined earlier in this chapter for the management of depressant poisoning. Particular attention to fluid replacement is especially important because of the potential risks of precipitating or aggravating cerebral edema. An initial formula of 1 ml/kg body weight to 1.5 ml/kg body weight per hour given as 5% dextrose solution with .5N saline is frequently acceptable but later details of volume and solute concentration must be monitored closely according to criteria that include neurologic course, central venous pressure, and urinary output. Placement of arterial lines for optimal blood gas assessment and of a central venous catheter are now standard practice for the patient with severe Reye's syndrome, whereas placement of a Swann-Ganz catheter is often advantageous. In all patients progressing to persistent obtundation, hyperventilation, and decortication (stage 3 Lovejoy), aggressive therapy should be instituted.[127] Nasotracheal intubation minimizes risks of aspiration and chemical pneumonitis and is followed by curarization. Pancuronium, 0.04 to 0.1 mg per kg body weight, followed by one-tenth of this dose hourly, is usually effective. The major advantage of this course is to allow optimal adjustment of blood gases, an important adjunct in management of intracranial hypertension. The main disadvantage is the sacrifice of clinical neurologic assessment. However, a combination of electroencephalogram (EEG) and intracranial pressure assessment provides satisfactory guides to the patient's response to therapy.[46,131] Blood PaO_2 maintained at 100 torr to 150 torr and pCO_2 at 20 torr to 30 torr represent optimal values. Small amounts of intravenous morphine (.05 mg/kg) can be used for sedation at this stage.

Although no controlled study of its overall benefit has been accomplished, intracranial pressure monitoring is almost universally accepted as an essential step in all patients receiving artificial ventilation and curarization. The outstanding advantages relate to the ability to detect immediately and to correct sudden increases in intracranial pressure. As a corollary, the intravenous administration of osmotic agents can be minimized and thereby complications of this mode of therapy such as hyperosmolality and hypovalemia can be reduced. Monitoring of intracranial pressure can be accomplished by a subarachnoid screw or by placement of an intraventricular catheter.[116,133] The advantage of the subarachnoid approach lies in a theoretically low risk of complications such as cerebritis or ventriculitis. Direct intraventricular monitoring offers the benefit of ventricular drainage as an extra mode for lowering of intracranial pressure as well as access to CSF for further diagnostic data.

Experience with intracranial pressure monitoring has revealed the frequent effectiveness of simple physical measures in combating sudden increases in intracranial pressure.[115,129] These measures include adjustment of patient's posture to avoid cervical venous constriction, manual hyperventilation, and adjustment of body temperature to 37° C if needed. These approaches have greatly reduced the need for osmotherapy. If needed, it is often effective to begin with relatively small doses (e.g., .25 g per kg) of mannitol by intravenous bolus.[66]

Beneficial results have been reported in the use of pentobarbital as an added therapy in severe Reye's syndrome.[81] Dose has been regulated according to various criteria e.g., cerebral perfusion pressure (50 torr or above), blood barbiturate levels of 2.5 mg/dl to 4 mg/dl or EEG findings of "burst suppression." The final assessment of this approach must await a controlled, multicenter trial of treatment results in Reye's syndrome populations treated with comparable supportive care and randomized as to the addition or withholding of barbiturates.

Several additional modes of therapy have been emphasized by individual groups but have not gained widespread acceptance. The approach of Haymond and associates involves continuous hypertonic glucose (700 mg/kg per hr), by intravenous administration.[50] This regime has a strong scientific rationale in view of the impairment of gluconeogenesis in Reye's syndrome, achieves excellent empirical results, and perhaps should be more widely adopted. Exchange transfusion to remove a hypothetical circulating toxin has been given a thorough clinical trial and has been strongly advocated by some but has not received uniform endorsement.[12,42] Hypothermic total washout has been proposed, whereas peritoneal dialysis was found to be of little value.[72,105]

PROGNOSIS

The mortality of Reye's syndrome has been greatly reduced by widespread use of intracranial pressure monitoring and the aggressive management procedures outlined in this chapter.[7,37] The earlier literature repeatedly indicates the potential for development of a severe encephalopathy in some survivors. Typical psychometric deficits range from severe global psychomotor retardation to mild specific perceptual or language impairments, and the motor involvement varies from mild dysarthria to decorticate posturing.[33] It is to be anticipated that a less severe and perhaps qualitatively different form of encephalopathy will result in survivors who receive modern treatment. Follow-up neurologic and psychometric studies of this group are awaited with great interest.

UREMIA

The term *uremia* refers to the symptom complex resulting from severe renal failure.

ETIOLOGY

The causes of renal failure may be classified into prerenal, renal, and postrenal groups. The majority of uremia cases in children fall into the renal group and are due to the late stages of intrinsic disease of the kidneys themselves, including infantile polycystic disease, congenital malformations of the kidneys, and the effects of obstructive lesions. Hereditary nephropathy (Alport's syndrome) is a familial disorder. Affected individuals appear to suffer from a form of glomerulonephropathy with pyelonephritis, as well as associated perceptive deafness and possibly defects of the ocular lens. It affects males more severely than females.[19,39,45]

PATHOLOGY

Following an acute renal illness the brain may appear morphologically normal or may show swelling with punctate hemorrhages. Histologically the neurons bear the brunt of the damage, changes varying from chromatolysis to profound disruption with vacuolation and pyknosis, the Purkinje cells being particularly vulnerable. Gliosis is not prominent. In subacute cases damage to the neurons may be mild. There may be diffuse perivascular myelin degeneration affecting especially the cerebral hemispheres with minimal alterations of other structures. In longstanding cases chronic alterations of neurons with pyknosis and shrinkage are seen, as is focal injury with formation of small cavities and glial nodules. The choroid plexuses show alteration with desquamation, swelling, and vacuolation. The effects of hypertension are superimposed upon these abnormalities. Damage to the peripheral nerves first affects the distal portions of the sensory neurons. The axon is first affected, presumably secondary to metabolic damage. Damage to the myelin sheath occurs secondarily, with segmental degeneration.[36]

The pathogenesis of uremic encephalopathy and polyneuropathy is obscure. The data suggest that they are the consequence of some abnormal metabolite, the nature of which remains to be elucidated. For example, the injection of CSF from uremic patients into the subarachnoid space of dogs produces central nervous system signs within a matter of minutes.

CLINICAL FEATURES

Generalized fatigue, lethargy, anorexia, and loss of weight are almost universal complaints. The patient may have periods of apathy and excessive drowsiness alternating with periods in which he is normally alert. There may be behavioral changes. These changes in the sensorium do not correlate well with the blood urea nitrogen level. Early morning vomiting and nausea are common, and a generalized, nonspecific headache may be present. Speech may be slurred, especially during periods of fatigue and confusion. Some patients develop uremic amaurosis. They rarely show changes in the optic fundi, and most recover their sight within 2 weeks to 3 weeks. Sixth nerve palsies are seen occasionally.

The patient looks chronically ill with a peculiar dirty pallor due in part to associated normo- or hypochromic anemia. In cases of longer duration the skin shows a yellowish brown coloration, with or without petechiae and ecchymoses. Itching may be severe, and excoriated and lichenified areas are sometimes seen where the child has scratched himself. The mouth and lips are dry and sordes may be present. The tongue is furred, and often there is a uremic fetor.

Muscle wasting and irritability manifested by fascicular and myokymic twitchings and intractable hiccups may be present; cramps are common. There may be asterixis or myoclonic jerks; epileptiform convulsions occur in a number of patients. Weakness is common and may show periodic exacerbations in patients whose blood potassium level falls to low levels. Some patients develop polyneuropathy, the incidence of this complication having increased since the advent of hemodialysis. Patients with milder cases of neuropathy may present with the restless legs syndrome in which the patient develops burning feet or an intolerable discomfort or feeling of weariness in the legs that obliges him to move them or walk about to obtain relief. Sensory loss may follow, and a mixture of sensory and motor involvement is seen in severe cases. The lower limbs are more severely involved than the upper ones.

Memory and ability to concentrate are nearly always impaired, and the latter fatigues rapidly (demonstrated by getting the patient to add serial twos.). Some patients show the picture of uremic psychosis, and coma may appear terminally. Acute psychotic episodes or coma may develop acutely after hemodialysis and may persist for hours or days despite maintenance of normal fluid and electrolyte values. Skeletal abnormalities such as a "rickety rosary" of the costochondral junctions and widening of the wrist with lipping and widening of the distal forearm metaphysis (seen on x-ray film) might be found along with the attenuated bone shadows of osteomalacia. Bone cysts from secondary hyperparathyroidism are infrequent. A bleeding diathesis may become manifest.

Hypertension is very common, and all of its complications are likely to be added to the picture. Retinal arterioles may be of uneven caliber and show an increased light reflex; there may be hemorrhages, exudates, and choked disks. Exudates appear, especially in renal disease, and may form an extensive peripapillary ring or a macular star. Terminal pericarditis may appear. Neck stiffness, Kernig's sign, and other signs of meningeal irritation are found in a number of patients.[109,132]

LABORATORY EXAMINATION

In renal failure the blood urea nitrogen (BUN) and serum creatinine are elevated and renal clearance is decreased. Certain anions are retained, particularly phosphate and sulfate, and this favors metabolic acidosis and hypocalcemia. Although the serum calcium may be as low as 6 mg/dl, overt tetany is uncommon. The serum potassium level is typically high in terminal uremia but may be normal or low in earlier phases. The urine is pale due to failure to excrete urochrome and shows a fixed osmolality with a specific gravity of about 1.010. Varying amounts of protein may be excreted. Cells, microorganisms, and casts may be found on microscopic examination.

The EEG remains unchanged in the early stages of renal failure; later the normal basic rhythms become disorganized and there is excessive slowing. Theta activity is the first to appear, but in the late stages generalized random delta waves predominate. Temporary worsening of the EEG may appear with rapid improvement of electrolyte concentrations in patients undergoing hemodialysis. Decreased nerve conduction velocity may antedate clinical neuropathy.

The CSF commonly shows some elevation of pressure and has a normal or elevated protein level. A lymphocytic reaction is found in a minority of cases showing signs of meningeal irritation. The nonprotein nitrogen level is elevated.

DIFFERENTIAL DIAGNOSIS

The diagnosis is usually obvious in uremic patients, but occasionally a different cause of the presenting symptoms may be thought likely; for example, patients have been diagnosed initially as suffering from acute gastroenteritis because of nausea and vomiting, or even from Addison's disease because of weakness, darkening of the skin, hyponatremia, and dehydration.

TREATMENT

The main approaches to the treatment of uremia are dietary control, dialysis, and kidney transplantation. It is inappropriate to discuss the details of management here apart from a few points of neurologic interest. The administration of alkalis in the presence of hypocalcemia leads to the risk of precipitating tetany or convulsions. Intravenous calcium gluconate is given to correct hypocalcemia, but this does not cure tremors, twitchings, or jactitations. The effect on convulsions is variable, and paraldehyde or intravenous dephenylhydantoin followed by oral maintenance are suitable drugs for their control. Patients undergoing hemodialysis have developed subdural hematomas from the use of heparin. Transplant recipients on immunosuppressive drugs may develop lymphomas involving the central nervous system, posterior subcapsular cataracts, increased intraocular pressure, or cytomegalovirus retinitis.[108]

PROGNOSIS

Formerly when the patient had reached the stage of chronic renal insufficiency with hypertension he rarely lived longer than 3 years, and the average life of a patient who remained anuric was about 3 weeks. The outlook has improved greatly since the development of hemodialysis and transplantation. With recovery of renal function after acute oliguric renal failure complete disappearance of all nervous system symptoms may be anticipated.

TETANUS

Tetanus is an infectious disease characterized by muscular rigidity and intermittent convulsive spasms. It is caused by the exotoxin of *Clostridium tetani*.

ETIOLOGY

Clostridium tetani is an obligatorily anaerobic spore-forming organism that inhabits the animal gut from whence it gains access to soil and dirt. It enters the body through contaminated wounds, although no obvious portal of entry is discovered in more than one-fourth of cases. Puncture wounds are particularly dangerous, especially if associated with introduction of a foreign body. Thus splinters, thorns, insect stings, rusty nails, particles of wadding from blank cartridges, and open fractures have been implicated in children. Burned areas are also liable to infection. Many cases occur in narcotic addicts (Fig. 11-4) who inject their drugs intravenously (mainliners) and more especially those who do so subcutaneously (skin poppers). Neonatal tetanus from infection of the umbilical stump is extremely

FIG. 11-4. Skin necrosis from intravenous and subcutaneous injection in a drug addict with tetanus.

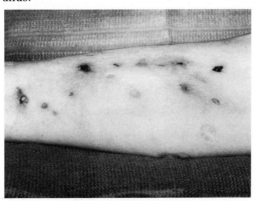

prevalent in socially backward countries and might account for more than half of infantile deaths from specific diseases.

PATHOLOGY

The bacilli produce two toxins: tetanolysin and tetanospasmin. The latter ascends the nerves to reach the central nervous system where it becomes fixed on the nerve cells of the anterior horns and brain stem, rendering the central nervous system hyperexcitable. The characteristic muscular rigidity and recruitment spasms are probably based on the suppression of spinal inhibitory mechanisms.

CLINICAL FEATURES

Cases of tetanus are conventionally categorized into six clinical groups: (1) localized tetanus, which is a relatively mild disease and occurs mainly in persons previously immunized (uncommon in children); (2) a generalized tonic form in which the rigidity eventually wanes without the appearance of convulsive spasms; (3) the fully developed form with genealized tonic rigidity and convulsive spasms; (4) the bulbar form with predominant involvement of the muscles of deglutition and respiration; (5) cephalic tetanus manifested by spasm or paralysis confined to the cranial nerve musculature without more generalized involvement; and (6) infantile tetanus.

In fully developed tetanus the incubation period varies from a few days to many months. The first symptoms are nonspecific and usually consist of vague malaise, restlessness, irritability, and headache followed by varying degrees of muscle aching. Pyrexia is not a feature of tetanus, the temperature being normal or only slightly raised unless secondary infection supervenes. The initial symptoms are followed by the more distinctive symptom of muscular rigidity. The muscles of mastication tend to be affected early, leading to trismus due to sustained contraction of the jaw-closing muscles. Involvement of the cranial nerves is common and can take the form of either paralysis or spasm. Thus the patient might show paralysis of the external ocular muscles, spasm or paralysis of the masseters, or spasm of one side of the face with paralysis of the opposite side. The pharyngeal and tongue muscles may also be involved. Spasm of the muscles innervated by the facial nerve leads to a sustained involuntary grin, the so-called risus sardonicus. Progressive hardening and boardlike rigidity of the muscles of the trunk and limbs ensues, leading to extension of the lower extremities, nuchal rigidity, opisthotonos (Fig. 11-5) with superimposition of severe convulsive muscle spasms. The deep tendon reflexes may be increased and spontaneous clonus elicited. All modalities of sensation are appreciated normally; the patient may suffer agonizing pain, which is very distressing because normal mentation is often maintained. Drug addicts who develop tetanus have a much more severe form of the disease than nonaddicts. Most develop spasms within 24 hours of admission to the hospital; their mortality rate, despite heroic measures, approaches 90%.[21]

Many patients develop overactivity of the sympathetic nervous system with labile hypertension, tachycardia, irregularities of cardiac rhythm, peripheral vasoconstriction, sweating, pyrexia, increased carbon dioxide output, and increased urinary catecholamine excretion.[64]

LABORATORY EXAMINATION

The diagnosis of tetanus is based on the clinical features of the illness. Attempts are made to confirm the diagnosis by anaerobic culture of the wound material or its debridement products; however, failure to grow C. tetani is common. Conversely, the organism is occasionally isolated from the wounds of patients not suffering from tetanus.

DIFFERENTIAL DIAGNOSIS

Trismus can be produced by peritonsillar abscess, retropharyngeal abscess, parotid infections, and hysteria. The fully developed picture could be confused with meningitis, rabies, strychnine poisoning (in which, however, the muscles relax between spasms), and tetany.

TREATMENT

Immunization is achieved by giving a series of tetanus toxoid injections, usually during early childhood. It has been customary to inject a booster dose of toxoid whenever an unclean wound or puncture wound is sustained. Recent work, however, has shown that children who have received four or more injections of toxoid do not lose their protective level of antibody for at least 12 years; thus additional emergency booster doses of toxoid are not recommended.[94]

It would be difficult to overemphasize the importance of skilled nursing care and experienced teamwork in reducing the mortality from tetanus. Elimination of toxin and prevention of its further fixation are promoted by full exploration and debridement of wounds; the wounds are sometimes irrigated with oxidizing solutions. The patient is isolated in a quiet, darkened room, and visitors are forbidden. Human antitetanus immune globulin is given. It is injected intramuscularly. The intravenous route must never be used because of the danger of anaphylaxis. Intrathecal antitoxin is not used. Full doses of penicillin should be given. Clostridium tetani is also sensitive to chloramphenicol and the tetracyclines. Sedation is usually required; either a medium-acting barbiturate or chlorpromazine is suitable for this, although chloral hydrate, meprobamate, and other drugs have been used. Lowering the mortality rate by using intravenous mephensin has been reported. The

FIG. 11-5. Tetanus: opisthotonos.

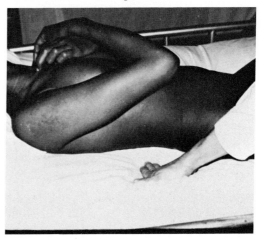

adrenergic blocking agents propranolol and bethanidine have been used in combination to counter sympathetic overactivity, but Cole and Youngman reported that paraldehyde is as effective as anesthetic agents in preventing this effect.[27,97] In severe cases a combination of muscle relaxants and intermittent positive pressure respiration, while monitoring blood gases, pH, and lung compliance to detect underventilation (with scrupulous attention paid to pulmonary toilet), has given the best results. Smythe describes a very low mortality in infantile cases by using these methods.[117] In older children tracheostomy should be undertaken early rather than late in order to avoid its performance as an emergency procedure. Tube feeding is used when possible and electrolyte balance undertaken by means of intravenous drip and strict laboratory control.

PROGNOSIS

In infantile cases the death rate used to be 75% to 90%. Skilled nursing teamwork and the use of chlorpromazine or mephenesin reduced it to about 50% and the introduction of curarization with intermittent positive pressure respiration to 11% to 20%.[62,68] In older children it probably lies between 20% to 50%, and in drug addicts it approaches 90%. As Hippocrates pointed out, the mortality is higher in cases with a short incubation period, but an even more accurate indicator is the "period of onset," which is the time between the onset of the first symptoms and the first reflex spasm. If the incubation period is less than 7 days or the period of onset less than 48 hours the prognosis is exceedingly grave.

Patients who recover usually show no abnormal aftereffects, but some have residual irritability, myoclonic jerks, convulsions, postural hypotension, or sphincter disturbances.[57] Recovery from tetanus does not confer protection against further attacks, and recurrent cases have been reported.

PREVENTION

The main hope for the final eradication of tetanus resides in the realm of public health care. The proportion of children receiving prophylactic inoculation with tetanus toxoid, usually in conjunction with diphtheria and pertussis toxoid, is rising. Such inoculation not only diminishes the number of cases of clinical tetanus, but those that do appear tend to be of the milder varieties such as the localized form. It is claimed that infantile tetanus does not occur when the mother has been actively immunized during pregnancy.

BOTULISM

ETIOLOGY AND PATHOGENESIS

Infant Botulism

Infant botulism, first recognized as a clinical entity in 1976, occurs when spores of *C. botulinum* germinate and then multiply in the gut and produce toxin *in vivo*. The intestinal tract of only some infants is susceptible to *C. botulinum* infection. In contrast with this, most infants and all older children and adults regularly ingest *C. botulinum* spores with no ill effects. All of the cases of infant botulism are caused either by type A or type B botulinal toxin. Approximately 250 cases needing hospital care occur annually.[4]

In children, botulism is a type of food poisoning that primarily affects the nervous system. It is caused by ingesting the exotoxin of *C. botulinum*, which is an anerobic, gram-positive, spore-forming rod. Seven types (A,B,C,D,E,F, and G) have been differentiated, each producing an antigenically distinct exotoxin. The majority of human cases are caused by types A and E. Type A spores are present in soil throughout the world; type E spores are found in the northern hemisphere particularly in lakeshore and seashore mud. The disease results from ingestion of toxin preformed in inadequately sterilized foods, particularly home-canned or home-bottled fruits and vegetables. Outbreaks have also occurred from commercially canned foods and from plastic-packaged foods, especially fish. The toxin produces its effects by inhibiting the release of acetylcholine from the synaptic vesicles.

In some outbreaks one or more individuals were severely affected whereas others who partook of the same food had mild cases or escaped disease. This is ascribed to patchy distribution of the organisms and toxin in the food. Mortality approaches 50% in type A poisoning but is less for type E. Rarely, cases of botulism result from wound infections. Wound botulism results when *C. botulinum* organisms infect and produce toxin in traumatized tissue.

CLINICAL FEATURES

Infant botulism occurs between 1 and 9 months of age; 98% of cases are between 1 and 6 months of age. Honey exposure is a significant risk factor for type B infant botulism. In one series 44% of cases and only 9% of controls had been fed honey. However, exposure to honey can only account for a minority of the cases because only one-third of all reported cases have been fed honey prior to onset of illness.

Infant botulism varies from a mild disorder, which may be considered as "failure to thrive," to a sudden infant death syndrome. In a fulminant case, paralysis of the pharyngeal muscles and tongue may produce obstruction of the airway with sudden death. Early clinical findings are constipation, lethargy, followed by a feeble cry, easy fatigability of the pupillary light reflex and of the extraocular muscles, and difficulty in sucking and swallowing with a weak gag reflex. Cranial nerve findings are followed by generalized flaccid muscular weakness or paralysis within a few hours or several days. Weakness becomes most severe within 1 week to 2 weeks and is then stationary for 2 weeks to 3 weeks before slow improvement begins.

In children the severity of disease varies from mild to fulminating. The first symptoms occur after a delay of 12 hours to several days. Lassitude, malaise, and feelings of disequilibrium are early complaints. Nausea and vomiting are particularly associated with type E intoxication and less frequently with the others. Paralysis of muscles supplied by the motor cranial nerves occurs early, with dysphagia, hoarseness, blurring of vision, diplopia, and usually loss of pupillary reactions. Gener-

alized weakness and respiratory failure follow in severe cases. The deep tendon reflexes are spared if the muscles are not paralyzed. Dryness of the mouth and pharynx and other effects of parasympathetic paralysis may be prominent. The level of consciousness varies from awake to lethargic. The intravenous edrophonium (Tensilon) test may be positive in mild cases.[104]

LABORATORY EXAMINATION

Electromyography frequently reveals a characteristic pattern of brief, small, abundant motor unit action potentials. In infant botulism the diagnosis is established by the identification of *C. botulinum* and also of botulinus toxin in the feces. Tests of toxicity are performed by injecting either the patient's serum or saline washings of suspected food into mice. If botulinus toxin is present the mice die; mice protected with specific antiserum survive.

DIFFERENTIAL DIAGNOSIS

Infant botulism is initially difficult to differentiate from septicemia, acute viral infections, dehydration, idiopathic hypotonia, and polyneuritis. If an infant develops constipation, weakness, difficulty in sucking, swallowing, crying or breathing, infant botulism is the most likely diagnosis.

TREATMENT

An infant with severe botulism is treated in the hospital intensive care unit with access to mechanical ventilation because aspiration or apnea may occur. Suction, mechanical respiration, and tube-feeding are used as needed. The infant is monitored until it can breathe, cough, and swallow adequately. Antitoxin and antibiotics are not currently recommended in the treatment of infant botulism.

When botulism occurs in children, artificial respiration and other supportive measures are undertaken in severe cases. Saline purgatives, enemas, and in early cases gastric lavage have been recommended. Specific equine antitoxin should be administered. The antitoxin may be trivalent (A,B,E) or bivalent (A,B), but the latter should be used only if the type is known because there is little or no cross protection. Skin tests to horse serum should be performed. Guanidine hydrochloride in an oral daily dose of 15 mg/kg body weight to 40 mg/kg body weight may help reverse the neuromuscular block. With modern intensive care the outlook has improved greatly.[104,106]

PREVENTION

It is recommended that honey not be fed to infants under 1 year of age since ingestion of honey is a significant risk factor for type B infant botulism.

REFERENCES

1. **Aoki Y, Lombroso CT:** Prognostic value of electroencephalography in Reye's syndrome. Neurology 23:333, 1973

2. **Aprille JR:** Reye's syndrome: patient serum alters mitochondrial function and morphology in vitro. Science 197:808, 1977

3. **Aprille JR, Austin J, Costello CE et al:** Identification of the Reye's syndrome serum factor. Biochem Biophys Res Commun 94:381, 1980

4. **Arnon SS:** Infant botulism. Ann Rev Med 31:541, 1980

5. **Atkins JN, Haponik EF:** Reye's syndrome in the adult patient. Am J Med 67:672, 1979

6. **Bakir F, Damluji SF, Amin-Zaki L et al:** Methylmercury poisoning in Iraq. An Interuniversity Report. Science 181:230, 1973

7. **Baliga RE, Fleishman LE, Chang C-H et al:** Acute renal failure in Reye's syndrome. Am J Dis Child 133:1009, 1979

8. **Barry P, Meysken SL, Becker CE:** Phenothiazine poisoning. A review of 48 cases. Calif Med 118:1, 1973

9. **Beaudoing A, Gachon L, Butin L et al:** Les consequences foetales de l'intoxication oxycarbonne de la mère. Pediatrie 24:539, 1969

10. **Berlin M, Jerksell LG, Nordberg G:** Accelerated uptake of mercury by brain caused by 2, 3-Dimercaptopropanol (BAL) after injection into the mouse of a methylmercuric compound. Acta Pharmacol et Toxicol 23:312, 1965

11. **Berlin M, Carson J, Norseth T:** Dose-dependence of methylmercury metabolism. A study of distribution, biotransformation and excretion in the squirrel monkey. Arch of Environ Hlth 30:307, 1975

12. **Bobo RC, Shubert WK, Partin JC et al:** Reye Syndrome: Treatment by exchange transfusion with special reference to the 1974 epidemic in Cincinnati. J Pediatr 87:881, 1975

13. **Booth CB, Swadey JG, Fiol RE:** Neurologic status of patients with liver disease. Arch Neurol 8:257, 1963

14. **Boutros AR, Esfandiari S, Orlowski JP et al:** Reye's syndrome: a predictably curable disease. Pediatric Clinics of North America 27(3):539, 1980

15. **Byers RK, Lord EE:** Late effects of lead poisoning on mental development. Am J Dis Child 66:471, 1943

16. **Cavanagh JB, Fuller NH, Johnson HRM et al:** The effects of thallium salts, with particular reference to the nervous system changes. Quarterly Journal of Medicine 43:293, 1974

17. **Chalmers RA, Langon AM:** Identification of 5-hydroxyhexanoic acid in the urine of twin siblings with a Reye's-like syndrome associated with dicarboxylic aciduria and hypoglycemia and with similarities to Jamaican vomiting sickness. Biomed Mass Spectrum 6:444, 1979

18. **Chamberlain P, Stavioha NB, Davis H et al:** Thallium poisoning. Pediatrics 22:1170, 1958

19. **Chappell JA, Kelsey WM:** Hereditary nephritis. J Dis Child 99:401, 1960

20. **Chernoff N, Rogers EH:** Fetal toxicity of kepone in rats and mice. Toxicology and Applied Pharmacology 38:189, 1976

21. **Cherubin CE:** Clinical severity of tetanus in narcotic addicts in New York City. Arch Intern Med 121:156, 1968

22. **Chisolm JJ, Barltrop D:** Recognition and management of children with increased lead absorption. Arch of Dis in Child 54:249, 1979

23. **Clarkson TW:** The pharmacology of mercury compounds. Ann Rev of Pharm 12:375, 1972

24. **Clarkson TW:** Mercury poisoning. In Brown SS (ed): Clinical Chemistry and Clinical Toxicology of metals, pp 189–200. Elsevier/North-Holland Biomedical Press, Amsterdam, 1977

25. **Cohen LS:** Clinical Pharmacology of acetylsalicylic acid. Current Cardiovascular Topics 2:166, 1976

26. **Cohen S:** Amphetamine abuse. JAMA 231:414, 1975

27. **Cole L, Youngman H:** Treatment of tetanus. Lancet 1:1017, 1969

28. **Conn HO:** A rational program for the management of hepatic coma. Gastroenterology 57:715, 1969

29. **Crocker JFS, Ozere RL:** The incidence and etiology of Reye's syndrome in Eastern Canada. In Crocker JFS (ed): Reye's Syndrome II, p 3. New York, Grune & Stratton, 1979

30. **Cumings JN:** Heavy Metals and the Brain. Oxford, Blackwell Scientific Publications, 1959

31. **Dales LG:** The neurotoxicity of alkyl mercury compounds. Am J Med 53:219, 1972

32. **David OJ, Hoffman SP, Sverd J et al:** Lead and hyperactivity. Behavioral response to chelation: a pilot study. Am J Psychiatr 133:1155, 1976

33. **Davidson PW, Willoughby RH, O'Tuama LA et al:** Neurological and intellectual sequelae of Reye's syndrome. Am J Ment Def 82:535, 1978

34. **Dhiensiri K, Sinavatana P, Lerksookprasert S:** Reye's syndrome in Northeastern Thailand. In Crocker, JFS (ed): Reye's Syndrome, p 77. New York, Grune & Stratton, 1979

35. **Dolcourt JL, Hamrick HJ, O'Tuama LA et al:** Increased lead burden in children of battery workers. Pediatrics 62:563, 1978

36. **Dyck PJ, Johnson WJ, Lambert EH et al:** Segmental demyelination secondary to axonal degeneration in uremic neuropathy. Mayo Clin Proc 46:400, 1971

37. **Ellis GH, Mirkin LD, Mills MC:** Pancreatitis and Reye's syndrome. Am J Dis Child 133:1014, 1979

38. **Erlickia, Rybalkin:** Ueber Arseniklähmung. Archiv Psychiatrie und Nervenkrankheiten 23:861, 1892

39. **Ferguson AC, Rance CP:** Hereditary nephropathy with nerve deafness (Alport's syndrome). Am J Dis Child 124:84, 1972

40. **Ganther, HE:** Modification of methyl-mercury toxicity and metabolism by selenium and vitamin E: Possible mechanisms. Environ. Health Perspect 25:71, 1978

41. **Gerber N, Dickinson RC, Harland RR et al:** Reye-like syndrome associated with valproic acid therapy. J Pediatr 95:142, 1979

42. **Glasgow AM, Claus HP:** Exchange transfusion to remove ammonia. Am J Dis Child 129:159, 1975

43. **Glasgow AM, Cotton RB, Dhiensiri K et al:** Reye's syndrome. Part I. Blood ammonia and consideration of the non-histologic diagnosis. Am J Dis Child 124:827, 1972

44. **Gocke DJ:** Fulminant hepatitis treated with serum containing antibody to Australia antigen. N Engl J Med 284:919, 1971

45. **Goldbloom RR, Fraser FC, Waugh D et al:** Hereditary renal disease associated with nerve deafness and ocular lesions. Pediatrics 20:241, 1957

46. **Haller J:** Intracranial pressure monitoring in Reye's syndrome. Hosp Pract 15(2):101, 1980

47. **Hanna TL, Ditzler DN, Smith CH et al:** Erythrocyte *porphyrin* analysis in the detection of lead poisoning in children. Clin Chem 22:161, 1976

48. **Hanson JW, Jones KL, Smith DW:** Fetal alcohol syndrome. JAMA 235:1458, 1976

49. **Hasan M, Chandra SV, Duer PR:** Biochemical and electrophysiologic effects of thallium poisoning on the rat corpus striatum. Toxicol Appl Pharmacol 41:353, 1977

50. **Haymond MW, Karl IE, DeVivo DC et al:** Sequential metabolic observations in Reyes's syndrome. In Pollack JD (ed): Reye's Syndrome, p 215. New York, Grune & Stratton, 1974

51. **Hilty MD, Romshe CA, Delamater PV:** Reye's syndrome and hyperaminoacidemia. J Pediatr 84:362, 1974

52. **Holinger PL, Klawans HL:** Reversal of tricyclic overdosage induced central anticholinergic syndrome by physostigmine. Am J Psychiatr 133:1018, 1976

53. **Hourani BT, Hamlin EM, Reynolds TB:** Cerebrospinal fluid glutamine as a measure of hepatic encephalopathy. Arch Intern Med 127:1033, 1971

54. **Hrdina PD, Hanin I, Dubas TC:** Neurochemical correlates of lead toxicity. In Singhal, RL, Thomas JA (eds): Lead Toxicity, pp 273–300. Baltimore-Munich, Urban and Schwarzenberg, 1980

55. **Huttenlocher PR, Schwartz AD, Klatskin G:** Reye's syndrome: ammonia intoxication as a possible factor in the encephalopathy. Pediatrics 43:443, 1969

56. **Iancu TC, Mason WH, Neustein HB:** Ultrastructural abnormalities of liver cells in Reye's syndrome. Human Path 8:421, 1977

57. **Illis LS, Taylor FM:** Neurologic and electroencephalographic sequelae of tetanus. Lancet 1:826, 1971

58. **Imbus CE, Warner J, Smith E et al:** Peripheral neuropathy in lead-intoxicated sickle cell patients. Muscle and Nerve 1:168, 1978

59. **Jenkins RB:** Inorganic arsenic and the nervous system. Brain 89:479, 1966

60. **Jenkins RB, Toole JF:** Polyneuropathy following exposure to insecticides. Arch Intern Med 113:691, 1964

61. **Jindal HR:** Bilateral retrobulbar neuritis due to insecticides. Postgrad Med 44:342, 1968

62. **Sopling WH:** Neonatal tetanus. Br Med J 1:818, 1963

63. **Juncja I, Yovic A:** Hepatic decerebration. Neurology (Minneap) 22:537, 1972

64. **Kerr JH, Corbett JL, Prys-Roberts C et al:** Involvement of the sympathetic nervous system in tetanus. Lancet 2:236, 1968

65. **Kerzner B:** Salicylate intoxication. Drug Ther Bul 6:94, 1976

66. **Kerzner B, Roberts R, Cramer J et al:** High dose glycerol therapy in the management of Reye's encephalopathy. In Crocker, JFS (ed): Reye's Syndrome II, p 177. New York, Grune & Stratton, 1979

67. **Kim CS, O'Tuama LA, Pick JR:** Ontogeny of anionic herbicide transport by choroid plexus and brain. Soc Neurosci Abst 6:291, 1980

68. **Klingler H:** Tetanus of the newborn. JAMA 218:1437, 1971

69. **Knowles JA:** Excretion of drugs in milk—a review. J Pediatr 66:1068, 1965

70. **Koos BJ, Longo LD:** Mercury toxicity in the pregnant woman, fetus and newborn infant. Am J Obs Gynec 126:390, 1976

71. **La Montagne JR:** Summary of a workshop on influenza B viruses and Reye's syndrome. J Infect Dis 142:452, 1980

72. **Lansky LL, Kalawsky SM, Brackett CE et al:** Hypothermia total body washout and intracranial pressure monitoring in Stage IV Reye syndrome. J Pediatr 90:639, 1977

73. **Lapresle J, Fardeaum:** The central nervous system and carbon monoxide poisoning. Part II. Anatomical study of brain lesions following intoxication with carbon monoxide (22 cases). Progress in Brain Research 24:31, 1967

74. **Lee JH, Turndorf H, Poppers PJ:** Physostigmine reversal of antihistamine-induced excitement and depression. Anesthesiology 43:683, 1975

75. **Leonard JV, Seakins JWT, Griffin NK:** B-hydroxy-B-methylglutaricaciduria presenting as Reye's syndrome. Lancet 1:680, 1979

76. **Longo LD:** The biological effects of carbon monoxide on the pregnant woman, fetus and newborn infant. Amer J of Obstet and Gynec 129:69, 1977

77. **Lovejoy FH, Smith AL, Bresnan MJ et al:** Anticerebral edema therapy in Reye's syndrome. Arch Dis Child 50:933, 1975

78. **Luscombe FA, Monto AS, Baublis JV:** Mortality due to Reye's syndrome in Michigan: distribution and longitudinal trends. J Infect Dis 142:363, 1980

79. **Mamunes P, DeVries GH, Miller CD et al:** Fatty acid quantitation in Reye's syndrome. In Pollack JD (ed): Reye's Syndrome, p 245. New York, Grune & Stratton, 1974

80. **Marsh DO, Myers GJ, Clarkson TW, et al:** Fetal methylmercury poisoning: clinical and toxicological data on 29 cases. Ann Neurol 7:348, 1980

81. **Marshall LF, Shapiro HM, Rauscher et al:** Pentobarbital therapy for intracranial hypertension in metabolic coma: Reye's syndrome. Crit Care Med 6:1, 1978

82. **Mitchell RA, Ram ML, Arcunue EL et al:** Comparison of cytosolic and mitochondrial hepatic enzyme alterations in Reye's syndrome. Pediatr Res 14:1216, 1980

83. **Montagos S, Genel M, Tonaka K:** Ethylmalonic - adipic aciduria. J Clin Invest 64:1580, 1979

84. **Muller PW:** Immunopharmacological considerations in Reye's syndrome: a possible xenobiotic initiated disorder? Biochem Pharmacol 27:145, 1978

85. **Munc JL, Guisburg HM, Nixon CE:** The 1932 thallotoxicosis outbreak in California. JAMA 100:1315, 1933

86. **National Academy of Sciences–National Research Council:** Drinking Water and Health. Washington, DC, National Academy Press, 1980

87. **Nelson DB, Kimbrough R, Landrigan PS et al:** Aflatoxin and Reye's syndrome: a case control study. Pediatrics 66:865, 1980

88. **Okinaka S, Yoshikawa M, Mozai T et al:** Encephalomyelopathy due to organic mercury compound. Neurology (Minneap) 14:69, 1964

89. **O'Tuama LA, Kim CS, Gatzy JT et al:** The distribution of inorganic lead in guinea pig brain and neural barrier tissues in control and lead poisoned animals. Toxicol Appl Pharmacol 36:1, 1976

90. **Papp JP, Gay PC, Dodson VN et al:** Potassium chloride treatment in thallotoxicosis. Ann Intern Med 71:119, 1969

91. **Parkes JD, Sharpstone P, Williams R:** Levodopa in hepatic coma. Lancet 2:1341, 1970

92. **Partin JC, Partin JS, Schubert WK et al:** Brain ultrastructure in Reye's syndrome. J Neuropathol Exp Neurol 34:425, 1975

93. **Partin JS, McAdams AJ, Partin JC et al:** Brain ultrastructure in Reye's disease. Part II. Acute injury and recovery processes in three children. J Neuropathol Exp. Neurol 37:796, 1978

94. **Peebles TC, Levine L, Eldred MC et al:** Tetanustoxoid emergency boosters. N Engl J Med 280:575, 1969

95. **Peterson RG, Rumack BH:** Pharmacokinetics of acetaminophen in children. Pediatrics 62:877, 1978

96. **Porter CA, Mowat AP, Cook PJL et al:** Antitrypsin deficiency and neonatal hepatitis. Br Med J 3:435, 1972

97. **Prys-Roberts C, Corbett JL, Kerr JH et al:** Treatment of sympathetic overactivity in tetanus. Lancet 2:542, 1969

98. **Reed O, Crawley J, Fado SN et al:** Thallotoxicosis, acute manifestations and sequelae. JAMA 183:516, 1963

99. **Reye RDK, Morgan G, Baral J:** Encephalopathy and fatty degeneration of the viscera—a disease entity in childhood. Lancet 2:749, 1963

100. **Robinson BH, Oei J, Sherwood WG et al:** Hydroxymethylglutaryl CoA lyase deficiency: features resembling Reye syndrome. Neurology 30:714, 1980

101. **Robinson RR, Gunnells JC, Clapp JR:** Treatment of acute barbiturate intoxication. Mod Treat 8:561, 1971

102. **Roe CR, Schonberger LB, Gehlbach SH:** Enzymatic alterations in Reye's syndrome: prognostic implications. Pediatrics 55:119, 1975

103. **Rogan WJ, Bagniewska A, Damstra T:** Current concepts. Pollutants in breast milk. New Engl J Med 302:1450, 1980

104. **Ryan DW, Cherington M:** Human type A botulism. JAMA 216:513, 1971

105. **Samaha FJ, Blau E:** The role of peritoneal dialysis in Reye's syndrome. In Pollack JD (ed): Reye's Syndrome, p 295. New York, Grune & Stratton, 1972

106. **Scaer RC, Tooker J, Cherington M:** Effect of guanidine on the neuromuscular block of botulism. Neurology (Minneap) 19:1107, 1969

107. **Schenker SF:** Hepatic coma: current concepts of pathogenesis. Viewpoints Dig Dis Vol 2, No 4, Sept 1970

108. **Schneck SA, Penn I:** De novo brain tumors in renal transplant recipients. Lancet 1:983, 1971

109. **Schreiner GE, Mahier JF:** Uremia. Springfield, Ill, Charles C Thomas, 1961

110. **Schubert WK:** Commentary: The diagnosis of Reye syndrome. J Pediatr 87:867, 1975

111. **Schwartz HS:** Acute meprobamate poisoning with gastrotomy and removal of a drug-containing mass. New Engl J Med 295:1177, 1976

112. **Seidel J:** Acute mercury poisoning after polyvinyl alcohol preservatives. Pediatrics 66:132, 1980

113. **Seto DSY, Freeman JM:** Lead neuropathy in children. Am J Dis Child 107:337, 1964

114. **Shankland DL, Schroeder ME:** Pharmacological evidence for a discrete neurologic action of dieldrin (HEOD) in the American cockroach, *Periplaneta americana.* Pesticide Biochemistry and Physiology 3:77, 1973

115. **Shaywitz BA:** Monitoring and management of increased intracranial pressure in Reye syndrome: results in 29 children. Pediatrics 66:198, 1980

116. **Shaywitz BA, Leventhal JM, Kramer MS:** Prolonged continuous monitoring of intracranial pressure in severe Reye's syndrome. Pediatrics 59:595, 1977

117. **Smythe PM:** Studies on neonatal tetanus and on pulmonary compliance of the totally relaxed infant. Br Med J 1:565, 1963

118. **Snyder RD:** The involuntary movements of chronic mercury poisoning. Arch Neurol 26:379, 1972

119. **Starko KM, Ray CG, Dominguez LB et al:** Reye's syndrome and salicylate use. Pediatrics 66:859, 1980

120. **Steinwall O, Snyder H:** Brain uptake of 14C-cyloleucine after damage to blood-brain barrier by mercuric ions. Acta Neurological Scand 45:369, 1969

121. **Stormont RT, Conley BE:** Pharmacologic and toxicologic aspects of DDT (chlorophenothane USP). JAMA 145:728, 1951

122. **Sweetman L, Nyhan W, Trauner DA et al:** Glutaric aciduria type II. J Pediatr 96:1020, 1980

123. **Syverson TLM:** Biotransformation of Hg-203 labelled methylmercuric chloride in rat brain measured by specific determinations of HG^{++}. Acta Pharmacologica et toxcologica 35:277, 1974

124. **Tanaka K, Kean EA, Johnson B:** Jamaican vomiting sickness. New Engl J Med 295:461, 1976

125. **Taylor JR, Selhorst JB, Houff SA et al:** Chlordecone intoxication in man. Neurology 28:626, 1978

126. **Tukuomi H, Okajima T, Kanai J et al:** Minamata disease. World Neurol 2:536, 1961

127. **Tomasi LG:** Treatment of Reye's syndrome—Importance of clinical staging. Ann Neurol 8:201, 1980

128. **Trauner DA:** Treatment of Reye syndrome. Ann Neurol 7:2, 1980

129. **Trauner DA, Broom F, Ganz E et al:** Treatment of elevated intracranial pressure in Reye syndrome. Ann Neurol 4:275, 1978

130. **Trauner DA, Huttenlocher PR:** Short-chain fatty acid-induced central hyperventilation in rabbits. Neurology 28:940, 1978

131. **Trauner DA, Stockard JJ, Sweetman L:** EEG correlations with biochemical abnormalities in Reye syndrome. Arch Neurol 34:116, 1977

132. **Tyler HR:** Neurologic disorders seen in the uremic patient. Arch Intern Med 126:781, 1970

133. **Vries JK, Baker DP, Young HF:** A subarachnoid screw for monitoring intracranial pressure: Technical Note. J Neurosurg 39:416, 1973

134. **Wall CD:** The determination of thallium in urine by atomic absorption spectroscopy and emission spectrography. Clinica Chimica Acta 76:259, 1977

135. **Watanabe I:** Organotins (triethyltin). In Spencer PS, Schaumburg HH (eds): Experimental and Clinical Neurotoxicology, p 545. Baltimore, Williams & Wilkins, 1980

136. **Yoshino Y, Neozar T, Nakao K:** Biochemical changes in the brain in rats poisoned with an alkylmercuric compound with special reference to the inhibition of protein synthesis in brain cortex slices. J of Neurochem 13:1223, 1966

Intracranial Infections

Thomas W. Farmer

In infants and children it is most important to consider the possibility that any acute systemic infection may be associated with an infection of the central nervous system. A delay in diagnosis with the resultant delay in treatment may result in irreparable brain damage, which might have been prevented.

If the history and the examination suggest the possibility of a meningeal or an encephalitic illness, then the major diagnostic possibilities are the following: (1) acute purulent meningitis; (2) subacute meningitis; (3) meningeal reaction secondary to extradural abscess, subdural empyema, septic thrombosis of venous sinuses, or brain abscess; (4) acute meningitis due to infection by a virus, *Leptospira,* or other cause; (5) some form of encephalitis.

Frequently the most important procedure to evaluate these diagnostic possibilities is examination of cerebrospinal fluid obtained by lumbar puncture (Table 12-1). Cloudy or purulent cerebrospinal fluid under increased pressure containing several hundred to several thousand leukocytes per cubic millimeter, mostly polymorphonuclear neutrophils (PMNs), is characteristic of acute purulent meningitis. Opalescent or clear fluid containing fewer than 500 leukocytes per cubic millimeter, predominantly mononuclear cells, with a decreased sugar content of 20 mg/dl to 40 mg/dl is characteristic of tuberculous and cryptococcal meningitis. Meningeal reactions secondary to intracranial infection, meningitis due to viral or leptospiral infections, and encephalitis are associated with a clear or opalescent cerebrospinal fluid. The fluid is under normal or increased pressure with a leukocyte count of 3/mm³ to 2000/mm³, which usually are predominantly mononuclear cells, and has a normal sugar content. Although the division of cerebrospinal fluid abnormalities into three broad categories (purulent cerebrospinal fluid, nonpurulent fluid with a cellular reaction associated with a decreased sugar content, and nonpurulent fluid associated with a cellular reaction and a normal sugar content) is of great value in the initial delineation of the diagnostic problem in children with infections of the central nervous system, cerebrospinal fluid findings must be evaluated in conjunction with the present illness and the findings on examination. They should also be correlated with additional laboratory studies of the cerebrospinal fluid and blood, and in some cases with radiologic and other studies.

ACUTE PURULENT MENINGITIS

Purulent meningitis includes a variety of acute bacterial infections of the meninges associated with a purulent reaction in the cerebrospinal fluid. Bacterial infections producing meningitis may occur in epidemic form or as sporadic cases in a community.

INFLUENZAL, MENINGOCOCCAL, AND OTHER TYPES

Etiology and Epidemiology. The relative incidence with which different bacteria produce purulent meningitis depends upon the presence or absence of epidemic spread and upon the age of the child. Thus if an epidemic of meningococcal meningitis oc-

TABLE 12-1. Usual Cerebrospinal Fluid Findings in Infections of the Central Nervous System

Clinical Picture	Initial Pressure (mm H$_2$O)	Appearance	Leukocytes No/mm^3	Leukocytes Predominant Cell Types	Sugar (mg/dl)
Normal	70–180	Clear	0–5	Mononuclear	50–80
Acute purulent meningitis	Elevated	Cloudy, purulent	400–40,000	Polymorpho-nuclear	Decreased or absent
Subacute meningitis due to tuberculosis or cryptococcosis	Elevated	Clear or opalescent	25–500	Mononuclear	Decreased
Meningeal reactions due to extradural abscess, subdural empyema, venous sinus thrombosis, brain abscess Acute meningitis due to viruses, leptospira, etc. Encephalitis	Normal or elevated	Clear or opalescent	5–2000	Mononuclear	Normal

curs during a given year, the majority of cases of purulent meningitis during that year will be due to *Neisseria meningitidis*. A number of different groups of meningococci are responsible for meningitis occurring at different times. These groups include the classical A, B, and C groups as well as the new X, Y, Z, W-135, and Z' groups.[21] However, the relative frequency of different types of bacterial meningitis in children over a number of years is relatively constant (Table 12-2).

More cases of purulent meningitis occur during the first month of life than during any other month, and most of these infections are due to *Escherichia coli* and the group B$_\beta$- hemolytic streptococcus.

Approximately half of the purulent

TABLE 12-2. Incidence of Infection and Mortality Rate in Purulent Meningitis

Bacteria	Cases of Known Etiology (%)	Mortality Rate Prior to Specific Therapy (%)	Mortality Rate With Current Specific Therapy (%)
Hemophilus influenzae	40	90	2–5
Neisseria meningitidis	25	50–90	2–5
Streptococcus pneumoniae	20	95–100	3–5
Escherichia coli	7	95–100	50–60
Streptococcus, Staphylococcus, Salmonella, Micrococcus, and *Pseudomonas*	8	90–100	10–50

meningitis cases in children occur during the first year of life, and almost all of the infections due to *E. coli* occur during the first year. Half of the children with pneumococcal meningitis develop it during the first year. Influenzal meningitis is the most common type of bacterial meningitis in children 6 months to 4 years of age. Pneumococcal meningitis is the most common etiologic agent in post-traumatic meningitis. The majority of meningitis cases following head injury develop within 2 weeks of head trauma.

Infection may spread from the upper respiratory tract, from the lungs, or from the middle ear to the bloodstream and thence to the meninges. In infants, enteric organisms may invade the bloodstream and then spread to the meninges. Two of the important factors in the pathogenesis of neonatal group B streptococcal meningitis are the initial transmission of the organism from the female genital tract to the infant and, secondly, the infant's lack of maternally acquired type-specific serum antibody. Purulent meningitis, particularly recurrent meningitis, may be associated with a dermoid sinus, which furnishes a path for extension of infection from the skin to the subarachnoid space. A dural tear resulting from a previous head injury may provide a pathway of infection from the nasopharynx to the subarachnoid space.

Pathology. With severe purulent meningitis the pia–arachnoid is thickened and white (Fig. 12-1). Microscopically there is a polymorphonuclear reaction associated with an acute inflammatory reaction surrounding blood vessels. Usually infection is restricted to the meninges. A dense exudate at the base may involve cranial nerves. With prolonged severe infection at the base of the brain, interference with cerebrospinal fluid circulation may occur with secondary dilatation of the ventricular system (Fig. 12-2). Severe leptomeningeal infection may be associated with thrombosis of cortical veins; focal areas of encephalomalacia may rarely occur, as may necrosis and demyelination of subcortical white matter. This may be due to vasculitis with ischemia and edema.[7] There may be associated subdural effusion with clear, yellow fluid present in the subdural space. Fatal

purulent meningitis may be associated with extradural abscess, subdural empyema (Fig. 12-1), venous sinus thrombosis, or brain abscess. Adrenal hemorrhage and necrosis complicate some cases of meningococcal and of other types of meningitis.

Symptoms. In infants the initial symptoms are poor feeding, vomiting, fever, and drowsiness. Convulsions frequently occur. In children the initial symptom may be headache followed by fever, sore throat, joint pains, drowsiness, and stiff neck. As the infection progresses, the patient becomes less responsive, confused, and eventually comatose.

Examination. A child with early meningitis is febrile and usually drowsy, with a staring expression. Examination of the skin may reveal petechiae, or purpura. An exanthem is present in two-thirds of children with meningococcal meningitis. Joint involvement occurs in 5% of cases of meningococcal meningitis. Increased tension of the fontanels may be noted. Infrequently

FIG. 12-1. Brain of an infant who died from *Hemophilus influenzae* meningitis complicated by a bilateral subdural empyema. Most of the exudate from the subdural space has been removed from the superior surface of the brain, and the clouding and thickening of the meninges are apparent.

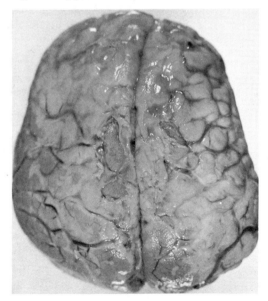

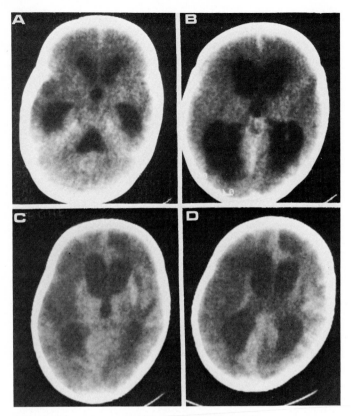

FIG. 12-2. Hydrocephalus and cerebral atrophy occurring in a 4-month-old boy after recovery from *Hemophilus Influenzae* meningitis. Treatment with ampicillin and chloramphenicol was begun on the first day of hospital admission, which was 10 days after the onset of frequent convulsions and fever. *A* and *B*, CT (computed tomography) sections with contrast enhancement on the day after admission reveal symmetric enlargement of the lateral, third, and fourth ventricles. *C* and *D*, CT sections without contrast enhancement three weeks later reveal persistent hydrocephalus with multiple areas of decreased density in both cerebral hemispheres consistent with infarctions and subsequent atrophy.

there may be evidence of a sinus tract leading from the scalp through the skull or from the skin in the midline of the back to the spine.

Infants under 6 months of age usually do not show definite stiffness of the neck early in the course of meningitis. However, in children nuchal rigidity is frequently present and Kernig's sign may be elicited. Neurologic examination may reveal evi-

dence of cranial nerve palsies. The most common paralyses are those of the sixth cranial nerve with weakness of the lateral rectus muscle of the eye, of the seventh cranial nerve with facial paralysis, or of the eighth cranial nerve with vertigo and deafness. Other cranial nerves are occasionally involved.

Coma, third cranial nerve dysfunction with persistent pupillary dilatation or respiratory arrest may be due to temporal lobe or cerebellar herniation.

Rarely a child suddenly develops acute shock, cyanosis, and prostration. This may be associated with a marked drop in blood pressure and a fast, feeble pulse. These signs of acute adrenal hemorrhage may be associated with meningococcal or other types of meningitis.

In addition to the initial examination and evaluation of a child with purulent meningitis, it is essential that he be reexamined carefully each day during the acute stage of the illness. If after 72 hours of antibiotic therapy the child has persistent fever, opisthotonos, increased head circumference, or bulging fontanels, or if he develops convulsions or focal neurologic signs, he should be evaluated for possible complications associated with acute meningitis. A common complication is subdural effusion, which may be uni- or bilateral. In any child in whom the clinical response to therapy is unsatisfactory after 72 hours of treatment, subdural tap should be done. Subdural empyema occasionally produces similar signs during the course of acute infection. Also the development of focal cerebral signs may be due to the presence of a cerebral abscess in association with purulent meningitis or may be related to an extensive exudate overlying one cerebral hemisphere with associated thrombosis of cerebral veins. Hemiparesis or homonymous hemianopia may develop in association with increased tendon reflexes, decreased abdominal reflexes, and an extensor plantar response on the same side. In some children focal cerebral defects associated with meningitis are due to occlusion of the internal carotid artery.[25] Transient cortical blindness, permanent cortical blindness, or quadriplegia with spinal cord involvement rarely occurs.[13,22,25,72]

Laboratory Examination. The cerebrospinal fluid pressure is frequently elevated (Table 12-1). The fluid is usually purulent but may be opalescent. It usually contains 400 leukocytes/mm³ to 40,000 leukocytes/mm³ of which 75% to 100% are PMNs. In early meningitis the fluid may appear clear and there may be fewer than 100 cells/mm³ in the cerebrospinal fluid. However, 75% to 100% of these cells are PMNs. Smears of the sediment of centrifuged cerebrospinal fluid stained by Gram's method reveal bacteria in approximately 80% of children with meningitis who have not had previous antibiotic or chemotherapy. *Hemophilus influenzae, Neisseria meningitidis,* and pneumococci can be identified with almost complete certainty by stained smears. Cultures of the cerebrospinal fluid from children with untreated purulent meningitis show a growth of the causative organisms in 95% of cases. Sensitivity tests are then done to determine *in vitro* which antibiotic drugs are most effective against the organism. Some strains of *Hemophilus influ-*

enzae are ampicillin-resistant. This is of great importance in planning appropriate antibiotic therapy. Early in the course of meningeal infection the glucose content of the cerebrospinal fluid may be normal or slightly reduced. However, with infection of several days' duration the glucose content is markedly decreased or absent. The cerebrospinal fluid protein is frequently elevated to 60 mg/dl to 500 mg/dl. Since many children already received antibiotic therapy for febrile illnesses before meningitis was suspected, smears and cultures of the cerebrospinal fluid may not reveal a causative organism. Diagnostic tests that depend on the presence in CSF of bacterial products rather than on whole, viable organisms are of definite value. The two main methods are the detection of specific polysaccharide antigens by countercurrent immunoelectrophoresis (CIE) and detection of endotoxin.[43] Countercurrent immunoelectrophoresis has a success rate of 70% to 90% in the diagnosis of meningococcal, pneumococcal, *Hemophilus influenzae*, and *E. coli* meningitis. Gram-negative bacteria multiplying within the CSF can produce enough endotoxin to cause gelation of limulus lysate, so the limulus test can be used to diagnose gram-negative bacterial meningitis with a success rate of nearly 100%. However, the limulus test cannot distinguish between different gram-negative organisms, so it does not provide an exact bacteriologic diagnosis. Detection of bacterial products in CSF is a supplement to routine bacteriologic investigation. The diagnostic success rate of culture and antigen detection combined is greater than that of either technique alone.

Blood cultures obtained prior to treatment may reveal the presence of bacteremia in association with purulent meningitis. In untreated patients with influenzal meningitis blood cultures are positive in three-fourths of the patients, whereas approximately 40% of patients with meningococcal meningitis have positive blood cultures. If meningitis is associated with a systemic infection in the middle ear, mastoids, throat, lungs, or elsewhere, cultures of material from these sites may reveal the same organism as is present in the CSF.

If subdural effusion or subdural empyema is suspected as a complication of

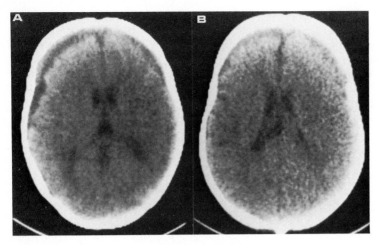

FIG. 12-3. Bilateral subdural effusion in a 6-month-old girl with *Hemophilus Influenzae* meningitis. *A*, CT section reveals crescent-shaped areas of decreased density overlying both cerebral hemispheres anteriorly with larger amounts of fluid in the left than the right subdural space. Subsequently daily subdural taps during the next 3 weeks yielded persistent accumulations of fluid. For this reason the child then had a subdural–pleural shunt. *B*, Repeat CT scan one week after shunt revealed marked decrease in accumulation of subdural fluid.

meningitis, subdural taps are done through the edge of the anterior fontanel or through the sutures in infants. Burr holes are made in children in whom the fontanels are closed. Fluid obtained from a subdural effusion is clear or slightly xanthochromic and usually contains 50 leukocytes/mm^3 to 500 leukocytes/mm^3 of which the majority are mononuclear cells. It may be free of cells. The protein content of the fluid is usually 60 mg/dl to 1000 mg/dl. The sugar content of the fluid is normal. Smears and cultures reveal no bacteria. Fluid obtained from a subdural empyema is cloudy or purulent with a cellular reaction that contains predominantly PMNs. The sugar content of the fluid is decreased. Smears and cultures of the fluid reveal bacteria unless previous treatment has suppressed the growth of organisms.

Radiographs of the skull may reveal a recent fracture consistent with a diagnosis of post-traumatic meningitis. Separation of the sutures of the skull suggests complications: subdural effusion, subdural empyema, or brain abscess. Rarely evidence of a midline bony defect in the skull may be noted. Radiographic evidence of acute mastoiditis or pneumonia may be demonstrated. A dermoid sinus tract in the spine may be demonstrated by radiographs. Computed tomography (CT) is very valuable in the early detection of complications of meningitis as well as in the evaluation of the extent of focal lesions. Computed tomography may reveal evidence of subdural effusion (Fig. 12-3). In some cases CT may reveal evidence of subdural empyema, brain abscess, areas of diminished attenuation in the brain parenchyma, or enlarged ventricles (Fig. 12-2).[5,11,66,75] In a child in whom the diagnosis of subdural effusion is suspected, an electroencephalogram may reveal a decrease in voltage or a difference in frequency over one cerebral hemisphere.

Differential Diagnosis. In infants and children with acute severe infections in whom no adequate diagnosis can be readily established, purulent meningitis is considered. Once the diagnosis of meningitis is suspected, lumbar puncture should be done to determine whether the child has a purulent meningitis. The association of purulent meningitis with a petechial rash strongly suggests meningococcal meningitis.[71]

If the child has had no previous antibiotic therapy, the diagnosis of purulent meningitis is usually apparent from the cloudy appearance of the CSF. If lumbar puncture is done very early in the course of meningeal infection, the fluid may still be clear even though it contains an increased number of leukocytes, predominantly PMNs. The bacteria producing meningitis can be identified by smears and cultures of the CSF in 95% of these children.

Antibiotic or chemotherapeutic agents administered to the child prior to lumbar puncture may alter the cellular reaction and the sugar content of the CSF, and organisms may not be cultured from the fluid. If, for example, the fluid contains 500 leukocytes/mm^3 with 50% PMNs and with a slightly decreased sugar content, these findings may be consistent with partially treated purulent meningitis or may be due to tuberculous meningitis. With antibiotic therapy prior to lumbar puncture, it may be difficult to distinguish purulent meningitis from early brain abscess. Brain abscess may initially result in a meningeal illness with headache, stiff neck, fever, and an increased cellular reaction in the CSF. The subsequent development of focal neurologic signs and increased intracranial pressure may strongly suggest brain abscess. During the acute phase of certain types of viral meningitis there may be a relatively high cellular reaction with a leukocyte count of 2000/mm^3 to 3000/mm^3, and there also may be a higher percentage of PMNs than mononuclear cells. The presence of a high percentage of PMNs in the fluid represents an acute inflammatory reaction but it does not necessarily imply a bacterial infection. Thus in many of the cases of eastern equine encephalitis the majority of the cells are PMNs.

Meningeal symptoms and signs including the acute onset of headache, stiff neck, and a positive Kernig's sign are rarely due to subarachnoid bleeding in a child. Lumbar puncture reveals grossly bloody CSF.

Treatment. The child should have bed rest in the hospital with adequate nursing care. With a temperature above 103°F (39°C) a sponge bath and acetylsalicylic acid in a dose of 10 mg/kg every 3 hours to 4 hours may be used to lower the temperature. If seizures occur, either phenobarbital in a daily dose of 2 mg/kg to 6 mg/kg or phenytoin in a daily dose of 5 mg/kg to 9 mg/kg is administered. Intravenous fluids are usu-

ally required to ensure proper intake of water, glucose, sodium, chloride, and potassium. Fluids are restricted to prevent cerebral edema, which occurs with excessive amounts of fluid. Mannitol is used to treat acute cerebral edema and cerebral herniation.[28] Care is taken to prevent edema, which occurs with excessive amounts of fluids. Blood pressure must be monitored frequently. An adequate airway must be maintained. Tracheostomy or assisted ventilation is occasionally necessary.

Each child with meningitis is evaluated carefully for the detection of inappropriate secretion of antidiuretic hormone. Body weight, serum electrolytes, urine volume, and specific gravity are measured on admission and the measurements repeated daily during the acute phase of infection. If fluid is retained in excess of solute, fluid administration is restricted until the serum sodium concentration increases and urinary specific gravity decreases. The syndrome of inappropriate secretion of antidiuretic hormone occurs in half of children with bacterial meningitis. Prompt treatment is essential because children with severe and prolonged hyponatremia are more likely to have complications of meningitis than those who maintain normal serum sodium concentration.[32]

If the organism responsible for meningitis is identified in smears of the sediment from the CSF, then antibiotic agents usually effective for this organism are immediately instituted (Table 12-3). The optimal aim of therapy is to obtain a bactericidal concentration in the CSF of a relatively nontoxic agent effective against the invading organism through the intravenous, intramuscular, or oral route.[3] Examination of the CSF is repeated 24 hours after the institution of therapy in order to be certain that the proper *in vivo* response has been obtained.

Influenzal meningitis is treated with ampicillin and chloramphenicol. If an ampicillin-resistant *Hemophilus influenzae* is identified, chloramphenicol must be continued, but the ampicillin may be stopped. If the strain is sensitive to ampicillin, chloramphenicol may be discontinued.[2,59,62] In infants under 1 week of age the daily dose of ampicillin is 100 mg/kg; in infants over 1 week of age and in children, the daily

TABLE 12-3. Drug Therapy of Purulent Meningitis

Type of Meningitis	Initial Drug Therapy	Minimal Duration of Therapy (Days)
Influenzal	Ampicillin and chloramphenicol	10
Meningococcal	Penicillin G or chloramphenicol	10–12
Pneumococcal	Penicillin G or chloramphenicol	14
Escherichia coli	Ampicillin or gentamicin or amikacin or kanamycin or colistin or tobramycin or carbenicillin or chloramphenicol	21
Streptococcal	Penicillin G	10
Staphylococcal	Methicillin or penicillin G or chloramphenicol	28
Etiology unknown	Infant less than 28 days of age: ampicillin & kanamycin or gentamicin	21
	Infant or child more than 28 days of age: ampicillin & chloramphenicol	14

dose is 200 mg/kg to 400 mg/kg intravenously. If the child is allergic to ampicillin, influenzal meningitis is treated with chloramphenicol. The daily dose in a premature infant or in a newborn is 25 mg/kg. In infants between 1 month and 1 year of age the maximal daily dose of 50 mg/kg is given intravenously or intramuscularly. In children over 1 year of age the daily dose is 50 mg/kg to 100 mg/kg (Table 12-4). It is important that these relatively smaller dosage schedules be used in infants, in contrast to the larger ones used in children, in order to avoid toxic concentrations of the drug in the blood. The incidences of death, relapse, subdural effusion, and neurologic sequelae are the same for treatment with ampicillin and with chloramphenicol.[2]

Meningococcal meningitis is treated with penicillin G or chloramphenicol. If penicillin G is used, it is administered intravenously or intramuscularly in a daily dose of 100,000 units/kg to 200,000 units/kg in divided doses given every 2 hours to 3 hours. With this dose of penicillin bactericidal levels are obtained in the CSF after 8 hours to 12 hours. A child sensitive to penicillin may be given chloramphenicol in a dose of 100 mg/kg daily.

Pneumococcal meningitis is treated with penicillin G or chloramphenicol. *Escherichia coli* meningitis may be treated initially with ampicillin or chloramphenicol. Other drugs to which the organism may be sensitive include kanamycin, gentamicin, amikacin, colistin, tobramycin, and

TABLE 12-4. Drugs Frequently Used in the Treatment of Purulent Meningitis

Drug	Daily Dose	Route of Administration	Adverse Reactions
Ampicillin	100 mg/kg (1 day–7 days old) 200 mg/kg–400 mg/kg (more than 7 days old)	Intravenous	Rash, anaphylaxis
Penicillin G	100,000 units/kg–200,000 units/kg	Intravenous or intramuscular	Fever, rash, mycotic stomatitis, anaphylaxis
Chloramphenicol	25 mg/kg–50 mg/kg (infants) 50 mg/kg–100 mg/kg (children)	Intravenous or intramuscular	Vomiting, diarrhea, stomatitis, glossitis, skin rash, aplastic anemia
Methicillin	100 mg/kg–300 mg/kg	Intravenous or intramuscular	Rash, anaphylaxis
Kanamycin	15 mg/kg	Intramuscular or intravenous	Ototoxic or nephrotoxic reaction, fever, rash

carbenicillin.[42] Streptococcal meningitis is treated initially with penicillin G, and staphylococcal meningitis with methicillin or penicillin G. Penicillin-resistant strains of staphylococci are treated with methicillin, which is administered intravenously or intramuscularly in a daily dose of 100 mg/kg to 300 mg/kg in divided doses every 6 hours.

Infants who develop meningitis during the first month of life and from whose CSF no causative organism can be initially identified should be treated with the presumptive diagnosis of *E. coli* or group B β-hemolytic streptococcus meningitis. Since many children receive antibiotic therapy prior to hospitalization with purulent meningitis, an etiologic diagnosis may not be established. If lumbar puncture reveals purulent fluid and no bacterial organisms, immediate therapy is begun. This includes antibiotic drugs effective against *Hemophilus influenzae, Streptococcus pneumoniae, Neisseria meningitidis, Staphylococcus,* and *Streptococcus.* Initially an infant under 28 days of age is treated with ampicillin and kanamycin or gentamicin; infants over 28 days of age and children are treated with ampicillin and chloramphenicol. Subsequently cultures may be positive for the causative organisms; the program of antibiotic therapy may be altered as soon as sensitivity test results are available. The patient is then treated with the single least toxic drug demonstrated to be effective against the organism *in vitro.*

If meningitis responds well to treatment, drug therapy in most forms of meningitis is continued for 10 days to 14 days. With staphylococcal infections treatment is usually continued for as long as 1 month. In overwhelming infections with a slow response to therapy, medications are continued until clinical recovery has occurred. Drug therapy is continued until the child is afebrile for 5 days, the CSF cell count is 30 leukocytes/mm^3 or less, and the sugar and protein contents have returned to normal. If these rigid criteria are followed relapse does not occur. In infants less than 2 months of age, therapy is continued for a minimum of 3 weeks.

At present, intrathecal therapy is not usually recommended in the treatment of purulent meningitis because the mortality rate is not significantly decreased by this method and toxic reactions may occur. Intrathecal therapy can result in optic atrophy and in transverse myelopathy. However, if *Pseudomonas* meningitis is treated with polymyxin B or other antibiotics that have similarly poor diffusibility, then the drug may be given both intramuscularly and intrathecally. Adrenal steroids offer no benefit to the usual patient with bacterial meningitis.[12]

The toxic reactions occurring with drugs used to treat meningitis are summarized in Table 12-4. Ampicillin may produce a skin rash, and rarely anaphylaxis occurs. Chloramphenicol may produce vomiting, diarrhea, stomatitis, glossitis, and skin rash; rarely, aplastic anemia occurs, which may be fatal. Frequent blood counts should be done on children given chloramphenicol. When counts show leukopenia, thrombocytopenia, or anemia, chloramphenicol should be discontinued and another appropriate antibiotic administered. Penicillin G is relatively nontoxic, although fever, skin rash, anaphylaxis, and mycotic stomatitis may occur. Methicillin may produce skin rash and rarely anaphylaxis. Kanamycin may produce fever and rash with associated ototoxic and nephrotoxic reactions. Gentamicin and tobramycin produce hearing loss of 15 decibels to 35 decibels at 4000 cycles per second to 8000 cycles per second in 10% of patients. Both of these drugs may produce nephrotoxicity in 10% to 20% of patients.[64]

If adrenal hemorrhage occurs as an acute complication of meningitis, an intravenous saline infusion is begun. If the child is in shock, norepinephrine, 4 ml containing 4 mg norepinephrine in 1000 ml 5% dextrose solution is given intravenously at a rate to maintain blood pressure and to prevent peripheral circulatory collapse. Hydrocortisone is administered intravenously in an initial dose of 50 mg to 100 mg; the dosage required depends not only on the age of the child but on the severity of adrenal damage. Doses of 50 mg to 100 mg are repeated intravenously at 4-hour intervals during the first day. Subsequently oral medication may be given in decreasing dosage. Although low plasma cortisol levels have been found in children with adrenal hemorrhage, clinical benefit from replacement therapy has not been clearly established.[44]

If subdural tap reveals a subdural effusion, repeated taps with removal of as much as 25 ml to 30 ml fluid each time are carried out every 1 day to 2 days. If a decrease in the amount of fluid removed does not occur after 2 weeks to 3 weeks, then surgical therapy with appropriate shunting of subdural fluid is necessary.[1] Surgical treatment of subdural effusion is required in approximately 1% of children with purulent meningitis. Antibiotic therapy is continued during surgery and for at least a week after surgery.

If meningitis is secondary to a dermoid cyst, the cyst should be removed surgically after the child has recovered from meningitis. If recurrent meningitis is due to a defect in the cribriform plate, this is treated surgically with closure of the defect in the dura. Recurrent meningococcal meningitis may be due to deficiency of the sixth, seventh, or eighth components of complement, and this possibility is explored by the determination of hemolytic complement titer.[49] Obstructive hydrocephaly occurring after meningitis may require a surgical procedure to shunt from the lateral ventricles to the cisterna magna or elsewhere.

Prognosis. Prior to the use of chemotherapeutic agents and antibiotic drugs meningitis was a fatal illness in the vast majority of children. The mortlaity rate in different epidemics of meningococcal meningitis varied from 50% to 90%. With other forms of purulent meningitis the mortality rate was 90% to 100% (Table 12-2).

Since the advent of chemotherapeutic and antibiotic agents there has been a dramatic fall in the mortality rate. Variations in this rate are related to many factors including the age of the child at the time of infection, duration of the infection at the time therapy is instituted, etiologic organism, and the presence of other complications. Half of the deaths in purulent meningitis occur during the first year of life. The chances of survival increase with age. The mortality rate varies with different causative organisms (Table 12-2); with influenzal and meningococcal meningitis it is approximately 2% to 5%.[40] The mortality rate in neonatal meningitis due to group B

-β hemolytic streptococcal infection is approximately 20%.[23] In contrast, approximately 50% to 60% of children with E. coli meningitis die.

The majority of children recover without residual damage to the nervous system. However, the sequelae sometimes observed after recovery from meningitis include recurrent convulsions, mental retardation, hydrocephaly (Fig. 12-2), hemiparesis, ataxia, blindness, deafness, aqueductal stenosis, and other significant complications.[20,35,60,61] One or more of these sequelae occur in approximately 25% to 40% of children after influenzal meningitis, in 4% after meningococcal meningitis, and in 50% after pneumococcal meningitis.[2,67] The incidence of sensorineural hearing loss among survivors of bacterial meningitis is approximately 20%. This may be unilateral or bilateral. Audiograms are done on children after recovery from meningitis because of this high incidence of deafness.[46,57] Recurrent meningitis may occur in a child with recurrent middle ear infection, mastoiditis, or rarely a dermoid cyst or a dural tear.

PRIMARY AMEBIC MENINGOENCEPHALITIS

Etiology. Primary amebic meningoencephalitis is an acute, fulminating, purulent meningoencephalitis caused by free-living amebas of the genus Naegleria. Infection is associated with a history of recent swimming in freshwater lakes or pools. Protozoa gain entry through the nasal mucosa and the cribriform plate to the central nervous system.

Pathology. The meninges are infiltrated with mononuclear and granulocytic cells with areas of perivascular necrosis.[58] Amebic trophozoites are seen in the meninges.

Examination. Children develop headache, stiff neck, and fever followed by drowsiness and stupor.

Laboratory Examination. Lumbar puncture reveals CSF that is under increased pressure. There is an increase in the number of cells that may be as high as several thousand cells per cubic millimeter with a predominance of PMNs. The protein content is increased and the sugar content is decreased. Mobile amebas may be seen on wet preparations of CSF.

Differential Diagnosis. Since primary amebic meningoencephalitis produces a purulent meningeal reaction, it must be differentiated from bacterial meningitis. A recent history of swimming or diving in a freshwater lake or pond may be obtained. If no bacteria are seen on smears of the CSF, a careful search for mobile amebas in the fluid may establish the diagnosis.

Treatment. Rarely recovery occurs following treatment with amphotericin B, rifampin, and miconazole nitrate.

Prognosis. The untreated mortality rate approaches 100%, usually within 7 days after the onset of meningitis.

Prevention. Identification of recreational swimming areas at specific risk and appropriate swimming restrictions will prevent infections.

SUBACUTE NONPURULENT MENINGITIS

TUBERCULOUS MENINGITIS

Tuberculous meningitis occurs as a complication of primary tuberculosis. From any primary site tubercle bacilli may spread through the bloodstream to the central nervous system and produce a subacute meningoencephalitis.

Etiology. *Mycobacterium tuberculosis*, the etiologic agent of tuberculous meningitis, is present in the CSF and in the meninges.

Pathology. In an untreated, fatal case the meninges are opaque and a yellow exudate surrounding cranial nerves is frequently present over the base of the brain (Fig. 12-4). Hydrocephaly with evidence of obstruction of the foramina of Luschka and Magendie may be present. Microscopic examination of the meninges (Fig. 12-5) and ependyma reveals miliary tubercles with a central necrotic zone surrounded by lym-

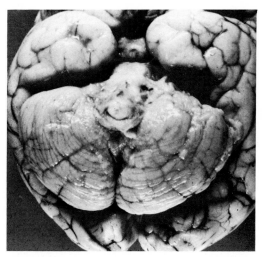

FIG. 12-4. Gross pathologic specimen of the base of the brain with severe basilar meningitis due to tuberculous infection.

phocytes, epithelioid cells, and multinucleated giant cells. A panarteritis of the pial vessels is present; and when these vessels become occluded areas of encephalomalacia develop. Thus a meningoencephalitis results.

If death occurs after several weeks of chemotherapy, the acute meningeal reaction may be minimal. Thickening of the meninges is present.

Miliary tuberculosis is also present in half of the cases. There may be lesions of the skin, lymph nodes, lungs, bones, gastrointestinal tract, or genitourinary tract.

Symptoms. Two-thirds of children who develop tuberculous meningitis are under 10 years of age, and most are in the first year of life. The onset of tuberculous meningitis is often gradual, with fever, irritability, headache, vomiting, and photophobia. In infants these symptoms may not be noted by the parents, a convulsion being the first symptom for which medical care is sought. With further progression diplopia, facial weakness, or deafness may be noted.

With careful inquiry a history of recent exposure to an active case of tuberculosis may be obtained in approximately 40% of cases.

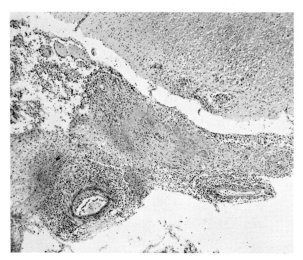

FIG. 12-5. Tuberculous meningitis, low power microscopic view. Meninges show lymphocytic inflammatory reaction, area of caseation, and arteritis. Beneath the surface of the cortex are small areas of inflammatory reaction.

Examination.   The temperature is in the range of 100° F to 103° F (38°C to 39°C). The pulse rate may be rapid. The child is frequently drowsy or stuporous. Stiff neck is frequently absent in infants, but it may be noted early in children. Bulging of the fontanels or early papilledema may be noted; and extraocular muscle paralyses involving the third, fourth or sixth cranial nerves may develop. Facial paralysis or deafness may occur; other cranial nerves are infrequently involved. Hemiparesis may be present.[73]

Laboratory Examination.   Lumbar puncture usually reveals increased initial pressure with clear or opalescent CSF. The leukocyte count varies from 25/mm³ to 500/mm³ usually predominantly mononuclear cells but rarely predominantly PMNs. In 90% of patients with advanced, untreated tuberculous meningitis, the sugar content in the CSF is 20 mg/dl to 40 mg/dl (Table 12-1), although early in the course of meningeal infection it may be normal. The protein content varies from 45 mg/dl to 500 mg/dl. When the fluid is allowed to stand, a fibrinous web or pellicle may form. Tubercle bacilli are sometimes attached to this web and can be identified on stained smears of the pellicle. The CSF may be centrifuged and the sediment stained for acid-fast organisms. A diligent search should be made on CSF smears for tubercle bacilli, even though they are identified in only 10% to 20% of fluids from children with tuberculous meningitis. In addition, cultures of CSF are made. Cultures are positive in 3 weeks to 4 weeks in fluids from children with untreated tuberculous meningitis.

The tuberculin test is initially carried out with 5 tuberculin units of purified protein derivative (PPD) and read at 48 hours. Nonreactors are then tested with 250 tuberculin units of PPD. Approximately 80% to 90% of children with tuberculous meningitis have a positive reaction to 5 or 250 tuberculin units shortly after admission. The remainder become positive reactors upon recovery after treatment. In contrast with this high incidence of a positive tuberculin test in these children, less than 10% of children in the general population have a positive test. A roentgenogram of the chest may reveal abnormal findings suggestive of tuberculous infection in approximately 50% to 70% of children with tuberculous meningitis. Smears and cultures of the sputum and gastric washings may reveal acid-fast organisms. Roentgenograms of the skull may demonstrate separation of the sutures.

In some patients CT scan shows contrast enhancement of the cisterns around the base of the brain and the brain stem as well as the cortical meninges. The ventricles may be enlarged. These findings are not specific for tuberculous meningitis because they have been observed in coccidioidal meningitis and central nervous system sarcoidosis.[9]

Differential Diagnosis.   In a patient with a progressive subacute meningoencephalitis associated with a CSF that has a leukocyte count of 25/mm[3] to 500/mm[3], predominantly lymphocytes, and a decreased sugar content, a presumptive diagnosis of tuberculous meningitis may be made. Occasionally cryptococcal meningitis presents a similar clinical course and CSF findings. In addition to acid-fast smears, India ink smears and cultures of the CSF for cryptococci should be carried out. Occasionally tumors involving the meninges may produce a similar clinical picture with the same findings in the CSF including a decrease in sugar content. The early course of a child with a brain abscess may be very similar to that observed in tuberculous meningitis. However, with brain abscess the CSF sugar content nearly always remains within normal limits.

Early in the course of tuberculous meningitis the cellular reaction may be associated with a normal sugar content. In this instance the clinical and CSF findings resemble those of viral meningitis. Also children with purulent meningitis who were treated with antibiotic and chemotherapeutic agents prior to lumbar puncture may present a clinical history and CSF findings similar to those in tuberculous meningitis.

Treatment.   If tubercle bacilli are found on smears of the CSF from a child with a subacute meningitis, the diagnosis is established and treatment immediately instituted. However, if no tubercle bacilli are demonstrated, then the clinical and laboratory findings are carefully evaluated to determine whether a presumptive diagnosis of tuberculous meningitis should be made and treatment started. If the clinical picture is that of a progressive form of meningitis and if the CSF reveals a lymphocytic reaction with a decreased sugar content, it is reasonable to institute therapy after cultures are obtained. If the clinical picture is that of nonpurulent meningitis without evidence of progression and if the CSF sugar is normal, it is advisable to investigate other etiologic possibilities prior to treatment with antituberculous drugs. The presence or absence of a positive tuberculin skin test, a pulmonary lesion, and a known tuberculous contact provide additional information for evaluation when deciding whether to initiate early therapy with a presumptive diagnosis of tuberculous meningitis.

Approximately 10% of M. tuberculosis strains are resistant to one or more of the therapeutic drugs, including isoniazid, streptomycin, paraaminosalicylic acid, cycloserine, and ethionamide. Because of this high incidence of resistant strains, it is currently recommended that children with tuberculous meningitis be treated initially with isoniazid, streptomycin, ethambutol, and rifampin (Table 12-5). All these drugs pass the blood–brain barrier when the meninges are inflamed. This four-drug regimen is subsequently altered, if necessary, to conform with the drug-susceptibility pattern of the source-case strain or of the patient's strain when available.

Isoniazid is included in all the therapeutic regimens, including those for isoniazid-resistant strains because of clinical and experimental observations that some isoniazid-resistant strains can revert to susceptible strains. In any therapeutic regimen at least two drugs to which the infecting strain is susceptible must be used to prevent the emergence of drug resistant strains. Treatment is continued for 2 years.

Isoniazid in a daily dose of 15 mg/kg to 30 mg/kg is given orally or intramuscularly. The optimal dose may be dependent upon the drug's rate of inactivation, which varies in different individuals. Simultaneously streptomycin sulfate solution in a daily dose of 20 mg/kg intramuscularly, ethambutol 15 mg/kg daily, and rifampin 10 mg/kg to 20 mg/kg daily are administered. After 1 month of therapy the streptomycin dosage is changed to 20 mg/kg two times per week for 1 month or more.

In addition to the five first-line drugs (Table 12-5) several second-line drugs are available, including ethionamide, pyrazinamide, and cycloserine. If indicated, one or more of these drugs may also be used, although they have more frequent and more severe side-effects than the first-line drugs.

TABLE 12-5. Drug Therapy of Tuberculous Meningitis: First-Line Drugs

Drug	Daily Dose	Route of Administration	Adverse Reactions
Isoniazid	15 mg/kg–30 mg/kg	Oral, intramuscular	Fever, rash, convulsions, vomiting, ataxia, somnolence, psychosis, polyneuropathy, hepatitis, optic neuritis, agranulocytosis, hyperglycemia, anemia, thrombocytopenia
Streptomycin	20 mg/kg	Intramuscular	Headache, vomiting, skin rash, fever, paresthesias of the face, vestibular damage, deafness, depressed bone marrow, depressed respiration, renal damage
Ethambutol	15 mg/kg	Oral	Rash, optic neuritis, anaphylaxis, vomiting, fever, headache, peripheral neuropathy, mental confusion
Rifampin	10 mg/kg–20 mg/kg to a maximum of 600 mg	Oral	Liver dysfunction, headache, ataxia, rash, thrombocytopenia, mental confusion
Sodium para-aminosalicylic acid	200 mg/kg	Intravenous, diluted in infusion; oral	Nausea, vomiting, diarrhea, fever, joint pains, skin rash, psychotic symptoms, hepatic coma

Toxicity to isoniazid has not been noted as frequently in children as in adults. Possible toxic manifestations include convulsions, ataxia, somnolence, psychosis, polyneuropathy, hepatitis, vomiting, fever, rash, optic neuritis, hyperglycemia, agranulocytosis, anemia, and thrombocytopenia. Transaminase levels may be mildly elevated. Pyridoxine, 25 mg to 50 mg, is given to reduce toxicity. Toxic symptoms associated with streptomycin include fever, skin rash, headache, vomiting, and paresthesias of the face. Vestibular damage may occur 3 weeks to 6 weeks after the onset of therapy, with the development of subsequent deafness. These toxic manifestations are usually permanent. Acute respiratory and central nervous system depression has also been reported in children treated with streptomycin in doses greater than 20 mg/kg per day. Preexisting renal impairment interferes with urinary excretion producing high blood levels of streptomycin and other antituberculous agents, which may increase toxicity. The blood concentration of streptomycin should not exceed 20 µg/ml plasma.

Ethambutol is of low toxicity. Optic neuritis can be avoided by a careful ocular history, funduscopic examinations, and determinations of visual acuity and visual fields. During therapy red green color discrimination and visual acuity are determined for both eyes each month. If color discrimination or acuity decreases significantly in either eye, the drug is stopped. Uni- and bilateral optic neuritis is reversible if the drug is discontinued. Other toxic reactions include rash, anaphylaxis, vomiting, fever, headache, peripheral neuropathy, and mental confusion.

Rifampin may produce liver dysfunction. It is essential that periodic liver function tests be performed. Rifampin may produce headache, ataxia, rash, thrombocytopenia, and mental confusion. Para-aminosalicylic acid therapy may be associated with nausea, vomiting, diarrhea, fever, joint pains, or skin rash. Occasionally psychotic symptoms may develop, and hepatic coma has been reported. Hepatic injury is not likely to occur unless the early warnings of toxicity are ignored. The early toxic symptoms usually appear between the third and fifth weeks of administration with fever occurring in almost every case.

Steroid therapy is of value in reducing cerebral edema and inflammatory exudate and preventing spinal block. In children with tuberculous meningitis treatment with antituberculous drugs in conjunction with prednisone in a dose of 1 mg/kg per day for 30 days results in a lower mortality rate than treatment with antituberculous drugs alone.[17]

Prognosis. The course of untreated tuberculous meningitis is progressive and uniformly fatal in 3 weeks to 6 weeks. With the treatment currently available the mortality rate is 15% to 30% in children who have received early treatment.[37] However, if the presumptive diagnosis is made and the treatment is begun late in the clinical course when the child is comatose, then the mortality rate rises to 50% to 90%.[30] In addition, severe residual neurologic deficits include recurrent convulsions, optic atrophy, and intellectual deterioration associated with obstructive hydrocephaly. The mortality rate and the rate of severe complications are increased when therapy is instituted late in the course of the illness. After successful prolonged chemotherapy, recurrence of tuberculous meningitis is unusual.

Prevention. It is recommended that infants and children under 3 years of age with a positive tuberculin test and children over 3 years of age who recently converted to a positive tuberculin test and who have roentgenographic evidence of primary tuberculosis receive prophylactic treatment to prevent tuberculous meningitis. Isoniazid in a daily dose of 10 mg/kg is administered for 1 year. Studies of alternately untreated and treated cases of primary tuberculosis have shown a reduction in extrapulmonary complications from 2.4% to 0.2%.

CRYPTOCOCCAL MENINGITIS

Etiology. The etiologic agent of cryptococcal meningitis is a budding yeast with a diameter of 2 μ to 40 μ. The portal of entry of the infection is probably through the lungs or the skin. Cryptococcal meningitis may occur in association with tuberculosis or Hodgkin's disease. It is the most common cause of meningitis due to mycotic infection. The sources of infection are the excreta of pigeons and chickens and soil containing such excreta.

Pathology. The meninges are thick and cloudy. Microscopically an inflammatory reaction involves the meninges and perivascular spaces. Small cysts containing cryptococci are seen in the cerebral cortex. (Fig. 12-6), and large cysts may form gross masses, particularly in the posterior fossa.

Symptoms. The onset is characterized by fever, headache, vomiting, and drowsiness. Convulsions may occur. The course is usually slowly progressive, although long remissions occasionally occur. Predisposing factors include steroid therapy, lymphoreticular malignancy, and sarcoid.

Examination. The child is febrile and drowsy. The head may enlarge, and papilledema may be present. There is usually stiff neck. Cranial nerves may be involved, and hemiparesis may develop. Focal weakness or hemianopia sometimes appears within a few days.

Laboratory Examination. Lumbar puncture reveals clear or cloudy CSF that may be under increased initial pressure. The leukocyte count varies from 25/mm³ to 500/mm³. Usually lymphocytes predominate, although occasionally there is a preponderance of PMNs. India ink preparations of the CSF may reveal cryptococci, which may show budding. Cultures of the fluid on Sabouraud's medium reveal the growth of cryptococci if they are present in the CSF at the time of examination. At times during the course of the illness organisms may not be present in the CSF, thus resulting in negative smears and cultures at that time, although subsequent examination of the CSF shows them to be present. The sugar content of the CSF is decreased to 20 mg/dl to 40 mg/dl. The protein content is usually elevated.

Differential Diagnosis. The clinical course of cryptococcal meningitis is very similar to that of tuberculous meningitis, although cryptococcal infections may have remis-

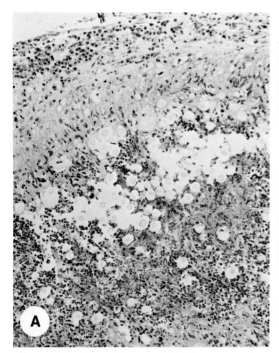
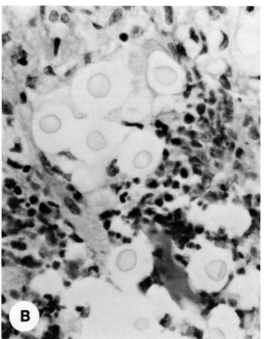

FIG. 12-6. Cryptococcal meningitis. *A*, Low power microscopic view shows multiple small cystic areas within the brain substance. Organisms are present within these small areas. The surrounding tissues show a lymphocytic infiltration. *B*, High power view taken from the center of the cystic area shown in the low power view. The encapsulated yeast *Cryptococcus neoformans* appears in the microscopic cystic areas.

sions, whereas tuberculous infections of the meninges do not. An etiologic diagnosis can be made only by isolating the organism from the CSF. In those cases in which meningeal illness is associated with focal cerebral signs one must exclude the possibility of brain abscess and also rarely the invasion of the central nervous system by other fungal infections, such as actinomycosis, nocardiosis, blastomycosis, histoplasmosis, aspergillosis, coccidioidomycosis, and mucormycosis.

Treatment. Amphotericin B is used to treat cryptococcal meningitis. Initially a daily dose of 0.25 mg/kg is given intravenously in a suspension of 5% dextrose in water over a period of 5 hours to 6 hours. The dosage is gradually increased to a level of

1.0 mg/kg body weight, if tolerated, and treatment is continued for approximately 6 weeks.

Febrile reactions may occur during the first few days of therapy. Subsequently headache, nausea, vomiting, and renal insufficiency may develop. If the blood urea nitrogen level (BUN) becomes elevated, medication should be stopped until it returns to normal. Toxic effects on the kidneys may be lessened by alternate-day intravenous therapy. It may be monitored by the creatinine clearance test.[41]

Prognosis. Without treatment cryptococcal meningitis is usually fatal within 3 months to 6 months, although there may be occasional prolonged remissions with eventual death occurring after 1 year to 3 years. Sixty percent of patients are cured with amphotericin B therapy, and residual neurological deficits are present in 20%.

OTHER TYPES OF FUNGAL MENINGITIS

Rarely actinomycosis due to *Actinomyces bovis* spreads from a primary site in the face or neck or in the cecum to the central nervous system. It then produces a chronic, purulent meningitis that may also be associated with brain abscess. The organism is sensitive to tetracycline and penicillin.

Blastomycosis produced by the yeast *Blastomyces dermatitidis* sometimes results in meningitis; this rare form responds to therapy with stilbamidine or amphotericin B.

Coccidioidomycosis due to the fungus *Coccidioides immitis* produces pulmonary infection, which may be complicated by a lymphocytic meningitis. Therapy with amphotericin B has been recommended.

Histoplasmosis due to *Histoplasma capsulatum* rarely produces a meningitis as part of a fatal systemic disorder. Amphotericin B is used in therapy.

Mucormycosis may produce a systemic infection with orbital cellulitis, thrombosis of the internal carotid artery, or meningitis. It usually occurs as a complication of diabetes mellitus. Treatment includes correction of ketoacidosis when present, surgical debridement, and amphotericin B therapy. The mortality rate is 30% to 80%.[6,51]

Nocardia and *Aspergillus* may rarely produce meningitis. Nocardiosis is treated with sulfadiazine. Aspergillosis is treated with amphotericin B.

MENINGEAL REACTIONS SECONDARY TO INTRACRANIAL INFECTIONS

Systemic bacterial infections that spread to the central nervous system may involve the meninges with resultant purulent meningitis, or they may produce infections of other intracranial structures, resulting in extradural abscess, subdural empyema, septic thrombosis of superior sagittal or transverse venous sinuses or of cerebral veins, or brain abscess (Fig.12-7).

The medial portion of each cerebral hemisphere is drained by the superior cerebral veins into the midline superior sagittal sinus (Fig. 12-8). Venous blood then flows into the transverse sinuses. In 4% of the normal population the transverse sinus is absent on one side. Thus one transverse sinus is adequate for the return of blood from the superior sagittal sinus. From each transverse sinus blood drains into the jugular bulb and thence into the internal jugular vein. The lateral half of the cerebral hemisphere is drained by inferior cerebral veins coursing downward and emptying into cavernous and transverse sinuses.

Since the sources of infection and the early clinical symptoms are similar in the pyogenic intracranial disorders, they are presented here as a group. Brain abscess is the most common type of infection in this group, although the other complications must be carefully considered in each child. In fact, more than one of these complications may be present in the same child.

EXTRADURAL ABSCESS, SUBDURAL EMPYEMA, SEPTIC THROMBOSIS, BRAIN ABSCESS

Etiology. The bacteria most commonly producing these infections are staphylococci, streptococci, and pneumococci. Intracranial infections may arise either by direct spread of infection through the skull or by indirect spread from a distant site through the bloodstream to the central nervous system. Direct extension may occur with spread of an acute or chronic sinusitis or mastoiditis. Infection of the face or scalp may result in septic thrombophlebitis, which can spread intracranially along emissary veins because these veins do not have valves. A compound skull fracture or a puncture wound of the skull may provide the path for bacterial invasion (Fig. 12-9). Infected embolic material may spread from chronic pyogenic lung disease, endocarditis, osteomyelitis, impetigo, or furunculosis. In a child with congenital heart disease associated with a septal defect, bacterial comtamination in the venous system may be shunted directly to the arterial system and thence to the brain.

With purulent sinusitis or mastoiditis the infection may be spread directly through draining veins into the diploic spaces of the frontal or temporal bone, resulting in osteomyelitis (Fig. 12-10). From here infection may spread into the extradural space and form an extradural abscess, a purulent mass lying between the inner table of the skull and the outer surface of the dura mater; or the infection may extend through the dura to the subdural space and form a subdural empyema (see Fig. 12-7). Extension of mastoiditis may result in lateral sinus thrombosis, or sinusitis may be followed by thrombosis of the cerebral veins and of the superior sagittal sinus. With direct spread of infection, a local or generalized meningitis may develop. A puncture wound of the skull or intracranial spread of infection from sinusitis or mastoiditis may result in a subsequent brain abscess (see Fig. 12-9). Infection of the extradural space, the subdural space, venous sinuses, or brain may result after spread from a distant site.

Subdural empyema in infants is usually a complication of bacterial meningitis. The bacteria cultured from the subdural empyemas are usually *H. influenzae, D. pneumoniae,* and *E. coli,* the same ones that produce meningitis in infants. Subdural

empyemas in infants probably reprsent infected subdural effusions and are often bilateral.[79] In contrast with this pathogenesis, subdural empyemas in children are usually secondary to infections of the paranasal sinuses and are not associated with meningitis. The pathogenic organisms are usually anaerobic streptococci and staphylococci.[19]

Pathology. An extradural abscess consists of a purulent mass lying beneath the inner table of the skull and frequently associated with osteomyelitis of the neighboring bone. A subdural empyema consists of a purulent exudate spreading beneath the dura and usually overlying most of the lateral surface of one or both cerebral hemispheres (Fig. 12-11), or lying between the hemispheres.

With thrombosis of cerebral veins, ve-

FIG. 12-7. Anatomic locations of different intracranial pyogenic infections.

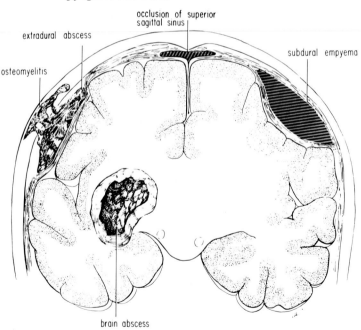

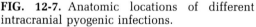

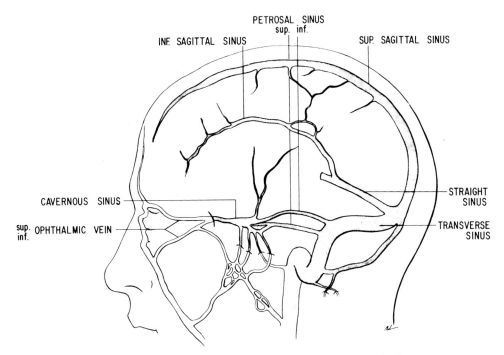

PETROSAL SINUS
sup. inf.

INF. SAGITTAL SINUS

SUP. SAGITTAL SINUS

CAVERNOUS SINUS

STRAIGHT SINUS

sup. OPHTHALMIC VEIN
inf.

TRANSVERSE SINUS

FIG. 12-8. The major cerebral venous sinuses. (Modified from Davies DV, Davies F (eds.): Gray's Anatomy, 33rd ed., p. 876. London, Longmans, 1962)

nous infarctions may occur with edema and tissue necrosis in the cerebral hemisphere. The veins are usually occluded by organized clot and surrounded by inflammatory reaction. A clot may also occlude the superior sagittal sinus or the transverse sinuses.

A brain abscess appears as an encapsulated mass within the brain substance (Fig. 12-12). The outer wall of the abscess is composed of glial cells, which surround a central, necrotic, purulent mass. An abscess usually develops over a period of several weeks. Initially infected embolic material lodges in a small arteriole and produces a microscopic area of suppurative necrosis. The necrotic area increases in size and is eventually encapsulated, the surrounding brain tissue becoming markedly edematous. Two-thirds of brain abscesses are single and one-third multiple. They may eventually contaminate the subarachnoid space or the ventricular system and then produce purulent meningitis.

Symptoms. There is a history of preceding focal systemic infection in the majority of children with intracranial pyogenic infections. An acute or chronic earache may be associated with pain behind the involved ear.[47] Acute frontal sinusitis is as-

FIG. 12-9. Brain abscess, left frontal lobe, secondary to a puncture wound of the skull. The defect in the frontal view produced by the old puncture wound is apparent on the x-ray film at the site of the *arrow.* The ventriculogram reveals displacement of the lateral ventricles and of the third ventricle to the right by a mass in the left frontal lobe. Separation of the sutures is also seen.

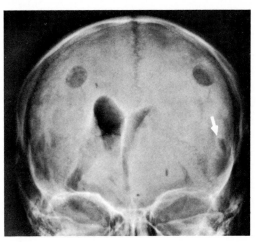

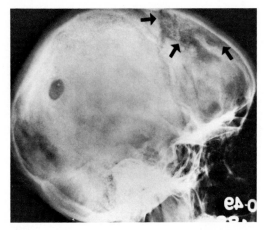

FIG. 12-10. Lateral skull film revealing osteomyelitis of the left frontal bone. The edges of the involved area are shown by the three *arrows.*

sociated with frontal headache and nasal obstruction. The history of an infection of the face or scalp or of a head injury may be obtained in some patients. The child may have productive cough, dyspnea, or cyanosis with associated heart or lung disease.[8]

The interval between the initial infection and the first manifestation of an acute extradural abscess, subdural empyema, or cerebral thrombophlebitis may be a few days to a few weeks. The average interval between initial infection and development of a brain abscess is 1 month, although it may vary from a few days to several months.

In some children with intracranial pyogenic disorders there is no history of a recent bacterial infection. This is true of one-fourth of patients with brain abscess.

The initial symptom of intracranial infection is frequently headache, localized or generalized. It may be associated with fever, nausea, vomiting, drowsiness, and mental confusion. Children may complain of pain or stiffness in the neck. Focal or generalized convulsions appear in two-thirds of children with subdural empyema, thrombosis of cerebral veins or sinuses, or brain abscess. They usually begin as unilateral seizures that may become generalized, and are often associated with progressive numbness and weakness of the arm and leg on the same side as the focal convulsion. The symptoms and signs are related

to: (1) focal or diffuse cerebral dysfunction, (2) meningeal irritation, and (3) increased intracranial pressure.

Examination. With extradural abscess the temperature and pulse are elevated. Stiff neck may or may not be present. Unless there are other central nervous system complications, no focal neurologic signs are seen.

Subdural empyema is associated with high fever of 103° F to 104° F (39° C to 40° C). The child may be drowsy, stuporous, or

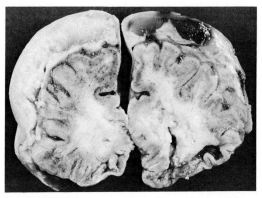

FIG. 12-11. Bilateral massive subdural empyema in an 8-month-old infant with initial purulent meningitis.

FIG. 12-12. An encapsulated brain abscess is present deep in the left cerebral hemisphere with resultant compression of the left lateral ventricle and displacement of the right lateral ventricle and the third ventricle to the right.

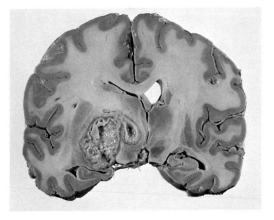

comatose, and may have a stiff neck. Hemiparesis or hemiplegia may develop, as may papilledema. With involvement of the dominant hemisphere, dysphasia may be present.

Papilledema occurs with superior sagittal sinus thrombosis, thrombosis involving both transverse sinuses, or transverse sinus thrombosis on one side associated with a congenitally absent transverse sinus on the opposite side. With extension of thrombosis to cerebral veins on one side, weakness of the opposite face, arm, and leg develops with or without disturbances of position sense, recognition of objects, and tactile localization. The tendon reflexes may be increased on the involved side, and the plantar response on that side may become extensor. Subsequently bilateral leg weakness may appear with bilateral superior cerebral vein thromboses.

In many children with subacute brain abscess the temperature, pulse, and respirations are normal. However, high fever may be present with an acute brain abscess of rapid onset or with brain abscess associated with purulent meningitis. A small percentage of patients may experience bradycardia. Examination may reveal an infection of the scalp or skin, tenderness of the paranasal sinuses or mastoids, cardiac murmurs, or signs of consolidation in the lungs. There may be acute swelling or tenderness of bones suggesting osteomyelitis. In one-fourth of patients there is no demonstrable site of a primary infection at the time the brain abscess develops.

Neurologic examination in children with brain abscess usually reveals stiff neck or a positive Kernig's sign. Most of the children show an altered state of consciousness beginning with irritability and disorientation, and progressing to stupor and coma. There may be unequal pupils or paralysis of extraocular muscles. One-third of the children have papilledema (Fig. 12-13). With an abscess in one cerebral hemisphere there may be dysphasia, homonymous hemianopia, hemiparesis, or sensory loss. These focal cerebral signs may be associated with increased deep tendon reflexes and extensor plantar response. Truncal ataxia or incoordination of one arm and leg may be noted in association with a posterior fossa abscess.

Laboratory Examination. The leukocyte count and erythrocyte sedimentation rate are usually elevated in all these infections. With brain abscess they are elevated in three-fourths of children.

Radiographs of the skull may reveal separation of the sutures due to increased intracranial pressure associated with subdural empyema or brain abscess (Figs. 12-9 and 12-14). With a chronic brain abscess in a child the radiographs may show demineralization of the sella turcica. A shift of the pineal gland, if calcified, suggests an intracranial mass. The skull may reveal a simple or depressed fracture or evidence of osteomyelitis (see Fig. 12-10). Radiographs may reveal evidence of mastoiditis or of frontal, ethmoidal, or maxillary sinusitis. Radiographs of the chest may reveal evidence of lung abscess, bronchiectasis, or congenital heart disease.

Computed tomography is the most valuable radiologic procedure in the diagnosis of brain abscess and subdural and extradural empyema.[82] A circular area of low density with peripheral rim-enhancement is characteristic of brain abscess. Multiple abscesses are demonstrated by CT scan (Fig. 12-15). Rim-enhancement is not specific for an abscess because it may be seen in neoplasms, infarcts, hematomas, or contusions. However, the combined clinical and CT findings usually will differentiate the patient with abscess.[33] The CT in a child with a unilateral subdural empyema over the convexity reveals a semilunar-shaped extracerebral lesion associated with a shift of the ventricular system to the opposite side (Fig. 12-16). The margins of the decreased density may be smooth or they may show varying degrees of irregularity or even loculation. The CT scan in a child with bilateral convexity subdural empyema reveals crescent-shaped areas of decreased density overlying both cerebral hemispheres. The inner subdural membrane and the adjacent cortical surface frequently show contrast enhancement (Fig. 12-17).[70] If the subdural empyema is located between the cerebral hemispheres, the CT scan shows an area of decreased density adjacent to the falx cerebri often associated with enhancement of its rim.[53] With extradural empyema the CT visualizes a well-localized nonhomogeneous, low-density, lenticular lesion

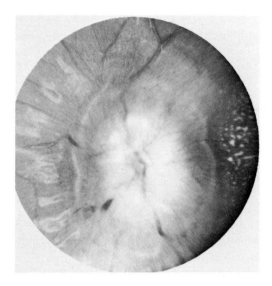

FIG. 12-13. Optic disk revealing secondary optic atrophy associated with prolonged papilledema. The elevation of the vessels at the edge of the disk is apparent. This 8-year-old child developed chronic mastoiditis following otitis media. During the subsequent 4 months she developed left-sided weakness associated with headache and vomiting. A brain abscess in the right temporal lobe was aspirated and then excised.

that may extend across the midline and appear contiguous with bone.[75]

The electroencephalogram reveals a focal slow-wave abnormality over all or a portion of one cerebral hemisphere in one-half to two-thirds of children with focal pyogenic intracranial infections. This may be of value in lateralization and at times in localization, although it does not differentiate subdural empyema, venous thrombosis, or abscess (Fig. 12-18).

Subdural punctures in infants with subdural empyemas overlying the lateral convexity of one or both cerebral hemispheres usually yield pus containing bacteria. However, failure to obtain fluid at subdural puncture does not completely exclude a subdural empyema, because failure may be due to thick subdural membranes, loculation of pus, or highly viscous pus.

Lumbar puncture in infants with subdural empyema usually reveals purulent fluid containing a predominance of PMNs, a sugar content of 0 to 40 mg/dl and bacteria on smear or culture. In children with subdural empyema the cellular reaction is frequently polymorphonuclear with normal sugar content and no organisms.

FIG. 12-14. Brain abscess in right parietal area. Lateral (A) and anteroposterior (B) skull radiographs reveal the abscess cavity filled with isophendylate (Pantopaque). Separation of the sutures is also seen. This 3-year-old boy developed a left hemiparesis 6 weeks after acute purulent tonsillitis.

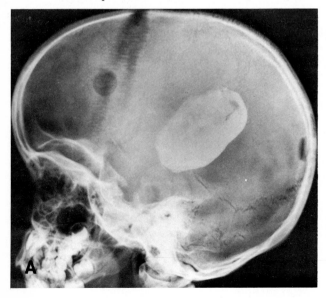

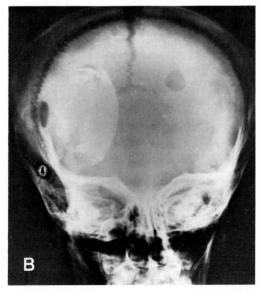

In children with brain abscess or cerebral thrombophlebitis lumbar puncture reveals clear or opalescent CSF. In the majority of cases the initial pressure is elevated. The fluid may contain no leukocytes or 50/mm³ to 500/mm³. In two-thirds of cases of brain abscess there is an increase in cellular reaction, lymphocytes usually predominating. Venous sinus thrombosis is often associated with a normal cell count and sugar content in the CSF. The protein varies from 50 mg/dl to 200 mg/dl. No organisms are present on smear or culture unless early meningitis is present.

Brain scans performed on children with brain abscess may show a local area of increased uptake. Those carried out on children with hemispheric subdural empyema and with cerebral thrombophlebitis usually show a focal increased uptake, often in a crescent pattern (Fig. 12-19). This pattern is not specific because it may be seen in patients with cerebral abscess, epidural abscess, osteomyelitis of the skull, subdural hematoma, cerebral infarction, or neoplasm.[26]

Echoencephalography may demon-

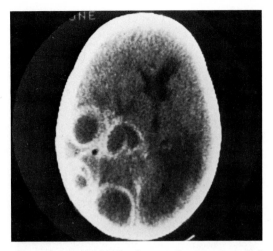

FIG. 12-15. Multiple brain abscesses in left temporal, parietal, and occipital lobes. CT scan reveals multiple areas of decreased density with ring enhancement in the left cerebral hemisphere posteriorly. The lateral and third ventricles are markedly shifted to the right. This 18-month-old boy was stuporous on admission. Cerebral abscesses were drained and subsequently excised during several operative procedures. Serial CT scans were done to plan this therapy. He recovered with mild residual deficits.

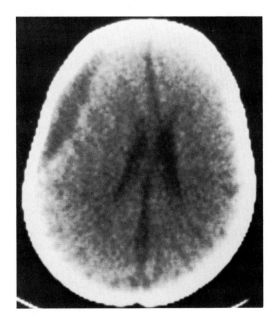

FIG. 12-16. Left convexity subdural empyema. Unenhanced CT scan in a 4-month-old boy with *Hemophilus influenzae* meningitis reveals a crescent-shaped hypodense area in the left frontal region with displacement of the lateral ventricles to the right. The subdural fluid was purulent.

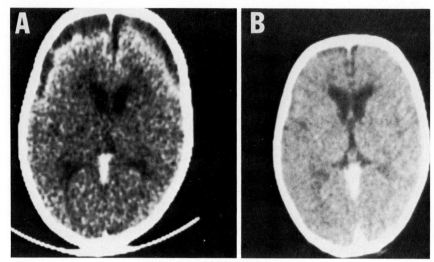

FIG. 12-17. Bilateral convexity subdural empyema. *A,* Enchanced CT scan in a 4-month-old girl with *Hemophilus parainfluenzae* meningitis reveals bifrontal hypodense areas with contrast enhancement of the inner subdural membrane and adjacent cortical surface. The ventricles are in the midline. *B,* Enhanced CT scan after drainage of subdural spaces is normal.

strate displacement of the midline echo toward the opposite side in children with brain abscess or subdural empyema. An abnormal finding may suggest the need for additional studies.

Brain abscess or subdural empyema is usually diagnosed by CT scan so that arteriography or ventriculography is not performed. In selected cases arteriography may provide additional information.[53]

Cerebral angiography in children with cerebral thrombophlebitis reveals no displacement of the major vessels. Delay in emptying of cerebral veins is seen occasionally.[80]

Differential Diagnosis. If the child has manifestations of increased intracranial pressure with headache and papilledema, thrombosis of the transverse sinuses or the superior sagittal sinus is a likely possibility. If he has focal or generalized convulsions with meningeal signs and focal neurologic signs, the differential diagnosis is between subdural empyema, thrombosis of the superior sagittal sinus associated with cerebral vein thrombosis, and brain ab-

scess. Subdural punctures are indicated in infants because they may establish the diagnosis of subdural empyema. Subdural empyema is usually associated with an acute, febrile illness and with the development of convulsions and hemiparesis within a week after onset. The cellular reaction in the CSF is frequently a preponderance of PMNs. The occurrence of bilateral neurologic signs, such as focal convulsions or paralysis appearing first on one side of the body and then the other, is suggestive of cerebral thrombophlebitis or of subdural empyema. A subacute cerebral abscess usually has an insidious onset with a longer course than that of subdural empyema. The temperature with abscess may be normal or slightly elevated. The CSF usually contains a small number of cells, predominantly lymphocytes. However, an acute cerebral abscess may have a clinical course identical with that of subdural empyema.

The same clinical findings may be due to herpes simplex encephalitis. If the presenting clinical picture is that of an expanding intracranial process with no antecedent history of infection, the differential diagnosis may relate primarily to the differentiation of brain abscess or subdural empyema from cerebral neoplasm or subdural hematoma.

After a detailed history and examination are completed, the most important laboratory study is the CT scan, which may

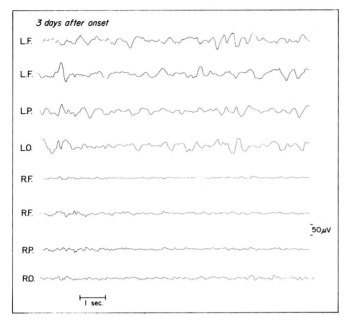

FIG. 12-18. Electroencephalogram of a 10-year-old boy with a subdural empyema overlying the left cerebral hemisphere. High voltage delta waves of 2 cycles per second–3 cycles per second are prominent over the left cerebral hemisphere.

FIG. 12-19. Brain scans with technetium-99m. Anteroposterior (*A*) and posteroanterior (*B*) scans done 3 days after onset of left facial seizures and left hemiparesis reveal a crescentic, peripheral increase in radioisotope uptake over the right cerebral convexity. Anteroposterior (*C*) and posteroanterior (*D*) scans 6 months after onset are normal. This 15-year-old boy developed left-sided convulsions and left hemiparesis due to cerebral thrombophlebitis. Cerebral angiograms were normal. (From Wise GR, Farmer TW: Bacterial cerebral vasculitis. Neurology 21:195, 1971).

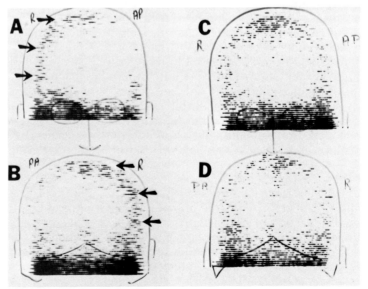

provide diagnostic information. Since the course of brain abscess or subdural empyema may be a rapid one with marked increase in symptoms and signs occurring within less than 24 hours, it is imperative that definitive diagnostic studies be performed on an emergency basis.[65]

Treatment. A pathogenic organism cultured from the initial site of systemic infection in the ears, sinuses, or elsewhere may be the same one producing the intracranial infection. Tests of antibiotic sensitivities to this organism may provide a guide to antibiotic and chemotherapy. Blood cultures are obtained, after which the patient is placed on systemic antibiotic and chemotherapeutic drugs. Since initial therapy is begun without bacteriologic information, a combination of antimicrobial drugs is used. Methicillin and chloramphenicol in full therapeutic dosage provide an effective combination. Currently ampicillin is the drug of choice for an unidentified bacterial leptomeningitis in a young child. Gram-negative bacteria must be treated in neonatal cases. Adequate systemic doses of appropriate antibiotics appear to be as effective as the combined use of subdural and systemic drug therapy. Antibacterial chemotherapy is continued for at least 3 weeks, and in selected cases for longer intervals (Table 12-4).

Extradural abscess is treated by direct surgical drainage, and the focal area of osteomyelitis is excised. Subdural empyema is treated by surgical drainage. If the subdural empyema is located over one frontal area, a burr hole is placed in the lateral frontal region for drainage. Multiple burr holes or craniotomy may be required to obtain adequate drainage of the empyema.[70] In some infants with subdural empyema serial four-quadrant subdural taps provide adequate drainage. The course is monitored with serial CT scans.

Brain abscess is initially treated with surgical aspiration and drainage.[16,81] Usually the abscess capsule is subsequently excised. Repeat CT scans are of value in the rapid detection of postoperative complications and in the treatment of multiloculated and multiple abscesses (see Fig. 12-15).[56,69] In a few patients on antibiotic therapy serial

CT scans have revealed resolution of an abscess.[56]

The purulent material obtained from the extradural abscess, subdural empyema, or brain abscess is cultured. If a pathogen is isolated, its sensitivity to different antimicrobial drugs is tested and subsequent antibiotic and chemotherapy are planned in accordance with these *in vitro* results.

When thrombosis of cerebral veins and sinuses is secondary to a pyogenic infection of the paranasal sinuses, middle ear, or mastoid, surgical drainage of purulent infection in these areas may be indicated. If bacterial infection is not controlled and if a penicillin-resistant staphylococcus has been isolated, methicillin or other antibiotic agents to which the organism is sensitive should be instituted. If seizures have occurred, anticonvulsant medications are continued after recovery.

Prognosis. An untreated extradural abscess is usually followed by extension of infection with subsequent meningitis and death. However, with early surgical drainage combined with chemotherapy the mortality rate is low. If the infection is controlled, healing occurs without residual signs.

The downhill course of a child with untreated subdural empyema is rapidly progressive. Since the subdural empyema is not encapsulated, meningitis rapidly ensues. Without chemotherapy and surgical intervention the course is uniformly fatal within 6 days to 20 days after the onset of headache and within 2 days to 5 days after the onset of focal neurologic signs. The CT scan has been a major advance in the early diagnosis of subdural empyema, and this has been associated with a decline in mortality rate following antibiotic and surgical therapy. The mortality rate has been reduced to 10% to 20%.[31] If focal neurologic signs develop prior to treatment, residual weakness may persist.

Septic thrombosis of cerebral veins and sinuses is usually associated with or followed by other intracranial infections. It is also preceded by a pyogenic infection elsewhere in the body, which may persist. If chemotherapy and appropriate surgical intervention are not instituted, the infection usually terminates fatally. However, with adequate control of infection associated with venous sinus thrombosis there is 90% recovery. Rapid recanalization of veins takes place. Since the cerebral veins have no valves, the blood flow may be reversed in these vessels. If severe neurologic deficit has resulted, it usually recovers within 1 month to 2 months, although serious residual effects may persist. Recurrent convulsive seizures sometimes follow adequate treatment.

Without therapy the course of a child with a brain abscess is uniformly fatal within 1 week to many months. However, with antibiotic and surgical therapy the mortality rate has been decreased to less than 10% in children with both single and multiloculated abscesses.[45,56,69] Computed tomography provides accurate early diagnosis and localization of abscesses. Serial CT scans also detect postoperative complications early. These scans provide important diagnostic information that results in a low mortality rate.

With early diagnosis when the child is still alert the operative mortality is less than 10%, whereas with late diagnosis when the child is in coma the mortality rate reaches 80%. After only simple drainage, a single brain abscess may recur. The drainage or removal of such an abscess may be unsuccessful due to the presence of one or more other brain abscesses. In a child with severe neurologic deficit due to a brain abscess, residual neurologic signs may be permanent after operation. Recurrent convulsive seizures occasionally follow adequate surgical management of brain abscess.

SEPTIC CAVERNOUS SINUS THROMBOSIS

Due to the characteristic clinical findings in cavernous sinus thrombosis, this disorder is presented separately from other types of sinus thrombosis.

Etiology. The most common organisms producing septic cavernous sinus thrombosis are staphylococci, streptococci, and pneumococci. Infections of the face, sinuses, orbit, mouth, throat, or middle ear may be associated with thrombophlebitis with subsequent extension along venous pathways to the cavernous sinus (see Fig. 12-8).

Pathology. The cavernous sinus and the ophthalmic veins are occluded by an organized clot associated with an acute inflammatory reaction. Cellulitis of the orbit is frequently present. Infection may spread to the meninges with purulent meningitis.

Symptoms. The child is acutely ill with fever, drowsiness, and confusion. Double vision may be noted initially followed by drooping of the eyelid on the affected side.

Examination. Thrombosis of the anterior cavernous sinus produces exophthalmos, chemosis, and edema of the eyelids on the affected side due to occlusion of the ophthalmic veins. Partial or complete paralysis of muscles supplied by the third, fourth, and sixth cranial nerves is noted (Fig. 12-20). Sensory loss in the ophthalmic division of the fifth cranial nerve with absent corneal reflex is observed, and the cornea may become clouded. These characteristic cranial nerve signs occur initially on one side, although thrombosis may spread through the intercavernous sinus to the opposite cavernous sinus with the development of similar signs on the opposite side (Fig. 12-21).

Laboratory Examination. Bacterial cultures are taken from the initial site of infection to isolate the pathogenic organism and to determine its sensitivities to antibiotic agents. Blood cultures are obtained. Lumbar puncture is done to exclude the possible spread of infection with resultant purulent meningitis.

Differential Diagnosis. The association of an acute systemic infection about the head with the development of swelling of one orbit associated with neurologic involvement of the third, fourth, fifth, and sixth cranial nerves is almost diagnostic of cavernous sinus thrombosis. Orbital cellulitis may produce the same findings with thrombosis of ophthalmic veins and involvement of the apex of the orbit. With orbital cellulitis the child may show less toxemia and

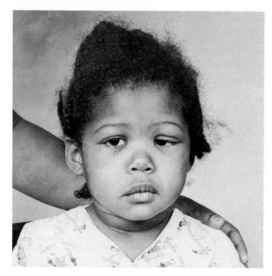

FIG. 12-20. A child recovering from left cavernous sinus thrombosis. Residual edema of the left orbit is apparent with slight ptosis and weakness of the lateral rectus muscle on the left.

the cranial nerve palsies may recover rapidly.

Treatment. As soon as bacterial cultures have been taken, antibiotic and chemotherapeutic drugs are administered. Ampicillin or a combination of penicillin, chloramphenicol, and sulfadiazine is used initially (Table 12-4). If there is no clinical response to therapy within 24 hours to 48 hours, additional antibiotic agents may be used. Subsequent therapy may be guided by the results of *in vitro* tests for antibiotic sensitivity if a pathogenic organism is isolated.

If a focal collection of pus is present in one of the paranasal sinuses, the middle ear, or mastoid, it is drained surgically and cultures are taken. If, in spite of apparent control of infection with a drop in temperature, there is nevertheless an increase of neurologic signs, then heparin and coumarin are used in an effort to prevent extension of thrombosis.

Prognosis. As a result of the use of chemotherapeutic and antibiotic agents the mortality rate in cavernous sinus throm-

FIG. 12-21. The cavernous sinuses and nerves that pass through them. The anatomic basis for the neurologic involvement with cavernous sinus thrombosis is apparent. Also the ease with which infection spreads from one cavernous sinus to the opposite cavernous sinus is clear from the presence of the intercavernous sinus.

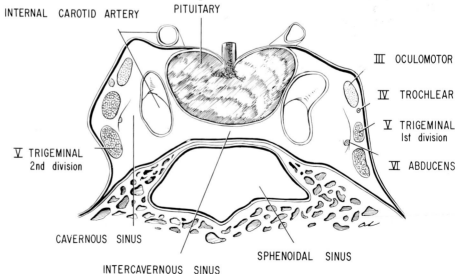

bosis has decreased from 95% to approximately 30%. Extraocular palsies and visual impairment resulting from cavernous sinus thrombosis may be permanent or they may clear.

VIRAL MENINGITIS

Mumps virus infections, Coxsackie virus infections, and infections with enteric cytopathic human orphan (ECHO) viruses account for 60% of the cases of "aseptic meningitis" (Table 12-6). The percentage due to poliomyelitis virus is now extremely small. Five percent of aseptic meningitis cases are due to the virus of lymphocytic choriomeningitis, and the remaining 35% to infrequently encountered viruses (or they are of unknown etiology).

Enteric viruses occur characteristically in the summer and fall months, whereas mumps meningitis and lymphocytic choriomeningitis occur frequently during the winter and spring months. (Table 12-6).

Epstein-Barr virus produces meningoencephalitis in some children as an additional manifestation of infectious mononucleosis. Meningoencephalitis in children occasionally occurs with adenovirus infections.[36]

ACUTE ANTERIOR POLIOMYELITIS

The virus of poliomyelitis initially invades the intestinal and respiratory tracts, and subsequently may invade the bloodstream producing a systemic infection. If the infection spreads to the central nervous system, meningeal reaction occurs. This may be followed by paralysis.

Etiology. Infection may be due to type I, II, or III poliomyelitis virus. The type I virus is the most common, then type III, and lastly type II. Virus isolations are performed on tissue culture. Infection with one type of virus does not completely protect against a second type so that reinfection may occur in the same individual.

Epidemiology. Poliomyelitis is usually an epidemic disease during the summer and fall months, although occasionally epidemics may occur during the winter. In addition, sporadic cases occur throughout the winter and spring.

Pathology. The meninges show an acute inflammatory reaction. The virus invades motor nerve cells and may produce necrosis of these cells with loss of innervation of the motor units supplied by them. Degenerative changes are most intense in the anterior horn cells of the spinal cord and in the motor nuclei of the medulla.

Symptoms. Approximately 10% of all poliomyelitis cases occur in children under 2 years of age and 70% in those under 10 years of age. Neonatal infection has been reported.

Since effective vaccines hve become widely available for the prevention of poliomyelitis, clinical infections are seen only where adequate preventive measures have not been used. The types of infections produced are (1) inapparent, (2) systemic, (3) meningitic, and (4) paralytic. With inap-

TABLE 12-6. Viral Infections Producing Nonpurulent Meningeal Reactions

Virus	Approximate Incidence (%)	Seasonal Occurrence
Coxsackie	20	Summer and fall
Enteric cytopathic human orphan	20	Summer and fall
Mumps	20	Winter and spring
Lymphocytic choriomeningitis	5	Winter and spring
Etiology unknown	35	

parent infection, which is the most common form, the virus invades the gastrointestinal tract and is excreted in the feces without producing apparent infection. With a systemic infection the symptoms are fever, poor appetite, diarrhea, and cough. Fever usually lasts 4 days to 7 days. A meningitic illness develops in a small percentage of infections due to poliomyelitis virus. In one-fourth of the children this is preceded by a prodromal illness consisting of fever and malaise. After a period of improvement for several days the child may become listless with headache, vomiting, and muscle soreness. There may be stiffness and pain in the neck as well as pain in the back muscles. In approximately 1% of all infections, paralysis develops during or shortly after acute meningeal illness. Weakness usually develops during the febrile meningeal phase of the disease, and paralysis may progress over a period of several days to a week. Occasionally the meningeal illness may subside and paralysis be delayed for 1 week to 2 weeks. In some children paralysis appears without definite meningeal symptoms. With bulbar involvement there is sometimes difficulty in swallowing or in breathing. Ulcerative lesions of the upper gastrointestinal tract with massive hemorrhage may develop, though rarely, in association with brain stem, probably hypothalamic, involvement.

A history of adenotonsillectomy within 1 month prior to clinical infection with poliomyelitis virus predisposes a child to involvement of motor nuclei in the medulla with bulbar poliomyelitis.

Examination. In the prodromal illness the temperature is elevated to 100°F to 104°F (38°C to 40°C) and the patient may appear mildly or moderately ill. There may be injection of the throat.

The patient usually appears acutely ill during the meningeal phase of the illness. The skin may be dry due to excessive loss of fluids with fever and vomiting. Neck flexion may be limited and a positive Kernig's sign present. The trunk may be hyperextended. If the child is asked to sit up, the trunk is supported by both hands and arms, and the back is arched in a tripod position. With nonparalytic infection there may be soreness of the neck, trunk, and thigh

muscles, but no definite weakness is present. During the meningeal illness daily brief neurologic examinations are done to search for the development of motor weakness, particularly respiratory weakness. As fever and meningeal signs subside a detailed examination of muscular strength is carried out.

With bulbar involvement, which occurs in approximately 10% to 30% of children with paralytic poliomyelitis, muscles supplied by cranial nerves are weakened. Occasionally there is extraocular muscle weakness and weakness of the upper and lower portions of the face. Uni- or bilateral weakness or paralysis of the palate may be present with a nasal voice, absent gag reflex, and difficulty in swallowing. The sternomastoid and trapezius muscles may be involved, and movement of the tongue may be weakened.

With involvement of the anterior horn cells in the spinal cord there may be weakness in the arms, trunk, or legs. Initially the muscular weakness may be associated with some fasciculations and soreness on palpation. Weakness progresses to flaccid paralysis. During the acute phase of the illness the strength in the extremities and trunk is tested only briefly to avoid overexerting the patient. The strength of the intercostal muscles and of the diaphragm is evaluated. The rate and depth of respirations are observed. A useful method of following the strength of respiratory muscles in older children is to have the patient take a deep breath, expire, and than count aloud as high as he can before a second inspiration. Intercostal movement can be evaluated by palpating the thoracic cage on deep inspiration. The descent of the diaphragm on inspiration can be palpated through the abdomen. The strength of abdominal and back muscles is also tested. Muscular involvement may be restricted to the muscles in one extremity or may involve the trunk and all extremities. Combined spinal and bulbar involvement may be present.

Involvement of the bladder occurs in 5% to 10% of children. The sensory examination reveals no abnormalities. The tendon reflexes are usually decreased or absent in the area of motor involvement.

A systematic evaluation of all skeletal musculature is necessary to determine which muscles are involved. The extent of weakness is graded on a scale of 0–5 (see Table 1-2). Muscle grading is of great value in following the course of the strength of each involved muscle.

In children with respiratory symptoms careful observations are required on rate and depth of respiration, blood pressure, pulse, temperature, presence of cyanosis, and mental confusion. Elevation of systolic and diastolic blood pressure may occur with hypoxia.

Laboratory Examination. *Cerebrospinal Fluid.* Lumbar puncture done at the time of the acute meningeal illness reveals clear or slightly turbid CSF under normal or slightly elevated initial pressure. In approximately 90% of patients the leukocyte count is 25/mm³ to 500/mm³. During the first 24 hours to 48 hours after the onset of meningeal signs there may be a predominance of PMNs in the CSF. After this initial period the cells in the CSF are predominantly lymphocytes. The sugar content is normal. In two-thirds of the patients the protein is normal and in one-third it is elevated to 50 mg/dl to 200 mg/dl. The virus of poliomyelitis cannot be isolated from the CSF.

Virus Isolation. The poliomyelitis virus may be isolated in tissue culture of monkey kidney or HeLa cells from stool suspensions treated with antibiotics and centrifugation, from throat washings, and rarely from blood (Table 12-7). Virus is usually present in the nasopharynx during the first week of infection only, whereas it persists in the feces for 1 month to 2 months. Cell destruction in tissue culture is indicative of virus growth. The type of virus is identified by demonstrating that specific immune serum neutralizes its effects in tissue culture. Under ideal circumstances the identification of a strain of poliomyelitis virus may be accomplished within 1 week. Poliomyelitis virus can be isolated from approximately 90% of patients with paralytic poliomyelitis. At the present time virus isolation is the most satisfactory method for diagnosing poliomyelitis.

Complement-Fixing and Neutralizing Antibodies. The titers of complement-fixing and neutralizing antibodies to each type of poliomyelitis virus may be simultaneously determined in acute and convalescent sera obtained from children during and subsequent to the acute infection (Table 12-8). A fourfold or greater rise in antibody titer to one type of poliomyelitis virus represents serologic evidence of a recent infection with this type of virus. However, since neutralizing antibody develops very early in the course of infection, the acute phase serum may already show an elevation in titer whereas the convalescent serum may have no further significant rise. The titer of complement-fixing antibody to poliomyelitis virus rises more slowly than that of the neutralizing antibody. However, complement-fixing antibody may never appear in detectable amounts in the serum as the result of infection. In approximately 50% of children it is possible to obtain serologic evidence of infection with a specific type of poliomyelitis virus.

TABLE 12-7.   Isolation of Viruses from Patients with Nonpurulent Meningeal Reactions

Virus	Sources of Virus				
	Blood	CSF	Stools	Nose and Throat Washings	Saliva
Poliomyelitis	Rarely	No	Yes	Yes	No
Coxsackie	Rarely	Yes	Yes	Yes	No
Enteric cytopathic human orphan	Rarely	Yes	Yes	Yes	No
Mumps	Rarely	Rarely	No	No	Yes
Lymphocytic choriomeningitis	Yes	Yes	No	Rarely	No

TABLE 12-8.   Specimens Collected for Viral Studies in Patients with Nonpurulent Meningeal Reactions

Viral cultures during acute illness
  Two fecal samples
  Throat swabs
  CSF
  Blood
  Saliva
Blood for antibody assay
  Acute serum on admission
  Convalescent serum (14 days–30 days after onset)

Differential Diagnosis.   The clinical picture produced by systemic infection with poliomyelitis virus is similar to that observed in many types of infections involving the upper respiratory and gastrointestinal tracts in children. Nonparalytic poliomyelitis must be differentiated from brain abscess, tuberculous or cryptococcal meningitis, and Coxsackie, ECHO, mumps, and other viral infections. Paralytic poliomyelitis sometimes must be distinguished from infectious polyneuropathy.

Treatment.   Poliomyelitis is treated symptomatically because there is no specific drug therapy for this infection. Respiratory weakness is treated with a respirator and subsequently with a rocking bed. Weakness of the trunk, arms, and legs is subsequently treated with physical and occupational therapy.

Prognosis.   The prognosis varies with the type of involvement by the infection. With systemic and nonparalytic virus infections all of the children recover without residual effects. The prognosis in paralytic infection varies with the site and severity of paralysis. In bulbar poliomyelitis the mortality rate is approximately 10% whereas in paralysis due to spinal cord involvement the mortality rate is approximately 1%. In bulbar poliomyelitis death is frequently related to involvement of centers controlling respiratory and cardiac function. Spinal poliomyelitis associated with paralysis of intercostal and diaphragmatic muscles may be associated with death in relation to pulmonary infections.

Patients with bulbar poliomyelitis who survive the acute illness usually recover completely. Recovery from paralysis of the trunk or extremities usually begins within 1 week. The rate of recovery is most rapid during the first 3 months. The probable extent of permanent disability can usually be estimated 3 months after the initial infection. Muscles that remain completely paralyzed after an interval of 3 months usually do not show return of function. Weakened muscles show slow, continued improvement over a period of 3 months to 12 months with minimal change between the first and second years. Approximately 20% of patients with spinal cord involvement require braces or reconstructive surgery.

Prevention.   Live, oral poliovirus vaccines are used for immunization. Adequate widespread vaccination programs of infants and children have almost eliminated paralytic poliomyelitis in those countries where it is effectively carried out.

COXSACKIE VIRUS INFECTIONS

Coxsackie virus was so named because it was first isolated from a patient from Coxsackie, New York. Infections with this virus may produce a wide variety of clinical syndromes, including aseptic meningitis, epidemic myalgia or pleurodynia, myocarditis of the newborn, and herpangina.

Etiology.   The Coxsackie viruses are classified into group A with more than 24 types and group B with 6 types. In newborn mice the group A viruses produce a generalized myositis, whereas the group B viruses produce fat necrosis, encephalomalacia, and patchy degeneration of striated muscle. The group A type 7 virus is characterized by pathogenicity for both monkeys and suckling mice. These viruses are prevalent in man during the summer months.

Pathology.   The only human pathologic studies of this disease are from fatal cases of myocarditis in newborns. With intrauterine or neonatal infection a widespread systemic disease occurs. Multiple organs are involved, and the changes of a viral encephalitis have been reported in fatal cases in these infants.

Symptoms. Those most commonly affected are 5 years to 9 years of age, although children of all ages are susceptible. The number of children with antibodies to these viruses gradually increases with age, from infancy to the age of 7 years to 9 years, at which time it reaches the same percentage as that among the adult population.

The types of infection produced are the following: (1) inapparent, (2) systemic, (3) meningitic, and (4) encephalitic. With inapparent infection the virus invades only the gastrointestinal tract. The symptoms of systemic infections, which develop after an incubation period of 2 days to 4 days, are malaise, loss of appetite, nausea, and fever of 101°F to 103°F (38°C to 39°C), which last 2 days to 6 days. Group A infections may also be associated with herpangina, skin rash, and rarely parotitis. Group B infections may produce myalgia or pleurodynia and infrequently myocarditis. In a small percentage of infections with group A and B viruses a meningitic illness develops (Table 12-9). In about half of these children fever and malaise precede the onset of meningitis; about 3% have associated pleurodynia. The child develops headache, stiff neck, vomiting, drowsiness, and photophobia. Muscular weakness, convulsions, and coma occur rarely.

Examination. Examination reveals stiff neck and Kernig's sign. Cranial nerve palsies, papilledema, irregular respirations, and motor paralysis sometimes occur with acute encephalitis.

Newborns with group B Coxsackie virus infection may rarely develop lethargy, grayish pallor, and icterus within the first 8 days to 9 days of life. Examination reveals tachycardia, dyspnea, and cyanosis with cardiac and hepatic enlargement.

Laboratory Examination. Examination of CSF reveals normal or increased initial pressure and an increase in leukocytes of $50/mm^3$ to $500/mm^3$ and occasionally as high as $2000/mm^3$. The differential count reveals 50% to 90% lymphocytes. The sugar content is normal and the protein normal or slightly elevated. In newborns with myocarditis chest x-rays reveal cardiac enlargement, and the electrocardiogram displays flat or inverted T waves during the acute phase of the illness. The virus may be recovered in tissue culture from the CSF or feces. Monkey kidney cells and human amnion cells are the best tissue for isolation of Coxsackie viruses. Rarely it is isolated from blood or oropharyngeal washings; finding it in CSF establishes the etiologic diagnosis of the meningitis. Isolation of virus from feces demonstrates only a viral enteric infection. Serologic tests may reveal a significant rise in homotypic neutralizing antibody titers during the period of convalescence.

Treatment. There is no specific treatment. Children should be seen 1 month after the acute illness to be certain that no additional symptoms have developed during convalescence.

TABLE 12-9. Clinical Manifestations of Viral Infections Producing Nonpurulent Meningeal Reactions

Virus	Systemic Illness		Central Nervous System Involvement	
	Fever, Malaise	Occasional Other Manifestations	Aseptic Meningitis	Severe Paralysis
Poliomyelitis	+	0	+	+
Coxsackie, group A	+	Herpangina, skin rash, rarely parotitis	+	0
Coxsackie, group B	+	Epidemic myalgia, myocarditis	+	Rarely encephalitis of the newborn
ECHO	+	Skin rash	+	0
Mumps	+	Parotitis, orchitis, ovaritis	+	0
Lymphocytic choriomeningitis	+	0	+	0

Prognosis. In most children acute aseptic meningitis due to Coxsackie virus is a mild infection followed by complete recovery within 1 week to 2 weeks, although occasionally mild weakness may occur in trunk or leg muscles either with the acute illness or during the convalescent period. Subjective complaints of fatigue, irritability, and difficulty in concentration occasionally prolong convalescence, although both subjective complaints and mild weakness subside with complete recovery in subsequent months.

Overwhelming infection associated with myocarditis and encephalitis in newborns may result in sudden death within a few hours or may progress to complete recovery in 1 week to 2 weeks. With pericarditis death may result from cardiac tamponade.

ENTERIC CYTOPATHIC HUMAN ORPHAN VIRUS

The ECHO viruses are a group of enteric pathogens of which more than 33 types have been identified. Thus far 24 of these have been demonstrated to produce aseptic meningitis in man, with or without skin rash.

Etiology. Enteric cytopathic human orphan viruses are found in the intestinal tract of man. The optimal medium for isolating them is monkey kidney tissue cultures. The vast majority of strains do not produce infection in laboratory animals on direct isolation from human material, although some strains of type 9 ECHO virus do produce paralysis in newborn mice.

Pathology. The pathologic findings produced by ECHO virus infections in man are not yet known.

Symptoms. The incubation period from the time of contact to the development of systemic illness is usually 3 days to 6 days. Most infections occur in the summer and fall. Infection may be characterized by an asymptomatic period during which the virus is present in the intestinal tract, a mild febrile illness, a systemic reaction associated with a skin rash, or an aseptic meningitis. The initial portion of the illness may consist of mild fever and malaise. This may then be associated with or followed by a skin eruption. The majority of children with types 9 and 16 ECHO virus infections show a generalized rash accompanied by fever. With type 16 infection rash develops after fever subsides. The rash is first noted over the cheeks and face and then spreads to the trunk and extremities. If rash occurs it usually lasts for a few days, occasionally as long as 10 days. The initial systemic illness may be followed by headache, stiff neck, lethargy, nausea, vomiting, and photophobia. In association with this, transitory motor weakness is occsionally seen.

Examination. Moderate fever is usually present and may last 2 days to 15 days. If skin rash is present, it is either macular, maculopapular, rubelliform, or sometimes petechial. Occasionally vesiculation and scaling occur. An enanthem with buccal lesions may be present, and the throat may be injected. Lymphadenopathy is occasionally noted. Mild to moderate stiffness of the neck against resistance is sometimes associated with Kernig's sign. Mild, transient muscular weakness has been observed. Extraocular muscle paralysis rarely occurs.[27]

Laboratory Examination. Lumbar puncture reveals clear or slightly cloudy fluid usually associated with a normal initial pressure. An increased cellular reaction is present in those patients with aseptic meningeal reaction. The leukocyte count is usually in the range of 50/mm³ to 1000/mm³, although higher counts are occasionally noted. During the first 24 hours to 48 hours after the onset of meningeal signs there may be a predominance of PMNs in the spinal fluid.[74] After this the predominant cell is the lymphocyte. The protein level is usually normal, although it may be slightly elevated, and the sugar content is normal. Inoculation of spinal fluid on monkey kidney tissue culture during the acute illness is positive in 50% to 80% of proved cases. In 85% of cases ECHO virus is isolated from stool specimens taken during the acute illness. Virus cultures of throat washings are positive in a small percentage of patients. Neutralizing antibodies are present in the serum 1 week after the onset of illness and persist for several months.

Differential Diagnosis. If a systemic illness develops with rash, the rash may resemble measles or rubella. If a rash is associated with a meningeal reaction, meningococcemia is suspected. The association of aseptic meningitis with a morbilliform skin eruption suggests the possibility of ECHO virus infection. Virus isolation is necessary to establish an etiologic diagnosis, however. Preferably CSF, stool specimens, and throat washings are cultured for virus (Tables 12-7 and 12-9).

Treatment. Acetylsalicylic acid or codeine sulfate may be ued to control severe headache. Bed rest during the acute febrile illness is advisable. No specific therapy is available.

Prognosis. The illness is uniformly followed by recovery within 1 week to 2 weeks without sequelae.

MUMPS VIRUS

Mumps is an acute viral infection usually associated with parotitis and occasionally with aseptic meningitis. An inflammatory reaction may also occur in the pancreas, testes, ovaries, and breasts.

Etiology. The etiologic agent is the filtrable myxovirus parotiditis, first isolated in 1934. The virus is readily isolated by tissue culture techniques.

Pathology. With meningoencephalitis the meninges are infiltrated with lymphocytes. Perivenous demyelination in the brain occurs with lymphocytic infiltration of the cerebral vessels.

Symptoms. The incubation period of mumps is 2 weeks to 3 weeks. Usually swelling or pain in the parotid gland is the first symptom, frequently associated with fever for 1 day to 3 days. In 70% of individuals swelling of the parotid gland is bilateral. Along with the parotid swelling, or at times preceding it, acute aseptic meningitis characterized by headache, drowsiness, vomiting, and stiff neck may occur. These symptoms usually subside along with the parotid swelling within 1 week. Some

children may have aseptic meningitis without parotid swelling. The incidence of aseptic meningitis associated with mumps varies with different epidemics, but it is usually approximately 10%.

Examination. Fever plus swelling and tenderness of one or both parotid glands are usual. The testes in adolescent boys and ovaries in adolescent girls may be inflamed. Abdominal tenderness may be associated with pancreatitis. With aseptic meningitis there is usually mild to moderate stiff neck, and frequently Kernig's sign is present. Occasionally mumps is associated with encephalitis, cranial or peripheral nerve palsies, or signs of spinal cord involvement. Optic neuritis and other cranial nerve palsies may develop 1 week to 2 weeks after onset of parotitis. Occasionally there is eighth nerve involvement with uni- or bilateral deafness; it is unilateral in two-thirds of patients affected.

Laboratory Examination. The peripheral blood usually reveals a slight leukopenia with a relative lymphocytosis. The initial pressure in the CSF is either normal or slightly increased. The fluid is clear or slightly cloudy, its leukocyte count being $5/mm^3$ to $2000/mm^3$, usually 90% to 100% lymphocytes. The protein content may be slightly increased and the sugar content normal. Mumps virus may be grown from CSF or saliva collected during the acute phase of the illness. The serologic diagnosis may be made from paired sera collected during the acute illness and 10 days to 14 days after the initial onset. Hemagglutinating and complement-fixing antibodies to mumps virus develop in the patient's serum within the first week after infection. If the child develops a meningoencephalitis, marked generalized slowing of the electroencephalogram to 2 cycles per second to 5 cycles per second may be observed (Fig. 12-22). These electroencephalographic abnormalities usually persist longer than clinical findings, but the pattern subsequently returns to normal.

Differential Diagnosis. In children who develop aseptic meningitis in association with acute parotitis the diagnosis is obvious clinically. To establish the diagnosis

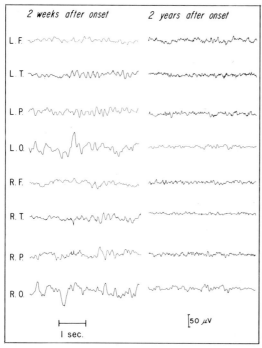

FIG. 12-22. Electroencephalographic changes associated wth mumps meningoencephalitis. This 12-year-old child had acute bilateral parotitis, fever, headache, vomiting, stiff neck, and lethargy. No focal neurologic signs were present. The leukocyte count in the cerebrospinal fluid was 889/mm³, all lymphocytes; the CSF protein level was 156 mg/dl. He was asymptomatic 3 weeks after the onset of his illness. Electroencephalogram 2 weeks after onset revealed a diffusely abnormal record with slowing anteriorly to 5 cycles per second and posteriorly to 2 cycles per second–4 cycles per second. Electroencephalogram 2 years after onset was within normal limits with occasional slowing to 4 cycles per second–7 cycles per second.

in those who develop aseptic meningitis without other manifestations of mumps it is necessary to isolate the virus or demonstrate a rise in antibodies to mumps virus.

Treatment.   No specific therapy is available. Symptomatic therapy for headache is frequently indicated. With high fever, alcohol sponges and acetylsalicylic acid may be needed to lower temperature.

Prognosis.   Although complete recovery is the rule, aseptic meningitis is occasionally associated with deafness, which may be permanent. If encephalomyelitis develops there may be residual deficits. Infection with

mumps provides permanent immunity in more than 95% of cases.

LYMPHOCYTIC CHORIOMENINGITIS

Etiology.   The name lymphocytic choriomeningitis, which is given to a specific infection with the virus of lymphocytic choriomeningitis, is derived from the striking lymphocytic infiltration in the choroid plexus seen with infections in susceptible animals. The virus has a wide range of pathogenicity among animals; monkeys, rats, mice, and guinea pigs are susceptible.[18]

Epidemiology.   A reservoir for the virus of lymphocytic choriomeningitis exists in gray house mice. The mice that acquire infection *in utero* or during the suckling period become carriers of the virus, which is found for long periods in the saliva, nasal washings, blood, urine, feces, and semen. Infection may be transferred to man by contact with infected mice, which are often found in the homes of patients with lymphocytic choriomeningitis. The exact portal of entry of the virus in man is not known. Lymphocytic choriomeningitis infections have also been transmitted from pet hamsters.[4]

Pathology.   The pathology of the human disease has not been clearly outlined.

Symptoms.   An initial systemic infection associated with fever may occur, followed by a remission of illness and the subsequent development of aseptic meningitis, with headache, vomiting, fever, and stiff neck.

Examination.   Stiffness of the neck and Kernig's sign are usually noted. Reflexes may be depressed; and rarely papilledema, oculomotor and facial paralyses, and signs of myelitis are reported.

Laboratory Examination.   Examination of the CSF reveals clear or slightly cloudy fluid with a leukocyte count of 5/mm³ to 1500/mm³. There is a predominance of lymphocytes. The protein content is normal or increased and the sugar content normal.
    Virus may be isolated from spinal fluid collected during the acute phase of the meningeal illness. Blood drawn very early

in the disease or during the systemic illness contains virus. Rarely virus is isolated from nose and throat washings, but it is not present in the stools (Table 12-7). Complement-fixing antibodies for the soluble antigen appear in the patient's serum about 4 weeks after the onset of infection and persist for several months. Neutralizing antibodies to the virus develop within 2 months after the onset and usually persist for several years. Antibody detectable by indirect immunofluorescence tests appears earlier after the onset of illness than complement-fixation antibody.

Differential Diagnosis.   The etiologic diagnosis is established either by isolating the virus from CSF or by demonstrating antibodies in the patient's convalescent serum.

Treatment.   No specific treatment is known.

Prognosis.   Although usually benign, the disease can produce obliteration of the subarachnoid space with hydrocephaly or cord symptoms.

MENINGITIS ASSOCIATED WITH INFECTIOUS MONONUCLEOSIS

Infectious mononucleosis due to Epstein-Barr virus (EBV) is a common disorder in children and adolescents. An initial acute systemic infection is characterized by fever, sore throat, and headache. A maculopapular eruption may occur. The lymph nodes, particularly cervical lymph nodes, are enlarged and the spleen is usually palpable.

In approximately 1% of children the systemic infection is associated with or followed by a meningeal reaction with stiff neck and a lymphocytic reaction in the CSF. Rarely encephalitis, myelitis, acute cerebellar ataxia, or polyneuropathy is associated with infectious mononucleosis. With encephalitis coma, convulsions and cranial nerve palsies appear. Myelitis results in weakness, sensory loss, and increased tendon reflexes. With polyneuropathy there is symmetrical weakness of all extremities usually associated with mild sensory loss. The tendon reflexes are decreased or absent in the involved extremities.

Laboratory examination usually reveals characteristic hematologic findings. The leukocyte count is usually elevated to $10,000/mm^3$ to $15,000/mm^3$ with an increase in lymphocytes including atypical lymphocytes with light-staining cytoplasm. The heterophile agglutination test is of confirmatory diagnostic value if a significant rise in titer is demonstrated in successive serum samples or if a late sample has a titer above 1:160. However, this is not specific and false–positive and false–negative results may occur. Specific EBV serologic determinations establish the etiologic diagnosis. The demonstration of antibody to early EBV antigen, particularly anti-D, because of its transitory character and early appearance, is useful in proving recent infections.[10] The CSF reveals a lymphocytic reaction in association with signs of meningitis, and also in some patients without meningeal signs. With polyneuropathy the cell count is normal but there is frequently an increase in protein.

No specific therapy is available. Complete recovery uniformly follows aseptic meningitis. With myelitis or polyneuropathy mild residual weakness may persist.

LEPTOSPIRAL MENINGITIS

There are more than 20 serologically identifiable strains of leptospiras, and at least 8 types are known to occur in North America, including *Leptospira icterohemorrhagiae*, *L. canicola*, *L. pomona*, and *L. mitis*. Human infection is usually acquired from bathing or swimming in water contaminated by urine from infected animals, including rats, mice, dogs, swine, cattle, horses, and foxes.

Leptospiral infection may result in an asymptomatic infection, a mild febrile illness, or a fatal disease. The incubation period is 6 days to 15 days. Infection with *L. icterohemorrhagiae* is characterized by fever, jaundice, oliguria, or anuria. Meningitis with headache, vomiting, and stiff neck may develop. Other strains of *Leptospira* may produce aseptic meningitis not associated with jaundice. Children with this form of infection may have fever of 102°F to 104°F (39°C to 40°C) with headache, nuchal rigidity, and conjunctival congestion. Occasionally nausea, vomiting, diarrhea, erythematous eruption over the pretibial regions, muscle pains, or mild weakness of the legs develops.

With aseptic meningitis the CSF has a leukocyte count of $10/mm^3$ to $250/mm^3$, predominantly lymphocytes. The sugar content is normal. Leptospiras may be cultured on artificial media from blood drawn from a patient during the acute illness. The serodiagnostic procedure of choice is the hemolysis test.

Tetracycline therapy during the acute phase of the illness is recommended, although most leptospiral infections subside without complications even without specific therapy.

MENINGOENCEPHALITIS ASSOCIATED WITH BEHÇET'S SYNDROME

A few cases of relapsing uveitis and keratitis with associated meningoencephalitis have been reported. This infection is of unknown (possibly viral) etiology. The pathologic findings are perivascular infiltration involving brain and spinal cord.

The systemic manifestations are chronic recurrent fever with conjunctivitis, keratitis, uveitis, and hemorrhages into the vitreous. Recurrent ulcers appear in the mouth and on the genitalia. With central nervous system involvement there may be confusion and convulsions, stiff neck, cranial nerve findings, motor weakness or ataxia, and spasticity.

Examination of the CSF may reveal a few or several hundred cells, predominantly lymphocytes. No specific therapy is available. The course is relapsing and may be fatal.

ENCEPHALITIS

Encephalitis is an inflammatory reaction in brain substance. It may result from a direct invasion by a virus, rickettsia, protozoa, spirochete, or other organisms, or it may represent an acute inflammatory reaction of the brain to a previous systemic infection or to previous vaccination. The inflammatory reaction may be restricted to the brain with encephalitis, or it may involve the brain and spinal cord with encephalomyelitis.

ACUTE VIRAL ENCEPHALITIS

Etiology.   Acute encephalitis due to direct invasion of the central nervous system may be produced by the following viruses: herpes simplex; eastern, western, and Venezuelan equine encephalitis; St Louis encephalitis; Japanese encephalitis; Russian tick-borne encephalitis; California encephalitis (CE); and rabies. Eastern and western equine encephalitis viruses are maintained in birds and are transmitted from birds to man, as well as to horses and other mammals, by the bite of an infected mosquito. St Louis encephalitis virus is maintained in domestic fowl and wild birds, and it is transmitted to man by mosquito vectors. The rabies virus is present in the saliva of infected dogs, cats, foxes, skunks, bats, and other domestic and wild animals. It is transmitted to man by the bite of a rabid animal. The most important vector of the CE virus is the woodland mosquito, *Aedes triseriatus*. The CE virus can be maintained from year-to-year in infected mosquito populations by way of transovarial passage of virus from parent mosquito to offspring.

The term *arbovirus*, a contraction of *arthropod-borne virus*, includes any one of over 250 arthropod-borne viruses transmitted between susceptible vertebrate hosts by blood-sucking arthropods. Arbovirus encephalitis in children is due to infection of the central nervous system with St Louis, western equine, eastern equine, Venezuelan equine, CE, or other arboviruses.

Pathology.   The pathologic findings are those of an acute inflammatory reaction involving meninges and blood vessels with degenerative changes in the nerve cells. Within the brain substance are focal accumulations of inflammatory and glial cells. Lesions occur in gray and white matter and involve the cerebral hemispheres, brain stem, and other areas. Although the distribution of lesions differs slightly depending on the encephalitic virus responsible, these are not diagnostic. With eastern equine encephalitis virus hippocampal lesions are pronounced. Encephalitis due to herpes simplex virus is associated with asymmetrical necrosis of the medial temporal and orbital regions with more damage to cortex than to white matter. With herpes simplex virus, type A inclusion bodies are present in nerve cells, astrocytes, and oligodendrocytes. These are large intranuclear masses surrounded by a clear halo. In rabies cytoplasmic inclusion bodies or Negri bodies are most common in the ganglion cells of Ammon's horn.

Symptoms.   Epidemics of equine, St Louis, and Japanese encephalitis have been reported. The incubation period is 5 days to 15 days. The onset of illness is usually sudden with fever, headache, stiff neck, and vomiting, sometimes followed by focal or generalized convulsions, drowsiness, stupor, or coma. With herpes simplex and St Louis encephalitis the illness is sometimes predominantly meningitic. Herpes simplex virus infection may be associated with bizarre behavior, olfactory or gustatory hallucinations, memory loss, and anosmia.[14] With acute encephalitis associated with rabies there are localized twitchings sometimes followed by generalized convulsions. California encephalitis occurs in 1 year to 14 year old children with the peak incidence in the 5 year to 9 year age group.

Examination.   With severe encephalitis the patient is usually drowsy, stuporous, or comatose. There may or may not be stiff neck. Cranial nerve palsies may be present. There may be evidence of hemiplegia, aphasia, or homonymous hemianopia. Motor and intellectual performance deteriorates. Focal signs may include cogwheel rigidity, cortical sensory loss, and asymmetry of tendon reflexes, extensor plantar responses, and grasp reflexes.

Laboratory Examination.   Examination of the CSF reveals increased or normal pressure with clear or opalescent fluid and a leukocyte count of $5/mm^3$ to $1500/mm^3$. Usually the reaction is predominantly lymphocytic, although early in the infection there may be a preponderance of PMNs. The protein content is frequently increased, and the sugar content is normal. The electroencephalogram usually reveals generalized slowing for the age level.

Computed tomography scans in patients with herpes simplex encephalitis reveal areas of decreased attenuation in the temporal lobes. These areas often extend to the insular cortex, and often to the frontal or parietal lobes. These changes develop between the third and 11th day of illness, so that they may be useful in suggesting that herpes simplex may be the etiology in a patient with an encephalitic illness.[34]

Computed tomography scans may indicate the most useful area for surgical biopsy so that preoperative angiography may not be needed. Angiography reveals nonspecific enlargement of the temporal or frontal lobes with early draining subcortical veins.[52] The CT changes in herpes simplex encephalitis are more accurate in localization than the changes found by isotopic brain scans, electroencephalogram (EEG), or cerebral angiograms.

An etiologic diagnosis can be established either by isolating the virus or by demonstrating the development of specific antibodies in the convalescent serum. In fatal cases virus can be isolated from brain tissue (Table 12-10). During the acute stage of the illness, however, virologic studies are quite limited. Rabies virus can be isolated from saliva. California encephalitis virus can be isolated from CSF. Herpes simplex virus infection can be diagnosed by brain biopsy with demonstration of inclusion bodies and virus isolation. An increase in specific antibody by neutralization, complement-fixation, or hemagglutination–inhibition techniques in the patient's convalescent serum may be demonstrated by performing serologic studies simultaneously on acute and convalescent sera. An etiologic diagnosis is usually not possible during the acute stage of the illness.

Differential Diagnosis.   In any patient with suspected viral encephalitis it is important to exclude the possibility of a postinfectious or postvaccinal encephalitis. It is also important to exclude tuberculous meningitis and brain abscess. The diagnosis of a virus etiology is usually based on serologic studies.

Treatment.   With difficulty in maintaining an adequate airway tracheostomy may be required. With respiratory difficulty the patient may need respirator care. In patients with herpes simplex encephalitis diag-

TABLE 12-10. Isolation of Viruses from Patients with Viral Encephalitis

Encephalitic Virus	Source of Virus			
	Blood	CSF	Saliva	Brain Tissue
Eastern and western equine	Rarely	Rarely	No	Yes
St Louis	Rarely	No	No	Yes
Japanese B	Rarely	No	No	Yes
Rabies	No	No	Yes	Yes
Herpes simplex	No	No	No	Yes

nosed by brain biopsy, vidarabine is effective in decreasing the mortality rate if administered early before coma develops. The dose is 15 mg/kg per day given intravenously for 10 days.[39,77] Vidarabine may occasionally produce nausea, vomiting, diarrhea, leukopenia, anemia, and thrombocytopenia. Dizziness, tremor, hallucinations, confusion, psychosis, and ataxia have been reported.

Prognosis. The mortality rate is 75% in eastern equine encephalitis, 20% in western equine encephalitis, 0 to 20% in St Louis encephalitis, 60% in Japanese B encephalitis, and 100% in rabies. Severe neurologic residual deficits may be present in patients who recover from viral encephalitis. Cranial nerve paralyses may be permanent. Residual hemiplegia, aphasia, impaired intellect, poor memory, and convulsive seizures may occur.[15,54]

The mortality rate in children with herpes simplex encephalitis who are not treated with vidarabine is 70%. In those treated early with vidarabine it is 30%. Half of those who recover have no or only moderately debilitating neurologic sequelae. However, postinfectious encephalomyelitis may occur as an early sequel of vidarabine-treated herpes simplex encephalitis.[38]

California encephalitis usually produces a brief illness, although neurologic residuals and death rarely occur.

Prevention. Since most cases of rabies develop from bites by rabid dogs, active immunization of dogs against rabies is a method of preventing the disease in man. If a child has been bitten by a rabid dog or

by a dog who develops signs of rabies during a 10-day period of observation, then vaccine is given. Active immunization is carried out with 5 doses of human diploid cell rabies vaccine (HDCV), which is an inactivated rabies vaccine grown on human diploid cell tissue culture. This is administered intramuscularly on each of days 0, 3, 7, 14, and 28. Rabies immune globulin in a dose of 20 units/kg is recommended with the first dose of HDCV.

Encephalitis transmitted by mosquitos may be controlled by destroying the larvae and eliminating mosquito breeding places.

ENCEPHALITIS DUE TO SALIVARY GLAND VIRUS OR GENERALIZED CYTOMEGALIC INCLUSION DISEASE

Etiology. This disorder is caused by the salivary gland virus, first isolated from an affected infant in 1957. Different strains of the virus are antigenically different and represent a cytomegalovirus group. Some or all of the strains are widely disseminated. Serologic studies have demonstrated a prevalence rate of 14% in 1-year to 2-year old children and in 81% in adults.

Pathology. The two categories of infection are generalized cytomegalic inclusion disease and a focal process confined to the salivary glands. Generalized infection is observed at autopsy in 1% of infants and in a smaller percentage of children. Inclusion bodies are found in the nuclei and less commonly in the cytoplasm of enlarged cells in the salivary glands, kidney, lungs, liver, and brain. Intranuclear inclusions limited to the salivary glands occur in about 10% of infants at autopsy.

Examination. Infection occurring prenatally may result in stillbirth or prematurity. If the child is born alive, there may be petechial hemorrhages, jaundice, or respiratory distress. The bleeding tendency disappears within a week. The liver and spleen are enlarged. Microcephaly, mental retardation, and motor disability are usually noted. Rarely megalocephaly occurs. Chorioretinitis, optic atrophy, epileptic seizures, and hemiparesis may be present.[76]

Laboratory Examination. In infants the isolation of virus from urine is a reliable diagnostic method, but in children virus isolation must be interpreted with caution. The demonstration of damaged renal cells containing inclusion bodies in the sediment of freshly collected urine is of diagnostic value. However, cytomegalic cells may be present only intermittently in the urine of affected infants, or they may be repeatedly absent even though virus is present in the urine. Serologic studies are of little diagnostic value.

Radiographs of the skull occasionally reveal periventricular cerebral calcification. In newborns with petechiae the platelet counts are decreased. With jaundice the bilirubin is elevated.

Differential Diagnosis. Cytomegalic inclusion disease may present a clinical picture similar to that of erythroblastosis or toxoplasmosis.

Treatment. Vidarabine may be used although its efficacy is not established.

Prognosis. With intrauterine infection death may occur before or shortly after birth. In other cases prolonged survival with mental retardation may be present.

SUBACUTE SCLEROSING PANENCEPHALITIS

Etiology. The measles virus or a measles-like virus plays a role in the production of this form of encephalitis. The interval from acute measles infection to encephalitis is usually 3 years to 9 years. Measles vaccination, by preventing measles, has a partially protective effect against subacute sclerosing panencephalitis (SSPE). Most of the children who have developed SSPE had measles when they were less than 3 years of age.

Pathology. There is perivascular infiltration of the cortex and white matter with mononuclear cells. There are patchy areas of gliosis and demyelination. Eosinophilic intranuclear inclusion bodies are found in the neurons and neuroglia in the areas of brain tissue destruction.

Symptoms. Symptoms include myoclonus, progressive dementia, paralysis, visual symptoms, and ataxia. The illness usually affects children under 12 years of age, and the symptoms progress over a period of weeks or months.

Examination. There is evidence of intellectual deterioration with loss of language function.. Cranial nerve palsies may occur, and there is bilateral weakness with increase in muscle tone in the motor system. Cerebellar ataxia may be present, and myoclonic jerks are frequently seen. The child develops severe dementia followed by coma and death.

Laboratory Examination. The measles antibody titers in the serum and CSF are elevated, and there is a marked increase of immunoglobulin in the CSF. The EEG usually shows recurring diffuse bursts of spike and slow wave complexes either with or without clinical evidence of myoclonic jerks. There is usually depression of electrical activity between the high voltage spike and wave complexes.

Differential Diagnosis. This disorder must be distinguished from other forms of progressive dementia in childhood.

Treatment. Isoprinosine does not alter the course of the acutely progressive form of SSPE nor is it a cure.[63] However, isoprinosine therapy in a dose of 100 mg/kg per day has been associated with remissions in a few cases and an increase in long-term survival in patients with slowly progressive SSPE.[29] Also amantadine therapy has been associated with prolonged survival and periods of remission in some cases of SSPE, although it does not have a permanent beneficial effect.[55] The dosage of amantadine is 5 mg/kg per day to 10 mg/kg per day, which is continued for many months unless serious side-effects develop.

Prognosis. The progression of the disease is variable. In 10% of children there is a fulminating course with death occurring within a few months. In approximately 80% of cases severe dementia followed by death occurs over a period of several years. Approximately 10% of children survive more than 4 years with an eventual fatal outcome. Younger children tend to survive longer than older children.

RICKETTSIAL ENCEPHALITIS

Etiology. The following rickettsial organisms are associated with the following clinical disorders: *Rickettsia prowazeki*—louse-borne typhus; *Rickettsia mooseri*—murine typhus; *Rickettsia rickettsii*—Rocky Mountain spotted fever; *Rickettsia tsutsugamushi*—scrub typhus. Dog, wood, and rabbit ticks infected with *Rickettsia rickettsii* transmit infection by attachment to the human host.

Pathology. In encephalitis associated with rickettsial infections the brain is swollen and petechial hemorrhages are present. Microglial nodules and perivascular infiltrations are seen microscopically. In Rocky Mountain spotted fever areas of focal necrosis in the brain are common.

Symptoms. The incubation period is 1 week to 2 weeks. The onset of symptoms is usually sudden with fever and generalized muscular aches. Skin eruption is usually present early in the disease. Headache, stiff neck, drowsiness, and confusion may develop rapidly, possibly followed by convulsive seizures, coma, and signs of focal cerebral lesions.

Examination. Examination may reveal a skin eruption. With typhus fever there is usually a macular eruption. With spotted fever the rash may appear first on the wrist and ankles and then spread to become hemorrhagic. The patient may be stuporous or comatose. The neck is stiff. There may be diplopia with extraocular muscle palsies, deafness, or dysarthria. Hemiplegia and aphasia may be present.

Laboratory Examination. *Proteus* agglutinations in the serum become positive after 5 days. The CSF may show an increase of cells to 25/mm^3 to 200/mm^3, usually with a predominance of lymphocytes. The protein may be increased, and the sugar content is normal.

Rickettsial organisms may be isolated by inoculating blood into guinea pigs. Specific complement fixation tests on acute and convalescent sera demonstrate a significant rise in antibody titer. The microimmunofluorescence test for Rocky Mountain spotted fever is both sensitive and specific. It provides a laboratory diagnosis 7 days to 10 days after the onset of illness.[50]

Differential Diagnosis. Typhus fever and spotted fever must be differentiated from meningococcic meningitis in which rash also occurs. Rocky Mountain spotted fever must be considered in any child who has fever and rash occurring in the season and geographic area in which ticks are prevalent.

Treatment. Chloramphenicol and tetracycline are effective in treating rickettsial infections. Chloramphenicol is administered intravenously or intramuscularly in an initial dose of 25 mg/kg to 50 mg/kg in infants and in 50 mg/kg to 100 mg/kg in children. Tetracycline is administered in a daily dose of 15 mg/kg to 50 mg/kg orally (Table 12-4).

In addition to specific antibiotic therapy, it is important to control excessive fever with cold packs and alcohol sponges. Severe headache may be controlled with acetylsalicylic acid and codeine.

Prognosis. Without specific therapy the mortality rate in young children with typhus fever is 5%, with murine typhus 5%, spotted fever 20%, and scrub typhus 50%. These mortality rates have greatly decreased with antibiotic therapy. The current mortality rate with Rocky Mountain spotted fever is 5%. Fatal cases are frequently related to a delay in diagnosis due to the late appearance of skin rash and the lack of a history of tick bite.[24]

The patient usually runs a febrile course for 1 week to 2 weeks, after which the temperature gradually subsides. The illness may be complicated by pneumonia or cardiac failure. With recovery there are few residual effects.

TOXOPLASMIC ENCEPHALITIS

Etiology. The etiologic agent of toxoplasmosis is *Toxoplasma gondii,* a protozoan organism, 2 μ to 3 μ, present in many mammals and birds. In congenital infections the source is the mother. The manner by which the acquired infection is spread is not known.

Pathology. When infection occurs in utero there is eye and central nervous system involvement; retinal lesions with chorioretinitis are frequent. Miliary granulomas are present in the brain, and they may become calcified. The *Toxoplasma* organisms are present in the epitheloid cells of granulomas. Either hydro- or microcephaly may be present.

Examination. The infant may present with convulsions. In congenital toxoplasmosis there may be rash, jaundice, and enlargement of liver and spleen during the neonatal period. During infancy and childhood there may be an increase or decrease in head size for the infant's age. Chorioretinitis and retarded development may appear.

Laboratory Examination. The CSF may show a slight increase in cells or protein. X-ray films of the skull may reveal small calcified foci in the cerebral hemispheres (Fig. 12-23). Dye tests and complement fixation tests establish the etiologic diagnosis. In suspected congenital toxoplasmosis sera from both mother and child should be tested. Lymphocyte transformation to toxoplasma antigen is useful in the diagnosis of congenital toxoplasma infection during infancy.[78]

Differential Diagnosis. About 80% of children with the tetrad of convulsions, chorioretinopathy, hydro- or microcephaly, and cerebral calcification have toxoplasmosis. Serologic tests are required to confirm the diagnosis.

Treatment. No specific therapy is of proved value, although sulfadiazine and pyrimethamine have been recommended for trial on the basis of their beneficial effect in mice.

Prognosis. The course is usually a progressive one with a high mortality rate.

TRYPANOSOMIASIS

American trypanosomiasis, which occurs in Central and South America, is due to infection with *Trypanosoma cruzi.* African trypanosomiasis is caused by *T. gambiense* and *T. rhodesiense.* The organisms are flagellated protozoa. Trypanosomiasis is transmitted to man from animals by bloodsucking insects. The brain from fatal human cases shows evidence of perivascular infiltration with lymphocytes. Miliary granulomas containing protozoa are present.

The clinical picture is characterized by prolonged fever with gradual enlargement of lymph nodes, liver, and spleen. Convulsions, stiff neck, and stupor develop with involvement of the central nervous system. Aphasia, extraocular palsies, choreiform movements, and hemiparesis may subsequently appear. The protozoa may be found in blood or CSF smears, or they may be cultured by inoculating the patient's blood into guinea pigs. The course is a chronic one with fatal termination after a year or more. Chemotherapeutic agents are effective in some forms of trypanosomiasis.

POSTVACCINAL AND POSTINFECTIOUS ENCEPHALITIS

Postvaccinal and postinfectious encephalitis and encephalomyelitis may follow measles, German measles, chicken pox, or mumps, or may appear after vaccination against smallpox or rabies. In these cases virus is not isolated from the central nervous system. The exact relationship of the preceding or concomitant infection or vaccination to the central nervous system disorder is not completely understood.

Pathology.   Lesions are present in the white matter of the brain, brain stem, cerebellum, and spinal cord. There is demyelination with preservation of the axis cylinders.

FIG. 12-23. Anteroposterior (A) and lateral (B) roentgenograms of the skull of a child with toxoplasmosis. Diffuse intracerebral calcification is visible.

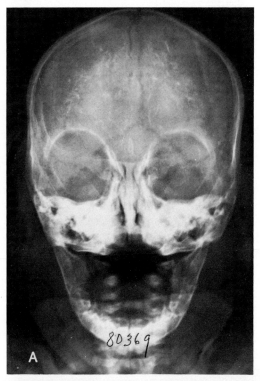

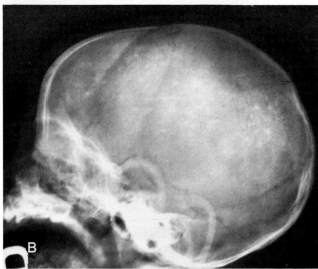

Symptoms.   Encephalomyelitis following vaccination against smallpox has an incidence of 1/10,000 vaccinations to 1/100,000 vaccinations. It is rare in infants. The onset of encephalitic symptoms usually occurs 10 days to 12 days after vaccination. Vaccination against rabies is associated with an incidence of encephalomyelitis of 1/6000 vaccinated persons. Measles is associated with encephalitis in approximately 1/500 cases to 1/1000 cases. The incidence following varicella, rubella, mumps, and smallpox is much less. Initial symptoms include high fever, headache, stiff neck, and drowsiness. These symptoms may be followed by convulsions, coma, paralysis, or speech disorder. Progressive weakness of the legs, trunk, and arms may develop with spinal cord involvement.

Examination.   The patient is drowsy or stuporous with evidence of stiff neck. There may be dysphasia, cranial nerve signs, hemiparesis, sensory loss, or increased tendon reflexes. If myelitis occurs, para- or quadriplegia usually results.

Laboratory Examination.   The CSF may reveal an increase in cells of 10/mm^3 to 200/mm^3, with a predominance of lymphocytes. There may be a slight increase in protein, and the sugar content is normal. The EEG reveals diffuse slowing for the child's age and may also show focal slowing and increased voltage (Fig. 12-24).

Differential Diagnosis. The diagnosis is based on the association of an encephalitic illness with a previous history of vaccination or the presence of one of the acute exanthemas.

Treatment. No specific therapy is available. Prednisone, 10 mg three times daily, has been recommended. This is based on

FIG. 12-24. Electroencephalographic changes associated with measles encephalitis. Four days after the onset of rash due to measles this 5-year-old boy developed lethargy, stiff neck, and twitching of the right face, arm, and leg, followed by a grand mal convulsion. No focal neurologic signs were present. Cerebrospinal fluid revealed an initial pressure of 220 mm water and had a leukocyte count of 380/mm³ with 90% lymphocytes. The protein content was 57 mg/dl. The child recovered rapidly and was discharged without residual signs after 8 days of hospitalization. Electroencephalogram 10 days after onset was abnormal with slowing bilaterally, but much greater on the left posteriorly. The voltage on the left was also increased. A second electroencephalogram 2 months after onset was within normal limits for the child's age.

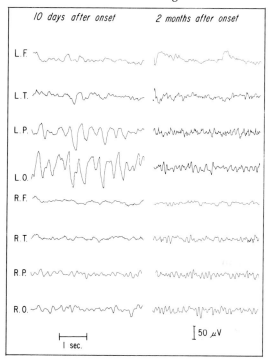

the possibility that the antiinflammatory effect of this drug might reduce disability. Steroid-responsive encephalomyelitis following a febrile illness does occur.[48]

Prognosis. In postmeasles encephalitis the mortality rate is 10% to 30% with an additional 30% having residual neurologic effects. The mortality rate in other forms of postinfectious encephalitis is approximately 10%. Residual neurologic deficits may include behavior disorders, convulsive seizures, and mental deterioration.

In order to prevent measles and its complications it is recommended that vaccine be given to children at 9 months to 12 months of age.

NEUROSYPHILIS

Neurosyphilis in children is usually due to congenital syphilis, which is now rare. Acquired syphilis with early neurosyphilis rarely occurs during adolescence.

Etiology. Infection of the fetus with *Treponema pallidum* by way of the placental circulation may occur if the mother has inadequately treated syphilis. Since early treatment with penicillin is now given to all pregnant women with untreated or inadequately treated syphilis who are seen for prenatal care, the only children with congenital syphilis are the offspring of infected mothers who have not been seen prenatally.

Symptoms. Infected infants are frequently asymptomatic at birth and may be seronegative if the maternal infection occurred late in gestation. If a child is born with congenital syphilis and is not treated during infancy or childhood, he may develop congenital paretic neurosyphilis at 6 years to 16 years of age. The early symptoms are those of intellectual deficiency. It may be noted that the child is not progressing satisfactorily in school, or he may exhibit forgetfulness and abnormal patterns of behavior. Subsequently hallucinations or delusions may occur. The usual pattern is one of progressive organic dementia. Convulsive seizures occur in about half of these patients.

Rarely, in untreated congenital syphilis an adolescent may develop failing vision, urinary incontinence, and lightning pains characteristic of tabes dorsalis. Acquired syphilis in children or adolescents is usually diagnosed by a positive serologic test for syphilis or by the presence of skin lesions. Latent or secondary syphilis may be associated with abnormalities of the CSF without any symptoms. Rarely syphilitic meningitis occurs.

Examination.   The pupils may be unequal and irregular in shape with loss of reaction to light and preservation of reaction in accommodation. Optic atrophy or chorioretinitis may be present. Examination of a child with juvenile paresis reveals evidence of intellectual deterioration. The tendon reflexes are usually hyperactive, and the plantar responses may be extensor. If tabetic neurosyphilis is present the knee and ankle jerks are absent; there is loss of position sense, vibratory sense, and deep pain; and the bladder may be atonic.

Laboratory Examination.   Blood serologic tests for syphilis are positive in all cases of untreated general paresis and in most cases of tabes dorsalis. The CSF reveals an increase in cells or protein with a positive serologic test for syphilis.

Treatment.   Neurosyphilis is treated with penicillin G, 50,000 units/kg intramuscularly or intravenously daily in two divided doses for 10 days. If the child is sensitive to penicillin, the alternative drugs are erythromycin or tetracycline given orally over a 10-day period. Tetracycline is not given to children less than 8 years of age. Repeat clinical evaluations and serological tests for syphilis on blood and CSF specimens are done at 6-month intervals for at least 3 years.

Prognosis.   The earlier the diagnosis of neurosyphilis is made and treatment administered, the better is the prognosis. If general paresis is untreated, it eventually terminates fatally. If treated adequately with penicillin, the central nervous system infection is arrested and CSF abnormalities gradually diminish. In subsequent months there is usually slight clinical improvement. However, if there has been extensive intellectual deterioration, recovery is only partial. Penicillin therapy in children with tabes dorsalis results in improvement of the CSF abnormalities, although the neurologic deficit usually remains unchanged.

REFERENCES

1.   **Arsalo A, Louhimo I, Santavuori P et al:** Subdural effusion: Results after treatment with subdural–pleural shunts. Child's Brain 3:79, 1977

2.   **Barrett FF, Taber LH, Morris CR et al:** A 12 year review of the antibiotic management of *Hemophilus influenzae* meningitis. J Pediatr 81:370, 1972

3.   **Bell WE:** Treatment of bacterial infections of the central nervous system. Ann Neurol 9:313, 1981

4.   **Biggar RJ, Woodall JP, Walter PD et al:** Lymphocytic choriomeningitis outbreak associated with pet hamsters. Fifty-seven cases from New York State. JAMA 232:494, 1975

5.   **Bilaniuk LT, Zimmerman RA, Brown L et al:** Computed tomography in meningitis. Neuroradiology 16:13, 1978

6.   **Blitzer A, Lawson W, Meyers BR et al:** Patient survival factors in paranasal sinus mucormycosis. Laryngoscope 90:635, 1980.

7.   **Buchan GC, Alvord EC Jr:** Diffuse necrosis of subcortical white matter associated with bacterial meningitis. Neurology (Minneap) 19:1, 1969.

8.   **Calkins RA, Bell WD:** Cerebral abscess and cyanotic congential heart disease. Lancet 87:403, 1967.

9.   **Chu N:** Tuberculous meningitis. Computerized tomographic manifestations. Arch Neurol 37:458, 1980

10.   **Cleary TG, Henle W, Pickering LK:** Acute cerebellar ataxia associated with Epstein-Barr virus infection. JAMA 243:148, 1980

11.   **Cockrill HH Jr, Dreisbach J, Lowe B et al:** Computed tomography in leptomeningeal infections. Am J Roentgenol 130:511, 1978

12.   **deLemos RA, Haggerty RJ:** Corticosteroids as an adjunct to treatment in bacterial meningitis: a controlled clinical trial. Pediatrics 44:30, 1969

13.   **DeSousa AL, Kleiman MB, Mealey J:** Quadriplegia and cortical blindness in *Hemophilus influenzae* meningitis. J Pediatrics 93:253, 1978

14.   **Drachman DA, Adams RD:** Herpes simplex and acute inclusion-body encephalitis. Arch Neurol 7:45, 1962

15.   **Earnest MP, Goolishian HA, Calverley JR et al:** Neurologic, intellectual, and psychologic sequelae following western encephalitis. Neurology (Minneap) 21:969, 1971

16.   **Eberhard SJ:** Diagnosis of brain abscess in infants and children. NC Med J 30:301, 363, 1969

17.   **Escobar JA, Belsey MA, Duenas A et al:** Mortality

from tuberculous meningitis reduced by steroid therapy. Pediatrics 56:1050, 1975

18. **Farmer TW, Janeway CA:** Infections with the virus of lymphocytic choriomeningitis. Medicine (Baltimore) 21:1, 1942

19. **Farmer TW, Wise GR:** Subdural empyema in infants, children, and adults. Neurology 23:254, 1973

20. **Fitzhardinge PM, Kazemi M, Ramsay M et al:** Long-term sequelae of neonatal meningitis. Develop Med Child Neurol 16:3, 1974

21. **Galaid EI, Cherubin CE, Marr JS et al:** Meningococcal disease in New York City, 1973 to 1978. Recognition of Groups Y and W-135 as frequent pathogens. JAMA 244:2167, 1980

22. **Glista GG, Sullivan TD, Brumlik J:** Spinal cord involvement in acute bacterial meningitis. JAMA 243:1362, 1980

23. **Haslam RGA, Allen JR, Dorsen MM et al:** The sequelae of Group B beta-hemolytic streptococcal meningitis in early infancy. Am J Dis Child 131:845, 1977

24. **Hattwick MAW, Retailliau H, O'Brien RJ et al:** Fatal Rocky Mountain spotted fever. JAMA 240:1499, 1978

25. **Headings DL, Glasgow LA:** Occlusion of the internal carotid artery complicating *Haemophilus influenzae* meningitis. Am J Dis Child 131:854, 1977

26. **Heiser WJ, Quinn JL, Mollihan WV:** The crescent pattern of increased radioactivity in brain scanning. Radiology 87:483, 1966

27. **Hertenstein JR, Sarnat HB, O'Connor DM:** Acute unilateral oculomotor palsy associated with ECHO 9 viral infection. J Pediatrics 89:79, 1976

28. **Horwitz SJ, Boxerbaum B, O'Bell J:** Cerebral herniation in bacterial meningitis in childhood. Ann Neurol 7:524, 1980

29. **Huttenlocher PR, Mattson RH:** Isoprinosine in subacute sclerosing panencephalitis. Neurology 29:763, 1979

30. **Idriss ZH, Sinno AA, Kronfol NM:** Tuberculous meningitis in childhood. Am J Dis Child 130:364, 1976

31. **Joubert MJ, Stephanov S:** Computerized tomography and surgical treatment in intracranial suppuration. J Neurosurg 47:73, 1977

32. **Kaplan SL, Feigin RD:** The syndrome of inappropriate secretion of antidiuretic hormone in children with bacterial meningitis. J Pediat 92:758, 1978

33. **Kaufman DM, Leeds NE:** Computed tomography (CT) in the diagnosis of intracranial abscesses. Neurology 27:1069, 1977

34. **Kaufman DM, Zimmerman RD, Leeds NE:** Computed tomography in Herpes simplex encephalitis. Neurology 29:1392, 1979

35. **Kaul S, D'Cruz J, Rapkin et al:** Ventriculitis, aqueductal stenosis and hydrocephalus in neonatal meningitis: diagnosis and treatment. Infection 6:8, 1978

36. **Kelsey DS:** Adenoviral meningoencephalitis. Pediatrics 61:291, 1978

37. **Kennedy DH, Fallon RJ:** Tuberculous meningitis. JAMA 241:264, 1979

38. **Koenig H, Rabinowitz SG, Day E et al:** Postinfectious encephalomyelitis after successful treatment of herpes simplex encephalitis with adenine arabinoside. N Engl J Med 300:1089, 1979

39. **Koshiniemi M, Vaheri A, Manninen V et al:** Herpes simplex virus encephalitis: new diagnostic and clinical features and results of therapy. Arch Neurol 37:763, 1980

40. **Laxer RM, Marks MI:** Pneumococcal meningitis in children. Am J Dis Child 131:850, 1977

41. **Littman ML, Walter JE:** Cryptococcosis: current status. Am J Med 45:922, 1968

42. **Mathies AW Jr, Lavetter A, Leedom JM et al:** Gentamicin in the treatment of meningitis. J Infect Dis 124(Suppl):S249, 1971

43. **McCracken GH Jr, Sarff LD:** Endotoxins in cerebrospinal fluid: detection in neonates with bacterial meningitis. JAMA 235:617, 1976

44. **Migeon CJ, Kenny FM, Hung W et al:** Study of adrenal function in children with meningitis. Pediatrics 40:163, 1967

45. **Moussa AH, Dawson BH:** Computed tomography and the mortality rate in brain abscess. Surg Neurol 10:301, 1978

46. **Nadol JB:** Hearing loss as a sequela of meningitis. The Laryngoscope 88:739, 1978

47. **Newlands WJ:** Otogenic brain abscess: a study of 80 cases. J Laryngol Otol 79:120, 1965

48. **Pasternak JF, DeVivo DC, Prensky AL:** Steroid-responsive encephalomyelitis in childhood. Neurology 30:481, 1980

49. **Petersen BH, Lee TJ, Snyderman R et al:** *Neisseria meningitidis* and *Neisseria gonorrhoeae* bacteremia associated with C6, C7 or C8 deficiency. Ann Intern Med 90:917, 1979

50. **Philip, RN, Casper EA, MacCormack JN et al:** A comparison of serologic methods for diagnosing of Rocky Mountain spotted fever. Am J Epidemiol 105:56, 1977

51. **Pillsbury HC, Fischer ND:** Rhinocerebral mucormycosis. Arch Otolaryngol 103:600, 1977

52. **Radcliffe, WB, Guinto FC Jr, Adcock DF et al:** Herpes simplex encephalitis. Am J Roentgenol 112:263, 1971

53. **Rao KCVG, Williams JP, Brenna TG et al:** Interhemispheric subdural empyema: neuroradiological diagnosis. Child's Brain 4:106, 1978

54. **Rennick PM, Nolan DC, Bauer RB et al:** Neuropsychologic and neurologic follow-up after herpesvirus hominis encephalitis. Neurology (Minneap) 23:42, 1973

55. **Robertson WC Jr, Clark DB, Markesbery WR:** Review of 38 cases of subacute sclerosing panencephalitis: effect of amantadine on the natural course of the disease. Ann Neurol 8:422, 1980

56. **Rosenblum ML, Hoff JT, Norman D et al:** Decreased mortality from brain abscesses since advent of computerized tomography. J Neurosurg 49:658, 1978

57. **Rosenhall U, Nylen O, Lindberg J et al:** Auditory

function after *Haemophilus influenzae* meningitis. Acta Otolaryngol 85:243, 1978

58. **Rothrock JF, Buchsbaum HW:** Primary amebic meningoencephalitis. JAMA 243:2329, 1980

59. **Schulkind ML, Altemeier WA III, Ayoub EM:** A comparison of ampicillin and chloramphenicol therapy in *Hemophilus influenzae* meningitis. Pediatrics 48:411, 1971

60. **Sell SHW, Merrill RE, Doyne EO et al:** Long-term sequelae of *Hemophilus influenzae* meningitis. Pediatrics 49:206, 1972

61. **Sell SHW, Webb WW, Pate JE et al:** Psychological sequelae to bacterial meningitis: two controlled studies. Pediatrics 49:212, 1972

62. **Shackelford PG, Bobinski JE, Feigin RD et al:** Therapy of *Haemophilus influenzae* meningitis reconsidered. N Engl J Med 287:634, 1972

63. **Silverberg R, Brenner T, Abramsky O:** Inosiplex in the treatment of subacute sclerosing panencephalitis. Arch Neurol 36:374, 1979

64. **Smith CR, Lipsky JJ, Laskin OL et al:** Double-blind comparison of the nephrotoxicity and auditory toxicity of gentamicin and tobramycin. N Engl J Med 302:1106, 1980

65. **Snyder BD, Farmer TW:** Brain abscess in children. South Med J 64:687, 1971

66. **Snyder RD, Stovring J:** The follow-up CT scan in childhood meningitis. Neuroradiology 16:22, 1978

67. **Sproles ET III, Azerrad J, Williamson C et al:** Meningitis due to *Hemophilus influenzae*: long-term sequelae. J Pediatr 75:782, 1969

68. **Steiner P, Portugaleza C:** Tuberculous meningitis in children. Am Rev Resp Dis 107:22, 1973

69. **Stephanov S:** Experience with multiloculated brain abscesses. J Neurosurg 49:199, 1978

70. **Stephanov S, Joubert MJ, Welchman JM:** Combined convexity and parafalx subdural empyema. Surg Neurol 11:147, 1979

71. **Swartz NM, Dodge PR:** Bacterial meningitis: a review of selected aspects. Part I. General clinical features, special problems and unusual meningeal reactions mimicking bacterial meningitis. N Engl J Med 272:725, 1965

72. **Tepperberg J, Nussbaum E, Feldman F:** Cortical blindness following meningitis due to *Hemophilus influenzae* Type B. J Pediatrics 91:434, 1977

73. **Udani PM, Perekh UC, Dastur DK:** Neurological and related syndromes in CNS tuberculosis: clinical features and pathogenesis. J Neurol Sci 14:341, 1971

74. **Varki AP, Puthuran P:** Value of second lumbar puncture in confirming a diagnosis of aseptic meningitis. A prospective study. Arch Neurol 36:581, 1979

75. **Weisberg LA:** Cerebral computerized tomography in intracranial inflammatory disorders. Arch Neurol 37:137, 1980

76. **Weller TH:** The cytomegaloviruses: ubiquitous agents with protean clinical manifestations. N Engl J Med 285:203, 267, 1971

77. **Whitley RJ, Soong SJ, Dolin R et al:** Adenine arabinoside therapy of biopsy-proved herpes simplex encephalitis. N Engl J Med 297:289, 1977

78. **Wilson CB, Desmonts G, Couvreur J et al:** Lymphocyte transformation in the diagnosis of congenital toxoplasma infection. N Engl J Med 302:785, 1980

79. **Wise GR, Farmer TW:** Subdural empyema in infants. In Locke S (ed): Modern Neurology, pp 515–526. Boston, Little, Brown, & Co 1969

80. **Wise GR, Farmer TW:** Bacterial cerebral vasculitis. Neurology (Minneap) 21:195, 1971

81. **Wright RL, Ballantine HT:** Management of the brain abscess in children and adolescents. Am J Dis Child 114:113, 1967

82. **Zimmerman RA, Patel S, Bilaniuk LT:** Demonstration of purulent bacterial intracranial infections by computed tomography. Roentgenol 127:155, 1976

Head Injury

Robert L. McLaurin

Head injury, as discussed here, includes the results of any mechanical force applied to the brain or its coverings. The most frequent causes of injury in this age group include falls of various types, vehicular accidents, and blows received during sports activities. Boys are affected much more frequently than girls. Less commonly, head injury may result from the process of birth or from penetrating foreign bodies. Finally, head trauma may result from intentional injury as one aspect of the "battered child" syndrome.

The basic mechanisms of head injury include impact by small objects (which is likely to produce localized damage to the brain and coverings) and impact against a relatively large surface (which is apt to cause more extensive intracranial commotion). The latter mechanism may in turn be subdivided into injuries resulting from sudden deceleration of a moving head (e.g., the impact sustained when the head strikes the ground in a fall) or to sudden acceleration of a stationary head (e.g., the blow received when struck by a vehicle). Intracranial damage that follows acceleration or deceleration injuries results from the relative inertia of the brain compared to the cranium and to actual deformation of the cranial vault.

The consequences of injury to the head are considered here in the following order: (1) scalp injuries, (2) skull fractures, and (3) injury to the intracranial contents, including direct damage to the brain and indirect damage owing to hematomas. It is apparent, however, that in any given instance of craniocerebral trauma, any combination of these injuries may be present. Fortunately, most head injuries are of no permanent consequence, and relatively few require surgical intervention. The majority of head injuries seen in any pediatric hospital include mild concussion and simple, uncomplicated skull fractures.

INITIAL EXAMINATION

Most children with head injuries are treated initially by persons who are not specialists and who may be inexperienced in dealing with neurosurgical problems. Yet it must be recognized that the ultimate mortality and morbidity of the child are largely dependent on the initial care.

Initial examination of the head-injured child should focus on considerations other than the direct effects of craniocerebral trauma. The first consideration should be the respiratory system. Establishment and maintenance of an adequate respiratory exchange is of paramount significance because (1) hypoxia enhances the severity of damaged brain tissue and (2) hypercarbia, if it exists, contributes to cerebral swelling. Thus, immediate evaluation and control of respiratory function is of top priority. Respiratory control may be achieved by simply placing the youngster in a lateral decubitus position, or it may require immediate intubation and mechanical respiratory control.

A second consideration concerns blood loss and the state of the vascular system. Any active blood loss must be immediately controlled. Excessive blood loss, as indicated by tachycardia and hypotension, must be dealt with immediately by replacement. Hypotension without overt blood loss suggests that some hidden blood loss must be occurring, either into the abdomen or chest or into the soft tissues. Head injury is rarely a cause of peripheral hypotension, so all other possible causes must be considered and appropriately treated.

A third priority is recognition of fractured extremities, which must be immobilized early. This not only prevents further soft tissue injury of the extremity, including nerves and vessels, but also reduces the likelihood of fat embolism, which may accentuate brain damage.

After the above aspects of the injured child have been appropriately dealt with, a neurologic examination (including examination of the brain and its coverings) is in order. The scalp should be examined for evidence of subgaleal hematoma and for lacerations. It must be noted that, in older children with considerable hair, a sizable laceration can be overlooked because of matting of the overlying hair with coagulated and dried blood. Hematomas beneath the scalp may obscure an underlying depressed fracture; conversely, a hematoma may feel like a depressed fracture because of peripheral firmness and elevation with central fluctuance. Examination of the scalp should also include a search for ecchymosis over the mastoid (Battle's sign), which indicates basal temporal fracture, and hemorrhage within the eyelids or subconjunctival region, which suggests either basal frontal fracture or direct impact to the eye.

During early infancy, the fontanelle tension is of great importance as an index of intracranial bleeding after birth or injury. If increased pressure has been present for several days, there may be actual separation of the sagittal suture to palpation. Tension of the fontanelle can best be evaluated when the infant is not crying and when his head is elevated.

External examination includes visualization of the tympanic membranes and external auditory canals. There may be blood behind the drum or the drum may be lacerated; bloody drainage from the ear may be mixed with cerebrospinal fluid. It should be remembered, however, that bleeding from

the ear does not invariably indicate a basal fracture. In the acute stage after injury, cerebrospinal fluid rhinorrhea is more difficult to detect because it is usually mixed with blood and tends to drip into the posterior nasopharynx.

Prior to specific neurologic examination, the neck should be tested for rigidity. If injury occurred within an hour or so, or if the child is deeply comatose from the injury, there may be false flaccidity of the cervical musculature, even though subarachnoid blood may be present.

Having completed evaluation of the brain coverings, the neurologic state should be examined. The most important aspect of this part of the examination is assessment of the conscious level. The most popular and practical grading system today is known as the Glasgow coma scale, described by Teasdale, Jennett, and associates.[11] The grading is on the basis of three parameters: eye opening, verbal response, and best motor response. These categories serve all age groups, although certain modifications may be made during infancy. Each parameter is graded on a range from normal (spontaneous and appropriate) to a condition of response to pain only to no response at all. The three parameters do not necessarily coincide in severity, hence the need for multiple parameters. The severity of coma, then, is expressed as a number which represents the summation of the three parameters.

The course of the conscious level may be even more significant than a single observation. The sequence of determinations may provide the most valuable information in the early evaluation of the patient. Certain types of patterns can be recognized, such as instant coma followed by recovery, instant coma occurring a definite period of time after the injury and precipitated by a seizure, or a lucid interval followed by progressive gradual improvement of the coma level. Delayed onset of coma strongly suggests the occurrence of cerebral swelling or hematoma, whereas slow recovery of the coma-scale grade usually denotes recovery of brain function and the absence of a traumatic hematoma.

Considerable neurologic evidence can be obtained from the eyes, regardless of the conscious level of the infant or child. This part of the examination includes evaluation of the pupils, extraocular movements, and fundi. The size, symmetry, and reactivity of the pupils must be assessed. With midbrain damage, the pupils are usually midposition in size and nonreactive to light. The ciliospinal reflex—homolateral pupillary dilatation evoked by pinching the skin of the neck—may be retained. With pontine injury, the pupils are likely to be pinpoint. Brain stem contusion frequently produces variability of pupillary size and symmetry, with changes occurring over periods of observation involving only a few minutes or hours. Unilateral consistent dilatation of a pupil with loss of light reflex must be interpreted to mean uncal herniation from cerebral swelling or hematoma, and is an indication for urgent intracranial investigation. Because of the importance of pupillary signs, drugs affecting pupils (e.g., opiates or atropine) should be avoided if possible during the early critical stage of observation.

Extraocular movements should be assessed by voluntary movements if the child is old enough and conscious. With infants who are awake, attention can usually be directed toward one side and then the other to test eye movements. In the unconscious patient, the presence of doll's eye movements are sought by passive rotation of the head from side to side while the eyelids are held open. A positive response is contraversive conjugate deviation. Specific extraocular paresis can be detected by this maneuver, and if no doll's eye movement is elicited, a serious brain stem injury must be suspected.

Funduscopic examination is important for two reasons. Even if papilledema is not present in the early period after injury, the examiner should attempt to establish a baseline against which future changes in the fundi can be compared. Secondly, subhyaloid hemorrhage may occur within a few minutes after sudden intracranial bleeding.

Facial nerve function can usually be tested regardless of the conscious state. This is done in the unconscious child by supraorbital compression, which causes grimacing on the homolateral side of the face. Symmetry of movement should be noted and an attempt should be made to distinguish central from peripheral facial paresis if such is present. The remaining cranial nerves can be tested with accuracy only in the awake child.

Peripheral motor and reflex functions are susceptible to gross testing regardless of the state of consciousness. Older, conscious children can be evaluated by usual motor testing maneuvers. Infants and unconscious children must be tested by observing spontaneous movements or movements evoked by noxious stimulation. Comparison of motor function on the two sides is most important. Motor tone of the extremities should also be noted by using passive manipulation.

Tendon reflexes are of less importance early after head injury than on later evaluation. Following a severe brain injury, there may be complete areflexia, so that the presence of tendon reflexes may be interpreted as a favorable sign. Plantar responses are important to note, as bilateral extensor responses are suggestive of brain stem damage. Sensory testing depends on a fully alert and cooperative child and has little usefulness after acute head injury.

The vital signs are valuable adjuncts to diagnosis and management after head injury. By far the most important of these signs are respiratory pattern and respiratory function. The pattern is significant in terms of localization and severity of injury, whereas the functional adequacy must be determined so that further brain damage does not occur from hypoxia or hypercarbia. Cheyne-Stokes breathing occurs with injuries of the cerebral hemisphere. Hyperventilation results from upper brain stem trauma, and ataxia breathing or prolonged periods of apnea are due to lower brain stem involvement.

Changes in blood pressure and pulse due to intracranial injury are usually late manifestations of intracranial hypertension and are generally preceded by alterations of conscious level and pupillary responses. The classic signs of increasing intracranial pressure are a slowed pulse and widened pulse pressure. The greater importance of these vital signs, however, is in their usefulness as an indication of blood loss and hypovolemia in the child with multiple injuries. Elevated temperature may occur with moderately severe brain injury, and hypothermia may result from more devastating damage, or in young infants.

SPECIAL DIAGNOSTIC PROCEDURES

Radiographic Examination

X-ray films of the skull should be made for every patient requiring hospitalization after head injury. Unfortunately, medicolegal pressures demand roentgenograms for many patients who do not need to be hospitalized, despite the lack of any contribution of these films to the patients' management. In cases of doubt concerning need of hospitalization, roentgenograms may be useful in demonstrating the force of impact depending on the presence or absence of fracture.

Although skull roentgenograms are considered important for any patient hospitalized for head injury, it does not follow that they must always be obtained in an emergency situation. Indeed, it is relatively seldom that they contribute to primary medical care. Thus, the patient admitted during the night with a mild to moderate closed head injury can usually wait until the following day for x-ray films to be taken. It should be added, however, that a single lateral roentgenogram of the cervical spine is considered part of the emergency evaluation of a person who is unconscious following injury, because of the incidence of associated head and cervical spine injuries.

In the acute stages after injury, x-ray films are used mainly to determine whether fracture is present and, if so, its location and extent. Linear fractures of the cranial vault are usually easily demonstrated, whereas fractures of the base are difficult to detect; in most instances, however, it is not necessary to subject the child with suspected basal fracture to extensive, time-consuming, expensive radiographic scrutiny. Depressed fractures are usually demonstrated by routine x-ray views, although the true depth of displacement can be determined only on tangential view of the injured area (Fig. 13-1). The presence of air within the cranial vault after injury (pneumocephalus) is rare, and signifies basal skull fracture. Foreign bodies that may have penetrated the skull in compound injuries are usually visible by roentgenogram (Fig. 13-2).

Plain radiography is also of value in diagnosing late effects or complications of head injury. Suture separation or pressure erosion of the sella or cranial vault may indicate chronic intracranial hypertension. Calcification may be seen within or outlining a hematoma, either intracerebral, subdural, or subgaleal. A growing skull fracture (leptomeningeal cyst) may be seen months or years after injury. Finally, evidence of cerebral atrophy or hemiatrophy may be indicated by the existence of abnormal thickness of the cranial vault and enlargement of the air-containing structures at the skull base. Although displacement of a calcified pineal gland is of diagnostic value in adults, it is rarely seen in childhood.

Angiography and air encephalography have been almost completely replaced by computerized tomography in post-traumatic diagnosis. Delineation of extracerebral or intracerebral hemorrhages is easily and accurately achieved, and contusion of brain tissue can usually be identified. The latter may include areas of decreased density (edema) intermixed with areas of increased density (hemorrhage). The extent of shift of the midline structures is easily seen on CT scan and is a useful parameter to follow in the course of treatment. It should be noted that, in the acute stage after trauma, contrast enhancement of the CT image is probably of no value because hemorrhage, edema, and shift may be properly seen and evaluated without enhancement. Later, enhancement may be of some value since a hematoma may become isodense relative to brain tissue and may be seen only by enhancement of the surrounding capsule. Finally, CT scanning is of great value in the late stages, particularly to identify porencephalic cavitation or hydrocephalus which may result from injury.

The role of angiography in pediatric head trauma has been reduced to evaluation of vascular trauma. Examples of the continued usefulness of angiography would include demonstration of direct injury of carotid arteries, including traumatic aneurysm and carotid-cavernous fistula, and visualization of obstruction or displacement of major dural sinus (Fig. 13-3).

Echoencephalography

Echoencephalography was first introduced as a diagnostic tool in 1955.[9] The A-mode scan assumed considerable importance in craniocerebral trauma because of its ease of application at the bedside and its ability to detect intracranial shifts (Fig. 13-4). With the advent of the CT scan, however, this form of echoencephalography has had less usefulness.

The B-mode scan, on the other hand, has assumed increasing value in pediatric diagnosis, including diagnosis of intracranial trauma. The development of gray-scale sonography enhanced its diagnostic value, and the recent advent of real-time scanning has further increased its precision and usefulness. The usefulness of sonography is limited to approximately the first year of life or until the fontanelle has closed. Its greatest usefulness currently seems to be in neonatal trauma and in demonstration of chronic infantile subdural hematomas. Sonography has certain advantages over the CT scan: avoidance of radiation, portable equipment which may be used in the nursery or ICU, and lower cost. The CT scan, on the other hand, carries the advantages of precision and resolution.

Electroencephalography

The electroencephalogram has limited usefulness in the acute stages of head injury, but becomes more valuable with certain late complications or sequelae.[4] Early after injury, electroencephalogram findings may range from a minor increase of theta activity to the ultimate injury effect of electrical silence (Fig. 13-5). Intermediate effects can be qualified by the frequency of the slow activity and the degree to which intrinsic rhythms are disrupted. Focal slow activity may be seen at the site of impact or on the opposite side of the head in contrecoup injury (Fig. 13-6). Although focal spiking is rarely seen in the acute stage, it occurs more

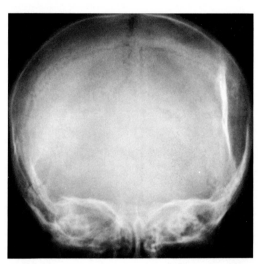

FIG. 13-1 Depressed fracture, left frontotemporal, showing characteristic linear density displaced inwardly.

FIG. 13-2. Frontal (A) and lateral (B) skull roentgenograms. Penetrating foreign body. Patient fell on the metallic object, which was part of a toy.

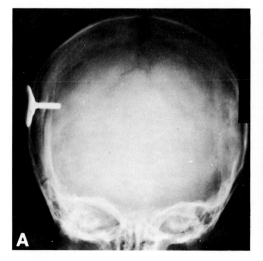

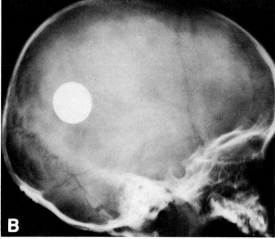

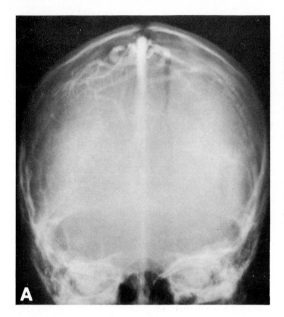

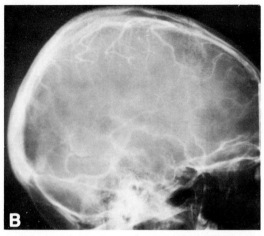

FIG. 13-3. Angiogram (venogram) frontal (A) and lateral (B) views showing displacement of sagittal sinus and parasagittal veins away from inner skull table, characteristic of extradural hematoma of venous origin.

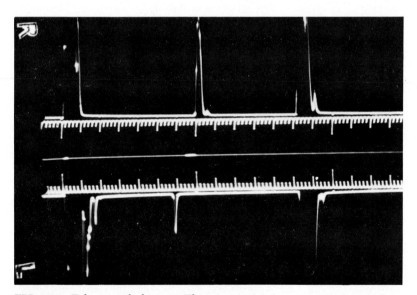

FIG. 13-4 Echoencephalogram. The upper tracing shows midline echo displaced away from transducer on right side. The lower tracing shows displacement toward transducer on left. The tracings are indicative of a mass lesion on the right, in this case a hematoma.

often in children than in adults. Resolution of the early abnormal activity may take place over a period varying from an hour or less to many months or years, depending on the intensity of the original disruption and injury. Slow-wave abnormality usually subsides within 1 to 3 months, whether focal or generalized. Restitution of intrinsic rhythms may lag behind the disappearance of slow waves.

In the later stages after injury, electroencephalography assumes more usefulness. Subdural hematomas are usually accompanied by abnormalities related to compression and distortion of the brain substance. Voltage depression is seen less commonly than would be anticipated by consideration of the damping effect between the cortex and the recording electrode. More commonly, the hematoma is indicated by focal slowing and loss of intrinsic rhythms. During the first week or so after injury electroencephalography is of no value in detecting a subdural hematoma. Although focal slowing may also be seen with epidural hematomas, there is no justification for using precious time to obtain a tracing if the patient is deteriorating neurologically.

The great majority of patients with post-traumatic epilepsy have abnormal electrical activity within weeks or months after injury. Focal spiking is characteristic of the post-traumatic epileptogenic focus, and occasionally paroxysmal discharges are seen (Fig. 13-7). In those rare cases of post-traumatic epilepsy uncontrolled by anticonvulsant therapy, electroencephalography is an essential part of surgical treatment because the spike focus must be delineated by direct recording from the exposed cortex and excised.

Nuclear Medicine Techniques

Three types of diagnostic procedures are done using radiopharmaceuticals, but only two of them have application to trauma. Radionuclide flow scans probably have no usefulness in the assessment of trauma, but brain scanning and cisternography do have application.[2]

The brain scan technique makes use of the impermeability the normal blood–brain barrier to the radioactive substance, whereas abnormal or injured tissue becomes permeable. However, the importance of isotope brain scan has declined with the availability of the CT scan.

Cisternography is the visualization of the movement of radionuclide injected into the cerebrospinal fluid compartment. In relation to trauma, there are two principal indications for performing cisternography. The first is hydrocephalus secondary to subarachnoid blockage due to traumatic hemorrhage. Because the blockage is usually in the basal cisterns and subarachnoid spaces over the hemispheres, the intrathecally injected substance flows into the lateral ventricles, whereas little or no activity passes over the cerebral surfaces toward the sagittal sinus. In addition, the ventricular size is characteristically enlarged.

The second use of intrathecal radionuclide is to demonstrate the site of cerebrospinal fluid leakage into the nose. In cases of late persistent rhinorrhea, the exact point of drainage, which may be difficult to detect clinically or by roentgenogram, can occasionally be demonstrated by this technique.

Lumbar Puncture

Tapping the spine to obtain cerebrospinal fluid is not indicated in the early phases of head injury management. It does not assist in establishing the intracranial pathology and, indeed, may be hazardous, because herniation may occur if a hematoma is present intracranially. Thus, spinal tap is mentioned only to be contraindicated in the early period after injury.

The principal indication for spinal fluid examination occurs later when infection is suspected, for example, meningitis resulting from spinal fluid leakage or contamination, with characteristic pleocytosis, glucose decrease, and positive bacteriologic culture. The other type of infectious process that may occur after injury is the development of a brain abscess with increased cerebrospinal fluid pressure and only moderate cellular reaction.

Subdural Tapping

The subdural tap is unique to pediatric practice. In older children and adults, the skull cannot be penetrated by percutaneous needling; in infants and young children, however, it is an extremely valuable method of detecting subdural accumulations of blood or fluid. The procedure is performed after the scalp is thoroughly shaved and sterilized. The needle is inserted through the lateral extent of the fontanelle or the coronal suture, not less than 1.5 cm from the midline. The dura is penetrated at right angles, and the needle is inserted no further. If a hydroma or a liquefied hematoma is present, it flows from the needle without aspiration.

SCALP INJURIES

Injuries of the scalp fall into two main categories: bruising and laceration. Bruising may include simply discoloration and may indicate the existence of fracture, for example, bruising over the mastoid area in relation to fractures of the middle fossa, or bruising around the eyes and into the subconjunctival layer in relation to anterior fossa fractures. Subgaleal collections of blood may be quite extensive, occurring more commonly in children than in adults (Fig. 13-8). The distinction between subgaleal and subperiosteal hematoma is made by the hematoma's distribution; subgaleal hematomas are not limited by the normal suture lines. Although there is always a temptation to tap a fluctuant subgaleal hematoma, this temptation should be resisted because of the possibility of introducing infection and the fact that the hematoma almost invariably is absorbed within a few days. It is very common for a hematoma of an infant's scalp to be noted by a mother, either without knowledge of previous injury or several days after a minor traumatic episode. Roentgenography usually discloses an undisplaced linear fracture of the skull.

It is worthwhile to recognize that scalp hematomas may be confused with depressed skull fractures on palpation. This occurs when there is a peripheral accumulation of firm hematoma surrounding a central fluctuant area.

The cephalohematoma of the newborn is usually in the subperiosteal space and occurs in the parietal region. As with older children, absorption is the rule and aspiration is not necessary. Rarely, calcification occurs in the wall of a hematoma and results in a firm, bony lump over the parietal bone (Fig. 13-9). As the skull thickens with growth, the lump becomes less prominent, but it can be easily removed surgically if it is objectionable to the parents.

Lacerations of the scalp vary from small puncture wounds to extensive avulsion injuries. Blunt blows to the head may cause stellate lacerations with some devitalization of skin edges. Because all lacerations are contaminated, meticulous care is advisable to prevent the spread of subgaleal infection, which of course may also be in contact with the intracranial space by way of skull fracture. Thus, wide shaving followed by irrigation, exploration for foreign mate-

FIG. 13-5. Electroencephalogram showing generalized slowing in a child 3 days after a moderately severe head injury.

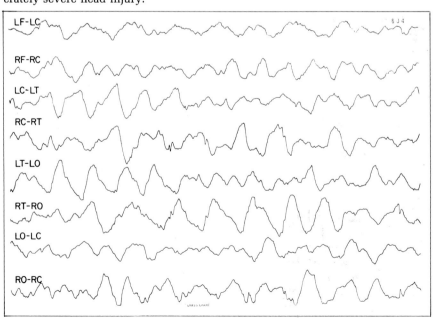

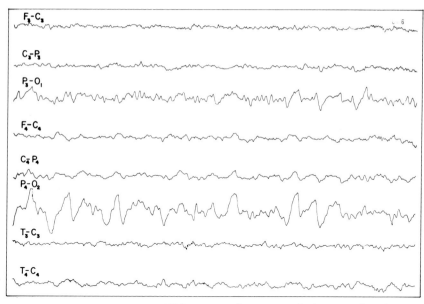

FIG. 13-6. Electroencephalogram, bipolar recording, showing post-traumatic slow wave focus, maximal in right occipital area (P_4-O_2).

rial, debridement, and closure are necessary. Antibiotics may be indicated if prolonged or excessive contamination has occurred. Avulsion injuries may result in actual loss of scalp, and rotation of scalp flaps or application of grafts from other areas may be necessary for repair.

SKULL FRACTURE

Popular opinion commonly equates the existence of skull fracture with severity of a head injury. This is an obvious fallacy, because fatal injury may occur without fracture, and extensive fractures may be seen in patients with minimal brain damage. Nevertheless, the existence of a fracture is of clinical significance in several ways: it is an index to the intensity of the blow received by the head; it may, because of its position, carry the risk of certain complications; and it may require surgery, as in the case of a depressed fracture.

The infant skull possesses certain physical characteristics different from those in older children and adults. It is composed of flexible, nonrigid plates of bone separated by membranous sutures, resulting in a malleable skull that absorbs considerable stress of any mechanical force and allows distortion to occur with a dampening effect on the transmission of the force to the intracranial contents. The older child's skull, like that of the adult, is a relatively rigid structure with very little ability to absorb or modify the force of an external blow.

Skull fractures may be classified in several ways according to their configuration, their location, and the break in continuity of the overlying soft tissues. Thus fractures may be linear, diastatic, or depressed; they may be of the cranial vault or basal; and they may be simple or compound. Certain combinations are seen more commonly than others.

Simple Linear Fracture

The simple linear fracture is the most common type of fracture and, fortunately, is usually the least hazardous (Fig. 13-10). The fracture line may vary from a narrow fissure barely distinguishable on x-ray examination to an extensive branching fracture involving both sides of the cranial vault. In the pediatric patient, the parietal and occipital bones are more frequently involved than the frontal bone. Because the skull is devoid of sensory nerve endings, the skull fracture itself is painless and therefore may

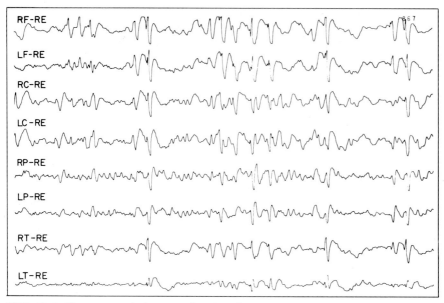

RF-RE

LF-RE

RC-RE

LC-RE

RP-RE

LP-RE

RT-RE

LT-RE

FIG. 13-7. Electroencephalogram, showing sharp waves diffuse but maximal in right temporal area. Patient was 6 years of age at the time of severe injury; seizures began 5 years later.

FIG. 13-8. Bilateral extensive subgaleal liquid hematomas, which subsided over a 10-day period.

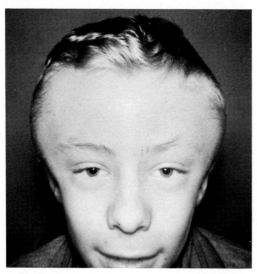

go unrecognized. Whatever discomfort does occur is due to contusion and spasm of adjacent muscles at the base of the skull, or to subperiosteal hematoma accumulation.

The only clinical manifestation of a linear parietal fracture is a subgaleal accumulation of blood that may not be noted by the injured child's mother for several days. The usual linear fracture can seldom be palpated, and the most accurate diagnostic method is by roentgenogram. There are limitations to this method also, however, and it is occasionally difficult to decide whether a fracture is indeed present. Clues that may distinguish fracture lines from other linear rarefactions include the double-linear appearance produced by obliquity of fractures involving the inner and outer skull tables in children, the darkness of a fracture line relative to its width as compared with vascular channels, and its angular branching course as compared with the gentler curves of vascular grooves.

Although simple linear fractures are not inherently dangerous, in certain locations they carry potential hazards. They may cross vascular channels and lead to intracranial bleeding from injury to the subjacent vessels; thus, a linear fracture in the temporal squama may cause laceration of the middle meningeal artery and consequent epidural hemorrhage. The fracture crossing the sagittal or lambdoid sutures may be associated with damage to the sagittal or lateral sinuses with ensuing subdural hemorrhage (Fig. 13-11). A linear fracture ex-

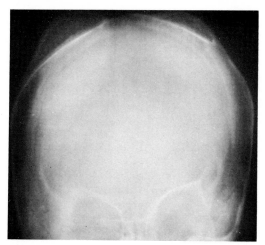

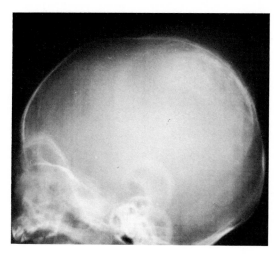

FIG. 13-9. Biparietal cephalhematomas, seen with early faint calcification in anteroposterior view and as increased density in lateral projection.

tending into the foramen magnum may be accompanied by considerable nuchal rigidity due partly to accompanying subarachnoid blood and partly to muscle spasm in the suboccipital area.

There is no treatment of the simple linear fracture as such. Functional healing probably occurs within about 3 months. The significance of linear fractures in children, therefore, lies in their implications concerning intracranial complications. In general, any infant or child with a fresh linear fracture should be hospitalized for observation, and this is particularly important if the fracture line crosses major vascular channels or extends into the foramen magnum.

Diastatic Fracture

The diastatic fracture is rarely seen after early childhood. Characterized by separation of the cranial bones at a normal suture, it may occur without any associated fracture or it may be accompanied by an adjacent linear fracture (Fig. 13-12). The linear fracture is frequently continuous with the diastatic suture line. The implications of a diastatic fracture are similar to those of linear fractures; if the lambdoid suture is involved, possible injury to the lateral venous sinus must be suspected.

Linear Fracture with Separation

A linear fracture characterized by separation (3 mm or more) of the fracture line usually occurs in infants and is the result of severe impact to the head. It is likely to be extensive and bilateral, and is commonly accompanied by evidence of brain injury. The significance of this type of fracture, other than its implication concerning the severity of the blow received, is that the underlying dura mater is apt to be torn. The dura, while flexible, is nonelastic and in infants is attached rather firmly to the skull at the sutures. Therefore, if separation of a fracture line occurs, there is almost certainly a corresponding tear of the subjacent dura. This may lead to herniation of the swollen brain beneath the fracture and compromise the circulation to the herniated brain tissue. In addition, the herniated brain and leptomeninges may prevent dural closure during the subsequent healing stage, and a leptomeningeal cyst may result (Fig. 13-13). Thus, a widely separated linear fracture, particularly if associated with clinical evidence of a corresponding neurologic deficit, is an indication for surgical exploration and repair of the lacerated dura mater.

Basal Fracture

The basal fracture is considered as a separate entity because it has specific complications and therapeutic indications.[5] It is usually a linear fracture that involves only the bones of the skull base or that extends

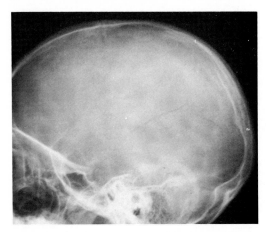

FIG. 13-10. Simple linear fracture, parietal. No displacement or separation of bones was noted.

into the base from the cranial vault. It rarely occurs in infants but is quite common after infancy. The significance of basal fractures derives from the danger of associated injury to cranial nerves, which exit through basal foramina, and from the fact that most basal fractures are "compound" because the fracture site and intracranial contents become exposed to air-containing spaces. Thus, intracranial infection is a threat after basal fracture.

FIG. 13-11. Frontal (A) and lateral (B) skull roentgenograms. Extensive linear fracture extending across the midline and a potential source of injury to the sagittal sinus and its tributaries.

The most frequent basal fracture involves the temporal bone. The patient presents with bloody drainage from the ear with ecchymosis over the mastoid region (Battle's sign). The same force that fractures the petrous portion of the temporal bone may cause laceration of the tympanic membrane and the meninges overlying the petrous pyramid. Thus, a communication is established between the intracranial space and the external auditory canal, and blood may become mixed with cerebrospinal fluid (CSF). The mixture can usually be identified by the appearance of a relatively clear ring surrounding the central blood stain when the bed linen absorbs the ear drainage. It must be emphasized that traumatic bleeding from the ear or appearance of blood behind the drum is not always due to basal fracture. Bloody drainage from the ear may result from laceration of the canal, from a rupture of the tympanic membrane alone, or from a compound fracture of the petrous bone and meninges. Therefore, bleeding from the ear is suggestive but not conclusive evidence of a basal fracture. Roentgenograms may be of assistance in demonstrating a petrous fracture, but special basal or tomographic views are usually necessary; in the acutely injured child, special views are rarely indicated. As a general rule, bleeding from the ear or hemotympanum after head injury is due to a basal fracture.

In early treatment of the temporal fracture, cover the draining ear loosely with

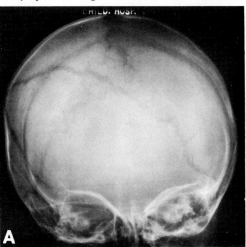

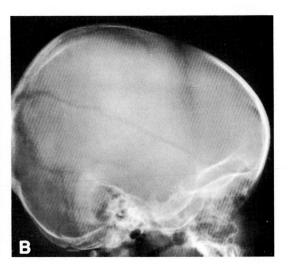

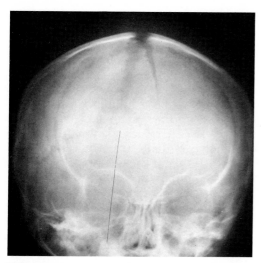

FIG. 13-12. Diastatic fracture. The sagittal suture is widely separated, and the fracture continues downward between the frontal bone plates along the metopic suture.

a sterile gauze but avoid extensive examination and manipulation within the external canal or plugging of the canal. It is preferable to permit free drainage, which usually stops spontaneously within 24 hours and rarely persists longer than 48 hours. The use of antibiotics routinely is a matter of some disagreement. Although the compound nature of the fracture creates a potential intracranial infection, CSF leakage usually stops quickly, and subarachnoid contamination apparently does not occur. Antibiotics are not used in our clinic unless otorrhea persists longer than 2 days or unless an upper respiratory infection was present at the time of the initial injury. The specific choice of antibiotics has also been a matter of debate because very few reach the normal CSF in any significant concentration. *Pneumococcus* is the organism most frequently involved, so penicillin is the antibiotic of choice. In the occasional case in which this is used, it is continued for at least 7 days, longer if the otorrhea persists. Intracranial infection following temporal bone fracture can be detected by clinical signs of meningitis, fever, and nuchal rigidity.

The other complication of the basal fracture is injury to the facial nerve (Fig. 13-14). This may be present as a peripheral type of facial paralysis immediately after injury, or it may occur within 3 days after trauma. When present immediately, it is likely that the nerve has been physically separated. It is necessary to protect the eye, which cannot be closed, from drying and corneal erosion. Additionally, the results of electromyographic studies reflect a reaction of degeneration, if present, after 10 days; if this is the case, surgical exploration and repair of the facial nerve may be indicated.

FIG. 13-13. Pneumoencephalogram. Frontal (*A*) and lateral (*B*) views. Widely separated linear fracture. The fracture line later widened, as shown, and there was porencephalic cavitation connected with the dilated right lateral ventricle.

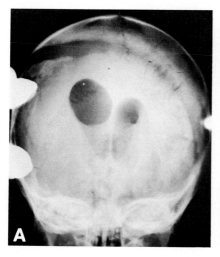

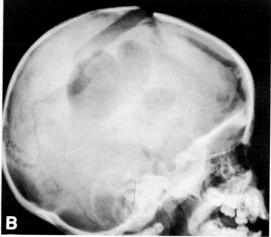

In the case of delayed facial palsy, presumably resulting from swelling of the nerve within its canal, recovery almost invariably occurs within 1 to 3 months and may be expedited by using corticosteroids during the acute stage to reduce nerve swelling.

Less common than basal fractures in the middle cranial fossa are those involving the anterior fossa. The floor of the anterior fossa is made up of portions of the frontal, ethmoid, and sphenoid bones. A common type of fracture in children is one that extends vertically in the frontal bone to the supraorbital ridge and then into the roof of the orbit. This fracture results in marked ecchymosis and swelling of the upper eyelid owing to bleeding from the supraorbital vessels into the loose areolar tissue. It rarely causes injury to the contents of the orbit except for occasional transient weakness of the muscles above the globe. No specific treatment is necessary.

Anterior basal fractures may extend across the midline and involve the roofs of both orbits. This results in the characteristic appearance of the patient who, shortly after injury, has ecchymosis involving both eyes but usually without other evidence of trauma to the forehead or face (Fig. 13-15). Regardless of whether a fracture is demonstrated by roentgenography, this appearance is pathognomonic of a basal frontal fracture of the orbital roof. No specific treatment is recommended unless there is accompanying evidence of CSF rhinorrhea.

Basal fractures involving the sphenoid and ethmoid bones may be complicated by injury to certain cranial nerves. The olfactory nerves may be damaged at the levels of the cribriform plate, resulting in partial or complete loss of olfaction. This cannot be detected in infants or toddlers, but in older children examination for this function should be done as soon as the patient's alertness and local soft tissue injury permit it. The optic nerve may be damaged at the optic foramen; it may not be due to actual bony laceration or compression of the nerve, but rather to damage to blood vessels supplying the nerve. An early sign of optic nerve damage in the patient with impaired consciousness is failure of pupillary response to direct light stimulation in the affected eye, with preservation of response on stimulation of the opposite eye (consensual reaction). Later, the optic nerve head becomes pale. There is no surgical treatment of benefit, and the prognosis for recovery of vision in the blind eye is quite poor.

The third, fourth, and sixth cranial nerves may also be injured by basal fractures involving the sphenoid bone. These injuries result in characteristic disturbances of pupillary size and reactivity, weakness or paralysis of extraocular movements, and impaired levator function of the lid. In contrast to the prognosis for injury of the optic nerve, the prognosis here is generally good for recovery. This may occur over a period of several months, so no corrective procedures should be undertaken until a prolonged period of observation has been completed.

In addition to cranial nerve injury, fractures of the floor of the frontal fossa may involve the paranasal air sinuses of the roof of the nasal cavity. The frontal, ethmoid, and sphenoid sinuses abut on the frontal fossa, and fractures may extend into these structures, creating a compound injury. The

FIG. 13-14. Paralysis of left abducens and facial paresis secondary to basal skull fracture. Both nerves recovered their function. (This is a retouched photograph.)

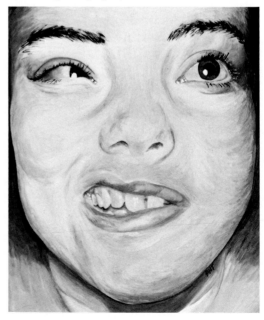

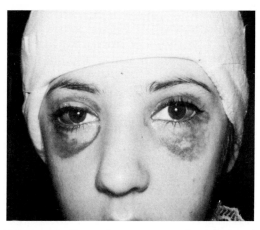

FIG. 13-15. Typical appearance of patient with basal fracture across frontal fossa. The discoloration affects the soft tissues around both eyes and the subconjunctival areas lateral to the pupils.

principles of treatments are similar to those that apply to temporal bone fractures, but there are certain unique features. Intracranial air (aerocele) is more likely to occur with fractures of the anterior fossa, probably because of the common occurrences of positive pressure within the nasal passages associated with sneezing or coughing. Air noted on the skull roentgenogram is proof of a basal fracture with meningeal tear, regardless of the ability to demonstrate a fracture line by roentgenogram or external CSF drainage. Whenever air is seen on the initial films, the roentgenograms should be repeated in several days to determine whether reabsorption has occurred. Meanwhile, antibiotic treatment should be instituted in an effort to prevent intracranial infection.

The most frequent sign of basal fracture into the paranasal air spaces is CSF rhinorrhea. As with temporal fractures, it can be distinguished by the watery appearance of the fluid and its sugar content. The drainage is usually mixed with blood initially and later becomes clear. Because it may drain into the nasopharynx and be swallowed, it can be especially difficult to recognize in growing children. Rhinorrhea is often delayed in onset and appears days or weeks after injury, presumably because of initial plugging of the fracture site by blood clot and swollen brain tissue. Because CSF rhinorrhea is more likely to per-

sist than CSF otorrhea, it is recommended that antibiotic therapy be routine. As stated previously, this treatment is directed mainly against pneumococci. In addition, surgical repair should be undertaken if the rhinorrhea persists longer than 10 to 14 days, as it is unlikely that spontaneous healing occurs after that time. It should be noted that recurrent bouts of meningitis with a history of significant head injury is presumptive evidence of basal fracture, calling for exploratory and reparative surgery.

Depressed Fracture

Depressed fractures may be simple or compound. They result from an impact of a relatively small object against the skull rather than a blow that causes abrupt acceleration or deceleration of the head. One of the more common types of depressed fracture occurs in newborns during the birth process. The fracture may result from forceps applied to the head or from vigorous grasping of the head by the obstetrician. The depression that results is called a "ping-pong" fracture, and when relatively small and shallow is of no significance (Fig. 13-16). Many such fractures correct themselves over a period of weeks or months. Large depressed fractures in newborns should be corrected electively. This can usually be achieved very quickly and easily by simply sliding a small instrument into the epidural space and forcing the depressed segment of bone outward to a normal contour. Antibiotics are unnec-

FIG. 13-16. Shallow depressed ping-pong fracture in a newborn, not accompanied by localized neurologic deficit or by seizures.

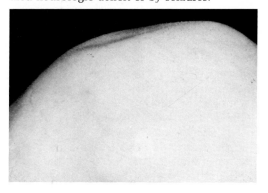

essary because these fractures are generally not compound.

Depressed fractures in older children may or may not require elevation, and, in general, the trend in recent years has been toward more conservative management. There is no definite way of establishing a diagnosis of a closed depressed fracture on clinical examination alone. There is frequently considerable swelling and hemorrhage in and beneath the scalp in the traumatized area, obscuring the contour of the underlying skull. In addition, hematoma beneath the scalp may be accompanied by a ring of firm, clotted hemorrhage, which on palpation feels like a depressed central area. Thus, x-ray examination is essential to establish the diagnosis of closed depressed fracture, and the minimal number of roentgenogram views include anteroposterior and lateral projection. The depressed segment frequently cannot be detected except when seen, at least partially, in tangential projection. Diagnosis of depressed fracture in the presence of an overlying scalp laceration can usually be done on direct inspection or palpation through the scalp wound, but roentgenograms should be obtained to determine the extent and depth of the skull deformity.

Not all depressed fractures need be treated surgically, and certain ones should not be operated on. The principal example of the latter type is the depressed fragment over a major dural venous channel. Although such an injury rarely leads to occlusion of the venous sinus, attempted repair is likely to lead to profuse hemorrhage with the inherent hazard of necessitating complete occlusion of the channel to control bleeding.

There is no universal agreement as to specific indications for repair of closed depressed fractures in children. In the past, the argument for correction of nearly all depressed areas centered mainly around the principle of progressive damage to the underlying cortex by pulsation of the growing brain against the indriven fragment, which presumably would lead to an epileptogenic focus. The evidence supporting this argument, however, has been lacking, and it appears likely that whatever irritable focus may occur at a later date is probably the result of the initial blow. The most obvious indication for surgical intervention is the existence of a neurologic deficit after injury corresponding to the area of cortex immediately beneath the depressed fracture. Although the deficit may be a result of initial cortical bruising, it is logical to believe that the best chance for rapid recovery of the damaged brain is afforded by removal of local pressure on the brain. This situation, then, constitutes an indication for immediate fracture elevation. Because of the frequent association of seizures with depressed fractures, anticonvulsant therapy should be started immediately and continued for several months until it can be established that there is no clinical or electroencephalographic evidence of a seizure disorder.

The depth of depression of a fracture must enter into the decision regarding elective surgery of depressed fractures. The most accurate assessment of the extent of deformity can be obtained from a tangential roentgenogram; because in most instances immediate surgical correction is not necessary, such radiologic evaluation can usually be done carefully at a later time. Although definite criteria cannot be proposed, it is the policy in this clinic to elevate fractures with depression greater than 3 mm over the sensorimotor area and greater than 5 mm over the rest of the brain. This can be done electively if there is no corresponding neurologic deficit. Fractures depressed greater than 5 mm are likely to be accompanied by laceration of the underlying dura, so this membrane must also be repaired. Such dural tear is more likely to occur if there has been comminution of the depressed fragment.

The most frequently occurring indication for immediate correction of depressed fracture is when it is associated with scalp laceration; this constitutes a compound depressed fracture, and repair of the fracture is part of the initial wound debridement. The extent of depression and comminution of the fragments is invariably greater than is usually presumed from clinical and x-ray examination. When the compound fracture is also comminuted, some fragments must be sacrificed; in most instances, however, bone can be salvaged and replaced, and subsequent cranioplasty can often be avoided (Fig. 13-17). Antibiotic and anticonvulsant therapy should be instituted immediately.

The final indication for elevation of a depressed fracture has a cosmetic or emotional basis. Any fracture, particularly frontal, that leaves a visible depression of the skull should be corrected fairly early before the fragments become fixed in an abnormal contour (Fig. 13-18). Certain depressions of the skull, regardless of visibility, may be a source of concern to the patient or his parents, and this also constitutes a valid reason for surgical treatment.

In summary, therefore, immediate

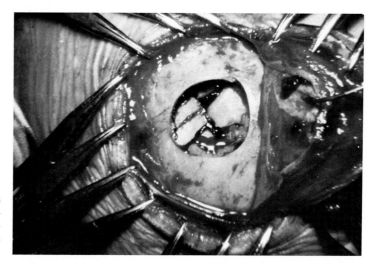

FIG. 13-17. Depressed fractures as seen at operation, showing indriven fragmented comminution of the bone. Such fragments can not be usefully salvaged.

FIG. 13-18. Lateral skull roentgenograms. Depressed fracture (frontal) (*A*) and postoperative restoration of normal skull contour (*B*).

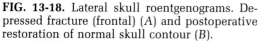

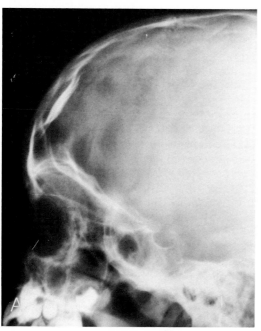

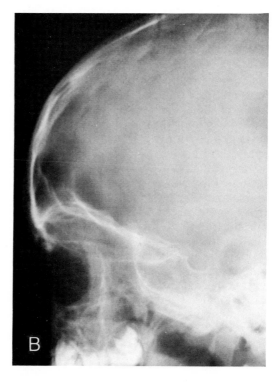

correction of a depressed fracture is undertaken if there is a corresponding neurologic deficit or compounding of the wound. Delayed correction may be done if there is depression greater than 3 to 5 mm (depending on location), or if there is sufficient concern about the cosmetic effect of the injury. Surgery consists in elevation of the bone fragments, inspection and repair of the underlying dura, investigation of the subdural space and brain if the dura has been torn, debridement of the comminuted fragments if there is compounding, and, finally, restoration of the normal skull contour if sufficient fragments can be salvaged.

BRAIN INJURY

Concussion

By definition, concussion is a mechanical impact that causes temporary disturbance of normal function of the affected tissue without structural damage. By usage, concussion implies a transient disruption of consciousness resulting from head injury. Because infants and young children cannot always indicate whether there was actual loss of contact and posttraumatic amnesia, some flexibility is allowed in the use of the term, and it has come to mean any mild, closed-head injury with transient residual neurologic effects.

The least severe type of concussion usually results from sudden acceleration or deceleration of the head and is not accompanied by overt evidence of unconsciousness. The classic example is the child who sustains an injury while playing football and continues playing the game, possibly with some evidence of confusion, but with no later recollection of participation. In such an instance, the transient neurologic deficit involves the mechanisms subserving recall, and there is posttraumatic amnesia for variable periods of time. The term *traumatic automatism* has been applied to this state, which usually runs its complete course within an hour or less.

A more severe type of concussion is accompanied by obvious impairment of consciousness.[10] This usually lasts only a few minutes and is associated with loss of postural tone, flaccidity of the extremities, and areflexia. This persists for seconds or minutes only and is followed by progressive recovery of function similar to that occurring after recovery from a minor epileptic attack. If the child is examined during the stage of flaccidity, there is pupillary dilatation, transient apnea, and bradycardia. These result from loss of neuronal function within the brain stem. As recovery progresses, there is a stage of confusion and automatic behavior. This may be followed by a period of restless activity, although in younger children it is usually replaced by lethargy. The child at that time is sleepy, behaves inappropriately in response to his parents, demonstrates pallor and a rapid pulse, and often vomits. Prolongation of this stage of recovery is unique to the pediatric age group and makes early evaluation of the seriousness of the injury quite difficult. Parents will often try frantically to keep the youngster awake during this stage. It may be noted that such efforts have no therapeutic benefit but have been popularized on the basis of the relationship between deepening coma and severity of intracranial injury. Evaluation of the early stage after injury is further complicated by the rather common appearance of spasticity, bordering on decerebrate rigidity, in the infant and young child. In the adult, this signifies serious brain stem injury, whereas in younger persons it probably is a reflection of an immature and undeveloped nervous system.

The child who has been momentarily stunned and then rapidly recovers to an apparently normal state need not necessarily be hospitalized. There are two specific circumstances, however, that indicate hospitalization. If there has been a definite period of unconsciousness followed by persistence of confusion or lethargy, it is essential that close neurologic observation be undertaken, and this can be done best in the hospital. The level of consciousness, pupillary equality and response, and motor activity should be observed and recorded at least once every hour for 6 hours after injury, and then at 2-hour intervals for 8 to 12 hours. Vital signs are of little help in the pediatric age group for detecting intracranial pathology.

The second reason for hospitalization is persistent vomiting, which may occur after only mild concussion. In the infant or young child, frequent vomiting may result in dehydration, which can often be controlled by the use of promethazine by suppository. The patient should be given nothing by mouth until approximately 4 hours after injury or after the most recent episode of vomiting. Clear liquids in small amounts are then given with progression to a regular diet as tolerated. The total period of hospitalization for simple concussion may be overnight or at most 2 days if vomiting is controlled and the child remains alert and responsive. There is no evidence that bed rest is of value, except during the stage of neurologic deficit or vomiting, and no indication that limitation of subsequent activity has any beneficial effect.

Contusion and Laceration

Severe closed head injuries result in bruising of the brain substance or actual tearing of the neural tissue.[7] These types of pathology result from various mechanical forces that occur intracranially after injury. The most common type of injury is due to sudden deceleration of the moving head, usually when the direction of movement is forward. The rate of deceleration of the brain is less than that of the skull, and the brain is then thrown forward intracranially and abuts against the frontal bone and sphenoid wing, resulting in contusion of the inferior frontal surface and the tip of the temporal lobe. Hence, the frontotemporal area is among the most frequent sites of contusion. The same forward motion of the brain results in impact of brain stem against the bony clivus, causing direct injury to that vital portion of the brain. Generalized widespread cerebral contusion may occur from penetrating missile injuries, owing to the explosive force liberated by the rapidly decelerating missile. Finally, brain bruises may occur at a site diametrically opposite to the site of impact—the so-called contrecoup injury.

Laceration of brain tissue results from at least two types of mechanical stress. First, as the brain is thrown forward, the sharp prominences of the sphenoid bone may cause actual disruption and tearing of the frontotemporal brain substance. A second mechanism is the production of shear stresses within the brain by different deceleration rates of the brain components; this may cause anatomic separation of neural tissue and also may lead to vascular injury and intracerebral hemorrhage.

Pathology associated with brain contusion and laceration consists basically of hemorrhage and edema (Fig. 13-19). Bleeding may be microscopic, petechial, or coalescent, resulting in gross mass hemorrhage within the brain substance. Edema occurs in and adjacent to the areas of impact and stress, and is a form of vasogenic edema, that is, edema due to damage to the blood–brain barrier and extravasation of protein-rich fluid into the extracellular space, especially the white matter. In addition to hemorrhage and edema, a third factor that contributes to cerebral swelling is vasoparalysis, which leads to hyperemia and actual enlargement of the vascular bed.

Clinical Features.   *Neurologic Signs.* There is invariably a loss of consciousness following severe closed head injury, and it may last from a few minutes to an indefinite length of time. Unconsciousness presumably results from damage to the reticular activating system whose functional integrity is necessary for maintenance of a conscious state. The depth of coma varies depending on the severity of injury; when first examined, the child may be totally unresponsive to painful stimuli, or he may have improved to a lighter stage of coma. As the unconscious state abates, the patient becomes responsive to pain with purposeless withdrawal of extremities; he then proceeds to a stage in which there is purposeful avoidance of noxious stimulation. Further recovery is characterized by responsiveness to verbal stimuli and commands; this is first associated with lethargy rather than hyperactivity, although the latter may appear later. The patient is confused and disoriented during this stage, and there is then gradual recovery of normal mental response and behavior.

The initial evaluation of the patient may be done according to the Glasgow coma scale. This scale has two advantages: it provides a common basis for comparison of observations between two examiners or between two separate assessments by the same examiner, and it has implications regarding

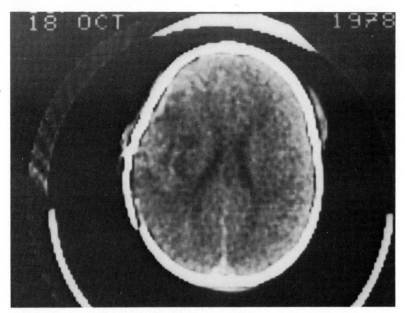

FIG. 13-19. CT scan showing shift of ventricles to right owing to edema and petechial hemorrhage of left frontotemporal areas resulting from contusion.

prognosis, although it must be recognized that such implications are less trustworthy in children than in adults.

The sequence of recovery is subject to many variations. The speed of improvement varies from minutes to weeks or months. The ultimate endpoint of recovery depends on the extent and location of irreversible brain damage. During the progress of recovery, there may be setbacks; these are of minor degree only, and if significant deterioration is noted, the possibility of an expanding compressing lesion must be sought.

Generalized cerebral contusion may be accompanied by features indicating that a particular portion of the brain has been most severely injured. In addition, there are syndromes characteristic of local contusion without evidence of generalized brain damage. Thus, contusion of the brain stem is characterized by respiratory irregularities; pupillary changes including irregularity, inequality, eccentricity, and impairment of reflex functions (light and ciliospinal); impairment of individual or conjugate extraocular movements; absence of doll's eye movements; bilateral Babinski reflexes; and decerebrate or decorticate postural responses on stimulation. Although all of these features are usually not found in the individual case, the presence of several of them localizes the site of major injury.

Hemiparesis usually implies focal contusion in the cerebral hemisphere. This may be present initially or may appear after 24 to 48 hours. Hemiparesis can be detected in all but the most deeply comatose or decerebrate child. It is usually accompanied by a unilateral Babinski sign. If there is an associated speech deficit, it will become apparent only as the level of contact improves, although aphasia can usually be detected long before full recovery of orientation occurs. Sensory disturbances usually cannot be determined during the early posttraumatic period.

The syndrome of temporal lobe contusion is unique. It may be accompanied by only brief initial impairment of consciousness, but after 24 to 48 hours, the child will become less alert and focal signs will appear (e.g., hemiparesis, with the face most severely involved and the leg relatively uninvolved). If the dominant temporal lobe is bruised, dysphasia will be evident. If the syndrome progresses to the point of herniation of the uncus, the pupil will dilate and there will be loss of light reflexes (Fig. 13-20).

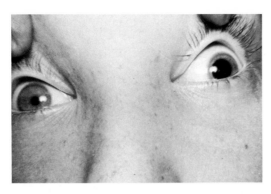

FIG. 13-20. Anisocoria due to uncal herniation. The left pupil is fixed and dilated, and there is outward deviation of the eye, that is, oculomotor nerve paresis.

Systemic Signs. Certain systemic features are commonly seen after cerebral contusion. Changes in respiration have been mentioned in relation to brain stem bruising. Cheyne-Stokes respiratory pattern may occur after an injury that primarily affects the diencephalon. Mesencephalic or pontine injury may be associated with central neurogenic hyperventilation, which results in hypocarbia and mild alkalosis (although there may also be an associated hypoxia). Damage to lower brain stem structures may produce ataxic irregular respiratory function progressing to apnea. Monitoring the respiratory pattern is therefore helpful in determining the level of maximal brain injury.

Hyperthermia after head injury is seen more frequently in children than in adults. It is presumably caused by damage to the thermoregulatory centers of the hypothalamus or to the presence of blood in the cerebrospinal fluid compartment. The body temperature may remain consistently elevated or may vary from hyper- to hypothermic levels spontaneously. The rise of body temperature is usually accompanied by a corresponding increase in pulse rate. Although temperature elevation to 101° to 102°F is quite common and not alarming, a rise to 104° to 105°F is ominous and usually a prelude to fatality.

Disturbances of water and salt metabolism occur after cerebral contusion in adults and children. The characteristic sequence of events includes a period of salt and water retention that lasts 2 to 3 days. A mild or moderate hyponatremia is usually seen despite the sodium retention; unless hyponatremia is severe or prolonged, excess salt should not be administered. Potassium loss is characteristically seen after head or bodily trauma, but unless there are extrarenal losses, as may occur from nasogastric suction, replacement is usually not necessary during the first few days.

Gastric ulceration occurs occasionally after brain stem injury and may lead to fatality owing to perforation or blood loss. The pathophysiology includes increased hydrochloric acid production, vascular changes in the gastric wall, and a decrease in protective mucin. It is imperative that this complication be recognized early and treated vigorously.

Treatment. *Respiratory Care.* Adequate respiratory exchange is of paramount importance for two reasons. Oxygenation is essential to reduce the tissue injury, particularly in those areas that may have marginal blood supply owing to vascular injury or spasm. Hypoxia may be due to alveolar hypoventilation, ventilation–perfusion abnormalities (shunting), or diffusion defects. The second reason for careful attention to pulmonary function is related to carbon dioxide exchange. The child with cerebral contusion and edema has very little if any residual margin of safety from the standpoint of intracranial pressure. Since CO_2 is a potent vasodilator, it is essential that the $PaCO_2$ be maintained at normal or slightly hypocarbic levels. It is recommended that the $PaCO_2$ be kept at about 30 mm Hg, as respiratory alkalosis does not occur at that level. CO_2 exchange is directly related to respiratory exchange; therefore, mechanical assistance or control is indicated in any child in a deeply comatose state or with an irregular respiratory pattern. Endotracheal intubation should be a routine part of early management of the child with contusion or laceration. Tracheostomy in children presents a greater risk of complications than it does in adults, and therefore tracheal intubation should be maintained for longer periods of time. With proper care, tubes have been left in place for 2 weeks or longer without apparent harm.

Neurogenic pulmonary edema occasionally occurs after acute head injury and is an ominous sign, because it usually signifies an acutely and severely elevated intracranial pressure. It can be treated by positive pressure ventilation, digitalization, and diuresis with furosemide.

Cerebral Edema. Cerebral contusion is accompanied by vasogenic edema, which is probably partly on an ischemic basis. The result is cerebral swelling, which leads to intracranial hypertension and possible herniation. Herniation may occur from one hemicranium to the other beneath the falx or from the supratentorial to the infratentorial compartment through the incisura of the tentorium. This latter form of herniation may result in signs of oculomotor and brain stem dysfunction.

Because herniation does not occur in the absence of intracranial hypertension, it is presently common practice to monitor intracranial pressure (ICP). Among the methods currently in use, the most commonly employed include direct pressure monitoring from a catheter inserted into the ventricle or from the subarachnoid space (Richmond screw), and monitoring from a pressure transducer inserted into the extradural space through a small burr hole. This last method has been in use in our clinic for several years; it is favored because it eliminates dural penetration, and there are fewer technical difficulties. Continuous pressure recordings are obtained, permitting visual evaluation of pressure trends and fluctuations.

Treatment of cerebral edema is undertaken, therefore, to reduce intracranial pressure, which, in turn, prevents herniation. Pharmacologic agents that reduce cerebral edema fall into four major categories: glucocorticoids, osmotic agents, diuretics, and barbiturates. The mechanisms of action of glucocorticoids and barbiturates are not defined precisely.

Glucocorticoids have been recommended for control of traumatic cerebral edema, mainly on the empirical basis of their known effectiveness in other forms of edema. It has not been possible to document their effect in traumatic edema. Their presumed mechanism of action is stabilization of the cell membrane and the blood-brain barrier. If glucocorticoids are to be used, dexameth-

asone is employed most often. In the child whose weight exceeds 50 kg, an initial intravenous loading dose of 10 mg is given followed by maintenance doses of 4 mg every 6 to 8 hours. Appropriate reductions of dosage are made for smaller children. Because of the increased likelihood of gastric ulceration occurring with steroid therapy, antacids are administered routinely through a nasogastric tube every 4 to 6 hours, and gastric suction is discontinued for 30 minutes. Gastric suction is employed for the first 2 to 4 days if coma remains deep.

The most commonly used osmotic agent is mannitol, which acts simply by raising the osmolarity of the intravascular compartment, and resulting in withdrawal of water from the extravascular compartment at a rate based on the resistence of the blood-brain barrier to its passage. It is administered intravenously as a 20% solution, and the recommended dose is 0.5 to 1.0 g/kg. Its effectiveness usually lasts approximately 4 hours, and it may then be necessary to repeat the dose depending on the ICP.

Because mannitol is not metabolized, it is excreted and therefore has a potent effect as a systemic dehydrating agent. Hypertonicity of the extracellular fluids of the body may occur after several doses, and it is imperative that serum sodium and total serum osmolarity be monitored. The systemic dehydrating effect of mannitol may be reduced by the use of glycerol. This osmotic agent is administered by nasogastric tube as a 50% solution, and is partially metabolized and only partially excreted. It is also given in doses of 0.5 to 1.0 g/kg. Glycerol has been used in this clinic for the past 3 years with satisfaction.

The most frequently used diuretic agent is furosemide. This substance functions principally through its effect on the distal renal tubules, although there is some evidence that it may have a specific inhibitory effect on the spread of cerebral edema.

Recently, barbiturates have been advocated in treatment of cerebral contusion because of the known reduction of metabolic requirements of the brain in barbiturate coma.[6] Also, barbiturates presumably reduce cerebral edema, by an unknown mechanism. Doses of intravenous pentobarbital (Nembutal) should range from 3 to 5 mg/kg, and the serum level should be maintained at 3 to 5 µg/ml. It is obvious that the child must be under continuous respiratory control accompanied by blood gas monitoring. It should be noted also that barbiturates in these doses may result in vascular hypotension.

Gastric Care. Because the normal cough reflexes are lost in a child with coma from cerebral contusion, aspiration of gastric contents and juice is common and probably contributes to a chemical pneumonitis. For this reason, a nasogastric tube should be inserted early and the gastric contents aspirated. The second reason for gastric aspiration and continued suction is the attempt to prevent gastric ulceration, which occurs as a consequence of hypothalamic injury; the use of glucocorticoids also favors ulceration. Thus, antacids are administered as indicated above. If evidence of peritoneal irritation is noted, the possibility of gastric or duodenal perforation must be considered, and if bleeding occurs blood replacement may be necessary.

Fluid Therapy. During the first few days of posttraumatic coma, it is not necessary to replace nitrogen losses or maintain a positive nitrogen balance. Careful attention should be directed, however, to fluid and electrolyte replacement. Because sodium and water retention are part of the normal metabolic response to injury, it is advisable to keep fluid maintenance fairly low during the first 3 days. Although overhydration does not lead to cerebral edema, hypotonicity of the body fluids does lead to cellular overhydration of the brain. Thus, fluid therapy in the child should be directed toward maintaining normal serum osmolality and pH. Total volume maintenance should be a normal 1200 to 1500 ml/m² to ensure adequate renal function, and the fluid should not be salt poor. In addition, the gastric aspirate should be replaced volume for volume with half-normal saline or a similar solution. Potassium is replaced cautiously and usually is not a critical part of metabolic balance.

Hyperosmolality and hypoosmolality are complications of cerebral trauma and its therapy. As indicated above, the commonest cause of hypertonicity is the frequent and repeated use of dehydrating (osmotic) agents. Another rare cause of excessive water loss is traumatic diabetes insipidus, which is a very uncommon complication of basilar skull fracture. Hypertonicity has its own harmful effect on the central nervous system, and therefore must be recognized early and prevented.

Hypoosmolality is generally the result of water retention. Although this is a normal response early after head injury, continuation of antidiuretic hormone output becomes inappropriate. Recently this has been recognized in neonates and premature infants as a complication of head trauma. For diagnosis, serum hypotonicity and hyponatremia in spite of urinary hypernatremia and disproportionate urine concentration must be present. There is still some question whether true "cerebral salt wasting" occurs, but the usual treatment is water restriction.

Hyperthermia. Children are more likely than adults to experience hyperthermia after head injury. It is important to control this fever because of the general metabolic stress it imposes and because it probably contributes to intracranial hypertension. The classic means of control employed antipyretic drugs and surface cooling with alcohol or water. At present, cooling blankets with constant-temperature monitoring and control seem to represent the most efficient means of temperature control. There is probably no advantage to hypothermia in the treatment of brain contusion, but a normothermic state is recommended.

Medications. In addition to the specific items already discussed, the infant or child with cerebral contusion should be given prophylactic anticonvulsant therapy. In most instances, a minimum sedative effect is advisable, and diphenylhydantoin is used in daily divided dosages totaling 5 to 8 mg/kg. The serum level should be monitored and maintained at 10 to 20 µg/ml. Although some evidence has suggested that routine use of anticonvulsants decreases the incidence of permanent posttraumatic epilepsy, this point is not firmly established. If sedation is required because of a restless, agitated state, phenobarbital is indicated; diazepam is also useful for this purpose.

Antibiotics are not used routinely after

severe head injury. However, the incidence of respiratory infection is high if the child remains comatose for longer than 3 to 5 days, and if such infection does occur, appropriate broad-spectrum agents are used.

Prognosis. Most patients who succumb to the immediate effects of the initial injury do so within 72 hours. Thus, the outlook for survival of the injury is good if death has not occurred during that period. Subsequently, survival of the comatose child depends on prevention or control of complications, particularly respiratory infection.

The ultimate neurologic recovery depends entirely on the extent and location of the initial brain damage. It is a well-recognized fact that children have considerably greater ability than adults to exhibit neurologic recovery and relearning. Hence, the most severely contused brain in a child deserves vigorous and heroic efforts at preservation and rehabilitation.

INTRACRANIAL HEMATOMAS

Extradural Hematomas

Extradural hemorrhage is less common in children than in adults and is rare in infants. The low incidence during early life is due to fixation of the dura to the suture lines so that the dura is more effectively anchored to the skull. In addition, the middle meningeal artery is less indented into the inner skull table in early life and is therefore less susceptible to trauma. Despite its rarity in infants, it occurs with sufficient frequency during childhood to constitute an incidence of 1% to 2% of patients admitted to the hospital because of head injury.

Hemorrhage into the extradural space almost invariably occurs from the middle meningeal artery or one of its major branches. Exceptions to this are the epidural bleeding from the sagittal sinus that follows extensive and usually comminuted fractures that cross the midline of the calvarium, and epidural bleeding from the lateral sinus following diastatic fracture of the lambdoid suture. Venous epidural bleeding

otherwise is probably extremely rare, and the chronic hematomas usually attributed to venous origin are probably the result of bleeding from a smaller arterial radicle in an aberrant location. The majority of epidural hematomas in childhood result from falls, in many instances the precipitating incident being quite trivial.

The hematoma begins with separation of the dura from the skull and a tear of the arterial channel.[3] The dural separation results from inbending of the skull in the temporal area. A potential space is thereby created into which bleeding occurs; as the hematoma enlarges, the dura is progressively stripped from the inner skull table. The hematoma rapidly increases in size and causes acute compression of the adjacent brain, the temporal lobe. Over the next few hours, there is molding of the brain, and displacement of the temporal lobe and adjacent brain stem toward the opposite side. At some point in this migration, uncal herniation occurs, leading to the characteristic signs of this critical event: ipsilateral pupillary dilatation and evidence of brain stem decompensation.

Extradural hemorrhage therefore constitutes a true neurosurgical emergency because of two contributing factors. Because bleeding is from an artery, it occurs under high pressure. Secondly, because the hemorrhage usually occurs fairly low in the temporal area, there is less cushioning between the hemorrhage and the uncus, and herniation occurs more quickly. The relative chronicity of extradural hemorrhage in aberrant locations is partly due to the greater expanse of the brain, which must be molded and moved before the critical herniation occurs.

Clinical Features. The classic case of extradural hemorrhage includes a history of head injury that frequently is considered rather trivial. It must be recalled, however, that although middle meningeal bleeding may be precipitated by a minor injury, it may also occur after more severe head trauma. Thus, the state of consciousness from the time of injury varies considerably. There may be an initial brief period of unconsciousness followed by a lucid interval before the secondary period of depressed consciousness supervenes. There may be definite loss of contact, or only momentary stunning, followed by an asymptomatic period of several hours' duration. Finally, there may be disturbed consciousness from the beginning, with either variable levels of confusion and coma or progressively decreasing contact leading to profound loss of responsiveness.

Examination of the child usually reveals some external evidence of trauma in the frontotemporal region. Characteristically, this consists of puffy swelling over the temporalis muscle accompanied by ecchymosis. When the skull injury extends to the posterior part of the squamous bone, the hematoma discolors the mastoid region (Battle's sign). Absence of local bruising and swelling does not exclude an underlying hematoma.

The neurologic picture depends entirely on the stage of progression of the intracranial pathophysiology. Headache is usually an early and continuous complaint as long as the child is alert. The normal conscious state gives way to lethargy or to a period of hyperirritability, which in turn is followed by decreasing awareness. While consciousness is being altered, there may be evidence of cortical dysfunction beneath the hematoma. This usually results in progressive hemiparesis (and speech disturbance if the dominant side is involved), but may be manifested by seizure activity of a focal nature. It is noteworthy that hemianopia occurs rarely with epidural hematoma.

When uncal herniation occurs, the child's condition suddenly becomes critical. This is characterized initially by evidence that the oculomotor nerve is compressed by traction and direct pressure. The earliest sign is usually dilatation of the ipsilateral pupil, which soon becomes fixed in a widely dilated position and is nonreactive (Fig. 13-20). The pupilloconstrictor loss is followed by paresis of extraocular and levator palpebrae function, which causes the eye to deviate laterally with a fixed, dilated pupil and a ptotic lid, but with evidence of intact vision as demonstrated by a consensual response of the opposite pupil. The eye signs are followed by motor and reflex evidence of brain stem compression. The hemiparesis, then, is superseded by decorticate or decerebrate response that first appears after painful stimulation, and later

spontaneously, accompanied by bilateral Babinski reflexes.

Changes in vital signs are usually late manifestations of intracranial hemorrhage, regardless of its precise location. The classic changes include a slowed pulse, widened pulse pressure, and slowed respiration followed by irregular breathing. In infants, intracranial bleeding may be of sufficient volume relative to the total blood volume so that the results of hypovolemia are superimposed on those of intracranial pressure. Thus, the pulse may be rapid and weak, and the blood pressure low and unobtainable.

In summary, the clinical manifestations of extradural hematoma include a head injury of variable severity, followed usually by a lucid interval that gives way to decreasing consciousness, ipsilateral oculomotor palsy, and contralateral hemiparesis, and that finally proceeds to a deeply comatose decerebrate state with changes in vital signs. Although this sequence of events usually occurs over 4 to 6 hours, it may be extended over a period of a day or more for reasons noted above.

The above description applies to supratentorial hematomas, but occasionally extradural bleeding occurs in the posterior fossa. This is notoriously difficult to diagnose. Upward herniation of the brain stem may lead to pupillary dilatation, suggesting a temporal hematoma. More specific localizing signs include ataxia of the ipsilateral limbs, nystagmus, and dysarthria. Because most extradural hematomas of the posterior fossa result from tear of dural venous sinus, the clinical course is more prolonged and not as critically demanding as that of extradural hematomas due to arterial bleeding in the temporal fossa.

Diagnostic Studies.   In rapidly progressive deterioration, no studies beyond the clinical examination are indicated because expediency in decompressing the intracranial space is of utmost urgency. In most instances, however, there is sufficient time to obtain a CT scan if the equipment is readily accessible (Fig. 13-21). The CT scan is usually easily diagnostic because of the characteristic lenticular configuration of the hematoma.

Roentgenograms of the skull are usu-

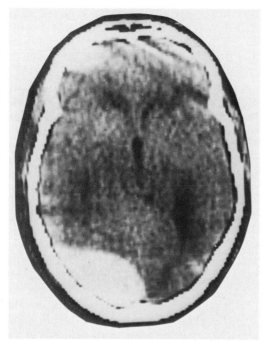

FIG. 13-21. CT scan showing typical picture of an extradural hematoma in left parieto-occipital area.

ally not helpful, but they reveal a linear fracture in approximately 75% of cases. Thus, absence of a fracture does not preclude the diagnosis.

Treatment. The ultimate objectives of treatment are removal of the hematoma, decompression of the underlying brain, and control of the arterial bleeding point. These should be done as expeditiously as possible to prevent irreversible brain damage. Quite often, however, some time must be expended in preparing the patient and the operating room, and certain measures are helpful in combating neurologic deterioration during this interval. These measures are designed to reduce the bulk of the normal brain and thereby temporarily forestall herniation. Hyperventilation achieves this end by producing hypocarbia, which decreases cerebral mass by vasoconstriction. Therefore, if the child is unconscious, intubation should be done rapidly so that effective hyperventilation can be accomplished. In addition, hypertonic agents (urea or mannitol) should be administered intra-

venously to cause dehydration and shrinkage of the cerebral mass. By these measures alone, the progress of neurologic deterioration can be delayed for an hour or so; this condition should not lead to a sense of security, however, and surgery should be performed with all dispatch.

Operation consists of placing a burr hole in the temporal region and enlarging the cranial opening beneath the temporalis muscle. The clotted hematoma is then evacuated and the bleeding point usually identified with ease. It is possible, however, for the patient to lose considerable blood during the brief period before bleeding is controlled, so transfusion may be necessary. After bleeding is controlled, the dura is held up against the inner skull table by several sutures to prevent recurrent accumulation of blood and fluid in the epidural space. The dura is then opened for a few millimeters only to exclude the remote possibility of an associated subdural hematoma.

Prognosis. Prognosis must be considered in terms of survival and residual deficit, and depends principally on the neurologic state at the time of actual decompression. If the child has reached the state of apnea and bilateral pupillary dilatation, survival or significant recovery are unlikely; if hematoma evacuation is accomplished before brain stem decompensation has occurred, survival and neurologic recovery are the rule. In most reported series, mortality in the pediatric age group is 5% to 10%; for those with residual neurologic deficit it is 5% to 10% higher.

Subdural Hematoma

Subdural hematomas have been arbitrarily classified as acute, subacute, or chronic depending on whether they are less than 3 days old, 3 to 10 days old, or older than 10 days. This classification may have merit in relation to pathophysiology, but it is somewhat artificial in that it delineates only the duration of the lesion before it becomes manifest rather than any basic difference in the disease process. In the pediatric patient, as with adults, chronic subdural hematomas are seen often as pure lesions, whereas acute hematomas are most apt to be associated with other intracranial injury. Although acute hematomas may occur at any pediatric age, chronic hematomas are more commonly encountered during infancy.

Acute Subdural Hematoma. Acute subdural hemorrhage may be difficult to distinguish from epidural hematoma because the time sequence of manifestations may be similar. Bleeding is most often from an arterial channel on the brain surface and is rarely of venous origin. Because a blow of sufficient force to tear a surface artery is likely also to cause considerable bruising and laceration of the brain tissue, the clinical features are a combination of these pathologic processes. The hematoma is usually a relatively thin layer of blood diffusely distributed over the cerebral convexity, in contrast to the thicker and more localized extradural hematoma. An acute subdural hematoma less than 5 mm thick is probably of little clinical significance.

Clinical Features. The initial injury in subdural hematoma is usually more severe than that which leads to extradural bleeding. The infant or child has usually had an extended period of unconsciousness or frequently may exhibit continuous lack of awareness with a superimposed, progressively deeper coma and signs of herniation. Intracranial pathophysiology involves an extracerebral expanding mass in combination with a bruised, swollen brain. Thus, although acute subdural hematomas may present with a lucid interval, the more common history is one of continuous unconsciousness from the time of injury. The ensuing manifestations include deterioration of the conscious level, evidence of progressive hemiplegia, and, finally, signs of uncal herniation. The last causes pupillary enlargement, changes in vital signs, development of the decerebrate state, and, finally, respiratory failure.

Diagnostic Studies. In general, acute subdural hematomas are not quite as critically emergent as extradural hematomas. The reason for the difference, since both are usually of arterial origin, is that the extradural hematoma's position low in the temporal fossa may lead to uncal herniation and brain stem decompensation more rapidly

than the hemorrhage that extends diffusely over the upper brain convexity. Because of this difference in urgency of management, more time is usually available for diagnostic studies of acute subdural hematomas.

Roentgenograms frequently show a fracture, although the absence of a fracture does not exclude subdural hemorrhage. CT scan is the most reliable noninvasive method of diagnosis (Fig. 13-22). The acute subdural hematoma, usually unilateral, is characteristically seen as a crescentic hyperdense surface lesion. Sonography may also demonstrate the surface lesion in infants less than 1 year old but is less effective than CT scanning. The diagnosis can usually be firmly established before any invasive diagnostic or therapeutic measures are undertaken.

Treatment. As with other hematomas, the ultimate aim of management is hematoma evacuation. If clinical deteriora-

FIG. 13-22. CT scan showing crescentic hyperdense area over left hemisphere (acute subdural hematoma) with marked shift of ventricular system to right.

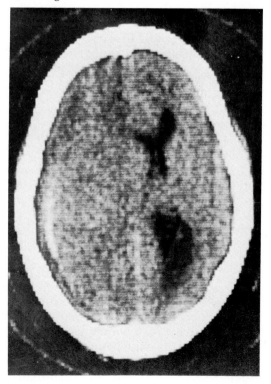

tion is rapidly progressive, hyperventilation and hypertonic agents are recommended to delay intracranial decompensation. As quickly as possible, multiple, bilateral burr holes are made (unless arteriography has demonstrated unilaterality of the lesion), and the hematoma is evacuated. A more extensive cranial opening may be necessary to evacuate a solid hematoma or to find and control bleeding sources on the brain surface. The underlying brain is frequently contused and swollen from the initial injury.

Chronic Subdural Hematoma. Although chronic subdural hematoma may occur at any age, it occurs with sufficient frequency during infancy to constitute a specific clinical entity. The peak incidence is seen at about 6 months, and few are seen after 1 year of age. The following remarks, therefore, are directed to a consideration of the unique diagnostic and therapeutic features of the chronic subdural hematoma as it occurs during the first few months of life.

Suspicion that a lesion is present generally comes from the family physician or the pediatrician. The initiating event is probably mechanical trauma to the head in nearly all instances. The specific event, however, is rarely documented by history, and it must be concluded that the average infant is subject to minor but potentially damaging head injury without necessarily showing external evidence of the trauma. Birth trauma rarely results in chronic hematoma, despite the head molding that frequently occurs and the incidence of subgaleal bleeding. The "battered" infant may present with subdural hematoma and is seen sufficiently often to permit the recommendation that all infants with subdural hematoma have thorough evaluation, including x-ray studies of long bones, for evidence of other trauma that may be old and healed.

Regardless of the mechanism of injury, the result is tearing of the veins connecting the brain to the major dural sinuses and consequent bleeding into the subdural space. Bleeding is under low pressure and does not accumulate rapidly. Because the subdural space is continuous over the hemisphere convexities and across the midline, the subdural accumulation is usually bilateral and widespread. The original attractive concept that a subdural hematoma gradually increases in size as a result of hemoglobin breakdown and osmotic attraction of water across the inner membrane has little support at present. It appears, however, that the original hematoma may cause some brain compression and also that it may stimulate membrane formation that encapsulates the hematoma. The encapsulated mass may actually enlarge, but this seems to be due to repeated bleeding from the fragile vessels of the neomembrane. The combination of reexpansion of the normal brain and the enlarging hematoma leads to the clinical consequence of chronic intracranial hypertension.

Clinical Features. The clinical picture is variable and often quite subtle during infancy. This is due to the chronicity of the pathophysiologic process and the flexibility of the infant's skull so that increased pressure of modest degree can be tolerated fairly well owing to accommodation of the cranial vault. One of the most common presenting symptoms is convulsions, usually generalized. Any infant who has onset of seizures after 3 months of age without evidence of fever or of abnormal calcium or carbohydrate metabolism must be considered as possibly harboring a subdural hematoma. Other presenting features may include hyperirritability or abnormal lethargy. Vomiting, poor feeding, and failure to gain weight are other commonly seen nonspecific symptoms.

The most important features are usually found on examination. There is often increased tone and hyperreflexia of the extremities. The evidence of intracranial hypertension is found in the presence of fullness or tightness of the fontanel, frequently with palpable separation of the sutures, and with a "crackpot" percussion note to the skull. Approximately one third of patients demonstrate definite macrocrania as indicated on standard charts of head growth (Fig. 13-23). This is usually of mild degree, rarely greater than 2 cm above the 90th percentile limit, in contrast to more extreme degrees of cranial enlargement seen with hydrocephalus. It has been stated that macrocrania characterized by biparietal enlargement is due to subdural hematoma, whereas fronto-occipital enlargement means hydrocephalus. Funduscopic examination is especially important in infantile macrocrania because of the frequency of hemorrhages when the offending lesion is a subdural hematoma. These hemorrhages are characteristically "subhyaloid" in type rather than small splinter or perivascular.

Special studies that may contribute to the diagnosis include blood count and roentgenograms. Subdural bleeding in the infant may be responsible for blood loss sufficient to account for anemia, which is accentuated by the nutritional impairment that results from poor feeding and vomiting. X-ray examination of the skull may demonstrate clear-cut evidence of trauma, or this may be suspected from evidence of healed injury elsewhere in the body.

Diagnosis can usually be established conclusively by noninvasive techniques, including ultrasonography (Fig. 13-24) and CT scan (Fig. 13-25). As noted earlier, ultrasonography is useful only during the period in which the fontanel is open, that is, the first 1 to 1½ years of age. Chronic subdural hematomas usually appear as bilateral vacant spaces between the brain tissue and the skull table. The CT scan also shows hypodense areas over the cerebral surfaces.

The final definitive diagnostic procedure, direct tapping of the subdural space, is actually a therapeutic maneuver. This is done by inserting a needle through a properly shaved and prepared scalp, through the lateral border of the fontanel or a coronal suture, and finally penetrating the dura. Bilateral tapping should always be done, each needle being inserted at least 1.5 to 2 cm from the midline. Subdural fluid should not be aspirated, but if a chronic hematoma is present, serosanguineous fluid drains spontaneously.

Treatment. The principles for treating infantile subdural hematomas have changed during the past few decades, and there is still not universal agreement. The problem has two components: proper management of the subdural accumulation, and whether there is need for removal of subdural membranes.

The original concept that there is functional restriction of the normal growth potential of the brain by neomembranes seems to have been largely abandoned. Although the concept was attractive, subsequent evidence accumulated in large series of cases has not borne out the need for membrane removal in order to achieve growth potential. Moreover, the argument is offered that if brain growth is sufficiently forceful under normal circumstances to enlarge the scalp, skull, and dura, the addition of a neomembrane to this list of restricting influences should not lead to limitation of growth. Thus, there is little enthusiasm at present for craniotomy performed purely for membrane removal (Fig. 13-26).

The main part of treatment consists in removal of the subdural fluid contents.[8] Treatment, therefore, is automatically initiated when the diagnosis is made and fluid is allowed to escape. Tapping may then be repeated at intervals of 1 day or more to achieve progressive depletion of the subdural accumulation (Fig. 13-27). Repeat taps

FIG. 13-23. Mild macrocrania, which is seen in some instances of infantile subdural hematomas. The infant developed normally after subdural tapping of the hematoma.

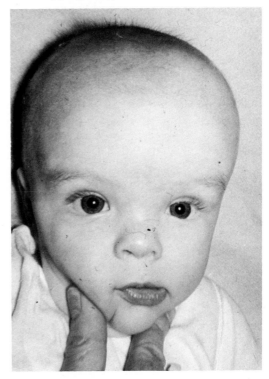

are indicated as long as there is clinical evidence of increased pressure (e.g., fontanelle tension or vomiting) but may be gradually discontinued when hypertension no longer exists. It is probably not essential to evacuate completely all subdural contents, because the subdural space has some reabsorptive potential.

In occasional instances, repeated intermittent tapping does not seem to control continued reaccumulation of fluid and pressure. Under such circumstances, some type of shunt procedure is indicated so that there is continued drainage of subdural fluid elsewhere in the body. Shunting is most frequently done to the vascular system by

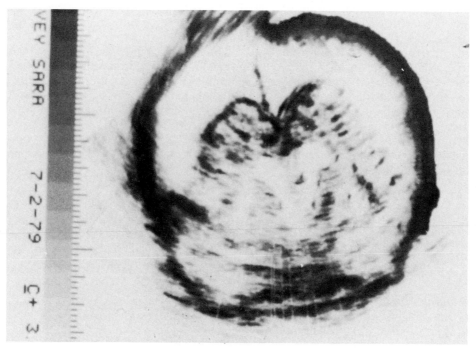

FIG. 13-24. Sonogram showing large bilateral subdural hematomas.

FIG. 13-25. Serial CT scans showing progressive decrease in infantile subdural hematomas and reexpansion of brain.

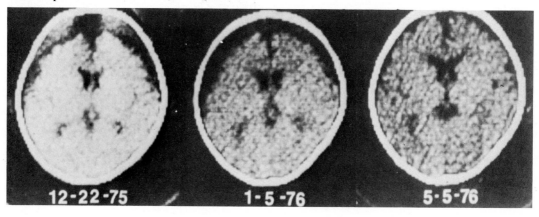

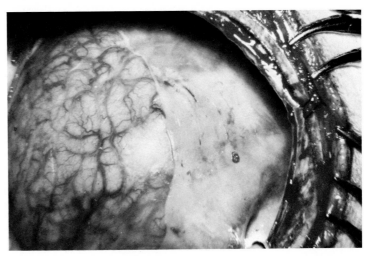

FIG. 13-26. Typical membrane associated with a subdural hematoma. The space between this inner membrane and the dura is seen.

way of the jugular vein, or to the peritoneal cavity.

When treating subdural hematoma, attention must also be paid to the seizure tendency and to anemia, if these exist. It is generally unnecessary to replace blood loss by transfusion, but administration of iron is advisable to compensate for that being depleted by way of the subdural fluid. If seizures have occurred as part of the presenting symptomatology, anticonvulsant therapy should be continued for several months after resolution of the hematoma.

Occasionally, subdural hematomas are accompanied by hydrocephalus, presumably owing to failure of the subarachnoid spaces to permit CSF reabsorption (Fig. 13-28). When hydrocephalus does occur, it must be treated separately, usually by some means of ventricular shunting. The prognosis for psychomotor development is greatly reduced when the combination of subdural hematoma and hydrocephalus coexist.

Prognosis. The prognosis depends mainly on the effect of the initial trauma on the brain; the secondary effects of the hematoma are usually reversible with early recognition and treatment. In nearly all reported series, the incidence of normal psychomotor development is approximately 75%. The remaining 25% of impaired children probably represent those whose brains were seriously damaged at the time of the initial trauma or by preceding injury. Re-

FIG. 13-27. Consecutive subdural taps produce gradual clearing of bloody fluid obtained initially.

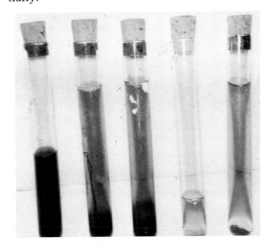

sidual convulsive tendency is extremely rare.

Calcified Subdural Hematoma. Occasionally, a subdural hematoma persists long enough to become partially calcified; this lesion can be visualized on plain radiographs (Fig. 13-29). The persistence of a hematoma is probably due to injury to the underlying brain sufficient to cause atrophy of the brain substance. This allows continued accumulation of surface hematoma, for if the brain is not simultaneously damaged, symptoms of intracranial hypertension and focal deficit occur earlier as described above.

The clinical manifestations accompanying calcified hematoma are principally those of underlying brain damage. Retardation is commonly present, and convulsions have been described in at least half the cases. In addition to the calcification, roentgenograms show evidence of cerebral or hemicerebral atrophy with thickened bone in the calvarium and enlargement of the air-containing spaces at the base of the skull. Electroencephalography is almost always abnormal with a generalized, slow dysrhythmia, and, in certain instances, a focal paroxysmal dysrhythmia.

Whether surgical removal should be recommended is still uncertain, because there is scant evidence of postoperative improvement in these children (Fig. 13-30). There has been no conclusive evidence to indicate improvement of psychomotor development of function, or a decrease of seizure tendency. This lack of benefit is consistent with the concept that the principal damage is to the brain and that the hematoma is an incidental accompaniment.

Subdural Hydroma. Subdural hydroma is a posttraumatic collection of blood-tinged or xanthochromic cerebrospinal fluid in the subdural space. The usually accepted explanation of its existence is that a tear of the arachnoid results in a valvelike action that allows fluid to escape from the subarachnoid compartment to the subdural compartment. The consequence is an accumulation that acts like any other expanding and compressing lesion. Thus, the symptoms and signs are similar to those of a subdural hematoma, and from the standpoint

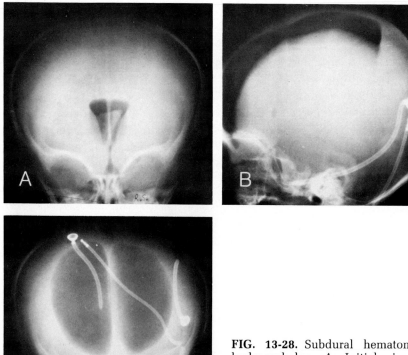

FIG. 13-28. Subdural hematoma associated with hydrocephalus. *A.* Initial size of ventricles and macrocrania. *B.* Air in subdural space showing depth of hematoma. Subdural shunt in place. *C.* Hydrocephalus, which occurred later. Ventricular shunt has been inserted.

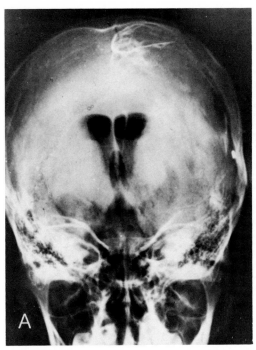
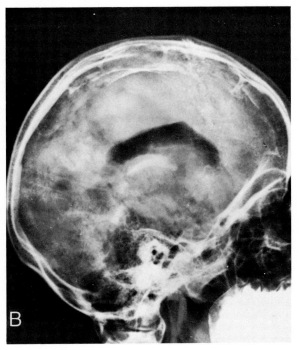
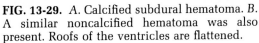

FIG. 13-29. *A.* Calcified subdural hematoma. *B.* A similar noncalcified hematoma was also present. Roofs of the ventricles are flattened.

of timing it compares to a subacute hematoma. It is possible that many subdural hydromas are unrecognized and undergo spontaneous resolution, because there is no question that fluid can be absorbed from the subdural space. If, however, there is evidence of progressive intracranial hypertension and neurologic deficit, the lesion is easily correctible by drainage through burr holes. For unknown reasons, this lesion is rare in infants but does occur in older children. The prognosis is excellent for complete recovery.

Intracerebral Hematoma

Intracerebral hematoma—bleeding within the parenchyma of the brain—is the result of shearing forces in the brain at the time of impact. The true incidence is difficult to define because it becomes a matter of definition concerning where contusion with multiple hemorrhages ends and localized hematoma begins. Thus, a localized intracerebral hemorrhage may be due to coalescence of small hemorrhages or to tearing

of a major vessel within the brain substance. The most common site is the temporal lobe, for the same reasons which make that part of the brain most susceptible to contusion.

The signs of intracerebral hematoma are similar to those of any other intracranial hematoma, and are usually indistinguishable from surface hematomas clinically. When the temporal lobe is the site of hemorrhage there is paresis of the opposite face and arm, and if the left temporal lobe is involved dysphasia is also present. A lucid interval may occur between the initial impact and the onset of localizing signs, or the child may be unconscious from the beginning. The signs of hematoma usually appear within 2 to 4 days after injury and therefore may be confused with a subacute subdural or a late extradural hemorrhage. As the hematoma expands, accompanied by swelling of surrounding brain substances, there eventually occurs uncal herniation with the characteristic signs of oculomotor paresis and brain stem dysfunction. Because the temporal lobe is commonly the site of hematoma, herniation often occurs fairly early in the clinical sequence.

Definitive diagnosis is usually made

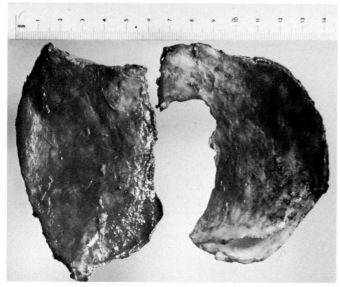

FIG. 13-30. Calcified subdural hematomas removed at operation.

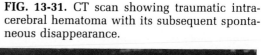

FIG. 13-31. CT scan showing traumatic intracerebral hematoma with its subsequent spontaneous disappearance.

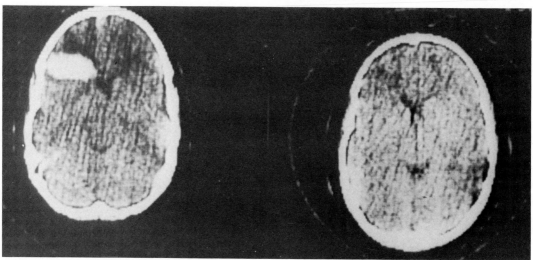

by CT scan if the equipment is available (Fig. 13-31). This usually defines accurately the location and extent of the hemorrhage as well as its relationship to the surface of the brain. The latter information may be of importance in planning the least destructive transcortical surgical approach to the hematoma. If any reasonable question ex-

ists about the traumatic origin of the hematoma, angiography may be necessary to determine whether a vascular malformation is present.

The prognosis following intracerebral hematoma removal is not as good as the prognosis after surface hemorrhage. This is understandable, because the brain parenchyma is necessarily destroyed in the process of hemorrhage rather than simply being compressed by a surface mass. Thus, permanent neurologic deficit and convulsive disorders frequently occur.

BIRTH INJURY

Birth injury is any injury to the brain or its coverings sustained during the process of birth.[1] The injury may result from application of forceps or from forces exerted on the skull during labor. The latter include compression of the skull during labor by a contracted pelvis, trauma to the skull against the pelvic floor during uterine contractions, breech delivery, and damage to the brain from pressure changes at the time of placental membrane rupture.

The factor of prematurity has been noted by many observers. Intracranial bleeding is several times more frequent in premature than in term infants. Intracerebral hemorrhage, specifically, is rare in term infants but not uncommon in premature babies. The exact basis for the role of prematurity is not clear, but it is probably related to the structural consistency of the premature skull and brain, which renders them more susceptible to the strains and forces of delivery. Birth injuries, as head injuries of later life, must be considered from the standpoint of injuries to the skull, the meninges, and the brain.

Skull Injuries

Skull fractures may be linear or depressed. Basal fractures do not result from birth trauma. Linear fractures may occur in any of the bones of the cranial vault. Depressed fractures may result from application of forceps or from forceful manipulation of the head by the obstetrician (see Fig. 13-16); these are "ping-pong" fractures and are easily corrected by simple surgery (Fig. 13-32). In many instances, small degrees of depression may be left alone because normal growth tends to correct them. No treatment is necessary for linear fracture. In general, skull injuries are of no consequence, and the more serious accompaniment is intracranial bleeding or brain damage.

Intracranial Hemorrhage

Hemorrhage may occur within the brain substance or ventricle, or on the surface of the brain from meningeal injury. While anoxia is thought to play a role as a contributory factor in intracranial hemorrhage, it seems likely that mechanical factors, such

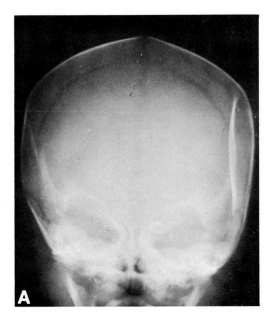

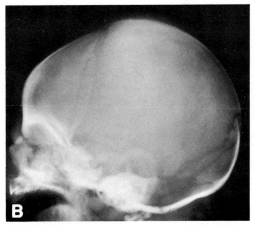

FIG. 13-32. Frontal (A) and lateral (B) skull roentgenograms. Ping-pong depressed fracture in left parietal bone of newborn.

as direct trauma, tentorial lacerations, and intracranial hypertension, are of primary importance. In the normal process of delivery, molding of the head occurs with overriding of the cranial bones. It is understandable that such molding may tear bridging veins between the brain and dural sinuses. Forceps also cause pressure on the cranial bones, and hemorrhage from meningeal tears. The incidence of fatality from intracranial injury is higher in term infants than in premature ones. It is noteworthy, however, that the incidence of birth trauma has markedly declined during the past few decades.

Tears of the tentorium at its junction with the falx have been recognized for years. The mechanism is presumably related to squeezing the head in a lateral or an anteroposterior direction; the consequent moldings lead to tears of the semirigid dural structures. The vein of Galen is torn when this injury occurs, and this leads to intracerebral and surface bleeding. Intracranial hypertension during labor is also thought to contribute to hemorrhage by raising the systemic blood pressure and causing ischemia with localized vascular necrosis.

Intracranial hemorrhage may consist principally of meningeal bleeding. Although the various locations of hemorrhage are similar to those occurring in older infants and children, the clinical distinction is less definite. Extradural hemorrhage due to birth trauma is quite rare, but when it occurs it is always associated with a fracture, frequently a depressed fracture. Subdural hemorrhage is much more common and is of the acute variety; rarely does the hematoma persist to a chronic stage. The symptoms of subdural hematoma due to birth trauma are irritability, convulsions, tight fontanelle, and frequently shock from intracranial blood loss. Tapping the subdural space is not a conclusive diagnostic test, because the blood may be in a semisolid state. Rarely is surgery necessary to remove neonatal subdural hemorrhage, and probably in most instances the subdural blood is reabsorbed if the infant survives.

Subarachnoid hemorrhage from birth trauma is not fatal in itself. Its incidence is probably fairly high (greater than 10%), but its only serious consequence is that it may contribute to a subsequent nonabsorptive hydrocephalus. The symptoms include irritability, nuchal resistence, fullness of the fontanelle, poor feeding, and convulsions. There is no specific treatment because the blood is invariably absorbed from the cerebrospinal fluid, but hydrocephalus must be sought.

Intraventricular hemorrhage occurs almost exclusively in premature infants and is presumed to be related to hypoxic changes. It is due to subependymal hemorrhage from terminal vein rupture and subsequent rupture into the ventrical. Intraventricular hemorrhage is probably fatal in most instances, and no effective treatment is available.

Intracerebral hemorrhage usually occurs in association with surface bleeding. When found alone, it is likely not due to mechanical trauma but to hypoxia. When intracerebral hemorrhage is due to a mechanical factor, it is usually a result of severe birth injury. The hemorrhage may consist in a single large hematoma within the white matter of the hemisphere with damage to basal ganglia. More commonly, it consists in petechial hemorrhages throughout the white matter and base of the brain. The petechiae are characteristically perivascular. The manifestations of intracerebral hemorrhage include lethargy or coma, respiratory irregularity, fever, convulsions, high-pitched cry, and fullness of the fontanelle. If the clinical diagnosis can be made, there is no specific treatment other than respiratory, nutritional, and temperature support.

The sequelae of birth injury are sometimes difficult to associate directly with the initial trauma. Nevertheless, they include specific neurologic deficits (hemiplegia, diplegia, etc.), psychomotor developmental retardation, porencephaly, hydrocephalus, and probably convulsive states.

LATE SEQUELAE OF HEAD INJURY

Certain late effects of head injury may become apparent within a few weeks following trauma or may not be recognized for several years. They must be anticipated and recognized, however, and their relationship to injury appreciated. Although head injury is generally thought of as an acute disease, there are certain late residual effects and complications that may make it a chronic illness.

Neurologic Deficits

Neurologic deficits may involve the brain or the cranial nerves. Certain cranial nerves are particularly susceptible to injury, either by direct trauma from a basal fracture or by stretching from deceleration or acceleration. The olfactory, optic, oculomotor, facial, and acoustic nerves are injured most often by fractures. Paralysis of the olfactory and optic nerves rarely improves; extraocular movement disorders usually recover over a period of several months. Facial nerve paralysis, especially if not immediate in onset, usually improves; however, if degeneration can be demonstrated electrically within 10 days after injury consideration should be given to exploration and attempted repair. Acceleration–deceleration injuries are most likely to damage the olfactory and abducens nerves. Falls on the back of the head may result in tearing of the olfactory fibers at the cribriform plate. The mechanism of abducens nerve paralysis is not clear but is presumably related to its long and circuitous intracranial course; it may be uni- or bilateral, but the prognosis is favorable for recovery.

Residual effects of brain damage may be focal or generalized. The most common deficits are motor dysfunctions, retardation of psychomotor development, and behavior disorders. Motor loss, either uni- or bilateral, is usually accompanied by permanent evidence of spasticity. There is improvement over a period of about 2 years, but little recovery can be expected thereafter; the major part of recovery occurs within the first 6 months after injury. Rehabilitation therapy is helpful in expediting the recovery process and minimizing the residual functional deficit.

Generalized cerebral damage may result in impaired intellectual development. After acute injury in infants, there may be slowing of the developmental motor milestones, usually followed by intellectual deficit and retardation as the child becomes older. In older children, impairment of memory, concentration, and analytic men-

tation may persist permanently. It should be noted that the "postconcussion syndrome," characterized by headache, dizziness, and nervous instability, is only rarely seen in children and, when it does occur, is usually temporary. It may be distinguished from permanent sequelae by psychometric evaluation, which is necessary for proper educational planning.

Behavior disorders are frequently difficult to evaluate in relation to head injury, particularly where litigation is involved. As with psychomotor impairment, behavior disturbance follows severe injury, usually cerebral contusion. It may appear during convalescence and subside over weeks or months, or it may persist indefinitely. It involves hyperactive, impulsive, destructive behavior with loss of inhibition or self-restraint. While drugs may be of symptomatic benefit, the ultimate prognosis is poor.

Posttraumatic Epilepsy

Epilepsy may be a complication of either closed or open head injury and may occur either early or late. The incidence of epilepsy varies considerably in different reports but is invariably higher after open head injury, especially following penetrating wounds. Approximate figures include an incidence of 4% to 6% after closed and 15% to 25% after open injury.

Early epilepsy is that which occurs within the first week after trauma; most early seizures occur within the first 24 hours. It is particularly significant that the incidence is about twice as high in children under 5 years of age as it is thereafter, a manifestation of the greater susceptibility of the young brain to seizure activity. Moreover, presence of a fracture or the development of an intracranial hematoma increases the incidence of seizures. The principal significance of early epilepsy is that it is associated with late seizures in about 25% of cases; hence, early seizures indicate the need for careful electroencephalographic and clinical observation during the ensuing years. It is recommended that anticonvulsant therapy be continued for a period of at least 2 years after an early seizure. Seizure onset rarely occurs later than 2 years after injury if there are no early attacks.

Seizures may be either focal or generalized, depending on the severity and extent of the epileptogenic focus. Focal seizures are likely to be accompanied by a spiking focus in the electroencephalogram in the appropriate brain area. It is also commonly associated with porencephalic cavitation within the brain substance as seen by air-contrast studies (Fig. 13-33) or CT scan. Epilepsia partialis continua, repeated focal epileptic attacks, may also occur. In most instances, posttraumatic seizures can be controlled by anticonvulsant medication, but occasionally surgical excision of a focus is necessary. This should be undertaken only after a conscientious and intensive trial of medication and when the focus is clearly delineated clinically and electroencephalographically.

It is occasionally difficult to distinguish epilepsy due to trauma from an idiopathic convulsive disorder with onset precipitated by trauma. This distinction becomes particularly important in medicolegal matters. True posttraumatic epilepsy should be preceded by a significantly severe injury, and the electroencephalographic focus and type of seizure should be consistent. There should be no history of pretrauma seizures, although a family history of epilepsy does not exclude posttraumatic epilepsy. It should be emphasized that true petit mal probably never occurs on a traumatic basis.

Posttraumatic Hydrocephalus

Occasionally, hydrocephalus follows head injury and is seemingly due to obstruction of the subarachnoid pathways. It is not likely to occur during the first few postnatal weeks or months, or following traumatic birth. Evidence supports the conclusion that intracranial bleeding, particularly of a repeated nature, leads to thickening of the arachnoid and obliteration of the subarachnoid pathways, especially at the base of the brain. This in turn leads to failure of CSF reabsorption and a communicating hydrocephalus.

Clinically, the evidence for hydrocephalus after birth trauma or head injury during early infancy consists in signs of intracranial hypertension, including increased fontanelle tension, cranial enlargement beyond the normal range, abnormal suture separation, irritability, and vomiting. Subdural hematoma may be excluded and ventriculomegaly demonstrated by the CT scan. Treatment consists of shunting the CSF, usually to the peritoneal cavity.

Hydrocephalus occasionally complicates infantile subdural hematoma. It can be recognized by persistent intracranial hypertension after the subdural accumulation has been evacuated; diagnosis and treatment are the same as above. The prognosis, however, appears to be considerably worse in this group of infants with respect to their ultimate psychomotor development.

Older children, like adults, may dem-

FIG. 13-33. Air-contrast studies. Frontal (A) and lateral (B) views. Porencephalic cavitation of left ventricle due to trauma.

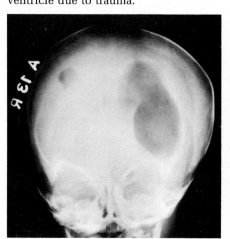
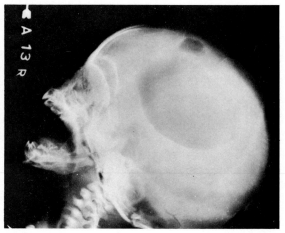

onstrate a type of ventricular dilatation after severe head injury that appears to be a form of hydrocephalus *ex vacuo*. There is no evidence of intracranial hypertension, but the ventricular enlargement is due to generalized loss of brain substance. It is extremely difficult in such cases to define precisely whether the pathogenesis may be partly due to subarachnoid blockage secondary to bleeding from the initial trauma. Although shunts in such patients should be considered, the outlook for significant improvement of cerebral function is usually disappointing.

Carotid-Cavernous Fistula

A rather rare complication of head injury, carotid-cavernous fistula occurs in children as well as in adults. The injury is usually frontal and on the same side as the subsequent arteriovenous fistula. Fractures of the sphenoid bone may cause direct tear of the carotid artery or shearing of some of the smaller intracavernous branches of the artery. In either event, the result is a direct communication between the carotid artery and the cavernous sinus. Symptoms and signs resulting from this fistula may be present within a few days after injury but more often are delayed several weeks or months.

The most characteristic sign is a bruit, which can nearly always be heard by the patient and usually by the examiner during auscultation over the affected eye. The bruit can be abolished by compressing the ipsilateral cervical carotid artery. A second sign is proptosis of the affected eye associated with chemosis and increased corneal and retinal vascularity. This is due to the arterial pressure within the draining venous system leading to marked venous distention of the orbit and eye. The proptosis is characteristically pulsatile. Extraocular motor nerves are often impaired, and the abducens nerve is more frequently involved than the oculomotor or trochlear nerve. Finally, there is often some impairment of vision. This may be due to direct injury to the optic nerve at the time of initial trauma or to a subsequent decrease in perfusion pressure of the retina resulting from the arteriovenous fistula. Occasionally, the proptosis and extraocular impair-

ment are seen also in the opposite eye, but visual impairment is confined to the side of the fistula.

Although the clinical picture is usually unmistakable, arteriography is necessary to confirm the lesion and the hemodynamics of the vascular supply (Fig. 13-34). Bilateral arteriography is essential because treatment usually includes sacrifice of the ipsilateral carotid artery.

Treatment is essential to eliminate the annoying bruit and to preserve remaining visual function in the affected eye. Treatment usually consists of clamping of the carotid artery above the fistula, embolization of the fistula from below, and, finally, occlusion of the internal carotid artery in the neck. This procedure obliterates most fistulas and is followed by cessation of bruit, subsidence of proptosis, and improved extraocular function.

Leptomeningeal Cyst

Skull fractures in infants and children usually heal without difficulty, but rarely there is progressive enlargement of the fracture site over a period of months and years. The syndrome accompanying the "growing skull fracture of childhood" is sufficiently frequent and reproducible to constitute a clinical entity. It occurs only during childhood or infancy, usually within the first year. The fracture site is predominantly in the parietal bone but rarely occurs in frontal or occipital bones. The fracture characteristically has some separation of the bone initially, which then progresses slowly with eburnation and erosion of the margins (Fig. 13-35). This is accompanied in most instances by soft, pulsatile swelling beneath the scalp and overlying the fracture site.

The pathogenesis of this lesion includes a tear of the dura, and herniation of the cerebral substance and leptomeninges through the dural defect (Fig. 13-36 and 13-37). The dura, then, does not close, but a cystic, fluid-filled herniation persists—hence the term *leptomeningeal cyst*. The pulsating cyst presumably erodes the cranial bone.

A fairly constant feature of the syndrome is the local brain injury beneath the skull lesion. This results in hemiparesis, hemiatrophy, or focal seizures. Porencephalic cavitation may extend outward from

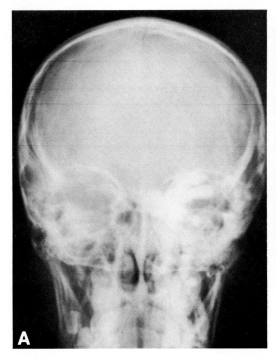

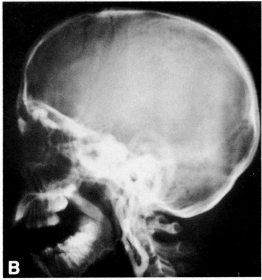

FIG. 13-34. Carotid–cavernous fistula. Cerebral angiogram. *A.* Frontal view. The carotid artery empties into a large collection of opaque substance at the level of the cavernous sinus. *B.* A dilated superior orbital vein is seen on the lateral view.

the ventricle toward the surface lesion, as seen on pneumoencephalography.

Treatment consists in operative repair of the defective dura by use of fascia or a dural substitute, followed by some type of cranioplasty to close the cranial defect.

Cranial Defects

There are several causes of cranial defects in children, but among the most common are those relating to trauma. The defect may result from debridement of a compound depressed fracture, craniectomy for removal of intracranial hematomas, or erosion of a growing fracture. Whatever the cause, cranioplasty is indicated for cosmetic reasons and for protection of the intracranial contents. Cranioplasty is done for smaller fractures in the supraorbital region most often for cosmetic reasons. Over the remaining part of the cranial vault, defects larger than 3 cm in diameter and not covered by muscle should be corrected by cranioplasty. The traditional concept that cranioplasty should not be done during early childhood or in-

fancy because the growing skull will result in an ill-fitting prosthesis seems to have no validity; the skull defect does not grow as the cranial vault enlarges. There are several types of cranioplasty substances, including plastic, metals, and autogenous bone, and the choice of materials is largely based on personal surgical preference.

Cerebrospinal Fluid Rhinorrhea

Although spinal fluid leakage is usually noted early after injury and stops within a week, it is occasionally recognized only as a late complication of head injury. In some instances, there appears to be late onset of the drainage owing to a temporary seal having been provided by blood clot, damaged brain tissue, or herniation of brain through a bony defect. In such cases, the onset of drainage may be precipitated by coughing or sneezing or by some sudden elevation of intracranial pressure. In other patients, the onset of rhinorrhea may not be delayed, but its recognition may depend on the occur-

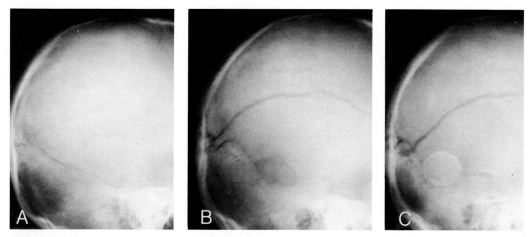

FIG. 13-35. *A.* Linear fracture. *B.* Subsequent erosion due to leptomeningeal cyst. *C.* Cranioplasty of the skull defect is shown after insertion of stainless steel mesh.

FIG. 13-36. A leptomeningeal cyst and a porencephalic cyst, each associated with a skull defect due to erosion.

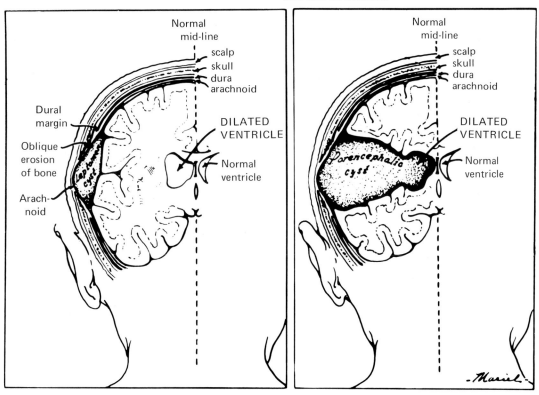

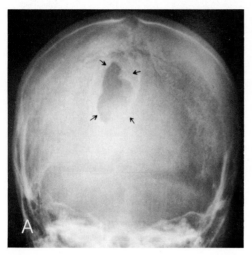
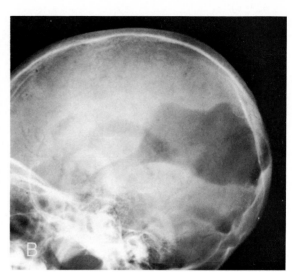

FIG. 13-37. *A.* Skull defect *(arrows)*. *B.* Underlying porencephalic cyst.

rence of intracranial infection. Thus, the first clue to long-standing leakage may be the onset of meningitis. A corollary of this is that, in cases of unexplained meningitis, particularly if recurrent, the possibility of an old basal injury should be suspected and sought. The organism most often responsible for meningitis secondary to cerebrospinal leakage through the skull is *Pneumococcus.*

Most fractures leading to persistent rhinorrhea involve the bony walls of the frontal or ethmoidal sinuses. By proper posturing, a few drops of fluid can be collected from the nose, and the presence of glucose distinguishes it as CSF. Occasionally, the usual radiographic techniques are inadequate to demonstrate the fracture site, and tomography may be necessary. If the fracture still is not detected, the point of leakage may be demonstrated by the use of dyes or radionuclides injected intrathecally, with subsequent retrieval from the nasal passages or visualization by scanning techniques.

Whatever the method used to delineate the point of drainage, the treatment consists in surgical repair by craniotomy. The operation is usually not difficult and is very often successful.

REFERENCES

1. **Alpers BJ, Berry RG:** Cerebral birth injuries. In Brock S (ed): Injuries of the Brain and Spinal Cord and Their Coverings, 4th ed, pp 225–284. New York, Springer-Verlag, 1960

2. **DeLand FH, Wagner HN Jr:** Atlas of Nuclear Medicine, Vol 1, Brain, pp 54–65, 177–211. Philadelphia, WB Saunders, 1969

3. **Ford LE, McLaurin RL:** Mechanisms of extradural hematomas. J Neurosurg 20:760, 1963

4. **Kooi KA:** Fundamentals of Electroencephalography, pp 198–205. New York, Harper & Row, 1971

5. **Lewin W:** The Management of Head Injuries, pp 155–187, 234–250. Baltimore, Williams & Wilkins, 1966

6. **Marshall LF, Bruce DA, Bruno L, Schut L:** Role of intracranial pressure monitoring and barbiturate therapy in malignant intracranial hypertension. Case report. J Neurosurg 47:481, 1977

7. **Matson DD:** Neurosurgery of Infancy and Childhood, 2nd ed, p 934. Springfield, Charles C Thomas, 1969

8. **McLaurin RL, Isaacs E, Lewis HP:** Results of nonoperative treatment in 15 cases of infantile subdural hematomas. J Neurosurg 34:753, 1971

9. **Schiefer W, Kazner E, Kunze S:** Clinical Echo-Encephalography, pp 87–88, 127–164. New York, Springer-Verlag, 1968

10. **Symonds C:** Concussion and contusion of the brain and their sequelae. In Brock S (ed): Injuries of the Brain and Spinal Cord and Their Coverings, 4th ed, pp 255–284. New York, Springer, 1960

11. **Teasdale G, Jennett B:** Assessment of coma and impaired consciousness. A practical scale. Lancet 2:81, 1974

Intracranial Tumors in Children

14

Ken R. Winston

It is best to not have an intracranial tumor, but given that such maladies befall children, it is important to recognize that nearly all can greatly benefit, both in terms of prolonging life (often achieving a cure) and improving its quality, from the services of a caring physician who is well informed on the subject. Almost nothing is known about the pathogenesis of tumors of the brain, and preventive medicine in this area, although a noble idea, has no foundation.

Tumor of the brain, after the leukemias and lymphomas, is the most common malignancy occurring in children under 15 years of age. The incidence is approximately 23.9 per one million children under 15 years of age per year.[53] Tumors of brain are rare in the first year of life and peak at 5 to 6 years of age. They occur more commonly in male children (approximately 56%); this is particularly true for medulloblastoma and ependymoma, which occur with approximately 66% and 69% male preponderance, respectively.[52]

The anatomic distribution of intracranial tumors in children is quite different from that in adults; 60% or more occur below the tentorium in children, and most involve the cerebellum. Three of the more common tumors of the central nervous system in children, all occurring below the tentorium, are very rare in adults: cerebellar microcystic astrocytoma, medulloblastoma, and brain stem glioma. Craniopharyngioma and optic gliomas are also more frequently diagnosed in children. Meningiomas and tumors of the pituitary gland are distinctly unusual in children.

INHERITED PROCLIVITY TO INTRACRANIAL TUMOR

There are several syndromes in which patients have an increased likelihood of intracranial tumor and a few less-well-defined patterns of apparent hereditary occurrence. The most common is von Recklinghausen's neurofibromatosis, which is inherited as an autosomal dominant trait. Regardless of criteria for diagnosis, only a very small proportion of patients with this disorder develop intracranial tumor; however, a high percentage of children with intracranial tumor have the cutaneous manifestations of this disorder, particularly *cafe-au-lait* spots. The most common intracranial tumor occurring in this syndrome is the schwannoma; however, this is quite uncommon in children. Probably all intracranial neoplasms in children occur more commonly in this syndrome, but this is particularly apparent with gliomas of the optic pathways and brain stem. The neoplasms occurring in children with neurofibromatosis are not fixed lesions, and malignancy is not uncommon.

Patients with tuberous sclerosis (Bourneville's disease), which is often familial, have a propensity for a particular type of intracranial tumor, the subependymal giant cell astrocytoma.[5] These tumors have a very characteristic histologic appearance and tend to occur near ventricular surfaces, often bulging into the ventricles. They should be distinguished from the subependymal tubers and from the gyral abnormalities. Multiple occurrence is not unusual. These tumors manifest themselves by very slow expansion and tend to be relatively benign, although malignant forms are known. The other manifestations of tuberous sclerosis are not reviewed here.

Lindau's syndrome includes hemangioblastoma of the cerebellum and some of the following: congenital cyst of the pancreas, renal tumors, von Hippel's disease (angiomatosis of the retinae), and capillary nevi of the skin. Erythrocythemia is often present with the cerebellar hemangioblastoma. Familial occurrence of this syndrome is clearly established.

CONFIDENCE IN DIAGNOSIS

Much misunderstanding surrounds the diagnostic labels for tumors of the brain. The diagnostic categories are not as distinct as the labels seem to indicate, and not even necessarily mutually exclusive. They are often so ambiguously described as to permit more than one interpretation. There is surprisingly broad latitude in the application of diagnostic labels by competent and experienced neuropatholgists. The recognition and identification of specific histologic features on a given microscopic slide varies among neuropathologists, and even with the same neuropathologist when presented with the same histologic slide on different occasions.[13] Also, many neuropathologists take into consideration a host of clinical features before assigning a diagnostic label, making their diagnosis a clinicopathologic diagnosis, and not purely a pathological diagnosis.

The clinical diagnosis of certain types of tumors has a high probability of accuracy (e.g., craniopharyngioma, glioma of optic pathways or brainstem, glioblastoma in the cerebral hemispheres, etc.). Although some children with such tumors may require surgery as a part of treatment, the acquisition of a piece of tissue for the sole purpose of making the diagnosis more certain is an overused rationalization for surgery. Although biopsy can prevent confusion of tumor with abscess, aneurysm, and demyelinating diseases, such distinctions can usually be made with high accuracy by an appropriate analysis of the clinical char-

acteristics and the results of appropriate neurodiagnostic tests. Also, the histologic appearance of a biopsy is often least ambiguous in those diagnostic categories that are least confusing from the clinical viewpoint.

MAKING A DIAGNOSIS

A thorough neurologic and general physical examination is essential, but perhaps not for the reasons some think. Intracranial tumor may be suspected, perhaps very strongly, from the clinical features, but should be diagnosed by the skillful correlation of these features with the results of neurodiagnostic tests. The clinical interpretation of symptoms and signs alone cannot be sufficiently precise for an accurate anatomic and pathologic diagnosis in a child suspected of harboring an intracranial tumor, and it is doubtful that any neurosurgeon or radiation therapist would treat a patient on purely clinical evidence. (Perhaps some extreme emergency would be an exception.) A thorough history and physical examination can give many clues to the diagnosis, but, from a practical standpoint, the history and examination are done to determine whether there is sufficient evidence to warrant neurodiagnostic tests and to determine which tests are appropriate. Still, knowledge of the patient's symptoms and signs is essential for directing the diagnostic efforts and planning the patient's treatment. Of particular usefulness in planning treatment is information on the patient's intracranial pressure, but this is often not helpful in localizing the lesion or determining its type.

The experienced clinician knows that symptoms and signs occur in recognizable patterns, not randomly. Therefore from knowledge and experience he can often suggest, with selective but remarkably little information, the correct diagnosis.

Committing to memory a list of symptoms and signs and their frequency of occurrence in children with brain tumors, whether in aggregate or by individual type, has probably never helped anyone make a diagnosis, and may do harm by distracting the inexperienced from the patterns of clinical features. Many of the reported statistics on the symptoms, signs, locations, and even incidence of some intracranial tumors, are changing because computed tomography allows earlier and more accurate detection of some tumors than was possible in the not-so-distant past. An indeterminate combination of symptoms and signs can be due to one or more non-neoplastic disorders. On the other hand, there is probably no pathognomonic clinical feature of an intracranial tumor. The clinician must be familiar with the patterns of clinical and laboratory manifestations of intracranial tumors, and we should strive to expand our knowledge of such patterns.

Tumors in the central nervous system make their presence known by symptoms and signs that result from dysfunction of nearby neural tissue and from the effects of elevated intracranial pressure. Although the rate varies, nearly all tumors expand, causing compression, destruction, or stimulation of nearby tissue; many also infiltrate, and are thereby even more harmful. As a generalization, focal symptoms are produced by alteration of function of tissue near the lesion and are therefore more useful for localization; the presence of intracranial hypertension is more indicative of the need for haste in diagnosis and treatment. Because intracranial tumors expand within a relatively confined space (the cranial vault), most tumors, particularly the rapidly growing, those obstructing the normal flow of cerebrospinal fluid, and those severely disrupting the blood-brain barrier, may get attention when relatively small. The younger the child, the less fixed this space, and the cranial vault of children may be able to compensate, in part, for the expansion of a tumor by expanding.

Headache

Elevated intracranial pressure is present in most children with intracranial tumors, and its most common symptom, headache, is also one of the least specific. The intensity varies greatly, and there is no typical headache pattern associated with tumor. Often, however, children with tumors, particularly tumors within the cerebellum or fourth ventricle, complain of headaches in the morning, and they are typically midfrontal.

It is not unusual for the headache to seem to be related to psychological or social stimuli, and it may even disappear for days or weeks. Usually, the intensity of the headaches increases and is associated later with nausea, vomiting, and finally anorexia.

Vomiting

Vomiting, particularly upon awakening in the morning, often indicates elevated intracranial pressure and is particularly common in children with large tumors in the posterior fossa. Because these episodes may clear quickly, and because the immediate result is often the missing of school or church, a psychological interpretation is commonly offered by family and physicians. Episodic vomiting without apparent cause followed by the onset of other neurologic symptoms strongly suggests tumor. The significance of "projectile vomiting" as indicative of elevated intracranial pressure has been greatly exaggerated, and it is not unusual for a parent, nurse, or even physician to describe any unexpected vomiting, particularly in an infant, as projectile. Persistent and unexplained vomiting, perhaps episodic, and particularly if *preceded* by headache, is far more characteristic of intracranial pathology. Vomiting associated with fever or diarrhea is rarely related to intracranial pathology.

Assessing Intracranial Pressure

In children with an open fontanelle, the intracranial pressure can be determined indirectly with impressive accuracy by the method of Welch.[50] With the child in the supine position, the head can be thought of as a manometer and tilted upward until the fontanelle is flat. In this position, the pressure immediately beneath the dura at the flat portion of the fontanelle is equal to atmospheric pressure. The intracranial pressure is determined by measuring the *vertical* distance between the anterior fontanelle and the point at which central venous pressure is zero, approximately the midpoint of the clavicle. Estimation of intracranial pressure by palpating the open fontanelle of a child lying flat in bed, or in any other one position, can be very misleading unless the pressure is very high. A taut fontanelle is indicative of very severely elevated pressure. The normal intracranial pressure in a child under 6 months of age is approximately 4 to 5 cm of water, and the pressure in a newborn may be much lower, even subatmospheric within the first 1 to 2 days of life.

Visual System

Papilledema is a very reliable sign of elevated intracranial pressure, but its identification requires a careful funduscopic examination which is difficult, occasionally impossible, in very young children unless they are sedated, and this may be contraindicated. Papilledema in a child under 2 years of age is unusual but does occur, particularly if intracranial pressure is very high or if it rose rapidly. Loss of visual acuity may result from chronically elevated intracranial pressure. Defects in the visual fields can often be documented, particularly in children with tumors in the sellar region (e.g., craniopharyngioma). Paresis of the abducens nerves, unilateral or bilateral, is a nonlocalizing sign of elevated intracranial pressure. Pupillary abnormalities may reflect pathology in the tectum. It has been said that the only intracranial structure that, when compressed, results in dilation of the pupil is the occulomotor nerve. Paralysis of conjugate gaze is often a sign of a lesion of the upper brain stem.

Ataxia and Dysmetria

Ataxia is a disturbance of range, rate, and direction of motion; dysmetria is the loss of ability to gauge the distance, speed, or power of a movement. Both are common in children with tumors of the posterior fossa, particularly if the tumor is within the cerebellum. If unilateral, the sign usually indicates the side of the cerebellum most severely affected. These signs are particularly characteristic of the most commonly occurring intracranial tumor of children, the type A cerebellar glioma.

Head Tilt

It is important to observe the position of the head and flexibility of the neck. Head tilt can be caused by herniation of cerebellum or the downward expansion of tumor into the foramen magnum, and is usually accompanied by stiffness of the neck. This must be distinguished from torticollis on the basis of muscular or skeletal abnormality and from a head tilt caused by a trochlear nerve palsy, the latter being relatively rare in children. As the severity of this situation becomes worse, patients may complain of pain in the neck and later maintain the neck in a strongly extended or rotated position. Typically, the head is tilted toward the more painful side and the child has suboccipital tenderness.

Cranial Nerves

Recognition of a pattern in the deficits of cranial nerves is often very useful diagnostically, and I shall mention some of these. Abducens paresis is rarely a localizing sign. Deficits in multiple cranial nerves arising from the brain stem, particularly if consecutive but not necessarily symmetric, suggests that tumor directly involves the brain stem. If the lower cranial nerves, particularly the seventh and eighth, are involved unilaterally, then there may be an extra-axial mass compressing the brain stem.

Seizures

Seizures occur in approximately 25% to 45% of children with supratentorial tumors, and in 12% of those with infratentorial tumors.[4,14] Information is sparse on the incidence of tumor in children who have seizures, and depends upon what population is examined (institutionalized patients, children who have had only one seizure, those who may have another cause for seizure such as meningitis, hemorrhage, or trauma, etc.). Location and type of tumor are the most important determinants of seizure activity. Tumors near the Rolandic fissure are particularly likely to cause seizures. Seizures caused by tumors may be of any type but tend to be focal, because they are often initiated in the neurons within or near the lesion; however, seizures can be caused by elevated intracranial pressure. It is not unusual for patients with infratentorial tumors and tight compression of the brain stem to have episodes of unresponsiveness, opisthotonos, and decerebrate posturing with clonic movements of the extremities. This is probably not a convulsive disorder, but is often so reported by inexperienced observers.

Unexpected Presentations

Sometimes intracranial tumors present in unexpected ways. Neoplastic cells in the cerebrospinal fluid can be mistaken for polymorphonuclear leukocytes or lymphocytes. By careful attention to the morphology of these cells you should avoid this mistake; however, this possibility should be considered whenever all cultures are negative and there is no response to antibiotics in a child thought to have meningitis, particularly if the case is atypical in some way.

Spontaneous subarachnoid hemorrhage may be the manner of presentation of intracranial tumor. Medulloblastoma, ependymoma, oligodendroglioma, choroid plexus papilloma, deposits of leukemic cells, and pineocytoma have presented in children in this way. The possibility of neoplasm must be considered in any child with spontaneous subarachnoid hemorrhage.

Rarely, a neurodiagnostic test done for the evaluation of a child with trauma identifies an intracranial neoplasm. Recognition of intracranial calcification in a child not suspected previously of having tumor is disturbing to all concerned, but such abnormality, once found, cannot be ignored. Not all abnormalities found in this way are tumors, and not all require treatment.

Other Clinical Manifestations of Intracranial Tumor

Other useful signs of elevated intracranial pressure include the presence of an abnormally large head, prominent veins in the scalp of young children, and the "cracked pot" sound on percussion of the head (Macewen's sign).

There are many other manifestations of intracranial neoplasia that are not reviewed here.

GUIDELINES FOR THE APPROPRIATE USE OF NEURODIAGNOSTIC TESTS

Neurodiagnostic tests are indispensable for diagnosing intracranial tumors, for planning treatment, and for predicting the prognosis of the tumor hosts, yet most are expensive, some not only in monetary terms but also in morbidity and mortality. The number of tests does *not* correlate with the quality or thoroughness of the investigation.

Examination of a child suspected of harboring a tumor within the brain is rarely, if ever, complete until the *computed tomography* is completed. This test has only a small risk of complication, is quick and relatively painless, and is both sensitive in detecting intracranial abnormality and selective in correctly identifying an abnormality as tumor. When the results are abnormal, this test alone often gives sufficient information for diagnosis and treatment. When results are normal, it strongly suggests, but does not prove, the absence of a tumor. This test is also valuable in monitoring the status of a tumor after treatment. This does not mean that the test should be done for frivolous indications, but the physician's threshold for requesting computed tomography should be low. To the chagrin of some of the best clinicians, both the very existence and the location of tumors, whose appearance on computed tomography was most obvious, have been missed.

Plain radiography of the skull is a very safe test, and about 80% of children with intracranial tumor will have some abnormality on radiographs of the skull. These abnormalities include separation of cranial sutures (usually coronal first), thinning of the posterior floor of the sella turcica, change in the shape of the dorsum sellae, demineralization of the posterior clinoid processes, accentuation of convolutional markings, local thinning of bone over a superficial mass or cyst, presence of abnormal calcification, and alteration in size or shape of cranial foramina. Radiography of the skull is a poor screening test and should not be routinely ordered in children suspected of harboring intracranial tumor. It should not be considered a prerequisite for computed tomography. *Tomography* (polytomography) of the sella or areas of calcification can be helpful occasionally.

Angiography is the only test that can detail the size, shape, and location of blood vessels. The interpretation of the study requires much skill and experience and frequent practice—more so than any other neurodiagnostic test. It is 'invasive' by nature and has significant associated complications, which should occur in less than 1% of patients when done by an experienced neuroradiologist or neurosurgeon. Since the advent of computed tomography, fewer cerebral angiograms are done each year, and, as a result, few of the younger (more recently trained) physicians gain experience in cerebral angiography; even those who are skilled and experienced get little practice.

Lumbar puncture is rarely helpful in the diagnosis of tumors but can contribute greatly to morbidity and mortality. Clinical evidence of elevated intracranial pressure in a child suspected of having a tumor should be apparent without lumbar puncture and is a strong, nearly absolute contraindication for lumbar puncture. In those rare cases in which there is strong evidence for the diffuse infiltration of the meninges by tumor, as may occur in some children with leukemia or advanced carcinomatosis (rare in children), then an examination of cerebrospinal fluid is important and can be diagnostic. Nearly all patients with elevated intracranial pressure for whom a lumbar puncture is being considered should have a prior examination with computed tomography to make certain that there is minimal risk of an intracranial herniation of brain when pressure relationships are altered.

Pneumoencephalography and *ventriculography* played a very important role in diagnostic neuroradiology in years past but are rarely indicated today. These tests demonstrate particularly well the size and shape of the ventricular system and much of the external surface of the brain, particularly when combined with polytomography. Metrizamide has nearly completely replaced gas (usually oxygen) as the agent injected for contrast. These tests continue to be useful in the evaluation of some difficult cases of suspected neoplasia that are not adequately demonstrated on computed tomography, for example, (1) evaluation of a small mass in the third ventricle (particularly near the foramina of Monro, the tuber cinereum, or the pineal gland); (2) evaluation of an occasional case of craniopharyngioma or other neoplasm within or near the sella turcica; (3) evaluation of a mass within any of the ventricles; and (4) eval-

uation of size and shape of the brain stem. In most of the foregoing, computed tomography can resolve the problem, and these more invasive tests are not necessary. Ventriculography and particularly pneumoencephalography (or any study requiring a lumbar puncture) may disrupt critical pressure relationships and allow intracranial herniations of brain (transtentorial [either upward or downward] transfalcial, or through the foramen magnum), and this must be kept in mind before a needle is inserted (see comments on lumbar puncture). For many such children, it is appropriate to have an operating room available when the test is done, particularly if gas is to be used. Ventriculography is often perceived by patients, families, and inexperienced physicians as a particularly dangerous test because it requires a needle through brain, but if done with proper precautions, it has little morbidity, usually less than in pneumoencephalography. Pneumoencephalography is often followed by significant headache and, not uncommonly, by nausea and vomiting.

Radionucleotide scans are rarely helpful in the evaluation of a child suspected of having an intracranial tumor, but in certain children they may be helpful. This test has proven useful in identifying some papillomas of the choroid plexus; however, the clinician must request that the scan be done before the agent (usually potassium perchlorate) is given to prevent the uptake of the radionucleotide by the choroid plexus. Exact localization of tumors in the cerebrum can be a difficult problem for the surgeon in patients in whom the lesion has been identified only on transverse computed tomography, and occasionally a lateral radionucleotide scan can be helpful.

Electroencephalography can identify electrical aberrations and give a rough indication of their location, but is rarely helpful today in diagnosing tumor. In patients in whom seizures are a significant part of the clinical picture (pre- or postoperatively), this test may be helpful. It is noninvasive and has no significant complications, but it may be an uncomfortable experience for some children. As a screening test for tumor and as a tool for following the status or progression of a known tumor, it is usually a waste of time and resources.

Tests of visual, auditory, and sensory evoked responses can detect functional abnormalities and are becoming increasingly popular. There is no appreciable risk of complication from these, but they have limited usefulness in diagnosing most tumors. Auditory evoked responses are being used with increasing frequency in evaluating patients with suspected abnormalities within the brain stem or in the cerebellopontine angle. Visual evoked responses and sensory evoked responses probably have a role in the evaluation of selected children with neoplasms of the optic pathways and the spinal cord, respectively. They also have been found useful for monitoring function during surgery.

The detection of tumors of the central nervous system by the detection of *chemical markers* in blood or cerebrospinal fluid continues to be an elusive yet enchanting goal.[43] Chorionic gonadotrophin, alphafetoprotein, and carcinoembryonic antigen are markers that have found some clinical application.[2] Also, the detection of polyamines in cerebrospinal fluid has been reported to be useful in detecting recurrence of medulloblastoma. The major problem with the use of information on these and a host of other chemical markers is their nonspecificity.

CHARACTERISTICS AND TREATMENT OF SPECIFIC TUMORS

Type A Cerebellar Glioma (Cerebellar Microcystic Astrocytoma)

Type A cerebellar glioma is the most common neoplasm of the nervous system in children and, if confined to the cerebellum, is, with rare exceptions, a benign lesion. There is a characteristic histologic appearance and, except in the occasional child in whom it coexists with features of other types of tumors, there should be little ambiguity in diagnosis. By definition, it is a neoplasm that is confined to the cerebellum and contains any one of the following histologic features: microcyst, Rosenthal fibers, leptomeningeal deposits of tumor, or focus of oligodendroglia.[51] The median age at diagnosis is 5 years, and it is rare beyond the teens; the median duration of symptoms before surgery was 5 months, but many have had suspicion of abnormality for several years. It usually presents with symptoms and signs of elevated intracranial pressure; however, headaches, dysmetria, and disturbance of gait tend to occur more frequently in children with this tumor than with the more malignant tumors of the cerebellum. Approximately 70% have a macrocyst, often eccentrically placed, and its appearance on computed tomography strongly suggests this diagnosis but does not prove it (Fig. 14-1). Rarely are other neurodiagnostic tests required or helpful.

Usually this lesion can be totally excised with low morbidity and mortality. The 5-year survival rate after surgery has been approximately 95%, and none of the deaths were from recurrent tumor. It is not unusual for more than one operative proce-

FIG. 14-1 Cerebellar glioma, type A. A 4-year-old child presented with headache, nausea, vomiting, ataxia, and papilledema. Computed tomography demonstrated a region of low density (a large cyst) in the cerebellum and dilated lateral and third ventricles. The tumor was surgically removed.

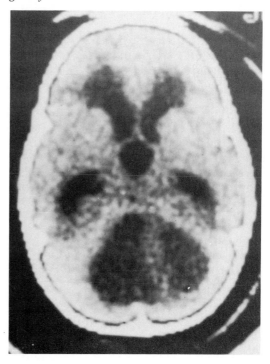

dure to be necessary to remove the lesion. Recurrence is rare except when the tumor is subtotally removed. Continued growth of an incompletely removed tumor is not a certainty and may not occur in more than 50% of such cases. Late tumor-related deaths are extremely rare and have usually been secondary to complications related to shunts. Recurrence years later as a malignant tumor has been reported but is quite rare. Radiation therapy has no role in treatment. If there is extension into brain stem, then it should be treated as a brain stem glioma. Preoperative clinical evidence of brain stem involvement is not conclusive evidence of invasion of this structure.

Type B Cerebellar Glioma

Cerebellar gliomas are designated as type B when they have perivascular pseudorosettes or any two of the following: necrosis, high cell density, or calcification in the absence of the type A features.[51] This category probably includes several tumor types (astrocytomas, ependymomas, glioblastomas, malignant undifferentiated tumors, *etc.*). The value in using the term *type B cerebellar glioma* lies in its distinction from the type A and its apparent correlation with survival.

The median age at diagnosis for the children with type B cerebellar gliomas is 3 years, and the median duration of symptoms before diagnosis is 2 months. Altered states of consciousness apparent at the time of presentation are characteristic of the type B glioma. A macrocyst occurs less commonly in type B (approximately 23%) than in the type A cerebellar gliomas. The lesion usually cannot be totally removed surgically. The median survival rate is just over 1 year, and the 5-year survival rate is 29%. Children with tumors of this type should be irradiated. Surgery for recurrence is usually not beneficial.

Medulloblastoma

Medulloblastoma is a very malignant tumor that occurs in the posterior fossa of children. These tumors account for 16% to 22% of intracranial tumors in children.[52] They often grow within the cerebellum and usually protrude into the fourth ventricle. They usually present between 3 and 9 years of age, but are not uncommon throughout childhood and, rarely, in young adults. This tumor usually appears on computed tomography as a noncystic mass within the fourth ventricle; other tests are rarely indicated (Fig. 14-2). The histology cannot be accurately determined from neurodiagnostic tests or clinical examination. These patients should be operated on immediately, with removal of as much of the tumor as is safely possible. No attempt should be made for radical removal, and pieces attached to the floor of the fourth ventricle should be left. Medulloblastoma is quite sensitive to ionizing radiation, and postoperatively all patients should receive radiation therapy.

The median survival rate is between 2 and 3 years, and the 5-year survival rate

FIG. 14-2. Medulloblastoma. Computed tomography of the brain of this 3-year-old child shows a densely staining solid mass in the region of the fourth ventricle and central portion of the cerebellum. Another area of dense uptake of contrast in the interpeduncular cistern identifies a metastasis. Much of the tumor within the fourth ventricle was removed and the patient received radiation therapy to the whole neuraxis.

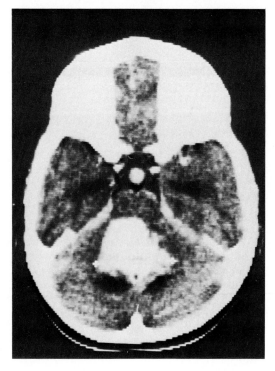

is about 35%.[8,30,38,39] Deaths from recurrent tumor have occurred even 15 years after diagnosis. There is some evidence that children in whom all visible tumor was removed live longer than those undergoing less complete removal. "Cure" of this tumor cannot be achieved by surgery. The results of treatment with chemotherapy have been disappointing.

Recurrence of medulloblastoma is common and may occur within the ventricular system, over the surface of the brain or spinal cord, or outside of the central nervous system. Recurrent medulloblastoma usually responds (shrinks) rapidly after the administration of additional ionizing radiation. In patients with recurrence of medulloblastoma, eventual death from the tumor is almost certain—perhaps it is certain—and physicians should not hesitate to exceed the usual safe limits for radiation therapy. Metastases outside the nervous system are known but usually occur through shunts that have been inserted for the diversion of cerebrospinal fluid. Metastases have been reported in lung and in bone.

Ependymoma

Ependymomas occur within the lateral ventricles and fourth ventricle of children, and there are no clinical features that distinguish this type of tumor from other tumors in similar locations. The peak age of occurrence is about 2 years.[7,11] In the posterior fossa, this tumor is usually solid (e.g., noncystic); it most often appears within the fourth ventricle but may occur as an intracerebellar tumor. The classic histologic feature is the true rosette that has the appearance of a section of the central canal of the spinal cord. The inconsistency with which neuropathologists require the presence of rosettes and weight the presence of pseudorosettes for assigning this diagnostic label may account for the wide variation in the reported incidence of ependymoma (often reported at 10 to 20% of intracranial tumors in children).[11,52] It is not unusual for these tumors to contain extensive regions of astrocytes or oligodendrocytes, and this has led some to assign the diagnosis "mixed glioma." A more malignant form of ependymal tumor is the ependymoblastoma.

Ependymomas are usually solid and cannot, on the basis of neurodiagnostic tests, be distinguished from other solid tumors such as medulloblastoma or noncystic astrocytoma. In most children, the only diagnostic test required to detect the lesion and determine its location is computed tomography.

The initial treatment is surgery; however, attachment to the floor of the fourth ventricle often makes complete removal impossible. Rarely, such tumors are attached to the brain by a small pedicle, and these can be completely surgically removed. Postoperatively, patients with incomplete removal should receive radiation therapy. Local recurrence is common and metastasis by way of the cerebrospinal fluid pathways is not unusual. Repeat operations are rarely beneficial. Some patients have survived for many years—were perhaps cured—after treatment of an ependymoma.

Ependymomas above the tentorium are less common in children, and may behave in a less malignant manner than those in the posterior fossa. These often appear as solid masses within the parenchyma of brain, but usually—perhaps always—have contact with an ependymal surface; however, this is not always apparent to the surgeon. Many of these (perhaps most) are accessible to excision, though usually subtotal. Those predominantly within thalamus should rarely be operated on. All of these patients should be treated with ionizing radiation. The median survival rate following surgery and radiation therapy is approximately 2 years.[11]

Hemangioblastoma (Capillary Hemangioblastoma, Lindau's Tumor)

Hemangioblastoma is a benign but relatively rare tumor occurring most commonly within the cerebellum.[37] Alternate locations include the brain stem and medulla oblongata. Multiple occurrence is not unusual. Histologically, this tumor is very similar to the angioblastic meningioma, and has been known to occur in more than one member of a family. Typically, the lesion appears as a cystic mass in the cerebellum with a "mural nodule" protruding into the cyst. Many, perhaps most, patients with this tumor will have at least some of the features of Lindau's syndrome. The tumor usually manifests itself as an expanding mass in the cerebellum. The treatment is surgical removal. Rarely, it is in an inaccessible location such as within the medulla oblongata. The expected result following the complete removal of tumor is cure.

Craniopharyngioma

Craniopharyngioma is a benign intracranial tumor that is diagnosed most often in childhood. It is of epithelial–ectodermal origin, probably arising from cells that migrated from Rathke's pouch and came to lie somewhere along the hypophyseal stalk. Craniopharyngioma has a very characteristic histologic appearance. Although it is the most common nonglial, primary, intracranial tumor in children, there are probably no more than 40 or 50 new pediatric cases per year in the United States. This lesion most often occurs as a suprasellar mass, but may appear to be predominantly intrasellar, within the third ventricle, parasellar, or even as a posterior fossa mass in close relation to the upper clivus and dorsum sellae.

The symptoms and signs are determined by the exact location and the rapidity of expansion. The clinical manifestations of the tumor may reflect (1) impairment of visual pathways, (2) dysfunction of the pituitary–hypothalamic axis, (3) obstruction of the normal pathways for cerebrospinal fluid, and (4) compression of frontal or temporal lobes. Visual symptoms include diminished acuity and field defects which are often asymmetric. Manifestations of endocrinologic disturbance are usually obvious on physical examination and can be confirmed by laboratory tests. Delay in onset and development of primary and secondary sexual development is particularly apparent in the teenagers. Most have a short stature, are moderately obese, and have very soft skin. Diabetes insipidus is uncommon before treatment. Many patients have mild to moderate organomegaly. Disturbances in memory may be related to impairment of the forniceal system or perhaps to compression of medial temporal lobes. Symptoms and signs of elevated intracranial pressure may result from occlusion of the basilar cisterns or from up-

ward expansion into the third ventricle with occlusion of the foramina of Monro.

The symptoms and signs can strongly suggest that a mass exists in the suprasellar region, but cannot establish the diagnosis. Any calcification in a suprasellar mass in a child strongly suggests craniopharyngioma, and the pattern of calcification can be pathognomonic (Fig. 14-3A). Occasionally, plain tomography can demonstrate more convincingly the characteristic pattern of calcification, but this is rarely necessary (Fig. 14-3B). Computed tomography can make the diagnosis by demonstrating the pattern of calcification and the cystic character of the mass (Fig. 14-3C). It can also reveal the relationships with other structures such as the third ventricle. Computed tomography may not show the location of the optic nerves and chiasm.

The treatment of craniopharyngioma is changing.[20,44] A decade ago, most neurosurgeons believed that the best treatment and the only hope for a cure was a surgical attempt to remove all of the lesion.[29] More recently, it has been learned that many children in whom all tumor was thought to have been removed experienced a recurrence.[25] Also, many children in whom such a radical removal was attempted, whether successful or not, received significant additional damage to the hypothalamus or the visual system. It is now apparent that radiation therapy can reduce the size and delay, or perhaps even arrest, the growth of these tumors.[27] Of course, radiation therapy is not without risks (see below). Still, many children, particularly those whose tumor contains a large cyst and those whose tumor is impairing vision, require a surgical procedure to reduce the size of the tumor. This may be as simple as the aspiration of a large cyst, or it may consist of a direct attack upon a solid tumor with removal of as much as easily possible, making certain that the visual pathways are well decompressed.

It is essential that an endocrinologist work closely with the patient before, during, and after treatment, regardless of the mode of treatment. These children should receive corticosteroids during and after surgical procedures. Very many will require replacement therapy for their pituitary–hypothalamic dysfunction. This is a complex issue that is not addressed further in this chapter.

Primary Tumors of Pituitary Gland

Primary tumors of the pituitary are not common in children but have been reported to account for 33% of parasellar masses in this age group.[40]

Some children, after adrenalectomy for Cushing's syndrome, develop a peculiar cutaneous hyperpigmentation and evidence of a tumor in the pituitary gland (Nelson's syndrome). Such patients probably had an ACTH-producing tumor of the pituitary that was mistakenly interpreted as a primary adrenal disorder.

Thalamic Tumors

Tumors of the thalamus account for approximately 1% of intracranial neoplasms. Approximately 25% of patients with thalamic tumors are less than 16 years old. It is common for these patients to present with elevated intracranial pressure or motor symptoms, and the latter is more common in the younger patients. Occasionally, because of gait disturbance and dysmetria, these patients may be thought to have cerebellar tumors. Tremor, chorea, and dystonic movements are often seen. Dysphasia and dysnomia have been described, as has anisocoria. Seizures occur in 11% to 30% of such patients. Some authors have thought the smaller pupil occurs on the side of the tumor, but this has not been a consistent finding.[19]

Thalamic tumors are glial, and when tissue is available for histologic examination, it often shows features of malignancy; these tumors are usually labeled astrocytoma, ependymoma, oligodendroglioma, or ganglioglioma.

The treatment of these tumors is usually considered to be palliative, and radiation therapy offers the best hope of achieving this. With the diagnostic tools available now (particularly computed tomography), it is rarely necessary to operate on these children to establish the diagnosis. A very small number of children have had relatively long survival rates following the "total" removal of a benign astrocytoma of this area. An extensive neurologic deficit would, of course, be expected after such surgery. Patients who develop hydrocephalus certainly benefit from a shunting procedure.

Gliomas of Cerebral Hemispheres

Tumors in the cerebral hemispheres of children may arise from astrocytes, oligodendrocytes, ependymal cells, less-well-differentiated cells,[26] or combinations thereof, but approximately 70% get classified as astrocytomas. These lesions are usually not truly benign, but the very malignant glioblastoma multiforme, which is so common in adults, is unusual in children.[29]

Children with tumors of the cerebral hemispheres usually present to the neurologist or neurosurgeon with severe headache or seizures, but a careful history often reveals the earliest symptom to have been a vague sense, both of the parent and the patient that "all is not well." This sense may have persisted for weeks or months, and may be described as lethargy, irritability, loss of ambition, indifference, or lack of interest in school or sports.[29] Elevated intracranial pressure is common, even though most of these tumors do not directly obstruct the flow of cerebrospinal fluid. The most common abnormalities apparent on physical examination involve the motor system and may be present when the lesion does not involve the precentral cortex. Also, abnormality of other specialized cortical functions (vision, speech, memory, motor function, etc.) may reflect (but not necessarily) the location of the tumor. Gait disturbance and abnormality in movements of the eyes, particularly conjugate gaze, may be apparent. The development of a strong preference for using one hand (handedness) before the age of 2 or a change in handedness is common.

The diagnosis of a tumor of the cerebral hemisphere can usually be made by computed tomography, and other neurodiagnostic tests are rarely helpful (Fig. 14-4). Except for glioblastoma multiforme, which has a characteristic appearance, the histologic diagnosis cannot be ascertained from neurodiagnostic tests; however, most are astrocytomas. Intracerebral neoplasms that have extensive mineralization are usually gliomas (often oligodendrogliomas). Occasionally, cerebral angiography may be help-

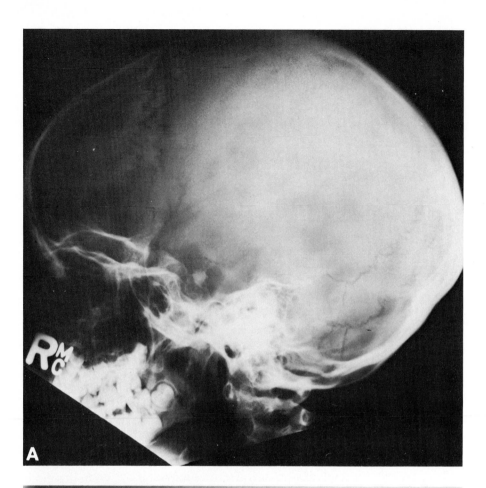

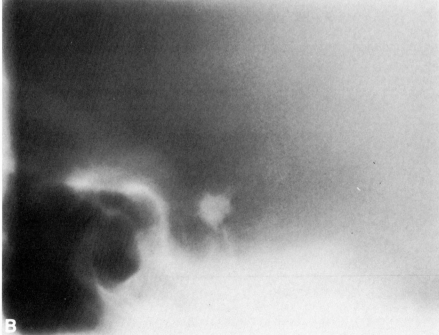

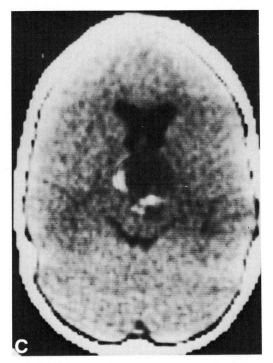

FIG. 14-3. Craniopharyngioma. This appearance of calcification above the dorsum sellae is probably pathognomonic for craniopharyngioma (*A* is a lateral radiograh, *B* a polytomograph in the same view). Computed tomogram of a different patient (*C*) shows a large cystic mass in the region of the third ventricle with calcification in part of the wall or solid portion of the lesion. This is strongly suggestive of craniopharyngioma.

ful in making the diagnosis of glioblastoma multiforme or in distinguishing a tumor from an arteriovenous malformation or other abnormality. Rarely, ventriculography may be the only way of identifying a mass that slightly deforms a temporal horn.

Most tumors of the cerebral hemispheres should be operated on, and an attempt should be made to remove as much of the tumor as safely possible. Some appear to have relatively distinct margins (some relatively benign astrocytomas, and a few glioblastomas and primitive neuroectodermal tumors; Fig. 14-5), and therefore much or all, by gross criteria, can be removed. Those that are severely infiltrative in nature cannot be totally removed. Those children who have good radiologic evidence of a glioblastoma multiforme, particularly if in the corpus callosum or crossing the midline, do not require surgery for diagnosis and, unless there is a very large mass of neoplastic tissue, do not benefit from surgery. If there is a large mass of tumor, then the patient often benefits greatly by the removal of a large part of this bulk. Such a "debulking" procedure allows the surrounding brain to return to a more normal position, and also may accomplish the removal of the source of cerebral edema. This may immediately improve the patient's condition and allow the patient to tolerate radiation therapy more safely and with less morbidity. The surgical removal of recurrent tumor is occasionally beneficial to the patient, but is not followed by long survival.[14]

Prognosis depends upon the biologic activity of the tumor, and this is best predicted by the histology and the location of the tumor. The prognosis is best for oligodendrogliomas and astrocytomas, and occasionally long survival occurs in children with some of the more malignant tumors, such as ependymoma. Glioblastoma has a particularly bad prognosis.[12,14]

Neuroblastoma

The neuroblastoma is quite rare as a primary intracranial neoplasm but does occur in the cerebral hemispheres. Its diagnosis below the tentorium is difficult because of its similarity to medulloblastoma. It usually occurs in children 5 years old or younger as a large solid mass. It acts as a very malignant tumor, metastasizing by way of cerebrospinal pathways, but some long-term survivals are known.[21]

Gliomas of Optic Pathways

Gliomas of the optic pathways can be considered in three categories: optic nerve gliomas, chiasmal gliomas and postchiasmal gliomas.[34] Many children with gliomas of the optic pathways (particularly gliomas of the optic nerves) have cutaneous manifestations of von Recklinghausen's neurofibromatosis. The diagnosis can be made with a high degree of accuracy using neurodiagnostic tests, and operations are rarely, if ever, required for diagnosis. Computed

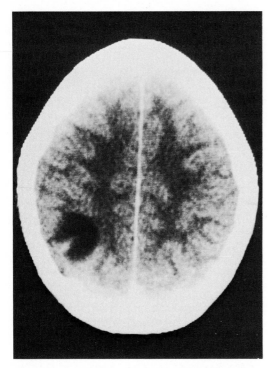

FIG. 14-4. Oligodendroglioma. This computed tomogram shows a radiolucent area with minimal "mass effect" in the parietal lobe of a 15-year-old girl who presented with seizures.

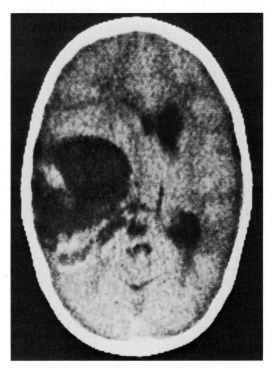

FIG. 14-5. Primitive neuroectodermal tumor. A 2-year-old girl presented with elevated intracranial pressure, seizures, and a mild hemiparesis. Computed tomography revealed this large mass within, and beyond, the temporal lobe. Six months after extensive surgical removal and radiation therapy, massive reexpansion of the tumor was apparent.

tomography, often with contrast material (metrizamide) in the subarachnoid or ventricular space may be the only test required.

Gliomas of the optic nerve present with unilateral decreased vision, axial proptosis of the globe without abnormality of the extraocular muscles, and edema of the optic disc. The median age at diagnosis is 7 years. Radiographs of the optic foramina may reveal an enlarged foramen on the symptomatic side, but this is not conclusive evidence of optic nerve glioma or even of neoplasm. The demonstration of an abnormally large optic nerve can usually be accomplished by computed tomography. Gliomas confined to the optic nerve, particularly those confined to the orbit, are thought to have a much better prognosis and may require no treatment.[22] It has been known for many years that an apparent cure can be achieved if the tumor is totally resected, and sometimes even when subtotally removed; of course, the lesions that could be so operated did not extend as far posteriorly as the optic chiasm. Rare cases in

which neoplasm involves optic nerve as well as brain suggests that none of the gliomas of the optic pathways can be considered, with confidence, to be benign. The efficacy of surgical excision of a glioma of the optic nerve that extends intracranially but not to the chiasm is not clear.[34]

Those gliomas of the optic pathways that involve the optic chiasm and tracts are really hypothalamic tumors. (The optic chiasm is a part of the hypothalamus and not just adherent to its surface.) These commonly present with bilateral loss of vision, bilateral optic atrophy, and visual defects suggestive of a chiasmal lesion. The median age at diagnosis is 4 years. Strabismus and nystagmus are also common. Some tumors involve only the anterior part of the chiasm and not the remainder of the hypothalamus; these are histologically similar to the tumors of the optic nerve, and they often behave in an equally benign manner.[34] They are not operable lesions, and the effectiveness of ionizing radiation is unclear.

The third category is that group in which the tumor clearly involves the hypothalamus. Patients with these tumors manifest both visual and hypothalamic symptoms. There is no diagnostic pattern of visual symptoms and signs; however, extensive and asymmetric defects in the visual fields are common. Histologically, these are quite different from the tumors of the more anterior parts of the visual pathways; they behave in a much more aggressive manner. Probably all of these should receive radiation therapy. These are not operable lesions.

Hypothalamic Glioma

Hypothalamic gliomas are usually astrocytic, and the range of their malignant characteristics varies extensively. Clinically, they may present with precocious puberty, diencephalic syndrome, or as gliomas of the optic pathways.[6,10] Vomiting unassociated with headache may occur in 30% of these children.[32] Children with diencephalic syndrome are usually severely emaciated and occasionally have hydrocephalus. Occasionally, sexual precocity is a presenting clinical feature of a hypothalamic tumor. In children beyond infancy, hyperphagia and obesity may be prominent features. Diagnosis of hypothalamic glioma can usually be established by computed tomography; however, if the mass is quite small, ventriculography with metrizamide may be required. The presence of two masses, one hypothalamic and one in the region of the pineal, suggests strongly the diagnosis of dysgerminoma. Radiation therapy may reduce the size of the tumor and may even result in improvement in visual signs. Surgery has little if any role in the diagnosis or treatment of this lesion.

Glioma of Brain Stem

Gliomas of the brain stem account for 13% to 18% of tumors of the posterior fossa and are most often diffusely infiltrating lesions. They are usually astrocytic neoplasms but are occasionally ependymomas or glioblastomas, though biopsy is rarely performed. They may appear to involve only one discrete portion of brain stem, or they may extend throughout the length and breadth of the brain stem. They may even extend to involve thalamus or spinal cord. Occasionally, these tumors appear to involve only one side of the brain, or they may present as a mass in the cerebellopontine angle. Gliomas of the brain stem have a peak incidence between the ages of 5 and 8 years. One of the most characteristic clinical features is the tendency for the development of multiple and progressive neurologic abnormalities without obstruction of the flow of cerebrospinal fluid. Therefore, symptoms and signs of elevated intracranial pressure are uncommon. Children with gliomas of the brain stem typically have bilateral, but not necessarily symmetric, cranial nerve abnormalities. Particularly, the abducens and facial nerves tend to be involved, and the corticospinal tracts are commonly involved. Many children present with an abnormal gait, and examination often demonstrates severe dysmetria. Stenosis of the aqueduct of Sylvius, which becomes apparent beyond infancy, is usually due to tumor involving the mesencephalon.

The clinical presentation often strongly suggests the diagnosis; however, because of the poor prognosis, it is important to be certain of the diagnosis. Several other lesions can be mistaken for brain stem glioma: demyelinating processes, extra-axial gliomas and other tumors compressing the brain stem, cerebellar tumors compressing the brain stem, and even epidermoid cysts or arteriovenous malformations within the brain stem. It is currently possible, with high resolution computed tomography, to demonstrate the size and shape of the brain stem with sufficient accuracy to firmly establish the diagnosis in most cases (Fig. 14-6). Sometimes it is necessary to introduce metrizamide into the subarachnoid space to assist in the computed tomographic examination. Also, sagittal and occasionally coronal reconstructions (computed tomography) from the usual coronal scans can prove particularly convincing in difficult cases. Angiography and pneumoencephalography are rarely, if ever, required. Very rarely, surgical exploration may be required to establish the diagnosis; this is usually in cases with strongly asymmetric presentations with an apparent extra-axial mass.

The only effective treatment, and one

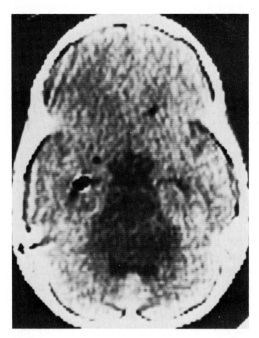

FIG. 14-6. Brain stem glioma. An 8-year-old boy with a 5-month history of progressively worsening ataxia and abnormalities involving multiple cranial nerves had this computed tomogram, which shows an area of abnormally low density throughout a massively enlarged brain stem. The posteriorly displaced fourth ventricle is also apparent on this view.

that should be considered palliative, is ionizing radiation. Surgery has no role except as mentioned above. The median survival rate following irradiation is approximately two years.[17,45] Survival for several years is possible, but often calls into question the accuracy of the diagnosis.

Choroid Plexus Papilloma

Papillomas may occur anywhere within choroid plexus: lateral ventricles, third ventricle, or fourth ventricle.[35] They usually act like benign neoplasms, even when they have some features suggestive of malignancy. Less often, they clearly act as malignant neoplasms. The presentation of these tumors follows, roughly, three patterns:

(1) They may present with hydrocephalus from overproduction of cerebrospinal fluid. This occurs most commonly in in-

fants, and the cerebrospinal fluid may be produced at three to four times the normal rate.

(2) Acute hemorrhage, often with a significant hematoma within or adjacent to the tumor, is a presentation more common in adolescents but is seen also in younger children. These tumors are often in the lateral ventricles and may appear to be within the parenchyma of brain.

(3) Choroid plexus papillomas may present with hydrocephalus caused by the tumor impairing the flow of cerebrospinal fluid. These are less prone to hemorrhage and do not produce an excessive amount of cerebrospinal fluid. They occur most commonly in the fourth ventricle. Occasionally, tumors of the choroid plexus are massive (Fig. 14-7).

Melanotic Progonoma

Melanotic progonomas (also called retinal anlage tumors and melanotic neuroectodermal tumors of infancy) are locally invasive

FIG. 14-7. Choroid plexus papilloma. This computed tomogram shows a very large mass with dense uptake of radiopaque contrast in a 15-month-old child with elevated intracranial pressure and a mild hemiparesis. The mass was surgically removed.

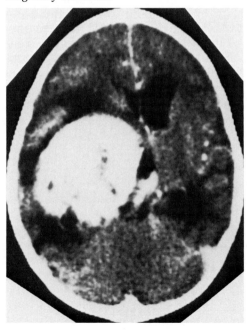

pigmented tumors of infancy thought to be of neural crest origin. Radiographs of the skull may be pathognomonic. This type of tumor grows very rapidly, and radiographs made a week apart may show dramatic progression. The tumor is primarily within bone, but may infiltrate the dura and compress brain. Histologically, the presence of melanin crystals with a shape characteristic of retinal melanin is the distinguishing feature. The treatment should consist of radical removal of all the tumor, and this may involve extensive removal of cranium and even part of the dura. If operated on early with gross total removal, cure is possible.

Third Ventricular Tumors

Tumors located anteriorly and superiorly in the third ventricle make their presence known by obstructing the foramina of Monro. Colloid cysts, ependymomas, astrocytomas, xanthogranulomas, and malignant gliomas may occur in this location. Astrocytomas are the most common tumors occurring *within* the third ventricle of children and may account for as many as 15% of astrocytomas in children. In general, those located anteriorly and inferiorly are not amenable to surgical removal. The same is true for those tumors that can be shown by appropriate neurodiagnostic studies to be arising from the lateral walls—that is, probably infiltrative tumors. Some astrocytomas in the third ventricle are discrete masses that can be easily separated from adjacent brain.[46] (See discussions of specific types of tumors that occur within the third ventricle.)

Pineal Tumors

Many types of tumors occur in the region of the pineal gland (dysgerminomas, teratomas, glial tumors, *etc.*), but tumors in this location account for 1% or less, of intracranial tumors in the U.S. In Japan, approximately 10% of intracranial tumors are in this region. As a generalization, pineal tumors make their presence known by symptoms and signs caused by obstruction of the flow of cerebrospinal fluid and compression of the tectum of the mesencephalon.[9] Pineal tumor compressing the tectum is one cause of aqueductal stenosis (see Glioma of Brain Stem). The hydrocephalus is usually caused by obstruction of the aqueduct of Sylvius, but the obstruction can occur in the posterior third ventricle when the mass is very large. Parinaud's syndrome is common, and the pupils tend to be small and asymmetric, and to react slowly to light. Also, the near reflex is commonly absent. Perhaps 10% of boys with tumors in the pineal region have precocious puberty. Every patient suspected of having a tumor in the pineal region should be studied thoroughly with appropriate neurodiagnostic tests, because the details of the anatomic relationships of the tumor determine not only the diagnosis, but also whether the tumor is amenable to surgical removal (Fig. 14-8).[36] The risks of operating upon a child with a tumor that is known, from neuroradiologic tests, to be nonresectable probably outweigh the benefits. Perhaps as many as 25% of tumors in the pineal region can be removed surgically.

FIG. 14-8. Pineal tumor. A 2-year-old child presented with elevated intracranial pressure and abnormalities of eye movements. Computed tomogram demonstrated a tumor within the posterior third ventricle. A high concentration of α-fetoprotein in the serum strongly suggested that the lesion was a dysgerminoma.

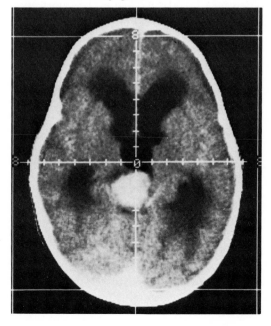

Dysgerminoma

The dysgerminoma (germinoma, pinea-loma, germinoma-type tumor, atypical teratoma) is the most common tumor in the pineal region; it is usually infiltrative, commonly metastatic by way of cerebrospinal fluid pathways, and responds favorably to radiation therapy. Diabetes insipidus is commonly an early symptom when there is also a hypothalamic mass.[23] Neurodiagnostic tests, particularly computed tomography, commonly demonstrate two masses, one in the region of the pineal body and one in the lower third ventricle involving the hypothalamus. Many clinicians consider this pattern sufficient evidence for diagnosis and do not require further neurodiagnostic tests.

It is usually possible to establish the diagnosis without surgery, at least to the extent of detecting the mass and determining if it is likely that it can be resected completely. This is particularly important because the pineal region is relatively difficult to approach surgically, and surgery has appreciable risk of morbidity and mortality.

Dysgerminoma is usually very responsive to ionizing radiation, and this is the treatment of choice.[24]

Teratoma

Teratomas are developmental tumors that contain tissue derived from all three germ layers. When intracranial, they usually become apparent in the neonate or infant, and are sometimes very large masses at the base of the brain and not necessarily in the midline. In the neonate, teratoma is the most commonly occurring intracranial tumor.[48] Calcification is usually apparent on plain radiographs of the skull. The very large teratomas are often benign and, depending upon their location, are often amenable to total surgical removal.

Malignant teratomas and lesions, which some neuropathologists have labeled teratoid tumors, may occur within brain, and these often infiltrate neural tissue. Their complete removal is usually impossible. Radiation therapy should be administered to the malignant teratomas unless there is good reason to think that all has been removed by surgery.

Endodermal Sinus Tumor

Endodermal sinus tumor (yolk sac tumor) is a highly malignant tumor that rarely ocurrs intracranially, but when it does it seems to prefer the pineal and hypothalamic locations.[1] Elevated concentrations of alpha-fetoprotein in serum and cerebrospinal fluid have been reported. Metastasis by way of cerebrospinal fluid pathways is common.

Dermoid and Epidermoid Tumors

Dermoid tumors contain tissue derived from mesoderm and ectoderm, whereas epidermoids (cholesteatomas) contain only the latter. Therefore, if hair follicles and sweat glands are present, the lesion is a dermoid. Dermoid and epidermoid tumors are cystic and contain desquamated epidermis. Both tumors are benign and are usually extra-axial lesions; and both commonly, but not necessarily, occur in or near the midline, particularly in pineal, suprasellar, and third ventricular regions (not mutually exclusive designations of location). Dermoid cysts, particularly if in the posterior fossa, tend to have a tubular stalk connecting them to the skin and therefore they may present with infection.[28] Usually these can be totally removed, and if this is accomplished recurrence is not expected. Rarely, occurrence in a relatively inaccessible location precludes surgical removal, but even some of these tumors can be decompressed. They present as mass lesions, and there is nothing characteristic about the clinical presentation. Computed tomography can demonstrate a cystic mass but cannot identify it further. When pneumoencephalography was more commonly used, an epidermoid tumor could be diagnosed by a characteristic appearance if the air entered the mass.

Colloid Cyst of Third Ventricle

Colloid cysts of the third ventricle (neuroepithelial cysts) probably arise from diencephalic cysts or from the paraphysis, but account for less than 1% of tumors of the brain in children. They are diagnosed more commonly in adults and are not infrequently an incidental finding at the autopsy of an adult— for example, the brain of Dr. Harvey Cushing. In general, the clinical presentations described for adults[3] are the same for children: (1) elevated intracranial pressure without localizing features, (2) syndrome of retardation or dementia, perhaps with occasional headaches, and (3) paroxysmal attacks, usually beginning with headache and rapidly progressing over minutes or hours, accompanied by neurologic deterioration. Effective treatment depends upon an understanding of the pathophysiology. The mass may obstruct one or both of the foramina of Monro by moving slightly or by steady growth in a critical position. If the obstruction is complete, then intracranial pressure will rise rapidly in the lateral ventricles until a normal pathway opens (e.g., the "ball valve" may move aside), or the pressure may be relieved by the insertion of ventricular needles or tubes into *both* ventricles. Any delay in treatment in those patients with acutely elevated intracranial pressure may result in the death of the patient. If a ventricular needle is inserted to relieve the elevated intracranial pressure—the only effective therapeutic measure in a patient *in extremis* from this lesion—both lateral ventricles should be tapped to prevent transfalcial herniation. Colloid cysts can usually be diagnosed by computed tomography, but ventriculography still has a role in the diagnosis of this lesion (Fig. 14-9). The preferred treatment is surgical removal through the corpus callosum, and this can be accomplished with small risk of additional permanent neurologic abnormality. The insertion of a biventricular shunt system can relieve symptoms but does not treat the lesion, and the same symptoms will appear if the shunt becomes obstructed, perhaps even more critically because the tumor may be larger. These tumors are never malignant, and radiation therapy has no role in their treatment.

Xanthogranuloma of Choroid Plexus

Xanthogranuloma of choroid plexus, a lesion that is usually an incidental finding at autopsy, can, in children, become symptomatic by obstructing the normal pathways for cerebrospinal fluid. They occur in the lateral and third ventricles, and in the lateral ventricles, they may be bilateral. Nearly all of the symptomatic cases reported have been in children. These lesions are ex-

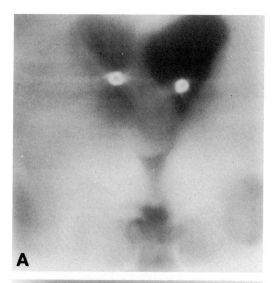

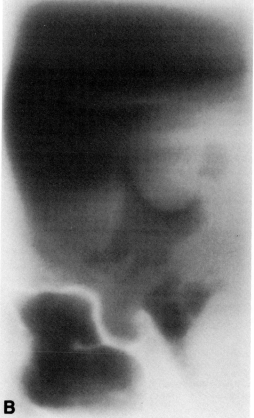

FIG. 14-9. Colloid cyst of third ventricle. A 5-year-old girl presented in a comatose and decerebrate state about 5 hours after the onset of headache. After a bilateral shunt was inserted, ventriculography (done with air) and pneumoencephalography demonstrated this lesion in the anterior third ventricle. *A.* Frontal view. *B.* Lateral view.

tremely slow growing and, if found accidentally, no treatment is required.[49]

Cerebellopontine Angle Tumors

Tumors in the cerebellopontine angle are not common in children, and when they do occur they are usually excrescences of astrocytomas of the brain stem or cerebellum but are occasionally astrocytomas without apparent connection to the brain. *Acoustic neurinoma* is a rare tumor in children but does occur, usually in association with von Reckinghausen's neurofibromatosis. Cholesteatomas in this location are not usually connected with the mastoid or middle ear.

Meningioma

Meningiomas are very rare in children[33] but have been known to occur, even in the very young,[31] in the lateral ventricles, in the third ventricle, and on the cerebral convexity. Intraventricular occurrence may be more common in children than in adults. Meningiomas in children have no histologic features distinguishing them from similar tumors in adults. When the tumor is accessible, as it usually is, the treatment is surgical excision. In relatively inaccessible locations (e.g., a large tumor within the third ventricle), treatment with radiation may be considered.

Chordoma

Chordomas, slowly growing intracranial tumors, are very rare but must be considered in the differential diagnosis of a mass which appears to arise within the basisphenoid and expand either upward against, but not into, the brain stem or laterally into the middle fossa. They occur about twice as frequently in males as in females.[42]

Chondrosarcoma

Chondrosarcomas are a rare type of tumor to involve the brain, but they may arise in the base of the skull, involve dura, and infiltrate brain.[18]

Lipoma

A lipoma within the brain is not a neoplasm in the usual sense of the term, but a malformation. Rarely if ever does the lipoma expand. Usually lipomas are near the midline and are often within or near the corpus callosum[47] or the tectum of the mesencephalon. They can be associated with other abnormalities in development of midline structures and may contain bone. Because of the low density of fat, these can usually be diagnosed by computed tomography and may occasionally be identifiable on plain radiographs of the skull. They rarely require treatment.

Metastases

Malignant tumors of the central nervous system commonly metastasize by way of the cerebrospinal fluid to sites over the external surface of the brain and spinal cord or the internal (ventricular) surface. Medulloblastoma is the most common tumor spreading in this way, but ependymomas, endodermal sinus tumors, and even astrocytomas and oligodendrogliomas have metastasized by way of cerebrospinal fluid pathways.

Tumors of the central nervous system only rarely metastasize outside of the central nervous system, and when this does occur, it usually follows surgery, often by way of a shunt. Distal metastasis is a particularly ominous sign. Medulloblastoma is the most common tumor to metastasize extracranially, but there are reports of ependymal tumors and malignant gliomas doing this as well as a few other isolated case reports. Skeletal bone and lung are the most common sites for these metastases.

Metastasis to brain from tumors originating outside of the central nervous system is uncommon in children. Exceptions are the metastatic deposits occasionally occurring in some children with leukemia and the metastases from Wilms's tumor; both are usually multiple. Children with multiple metastases, regardless of origin, should be treated with radiation therapy, and those with leukemia will require special attention to their chemotherapeutic regimen. An intraventricular catheter can be inserted for the administration of chemotherapeutic agents. Surgical removal should be seriously considered in the rare situation in which a child who is otherwise in relatively good condition has a single intracranial mass in an accessible location.

GENERALIZATIONS CONCERNING TREATMENT

Physicians treat patients, not tumors of the brain, and this is more than a semantic point. Some of the considerations for treatment have been addressed above, but, to emphasize the obvious, knowing how to best treat children with such lesions requires far more than memorizing the treatment(s) for each type of tumor. Not only does each type of tumor require special consideration and knowledge, but, perhaps more importantly, each child with tumor of the brain is a unique entity. The terms "conservative treatment" and "radical treatment" are not clearly defined, and that which is radical for one patient may be conservative for another. "Treating the patient expectantly" is usually a euphemism for not treating the patient but may be occasionally the best "treatment." Although generalization may be essential for the learning process, individualization is essential in the care of a specific child.

Prognosis

There is an artificial quality to any discussion that groups all intracranial tumors (i.e., ignores histologic and clinical classification); however, it is, perhaps, valuable to know that 40% of all children who survive for one month following an operation for intracranial tumor will live for at least 15 years. In general, prognosis depends upon histology, location of the tumor, age of the patient, sex, and, of course, treatment. In general, a better prognosis is correlated with a long duration of symptoms before diagnosis, with advancing years, and with being female.[15]

Management of Elevated Intracranial Pressure

Patients with elevated intracranial pressure related to tumor of the brain should be hospitalized immediately and started on steroids (usually dexamethasone). This medication may relieve all symptoms and thereby suggest to parents that no further treatment is needed. The ideal treatment is the removal of the cause, (i.e., the tumor), but this is not always immediately possible, and sometimes it is not possible at all.

Children with elevated intracranial pressure due to mechanical obstruction to the flow of cerebrospinal fluid must be observed particularly closely because they can suddenly become much worse. Herniation of the brain with cardiorespiratory arrest and death can occur. For such children (those at risk for complete obstruction of the outflow of cerebrospinal fluid), appropriate instruments for ventricular puncture should be at the bedside and a physician familiar with the procedure should be available on very short notice. Some children with severe or immediately life-threatening intracranial hypertension may require the diversion of cerebrospinal fluid by way of a shunt or a system for continuous external drainage. In the case of tumors with extensive surrounding edema, the only effective treatment, when they are not controlled by steroids, may be the removal of the tumor.

Generalization Concerning Modes of Treatment

Treatments of children with tumors of the brain can be considered in three categories: surgery, ionizing radiation, and chemotherapy. The management for a particular patient with brain tumor must be highly individualized and often requires more than one type of treatment. It is most important that no physician, regardless of specialty, become an advocate of a particular mode of therapy; every physician involved in the care of the child should be an advocate of the child's well being.

Surgery

Surgery can accomplish the total removal of most non-infiltrating tumors, the reduction in the bulk of most tumors that are infiltrating and expanding within relatively noncritical regions, and the reduction or elimination of the edema (if the tumor is removed). Also, tissue for histologic examination of most tumors can be obtained through surgery. But feasibility does not imply best treatment for a specific child. Surgery necessarily has risks of anesthetic complications, infection, hemorrhage, and more extensive damage to the nervous system than planned. Under ideal circumstances, only the tumor and the immediately surrounding brain are affected by this form of treatment.

Radiation Therapy

Ionizing radiation is harmful to all tissue in its path, but its therapeutic usefulness is based upon the fact that it is more harmful to neoplastic than to non-neoplastic tissue. The effects continue for months and years in all tissue in the irradiated field. The therapeutic effect can be delivered to extensive volumes of tissue, including infiltrating and multifocal tumors as well as cerebrospinal fluid containing malignant cells. Epilation and other effects on epidermis are often major sources of concern to patients and parents. The details of the morbidity associated with radiation therapy are appreciable but are not to be reviewed here.

Chemotherapy

Chemotherapy is, in the view of some, the hope of the future for children with malignant tumors of the brain, but it has not yet proven to be an effective and reliable mode of treatment. A few agents have been developed that, at least in adults with glioblastoma multiforme, may prolong survival by a few weeks. There are also several titillating reports of the beneficial effect of certain other agents on children with brain tumors. It should not be overlooked that the whole body is necessarily treated, at least to some extent, and in this respect chemotherapy is unlike surgery or radiation therapy. More recently, several techniques for delivery have been developed that minimize the effect outside of the central nervous system. Rarely emphasized, but extremely important to children and their parents, is the very high morbidity associated with chemotherapy. Anorexia, lethargy, epilation, peripheral neuropathy, and the requirement for multiple venipunctures over many months are commonly part of the price paid and must be weighed against the unlikely, but wished for, beneficial effect of chemotherapy before it can be recommended in a child with a brain tumor.

Long-Term Management

Post-treatment management consists of trying to detect recurrence as early as reasonably possible, looking for evidence of hydrocephalus, and helping the patient and family deal with anxiety about the future and about any neurologic deficits that are present. Computed tomography is an unparalleled test for monitoring the site of the tumor for reappearance or expansion, regardless of mode of therapy. Also this test is ideal for monitoring the size and shape of the ventricles. Assay for certain chemical markers in serum or cerebrospinal fluid which herald the presence or the recurrence of tumor is an exciting prospect, and there appears to be some progress in this field.

Children with intracranial tumors that are clearly not curable (this includes both malignant tumors and certain benign tumors such as an inoperable craniopharyngioma that has regrown after irradiation) require a great amount of the physician's time and often tax his resourcefulness, but nearly all can be helped tremendously. Hydrocephalus can be treated, tumors reirradiated, cysts drained, additional tumor removed, steroids used to reduce cerebral edema, and inquiries of patient and families answered. In summary, much can be done to prevent or relieve suffering.

Talking with Parents

Parents of children with intracranial tumors are understandably anxious, and their manner of coping with this threat to their child varies greatly. Physicians should not attempt to prevent parental anxiety; however, there are ways of reducing the severity of this normal reaction and of channeling it in an appropriate direction. Frequent contact with parents and the transmission by physicians of information that is complete and honest goes a long way toward achieving this goal. It is equally important for physicians to make it overwhelmingly apparent that everything reasonable is being done in a thoughtful manner and that no information, favorable or unfavorable, is being withheld.

Incorrect information concerning brain tumors comes to parents from many sources: parents of other children with brain tumors, friends, and, unfortunately, from poorly informed physicians. Also there is a surfeit of novels, short stories, and even television programs that tends to group all patients with brain tumors and depict a painful, humiliating, and agonizingly hopeless existence that finally and mercifully is relieved by death. Such information has a particularly harmful influence on parents and makes even more important the dissemination of accurate and individualized information by the patient's physician. No one else can speak with such authority about a particular case, and therefore this part of management of the case cannot be delegated.

Talking with the Children

All children old enough to understand speech should be given, in language they understand, an explanation for the symptoms of which they are aware, and for the examinations, tests, and treatments they must undergo. Children, not unlike adults, should be reassured that pain is not expected to be a serious problem and that the treatment plan includes their returning home after their condition improves. If any diagnostic or therapeutic endeavor will alter a child's physical appearance (*e.g.*, loss of hair, scarring, *etc.*), he should be informed of this *in advance*. Some parents, wishing to "protect" their children from a truth they find painful to accept, enjoin the physician to participate in an elaborate plot to deceive the patient about diagnosis, treatment, or prognosis. Physicians should not participate in this and should discourage the entire scheme. All children should be encouraged to ask questions and should receive honest answers. Except when death is imminent, the most accurate and honest assessment of any child with tumor of the brain is rarely, if ever, one of utter hopelessness. It is important, in the course of answering questions honestly, never to remove all hope.

REFERENCES

1. **Albrechtsen R, Klee JG, Moller JE:** Primary intracranial germ cell tumours including five cases of endodermal sinus tumour. Acta Pathol Microbiol Scand [A] [Suppl] 233:32–38, 1972

2. **Allen JC, Nisselbaum J, Epstein F, Rosen G, Schwartz MK:** Alphafetoprotein and human chorionic gonadotropin determination in cerebrospinal fluid. J Neurosurg 51:368–374, 1979

3. **Antunes JL, Louis KM, Ganti SR:** Colloid cysts of the third ventricle. Neurosurgery 7:450–455, 1980

4. **Backus RE, Millichap JG:** The seizure as a manifestation of intracranial tumor in childhood. Pediatrics 29:978–984, 1962

5. **Boesel CP, Paulson GW, Kosnik EJ, Earle KM:** Brain hamartomas and tumors associated with tuberous sclerosis. Neurosurgery 4:410–417, 1979

6. **Costin G:** Endocrine disorders associated with tumor of the pituitary and hypothalamus. Pediatr Clin North Am 26:15–31, 1979

7. **Coulon RA, Till K:** Intracranial ependymomas in children. Childs Brain 3:154–168, 1977

8. **Cumberlin RL, Luk KH, Wara WM, Sheline GE, Wilson CB:** Medulloblastoma: Treatment results and effect on normal tissue. Cancer 43:1014–1020, 1979

9. **DeGirolami U, Schmidek HH:** Clinicopathological studies of 53 tumors of the pineal region. J Neurosurg 39:455–462, 1973

10. **DeSousa AL, Kalsbeck JE, Mealey J, Fitzgerald J:** Diencephalic syndrome and its relation to opticochiasmatic glioma: Review of twelve cases. Neurosurgery 4:207–209, 1979

11. **Dohrmann GJ, Farwell JR, Flannery JT:** Ependymomas and ependymoblastomas in children. J Neurosurg 45:273–283, 1976

12. **Dohrmann GJ, Farwell JR, Flannery JT:** Glioblastoma multiforme in children. J Neurosurg 44:442–448, 1976

13. **Gilles FH, Winston K, Fulchiero A, Leviton A:** Histologic features and observational variation in cerebellar gliomas in children. J Natl Cancer Inst 58:175–181, 1977

14. **Gjerris F:** Clinical aspects and long-term prognosis in supratentorial tumors in infancy and childhood. Acta Neurol Scand 57:445–470, 1978

15. **Gjerris F:** Clinical aspects and long-term prognosis of intracranial tumours in infancy and childhood. Dev Med Child Neurol 18:145–159, 1976

16. **Glasauer FE, Yuan HP:** Intracranial tumors with extracranial metastases. J Neurosurg 20:474–493, 1963

17. **Greenberger JS, Cassady JR, Levene MB:** Radiation therapy of thalamic, midbrain and brain stem gliomas. Radiology 122:463–468, 1977

18. **Heros RC, Martinez AJ, Ahn HS:** Intracranial mesenchymal chondrosarcoma. Surg Neurol 14:311–317, 1980

19. **Hirose G, Lombroso CT, Eisenberg H:** Thalamic tumors in childhood, clinical laboratory and therapeutic consideration. Arch Neurol 32:740–744, 1975

20. **Hoffman HJ, Hendrick EB, Humphreys RP, Buncic JR, Armstrong DL, Jenkin RDT:** Management of craniopharyngioma in children. J Neurosurg 47:218–227, 1977

21. **Horten BC, Rubinstein LJ:** Primary cerebral neuroblastoma, a clinicopathological study of 35 cases. Brain 99:735–756, 1976

22. **Hoyt WF, Baghdassarian SA:** Optic glioma of childhood: Natural history and rationale for con-

servative management. Br J Ophthalmol 53:793–798, 1969

23. **Izquierdo JM, Rougerie J, Lapras C, Sanz F:** The so-called ectopic pinealomas: A cooperative study of 15 cases. Childs Brain 5:505–512, 1979

24. **Jenkin RDT, Simpson WJK, Keen CW:** Pineal and suprasellar germinomas: Results of radiation treatment. J Neurosurg 48:99–107, 1978

25. **Katz EL:** Late results of radical excision of craniopharyngiomas in children. J Neurosurg 42:86–90, 1975

26. **Kosnik EJ, Boesel CP, Bay J, Sayer MP:** Primitive neuroectodermal tumors of the central nervous system in children. J Neurosurg 48:741–746, 1978

27. **Kramer S:** The value of radiation therapy for pituitary and parapituitary tumors. Can Med Assoc J 99:1120–1127, 1968

28. **Logue V, Till K:** Posterior fossa dermoid cysts with special reference to intracranial infection. J Neurol Neurosurg Psychiatry 15:1–12, 1952

29. **Matson DD:** Neurosurgery of Infancy and Childhood, 2nd ed. Springfield, Charles C Thomas, 1969

30. **McIntosh N:** Medulloblastoma—A changing prognosis? Arch Dis Child 54:200–203, 1979

31. **Mendiratta SS, Rosenblum JA, Strobos RJ:** Congenital meningioma. Neurology 17:914–918, 1967

32. **Menezes AH, Bell WE, Perret GE:** Hypothalamic tumors in children. Their diagnosis and management. Childs Brain 3:265–280, 1977

33. **Merten DF, Gooding CA, Newton TH, Malamud N:** Meningioma of childhood and adolescence. J Pediatr 84:696–700, 1974

34. **Miller NR, Iliff WJ, Green WR:** Evaluation and management of gliomas of the anterior visual pathways. Brain 97:743–754, 1974

35. **Nassar SI, Mount LA:** Papillomas of the choroid plexus. J Neurosurg 29:73–77, 1968

36. **Neuwelt EA, Glasberg M, Frenkel E, Clark WK:** Malignant pineal region tumors. J Neurosurg 51:597–607, 1979

37. **Obrador S, Martin-Rodriguez JG:** Biological factors involved in the clinical features and surgical management of cerebellar hemangioblastoma. Surg Neurol 7:79–85, 1977

38. **Quest DO, Brisman R, Antunes JL, Housepian**

EM: Period of risk for recurrence in medulloblastoma. J Neurosurg 48:159–163, 1978

39. **Raimondi AJ, Tomita T:** Medulloblastoma in children: Comparative results of partial and total resection. Childs Brain 5:310–328, 1979

40. **Richmond IL, Wilson CB:** Pituitary adenoma in childhood and adolescence. J Neurosurg 49:163–168, 1978

41. **Rubinstein LJ:** Tumors of the Central Nervous System, Atlas of Tumor Pathology, Second Series, Fascicle 6. Washington DC, Armed Forces Institute of Pathology, 1972

42. **Sassin JF, Chutorian AM:** Intracranial chordoma in children. Arch Neurol 17:89–93, 1967

43. **Seidenfeld J, Marton LJ:** Biochemical markers of central nervous system tumors in cerebrospinal fluid. Assoc Clin Lab Sci 8:456–466, 1978

44. **Shapiro K, Till K, Grant DN:** Craniopharyngiomas in childhood. J Neurosurg 50:617–623, 1979

45. **Shin KH, Fisher G, Webster JH:** Brain stem tumors in children. J Can Assoc Radiol 30:77–78, 1979

46. **Stein BM, Fraser RAR, Tenner MS:** Tumours of the third ventricle in children. J Neurol Neurosurg Psychiatry 35:776–788, 1972

47. **Suemitsu T, Nakajima S, Kuwajima K, Nihei K, Kamoshita S:** Lipoma of the corpus callosum: Report of a case and review of the literature. Childs Brain 5:476–483, 1979

48. **Takaku A, Kodama N, Ohara H, Hori S:** Brain tumor in newborn babies. Childs Brain 4:365–375, 1978

49. **Terao H, Kobayashi S, Teraoka A, Okeda R:** Xanthogranulomas of the choroid plexus in a neuro-epileptic child. J Neurosurg 48:649–653, 1978

50. **Welch K:** The intracranial pressure in infants. J Neurosurg 52:693–699, 1980

51. **Winston K, Gilles FH, Leviton A, Fulchiero A:** Cerebellar gliomas in children. J Natl Cancer Inst 58:833–838, 1977

52. **Yates AJ, Becker LE, and Sachs LA:** Brain tumors in childhood. Childs Brain 5:31–39, 1979

53. **Young JL, Miller RW:** Incidence of malignant tumors in U.S. children. J Pediatr 86:254–258, 1975

Cerebrovascular Diseases

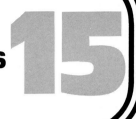

Arnold P. Gold
James F. Hammill
Sidney Carter

The group of disease entities classified as cerebrovascular include all morbid processes, primary or secondary, in which the blood vessels of the brain are involved. All are characterized by loss of or damage to neural parenchyma when its arterial blood supply or venous drainage is abnormal or interrupted. They include congenital anomalies; occlusive vascular disease caused by thrombus, embolus, or dissecting aneurysm; hemorrhage; entities that alter the permeability of the vascular wall; and the blood dyscrasias. Cerebrovascular disease in childhood was thoroughly reviewed by the Strokes in Children Study Group of the Joint Committee for Stroke Facilities.[28,29]

INCIDENCE

Incidence figures for cerebrovascular disease in the pediatric age group have changed significantly during the past 2 decades, and in large part this is due to improved diagnostic techniques. Initially, cerebral angiography with echoencephalography and the radioisotope brain scan enabled physicians to define and treat many clinical entities, and during the past decade, noninvasive computerized tomography (CT scan) revolutionized clinical pediatric neurology. Prior to this period, entities such as subependymal hemorrhage or intraventricular hemorrhage that occurs in a significant number of premature infants were rarely recognized, and epidemiologic data from two decades ago reflect this.

It is difficult to obtain accurate information about the relative frequency of the various types of cerebrovascular lesions because of deficient clinical recognition, inadequate epidemiologic facilities for reporting pediatric cases, and incidence reports frequently based on autopsy data.[28] Kurtzkes' epidemiologic monograph obtained from mortality data emphasizes that children are more likely to die from a subarachnoid or parenchymal hemorrhage than a thrombosis or embolism. Occlusive vascular diseases are those most commonly seen, with arterial involvement more frequent than venous.[47,7] At our medical center, the single most commonly associated disorder with occlusive vascular phenomena was congenital heart disease; 25% of the autopsied cardiac cases had evidence of cerebrovascular occlusion. In more than 500 unselected pediatric autopsies, Banker reported an 8.7% incidence of occlusive vascular disease, congenital heart disease being the most frequently associated condition.[6] All of her patients with the dual lesion had evidence of a left-to-right shunt, with tetralogy of Fallot or transposition of the great vessels present in over 80%.

Incidence of cerebrovascular disease in a well-delineated pediatric population in Rochester, Minnesota, revealed an annual incidence rate of 2.52 cases per 100,000 per year, which is about half the incidence for primary intracranial neoplasm. The data did not include conditions associated with birth, infection, or trauma; the population studied did not include many blacks, and therefore no children with sickle cell anemia.

For these reasons, the incidence of cerebrovascular disease is much higher than reported in this study.[79]

Subependymal hemorrhage or intraventricular hemorrhage occurs in approximately 50% of premature babies weighing less than 1500 g and in 50% of infants of less than 35 weeks gestation who require intensive care for more than 24 hours.[99,52,86]

Cerebrovascular complications are commonly associated with sickle cell disease, with an incidence of approximately 6% to 25%, the overwhelming majority of complications occurring in children less than 15 years. The untreated child with cerebrovascular complications has a 67% risk of additional vascular problems.[71,72,85]

During a 12-year period, 110 children with cerebrovascular disease were seen at the St. Louis Children's Hospital. Twenty-nine had subarachnoid or intraventricular hemorrhage during the first 30 days of life, and 58 (53%) of these cases occurred during the first 2 years. Twenty-three percent had cerebral arterial occlusion, 10% had venous sinus occlusion, 10% had intracerebral hemorrhage, 41% had subarachnoid hemorrhage without an identifiable etiology, and 16% had subarachnoid hemorrhage secondary to a defined etiology.[28]

Acute acquired hemiplegia in childhood caused by cerebrovascular disease was the subject of a report on 86 children. Sixty had evidence of a cerebrovascular disease; occlusive vascular disease was angiographically documented in 16 children, 10 had cardiac disease, 5, sickle cell disease, and 4, a vascular malformation of the brain.[87]

Intracranial bleeding is associated with a variety of disorders. Blood dyscrasias have a high incidence of central nervous system complications. Spontaneous cerebral hemorrhage occurs more frequently than is suspected clinically; it is found in 50% of leukemic patients at necropsy. In children, arteriovenous malformations are ten times as common as intracranial aneurysms and constitute the most common cause of primary subarachnoid hemorrhage. In the adult, these frequencies are reversed.

Trauma is an important risk factor in the pediatric age group, which is unusually prone to head injuries. Three percent of children during the first 7 years of life will have a significant head injury with possible cerebrovascular complications.

CLASSIFICATION

There is no fully acceptable classification of cerebrovascular disease.[1] Conditions that produce thrombosis in one patient may result in hemorrhage in another. Etiologic factors associated with cerebrovascular disease during childhood are often obscure. Hypertension and arteriosclerosis, the major risk factors in adults, are rare in the child. A clinically useful classification of the commonly identified associated conditions is listed below.

Classification of Cerebrovascular Disease

Occlusive vascular disease
  Dural sinus and cerebral venous thrombosis,[3,5,9,10,43,46,82] *associated with:*
    Meningitis
    Infections of face, ears, or paranasal sinuses[45,93]
    Dehydration
    Debilitating states (Marantic)
    Blood dyscrasias: leukemia[19] sickle cell disease,[32] polycythemia, thrombotic thrombocytopenia,[61] thrombocytosis
    Metastatic neoplasms, e.g., neuroblastoma
    Congenital heart disease[19]
    Lead encephalopathy
    Sturge-Weber-Dimitri syndrome (trigeminal encephaloangiomatosis)
    Pregnancy[13]
    Oral contraceptives[3]
  Arterial thrombosis[6,11,14,25,34,41,42,102] *with:*
    Idiopathic or spontaneous[102]
    Dissecting cerebral aneurysm[104]
    Arteriosclerosis: progeria
    Cyanotic congenital heart disease[18,95,96]
    Cerebral arteritis
      Acute infectious diseases
      Granulomatous (Takayasu's disease)[48]
      Syphilis
      Tuberculosis
    Collagen disease
      Polyarteritis nodosa[55]
      Systemic lupus erythematosus[31]
      Dermatomyositis
    Drug abuse[27]
    Trauma to the carotid or cerebral arteries[26]
    Complication of arteriography
    Extraarterial diseases
      Retropharyngeal abscess
      Mucormycosis[103]
      Tumors of the base of the skull
      Craniometaphyseal dysplasia[42]
    Tortuosity and kinking
    Terminal arterial bed phenomenon
    Sickle cell disease[71,72,84,85,90,101]
    Oral contraceptives[37]
    Radiation[64,106]
    Inflammatory bowel disease[57,78]
    Diabetes mellitus[54]

Cerebral embolism[100] *associated with:*
 Atrial fibrillation or other arrhythmias
 Rheumatic heart disease
 Congenital heart disease: right-to-left shunt
 Coronary thrombosis
 Acute or subacute bacterial endocarditis
 Infarcted necrotic placental tissue
 Air complications of cardiac, neck, or thoracic
  surgery[17,98]
 Septic pneumonia or lung abscess
 Parasitic disease[63]
 Fat complications of long-bone
  fractures[7,24,36,52,68,77]
 Tumor[76,81]
 Drug abuse[4,74]
Intracranial (intracerebral and subarachnoid)
  hemorrhage
 Neonatal hemorrhage
  Subdural hematoma
  Intraventricular and subependymal
   hemorrhage[97,101,104]
 Arteriovenous malformation or
  angioma[8,30,40,44,49,50,58,60,67,69,75]
 Intracranial aneurysm[89,2,20,35,56,66,73,83]
 Trauma
  Cavernous sinus fistula
  Subdural hemorrhage
  Epidural hemorrhage
 Blood dyscrasias[83]
  Leukemia[15,33,65]
  Thrombocytopenic purpura
  Aplastic anemia
  Hemophilia[59]
  Anaphylactoid purpura[23]
  Thrombocytosis
  Hemolytic-uremic syndrome
 Hypertension
 Liver disease
 Complications of anticoagulant therapy
 Intracranial neoplasms
 Deficiency syndromes
  Vitamin B_1 deficiency: Wernicke
   encephalopathy
  Vitamin C deficiency: scurvy
  Vitamin K deficiency: hemorrhagic disease of
   the newborn
 Toxic or infectious encephalopathy

OCCLUSIVE VASCULAR DISEASE

In occlusive vascular disease, the brain is
deprived of oxygen by either arterial or venous occlusion, and there is degeneration
of its neurons and its supporting structure,
the glia. Accompanying the necrosis (encephalomalacia) of the tissue is swelling of
surrounding areas. The process of repair that
occurs over the subsequent months is characterized by phagocytosis of the necrotic
tissue by macrophages and the formation of
an astrocytic and fibroblastic scar. This ischemic area, or infarct, may be pale, red, or
mixed. A red infarct, usually seen in venous occlusion, is hemorrhagic owing to loss
of endothelial integrity. The infarct is the
nonspecific end result of any type of occlusion; however, the changes in the blood
vessels or the surrounding brain may be
highly specific. Arteriosclerosis in progeria
and the vascular changes found with granulomatous arteritis (Takayasu's disease),
blood dyscrasias, and neoplasms all have
characteristic anatomic changes. A dissecting aneurysm of a cerebral artery with subsequent intramural thrombosis has been
identified as the cause of occlusion in some
cases of acute infantile hemiplegia.

DURAL SINUS AND CEREBRAL VENOUS THROMBOSIS

Thrombosis of dural venous sinuses and
cerebral veins may cause obstruction of venous drainage and lead to cerebral edema
and hemorrhagic infarction of the brain.
Thrombosis of venous sinuses may occur
without causing any gross cerebral lesion
because anastomoses of the cerebral venous
system (collateral venous circulation) are
often effective in bypassing the obstruction,
and the integrity of the venous circulation
may be maintained. The lateral dural sinuses
are unequal in size, with the larger vessel
carrying the major drainage. Obstruction of
the minor sinus may therefore be asymptomatic.

The incidence of venous and dural
sinus thrombosis has decreased during the
past century. This is attributed to reduced
frequency of infantile dehydration and
malnutrition. Kalbag and Wolff's monograph contains a detailed review on the
subject of cerebral venous thrombosis.[43]

Venous occlusion is most often secondary to pyogenic infections of the face,
mouth, mastoids, or leptomeninges. In addition to infection, children commonly develop cerebral venous thrombosis in association with congenital heart disease,
trauma, dehydration, debilitating and ca-
chectic states, sickle cell disease, polycythemia, or leukemia.[53] This complication is
less frequently observed in thrombotic
thrombocytopenia, metastatic neoplasia,
lead encephalopathy, or the Sturge-Weber-
Dimitri syndrome. During adolescence, ve-

nous occlusion may be associated with pregnancy or the use of oral contraceptive agents.

Cerebral venous or dural sinus thrombosis is the most frequent central nervous system complication of cyanotic congenital heart disease. Cyanotic children under 4 years of age, particularly those whose hematologic indices indicate a hypochromic microcytic anemia (iron deficiency anemia), are at risk for this complication.[19]

Clinical Findings. The clinical picture in patients with cerebral venous thrombosis is generally less dramatic and more difficult to recognize than that seen with arterial occlusive vascular disease. Clinical findings are related to the extent of cerebral vein involvement, the rapidity of occlusion, and the nature of the primary disease.[5]

The common manifestations of dural sinus and cerebral venous thrombosis are increased intracranial pressure, focal motor deficits, seizures, altered states of consciousness, and signs of circulatory stasis. Occlusion of the major lateral dural sinus may result in a clinical picture of increased intracranial pressure without focal neurologic deficit (pseudotumor cerebri). Those children who develop focal signs may slowly recover but may be left with a residual hemiparesis, seizures, or mental retardation. Prolonged convulsions, profound coma, and a febrile reaction are often associated with rapid and complete occlusion of the superior sagittal sinus, which usually leads to death within a short time.

Superior sagittal sinus thrombosis is suggested by alternating hemiplegias and multifocal seizures. Focal or generalized convulsions may occur alone, before, or after the motor deficit is evident. Local signs of circulatory stasis are rare, but when present are pathognomonic for involvement of a specific vessel. Cavernous sinus thrombosis results in a typical picture characterized by exophthalmos of the homolateral eye, palpebral and conjunctival edema, and involvement of the third, fourth, and sixth cranial nerves and the first two branches of the fifth cranial nerve. Lateral sinus thrombosis may be accompanied by painful swelling of the mastoid region. Superior sagittal sinus thrombosis frequently results in dilatation of scalp and eyelid veins as well as edema of the forehead.

Laboratory Findings. Examination of the peripheral blood may yield normal findings, but more commonly there is moderate polymorphonuclear leukocytosis and an elevated erythrocyte sedimentation rate. The urine is normal.

Changes in the cerebrospinal fluid vary according to the pathologic process. The fluid may be under increased pressure but clear and colorless with little or no pleocytosis. Rapid and complete thrombosis of a major vessel may result in xanthochromic cerebrospinal fluid with red blood cells or even frank hemorrhage under markedly increased pressure. Extension of infection from contiguous areas with the production of cortical thrombophlebitis causes pleocytosis in the cerebrospinal fluid, but the sugar content is normal and the fluid is sterile unless there is associated meningitis. This is in contrast to venous thrombosis secondary to pyogenic meningitis, in which case there is leukocyte pleocytosis, a low sugar content, and positive cultures. The Tobey-Ayer test, although not always reliable, may be of some value in the diagnosis of lateral sinus or jugular vein thrombosis. With this maneuver, compression of the jugular vein on the affected side produces no rise in the cerebrospinal fluid pressure. Compression of the normal side results in a brisk response. The electroencephalogram may be normal, particularly when the clinical signs are limited to only those of increased intracranial pressure as is often encountered in lateral sinus thrombosis. When focal neurologic signs and seizures are part of the clinical picture, marked focal and general abnormalities are seen.

Skull roentgenograms may show signs of increased intracranial pressure and mastoid disease. It is often possible to estimate the relative size of the lateral sinuses by their imprint on the bony occiput. CT scan demonstrates a lucent lesion in the area drained by the occluded dural sinus.[46] The site of the thrombosis can often be confirmed in the venous phase of a cerebral arteriogram.[82]

ARTERIAL THROMBOSIS

Arterial thrombosis produces stenosis or occlusion of a cerebral artery. The effect of such occlusion is extremely variable because it depends upon the rapidity of occlusion, the collateral circulation, and the maintenance of systemic blood pressure.

Cerebral artery thrombosis in children is frequently a complication of certain systemic disease entities, including the collagen diseases and the cerebral arteritides. Lupus erythematosus may involve almost any portion of the nervous system. The most common site of involvement is the cerebral cortex, although the spinal cord and peripheral nerves may be affected. Neurologic manifestations depend upon the area involved. Ninety percent of the children with systemic lupus at the Babies Hospital in New York developed manifestations related to central nervous system involvement. Convulsions were the most frequently observed phenomena, but organic psychotic states, hemiplegia, cortical sensory changes, and other focal signs were also evident. Nervous system involvement with lupus erythematosus in the adult has been assumed to be secondary to arteritis of small vessels with resultant occlusion. The absence of such small vessel involvement is quite striking in children, although the appearance and distribution of lesions suggest a cerebral arterial lesion.[26] Polyarteritis nodosa rarely involves the cerebral arteries, but when such involvement does occur the small vessels are affected with a resultant slowly progressive deficit.

Delayed radiation vasculopathy is occasionally seen in children.[64,106] Primarily occluding the large basal arteries with or without telangiectasia, radiation may also result in branch occlusion. The amount of radiation required to produce arterial occlusion ranges between 1000 and 8500 rads, and the final effects of radiation on blood vessels may not be clinically apparent for many years, with a range of 2 to 22 years. Relatively small radiation doses in the infant may produce occlusion of the large basal arteries, whereas greater radiation to the neck, face, and brain is usually required to produce this vasculopathy in the older child.

Inflammatory bowel disease may be complicated by cerebral arterial or venous thrombosis.[57,78] A hypercoagulable state with or without thrombocytosis may be associated with the intestinal inflammation and predispose the child to a stroke.

Juvenile diabetes may be complicated by acute hemiplegia secondary to a branch occlusion in some children, whereas others fail to demonstrate a vascular lesion with detailed cerebral angiography.[54] Characteristically, this produces a transient neurologic deficit, and complete recovery is anticipated.

Oral contraceptive use increases the risk of thrombotic cerebrovascular disease in adolescent girls and young adults.[37] The relative risk is approximately nine times greater for girls who use oral contraceptives than for those who do not. Because oral contraceptives accelerate clotting, it is not surprising that cerebral arteries as well as veins may be involved.

Drug abuse has been shown to produce a necrotizing angiitis and clinical manifestations indistinguishable from periarteritis nodosa. Phencyclidine intoxication may result in an altered state of consciousness and seizures, or focal manifestations suggestive of a stroke.[21]

Cerebral arteritis may result from any of various factors. Infectious diseases, usually bacterial, may be systemic or may involve only the meninges. There may be a direct inflammatory effect on the artery, or bacterial toxins may damage the vessel wall, which subsequently develops a thrombosis. Idiopathic granulomatous arteritis (Takayasu's disease), recently described in adolescents, involves the aorta and its major branches with occlusion of intracranial and limb arteries. This results in neurologic manifestations of arterial thrombosis and a pulseless state.[48] Mucormycosis infection of the paranasal sinuses, occasionally seen in association with uncontrolled diabetes, may extend into the cranium with involvement of arteries in the region of the frontal lobe.[103] Meningovascular syphilis and tuberculosis may be causes of cerebral thrombosis in children as well as in adults.

Extrinsic conditions may either directly traumatize or compress the cerebral vessels. Damage to the vessel wall by either mechanism may result in thrombosis. Tumors of the base of the skull, retropharyngeal abscesses, and craniometaphyseal dysplasia are capable of compressing the arteries. Children with craniometaphyseal dysplasia have involvement of the skull and long bones. There is a bony overgrowth of the facial bones and the base of the skull, and narrowing of the foramina of the internal carotid artery and cranial nerves.[42]

Atherosclerosis, commonly seen in adults, is rarely observed in the pathogenesis of arterial thrombosis in children. Progerics characteristically develop atherosclerosis, and the affected child with normal intelligence resembles a dwarfed elderly person with a large alopecic cranium, a small face with a beak-like nose, underdeveloped maxillae, absent earlobes, and marked loss of subcutaneous and muscle mass. Neurologic manifestations and even death may result from carotid artery thrombosis.

The majority of children with cerebral artery thrombosis are apparently healthy prior to the occlusion.[102] It is conceivable that the entities referred to as idiopathic or spontaneous infantile hemiplegia (Marie-Strümpell disease, polioencephalitis) are the result of cerebral artery thrombosis. A dissecting aneurysm caused by a congenital defect of the arterial wall has been implicated in some of these cases.[104]

Clinical Findings. Depending upon etiology, the child demonstrates clinical manifestations of the underlying disorder as well as neurologic changes to the area involved. Solomon and her associates clarified the natural history of acute hemiplegia of childhood.[87] It characteristically appears during the first year or two of life. Unexplained or idiopathic hemiplegia rarely develops after the preschool period. The previously well youngster suddenly develops fever, has a series of convulsions, and is left with a hemiplegia that may partially clear. In addition to the hemiplegia, there may be a cortical hemisensory defect, hemianopia, and aphasia. Recurrent focal motor seizures may complicate the subsequent course and can be resistant to anticonvulsant medications.

Classically, the episode of hemiplegia is an isolated clinical phenomenon. Most otherwise healthy children with cerebral artery thrombosis rarely have subsequent strokes or transient ischemic attacks.[27] In contrast, children with systemic disorders may develop subsequent cerebrovascular complications. Alternating hemiplegia (from one side to another) indicates diffuse vascular disease. Basal occlusive disease of the internal carotid artery with telangiectasia (moyamoya) is often preceded by a headache and typically is manifested by alternating hemiplegia. Subarachnoid hemorrhage occasionally occurs at the onset. The infant and young child have a clinical course that is usually progressive and fatal, whereas the older child has a progressive course with permanent motor and intellectual deficits.[12]

Sickle cell disease is not uncommonly associated with cerebrovascular complications, with an incidence of approximately 6% to 25%, and with the overwhelming majority occurring in children less than 15 years of age.[71,72] Small blood vessel thrombosis or, less commonly, dural sinus thrombosis has been identified as the most common pathologic lesion. Recently, large cerebral artery thrombosis, often with telangiectasia (moyamoya), has been reported in children presenting with an acute hemiplegia. Although improvement of the hemiplegia is anticipated, recurrent episodes of hemiplegia, often with contralateral involvement, occur in 67% of untreated children.[71,101] Other neurologic manifestations, often secondary to small vessel thrombosis, include an altered state of consciousness with stupor or coma, convulsions, visual disturbances, and meningeal signs. After each cerebrovascular episode, there is often further impairment, above all in motor and intellectual functions. Cerebrovascular complications are far less common in children with sickle cell–hemoglobin C disease.

Arterial thrombosis in children usually occurs in the internal carotid or anterior circulation.[70,94] Vertebral–basilar artery occlusion, rarely seen in children, is manifested by recurrent vertigo and ataxia as well as extraocular palsies, nystagmus, and dysarthria.

Palpation of the carotid artery or measurement of the retinal arterial pressure (ophthalmodynamometry) has not been useful in diagnosing childhood arterial thrombosis. When the child is seen years after the onset of the acute episode, the involved extremities may be short, atrophic, and spastic.

Laboratory Findings. The blood count, urinalysis, and erythrocyte sedimentation rate are normal. The cerebrospinal fluid during the acute period is normal, but a slight leukocytic pleocytosis may be found a few weeks later. Electroencephalograms, sometimes normal, are characterized by slow-wave foci over the involved area. With major artery occlusion, a general decrease in amplitude of background activity is also sometimes encountered and on rare occasions is the only abnormality seen. Thermograms may be useful in arterial thrombosis; a "cold area" indicates poor perfusion in the distribution of the occluded internal carotid artery.[105]

Radiologic findings are frequently of diagnostic importance. Early plain skull roentgenograms are normal, but after a period of years they may show the characteristic features as described by Dyke et al, with thickening of the cranial vault, overdevelopment of the frontal and ethmoid sinuses, and elevation of the petrous pyramid of the temporal bone on the ipsilateral side. Coincident with the appearance of cerebral atrophy, CT scan (Fig. 15-1) and air contrast studies may show porencephaly or a dilated lateral ventricle on the affected side.[22]

CT scan supplies the anatomic localization and the "age" of the lesion; serial scans define pathologic changes. Angiography may delineate specific vascular changes. CT scan following a transient ischemic attack is often normal, whereas cerebral arterial thrombosis produces an infarct in the area supplied by the occluded artery. Within 24 hours (Fig. 15-2) there is a nonhomogenous decreased density lesion secondary to cerebral edema. By the end of one week (Fig. 15-3), liquifaction necrosis develops, and the lesion becomes homogenous with well-defined margins. Within 2 to 4 months (Fig. 15-4), necrosis is replaced by a cystic cavity, and the lesion has the homogenous appearance of cerebrospinal fluid.

Angiography early in the course of the illness may demonstrate complete occlusion of the artery, but later there may be recanalization of the occluded vessel or the presence of collateral circulation (Figs. 15-5 and 15-6). A very practical angiographic classification for primary arterial thrombotic occlusions was formulated by Hilal and associates[38,39]:

1. Extracranial occlusions
2. Basal occlusive disease without telangiectasia
   a. Congenital or perinatal
   b. Acquired
3. Basal occlusive disease with telangiectasia
4. Peripheral leptomeningeal artery occlusions
5. Perforating arterial occlusions

The angiographic findings are not only important diagnostically but also often supply important prognostic information.

Extracranial Occlusive Lesions. Trauma is the most common cause of occlusion of the cervical portion of the carotid artery in a child. Occlusion can result either from an external impact of the internal carotid artery against the transverse process of C_2 or from blunt trauma, usually to the oropharynx. Clinically, there is usually a delay of up to 24 hours between the traumatic episode and the development of neurologic deficit. Rare nontraumatic etiologies include infection and an atheromatous plaque. Tortuosity and kinking of the cervical carotid artery, common in children, has yet to be established as a definitive factor related to arterial thrombosis. Figure 15-7 demonstrates this clinical entity.

Basal Occlusive Disease Without Telangiectasia. The primary lesion in basal occlusive disease without telangiectasia is in the major arteries at the base of the brain (i.e., the supraclinoid internal carotid artery; Fig. 15-8), the anterior and middle cerebral arteries, and the basilar artery. The condition is unilateral and so does not recur. The congenital or perinatal basal occlusions are usually associated with large porencephalic cysts, and the acquired variety has cerebral atrophy as a late sequela. Motor deficit is the most common manifestation. These children do not usually develop epilepsy, hyperkinetic behavior, or an intellectual deficit.

Basal Occlusive Disease With Telangiectasia (moyamoya). The occlusive lesion in basal occlusive disease with telangiectasia involves the arteries at the base of the brain, but there is also marked telangiectasia in the region of the basal ganglia (Fig. 15-9). It is much more common in girls and is usually progressive and bilateral. It has been associated with bacterial and tubercular meningitis and has been seen with neurofibromatosis, tuberous sclerosis, sic-

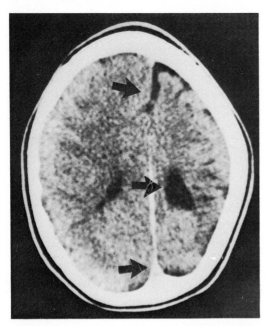

FIG. 15-1. Old carotid artery occlusion. Child with infantile hemiplegia secondary to internal carotid artery occlusion that occurred 5 years previously. CT scan demonstrates a small atrophic cerebral hemisphere (*black arrows*) with a dilated lateral ventricle and an enlarged subarachnoid space. The cranium over the atrophic hemisphere is thickened when compared to the normal contralateral side.

FIG. 15-2. Middle cerebral artery occlusion of 24 hours duration in a two-year-old child with middle cerebral artery thrombosis. CT scan reveals a nonhomogenous decreased density lesion with hazy margins in the parieto-occipital area.

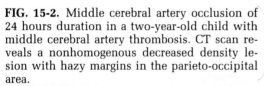

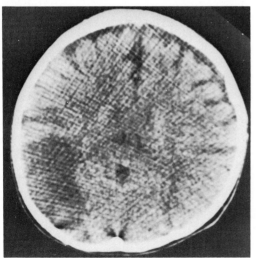

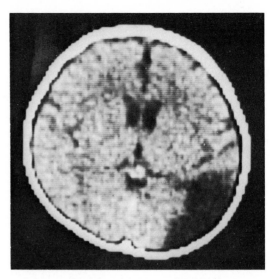

FIG. 15-3. Middle cerebral artery occlusion of 3 weeks duration. CT scan reveals a homogenous lucency with well-defined margins.

FIG. 15-4. Middle cerebral artery thrombosis of 4 months duration. CT scan reveals a well-defined cystic lucency having the appearance of cerebrospinal fluid.

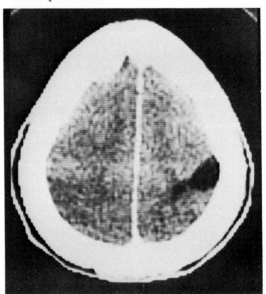

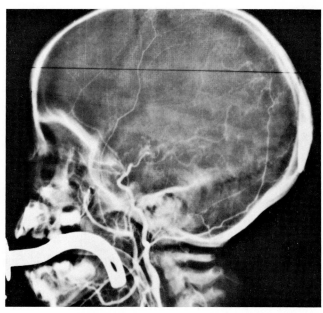

FIG. 15-5. Basal occlusion without telangiectasia. Lateral view of a carotid angiogram showing the occlusion of the internal carotid artery distal to the origin of the posterior communicating and anterior choroidal arteries. The collaterals on the surface of the brain are between the terminal branches of the posterior cerebral and the middle cerebral arteries.

kle cell disease, and an optic nerve glioma treated with radiotherapy. Epilepsy, behavioral problems, and intellectual deficits are commonly observed in addition to the alternating hemiparesis.

Peripheral Leptomeningeal Artery Occlusions. The occlusive lesions in the distal leptomeningeal arteries are best demonstrated with magnification angiography. (Fig. 15-10). Diabetes mellitus, sickle cell disease, intravenous drug abuse, and the neurocutaneous syndromes are some of the known primary etiologic conditions. Similar occlusions can occur secondary to cerebral abscesses, trauma, or tumor encasement. Recovery from the hemiparesis is anticipated because of the excellent collateral circulation in children.

Perforating Artery Occlusions. Periarteritis nodosa and homocystinuria can both exclusively involve the small perforating arteries, most commonly the striate arteries and result in progressive neurologic disease with alternating hemiplegia, subarachnoid hemorrhage, and often death.

FIG. 15-6. Stenosis of the peripheral leptomeningeal branches. Lateral view of a carotid angiogram showing the attenuated branches of the middle cerebral artery. The narrowed arterial lumen probably resulted from an occlusion and subsequent canalization of the middle cerebral artery branches.

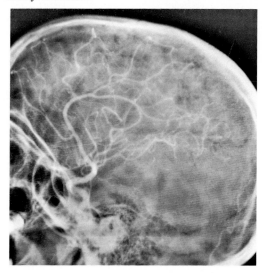

CEREBRAL EMBOLISM

In cerebral embolism, a cerebral artery is occluded by bacteria, parasites, air, fat, tumor, foreign bodies or a fragment of organized thrombus. An embolus lodges most commonly in a small peripheral vessel at a point of bifurcation. The middle cerebral artery or one of its branches is the vessel most frequently occluded, although no artery is exempt. The speed of occlusion is so rapid that compensatory collateral circulation usually cannot be established, and a cerebral infarct results.[100]

Cerebral embolic phenomena during childhood are usually of cardiac origin. Atrial fibrillation and other arrhythmias favor the formation of mural thrombi, fragments of which may then become detached. The phenomenon is seen in patients with cyanotic congenital heart and rheumatic valvular disease. Emboli may result from the vegetations of bacterial endocarditis or from lesions produced by cardiac, pulmonary, or neck surgery. During the newborn period, cerebral emboli may result from liberation of infarcted placental tissue. In adults, coronary thrombosis and atrial fibrillation associated with atherosclerotic or rheumatic heart disease are common causes of cerebral emboli.

Air embolism may be either venous or arterial.[17,98] Air introduced into a vein is usually arrested in the right cardiac chambers and rarely reaches the brain. Less commonly, paradoxical embolism may result from bypassing the pulmonary circulation. Although not fully understood, this is best explained by transit through a patent foramen ovale or other communication between the right and left sides of the heart. The paravertebral venous system may be the pathway of some of these paradoxical emboli. Arterial embolism commonly results in cerebral manifestations and occurs after the entrance of air into the pulmonary veins, left cardiac chambers, or carotid artery. Air embolism has been encountered with greater

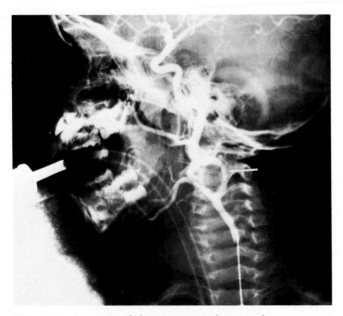

FIG. 15-7. Stenosis of the extracranial internal carotid artery. The lateral view shows a marked stenosis of the internal carotid artery (*arrow*) about 1.5 cm distal to the carotid bifurcation. There was no clinically detectable inflammatory process in the neck of this patient and no history of trauma. The facial thermogram indicated an area of coolness on the medial canthus of the eye corresponding to the site.

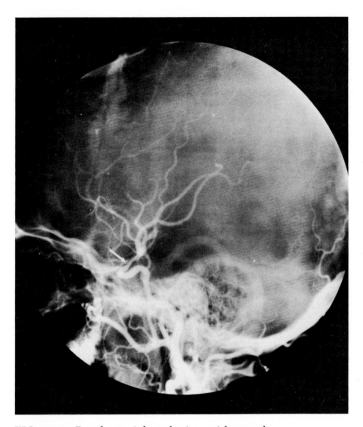

FIG. 15-8. Basal arterial occlusion without telangiectasia. The lateral view of the carotid arteriogram shows a narrowing of the supraclinoid portion of the internal carotid artery (*arrow*). The internal carotid artery on the opposite side (not illustrated) is normal.

frequency since the advent of newer techniques in thoracic surgery, but this condition may originate from diverse etiologies: sudden reduction in barometric pressure with liberation of nitrogen bubbles in the bloodstream (Caisson disease); therapeutic procedures, such as puncture and irrigation of the maxillary antrum; cardiac surgery or catheterization; therapeutic pneumothorax; lung puncture; and neck surgery.

Fat embolism is usually associated with fractures of long bones. Fat particles are carried to the pulmonary capillaries and forced through to the pulmonary vein whence they may ultimately reach the brain by way of the left side of the heart.[7,24,36,52,68,77]

Septic embolism is commonly asso-ciated with pulmonary inflammatory conditions such as nonsuppurative pneumonia or lung abscess, and may result in brain abscesses or mycotic aneurysms. Rarely, parasitic embolism has been observed.[63]

Tumor embolism, other than that secondary to atrial myxoma, is rarely observed because the cells are too small to occlude a cerebral artery rapidly. Multiple small aneurysms of the leptomeningeal vessels can be caused by emboli from an atrial myxoma.[95]

Clinical Findings. Cerebral embolism is characterized by acute onset without significant prodromata. Occasionally, premonitory symptoms (headache, vomiting, lassitude) occur. The clinical picture may be complete within seconds to minutes and may appear at any time of the day unrelated to physical activity. Convulsions, transient loss of consciousness, and headache may be observed at the onset. Focal neurologic findings depend upon the cerebral artery

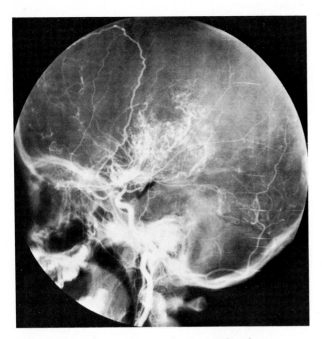

FIG. 15-9. Basal arterial occlusion with telangiectasia. Lateral view of the carotid arteriogram showing complete occlusion of the internal carotid artery distal to the origin of the anterior choroidal. There is a large telangiectatic formation in the basal ganglia supplied by the thalamoperforate vessels arising from the posterior communicating artery and by the lenticulostriate branches of the internal carotid. The anterior choroidal artery is also supplying this large telangiectatic formation. Note also a large middle meningeal artery reaching to the top of the convexity and providing collaterals to the anterior cerebral branches over the frontal lobe across the subarachnoid space (rete mirabile anastomosis). The ophthalmic artery is large and contributes to the supply of the undersurface of the frontal lobe through its ethmoidal and meningeal branches.

occluded and may take the form of hemiplegia, hemianesthesia, hemianopia, and aphasia. Transient blindness is the most characteristic manifestation of air embolism.[17,98]

Fat embolism is rarely encountered. Usually associated with long bone fractures, this central nervous system complication can also occur after intravenous fat infusions (infant fat overloading syndrome).[7] Fat embolism has a characteristic clinical picture. Initially, there is a lucid interval after the injury, and then at 12 to 48 hours (after a long-bone fracture, for example), pulmonary symptoms and signs occur with fever, respiratory distress, cyanosis, and blood-tinged sputum. This is then followed in a few hours by neurologic manifestations. The symptoms may be mild, including headache, restlessness, or irritability; the process can progress to a focal neurologic deficit, which may include diabetes insipidus, delirium, stupor, or coma; if severe, it results in shock or death. In addition, there may be petechial hemorrhages of the skin, fat in the retinal vessels, and free fat droplets in the urine.[7,24,36,52,68,77]

Tumor emboli associated with atrial myxoma present with a characteristic clinical picture of heart murmurs that change with time or body posture, systemic manifestations of fever and weight loss, and neurologic syndromes that include transient

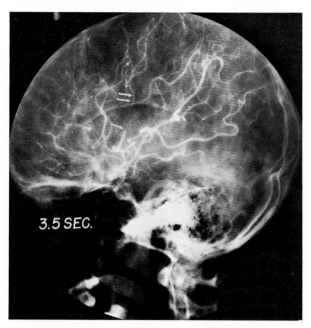

FIG. 15-10. Peripheral leptomeningeal arterial occlusion. The lateral carotid arteriogram shows an occlusion of one of the branches of the middle cerebral artery (*arrow*) and retrograde filling through collaterals (*double arrows*).

neurologic deficits, multiple cerebral aneurysm formation, spinal cord embolization, and cerebral embolization with focal neurologic deficits, seizures, syncope, and even death.[76,81]

Foreign body emboli, most commonly a complication of intravenous drug abuse, are rare. Unknown to the recipient, the drug may be diluted with foreign materials (e.g., starch or talc), or the diluent for illicit intravenous drug administration may be the source of cerebral emboli.[4,74]

Laboratory Findings. A polymorphonuclear leukocytosis (less than 20,000/cu mm) is usually present. The erythrocyte sedimentation rate, urinalysis, and skull roentgenograms are generally normal. The cerebrospinal fluid is generally under normal pressure, clear, and contains a normal or slightly elevated concentration of protein with a normal number of cells. Atrial myxomas are associated with leukocytosis, an elevated erythrocyte sedimentation rate, hyperglobulinemia, anemia, or more rarely polycythemia. Pleocytosis and elevated protein content may be found in children with bacterial endocarditis. The electroencephalogram in most cases of symptomatic embolism shows a slow-wave abnormality which tends to be persistent.

CT scan with contrast is often characteristic in that there are often multiple lesions (Fig. 15-11). The CT findings of a hemorrhagic infarct include high-density lesions with enhancement, which may suggest a metastatic neoplasm, hemorrhage, or an intracerebral hematoma. Two to three months later, lesions on CT scan will be lucent and sharply defined.

Cerebral angiography is often diagnostic. Cerebral emboli commonly lodge in the supraclinoid segment of the internal carotid artery or the middle cerebral artery, typically sparing the anterior cerebral artery. Angiographically, the occluded artery is of normal caliber up to the level of the obstruction, where the contrast media outlines a cup-shaped defect.

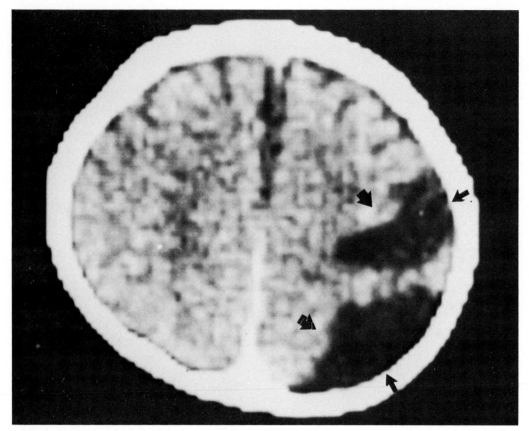

FIG. 15-11. CT scan performed on a child 3 months after cerebral embolism reveals multiple infarcts (*black arrows*). This child had congenital heart disease and developed a hemiplegia related to cerebral embolism at the time of cardiac catheterization.

INTRACRANIAL HEMORRHAGE

Intracranial hemorrhage, either intracerebral or subarachnoid, results from a defect in the integrity of cerebral blood vessels with extravasation of blood into one or more of the following: brain, ventricles, subarachnoid, and subdural spaces. Intracranial hemorrhage most frequently results from trauma, but not infrequently occurs in children with vascular malformation, aneurysm, blood dyscrasia, toxic or infectious encephalopathy, systemic hypertension, intracranial neoplasm, liver disease, or vitamin deficiencies, or as a complication of anticoagulant therapy.

Despite the varied etiologies, clinical manifestations are similar in the different conditions, and identification of the cause is further complicated by the nonspecific finding of blood in the cerebrospinal fluid. Proper management is largely dependent upon delineation of the specific etiologic process, and this is possible only with a complete clinical history and adequate laboratory facilities.

The child with a subarachnoid hemorrhage shows signs of increased intracranial pressure and meningeal irritation. The onset is usually dramatic, with severe headache, vomiting, loss of consciousness, and convulsions. Evidence of meningeal irritation is an early clinical manifestation with nuchal rigidity and Brudzinski and Kernig signs. Extensor plantar responses may be noted early, and funduscopic evaluation may reveal subhyaloid hemorrhages. Fever may be a prominent and often misleading feature. There is usually systemic hypertension, although the blood pressure may be normal. The patient with intracerebral bleeding may have evidence of blood in the subarachnoid space, in which case there may be the symptoms and signs previously mentioned as well as focal neurologic deficit.

Intracranial hemorrhage is the most common neurologic problem in the neonate, with subependymal and intraventricular hemorrhage being diagnosed with increased frequency in the premature baby.[23,65,97] CT and, more recently, ultrasound studies have enabled the physician, even with a critically ill neonate, to define with precision the site and extent of the hemorrhage. The other hemorrhagic complications in the newborn include subdural hematoma, primary subarachnoid hemorrhage, and posterior fossa or intracerebellar hematoma. Subdural hematoma, a complication of obstetric trauma in the full-term neonate, is now uncommon owing to improved obstetrical management. Primary subarachnoid hemorrhage is common, but unless massive rarely presents as a clinical problem. Posterior fossa hematoma, often associated with a difficult delivery, has an acute onset within the first 24 hours of life, and is characterized by apnea, lethargy, increased pressure with a bulging fontanel, bloody cerebrospinal fluid, and a falling hematocrit. Intracerebellar hematoma may be present in an asymptomatic small premature, and its presence is of uncertain clinical significance. Surgical evacuation of a posterior fossa subdural hematoma is often lifesaving.

The neonate with intracranial bleeding may be asymptomatic or may show a more varied picture, including apathy or restlessness, cyanosis or pallor, bulging of the fontanels, respiratory distress, convulsions, a high-pitched cry, vomiting, poor suck, a failure to thrive, and an exaggerated or absent Moro's reflex. Secondary hydrocephalus may be a complication in those children who survive subarachnoid bleeding. This is due to partial obliteration of the subarachnoid space or to incisural block.

The premature infant who has sustained a significant hypoxic–ischemic event 24 to 48 hours previously is at risk for the development of a periventricular hemorrhage. Fifty percent of all premature infants weighing less than 1500 g had CT evidence of this hemorrhagic lesion.[65] The hemorrhage consists of bleeding into the subependymal germinal matrix, usually at the level of the foramen of Monro and the head of the caudate nucleus, and if extensive may extend through the ependyma into the ventricle. Clinical manifestations of periventricular hemorrhage vary from a completely asymptomatic premature infant to a severely and acutely ill infant. The symptomatic premature infant may present with either a catastrophic, often fatal, condition or a milder progression of neurologic manifestations consistent with survival. The acute or catastrophic syndrome develops rapidly over a period of minutes to hours and is characterized by an alteration of the state of consciousness progressing to coma, a bulging fontanel, apneic episodes, generalized seizures, flaccid quadriparesis, unresponsive pupils, and eyes that do not respond to light stimulation. The milder or subacute syndrome follows an uneven course for a period of days, with stupor, hypotonia with decreased spontaneous movements, and eyes that are in an abnormal position or have incomplete horizontal movements. Prognosis is dependent on the size of the hemorrhage as defined by CT (Fig. 15-12), with a 10% to 25% mortality rate in cases of subependymal blood or small amounts of intraventricular blood, and a 50% to 70% mortality rate with large intracortical or intraventricular hemorrhages. Survivors may have a neurologic residual deficit secondary to the hemorrhage or may develop a posthemorrhagic hydrocephalus. The risk of hydrocephalus is related to the size of the hemorrhage, with a 25% risk in mild to moderate hemorrhages and a 50% to 75% risk in moderate to severe hemorrhages.

Blood studies may be helpful in the diagnosis of blood dyscrasias, but patients with intracranial bleeding from other causes may show a polymorphonuclear leukocytosis greater than 20,000/cu mm. The erythrocyte sedimentation rate may be normal or only moderately elevated (to 30–40 mm/hr). Transient albuminuria, hyperglycemia, or glycosuria may be found shortly after the hemorrhage. The electrocardiogram is usually normal in the absence of underlying cardiac disease, but transient T wave and S-T segment changes may be noted. Focal

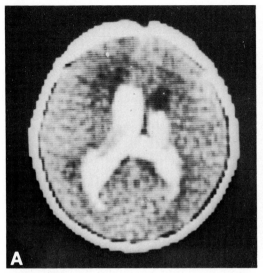
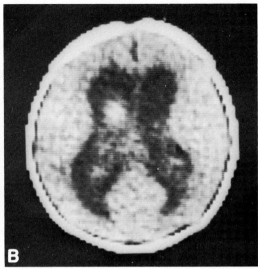

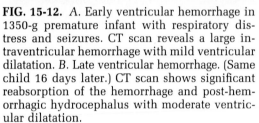

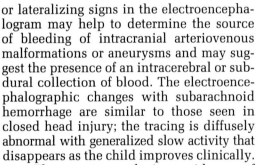

FIG. 15-12. *A.* Early ventricular hemorrhage in 1350-g premature infant with respiratory distress and seizures. CT scan reveals a large intraventricular hemorrhage with mild ventricular dilatation. *B.* Late ventricular hemorrhage. (Same child 16 days later.) CT scan shows significant reabsorption of the hemorrhage and post-hemorrhagic hydrocephalus with moderate ventricular dilatation.

or lateralizing signs in the electroencephalogram may help to determine the source of bleeding of intracranial arteriovenous malformations or aneurysms and may suggest the presence of an intracerebral or subdural collection of blood. The electroencephalographic changes with subarachnoid hemorrhage are similar to those seen in closed head injury; the tracing is diffusely abnormal with generalized slow activity that disappears as the child improves clinically.

The most conclusive evidence of intracranial bleeding is the presence of blood in the cerebrospinal fluid. This must be clearly differentiated from hemorrhage due to a traumatic lumbar puncture. Failure of the fluid to clear in successive test tubes, or a xanthochromic supernatant in a hemorrhage older than 2 hours is diagnostic of bleeding antedating the lumbar puncture. The cerebrospinal fluid is usually under increased pressure with an elevated protein content; leukocytes are present in proportion to the red cells, although great variation may occur.

Noninvasive diagnostic techniques, including CT scan and ultrasound studies, have proven invaluable in the diagnosis of hemorrhage and its major complication, posthemorrhagic hydrocephalus, as well as in determining the site and size of the hemorrhage.

Intracerebral hematomas are slowly resorbed over months by both diffusion and macrophages, and protein changes in the cerebrospinal fluid may be evident during this period. Hemorrhage into the subarachnoid space may be completely cleared of xanthochromic discoloration, pleocytosis, or elevated protein concentration in a period as short as 7 days. Three pigments may be detected in the cerebrospinal fluid following a subarachnoid hemorrhage: oxyhemoglobin, bilirubin, and methemoglobin. Oxyhemoglobin released during red cell lysis is red, but with dilution appears xanthochromic, and may be present in the cerebrospinal fluid supernatant 2 hours after a subarachnoid hemorrhage. It reaches its maximum concentration in 36 hours and gradually disappears within 1 week. In addition to visual or spectroscopic determination, it may also be detected with the benzidine test. Bilirubin (yellow) is first detected about 10 hours after hemorrhage, reaches a maximum concentration at 48 to

72 hours, and may persist in the fluid for 2 to 3 weeks. The severity of the meningeal signs associated with subarachnoid hemorrhage may be roughly correlated with the cerebrospinal fluid bilirubin concentration. Methemoglobin, a brown pigment that is dark yellow with dilution, is a reduction product of bilirubin and may be found in the cerebrospinal fluid with encapsulated hematomas or old intracerebral hematomas. Other changes in the cerebrospinal fluid following bleeding are a pleocytosis, initially polymorphonuclear and subsequently lymphocytic, and an elevated protein concentration. In some patients, the cerebrospinal fluid sugar is low and out of proportion to the blood sugar level, which may even be elevated. These phenomena, though their mechanisms are unknown, should not cloud the diagnostic evaluation.

VASCULAR MALFORMATIONS

Vascular anomalies are the most common cause of primary subarachnoid hemorrhage in children and are at least ten times as common as intracranial aneurysms.[44,58,60,67,88,89] The vascular malformations are usually classified as traumatic, infectious, or congenital. Traumatic or infectious etiologies are rarely seen because anatomically the cerebral vessels are unique and the principal cerebral arteries and veins are not in juxtaposition. The sole exception is the internal carotid artery in the cavernous sinus, which, due to this unique anatomic arrangement, may be considered extracranial. Spontaneous carotid–cavernous fistulas can occur in association with the Ehlers-Danlos syndrome.[80] The malformations of congenital origin are due to failure of maturation with persistence of a more primitive vascular system or to lack of capillary development between the arterial and venous systems. The former is frequently referred to as an angioma and is the result of a network of poorly differentiated noncapillary vessels situated between artery and vein, forming a nonneoplastic mass. The latter type is more common and involves direct anastomosis between one or more enlarged feeding arteries and thinwalled, dilated veins.

Arteriovenous malformations range in size from angiographically occult or cryptic lesions to massive malformations that involve a lobe or even an entire hemisphere of the brain. The malformation may change in size over a period of years; approximately one third enlarge, one third remain unchanged, and one third become smaller.

Arteriovenous malformations are of two major types: deep midline (occurring in the great vein of Galen) and hemispheric (occurring in the area supplied by major branches of the internal carotid artery). On rare occasions, a vascular malformation may involve the brain stem[75] or the spinal cord.[60] The malformation involving the Galenic system is usually a direct anastomosis between the posterior cerebral or the superior cerebellar artery and the great vein. The feeding arteries in this direct type of anastomosis may divide and recombine with themselves or other arteries to form a lacelike network prior to communication with the vein of Galen. There is dilatation of the feeding arteries and marked enlargement of the vein and the draining dural sinuses. The midline aneurysmal dilatation not infrequently compresses and displaces the aqueduct, third ventricle, and quadrigeminal plate.

The hemispheric malformation involving branches of the internal carotid artery is most frequently found over the convexity of the brain in the territory of the middle cerebral artery. This vascular malformation is also seen in other areas of the brain including the basal ganglia, brain stem, and cerebellum. The lesion usually consists of an enlarged feeding artery and a mass of dilated, tortuous veins. Other types of cerebral vascular malformations include capillary telangiectasis, cavernous hemangiomas, and leptomeningeal venous and capillary malformations. They are without a direct shunt between artery and vein, and are difficult to visualize by angiography.

Deep Midline Arteriovenous Malformation (Great Vein of Galen)

Clinical Findings. The manifestations can be placed into three groups, depending upon the size of the vascular shunt and the corresponding age at which symptoms first appear.

1. The symptomatic newborn has a shunt of arterial blood into the venous circulation of such magnitude that it results in peripheral congestion and congestive heart failure.[30,40,50] In addition there may be hydrocephalus and convulsions.

2. During infancy there is less blood shunted with a paucity of clinical cardiac manifestations; however, cardiomegaly and other evidence of abnormal circulatory function may be present. In this group, the arteriovenous shunt produces marked dilatation of the vein of Galen, causing compression of surrounding structures and often leading to aqueductal stenosis with secondary hydrocephalus. An important sign in this age group is an intracranial bruit. There may also be convulsions, subarachnoid hemorrhage, scalp hemangiomas, psychomotor retardation, pyramidal tract involvement, proptosis, epistaxis, a pulsatile retromastoid mass, or papilledema.

3. The older child has a still smaller effective shunt, and dilatation of the vein of Galen is only moderate. There is neither cardiovascular dysfunction nor hydrocephalus, but headaches and subarachnoid hemorrhage are common. Neurologic manifestations may include hemiparesis, cranial nerve palsies, vertigo, convulsions, aphasia, or organic psychosis. Visual and ocular symptoms may take the form of decreased visual acuity, paralysis of upward gaze, proptosis, ptosis, strabismus, loss of pupillary reflex, or papilledema. Because of the small size of the shunt, an intracranial bruit is rarely heard in this age group.

Laboratory Findings. Blood count, erythrocyte sedimentation rate, and urinalysis results are usually normal. The electrocardiogram, especially in the younger patients, shows an intermediate axis or left axis deviation, which is unusual for this age group. According to the magnitude of the arteriovenous shunt, the blood volume is increased; cardiac output may be twice normal.

Electroencephalography is generally not helpful and shows nonspecific slow-wave changes with a temporal or occipital accentuation. The cerebrospinal fluid is usually under increased pressure and not infrequently shows evidence of recent or old hemorrhage. The presence of increased oxygen tension in jugular venous blood is an important simple diagnostic test and is indicative of a large cerebral arteriovenous shunt.

Radiologic findings are frequently of diagnostic importance and may show cardiomegaly or evidence of increased intracranial pressure. In all patients over 15 years of age with a vein of Galen aneurysm, a characteristic curvilinear calcification in the aneurysm's wall may be seen. CT scan (Fig. 15-13) with contrast will demonstrate the midline aneurysmal dilated vein of Galen as well as the enlarged feeding arteries and the draining sinuses.[40] Air contrast studies suggest a vein of Galen malformation by demonstrating a posterior midline mass

FIG. 15-13. Deep midline arteriovenous malformation in 4-year-old boy with chronic headaches. CT scan with contrast shows a large midline malformation involving the veins of Galen and Rosenthal and a hydrocephalus with moderate dilatation of the lateral and third ventricles.

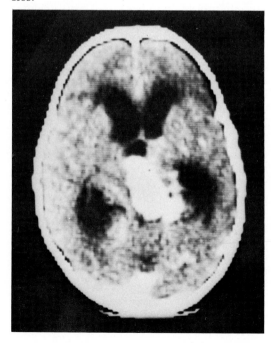

displacing the aqueduct downward and the third ventricle anteriorly with accompanying dilatation of the lateral and third ventricles. Cerebral angiography is the definitive diagnostic tool (Fig. 15-14). There is a midline collection of contrast material outlining the vein of Galen, enlargement of the feeding arteries (usually the posterior cerebral), and marked dilatation of the draining venous sinuses.

Hemispheric Malformations

Clinical Findings. The onset of clinical manifestations occurs most commonly during late childhood, adolescence, or early adult life. The average age of onset is in the early twenties, but patients may remain asymptomatic until late in life.

Although the child may complain of periodic migrainoid headaches for many years, diagnosis is frequently not made until the acute onset of subarachnoid hemorrhage. The cardinal clinical manifestations are related to the site of the malformation. Involvement of branches of the middle cerebral artery is most common, and the clinical features are usually referable to the motor cortex. Focal (motor or sensory) and generalized convulsions may be the initial symptoms, and perhaps the only ones for many years. When focal, the seizures are often confined to one limb and are contralateral to the site of the malformation. The attack is frequently followed by a transient postictal paralysis that gradually becomes a permanent lateralizing sign. Involvement of the parietal lobe is suggested by contralateral sensory seizures and hemisensory deficit involving position, stereognosis, discrimination of tactile stimuli, localization of stimuli, and body image. Posterior fossa malformations produce signs of cerebellar dysfunction and evidence of increased intracranial pressure. The clinical picture is sometimes seen in children with Sturge-Weber-Dimitri syndrome.

Infants and children may have intracerebral hemorrhage without bleeding into the subarachnoid space. There is no obvious trauma or vascular disease, but careful pathologic study shows that many such cases result from a small single angioma or vascular hamartoma. Clinically, there are signs and symptoms of progressive increase of intracranial pressure owing to an intracortical clot.

The child with a hemispheric malformation may complain of and localize a pulsatile sound in the head, and a pathologic intracranial bruit may be heard on auscultation. Physiologic bruits may be found in 50% to 60% of normal children. This sound is faint, soft, somewhat blurred, frequently disappears during auscultation, and is best heard over the orbits or the fontanel. It must be clearly differentiated from the pathologic sound, which is sharp, sonorous with a pronounced resonance, always synchronous with the pulse, and immediately obliterated by compression of the carotid artery. This pathologic bruit is most commonly found in large shunts, in patients who complain of migrainoid headaches, and in posteriorly situated lesions. It is unusual to have a bruit when hemorrhage is the initial clinical feature.

Hemangiomas of the scalp or localized pulsatile, dilated, tortuous scalp veins may be an aid in the diagnosis of an underlying intracranial vascular malformation. Cardiovascular changes are only rarely observed, but large shunts may result in cardiomegaly and even congestive heart failure.

Laboratory Findings. Blood count, erythrocyte sedimentation rate, and urinalysis results are seldom abnormal unless examined shortly after a hemorrhage. Electrocardiogram, blood volume, and cardiac output levels are usually normal because of the relatively small size of a hemispheric arteriovenous shunt. The electroencephalogram is often normal and usually does not show signs of a space-occupying lesion. Paroxysmal electroencephalographic changes may be seen when there is an associated convulsive disorder, and focal slowing may be demonstrable with recent bleeding or rapid growth. The cerebrospinal fluid may be normal or show evidence of old or recent hemorrhage. Plain skull roentgenograms are seldom helpful; they may show changes compatible with increased pressure or a deep groove in the inner table due to an enlarged vein. Intracranial calcifications associated with vascular anomalies are rarely seen in the pediatric age group. This is in contrast to adults, for whom the plain skull roent-

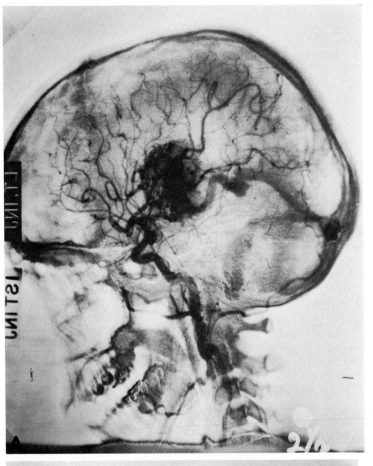

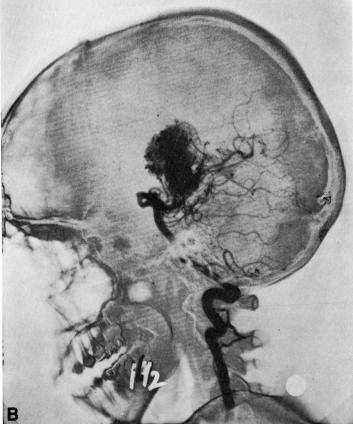

◄FIG. 15-14. *A.* Deep midline arteriovenous malformation. Lateral view of a carotid angiogram with branches of the middle cerebral artery draining into a dilated vein of Galen. *B.* Deep midline arteriovenous malformation (same child as in *A*). Lateral view of a vertebral angiogram with branches of the posterior cerebral artery feeding the malformation.

genograms are often diagnostic, with a significant number having radiologic evidence of calcification within the malformation. Brain scan may identify an arteriovenous malformation by immediate early uptake of the radioisotope. The diagnosis is often confirmed by CT scan[49] and cerebral angiographic study[69] (Fig. 15-15). Even in the young child, the angiogram should be a femoral catheter four-vessel study.

Corpus Callosum Malformation

Corpus callosum malformations, supplied primarily by the anterior and posterior pericallosal arteries, produce symptoms by rupture and hemorrhage. Neurologic deficits include lower extremity involvement or bladder disturbances, whereas seizures and headaches are rare.

Spinal Cord Malformation

Arteriovenous malformations of the spinal cord usually become symptomatic during childhood.[60] The malformation is most commonly localized to the middle or lower thoracic and upper lumbar spinal cord. Pathologically varied, it can consist of a single coiled long vessel, a localized plexus of coiled vessels (glomus type), or multiple large arteries supplying markedly dilated veins (juvenile type).

Clinical manifestations result either from the compressive effect of the malformation, from ischemia with infarction, or from hemorrhage. The corresponding clinical presentations are multiple transient ischemic attacks, progressively increasing deficit, or sudden severe deficit. The symp-

FIG. 15-15. Lateral view of a carotid angiogram showing a hemispheric arteriovenous malformation involving branches of the middle cerebral artery. As shown in this film these malformations frequently have a typical wedge-shape configuration.

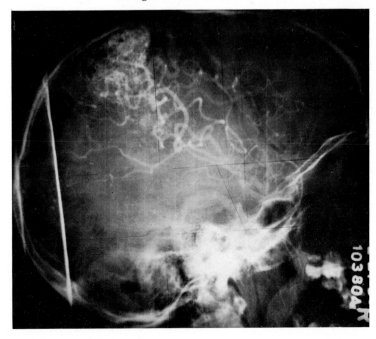

tomatic child often complains of a constant unpleasant burning pain at the site of the malformation or in the lower extremities, and this is frequently associated with meningeal signs secondary to a subarachnoid hemorrhage. Clinically, there may be a cutaneous hemangioma overlying the malformation; a bruit on auscultation; and a neurologic deficit consisting of motor impairment of the lower extremities, a transverse or segmental sensory loss, and deficient bowel or bladder sphincter function. Diagnosis can be accomplished with visualization of the malformation by myelography and definitive delineation with selective spinal angiography.

Spinal cord vascular malformations can be associated with Klippel-Trenaunay syndrome. In this condition, there is a classical triad of a cutaneous hemangioma, often with a metameric distribution, varices of an extremity dating from birth, and hypertrophy of the involved extremity.

TRAUMATIC ARTERIOVENOUS FISTULA

Because of the anatomic relationships, traumatic arteriovenous fistula can occur only in the region of the cavernous sinus where artery and vein are in juxtaposition. The fistula results from a fracture of the base of the skull with tearing of the internal carotid artery within the cavernous sinus. In children, trauma is the most common etiology of this acquired arteriovenous malformation, whereas in the adult a similar malformation results from rupture of an aneurysm in the intracavernous portion of the internal carotid artery. Spontaneous rupture, often bilateral, can occur in Ehlers-Danlos syndrome.[80]

Clinical Findings. The clinical manifestations are highly characteristic; within hours of a head injury there develops a pulsating exophthalmos and an associated intracranial bruit. The ophthalmic and maxillary divisions of the trigeminal nerve and the oculomotor, trochlear, and abducens nerves normally pass through the cavernous sinus, and pressure from the fistula on these structures results in facial sensory loss, diminished corneal reflex, dilated and fixed pupil, and diplopia with extraocular muscle palsies. Pressure on the optic nerve results in decreased visual acuity, which may progress to blindness and optic atrophy.

Laboratory Findings. The CT scan and carotid arteriogram are diagnostic, with the arterial phase demonstrating the cavernous sinus and the enlarged ophthalmic and internal jugular veins.

INTRACRANIAL ANEURYSM

Ruptured saccular aneurysms are a rare cause of subarachnoid hemorrhage in children.[2,35,56,66,73,83] This is in contrast to the adult, in whom this is the most common cause of primary subarachnoid hemorrhage. Because of the unusual location of some aneurysms in the younger age group, many cases go unrecognized.

Aneurysms in the pediatric age group have features that are characteristic of this age group: a greater percentage of peripheral aneurysms involving branches of the middle cerebral artery and the vertebrobasilar arteries,[73] aneurysms of greater size (giant aneurysms), and frequent pseudotumor syndromes.

The symptomatic aneurysm in adults originates from one of the bifurcations of the circle of Willis or the adjacent arteries. The child more commonly shows involvement at the bifurcation of the smaller peripherally placed arteries (Fig. 15-16). This contrast in sites (Table 15-1) results in distinct clinical syndromes for the two age groups.

The pathogenesis of intracranial aneurysms is varied.[20] Most commonly there are developmental defects in the media of cerebral arteries at the points of bifurcation, leaving gaps of varying size. These weakened areas can produce aneurysms with the assistance of two other factors: elevated blood pressure and atherosclerosis. In children, these two factors rarely play a role. Although saccular aneurysms may be associated with coarctation of the aorta, congenital polycystic kidney, or generalized connective tissue disease, they seldom cause symptoms in the pediatric age group. Aneurysms termed "septic" or "mycotic" can result from infected emboli associated

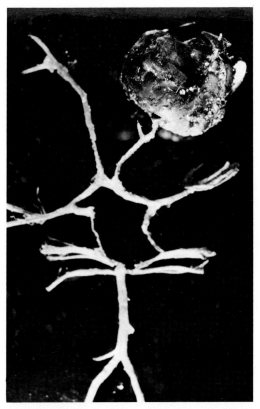

FIG. 15-16. Pathologic specimen showing a large aneurysm arising from a peripheral branch of the anterior cerebral artery.

TABLE 15-1. Distribution of Intracranial Aneurysms

Type of Aneurysm	Children, 26 Cases (%)	Adults, 149 Cases (%)
Middle cerebral	32	18
Internal carotid	32	45
Anterior cerebral	20	6
Basilar and vertebral	12	3
Anterior communicating	4	27
Posterior cerebral	0	1
Total	*100*	*100*

with bacterial endocarditis or with cerebral arteritis.

Rupture, usually at the fundus of the aneurysm may occur when the aneurysm has attained a diameter of 6 to 15 mm. The resultant hemorrhage may involve the subarachnoid space, subdural space, brain substance, or ventricular cavity.

Clinical Findings. Clinical manifestations are due to direct pressure of the aneurysm on surrounding structures or to hemorrhage from rupture. Children typically present with acute manifestations of rupture following strenuous physical activities. The onset is sudden, without warning, and is characterized by severe fronto-occipital headache, vomiting, mental confusion, loss of consciousness, and often convulsions, hemiplegia, monoplegia, or aphasia. Death may result promptly from massive hemor-

rhage, but more commonly consciousness is regained accompanied by confused sensorium, stiff neck, and headache.

If hemorrhage is restricted to the subarachnoid space, there are no lateralizing signs—only the signs of meningeal irritation with fever, subhyaloid retinal hemorrhages, and, in the young infant, a tense, bulging fontanel. Hemorrhage into the brain or surrounding areas rarely produces the cranial nerve palsies commonly seen in the adult. Intracerebral and subdural hematomas may give rise to focal neurologic signs depending on the areas involved, or they may produce a paucity of clinical manifestations if confined to "silent" areas.

Vital signs may be normal if the hemorrhage is a small one. More commonly, there is a moderate febrile reaction and slightly elevated blood pressure, pulse, and respiratory rates. In patients who make a partial or complete recovery from the initial hemorrhage, there is always the possibility of subsequent recurrence of bleeding. In contrast to what occurs in adults, subsequent hemorrhage within the first 2 weeks is very uncommon in children.

Laboratory Findings. Following rupture there is usually a moderate to marked polymorphonuclear leukocytosis, an elevated erythrocyte sedimentation rate, and a transient hyperglycemia and glycosuria in the absence of diabetes mellitus. The urine may also have casts and albumin. Before rupture, the electroencephalogram is usually normal unless the aneurysm is unusually large and acts as a mass lesion. Rupture is usually followed by diffuse generalized slowing or depression of activity. After a few days, the site of the bleeding may be indicated by lateral slowing or decrease in the amplitude of the electrical activity. The most significant laboratory procedure is evaluation of the cerebrospinal fluid. There is evidence of increased intracranial pressure and a uniformly bloody fluid with xanthochromic supernatant when the hemorrhage has occurred 2 hours or more before the diagnostic lumbar puncture. The leukocyte count and protein content of the fluid are proportional to the erythrocytes shortly after the rupture, but later there may be leukocytic pleocytosis and elevated protein content from the irritating effect of the blood. The sugar content of the fluid may be depressed and out of proportion to the blood sugar level, which not infrequently is elevated.

CT scan [99] has become the most important diagnostic aid in the delineation of subarachnoid and intraventricular hemorrhage. In addition, this noninvasive scan can define with precision many of the complications of a ruptured cerebral aneurysm, including an intracortical hematoma, edema, infarction, and delayed hydrocephalus. At times, larger or giant aneurysms can be identified, but precise anatomic localization requires a cerebral angiogram. Unless the aneurysm is occluded by a thrombus, it can often be demonstrated by cerebral angiography (Fig. 15-17). By this study, the aneurysm can be localized, its size and shape determined, and the adequacy of the collateral circulation and the complications of

FIG. 15-17. Cerebral artery aneurysm. Lateral view of a carotid angiogram showing multiple aneurysms arising from the internal carotid artery.

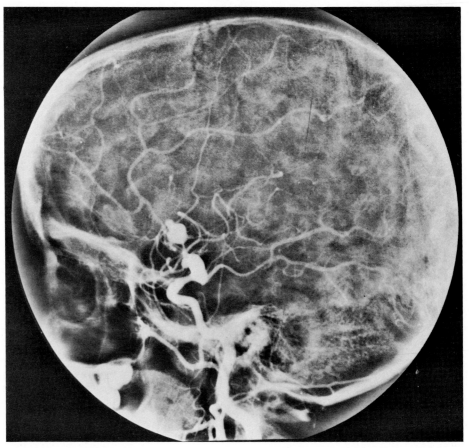

rupture (subdural or intracerebral) delineated. Early angiography is indicated except in the presence of coma with fluctuating vital signs.

HEMMORRHAGIC DIATHESIS

Any of the hemorrhagic hematologic disorders may result in central nervous system hemorrhage.[15] This complication occurs more commonly in leukemia[33,59,91] and aplastic anemia, and less commonly in hemophilia,[86,81] and is only rarely found in idiopathic thrombocytopenia, anaphylactoid purpura,[51] or with an abnormal blood clotting mechanism as seen in chronic liver disease or with anticoagulant therapy. Intracranial hemorrhage in leukemia and aplastic anemia probably results from thrombocytopenia, which then leads to increased permeability of blood vessels; the diapedesis of blood cells is enhanced by defects of the clotting mechanism.

Clinical Findings. The neurologic manifestations of an intracranial hemorrhage are similar for the various etiologies. Intracranial hemorrhage occurs more frequently than it is suspected clinically, being found in approximately 50% of leukemic patients who come to autopsy. Cerebral hemorrhage tends to be multiple, and there is often a propensity for the subcortical white matter to be involved. Severe headache, stupor or coma, and hemiparesis are the most common neurologic manifestations, but the signs and symptoms are highly variable and are dependent upon the site and volume of hemorrhage. Intracranial hemorrhage in patients with altered coagulation may be the immediate cause of death. Diagnosis is not difficult, for there may be a history of a familial bleeding tendency as in hemophilia, evidence of hemorrhage in other organ systems, and laboratory confirmation of the specific hematologic defect.

Laboratory Findings. The cerebrospinal fluid shows evidence of hemorrhage, which must be differentiated from a traumatic lumbar puncture. Hematologically there is evidence of the underlying hemorrhagic disorder.

DIAGNOSIS

The differential diagnosis of cerebrovascular disease is complex and difficult. Not only must these entities be distinguished from other conditions involving the central nervous system, but they must also be differentiated from one another. The distinction from other conditions involving the nervous system is facilitated by a good history, a thorough examination, and ancillary laboratory tests, especially evaluation of the cerebrospinal fluid. CT scan has proven to be a highly reliable diagnostic test for most cerebrovascular diseases. This noninvasive procedure supplies information concerning infarcts, hematoma, intraventricular hemorrhages, cerebral edema, ventricular size, hemispheric shifts, and porencephaly. CT identifies most arteriovenous malformations, and significant enhancement occurs after contrast administration; however, only the larger aneurysms can be documented with this procedure. Cerebral angiography is the definitive study for both malformations and aneurysms, and in addition supplies precise anatomical localization.

Brain abscess must be differentiated from cerebral occlusive vascular disease. It is relatively slow in evolution and is most commonly found in children with cyanotic heart disease. Cerebral abscess in congenital heart disease rarely occurs before 2 years of age, whereas the majority of vascular diseases associated with cyanotic heart disease have occurred by that time. Signs and symptoms of increased intracranial pressure are frequent in brain abscess. The onset of focal neurologic deficit is sudden in the vascular disease, gradual in abscess. Cerebrospinal fluid changes are important; brain abscess is accompanied by clear or slightly xanthochromic fluid that is under increased pressure with a mild to moderate lymphocytic pleocytosis and an increased protein content.

Cerebral tumors present a clinical picture similar to that of an abscess but with more gradual development of neurologic signs that are generally preceded by manifestations of increased intracranial pressure with headaches, vomiting, and papilledema. Cerebrospinal fluid usually has a normal cell count but is otherwise similar to the fluid found with an abscess.

Trauma should always be suspected, and the child must be examined for the presence of contusions and lacerations of the scalp. Extradural hematoma must be differentiated from vascular disease because the hematoma requires immediate surgical evacuation. The diagnosis of an extradural hemorrhage is suggested by the history of trauma, rapid development of a fluctuating state of consciousness, and evidence of skull fracture, particularly in the region of the middle meningeal artery.

Subdural hematoma may present a difficult differential diagnosis because the injury, which occurred days or weeks before, may have been trivial and forgotten. This is further complicated by the "normal" occurrence of head trauma in preschool-age children. Its presence is suggested by the subacute evolution of focal signs and by depression in the state of consciousness. Skull roentgenograms showing a fracture, demonstration of bloody or xanthochromic spinal fluid, and depression of electrical activity over the affected hemisphere differentiates a subdural collection of blood from vascular disease. CT scan and carotid arteriography distinguishes these conditions with certainty.

Epilepsy is suggested by a history of previous convulsions. The paralysis or coma, when present, always follows the seizure. Cerebrospinal fluid analysis is normal, and the electroencephalogram shows evidence of paroxysmal activity.

Subarachnoid hemorrhage has a sudden and dramatic onset, with signs of meningeal irritation. It must be differentiated from meningitis. In many cases, this can be accomplished only by cerebrospinal fluid examination, the diagnosis of subarachnoid hemorrhage being confirmed by the presence of blood. There may be an associated intracerebral hematoma, as suggested by hemiplegia, hemianopia, or aphasia.

Differentiation of cerebral arterial thrombosis from cerebral embolism is difficult because the resultant clinical picture with its rapid onset may be identical in both conditions. The diagnosis of an embolus is suggested when the neurologic episode is of acute onset in a child with bacterial endocarditis, sepsis, atrial fibrillation, or rheumatic fever.

Cerebral venous thrombosis rarely has the acute onset that is so characteristic of arterial occlusive disease or primary subarachnoid hemorrhage. Thorough history-taking and examination generally uncover the etiology of the venous thrombosis.

The symptomatic child with sickle cell disease may require angiography to distinguish thrombotic lesions from coincidental surgical remedial lesions. Special precautions are necessary to reduce the hazards of angiography. When implemented the risks of this procedure are small, and at the same time the effects may be therapeutic. The child should receive either a partial exchange transfusion or repeated transfusions of sedimented red blood cells to achieve a hemoglobin level of at least 10 g/dl and a reduction of hemoglobin S to less that 20%. For at least 12 hours prior to the procedure, the child should be well hydrated by intravenous administration of twice the usual fluid requirement.

PROGNOSIS

Prognosis of cerebrovascular diseases in children is highly variable. The prognosis differs with each clinical entity and may be significantly modified with proper management and therapy. Children differ from adults in their clinical responses to cerebrovascular disease. The young child recovers more rapidly than the adult from motor and speech deficits but is at greater risk of intellectual and behavioral problems and the subsequent development of epilepsy. Permanent aphasia is rare, particularly when the age of onset is less than 4 years.

Venous and dural sinus thromboses, often considered to have a poor prognosis, may vary in their outcome according to the thrombosis site. Superior sagittal sinus thrombosis usually results in early death. The few surviving children are left with a serious neurologic deficit characterized by hemiplegia, seizures, and mental retardation. Lateral sinus thrombosis rarely leads to early death, and the manifestations of increased intracranial pressure may be reversible with antibiotics and mastoidectomy. Cavernous sinus thrombosis is usually responsive to antibiotics, and fatalities have been reduced from 90% to less than 25% since the introduction of these agents.

Cerebral arterial thromboses may lead to immediate death. In general, infants less than 2 years of age at the onset of the arterial thrombosis have a poor prognosis. The prognosis for survival is often dependent upon the primary etiology. Cerebral angiography with delineation of the arterial lesion may produce definitive prognostic data on recurrence of episodes and the risk of a residual neurologic deficit.[38,39,87] Twenty-five percent of patients with the acute infantile hemiplegic syndrome die during the early phase of the illness, and more than 50% of the survivors have a residual hemiparesis or convulsions. The onset of hemiparesis with status epilepticus has a more ominous prognosis for future epilepsy. Twenty percent of the children surviving thrombosis associated with cyanotic heart disease are mentally retarded, 10% have seizures, and more than 25% have hemiparesis. Central nervous system involvement in lupus erythematosus is a poor prognostic sign and is frequently followed by death. Atherosclerosis in progeria often produces a progressive neurologic deficit, whereas the extra-arterial conditions if surgically corrected may produce a static neurologic deficit or even be reversible. Cerebrovascular complications with sickle cell disease, unless treated with chronic transfusions, are likely to recur with each episode, resulting in an increased neurologic deficit. In one study, there was a 67% recurrence rate in untreated children.[71]

Cerebral embolism in children has a mortality rate of approximately 25%; 50% of the survivors may have severe neurologic residua. Children whose embolic episodes are manifested by seizures, prolonged coma, or Cheyne-Stokes respiration are more likely to have a poor prognosis.

Intracranial hemorrhage varies in its prognosis, being dependent upon the etiology, magnitude, and location of the bleeding. Ruptured intracranial aneurysm often produces massive bleeding, and in more than half of the cases, early death. After recovery from an initial attack, bleeding recurs in an unknown number of patients and they die. Subarachnoid hemorrhage secondary to a hemispheric arteriovenous malformation seldom results in immediate death. The clinical course usually extends over many years, with multiple small hemorrhages, seizures, and a progressive neurologic deficit. Vein of Galen arteriovenous malformation has a prognosis correlated with the age of onset of symptoms. Most neonates die of cardiac decompensation. The symptomatic infant has a poor prognosis because of cardiovascular changes, poor operative results, and the high incidence of hydrocephalus with psychomotor retardation. The older child has the most favorable prognosis, the small size of the shunt resulting in a less significant cardiovascular problem. Subarachnoid hemorrhage unrelated to a specific etiology and unassociated with demonstrable vascular pathology has a better prognosis than that associated with intracranial aneurysm or arteriovenous malformations. Intracranial bleeding due to blood dyscrasia has a poor prognosis. Neurologic involvement is more often a late than an early complication of hematologic disorders.

TREATMENT

The problems of therapy are complex, and the literature is replete with uncritical evaluations of varied forms of treatment. A rational therapeutic approach consists of a complete understanding of the pathologic process and its resultant alteration of function. For a given disease entity there are nonspecific as well as specific therapeutic measures.

Nonspecific therapy consists of administering oral and parenteral fluid to prevent dehydration and maintain circulation, antibiotics to combat infections, anticonvulsants to control seizures, and anticoagulants when indicated to prevent extension of the thrombosis, as well as management of increased intracranial pressure.

Oral or parental fluids should fulfill maintenance requirements as well as provide supplementary hydration in the presence of fever or abnormal fluid loss. Maintenance fluids are calculated at 2000 ml/sq m/24 h; this should include sodium 50 mEq/sq m/24 h and potassium 40 mEq/sq m/24 h. When the condition of the child is satisfactory, oral feedings are preferable. Nasogastric administration of fluids and medications should be considered for the unconscious patients.

Infection is treated with parenteral antibiotics. Specific therapy is used when the infecting agent is known; with an infection of unknown etiology, ampicillin, 200 to 400 mg/kg/24 h is given in divided doses at 4- to 6-hour intervals. These medications are maintained for a period of 7 to 10 days.

Convulsions must be promptly controlled. Initially, this is best done with diazepam (Valium), barbiturates, or paraldehyde, but at times prompt control requires ether or chloroform inhalation. Diazepam in a dose of 0.1 to 0.2 mg/kg body weight, with a maximum dose of 10 mg, is administered intravenously over a period of 1 to 2 min. During administration, respiration and cardiac rate must be monitored and the physician should be prepared to intubate the child. A second dose, if necessary, may be administered after 30 min has elapsed. Phenobarbital is administered intravenously in a dosage large enough to control seizures but not to suppress respiration. An initial dose of intravenous phenobarbital is 5 mg/kg. If either diazepam or phenobarbital is used alone, the other should not be given intravenously because there may be an unpredictable synergistic effect with suppression of respiration. Paraldehyde is diluted with 2 ml added to 50 ml normal saline; this suspension is given intravenously as a rapid infusion until seizures are controlled. Phenobarbital or diphenylhydantoin (Dilantin) is then administered for long-term maintenance therapy.

Anticoagulation initiated with heparin and maintained with dicumarol is potentially dangerous, and strict hematologic control is mandatory to prevent hemorrhage.

Increased intracranial pressure secondary to cerebral edema may at times be difficult to evaluate and control. Intracranial pressure monitoring offers a rational approach in the management of this problem. Supportive measures, such as, maintaining an airway, controlling blood pressure, and elevating the child's head to an angle of 45°, which enhances venous outflow from the brain, are essential. Hyperventilation, light hypothermia, mannitol, and corticosteroids are often used to lower increased pressure. Barbiturates, in doses producing so-called barbiturate coma, are less commonly used, and their effectiveness is still in question. Hyperventilation is the most effective and rapid treatment of acute increased intracranial pressure. Lowering the PCO_2 to 25 or even 20 will significantly reduce cerebral blood flow and thereby reduce intracranial pressure. Light hypothermia maintains the body temperature at 31° to 32°C.

In this manner, the brain volume is reduced and oxygen uptake by the brain is decreased. The desired temperature may be obtained by exposing the nude child to room air and applying ice bags to a large part of the body (or preferably by using a mechanical refrigeration device or cooling blankets). Shivering, often observed with hypothermia, must be controlled if the temperature is to be maintained. Chlorpromazine is the most effective agent in controlling this side-effect and is most often given intramuscularly or intravenously; the dosage varies with the age of the child and the route by which the drug is administered. Intramuscular doses may be repeated every 4 hours with a dosage of 5 mg up to 1 year of age, 10 mg at 1 to 5 years, 20 mg at 5 to 10 years, and 25 to 35 mg in older children. The drug is administered intravenously and should be given slowly in a dilute solution with 1 to 3 mg chlorpromazine added to 50 or 100 ml of 5% glucose in water. Mannitol effectively decreases raised intracranial pressure but has the undesirable side effect of rebound, that is, a secondary increase in pressure approximately 8 to 12 hours after administration. Mannitol 20% in the dosage of 0.5 to 1.0 g/kg is administered intravenously over a period of 30 minutes and repeated at 8- to 12-hour intervals. An indwelling catheter must be inserted prior to introduction of the drug, and the serum electrolytes must be carefully controlled. Therapy of this type is reserved for the child with acute increased pressure and is best accomplished in acute treatment units where the necessary equipment and nursing and surgical personnel are available.

Although highly effective in the treatment of cerebral edema associated with intracranial neoplasms, it is questionable whether glucocorticoids are effective in the management of increased intracranial pressure. Corticosteroids reduce pressure less rapidly than the osmotic diuretics; their efficacy is noted within hours, but they have the advantage of long-term use without rebound or major side-effects. Most of the parenteral preparations have the same therapeutic effect in equivalent doses. Dexamethasone (Decadron) is administered parenterally to a child whose weight exceeds 50 kg in an initial dose of 10 mg, then in a maintenance dose of 4 mg/day in four divided doses; it is subsequently tapered and discontinued within 7 to 10 days. Appropriate reductions of dosage are made for smaller children. A constant state of alertness for the varied and complex side-effects, especially electrolyte disturbances, is essential whenever steroids are employed.

Venous and dural sinus thromboses are managed by strict control of fluids and electrolytes, and, when indicated, by antibiotics and anticoagulants. Anticoagulants are rarely used and do not seem to improve the clinical course. Mastoidectomy with decompression of the lateral sinus is the treatment of choice in managing increased intracranial pressure associated with that condition. Repeated and often daily lumbar punctures may be necessary to reduce the pressure; if these are ineffective, a lumbo-peritoneal shunt is the preferred neurosurgical procedure to preserve vision. Correction of iron deficiency anemia may prevent the development of cerebral venous thrombosis in children with cyanotic congenital heart disease.

Arterial thromboses are treated symptomatically. Anticoagulation is contraindicated. It may result in the conversion of a pale infarct to a hemorrhagic infarct or may actually extend one that is primarily hemorrhagic. Stellate ganglion block or inhalation of 5% carbon dioxide to increase cerebral blood flow has been clinically unrewarding. Newer therapeutic methods using proteolytic enzymes to lyse the thrombus have not been adequately investigated. An indication for vascular surgery is thrombosis of the extracranial portion of the internal carotid artery. It is rare for the pediatric patient to meet this criterion. Bilateral cervical sympathectomies have been carried out to increase regional blood flow in arterial thrombosis with telangiectasia

(moyamoya) with questionable results.[92] Recurrent cerebral arterial thrombosis with or without telangiectasia has been treated with a surgical anastomosis between the external and internal carotid arteries.

Physiotherapy and occupational therapy are indicated in the management of residual hemiplegia, as is the use of anticonvulsants for seizures. Hemispherectomy may be considered in hemiplegic patients with medically refractory seizures, often with an associated behavior disorder. Sickle cell disease is best treated by repeated blood transfusions to reduce the percentage of hemoglobin S. Future cerebrovascular complications are prevented as long as transfusions are continued and hemoglobin S is maintained at levels below 20%.

The management of arterial emboli is mainly symptomatic, consisting of skillful nursing care, treatment and prevention of infections, and, if indicated, administration of anticonvulsants. Anticoagulation agents may be used to prevent the formation of future emboli. Corticosteroids in dosages used to treat increased intracranial pressure are most effective in fat embolism with resultant dramatic reversal of the respiratory distress.

The management of intracranial hemorrhage is largely dependent upon the primary pathologic process. The beneficial results obtained with hypothermia, mannital, steroids, and repeated lumbar punctures are highly controversial. Lumbar puncture is initially indicated as a diagnostic procedure, and it may be repeated at intervals of 12 to 24 hours. Intracranial aneurysms are the subject of many reviews, with controversy between the adherents of medical and surgical therapy. Certainly, good medical and nursing care is mandatory, but unless the patient is in coma or has medical contraindications a direct intracranial approach with clipping of the aneurysm offers the best prognosis. The occurrence of a second hemorrhage following shortly after the initial one is uncommon in children. For this reason, surgery should be delayed until the child is in optimal condition.

Arteriovenous malformations are treated both medically and surgically. Medical management consists largely of support for a decompensated cardiovascular system with cardiotonics, rigid control of blood volume with phlebotomy, careful management of fluids and electrolytes, and control of seizures. Surgical extirpation should be performed whenever possible, even with arteriovenous malformations that involve the dominant hemisphere or motor and speech areas. Embolization with Silastic spheres must be done preoperatively to reduce the size of a malformation or may be used alone in deep midline or inaccessible lesions. Anterior temporal lobe malformations are best treated by temporal lobectomy. Traumatic arteriovenous fistulas are treated by ligation of the fistula, embolization, or implanting detachable balloon catheters. Spinal malformations should, if at all possible, be surgically extirpated or embolized with a liquid plastic.

REFERENCES

1. A classification and outline of cerebrovascular diseases. Neurology (Minneap) 8:395, 1958
2. **Amacher AL, Drake CG:** Cerebral artery aneurysms in infancy, childhood and adolescence. Childs Brain 1:72, 1975
3. **Atkinson EA, Fairburn B, Heathfield KWG:** Intracranial venous thrombosis as complication of oral contraception. Lancet 1:914, 1970
4. **Atlee WE Jr:** Talc and cornstarch emboli in eyes of drug users. JAMA 219:49, 1972
5. **Averback P:** Primary cerebral venous thrombosis in young adults: The diverse manifestations of an unrecognized disease. Ann Neurol 3:81, 1978
6. **Banker BQ:** Cerebral vascular disease in infancy and childhood: I. Occlusive vascular diseases. J Neuropathol Exp Neurol 20:127, 1961
7. **Barson AJ, Chisturck ML:** Fat embolism in infancy after intravenous fat infusions. Arch Dis Child 53:218, 1978
8. **Boulos R, Kricheff II, Chase NE:** Value of cerebral angiography in the embolization treatment of cerebral arteriovenous malformations. Radiology 97:65, 1970
9. **Buchanan LS, Brazinsky JH:** Dural sinus and cerebral venous thrombosis. Arch Neurol 22:440, 1970
10. **Byers RK, Hass GM:** Thrombosis of the dural venous sinuses in infancy and in childhood. Am J Dis Child 45:1161, 1933
11. **Byers RK, McLean WT:** Etiology and course of certain hemiplegias with aphasia in childhood. Pediatrics 29:376, 1962
12. **Carlson CB, Harvey FH, Loop J:** Progressive alternating hemiplegia in early childhood with basal arterial stenosis and telangiectasia (moyamoya syndrome). Neurology (Minneap) 23:734, 1973
13. **Carroll JD, Leak D, Lee HA:** Cerebral thrombophlebitis in pregnancy and the puerperium. Q J Med 35:347, 1966
14. **Carter S, Gold AP:** Acute infantile hemiplegia. Pediatr Clin North Am 14:851, 1964
15. **Chalgren WS:** Neurologic complications of the hemorrhagic diseases. Neurology (Minneap) 3:126, 1953
16. **Clark RM, Linell EA:** Case report: Prenatal occlusion of the internal carotid artery. J Neurol Neurosurg Psychiatry 17:295, 1954
17. **Cohen AC, Glinsky GC, Martin GE et al:** Air embolism. Ann Intern Med 35:779, 1951
18. **Cohen MM:** Central nervous system in congenital heart disease. Neurology (Minneap) 10:452, 1960
19. **Cottrill CM, Kaplan S:** Cerebral vascular accidents in cyanotic congenital heart disease. Am J Dis Child 125:484, 1973
20. **Crawford T:** Some observations on the pathogenesis and natural history of intracranial aneurysms. J Neurol Neurosurg Psychiatry 22:259, 1959
21. **Crosley CJ, Binet EF:** Cerebrovascular complications in phencyclidine intoxication. J Pediatr 94:316, 1979
22. **Dyke CG, Davidoff LM, Masson CB:** Cerebral hemiatrophy with homolateral hypertrophy of the skull and sinuses. Surg Gynecol Obstet 57:588, 1933
23. **Dykes FD, Lazarra A, Ahmann P et al:** Intraventricular hemorrhage: A prospective evaluation of etiopathogenesis. Pediatrics 66:42, 1980
24. **Evarts CM:** The fat embolism syndrome: A review. Surg Clin North Am 50:493, 1970
25. **Fisher RG, Friedmann KR:** Carotid artery thrombosis in persons fifteen years of age or younger. JAMA 170:1918, 1959
26. **Frantzen E, Jacobsen HH, Therkelsen J:** Cerebral artery occlusions in children due to trauma to the head and neck: A report of 6 cases verified by cerebral angiography. Neurology (Minneap) 11:695, 1961
27. **Furlan AJ, Whisnant JP, Baker HL Jr:** Long-term prognosis after carotid artery occlusion. Neurology 30:986, 1980
28. **Gold AP, Challenor YB, Gilles FH et al:** IX. Strokes in Children (part 1). Stroke 4: Sept-Oct, 1973
29. **Gold AP, Challenor YB, Gilles FH et al:** IX. Strokes in children (part 2) Stroke 4: Nov-Dec, 1973
30. **Gold AP, Ransohoff J, Carter S:** Arteriovenous malformation of the vein of Galen in children. Acta Neurol Scand [Suppl] 11:1, 1964
31. **Gold AP, Yahr MD:** Childhood lupus erythematosus: A clinical and pathological study of the neurological manifestations. Trans Am Neurol Assoc 85:96, 1960
32. **Greer M, Schotland D:** Abnormal hemoglobin as a cause of neurologic disease. Neurology (Minneap) 12:114, 1962
33. **Groch SN, Sayre GP, Heck FJ:** Cerebral hemorrhage in leukemia. Arch Neurol 2:439, 1960
34. **Gross RE:** Arterial embolism and thrombosis in infancy. Am J Dis Child 70:61, 1945

35. **Hamby WB:** Intracranial Aneurysms. Springfield, Ill, Charles C Thomas, 1952

36. **Herndon JH, Riseborough EJ, Fisher JE:** Fat embolism: A review of current concepts. J Trauma 2:673, 1971

37. **Heyman A:** Oral contraception and increased risk of cerebral ischemia or thrombosis: Collaborative group for the study of stroke in young women. N Engl J Med 288:871, 1973

38. **Hilal SK, Solomon GE, Gold AP et al:** Primary cerebral arterial occlusive disease in children. Part I. Acute acquired hemiplegia. Radiology 99:71, 1971

39. **Hilal SK, Solomon GE, Gold AP et al:** Primary cerebral arterial occlusive disease in children. Part II. Neurocutaneous syndromes. Radiology 99:87, 1971

40. **Holden AM, Fyler DC, Shillito J et al:** Congestive heart failure from intracranial arteriovenous fistula in infancy. Pediatrics 49:30, 1972

41. **Isler W:** Acute Hemiplegias and Hemisyndromes in Childhood. Burrows EH (trans): London, Clinics in Developmental Medicine Nos. 41/42, Heinemann, 1971

42. **Jackson WPU, Hanelin J, Albright F:** Metaphyseal dysplasia, epiphyseal dysplasia, diaphyseal dyplasia, and related conditions: Familial metaphyseal dysplasia and craniometaphyseal displasia; their relation to leontiasis ossea and osteopetrosis; disorders of "bone remodeling." Arch Intern Med 94:871, 1954

43. **Kalbag RM, Woolf AL:** Cerebral Venous Thrombosis. London, Oxford University Press, 1967

44. **Kelly JJ, Mellinger JF, Sundt TM:** Intracranial arteriovenous malformations in childhood. Ann Neurol 3:338, 1978

45. **Kinal ME, Jaeger RM:** Thrombophlebitis of dural venous sinuses following otitis media. J Neurosurg 17:81, 1960

46. **Kingsley DPE, Kendall BE, Moseley IF:** Superior sagittal sinus thrombosis: An evaluation of the changes demonstrated on computed tomography. J Neurol Neurosurg Psychiatry 41:1065, 1978

47. **Kurtzke J:** Epidemiology of Cerebrovascular Diseases. Berlin, Springer-Verlag, 1969

48. **Lande A, Bard R, Rossi P, Passariello R, Castrucci A:** Takayasu's arteritis: A worldwide entity. N Y State J Med 76:1477, 1976

49. **LeBlanc R, Ethier R, Little JR:** Computerized tomography findings in arteriovenous malformations of the brain. J Neurosurg 51:765, 1979

50. **Levine OR, Jameson AG, Nellhaus G et al:** Cardiac complication of cerebral arteriovenous fistulas. Pediatrics 30:563, 1962

51. **Lewis IC, Philpott MG:** Neurological complications of Schönlein-Henoch syndrome. Arch Dis Child 31:369, 1956

52. **Limbord TG, Ruderman RJ:** Fat embolism in children. Clin Orthop 138:267, 1978

53. **Lockman LA, Mastri A, Priest JR, Nesbit M:** Dural venous sinus thrombosis in acute lymphoblastic leukemia. Pediatrics 66:943, 1980

54. **MacDonald JT, Brown DR:** Acute hemiparesis in juvenile insulin-dependent diabetes mellitus (JIDDM). Neurology 29:893, 1979

55. **Malamud N:** A case of periarteritis nodosa with decerebrate rigidity and extensive encephalomalacia in a five-year-old child. J Neuropathol Exp Neurol 4:88, 1945

56. **Matson DD:** Intracranial aneurysms in childhood. J Neurosurg 23:578, 1965

57. **Mayeux R, Fahn S:** Strokes and ulcerative colitis. Neurology 28:571, 1978

58. **Mickelsen WJ:** Natural history and pathophysiology of arteriovenous malformations. Clin Neurosurg 26:307, 1979

59. **Moore EW, Thomas LB, Shaw RK et al:** The central nervous system in acute leukemia: A postmortem study of 117 consecutive cases, with particular reference to hemorrhages, leukemic infiltrations, and the syndrome of meningeal leukemia. Arch intern Med 105:451, 1960

60. **Moyes PD:** Intracranial and intraspinal vascular anomalies in children. J Neurosurg 31:271, 1969

61. **O'Brien JL, Sibley WA:** Neurologic manifestations of thrombotic thrombocytopenic purpura. Neurology (Minneap) 8:55, 1958

62. **Ouvrier RA, Hopkins IJ:** Occlusive disease of the vertebrobasilar arterial system in childhood. Dev Med Child Neurol 12:186, 1970

63. **Paillas J, Bonnal J, Payan H et al:** Thrombose de l'artère carotide interne révélatrice d'echinonoccose cardiaque rompue et suivie d'hydatidose intracranio-orbitaire. Rev Neurol (Paris) 101:188, 1959

64. **Painter MJ, Chutorian AM, Hilal SK:** Cerebrovasculopathy following irradiation in childhood. Neurology 25:189, 1975

65. **Papile L, Burstein J, Burstein R et al:** Incidence and evolution of subependymal intraventricular hemorrhage: A study of infants with birth weights less than 1500 grams. J Pediatr 92:529, 1978

66. **Patel AN, Richardson AE:** Ruptured intracranial aneurysm in the first two decades of life: A study of 58 patients. J Neurosurg 35:571, 1971

67. **Patterson JH, McKissock W:** A clinical survey of intracranial angiomas with special reference to their mode of progression and surgical treatment: A report of 110 cases. Brain 79:233, 1956

68. **Peltier LF:** Fat embolism: A current concept. Clin Orthop 66:241, 1969

69. **Poser CM, Taveras JM:** Cerebral angiography in encephalotrigeminal angiomatosis. Radiology 68:327, 1957

70. **Poser CM, Taveras JM:** Clinical aspects of cerebral angiography in children. Pediatrics 16:73, 1955

71. **Powars D, Wilson B, Imbus C, Pegelow C, Allen J:** The natural history of stroke in sickle cell disease. Am J Med 65:461, 1978

72. **Powars DR:** Natural history of sickle cell disease: The first ten years. Semin Hematol 12:267, 1975

73. **Read D, Esire MM:** Fusiform basilar artery aneurysm in a child. Neurology 29:1045, 1979

74. **Richter RW, Baden MM:** Neurologic complica-

tions of heroin addiction. Trans Am Neurol Assoc 94:330, 1969

75. **Russo RH, Dicks RE III:** Arteriovenous malformations of the brain stem in childhood. Surg Neurol 8:167, 1977

76. **Sandok BA, VonEstorff I, Guiliani ER:** CNS embolism due to atrial myxoma: Clinical features and diagnosis. Arch Neurol 37:485, 1980

77. **Schneider RC:** Fat embolism: A problem in the differential diagnosis of craniocerebral trauma. J Neurosurg 9:1, 1952

78. **Schneiderman JH, Sharpe JA, Sutton DMC:** Cerebral and retinal vascular complications of inflammatory bowel disease. Ann Neurol 5:331, 1979

79. **Schoenberg BS, Mellinger JF, Schoenberg DG:** Cerebrovascular disease in infants and children: A study of incidence, clinical features, and survival. Neurology 28:763, 1978

80. **Schoolman A, Kepes JJ:** Bilateral spontaneous carotid cavernous fistulae in Ehlers-Danlos syndrome. J Neurosurg 26:82, 1967

81. **Schwarz GA, Schwartzman RJ, Joyner CR:** Atrial myxoma: Cause of embolic stroke. Neurology (Minneap) 22:1112, 1972

82. **Scotti LN, Goldman RL, Hardman DR et al:** Venous thrombosis in infants and children. Radiology 112:393, 1974

83. **Sedzimir CB, Robinson J:** Intracranial hemorrhage in children and adolescents. J Neurosurg 38:269, 1973

84. **Seeler RA, Royal JE:** Commentary: Sickle cell anemia, stroke and transfusion. J Pediatr 96:243, 1980

85. **Seeler RA, Royal JE, Powe MD, Goldberg HR:** Moyamoya in children with sickle cell anemia and cerebrovascular occlusion. J Pediatr 93:808, 1978

86. **Silverstein A:** Intracranial bleeding in hemophilia. Arch Neurol 3:141, 1960

87. **Solomon GE, Hilal SK, Gold AP et al:** Natural history of acute hemiplegia of childhood. Brain 93:107, 1970

88. **Stein BM, Wolpert SM:** Arteriovenous malformations of the brain. I. Current concepts and treatment. Arch Neurol 37:1, 1980

89. **Stein BM, Wolpert SM:** Arteriovenous malformations of the brain. II. Current concepts and treatment. Arch Neurol 37:69, 1980

90. **Stockman JA, Nigro MA, Mishkin MM, Oski FA:** Occlusion of large cerebral vessels in sickle-cell anemia. N Engl J Med 287:846, 1972

91. **Sullivan MP:** Intracranial complications of leukemia in children. Pediatrics 20:757, 1957

92. **Suzuki J et al:** An attempt to treat cerebrovascular "Moyamoya" disease in children. Childs Brain 1:193, 1975

93. **Symonds CP:** Otitic hydrocephalus. Neurology (Minneap) 6:681, 1956

94. **Taveras JM, Poser CM:** Roentgenologic aspects of cerebral angiography in children. Am J Roentgenol Radium Ther Nucl Med 82:371, 1959

95. **Tyler HR, Clark DB:** Cerebrovascular accidents in patients with congenital heart disease. Arch Neurol Psychiatry 77:483, 1957

96. **Tyler HR, Clark DB:** Incidence of neurological complications in congenital heart disease. Arch Neurol Psychiatry 77:17, 1957

97. **Volpe JJ:** Neonatal periventricular hemorrhage: Past, present, and future. J Pediatr 92:693, 1978

98. **Walsh FB, Goldberg HK:** Blindness due to air embolism: Complication of extrapleural pneumolysis. JAMA 114:654, 1940

99. **Weisberg LA:** Computed tomography in aneurysmal subarachnoid hemorrhage. Neurology 29:802, 1979

100. **Wells CE:** Cerebral embolism: The natural history, prognostic signs, and effects of anticoagulation. Arch Neurol Psychiatry 81:667, 1959

101. **Wilimas J, Goff JR, Anderson HR, Langston JW, Thompson E:** Efficacy of transfusion therapy for one to two years in patients with sickle cell disease and cerebrovascular accidents. J Pediatr 96:205, 1980

102. **Wisoff HS, Rothballer AB:** Cerebral arterial thrombosis in children: Review of literature and addition of two cases in apparently healthy children. Arch Neurol 4:258, 1961

103. **Wolf A, Cowen D:** Mucormycosis of central nervous system. J Neuropathol Exp Neurol 8:107, 1949

104. **Wolman L:** Cerebral dissecting aneurysms. Brain 82:276, 1959

105. **Wood EH:** Thermography in the diagnosis of cerebrovascular disease. Radiology 86:270, 1965

106. **Wright TL, Bresnan MJ:** Radiation-induced cerebrovascular disease in children. Neurology 26:540, 1976

Disorders of Basal Ganglia, Cerebellum, Brain Stem, and Cranial Nerves

16

Enrique Chaves
L. Matthew Frank

DISORDERS OF BASAL GANGLIA

Dystonia Musculorum Deformans (Torsion Dystonia)

Dystonia musculorum deformans is the name given by Oppenheim[123] to a disorder characterized clinically by prolonged, writhing, involuntary movements. These movements involve the trunk, neck, arms, and legs, and result in grossly disturbed postures.

Etiology. The etiology is unknown. The pattern of inheritance of this genetic disorder is usually autosomal recessive among Ashkenazi Jews and autosomal dominant among non-Jewish populations. Variable patterns of inheritance and different clinical courses suggest that dystonia musculorum deformans represents a group of related disorders rather than a single entity.[160] Absence of specific pathologic changes in the central nervous system raises the possibility that this may be a disorder of neurotransmitter function. Abnormal serum dopamine-β-hydroxylase concentrations have been found in some patients but not in others.[80]

Pathology. Neuronal degeneration has been described in the caudate nucleus, putamen, thalamus, corpus Luysii, substantia nigra, dentate, and olivary nuclei in some cases. However, when secondary cases are excluded, no specific neuropathologic lesions are associated with dystonia musculorum deformans.[161]

Symptoms. In two thirds of affected children, the onset is between 6 to 12 years of age,[103] although occasionally symptoms may be present during infancy. In more than 80% of affected children, involuntary movements begin first in one foot with plantar flexion and inversion at the ankle. In the remainder, the disorder begins with involuntary movements at the wrist. Spasmodic plantar flexion of the feet may make it impossible for the child to stand without support. The child may complain of muscle spasms, which are frequently aggravated by emotional upset.

Examination. Observation of the child while he is sitting, standing, walking, or running reveals involuntary movements of the legs, arms, or trunk. Involuntary movements may interfere with writing. Spasms in the muscles of the spine produce an increase in lumbar lordosis and a tilting of the pelvis. Dysarthria, facial grimacing, and torticollis may be present. With severe involvement, the typical position of the leg is that of plantar flexion and inversion at the ankle, extension at the knee, and mild flexion of the hip. In the hands there is flexion or extension of the interphalangeal joints, flexion at the metacarpophalangeal joints, and adduction and flexion of the thumb. Involuntary flexion of the wrist, extension of the elbow, and adduction at the shoulder produce a characteristic posture. These involuntary movements disappear during sleep. Motor strength and coordination are otherwise normal. Sensory and reflex examinations are normal.

Differential Diagnosis. The clinical diagnosis is based upon the appearance of the characteristic dystonic movements of the arms, trunk, and legs. The sustained involuntary muscle contractions produce writhing movements involving proximal and distal musculature. Similar sustained movements appear distally in the arms and legs in athetosis, although the severe proximal torsion spasms are not present. The involuntary movements seen in chorea minor are rapid movements occurring primarily in the hands and feet. Two factors important in the clinical diagnosis are the gradual development, without recognizable etiologic factors at the onset, and the characteristic dystonic movements and postures. Other conditions associated with dystonia may need to be excluded, such as perinatal hypoxia, kernicterus, paroxysmal choreoathetosis, rumination (Sandifer) syndrome, phenothiazine reactions, and hysteria.

Treatment. There is no effective medical treatment. Drugs such as reserpine, chlorpromazine, or levodopa usually produce little change in the amount of involuntary movements. Surgical lesions placed in the thalamus centered in the ventrolateral nucleus have produced a marked decrease or a complete abolition of involuntary movements in three fourths of patients. This reversal of symptoms has been maintained in patients followed as long as 20 years[29] (Fig. 16-1). Others have not been able to obtain comparable results with stereotactic surgery.

Prognosis. The course is slowly progressive. It progresses most rapidly when involvement is early and the onset is in the lower extremities. The usual progression of symptoms is from the distal portion of the arm or leg proximally with subsequent involvement of trunk and neck muscles. The course is variable but relentlessly progressive.[103] One child may become bedridden within 5 years; at the other extreme, another child may reach adult life and not become incapacitated until 40 to 50 years of age. Nearly half of the patients are unable to ambulate within 5 to 10 years after onset of the disorder.[103] The majority of affected persons live a normal life span with preserved intellect even if severely disabled.

Pigmentary Degeneration of the Globus Pallidus (Hallervorden-Spatz Disease)

Hallervorden-Spatz disease is a rare hereditary movement disorder characterized by progressive stiffness of the extremities, intellectual deterioration, athetosis, and retinitis pigmentosa.[157]

Etiology. The etiology is unknown. The pigmentary changes in the globus pallidus and substantia nigra suggest a disturbance of iron metabolism or lipid peroxidation, but none has been found. The pattern of inheritance is autosomal recessive.

Pathology. The globus pallidus and pars reticulata of the substantia nigra have deposits of greenish-blue or brown iron-containing pigment. Myelin is decreased in the globus pallidus and focal neuroaxonal swellings (spheroids) are seen in the pallidonigral system and cortex.[40] The presence of spheroids suggests that Hallervorden-Spatz disease and infantile neuroaxonal dystrophy (Seitelberger's disease) may be related conditions.[57]

Symptoms. The usual presenting symptoms are abnormalities of the lower extremities with foot dystonia and deformity, gait difficulty, and leg rigidity. Progressive intellectual deterioration and speech involvement eventually halt communication. A grimacing face caused by contraction of facial muscles may be present.[42] Seizures occur only rarely. Retinitis pigmentosa, optic atrophy, emotional incontinence, and occasionally extensor plantar responses may be noted. Symptoms usually begin between 8 and 10 years of age and progress to a fatal outcome 5 to 20 years later.

Computerized tomography may show intercaudate distance abnormalities distinctive from those seen in Huntington's disease.[39]

Juvenile Parkinsonism (Paralysis Agitans)

Juvenile parkinsonism is a rare disorder of children consisting of tremor, rigidity, bradykinesia, and impaired postural stability.[105]

Etiology. Parkinsonism in adults is associated with decreased levels of dopamine and its major metabolites in the substantia nigra and striatum. Serotonin levels in the globus pallidus, thalamus, and hypothalamus are also decreased. Cerebrospinal fluid homovanillic acid concentrations have been measured in patients with juvenile parkinsonism, with conflicting results.[114,132] Tardive dyskinesia is a parkinsonian syndrome induced in children as well as in adults by the administration of reserpine, phenothiazines, and butyrophenones. Rarely, juvenile parkinsonism follows an encephalitic process.[86,132]

Pathology.   A decreased number of neurons and an increased number of glial cells are seen in the globus pallidus, putamen, and caudate nucleus. The substantia nigra appears normal in some cases, whereas in other cases it appears shrunken, depigmented, and with extensive cellular loss.[97]

Symptoms.   The disorder begins in childhood with a rhythmic resting tremor at approximately 6 Hz that is diminished by volitional movement. The tremor begins in one arm and spreads to the other arm and to the legs. The handwriting is slow with small letters. Occasionally there is dystonic posturing of the neck, shoulder, or extremities.

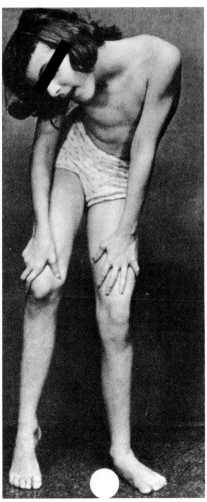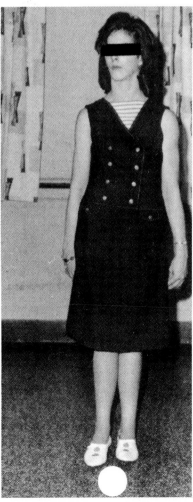

FIG. 16-1. Dystonia musculorum deformans. *A.* A 9-year-old girl with torsion dystonia involving cervical, thoracic, and lumbar musculature prior to operation. *B.* Seven years after bilateral thalamic surgery. Persistent relief of previously incapacitating scoliosis is noted. (From Cooper: Involuntary Movement Disorders. New York, Harper & Row, 1969)

Eventually bradykinesia, rigidity, postural instability, and other features characteristic of adult parkinsonism develop.

Examination.   The child's facial expression is masked and the volume of the voice is decreased. The gait is slow with ventral flexion and loss of associated arm movements. The characteristic tremor, rigidity, and bradykinesia may be associated with impaired ocular convergence, blepharospasm, and seborrhea.

Differential Diagnosis.   Parkinsonism must be differentiated from essential tremor, the rigid form of Huntington's disease seen in children, hepatolenticular degeneration, and pigmentary degeneration of the globus pallidus.

Treatment.   Levodopa, which is able to pass the blood–brain barrier and is then converted into dopamine, reverses the clinical signs of rigidity, tremor, and bradykinesia.[30] It has been effective in adults, alone or in combination with decarboxylase inhibitors, and has also been used in older children.[86] The usual initial dose is 0.5 g, which is then gradually increased over a period of 6 to 8 weeks to determine the optimal dose producing the maximal improvement in symptoms with tolerated side-effects. In adults this dose is 1.5 to 8 g daily, administered in three or more divided doses with food. The safety of levodopa in children under 12 years of age has not been established. Periodic evaluation of hepatic, renal, hematopoietic, cardiovascular, and renal function is recommended during extended therapy. The most frequently occurring side-effects of levodopa are vomiting, cardiac irregularities, orthostatic hypotension, dystonic movements, and psychiatric symptoms. Amantadine and bromocriptine may be useful in patients who are unable to tolerate levodopa.

Prognosis.   The course is slowly progressive over a period of 20 years or more.

Familial Calcification in the Basal Ganglia

A rare familial disorder characterized by calcification in the basal ganglia has been reported and referred to inaccurately as Fahr disease.[109] The calcification affects mainly the putamen and globus pallidus, but is also found in the dentate nucleus of the cerebellum. Patchy calcification of the cerebral and cerebellar cortex is also present. Calcium is deposited in the walls of cerebral vessels, in perivascular spaces, and in surrounding capillaries. However, the relationship of the calcification to vascular structures is less clear in the basal ganglia than it is in the cortical areas,[108] perhaps because of its greater confluency in more severely affected regions of the brain. Bilateral symmetrical calcification in the basal ganglia can be detected by skull radiographs or by computerized tomography.[112]

The observed variability of clinical features among families may be related to location and extent of the calcification as well as the maturational stage of the central nervous system at the time the calcification occurs. Children with this disorder develop intellectual impairment and speech impediment.[19] Less frequently, seizures, pyramidal tract signs such as weakness, spasticity, and hyperreflexia, and extrapyramidal signs such as tremor, chorea, rigidity, parkinsonism, athetosis, and ataxia may be present. The course is slowly progressive and no specific therapy is available.

In nonfamilial cases, calcification in the basal ganglia is more commonly associated with endocrinopathies such as hypoparathyroidism and pseudohypoparathyroidism, prior cranial irradiation, intrathecal methotrexate, or deep-seated arterio-venous malformations.[110]

Chronic Progressive Chorea (Huntington's Disease)

Chronic progressive chorea is a hereditary disorder of the cerebral cortex and basal ganglia associated in children with muscular rigidity, intellectual deterioration, and seizures.[22] It is inherited as an autosomal dominant gene with almost complete penetrance. In three fourths of cases, the father is the affected parent. This is a rare disorder that occurs primarily in adults; only 1% to 5% of cases occur in children.

Etiology.   The etiology is unknown. Gamma-aminobutyric acid (GABA) has been found to be decreased in postmortem brain samples from patients with Huntington's disease. Available evidence suggests that the pathophysiology of this disorder may be a heightened response of striatal cells to dopamine. Specific receptors for dopamine and serotonin may have increased sensitivity, whereas acetylcholine receptor sensitivity may be decreased. It has also been hypothesized that Huntington's disease is the result of a deficit in caudate-nigral and caudate-pallidal gabaminergic pathways.[9,88]

Pathology. Degenerative changes are found throughout the brain, with severe shrinkage and loss of cells in the caudate and putamen, cerebral atrophy, and rarely cerebellar atrophy associated with loss of Purkinje cells. Less severe changes are seen in the globus pallidus and substantia nigra. Severe gliosis of the globus pallidus may be more frequent in children than in adults with this disorder.

Symptoms. Within affected families, symptoms may appear as early as 3 years of age. After normal early development the child becomes clumsy and unsteady. The initial symptoms are usually grand mal convulsions and deterioration of schoolwork. Convulsions occur in two thirds of children in some families, in contrast with their infrequent occurrence in affected adults.[102]

Examination. Children may have difficulty with rapid eye movements, resulting in only slow movements on voluntary gaze, on reading, and in response to optokinetic nystagmus and vestibular stimulation.[15] Examination may reveal grimacing and dysarthric speech. Blank facies or twitchings of facial muscles are usually present. The protruded tongue is usually retracted within 5 seconds. Choreic movements of the arms and legs occur in only one third of affected children in contrast with their much more frequent appearance in adults. Muscular rigidity of the arms and legs and bradykinesia are present in two thirds of cases, producing progressive motor disability.[16] Occasionally, rigidity is severe enough to produce hyperextension of the head with stiffness of the neck. Cerebellar ataxia occurs rarely. Progressive intellectual impairment results in defective memory and emotional instability.[78,122]

Laboratory Examination. The electroencephalogram usually reveals spike discharges. The cerebrospinal fluid is usually normal, although the protein content is occasionally elevated. Pneumoencephalography or computerized tomography usually reveals dilatation of the anterior horns of the lateral ventricles with rounding of their lateral borders due to atrophy of the caudate nuclei.[11] Although these findings are not diagnostic of Huntington's disease, they may suggest that this is the most likely diagnosis.[22]

Differential Diagnosis. The clinical picture in children is similar to that of hepatolenticular degeneration, although no corneal ring is present and the serum ceruloplasmin content is normal. Other differential diagnoses include Friedreich's ataxia, Hallervorden-Spatz disease, postencephalitic parkinsonism, striatonigral degeneration,[44,129] and Gilles de la Tourette's syndrome.

Treatment. No specific treatment is available. Anticonvulsant medications are usually partially effective in the control of convulsive seizures. Levodopa decreases bradykinesia and rigidity, but it may produce choreic symptoms.[15]

Prognosis. As muscular rigidity increases, the child becomes more disabled and is eventually bedridden. There is associated progressive intellectual impairment. Frequent convulsions usually persist. For these reasons, institutional care is often required. Death usually occurs 3 to 10 years after the onset of disability.

Genetic Counseling. Genetic counseling of asymptomatic offspring of affected parents is difficult owing to the lack of a predictive test. Levodopa and amantadine may induce choreic symptoms in an asymptomatic person with a positive family history. The predictive value of oral dopamine for early detection of Huntington's disease in presymptomatic persons has been reported in an 8-year follow-up study.[88] However, a positive result does not prove that the person has Huntington's disease, and the significance of a negative result is not known.

Fetal Erythroblastosis, Hyperbilirubinemia, and Kernicterus

Fetal erythroblastosis is a hemolytic anemia caused by the destruction of fetal erythrocytes by maternal antibody. This results in hyperbilirubinemia and an increased number of circulating nucleated red blood cells. Ultimately there may be failure to compensate for the continuing hemolysis, with increasing anemia, hypoalbuminemia, cardiac failure, anasarca, and death.

Neonatal hyperbilirubinemia above 20 mg/dl may be associated with a distinct clinical syndrome followed by the classic neurologic picture of athetosis or deafness. These characteristic neurologic findings are correlated with the pathologic picture of kernicterus, which consists of abnormal findings in the basal ganglia, hippocampus, and other cerebral structures. In addition, neonatal hyperbilirubinemia may subsequently be associated with mild intellectual impairment and spasticity without the classic signs of athetosis or deafness.[93]

Etiology. Fetal erythroblastosis is usually caused by an incompatibility of Rh factor, notably the D antigens, between mother and fetus. It is the result of maternal sensitization by a fetal erythrocyte antigen. It may be related also to an A or B incompatibility.

Pathology. The hydropic fetus with hemolytic disease shows anasarca, serous effusions, hepatomegaly, splenomegaly, and cardiomegaly associated with an enlarged placenta. If death occurs during the neonatal period, the brain reveals intense yellow pigmentation of the lenticular and caudate nuclei with less intense discoloration of other nuclei of the basal ganglia. The ganglion cells in the pigmented regions are damaged. If the child dies 1 month or more after birth, the yellow stain is no longer present, but there is gliosis in the involved areas. The hippocampus is frequently involved.

Examination. Jaundice develops on the first day after birth and becomes more intense within a few days. The face and neck are swollen, and the liver and spleen are enlarged. During the initial neonatal period, hypotonia, lethargy, and a poor sucking reflex are usually noted, followed by spasticity, opisthotonos, and fever. After this there is a decrease or disappearance of spasticity. Neurologic signs usually develop between the second and the fifth day, and death may occur after a few days. If the infant survives, paralysis of upward gaze, head retraction, weakness, and hypotonia appear by 3 months of age. Between 18 months and 8 years of age, involuntary choreiform and athetotic movements develop. The child usually learns to walk between 2 and 3 years of age, but the gait is ataxic. Speech is usually dysarthric. Approximately one third of patients are partially or completely deaf. The child may be of normal intelligence or mentally defective. Athetosis and neural hearing loss are the most frequent findings after the neonatal bilirubin level exceeds 20 mg/dl.[73]

Laboratory Examination. Anemia is present at birth, and an excessive number of nucleated red blood cells is usually seen on peripheral blood smears. The indirect antiglobulin or Coombs' test is positive, and the serum bilirubin level rises each day if exchange transfusions are not given. Kernicterus rarely occurs in term healthy infants unless the serum level of indirect bilirubin exceeds 20 mg/dl. However, infants with low birth weights and short gestational periods, frequently associated with hypoxia, acidosis, or septicemia, may develop kernicterus with a bilirubin level as low as 10 to 15 mg/dl.[52] Although the indirect serum bilirubin provides a laboratory aid for clinical evaluation, it is only the fraction of the serum bilirubin that is dissociated from albumin which is then free to diffuse into cells. The urine becomes bile-tinged between the first and fourth weeks of life.

The laboratory diagnosis of hemolytic disease of the newborn is based upon demonstration of an abnormal maternal agglutinin, which has specific activity for the infant's erythrocytes. When erythroblastosis is due to Rh incompatibility, it is found that the mother is Rh-negative and the father and baby are Rh-positive.

Assessment of neural hearing loss may be facilitated by determining brain stem auditory evoked responses.

Differential Diagnosis. Erythroblastosis must be distinguished from physiologic jaundice, which occurs in one third of normal infants. With physiologic jaundice, the degree of jaundice decreases after the first week of life. Jaundice during the newborn period may also occur with congenital atresia of the bile ducts and other disorders.

Treatment. When erythroblastosis in a newborn is diagnosed, multiple exchange transfusions are given. If erythroblastosis is due to Rh incompatibility, Rh-negative blood is given. In term infants, a bilirubin level well below 20 mg/dl is maintained. In premature infants, the bilirubin level is maintained below 10 mg/dl. Phototherapy is used early in the course in premature infants.[137] If the process is related to A or B incompatibility, exchange transfusions are given with blood in which the anti-A and anti-B antibodies were neutralized by A and B substances.

Prognosis. Among first infants born after maternal sensitization, 90% recover with adequate treatment and 10% are stillborn. With subsequent pregnancies the stillbirth rate increases to 30%. Premature birth carries a high risk of kernicterus in affected infants. The incidence in affected infants treated by adequate transfusions is less than 1%. Half of the babies who do develop kernicterus die during the first month of life. In children who survive, there is residual damage chiefly to the basal ganglia with resultant choreoathetosis and other signs.

Prevention. During pregnancy, the Rh status of both mother and father is determined. If the mother is Rh-negative, the tentative diagnosis is made before the birth of the infant by demonstrating anti-Rh antibody in the mother's blood. If the initial sample from an Rh-negative mother contains no anti-Rh antibodies, blood tests are repeated at 4-week intervals until term and 6 weeks postpartum. If an antibody titer in excess of 8 by the indirect Coombs' test is demonstrated and if there is a history of stillbirth or previous births in which the baby required exchange transfusions, then amniocentesis is done. This technique provides a safe and valuable means of assessing the presence and severity of hemolytic disease in the fetus. The presence in amniotic fluid of bilirubin pigments derived from hemolysis of fetal blood raises the optic density of amniotic fluid at 450 nm above that of fluid from normal gestations of the same age. The spectrophotometric estimation of bile pigment concentration distinguishes between an uninvolved Rh-negative fetus and an affected Rh-positive fetus in a mother with circulating Rh antibodies.

Analyses of amniotic fluid of Rh-sensitized fetuses have improved the criteria for administering intrauterine transfusions. These are recommended to correct anemia and to prevent imminent fetal demise. If gross ascites is not present by ultrasonography and if the change in optical density at 450 nm (OD_{450}) is above 0.25, intrauterine transfusions are recommended, even though they are occasionally followed by fetal death. After three or more successful intrauterine transfusions of adult, packed red blood cells, fetal blood is almost completely replaced by adult blood. When intrauterine transfusions are combined with excellent prenatal care in these cases, the survival rate is approximately 50%. Follow-up of surviving infants has shown normal development thus far in the vast majority of children. Administration of immune globulin to unsensitized Rh-negative women following elective and spontaneous abortion, amniocentesis, or the delivery of an Rh-positive infant has resulted in further decline in the incidence of hemolytic disease of the newborn.[26,48]

Hepatolenticular Degeneration (Wilson's Disease)

Hepatolenticular degeneration is a hereditary, progressive, fatal disorder characterized by slowly progressing liver disease, by dysfunction of the lenticular nucleus, or by both.[104]

Etiology. The disorder is transmitted as an autosomal recessive gene, and it is probably due to chronic copper toxicity. There is an increased absorption of copper from the intestine; increased content of copper in liver, brain, cornea, and kidney; increased urinary excretion of copper; decreased level of copper in the plasma; and a decreased level of the plasma protein ceruloplasmin.

Pathology. Pathologic changes occur in the basal ganglia and to some extent in the cerebral cortex and the cerebellum. The size of the caudate and putamen is decreased and there may be cavitation. Microscopically, Alzheimer type II cells and Opalski cells are seen, and there is a loss of nerve cells. The liver is usually small with nodular cirrhosis. Microscopic sections of the cornea reveal yellow granules in Descemet's membrane.

Symptoms. The age of onset of hepatolenticular degeneration in children is usually between 8 and 16 years. An early symptom is tremor of the hands. The child may stumble and fall owing to unsteadiness in walking. He may also have difficulty in speaking clearly.

With subsequent involvement of the liver, symptoms may include nausea, jaundice, hemolytic anemia, abdominal pain, swelling of the abdomen and legs, and drowsiness. Symptoms relating to liver damage may appear before or after the symptoms related to neurologic disorder.[36]

Examination. Physical examination may reveal a greenish brown ring of pigment in the cornea at the junction of the sclera. This occurs in more than half the patients. In some patients it can be identified only by slit-lamp examination. Jaundice may be present, and diffuse pigmentation of the skin may appear. The liver and spleen may be palpable, and there may be ascites or peripheral edema. Hyperpigmented lesions on the anterior aspect of the lower legs due to melanin deposition are commonly associated.[96]

Neurologic examination frequently reveals dysarthria of cerebellar type. The patient may have difficulty in swallowing. Drooping of the lower jaw and excessive salivation frequently occur. The motor system reveals involuntary movements which may appear in several different patterns. Titubation of the head is usually present. A rhythmic tremor at rest may occur in the arms or legs, or an intention type of action tremor may develop with voluntary activities. With extension of the arms there may be beating movements seen at the wrist. More proximal sustained writhing movements of dystonia may occur. The muscle tone is increased with rigidity. Sensory examination is normal. The tendon reflexes may be increased, and occasionally the plantar responses may be extensor.

Laboratory Examination. A decrease of serum ceruloplasmin occurs in the vast majority of patients with hepatolenticular degeneration. Only those patients with marked liver disease have a normal ceruloplasmin level (25 mg/dl). A plasma ceruloplasmin level below 20 mg/dl in a child who is not suffering from the nephrotic syndrome is characteristic of hepatolenticular degeneration. The urinary copper excretion is above 100 µg/24 hours and hepatic copper concentration is in excess of 100 µg/g dry liver. Aminoaciduria is an associated finding. Computerized cranial tomography may show atrophic changes in the basal ganglia.[117] Electroencephalographic studies may show nonspecific slowing in theta or delta frequencies if neurologic or hepatic dysfunction is severe. Evoked potentials in response to visual, auditory, and somatosensory stimuli are within normal limits.[155]

Differential Diagnosis. A clinical diagnosis can be established in a child who has the classic picture, including tremor, rigidity, corneal pigmentation (Kayser-Fleischer ring), evidence of liver disease, and a familial incidence. However, early in the course of the disorder the child may have evidence of an extrapyramidal disorder without changes in the cornea, without liver disease, and without a history of a similar disorder in another family member. Demonstration of a low serum ceruloplasmin level in these children establishes the diagnosis. The pattern of involuntary movements seen in dystonia musculorum deformans may be very similar to that seen in some patients with hepatolenticular degeneration. Children with juvenile paralysis agitans or striatal degeneration may have a neurologic picture of rhythmic tremor similar to that which occurs in patients with hepatolenticular degeneration. The signs of athetosis and deafness with kernicterus are associated with hyperbilirubinemia at birth. Huntington's disease presents with rigidity, convulsions, and often a positive family history of a similar disorder. Sydenham's chorea has a subacute onset with choreic movements followed by complete recovery.

Treatment. The urinary excretion of copper is increased by the administration of penicillamine (β,β-dimethylcysteine). Penicillamine combined with a low copper diet is used in the treatment of hepatolenticular degeneration.[36] Penicillamine (Cuprimine), a sulfhydryl-bearing compound that binds copper, is given orally in a dosage of 15 to 30 mg/kg/day in three divided doses. Initially, this therapy produces an increase in the urinary excretion of copper of 2 to 5 mg of copper daily. Within a few months after initiation of daily treatment, the daily urinary excretion of copper decreases, and after 1 year the excretion may approach the pretreatment range. A low copper diet high in calories, protein, and carbohydrate is a very important part of therapy.[60]

With penicillamine therapy, most children show limited improvement in neurologic signs and extent of disability, although some may not respond to therapy. Those with minimal tremor, ataxia, and dysarthria may regain almost normal motor function. Those with moderate involvement may show definite improvement, although neurologic signs persist. Those with severe involvement who are unable to care for themselves may improve sufficiently to carry out the activities of daily living independently.

Prognosis. Untreated, the disorder is progressive, with death usually occurring within 4 to 6 years. It may progress rapidly with death occurring within a few weeks, or more slowly with death occurring in adult life. Death is generally due to intercurrent infection or acute hepatic failure.

Prevention. In an asymptomatic child suspected by family history of being destined to develop hepatolenticular degeneration or in a child with idiopathic juvenile cirrhosis, specific laboratory findings may be considered adequate to establish that the child is homozygously abnormal. The necessary findings include both of the following abnormalities: (1) There is a decrease in the serum ceruloplasmin concentration (less than 20 mg/dl). This determination is made after the child is more than 6 months of age at a time when the physiologic hypoceruloplasminemia of the newborn is no longer present. (2) There is an elevation of hepatic copper concentration (greater than 250 μg/g dry weight) associated with nonspecific histologic changes in the liver. It is proposed that penicillamine therapy to increase copper excretion in these children will prevent the disorder. However, because of the toxicity of penicillamine and the lack of controlled studies, use of this agent in these asymptomatic patients remains controversial.

Chorea Minor (Sydenham's Chorea)

Chorea minor, or Sydenham's chorea, is a disorder characterized by abrupt spontaneous movements of the face and extremities associated with incoordination and muscular weakness. The word *chorea*, meaning dance, describes the involuntary movements of the hands and feet, which frequently suggest a dancing type of gait.

Etiology. The etiology of chorea minor is not definitely established. Approximately half of patients with chorea develop evidence of rheumatic arthritis or carditis either before, during, or subsequent to an attack of chorea. The evidence suggests that chorea, like rheumatic fever, is a manifestation of an antigen–antibody reaction following streptococcus group A infection. If patients with pure chorea and no rheumatic manifestations are studied within 1 month of the onset of chorea, 73% have elevated antistreptolysin O titers. This is in contrast with positive antistreptolysin O titers in 95% of patients with acute rheumatic fever. It has been hypothesized that, whereas arthritis and carditis develop 1 to 2 months after a streptococcus group A infection, chorea is a later manifestation occurring within 2 to 3 months, or as late as 6 to 8 months, after a streptococcal infection. About half of tested children have immunoglobulin G antibodies that react with neuronal cytoplasm of human caudate and subthalamic nuclei.[72] Sydenham's chorea may result from functional overactivity of dopamine on striatal neurons.[113] The number of reported cases of Sydenham's chorea in the United States has declined steadily since 1968.[115]

Pathology. The pathologic findings are those of a difuse encephalopathy. The involvement of the gray matter is more intense than that of the white matter. Inflammatory, vascular, and degenerative lesions may be found in the cortex, cerebellum, basal ganglia, medulla, and meninges.[92,149]

Symptoms. Approximately 80% of patients with chorea minor develop symptoms between 2 and 15 years of age. Rarely, the disease occurs during early childhood or late adolescence. About twice as many cases are seen in girls as in boys. The child may show irritability and easy fatigability. Difficulty may be noted in using one or both arms when writing, eating, or playing games, and the child may complain of weakness.

Examination. Characteristically, the child shows spontaneous movements, incoordination, and muscular weakness. When the muscles of facial expression are involved, there is frequent grimacing. Sudden movements of the corner of the mouth, the cheeks, or the eyelids, usually bilateral, may be seen. When the child is asked to move various facial muscles, it is difficult for him to maintain voluntary movements because they are interrupted by involuntary ones. There may be dysarthria or difficulty in swallowing. The "jack-in-the-box" tongue is characterized by difficulty in maintaining the tongue in an extended position. Spontaneous movements of the jaw may also occur, so the tongue is withdrawn into the mouth to prevent biting it. Frequently, spontaneous movements occur in the arms and legs. In one third of the cases, these movements are more prominent on one side of the body than on the other, whereas in the majority of the children the involuntary movements are bilateral but not synchronous. Rarely, these involuntary movements are confined to one side and produce the picture of hemichorea. Frequently there are spontaneous movements involving the small muscles of the fingers and the forearm muscles. When the arms are extended, there may be sudden flexion at the wrist with return of the hand to a more normal position. In this position, the hands are frequently flexed at the wrist and hyperextended at the metacarpophalangeal joints in a "silver fork" posture. Occasionally, with lapses in posture, the entire arm may suddenly drop to the patient's side. Frequently, if the arms are extended above the head, the palms face laterally owing to internal rotation of the shoulder and pronation of the forearm (pronator sign). Spontaneous movements in the legs and feet also occur. If the involvement of proximal muscles becomes marked, then flinging movements of the involved extremity appear, which may result in bruises. In addition to involuntary movements, incoordination is frequently marked. The finger-to-nose and heel-to-shin tests may reveal an action tremor, which may be more prominent at the end of the voluntary movement. If the right arm is involved, the child may notice great difficulty in writing (Fig. 16-2) or in feeding himself. Also, there is usually motor weakness. When the arms are extended, one arm may drift downward due to weakness. The grip may be weak and it may be difficult to maintain sustained contraction of muscles. With severe weakness, spontaneous movements are infrequent. Hypotonia may be present. The motor findings are less prominent when the child is alone in a quiet room, and they decrease markedly during sleep. They also vary from day to day.

Some patients show irritability. Occasionally transient intellectual impairment is noted.[53] On rare occasions the patients develop psychotic manifestations. Sensory examination is normal. The tendon reflexes may be normal or may reveal a sustained contraction to repeated stimulation. Abdominal and cremasteric reflexes are frequently hyperactive. The plantar responses are flexor.

Examination reveals evidence of cardiac involvement in about half of the cases. Rarely, central retinal artery occlusion occurs, probably as an embolic complication of carditis.[98]

Laboratory Examination. The erythrocyte sedimentation rate may be elevated or normal. Abnormal C-reactive protein may be present. During the first month of chorea, the antistreptolysin O titer is elevated in approximately three fourths of children. In those patients who have chorea associated with arthritis or carditis, abnormalities may be noted in the electrocardiogram, and radiographs of the chest may reveal cardiac

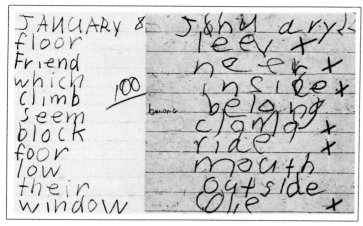

FIG. 16-2. Chorea minor (Sydenham's chorea). Rapid deterioration of handwriting in a 9-year-old child between January 8 (*left*), and January 22 (*right*). Involuntary movements in the hand prevented normal coordination in writing.

enlargement. Results of lumbar puncture are normal. The electroencephalogram may show increased slowing for the child's age.

Differential Diagnosis.   Chorea is a clinical diagnosis based on the findings of explosive, abrupt, spontaneous movements involving various muscle groups associated with weakness, lapses in movement, and incoordination. In contrast, tics involving the face, shoulders, arms and legs occur in a uniform repetitive manner and are not associated with weakness.

Children with choreoathetosis related to congenital maldevelopment of the cerebrum or to cerebral damage at birth show choreiform movements similar to those in Sydenham's chorea. These spontaneous movements are present from the time of onset of the symptoms and signs and do not disappear as do those in Sydenham's chorea. Frequently, pyramidal tract signs are present with spasticity, weakness, increased reflexes, and extensor plantar responses.

Chorea may be the initial manifestation of lupus erythematosus in children.[62,65] Other disorders in which chorea may be a prominent feature are benign familial chorea[27] and paroxysmal choreoathetosis of Mount and Rebuck.[87]

Treatment.   There is no specific therapy for chorea. If the spontaneous movements are violent, involving large muscle groups, it is important to decrease them. Phenobarbital, diazepam, chlorpromazine, chloral hydrate, or paraldehyde may be used for their sedative effects. Frequently, large dosages of hypnotic drugs are required. In severe cases, reserpine has been used to decrease the choreiform movements. There is no evidence that any of these drugs decreases the duration of the choreic manifestations. Also, amphetamine sulfate in a dose of 10 mg is reported to be effective in controlling spontaneous movements. There is no controlled study to demonstrate that cortisone is of value in chorea, although its use has been reported. Haloperidol may be effective in controlling choreatic movements in some patients.[141]

Prognosis.   The mortality rate from chorea is extremely low; approximately one patient in 1000 may die during the course of severe chorea. In a few children, minor neurologic residua persist.[14] With this exception, the symptoms of chorea are self-limited and disappear after an interval, which may vary from 1 week to 2 years with a mean of 19 weeks. Approximately half of the children with chorea also have rheumatic carditis, which is fatal in 2% of cases.

One fourth of a group of children with chorea not associated with cardiac abnormalities developed valvular heart disease within a follow-up period of 30 years.[8] Chorea recurs in one third of children.

Prevention. Due to the high incidence of rheumatic fever attacks in children who have had chorea, it is recommended that patients be placed on a prophylactic regimen of penicillin therapy to prevent recurrence of rheumatic infection with or without chorea. Prophylaxis with penicillin is continued over many years.

X-Linked Recessive Hypoxanthine-Guanine Phosphoribosyl Transferase Deficiency (Lesch-Nyhan Syndrome)

Lesch-Nyhan syndrome, a rare, sex-linked recessive disorder of purine metabolism, is characterized by choreoathetosis, mental retardation, compulsive self-mutilation, aggressive behavior, and hyperuricemia. Over 90 cases from 74 families have been reported[138] since Lesch and Nyhan[95] described this condition in 1964.

Etiology. A deficiency of hypoxanthine-guanine phosphoribosyl transferase enzymatic activity has been found in the cells of virtually all patients studied with this disorder. The activity of this enzyme is determined by a gene on the X chromosome. The enzyme regenerates inosine and guanylic acids from the purine bases hypoxanthine and guanine. Patients with the complete syndrome have less than 0.1% of normal enzyme activity in hemolysates of washed erythrocytes.[138] The enzyme defect appears to explain the hyperuricemia and its consequences, such as hematuria, renal calculi, and tophi, but does not clarify the neurologic manifestations. A favorable response has been observed in some patients treated with a serotonin precursor.[121] Neurotransmitter function studies in patients with Lesch-Nyhan syndrome may improve understanding of this complex disorder.

Pathology. Routine pathologic studies in about ten cases of Lesch-Nyhan syndrome have failed to show any abnormality in brain tissue by conventional histologic studies.

Symptoms. The disorder has been found only in boys. Affected infants appear normal at birth and develop normally for 6 to 8 months. Uricosuria in the form of orange sand may be noted early but is seldom given the significance it deserves. More commonly, the first recognized manifestations are those that affect the central nervous system. Infants who have been sitting up and holding their head up lose this ability. At 6 to 8 months of age, there is evident hypertonicity (usually preceded by hypotonia), hyperreflexia, and Babinski responses. These progress to spasticity, involuntary athetoid movements, and often bilateral dislocation of the hips. None of the reported patients has been able to walk. Mental retardation becomes evident and measured intelligent quotients are usually less than 50.[121] At 2 to 3 years of age or later childhood, aggressive and mutilating behavior appears. The children may be self-destructive in other ways and demonstrate irrepressible behavior against others.[121] Growth failure occurs and there are constant torsion spasms.

Examination. When the clinical picture is fully developed, destruction of the terminal portions of fingers and mutilation of the lips result. The boys are severely retarded, but are alert, responsive, and very aggressive in their behavior and in their language. Dysarthria is marked and there may be difficulty in swallowing. The motor system examination reveals severe choreoathetosis and dystonic movements. Cerebellar signs may be present. Muscle tone is increased with crossing of the extended legs. There is no sensory loss. Tendon reflexes are hyperactive and plantar responses may be extensor. Gouty arthritis, tophi, and uric acid calculi may develop during childhood or adult life.

Laboratory Examination. Hyperuricemia in affected patients usually exceeds 6 mg/dl and generally approximates 9 to 11 mg/dl. The 24-hour urinary excretion of uric acid usually exceeds 600 mg beyond infancy or 40 to 70 mg/kg of body weight. A more convenient measurement is that of urate excretion per mg of creatinine. Patients with Lesch-Nyhan syndrome usually excrete 3 to 4 mg of uric acid per mg of creatinine, whereas control patients excrete less than 1.[121]

Hypoxanthine-guanine phosphoribosyl transferase activity is nearly absent in every tissue in the body of these patients. Erythrocytes and cultured fibroblasts provide a convenient source for measuring the enzyme activity in suspected patients. Cerebrospinal fluid hypoxanthine concentrations are increased to four times those of controls. Purines other than uric acid may also accumulate. Megaloblastic anemia may be present.

Differential Diagnosis. This disorder must be distinguished from other extrapyramidal disorders of childhood (Table 16-1). Among the disorders that produce mental retardation, Down's syndrome may be associated with hyperuricemia.

Treatment. The most important aspect of management is protecting the patient from injuring himself. The use of elbow restraints allows the patient to use his hands without permitting finger mutilation. Removal of primary teeth to prevent early disfigurement is advocated. Behavior modification may not be as effective in these patients as with other forms of mental retardation.[121]

Allopurinol (Zyloprim) in a daily dosage of up to 8 mg/kg body weight in divided doses blocks the formation of uric acid and is effective in arresting all those features of the syndrome that are common to gout (arthropathy, nephropathy, tophi). Unfortunately, allopurinol does not alter the neurologic or behavioral manifestations of the disease. Oral administration of 5-hydroxy-tryptophan has been reported to induce almost complete reduction of self-mutilative behavior in some patients but not in others.[49]

Prognosis. The neurologic disorder is slowly progressive, and institutional care is usually required. Death may be associated with malnutrition due to dysphagia and vomiting, gouty nephropathy, or bronchopneumonia and other infections.

Prevention. Heterozygous women can be detected and informed of their chances of having affected children. In heterozygous women who become pregnant, the sex and the mutant or normal status of the fetus can be established by amniocentesis and by demonstrating in cultured fibroblasts the enzyme defect.

TABLE 16-1.   Differential Diagnosis of Extrapyramidal Disorders

Disorder	Familial	Signs	Associated Findings
Hepatolenticular degeneration	Autosomal recessive	Rigidity, tremor, dystonia, dementia, corneal ring, jaundice	Increased urinary and hepatic copper, low serum ceruloplasmin
Juvenile parkinsonism	Rarely	Resting tremor, rigidity, bradykinesia	Decreased dopamine level in substantia nigra
Kernicterus	No	Athetosis, deafness, occasional intellectual impairment	Neonatal hyperbilirubinemia
Huntington's disease	Autosomal dominant	Rigidity, chorea, convulsions, dementia	
Torsion dystonia	Autosomal dominant or recessive	Dystonia, involuntary movements, normal intellect	
Chorea minor	No	Involuntary choreic movements, possibly carditis	Group A streptococcal infections
Absence of hypoxanthine-guanine phosphoribosyl transferase	X-linked recessive	Choreoathetosis, mental retardation, self-mutilation	Increased urinary and blood uric acid

DISORDERS OF THE CEREBELLUM

Disorders of the cerebellum result in ataxia and other symptoms, which may be initially classified from the history as follows: (1) relatively stationary ataxia since infancy, (2) chronic progressive ataxia, (3) acute ataxia with partial or complete recovery, and (4) acute, intermittent ataxia. Some of these disorders are restricted primarily to the cerebellum, whereas in others cerebellar dysfunction is part of a more widespread disorder of the central nervous system.

DISORDER OF THE CEREBELLUM PRESENTING AS STATIONARY ATAXIA: HYPOPLASIA, OR AGENESIS OF THE CEREBELLUM

Congenital cerebellar hypoplasia is a rare, autosomal recessive disorder characterized clinically by hypotonia, ataxia, and developmental delay, and pathologically by severe loss of granule cells in the cerebellum.[77] This disorder is distinct from cerebellar hypoplasia associated with other neurologic conditions such as spinal muscular atrophy, Tay-Sachs disease, Menkes disease, and Arnold-Chiari malformation.[135] It must also be differentiated from sclerotic atrophy of the cerebellum occurring as a secondary alteration in previously normal cerebellar tissue.[130]

Etiology.   The etiology of congenital cerebellar hypoplasia is unknown. Cerebellar granule cell atrophy due to panleukopenia virus occurs in kittens. Depletion of granule cells may be induced by cytotoxic agents and ionizing radiation.

Pathology.   Diffuse and severe degeneration of granule cells is the main pathologic finding. Neuronal loss is evident in Sommer sector of the hippocampus. Focal dendritic swellings referred to as asteroid bodies may be found in Purkinje cells.[119,135]

Symptoms.   During infancy, poor muscle tone and developmental delay may be the first abnormalities noted by the parents. Sitting, standing, and walking may be delayed. Poor coordination is evident during voluntary movements of the extremities.

Examination.   Hypotonia is a prominent feature during infancy. Titubation of the trunk interferes with sitting unsupported, which may not be accomplished until 1 to 4 years of age. Walking alone may not be possible until 2 to 5 years of age. The gait is ataxic. Nystagmus and dysarthria are associated findings. The head size may be small, and sometimes there is mental retardation.

Laboratory Examination.   Skull roentgenograms frequently show evidence of a shallow posterior fossa. Computerized tomography or pneumoencephalography may demonstrate an increase in the size of the fourth ventricle, vallecula, and cisterna magna surrounding the rudimentary cerebellar hemispheres.[135]

Treatment.   No specific treatment is available.

DISORDERS OF THE CEREBELLUM PRESENTING AS CHRONIC PROGRESSIVE ATAXIA

Arnold-Chiari Malformation

A congenital anomaly of the hindbrain, Arnold-Chiari malformation (Chiari type 2) is characterized by varying degrees of herniation of the cerebellum, kinking of the medulla oblongata, and spina bifida.[43,51] The malformation probably originates in the first 4 to 5 weeks of embryonic development.[51]

Pathology.   The cerebellar tonsils extend through the foramen magnum in tonguelike projections. The lower portion of the medulla is below the level of the foramen magnum, and the lower cranial nerves are stretched. This malformation is almost always associated with spina bifida occulta or with a myelomeningocele in the thoracic or lumbosacral region. Hydrocephalus is usually present, and there may be microgyria and defects in the spinal cord.

Symptoms.   In the infant born with spina bifida cystica, subsequent development of hydrocephalus is indicative of associated Arnold-Chiari malformation. When manifestations appear later in life, headache is sometimes an early symptom in association with increased intracranial pressure. There may be difficulty in swallowing or difficulty with speech, and laryngeal stridor may develop. Unsteadiness in walking may be present.

Examination.   Older children may have papilledema. Rarely, third, fourth, sixth, seventh, or eighth cranial nerve palsies appear.[142] The gag reflex may be absent with weakness of the soft palate. Vocal cord paralysis may occur, as may weakness of the sternomastoid and trapezius muscles and weakness or atrophy of the tongue. There may also be unsteadiness in walking, and horizontal or vertical nystagmus. The tendon reflexes may be hyperactive with extensor plantar responses. Weakness and spasticity of the arms and legs may appear.

Laboratory Examination.   Skull roentgenograms may show evidence of hydrocephalus, and computerized tomography or pneumoencephalography reveals dilatation of the lateral and third ventricles. Roentgenograms of the lumbosacral spine frequently demonstrate associated spina bifida.

Differential Diagnosis.   The presence of hydrocephalus with lower cranial nerve involvement, cerebellar ataxia, and associated spina bifida suggests the possible presence of the Arnold-Chiari malformation. Skeletal deformities at the level of the foramen magnum may also be present. Cranium bifidum may be found in association with the Arnold-Chiari deformity. Also, basilar impression, occipitalization of the atlas, or maldevelopment of the central cervical vertebrae may be present (Table 16-2).

Treatment.   The treatment is surgical. The posterior portion of the foramen magnum and the arches of the first four cervical vertebrae are removed.

Prognosis.   The symptoms produced by compression of the inferior lobes of the cerebellum and of the medulla are usually relieved by surgery.

Hereditary Spinocerebellar Ataxia (Friedreich's Ataxia)

Friedreich's ataxia, the commonest of the spinocerebellar degenerations, is an inherited, progressive degeneration of the spinal cord, characterized by degeneration of the spinocerebellar tracts, posterior columns, and corticospinal tracts. Commonly associated defects are pes cavus, kyphoscoliosis, and myocardial abnormalities.[150]

Etiology.   The etiology of hereditary spinocerebellar ataxia is unknown. It is transmitted as an autosomal recessive gene in 75% of cases. It affects males and females equally. Other members of the family in which Friedreich's ataxia occurs may show only skeletal deformities, such as Friedreich's foot. In some families, a mild and incomplete form may occur, with ataxia associated with muscular atrophy (Roussy-Lévy syndrome). Pyruvate metabolism may be defective in patients with Friedreich's ataxia. A deficiency of one or another component of the pyruvate dehydrogenase complex, the enzyme group that oxidizes pyruvate to acetyl-CoA, has been found in some, but not all, patients with Friedreich's ataxia.[10,17,81]

Pathology.   In the spinal cord, there is degeneration of the dorsal and ventral spinocerebellar tracts, the corticospinal tracts, and the posterior columns. Changes may occur in the cerebellum, brain stem, and cerebral cortex. Atrophy of the Purkinje cells and the dentate nuclei in the cerebellum has been described. In advanced cases, the degeneration may extend into the dorsal roots and the peripheral nerves. The anterior horn cells are usually normal. Rarely does the degeneration in the corticospinal tract extend above the level of the medulla and involve the cerebral cortex. The heart usually reveals myocardial fibrosis or hypertrophic obstuctive cardiomyopathy.[13]

Symptoms.   Unsteadiness in walking and easy fatigability appear, usually between 7 and 15 years of age. In half the cases, the onset occurs before the child is 10 years old. He may have difficulty in making sudden turns and may fall while running. Over a period of a few years, these symptoms

TABLE 16-2. Differential Diagnosis of Chronic Progressive Ataxia

Clinical Disorder	Preceding History	Usual Year of Onset in Children	Examination	Usual Laboratory Examination	Usual Prognosis
Arnold-Chiari malformation	Headache, dysphagia		Palatal and tongue weakness, pyramidal signs, ataxia	May have hydrocephalus, spina bifida	Slowly progressive; stationary after surgery
Hereditary spinocerebellar ataxia	Stumbling, dizziness, familial incidence	7–10	Ataxia, loss of position sense, extensor plantar responses, kyphoscoliosis, pes cavus	Frequent associated ECG changes	Progressive, with death usually by 30 years of age
A-β-lipoproteinemia	Fatty diarrhea at 6 weeks to 2 years of age	2–17	Cerebellar ataxia, posterior column signs, retinitis pigmentosa, scoliosis, pes cavus	Acanthocytosis, lack of β-lipoprotein in serum	Slowly progressive
Dentate cerebellar ataxia	Myclonus, convulsions	7–17	Ataxia with severe intention tremor		Slowly progressive
Hereditary cerebellar ataxia	Familial incidence	3–17	Ataxia, optic atrophy, occasionally associated posterior column and pyramidal tract signs	Pneumoencephalo-gram: small cerebellar folia	Slowly progressive
Ataxia telangiectasia	Recurrent sinopulmonary infections in two thirds of cases; familial incidence	1–3	Oculocutaneous telangiectasia at 4–6 years; ataxia, choreoathetosis, dysarthria	Chest roentgenogram indicates brochiectasis; absence of IgA in serum	Death before 25 years of age
Cerebellar tumors	Headache, vomiting		Papilledema, ataxia, nystagmus	Skull roentgenograms indicate separation of sutures	Progressive until operated
Heredopathia atactica polyneuriti-formis	Anorexia, failing vision, unsteady, familial incidence	4–7	Retinitis pigmentosa, ataxia, deafness, polyneuropathy, ichthyosis	Elevated phytanic acid in blood, increased spinal fluid protein	Slowly progressive with death
Multiple sclerosis	Preceding neurologic symptoms	14–17	Optic neuritis; brain stem, cerebellar, pyramidal, or sensory signs	Spinal fluid may reveal increased cells, protein, or γ-globulin	Exacerbations and remissions
Spinal cord tumor	May have numbness or bladder disorder		Ataxia with weakness or sensory loss	Defect on myelography	Progressive until operated on

progress, and unsteadiness in the hands and arms also develops. Vertigo is frequently noted early in the course of the illness. With progression, the patient is unable to walk without support.

Cardiac involvement occurs in more than half of the cases. In patients with heart disease, dyspnea and palpitation on effort occur several years after the onset of the neurologic symptoms. Severe chest pain may occur late in the course of the disease.

Diabetes mellitus develops in 10% to 20% of the patients; nearly all of these are insulin-dependent, and two thirds are female. Diabetes usually develops late in the course of the disease.[127]

Examination.   Physical examination usually reveals characteristic deformities of the skeleton. Kyphosis or scoliosis in the thoracic region is present in 80% of cases (Fig. 16-3A). Kyphoscoliosis develops early or late and progresses slowly. Deformity of the feet occurs in 75% of patients, consisting of a highly arched instep with extension of the proximal phalanx and flexion of the distal phalanges (Fig. 16-3B). The foot deformity may appear before the onset of neurologic signs, or it may develop during the course of the disease. Tachycardia and evidence of cardiac failure may be late manifestations.

Usually the child has horizontal or rotatory nystagmus. Caloric tests may reveal loss of vestibular function uni- or bilaterally. Decreased vision, optic atrophy, or extraocular muscle palsies may be found.[23] The speech is staccato, explosive, and slurred. Head tremor may be present.

The gait is unsteady with a wide base. The child is usually unable to walk heel to toe. Heel-to-shin ataxia and, later, finger-to-nose ataxia may be present. Alternating movements of the hands are frequently slowed. Fine movements may be difficult to perform, and handwriting may be unsteady. Hypotonia and rebound phenomenon are seen. With root involvement, distal weakness in the legs occurs.

There is usually loss of position and vibration sense and of two-point discrimination in the feet and later in the hands. Sensations of touch, pain, and temperature are preserved. The jaw jerk is brisk.[133] The knee and ankle jerks are usually absent early in the course of the disease, and subsequently the tendon reflexes in the arms may

be lost. The plantar responses are extensor. Abdominal and cremasteric reflexes are usually present. A midsystolic murmur frequently heard at the left sternal border may appear in cases with cardiac manifestations.

Laboratory Examination.   There are no diagnostic laboratory findings. Examination of the cerebrospinal fluid is usually normal, although rarely there may be an increase in the protein content. The electrocardiogram is abnormal in the vast majority of patients. It may show disorders of rhythm including atrial fibrillation, T wave inversion, conduction defects with bundle branch block, or complete heart block in association with myocardial fibrosis. Also the electrocardiogram may occcasionally show changes associated with acute or chronic occlusive coronary artery disease. Roentgenograms of the chest reveal cardiac enlargement in half of those patients with cardiac involvement. Radiographs of the spine may reveal scoliosis (Fig. 16-3C,D). The fasting blood sugar may be elevated. In some cases, glucose administration may result in hyperglycemia and a marked increase in the plasma insulin level. Nerve conduction studies show normal or slightly low conduction velocity in motor fibers, and they usually demonstrate a marked depression of sensory action potentials. Visual and somatosensory evoked potentials may show prolonged latencies.[23]

Differential Diagnosis.   The diagnosis is readily apparent in a child with clubfeet, kyphoscoliosis, and signs of involvement of the tracts in the posterior half of the spinal cord. The additional finding of one or more similar cases in the family pedigree assures a conclusive clinical diagnosis. If there is no family history of a similar disorder and if skeletal deformities are not present, then the neurologic signs may be quite similar to those found in multiple sclerosis. Friedreich's ataxia usually first appears during childhood, whereas multiple sclerosis rarely begins before 14 years of age. Involvement of other areas of the central nervous system, such as the occurrence of retrobulbar neuritis, helps to establish a diagnosis of multiple sclerosis. The slowly progressive course of Friedreich's ataxia is frequently distinguishable from the exacerbations and re-

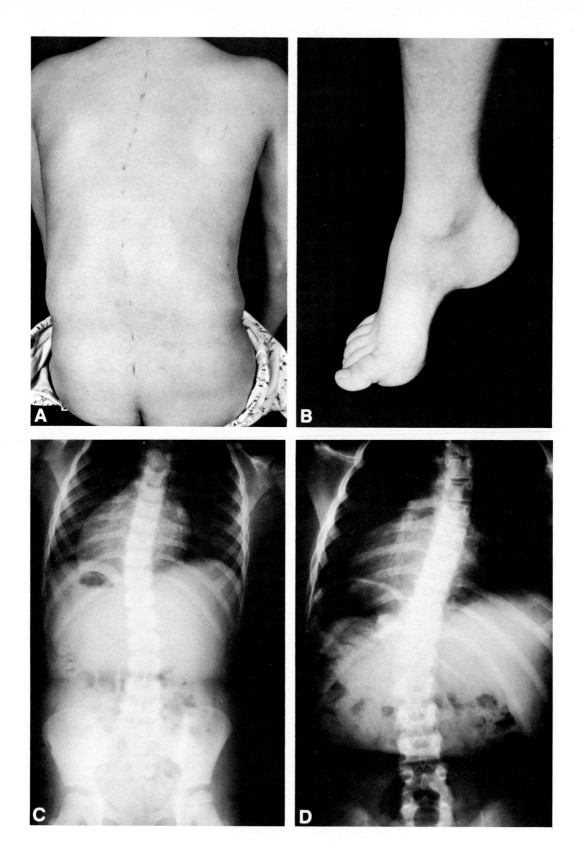

missions that often occur in multiple sclerosis. Spinocerebellar ataxia must be distinguished from the childhood forms of familial amaurotic idiocy.[79] Other familial cerebellar diseases are very similar to Friedreich's ataxia and may be indistinguishable. Cardiac manifestations may suggest the likelihood of Friedreich's ataxia in dubious cases (Table 16-2).

Treatment. There is no therapy that favorably alters the course of the disease. Symptomatic treatment includes physical therapy, the use of a walker, tenotomies, and other orthopedic procedures for correction of the foot deformity.

Prognosis. The course is slowly progressive, with incapacity by 20 to 30 years of age. Most patients are not able to walk without aid 5 years after the onset of symptoms. The duration of the disease from its onset until death averages 24 years. Death is usually due to heart failure associated with interstitial myocarditis or secondary pulmonary infection. Patients with diabetes mellitus may develop ketosis terminally.[127] In that form of spinocerebellar ataxia associated with distal muscular atrophy, progressive disability occurs more slowly than in classic Friedreich's ataxia, and more patients may live a normal life span.

Abetalipoproteinemia (Bassen-Kornzweig Syndrome)

Abetalipoproteinemia, or Bassen-Kornzweig syndrome, is a rare disorder characterized by ataxia, retinitis pigmentosa,

FIG. 16-3. Hereditary spinocerebellar ataxia. This 12-year-old girl developed unsteadiness in walking at 7 years of age with progressive signs of cerebellar, posterior column, and corticospinal tract disorder associated with scoliosis and pes cavus. *A.* Thoracolumbar scoliosis. The locations of the spinous processes are indicated by skin markers. *B.* Pes cavus. *C.* Radiograph of the spine (posterior view) at 4 years of age reveals moderate mild scoliosis with convexity to the left at the 12th thoracic level. *D.* Radiograph of the spine (posterior view) at 12 years of age reveals a moderate increase in scoliosis during the 8-year interval.

acanthocytosis, steatorrhea, and an absence of circulating low-density lipoproteins (LDL, β-lipoproteins, or apoprotein B). More than 40 patients with this disorder have been identified[64] since it was described by Bassen and Kornzweig[12] in 1950.

Etiology. The limited data available are consistent with an autosomal recessive mode of inheritance. About one fourth of the cases have been reported among Ashkenazi Jews. Nearly half of affected persons were the offspring of consanguineous marriages.

The initial observation[137] that β-lipoproteins were absent in these patients has been studied by more modern techniques of lipoprotein analysis.[59] Low-density lipoproteins (LDL) are absent in plasma subjected to analysis by ultracentrifugation, and apoprotein B is absent when tested by radioimmunochemical assay. Furthermore, plasma high-density lipoproteins (HDL), cholesteryl esters, and lecithin–cholesterol acyltransferase activity are decreased in patients with abetalipoproteinemia. Because LDL are the main carriers of cholesterol in plasma, the absence of this fraction may account for the malabsorption of fat and the morphologic abnormality of the erythrocytes. The central nervous system abnormalities are more difficult to explain. Defective absorption of fat-soluble vitamins, particularly vitamin E, may play a major role in the neurologic disabilities.[111]

Pathology. Detailed neuropathologic studies have not been reported. A demyelinating process involves the posterior columns severely, the dorsal and ventral spinocerebellar tracts to a lesser degree, and the corticospinal tracts only slightly.[35] Loss of Purkinje cells and granular layer neurons was evident in one reported case but not in another.[35] Peripheral nerve studies show focal areas of demyelination.[136,143]

Symptoms. The infant appears normal at birth and the neonatal period is rarely complicated. Later on the infant grows and gains weight more slowly than normal infants. Steatorrhea and abdominal distention appear between 6 weeks and 2 years of age.

Neurologic symptoms present later, between 2 and 17 years of age, with gradual unsteadiness in walking associated with progressive weakness. During this phase, patients are frequently misdiagnosed as cases of Friedreich's ataxia. Decreased visual acuity and scotomas become evident at about puberty. Some patients develop cardiovascular abnormalities in early adult life, including arrhythmias and congestive heart failure.[35]

Examination. The examination may reveal findings consistent with an atypical form of spinocerebellar degeneration. Ataxia, extensive loss of proprioception, and, in some patients, associated skeletal abnormalities such as pes cavus, scoliosis, and increased lordosis may suggest a spinocerebellar degeneration. An early finding is the loss of deep tendon reflexes. Pyramidal tract involvement is not prominent because spasticity is not usually present and Babinski response is not always elicited. Ocular abnormalities may present early or late in the course of the illness, depending upon the degree of macular degeneration. Night blindness, decreased vision, and nystagmus are eventually found in all patients. The retinal pigmentary changes develop later, usually in the second decade of life, and are described as retinitis pigmentosa or retinitis punctata albescens. Plotting of the visual fields reveals complete or partial ring scotomas. The electroretinogram frequently shows scotopic impairment or complete extinction.

Somatic abnormalities may be prominent in some patients and include epicanthal folds, high, arched palate, low hairline, webbed neck, small external ears, thoracic scoliosis, thin arms and legs, and pes cavus.

Laboratory Examination. At least half of the erythrocytes have spines projecting from their surfaces (acanthocytes) in the peripheral blood smear. Another useful clue to the diagnosis is a clear serum or plasma due to the absence of chylomicrons. Low serum cholesterol and triglyceride concentrations may also be helpful in suspecting the diagnosis. The diagnosis may be confirmed by demonstration of absent circulating β-lipoproteins, low-density lipoproteins (LDL) or apoprotein B, depending on the availability of these laboratory tests.

Gastrointestinal radiographic studies may show nonspecific findings such as mild small bowel dilatation and thickened mucosal folds. Jejunal biopsy is considered to be diagnostic if it shows unblunted, well-formed villi that have apical mucosal cells laden with lipid vacuoles.[84]

Differential Diagnosis. The neurologic signs are similar to those observed in Friedreich's ataxia and in Refsum's syndrome, although the changes in the red blood cells and in the serum lipids are not present in the latter disorders (Table 16-2).

Treatment. No specific therapy is available. Steatorrhea is diminished by giving affected children a low-fat diet. Supplementation with fat-soluble vitamins A and K has long been advocated.[74] More recently, prolonged therapy with vitamin E at doses of 100 mg/kg daily has resulted in neurologic improvement and regression of the retinal abnormalities.[111]

Prognosis. The neurologic signs are usually progressive with eventual severe disability in young adult life. Visual impairment gradually progresses until there is complete loss of useful vision. No data on life expectancy are available, although long-term therapy with vitamin E appears encouraging.

Dentate Cerebellar Ataxia (Dyssynergia Cerebellaris Myoclonica or Ramsay Hunt Syndrome)

Dentate cerebellar ataxia is a familial disorder characterized by ataxia, cerebellar intention tremor, and myoclonus. Nearly 50 cases have been reported[55] since Ramsay Hunt[71] described his cases in 1921.

Etiology. A genetic factor is recognized in dentate cerebellar ataxia, although the etiology is unknown. In those cases associated with spinocerebellar ataxia of Friedreich, there is a marked familial incidence.

Pathology. The dentate nuclei are grossly degenerated with almost complete loss of cells. Demyelination of the brachium conjunctivum is present, and there is degeneration of small cells of the red nucleus. The remaining parts of the nervous system are normal, except in those cases associated clinically with Friedreich's spinocerebellar ataxia.

Symptoms.   When this disorder occurs in children, it may begin anytime from 7 to 16 years of age. Initially the child develops a generalized convulsion as well as myoclonic jerks, followed after an interval of several years by incoordination in the use of one and then both hands and arms. Marked tremor develops in the arms and legs, interfering with walking.

Examination.   The motor system reveals severe intention tremor noted on finger-to-nose testing. Movements of the arms and hands are erratic with inability to perform fine coordinated movements and with marked tremor. Alternating movements are poorly performed with overshooting. There is hypotonia. The gait is unsteady, and the heel-to-shin test usually shows some ataxia, although less marked than that in the arms. Myoclonic jerks are present in half of the patients. If the disorder is associated with spinocerebellar ataxia, then there are the additional findings of loss of position and vibration sense, absence of tendon reflexes, and extensor plantar responses.

Laboratory Examination.   Electroencephalography may reveal a paroxysmal dysrhythmia associated with clinical seizures. Electrical abnormalities may also be noted in association with myoclonic jerks. Skull roentgenograms and lumbar puncture results are normal.

Treatment.   Diphenylhydantoin (Dilantin) or phenobarbital are indicated for the control of generalized motor seizures. Valproate or clonazepam may decrease the frequency of myoclonic jerks. For detailed treatment of seizures, see Chapter 7.

Hereditary Cerebellar Ataxia

The diagnostic category hereditary cerebellar ataxia includes a variety of clinical pictures in which cerebellar signs are the only or the most prominent findings.

Etiology.   Although the etiology of this group of disorders is not known, a genetic factor is present; 15% of children with cerebellar ataxia are found on routine history-taking to have a close relative with a similar cerebellar disorder. Genetic factors are probably of importance in more than half of these patients, although the nature of the presumed metabolic defect is unknown.

Pathology.   Atrophy of the cerebellum is usually marked with small folia and widened sulci, and there is generally a marked loss of Purkinje cells. There may be associated atrophy of the inferior olives and of spinocerebellar tracts. Occasionally the disorder may be associated with atrophy of the optic nerves or with lesions of the brain stem or spinal cord.

Symptoms.   The first symptom of hereditary cerebellar atrophy in children may occur at any time between 3 and 17 years of age. Initially, an unsteady gait and impaired balance are noted. The hands become unsteady, apparent when the child is playing with toys, crayoning, and writing. Dysarthria may be noted.

Examination.   Occasionally, optic atrophy, retinitis pigmentosa, or cataract may be present. Nystagmus, dysarthria, or deafness may be noted. The gait is ataxic and wide-based with an inability to walk heel-to-toe. An action tremor may be present on the finger-to-nose or heel-to-shin test, and the muscles may be hypotonic. In some of these patients, there may be associated loss of position and vibratory sense. The tendon reflexes may be hyperactive, normal, or absent, and the plantar responses may be flexor or extensor. Occasionally, mental retardation is present.

Laboratory Examination.   Radiographs of the skull are normal. Cerebrospinal fluid examination is usually normal, although a slight increase in protein (to 50–100 mg/dl) occasionally occurs. Computerized tomography or pneumoencephalography may reveal an increase in the air surrounding small cerebellar folia with an increase in sulcal markings.

Differential Diagnosis. Hereditary cerebellar ataxias must be distinguished from the group of spinocerebellar ataxias, posterior fossa tumor, and multiple sclerosis (Table 16-2).

Treatment. No specific therapy is available. With progressive difficulty in gait, the use of a walker is helpful.

Prognosis. The course is usually slowly progressive over many years.

Ataxia-Telangiectasia

Ataxia-telangiectasia is a rare hereditary disorder associated with progressive cerebellar ataxia, oculocutaneous telangiectasia, and frequent sinopulmonary infections.[106]

Etiology. This is a familial syndrome, and the mode of inheritance is by an autosomal recessive gene. In addition to the clinical features of ataxia, telangiectasia, and frequent infections, ataxia-telangiectasia is associated with immune defects of the humoral and cellular systems, as evidenced by decreased immunoglobulin A and E concentrations, underdeveloped thymus, lymphoreticular malignancies, abnormal response to ionizing radiation, and increased serum α-fetoprotein concentrations. As more information on this disorder becomes known, a satisfactory explanation for the relationship of the eye, skin, lungs, thymus, and other organ findings is more difficult to find. Three hypotheses have been proposed to unify the multisystem involvement in ataxia-telangiectasia: a faulty mesoderm hypothesis, a suppressed or retarded multisystem hypothesis, and an autoimmune hypothesis.[148] The demonstration of cytotoxic antibodies to brain and thymus in patients with ataxia-telangiectasia supports the autoimmune hypothesis.[82]

Pathology. The characteristic neuropathologic features are severe degeneration of the cerebellum with loss of Purkinje cells and granulosa cells involving all cortical layers.[94] Other described findings are severe degeneration of the spinal cord involving the posterior columns and occa-sionally the anterior horn cells, neurogenic amyotrophy, and dystrophic changes in the dorsal root and sympathetic ganglia, and in peripheral nerves.[1,94]

The thymus is small or absent and lymphoid tissues are abnormal. Lymphoreticular malignancies such as lymphoma and leukemia are increased in incidence in affected persons. Abnormalities of the endocrine systems may include ovaries and anterior pituitary acidophils. The leading cause of death is recurrent respiratory infections.[125]

Symptoms. Ataxia usually develops at 1 to 3 years of age, and telangiectasia appear initially by 4 to 6 years of age. An unsteady gait generally becomes apparent by 18 months of age and progresses until the patient is confined to a wheelchair by early adolescence.[125] After symptoms have progressed over several years, recurrent ear infections, sinusitis, and cough are noted in most patients. Sinopulmonary infections have not been as prominent in certain series.[75]

Examination. Telangiectasia first appears on the exposed bulbar conjunctivae and is primarily arterial. The spread is characteristic, with involvement in a butterfly area over the bridge of the nose and over the upper cheeks. Subsequently, dilated vessels may appear on the external ears, palate, neck, antecubital and popliteal fossae, and the dorsum of the hands and feet. Areas of depigmentation and *café au lait* spots are sometimes noted. Scleroderma, atopic dermatitis, eczema, and cutaneous malignancy occur rarely. The eardrums may reveal evidence of chronic middle ear disease, and the sinuses may be clouded on transillumination. Examination of the chest may reveal rales or localized areas of dullness. Eye movements are initiated with difficulty and then are quite slow; they are often jerky and may halt before the movement is completed. The eyes may show fixation nystagmus. Shortness of stature is a common feature.

The predominant neurologic finding is usually that of a progressive cerebellar ataxia with difficulty on walking heel to toe. The gait is wide based and unsteady. Subsequently, difficulty with coordination in the arms develops. In some patients, choreoathetosis may also be present, and occasionally this may be the major neurologic disability. Progressive dystonia may rarely mask the ataxia.[18] The speech is dysarthric, the face expressionless, and growth retarded. The tendon reflexes may be diminished or absent. As the disease progresses, the previously normal intellectual function falls below the normal range.[107]

Laboratory Examination.   There is a deficiency of immunoglobulin A in most patients, and in half of the children there is an immunoglobulin E deficiency (Table 16-3). Children with deficiencies of both immunoglobulin A and immunoglobulin E have frequent sinopulmonary infections. Leukopenia often is noted. Roentgenograms of the sinuses and of the thorax may show evidence of chronic infection. Computerized tomography or pneumoencephalography may show evidence of cerebellar atrophy.

Approximately half of affected children have hyperglycemia without glycosuria, and marked elevation of plasma insulin levels in response to the administration of glucose. These children may have evidence of liver disease in addition to diabetes mellitus.

Serum α-fetoprotein concentrations are usually elevated 2 to 10 times.[125,152] About one in ten patients develops malignancies such as lymphoma or leukemia. Cultured cells from patients with ataxia-telangiectasia exhibit increased chromosomal breakage and hypersensitivity to DNA-damaging agents such as ionizing radiation.[125]

Differential Diagnosis.   Ataxia-telangiectasia is the only form of progressive cerebellar ataxia that has its onset during infancy. This disorder, nevertheless, must be differentiated from an Arnold-Chiari (Chiari type 2) malformation associated with lower cranial nerve signs and pyramidal tract signs. Progressive cerebellar ataxia in children may be due to a neoplasm in the posterior fossa, and it is essential that this possibility be excluded. In fact, ocular telangiectasia may be an incidental finding in a child with ataxia due to a neoplasm or a vascular malformation (Table 16-2).

TABLE 16-3.   Cerebellar Disorders with Metabolic Defects

Disorder	Laboratory Findings	Metabolic Defect
Heredopathia atactica polyneuritiformis (Refsum's disease)	Increased blood phytanic acid	Defect of metabolism of exogenous phytanic acid
Hartnup's disease	Aminoaciduria, high urinary indolic acid, impaired absorption of tryptophan	Defect of intestinal and renal transport of neutral α-amino acids
A-β-lipoproteinemia (Bassen-Kornzweig disease)	Impaired gastrointestinal absorption of fat, a-β-lipoproteinemia, acanthocytosis	Defect of lipid-transporting peptides (apoLP-ser)
Ataxia telangiectasia	Absence of IgA; deficiency of IgE	Defect in serum immunoglobulins
Intermittent branched-chain ketonuria with intermittent cerebellar ataxia	Intermittent maple syrup urine; increased valine, leucine, isoleucine, and α-ketoacids in serum and urine	Decreased oxidation of branched-chain α-ketoacids
Pyruvate decarboxylase deficiency with intermittent cerebellar ataxia	Increased serum pyruvate and urinary alanine; flat oral glucose tolerance test	Pyruvate decarboxylase deficiency
Partial deficiency of hypoxanthine-guanine phosphoribosyl transferase: spinocerebellar ataxia	Increased uric acid in blood and urine	Partial deficiency of hypoxanthine-guanine phosphoribosyl transferase

Hartnup disease is distinguished by characteristic amino-aciduria. When extrapyramidal signs are prominent in ataxia-telangiectasia, the disease must be distinguished from hepatolenticular degeneration and from pigmentary degeneration of the globus pallidus.

Treatment. Antibiotics and chemotherapy may be indicated for specific sinus, ear, and pulmonary infections.

Prognosis. Most of the patients are confined to wheelchairs before adolescence. The disease is slowly progressive with death occurring 10 to 25 years after onset. More than half of the patients die from chronic pulmonary disease, and many others from malignant tumors of lymphatic tissue including lymphosarcoma, Hodgkin's disease, reticulum cell sarcoma, and undifferentiated round cell sarcoma.

Heredopathia Atactica Polyneuritiformis (Refsum's Disease or Phytanic Acid Storage Disease)

The salient features of heredopathia atactica polyneuritiformis, or Refsum's disease, are retinitis pigmentosa, nerve deafness, ataxia, polyneuropathy, and ichthyosis. Since Refsum[128] described the condition in 1944, more than 50 cases have been identified and the biochemical defect has been defined.[146]

Etiology. The disease is transmitted as an autosomal recessive gene. Many of the cases described have been of Scandinavian origin. High concentrations of phytanic acid (3,7,11,15-tetramethylhexadecanoic acid) are present in blood and tissue of most affected patients (Table 16-3). The same clinical syndrome occurs rarely without the accumulation of phytanic acid. A deficiency of phytanic acid α-hydroxylase has been found in cultured fibroblasts from affected children.[145]

Pathology. Large globules of fat are present in excess in the globus pallidus. Degenerative changes in the olivocerebellar tracts, anterior horn cells, and peripheral nerves have been described.

Symptoms. In children, symptoms occur at 4 to 7 years of age. Anorexia, lassitude, failing vision with night blindness, and loss of hearing are noted early. The gait becomes unsteady with a nodding tremor of the head. Lightning pains in the legs have been described.

Examination. The skin is dry with hyperkeratosis of the limbs. Anosmia may be present. Visual acuity is reduced, and visual fields may be constricted. Retinitis pigmentosa, nystagmus, and nerve deafness are usually observed. Intention tremor and ataxia of gait are evident, as are also distal weakness and hypotonia in arms and legs. Sensation is decreased to all modalities with the presence of Romberg's sign. The tendon reflexes are decreased or absent.[50]

Laboratory Examination. The cerebrospinal fluid protein is frequently elevated and may be as high as 500 mg/dl. Phytanic acid plasma concentrations are increased as determined by gas chromatography and may constitute as much as 5% to 30% of total plasma fatty acids.[145]

Differential Diagnosis. The disorder has several features in common with Bassen-Kornzweig syndrome and with Roussy-Lévy syndrome. The presence of increased phytanic acid in blood establishes the diagnosis.

Treatment. A diet containing only a minimal amount of phytol has been used in an attempt to prevent further accumulation of phytanic acid in tissues of affected patients. Dietary restriction may result in improvement in the cutaneous, cardiac, and peripheral nerve abnormalities, but usually the retinitis pigmentosa remains unchanged.[54,147]

Prognosis. The course is fluctuating with gradual progression and fatal termination.

Cerebellar Tumors

See Chapter 14.

DISORDERS OF THE CEREBELLUM PRESENTING AS ACUTE ATAXIA

Acute Cerebellar Ataxia

Acute cerebellar ataxia is a clinically defined entity that occurs rarely in children and is usually followed by complete recovery in 6 months.

Etiology. The etiology is usually unknown. Half of the children with acute cerebellar ataxia have had an acute prodromal illness with fever, respiratory symptoms, or gastrointestinal symptoms at some time during the 3 weeks preceding the onset of acute ataxia. However, the etiologic agent that might produce this prodromal illness and its possible relation to the subsequent ataxia are not known. Occasional cases are associated with varicella infection, infectious mononucleosis, Coxsackie virus, herpes simplex virus, and *Mycoplasma pneumoniae*.[144] The isolation of ECHO virus type 9 from the cerebrospinal fluid in association with acute cerebellar ataxia has been reported. In several children with acute cerebellar ataxia, poliomyelitis virus has been isolated from the stools, and neutralizing antibodies to the same type of virus have been demonstrated in the patients' sera. The possibility that poliomyelitis virus is one of the etiologic agents producing this syndrome has been suggested. An occasional association with neuroblastoma has been noted.[4,140]

Pathology. Because this disorder is a nonfatal one, the pathologic findings are unknown.

Symptoms. The age of onset in the majority of childen is at 1 to 2 years of age, with occasional cases occurring throughout childhood. The initial symptoms develop acutely with rapid deterioration of gait, which may range from mild unsteadiness to complete inability to walk. In some children, tremors of the head, trunk, or extremities are noted.

Examination. In some of the patients, horizontal nystagmus on lateral gaze is noted. Occasionally there is opsoclonus (spontaneous, chaotic, jerking movements of the eyes). Dancing eye movements and myoclonic ataxia are characteristic of infantile polymyoclonia. The gait, often associated with occult neuroblastoma,[4,140] is ataxic with staggering and reeling from side to side. With severe involvement the child is unable to walk or even to sit without support. Incoordination of the arms and legs is noted, with marked rhythmic tremor on voluntary movement. The finger-to-nose and heel-to-shin tests reveal an action tremor. Alternating movements of the hand are poorly performed. A rhythmic tremor of the head or trunk sometimes occurs. Cerebellar incoordination may at times be associated with hypotonia. Sensory and reflex examinations are usually within normal limits.

Laboratory Examination. Examination of the cerebrospinal fluid usually reveals normal initial pressure with a normal cell count and normal protein content. Occasionally, a slight lymphocytic pleocytosis of 7 to 25/cu mm does occur. The electroencephalogram is usually normal, although occasionally there may be nonspecific slowing. Skull roentgenograms are normal.

Because neuroblastoma occurs in some children with acute cerebellar ataxia, a careful search for tumor is recommended. This includes chest, skull, and spine roentgenograms, intravenous urograms, bone marrow examination for malignant cells, and determination of the urinary excretion of catecholamines.

Differential Diagnosis. On rare occasions, this clinical picture develops following exanthems, especially varicella. In these children there is usually a history of infection, and the skin rash persists. With a large dose of diphenylhydantoin (Dilantin), toxic symptoms may develop, consisting of acute truncal ataxia, which may be severe enough to prevent walking and may be associated with nystagmus (Table 16-4). In these children, the history of a convulsive disorder and of therapy with diphenylhydantoin is usually readily available from the parents. Acute cerebellar ataxia also occurs occasionally in association with more diffuse and severe encephalitis due to many different etiologies. In these cases, neurologic

TABLE 16-4.   Differential Diagnosis of Acute Ataxia

Disorder	Preceding History	Examination	Laboratory Examination	Usual Prognosis
Acute cerebellar ataxia	Half have had a prodromal systemic illness, occasionally exanthems	Cerebellar ataxia	Spinal fluid usually normal	Recovery
Dilantin intoxication	Convulsions treated with diphenyl-hydantoin	Cerebellar ataxia, nystagmus	High serum diphenyl-hydantoin level	Recovery
Cerebellar tumor or abscess	Headache, vomiting	Papilledema, ataxia, nystagmus	Separation of cranial sutures	Progressive until operated on
Hartnup syndrome	Skin eruptions on exposure to sun; familial incidence	Skin lesions, ataxia, nystagmus, mental disturbances	Aminoaciduria, increased indole in urine	Recurrent ataxia
Multiple sclerosis	Preceding neurologic symptoms	Optic neuritis; brain stem, cerebellar, pyramidal, or sensory signs	Spinal fluid may reveal increased cells, protein or γ-globulin	Exacerbations and remissions
Encephalitides	Headache, stiff neck, fever	Cerebral and brain stem signs; also may have ataxia	Spinal fluid: lymphocytosis; possible virus isolation or rise in antibody titer	May be fatal, or slow recovery with or without residual effects
Spinal cord tumor	May have numbness or bladder disorder	Ataxia with weakness or sensory loss	Defect on myelography	Progressive until operated on
Infectious polyneuropathy	Half have a prodromal systemic illness	Ataxia with motor and sensory loss	Spinal fluid: normal cells, increased protein	May be fatal, recovery usually complete

examination shows involvement of other portions of the central nervous system in addition to the cerebellum. Also, in these children the acute onset is frequently associated with meningeal signs and with a marked lymphocytosis in the cerebrospinal fluid. A virus may be demonstrated by culture of cerebrospinal fluid, stools, or throat washings, or evidence of viral infection may be obtained from serologic study. This disorder must be distinguished from the rapid onset of cerebellar signs which may develop in children with neoplasm in the posterior fossa and occasionally with meningococcal meningitis.

Treatment.   There is no specific therapy for acute cerebellar ataxia of unknown etiology. With severe ataxia, it is important to prevent any injury to the child that could occur as a result of falling from the crib or repeated blows of the head or arm against the crib. The crib can be padded with pillows, and support can be provided. Adequate intake of food and fluid should be carefully maintained.

Myoclonic encephalopathy of infants with ataxia and opsoclonus has been treated with steroids. This produces in some infants dramatic immediate improvement of the neurologic symptoms, but the subsequent course of the illness is not definitely altered.

Prognosis.   The disorder is a nonfatal one. However, the presence of severe cerebellar deficit at the onset of illness is correlated with slow or incomplete recovery. Two thirds of children regain normal cerebellar function within a week to 12 months. Among the others, some may show sufficient improvement during the next several years so that they are able to walk but still have residual cerebellar signs. A few children who have been followed for several years have persistent ataxia of the trunk and extremities with tremors and abnormal arm movements. In addition, these children have evidence of organic brain damage with short attention spans, difficulty with speech, limited vocabulary, and inability to handle abstract concepts. In these few children, recovery was slower than in the majority of cases and remained incomplete.[154]

Injury of the Cerebellum

The cerebellum is rarely traumatized in closed head injuries. Laceration or contusion of the cerebellum may accompany fractures of the occipital bone. Along with the laceration, there commonly is hemorrhage into one or occasionally both of the cerebellar hemispheres, and there may be an associated acute subdural hematoma. Most children with intracerebellar hematomas are stuporous, and many are in coma when they are first seen. This makes detection of the lesion difficult. If the child is sufficiently alert to be examined, ataxia and hypotonia of the extremities on the side of the lesion may be seen. The lesion should be suspected in a child with a deepening level of consciousness who has a fracture over the occipital bone. It also should be suspected in children with head injuries who are deteriorating but in whom intracranial hemorrhage above the tentorium has not been found.

If an intracerebellar hematoma is present, then respiratory and vasomotor centers in the medulla may be rapidly compressed; therefore, surgical treatment is urgent. This consists of evacuating the hematoma and the surrounding lacerated necrotic cerebellum. Children who survive often have residual cerebellar disorder.

DISORDERS OF THE CEREBELLUM PRESENTING AS ACUTE INTERMITTENT ATAXIA

Acute Intermittent Cerebellar Ataxia

Etiology. Acute intermittent cerebellar ataxia, a rare disorder, has been described in children as an autosomal dominant trait and as a recessive gene. In some cases, a hereditary defect of pyruvate decarboxylase has been demonstrated. In other cases, the etiology is unknown.

Symptoms. An initial episode of ataxia may occur as early as 12 months to 2 years of age. The child suddenly becomes unsteady in walking and develops slurred speech. This may follow a febrile illness, fatigue, excitement, or minor head trauma,[68] or it may occur with no known precipitating factors. Ataxia lasts for a few hours to as long as a month and then clears completely. Identical episodes may occur after intervals of hours, days, or weeks. These intermittent attacks recur throughout childhood and may be associated with double vision.

Examination. During an acute attack, the child's speech is dysarthric. Horizontal or vertical nystagmus may be present. Ataxia may be mild with an unsteady gait and intention tremor, or it may be so severe that the child has to crawl instead of walk. Choreiform movements are sometimes present. After an attack has subsided, the neurologic examination results are usually normal. Nystagmus or mild clumsiness may persist. Caloric tests are normal, and hearing is not impaired. Optic atrophy is occasionally found.

Laboratory Examination. An increase in serum pyruvic acid and in urinary pyruvate and alanine are noted.[100] The oral glucose tolerance curve is frequently abnormal. Studies of cultured skin fibroblasts may show a deficiency of pyruvate decarboxylase (Table 16-3). The cerebrospinal fluid is normal.

Differential Diagnosis. Similar episodes of ataxia occur in Hartnup disease in which aminoaciduria is evident and in which there is an inherited defect in the transport of tryptophan. Intermittent ataxia occurs in patients with intermittent branched-chain ketoaciduria, benign paroxysmal vertigo, vertebrobasilar migraine, and familial periodic ataxia.[38]

Treatment. Thiamine has been given without cessation of attacks. The frequency of attacks decreased during a brief course of dexamethasone. Dimenhydrinate[156] and acetazolamide[38,45] have been more effective than other medications in certain patients.

Prognosis. Episodes of ataxia may become milder and less frequent in adult life.

Intermittent Branched-Chain Ketonuria

Etiology. Intermittent branched-chain ketonuria is a rare disorder related to decreased oxidation of branched-chain α-ketoacids due to a marked reduction in decarboxylase activity.[31]

Pathology. Spongy degeneration of the cerebral cortex and necrosis of the granule cell layer of the cerebellum occurs.

Examination. Attacks of anorexia, lethargy, ataxia, and convulsions occur at 1 to 8 years of age. These episodes clear completely but may recur after an interval of a few months or a few years. A severe unrecognized attack may be fatal.

Laboratory Examination. At the time of attacks, the urine has the odor of maple syrup, and there is an increase in valine, leucine, isoleucine, and α-ketoacids in the serum and urine. Between attacks, the diagnosis can be established by demonstrating a reduction in the ability of peripheral leukocytes to metabolize branched-chain ketoacids (Table 16-3).

Differential Diagnosis. This disorder must be distinguished from acute encephalopathy related to infections.

Treatment. With an acute attack, intravenous glucose is administered, and a diet low in branched-chain amino acids is implemented to produce a remission.

Prognosis. With proper therapy an acute attack subsides. Recurrences may be prevented by giving the patient a low protein diet.

Hartnup Disease

See Chapter 9.

TREATMENT OF ATAXIA

There is no specific therapy for acute or chronic cerebellar disorders. In a child with acute cerebellar ataxia or one with mild chronic ataxia, a program of symptomatic treatment with physical therapy is indicated. Efforts to improve the gait are made with balancing and foot placement exercises while the child is standing. With mild ataxia, independent walking is practiced before a mirror. With more severe ataxia, gait training is carried out with the assistance of canes, crutches, or parallel bars. The exercise program should include foot placement in climbing stairs if the child is able to walk. Resistance and coordination exercises are of additional help. Occupational therapy is of symptomatic value in using visual cues to develop improvement in motor skills. In retraining children with acute ataxia who are showing spontaneous improvement, physical therapy and occupational therapy may accelerate this improvement. In chronic progressive ataxias, these measures may be of value in helping the child continue with functions relating to activities of daily living, which he might otherwise cease doing at an earlier date. With severe involvement, spoon or tube feeding may be necessary.

ESSENTIAL TREMOR

Etiology. Essential tremor occurs in children as well as in adults as an autosomal dominant gene or as a sporadic disorder. The etiology and pathology are unknown.[67]

Symptoms. This benign form of action tremor may develop in children 4 to 16 years of age. During infancy and early childhood, brief, frequent episodes of shuddering may precede the onset of essential tremor.[151] The child may complain of unsteadiness in writing or in drinking from a glass or cup. These symptoms progress gradually over many years.

Examination. There is usually no tremor at rest. With voluntary movement a rhythmic tremor develops at a rate of 4 to 10 Hz, beginning in the fingers and spreading to the hands. On finger-to-nose testing there is slight ataxia. Handwriting may show jerky movements, and the child may steady the pencil by holding it tightly and using finger movements with no arm movement. Occasionally there is an associated tremor of the head, tongue, or legs. Motion and fatigue accentuate the tremor. There is no rigidity or akinesia.

Differential Diagnosis. Essential tremor must be distinguished from physiologic tremor and from a similar action tremor occurring in thyrotoxicosis and with anxiety. Cerebellar hypoplasia may produce similar mild intention tremor. Dentatocerebellar ataxia produces progressive cerebellar signs with dysarthria and gait disorder.

Extrapyramidal tremor is characteristically present at rest and may be decreased with voluntary movement, whereas essential tremor is usually absent at rest and occurs on voluntary movement. Hepatolenticular degeneration is associated with progressive cerebellar and extrapyramidal signs and with liver disease. Juvenile paralysis agitans is associated with a resting tremor, rigidity, and difficulty initiating movements.

Treatment. There is no specific therapy. Mild tranquilizing drugs may decrease tremor slightly. Propanolol may be effective in some patients.[158]

Prognosis. Over a period of decades, essential tremor does progress, and it may produce mild to moderate disability due to limitations in manual dexterity.

DISORDERS OF THE BRAIN STEM AND CRANIAL NERVES

Congenital Defects of Motor Cranial Nerves

Etiology. The etiology of congenital defects of motor cranial nerves, which develop during intrauterine life, is frequently not known. Ingestion of thalidomide during the first trimester of pregnancy may result in facial paralysis and ear defects. Ir-

radiation, virus infection, and hypoxia may be etiologic factors. A genetic cause is present in some cases.

Pathology. With involvement of motor cranial nerves, it has been established in some patients that the nucleus in the brain stem is defective and that this is associated with an absent or atrophic muscle.

Examination. The neurologic signs may relate to any one or several of the cranial nerves, and the findings may be uni- or bilateral. Uni- or bilateral ptosis is probably the most common congenital defect of cranial nerves. Paralysis of extraocular muscles occurs less frequently than ptosis (Fig. 16-4). Involvement of the extraocular muscles supplied by the third nerve may be partial or complete. Congenital paralysis of the lateral recti may be associated with congenital aplasia of the sixth nerve. Rarely difficulty in jaw movement is related to aplasia of the motor portion of the fifth cranial nerve. Congenital weakness of facial muscles due to aplasia of the seventh nerve nuclei is usually bilateral (Fig. 16-4). The facial skin appears smooth with no wrin-

FIG. 16-4. Aplasia of cranial nerves. This 14-month-old boy has bilateral facial paralysis. The eyes deviate laterally. Examination of the extraocular muscles reveals no function of medial recti or superior or inferior recti muscles in either eye. Weak lateral rectus function is present bilaterally.

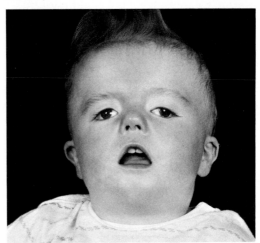

kles. Paralysis of pharynx, larynx, and tongue may also be infrequently observed in infants. Rarely, sternomastoids and trapezius muscles are absent.

These cranial nerve defects may be single or multiple, and they may or may not be associated with other congenital defects involving other systems of the body. Congenital bilateral facial and abducens paralysis—Moebius' syndrome—may be associated with other cranial nerve palsies producing weakness of extraocular muscles, jaw muscles, palate, and tongue, and also with congenital anomalies of the arms and legs including absence of fingers and toes, syndactylism, supernumerary digits, and clubfoot.

Differential Diagnosis. The congenital basis of paralysis of a cranial nerve is usually suggested by its occurrence during early infancy. The same defect may occur in one or more members of the same family.

Prognosis. The neurologic signs remain stationary.

Progressive Bulbar Palsy (Fazio-Londe Disease)

Etiology. The cause of progressive bulbar palsy, a rare disorder, is unknown.

Pathology. Although neuropathologic studies are few, those available correlate well with the clinical features. There is virtual absence of neurons in affected motor nuclei of the brain stem. Anterior horn cell degeneration has also been observed in the upper cervical spinal cord.[2]

Examination. Onset of symptoms is variable. These may begin between 2 to 12 years of age. Progressive weakness usually affects facial muscles, palate and tongue, and less frequently the ocular muscles. Weakness, atrophy, fasciculations, and spasticity may develop later in the arms and legs.[58]

Differential Diagnosis. Progressive involvement of multiple cranial nerves in children is nearly always due to a neoplasm. This diagnosis is established by computerized tomography or by pneu-moencephalography. Other diagnostic considerations include botulism, myasthenia gravis, progressive ocular myopathy, and cranial polyneuropathy.

The rare occurrence of a degenerative disorder in childhood, which begins in the motor nuclei of cranial nerves and which later may spread to anterior horn cells, is very similar to the picture of infantile progressive muscular atrophy or Werdnig-Hoffmann disease. Progressive bulbar palsy may belong to a group of neurologic disorders of infancy and childhood characterized by degeneration of anterior horn cells in the spinal cord and of motor nuclei neurons in the brain stem. Among these disorders are included progressive muscular atrophy, chronic proximal spinal muscular atrophy (Kugelberg-Welander disease), and juvenile amyotrophic lateral sclerosis.

Treatment. There is no specific therapy.

Prognosis. The course is progressive, and death occurs after 2 to 7 years.

Diencephalic Syndrome

The association of a diencephalic tumor with emaciation during infancy was described by Russell in 1951.[131] The onset is typically in the first year of life, with rapid and severe loss of subcutaneous fat despite normal appetite and caloric intake. Linear growth is not affected, but weight gain is poor. Pallor is prominent.[34] The clinical feature of failure to thrive combined with a characteristic state of euphoria manifested by overactivity, friendliness, and alertness is striking.[37] Examination of the eyes reveals abnormalities, including poor pupillary reaction to light, rotatory nystagmus, and strabismus. Funduscopic examination usually identifies the presence of optic atrophy. Radiographic studies reveal displacement of the third ventricle by an optochiasmatic tumor. Occasionally, the neoplasm may be located more posteriorly.[21] Histologic diagnosis is usually that of a low-grade astrocytoma.[34] Survival in untreated cases averages 12 months, whereas treatment with radiotherapy alone or in combination with surgery may result in over 90% survival at least 24 months after treatment.[21] A satisfactory explanation for this clinical syndrome is still forthcoming. Compression of the hypothalamus by a neoplasm at a vulnerable period may explain why other tumors in the same region but presenting at later ages do not cause a diencephalic syndrome. Abnormalities of plasma growth-hormone and cortisol levels have been reported in some patients.

Congenital Blindness of Retinal Origin (Leber's Congenital Amaurosis)

Congenital blindness of retinal origin is characterized by congenital blindness, pendular nystagmus, and a markedly reduced or absent electroretinogram response.[33,118]

Etiology. The etiology is unknown. An autosomal recessive pattern of inheritance has been established for most cases.

Pathology. The usual histopathologic finding is a primary degeneration of the outer photoreceptor layer in the retina. Degenerative changes are also found in the ganglion cells, papulomacular bundle, and optic nerve. Pigmentary dispersion occurs.[118]

Examination. Reduced visual acuity is evident in all affected children at the time of birth or shortly thereafter. Pendular nystagmus is present in 75% of cases. The appearance of the fundus is variable, from normal to generalized retinal atrophy and pigmentary changes. The more common findings at funduscopy include arteriolar narrowing, "salt-and-pepper" or spicule pigmentation, macular granularity, choroidal atrophy, and optic nerve pallor. Associated ocular findings are strabismus and refractive errors. A high incidence of neurologic abnormalities is found in these patients, including mental retardation, neuromuscular dysfunction, deafness, and electroencephalographic abnormalities.[33]

Laboratory Examination. The electroretinogram response is markedly abnormal in all patients with congenital blindness of retinal origin. The response is absent in 75% of cases, indicating a diffuse photoreceptor dysfunction. The electroretinogram is useful in differentiating this form of blindness from others, such as congenital optic atrophy, aniridia, congenital cataracts, macular coloboma, and achromatopsia.[118]

Hereditary Optic Atrophy (Leber's Optic Atrophy)

Etiology. This hereditary disorder is usually sex-linked and occurs six times as frequently in males as in females.[24] Transmission as a simple recessive or dominant trait has also been reported. The etiology is not known. It has also been postulated that this is a viral illness with vertical transmission from mother to children in which the expression of the disease is dependent upon the genetically determined resistance of the child.[153]

Pathology. There is selective degeneration of the papulomacular bundle of the optic nerve, as well as primary neuronal degeneration of the retina and optic nerve with secondary degenerative changes in the optic tracts.

Symptoms. The onset may occur any time during childhood, frequently with sudden loss of vision. Usually both eyes are affected simultaneously, although one eye may be involved several months before the other. The onset may be associated with headache, dyspnea, lassitude, and occasionally convulsions. Vision deteriorates over a period of several weeks or months, then the visual loss becomes stationary. The onset of neurologic symptoms occurs at 1 to 15 years of age with the appearance of unsteadiness.

Examination. The visual acuity is reduced, and the visual fields reveal a central scotoma. The optic disk at the onset of the disorder usually appears normal, although there may be blurring of the disk margins. In about 40% of cases, other neurologic signs may develop,[153] including nystagmus, dysarthria, spasticity, occasional athetosis, occasional mild distal atrophy, increased tendon reflexes, and extensor plantar responses. There is marked variability in the severity of neurologic disability. Kyphosis is occasionally an associated finding.

Treatment. No therapy is available.

Prognosis. Visual acuity declines rapidly during the first few months of disability, and then the process becomes stationary. In some patients there is progression to complete blindness, and in some remissions in neurologic disability occur. However, a few patients have shown progressive neurologic disease with subsequent death.

Congenital Nystagmus

Congenital, pendular, or searching nystagmus is observed in the newborn or during the first few weeks or months of life. Usually there is a family history of a similar disorder. Congenital nystagmus also appears in albinism. Rapid horizontal movements occur equally in the two eyes and are present on looking straight ahead as well as laterally. Horizontal movements of the head may be associated with nystagmus, but no other neurologic signs are usually present. With increase in the age of the child, head movements usually decrease and nystagmus either remains the same or becomes slightly less marked. No therapy is available.

Spasmus Nutans (Nodding Spasm)

Spasmus nutans is a rare, transient, nonfamilial disorder characterized by nystagmus, head nodding, and tilting of the head.[69]

Etiology. The etiology is unknown. Earlier reports stressed an association of spasmus nutans with rickets or poor illumination in the infant's home.[66] This association has not been found in cases reported more recently.[120]

Examination. The three cardinal signs of spasmus nutans are nystagmus, head nodding, and tilting of the head. These signs appear at 4 to 18 months of age, and any one of the signs may precede the others. The nystagmus is a characteristic feature and its presence may facilitate diagnosis when other features are absent. The nystagmus is described as being asymmetric, usually involving prominently one eye and barely discernible in the other eye, fine and rapid (6–8 Hz), and variable in its direction. The direction may change spontaneously or in response to change in direction of gaze or change in head position.[120] Head movement may be horizontal, vertical, or a combination of both. It may diminish when the child lies down and disappears during sleep. The direction and rhythmicity of the head movement are also in an unpredictable pattern.[69]

Differential Diagnosis. The main condition to be differentiated is congenital nystagmus. Although congenital nystagmus may be accompanied by head nodding, making the distinction from spasmus nutans more difficult, the age at onset as well as rhythmicity and direction of the eye movements help distinguish spasmus nutans from congenital nystagmus. Other abnormal eye movements seen during infancy, such as ocular bobbing, opsoclonus, oscillopsia, and lightning eye movements, are frequently associated with neurologic abnormalities involving brain stem function. An erroneous diagnosis of spasmus nutans is not infrequently made in patients with hypothalamic tumors or diencephalic syndrome.[6] Poor weight gain, failure to thrive, or frank emaciation should raise suspicion about the presence of a hypothalamic neoplasm.

Treatment. No treatment is available.

Prognosis. In the absence of other neurologic abnormalities, spasmus nutans is regarded as a transient condition with cessation of symptoms by 2 to 5 years of age.[76]

Neuromyelitis Optica (Devic's Syndrome)

Devic's syndrome is characterized by the combined occurrence of optic neuritis and transverse myelitis. It is a demyelinating disorder that probably represents a form of acute multiple sclerosis.

Etiology. The etiology is unknown. Demyelinating lesions are seen in the optic nerve, brain, and spinal cord. In small lesions there is a loss of myelin with preservation of axis cylinders. In extensive lesions both myelin and axis cylinders are destroyed.

Symptoms. This is a rare disorder that occurs in children and in adults. The initial symptoms may relate either to the onset of an acute optic neuritis or to the onset of an acute transverse myelitis. If visual symptoms appear first, they consist of an acute loss of visual acuity, usually in both eyes. This may then be followed after an interval of a few days or weeks by the onset of numbness and weakness in the legs and possibly in the arms. Urinary retention and incontinence may occur. The symptoms may also appear in the reverse order, with the initial onset of numbness and weakness in the arms followed after an interval of a few days or weeks by the development of failing vision.

Examination. The ocular findings are those of acute optic neuritis or retrobulbar neuritis, with a marked decrease in visual acuity, usually noted bilaterally, and a loss of color vision associated with a large central scotoma. The optic disk may be normal or show evidence of edema with venous engorgement. Within a few days, the size of the scotoma may increase and visual acuity may decrease to blindness. Motor examination reveals weakness or complete paralysis of the legs, sometimes associated with weakness or paralysis of the trunk and arms. Sensory examination usually reveals a sensory level in the cervical or thoracic region with loss of sensation below this level. Initially, the tendon reflexes are frequently absent. Subsequently, the tendon reflexes are increased and the plantar responses become extensor. Paralysis of the bladder and rectal sphincter may occur.

Laboratory Examination. Examination of the cerebrospinal fluid usually reveals a pleocytosis of 20 to 50/cu mm, mostly lymphocytes; the total protein content is elevated.[47] Myelin basic protein[28] and oligoclonal bands[99] may be detected in the cerebrospinal fluid. Visual and somatosensory evoked potentials are often abnormal.

Differential Diagnosis. The clinical diagnosis of neuromyelitis optica is based on the acute occurrence of transverse myelitis associated with optic neuritis. A similar clinical disorder may occur with encephalomyelitis following measles or vaccinia. If the illness begins with the transverse myelitis, it may not be possible to distinguish this disorder from other spinal cord disorders until optic neuritis develops. In these cases, presence of prolonged latencies and decreased amplitude of visual evoked response to pattern reversal may help to detect early neuromyelitis optica.[63]

Treatment. No specific therapy is available. Steroid therapy is usually given, particularly if optic nerve involvement is bilateral. Good nursing care is essential to prevent bedsores. Periodic catheterization or tidal drainage may be required. Chemotherapeutic or antibiotic therapy may be required for urinary tract infection. Physical therapy initially with passive motion and subsequently with active motion is of value.

Prognosis. After the acute onset there is usually improvement both in visual symptoms and paralysis. During the acute stage, death may occur due to respiratory paralysis or to uncontrollable infection. If the child survives the initial acute transverse myelitis, improvement in motor and sensory function usually begins within a few weeks. Within 1 to 2 months after onset, there is a marked improvement in visual acuity. Frequently, residual decrease in visual acuity and residual motor, sensory, and reflex findings persist. Attacks may recur and result in blindness and paraplegia.

Multiple Sclerosis (Disseminated Sclerosis)

Multiple sclerosis is characterized clinically by widespread neurologic symptoms and signs that develop subacutely, improve, and recur, and that are due to demyelinating lesions spread in space and time.

Etiology. Although the cause of multiple sclerosis is not known, current hypotheses suggest that viruses and immune responses[7] play an etiologic role. Virus antibody titers for rubeola, type C influenza, herpes simplex, parainfluenza 3, mumps, and varicella-zoster are higher in the sera of patients with multiple sclerosis than in controls. However, these titers are the same as those in unaffected siblings.[20] An abnormal humoral immune response within the central nervous system is demonstrated by the finding of oligoclonal immunoglobulin

G in cerebrospinal fluid.[99] Abnormal cell-mediated immune response has been more difficult to define in patients with multiple sclerosis. Studies of histocompatibility antigen system (HLA) reveal that certain haplotypes are associated with increased susceptibility to multiple sclerosis, notably HLA-A3 and HLA-A7.[106] Occasional familial occurrence suggests that first-degree relatives may be at increased risk of acquiring multiple sclerosis.[56] Migration studies[91] reveal ethnic and geographic predisposition to multiple sclerosis and suggest that exposure to an environmental factor at an early age may be important.

Pathology.   Gross sections reveal multiple gray plaques in the white matter of the cerebrum, cerebellum, brain stem, or spinal cord. Myelin sheath stains reveal multiple large and small areas of demyelination, which is the most significant pathologic change. Lesions are frequently located in the optic nerves, in the white matter near the lateral and third ventricles, and in the white matter in the brain stem. In contrast with the complete loss of myelin in areas of involvement, there may be little damage to axis cylinders. Proliferation of glial cells is also seen.

Symptoms.   Multiple sclerosis is much less common in children than in adults, although rarely the first attack occurs at 5 to 10 years of age. When it occurs in children, the usual age of onset is between 10 and 16 years. The symptoms may relate to many different parts of the central nervous system, and they usually develop acutely or subacutely. A common early symptom in affected children is the acute onset of blurred vision in one or both eyes, which may be associated with orbital pain.[85] Acute diplopia or sudden vertigo may be the initial symptom. Weakness of one arm and leg may appear suddenly or over a period of weeks. The child may be clumsy in using his hands or in walking. Numbness may develop with tingling, burning, sensations of coldness, and feelings of deadness or tightness of the skin in one arm and leg, or in both legs. Electric shock-like sensations in the arms or legs may be noted on neck flexion. Paroxysmal brief local pains may recur in one portion of an arm or leg. A band of tightness or numbness may extend across the chest or abdomen. Also, frequency and urgency of urination or urinary incontinence may develop.

After an initial episode of neurologic symptoms, which usually lasts a few weeks or months, the child may recover completely or nearly completely. Then, after an interval of months or several years or even later in adult life, another cluster of symptoms relating to the same or a different portion of the central nervous system may appear. For example, visual impairment may occur acutely for a period of a few weeks at 13 years of age and recur in a second episode at 16 years of age, and then signs suggesting spinal cord disease may appear after an interval of several years. The temporal profiles of the symptoms of children with multiple sclerosis vary from a rapidly progressive course over a period of months or a few years to a mild course with exacerbations and remissions extending over many years.

Examination.   Examination of the cranial nerves may reveal a decrease in visual acuity associated with a visual field defect, frequently a paracentral scotoma, in one or both eyes. Decreased color vision may be the earliest detectable evidence of optic neuritis. Ophthalmoscopic examination of the optic disks in a child with an acute optic neuritis located distally along the nerve may reveal swelling of the optic disks with blurred margins, dilated veins, and occasionally hemorrhages in the surrounding retina. If the visual symptoms are related to a demyelinating process in the proximal part of the optic nerve, the optic disk may appear normal. Eye examination several months or years after an acute optic neuritis has subsided may reveal residual findings, possibly including a slight residual decrease in visual acuity, a small paracentral scotoma, or pallor of the temporal portion of the disk. There may be weakness of extraocular muscles and an internuclear ophthalmoplegia. The latter is noted on lateral gaze and consists of horizontal monocular nystagmus in the abducting eye and limited medial movement of the adducting eye. Convergence is normal. Internuclear ophthalmoplegia is due to a lesion in the region of the medial longitudinal fasciculus. Horizontal, vertical, or rotatory nystagmus is a common finding. Decrease in sensation on one side of the face occurs rarely, and facial weakness occasionally. Dysarthria and scanning speech are common findings.

The motor system may reveal mono-, hemi-, or paraparesis. Cerebellar ataxia with intention tremor may be present in the arms, and the child may walk with a wide base and marked unsteadiness. Finger-to-nose and heel-to-shin tests may reveal incoordinated movements with intention tremor.

Sensory examination may show mild loss to pinprick and temperature in areas of numbness and tingling. The objective findings may be minimal in spite of severe complaints from the child. Position and vibratory sense may be disturbed in the arms or legs. The impairment of position and vibratory sense may be dissociated, with loss of position sense but not vibratory sense in one area or with loss of vibratory sense but not position sense in another area. Loss of position sense in the hands results in awkwardness in movements, and in the legs results in unsteady gait.

The tendon reflexes are frequently hyperactive and may be asymmetrical. Ankle clonus may be present. The abdominal reflexes are usually absent, and the plantar responses may be extensor. The bladder may be hypertonic in association with incontinence. Occasionally, organic cerebral involvement occurs with intellectual impairment and personality change.

Laboratory Examination. Examination of the cerebrospinal fluid may reveal abnormalities of one or more of the following constituents: cell count, total protein, colloidal gold curve, myelin basic protein, oligoclonal bands and γ-globulin. In one third of fluids there is a slight lymphocytic pleocytosis of 5 to 40/cu mm. The total protein is increased to 50 to 100 mg/dl in one third of fluids. Also, in one third to one half of fluids, the colloidal gold curve is either first zone or midzone. An increase in γ-globulin greater than 14% of total protein is present in half of the fluids from patients during the first episode, and in the vast majority of fluids from patients who have had recurrent attacks.[47]

Visual,[63] auditory, and somatosensory[61] evoked responses may help to define the site and the extent of the lesions in multiple sclerosis.

Differential Diagnosis. The clinical diagnosis depends upon the appearance of multiple symptoms and signs of central nervous system involvement separated in time and space and usually associated with exacerbations and remissions. The combination of an initial episode of optic neuritis followed by sensory, motor, and reflex signs suggesting cerebellar, brain stem, or spinal cord disease is very frequently due to multiple sclerosis. However, with the first episode and occasionally even with the second, the clinical diagnosis cannot be assured. All efforts should be made to exclude any treatable lesion of the brain or spinal cord that might be producing the symptoms and signs.

The groups of disorders to be considered in the differential diagnosis of an individual child relate to the site of the lesions. If the signs relate to dysfunction of the cerebellum and brain stem, then the disorders to be excluded include the cerebellar ataxias, Arnold-Chiari malformation, basilar impression, meningioma at the foramen magnum, and fracture of the odontoid process. If the signs are those of spinal cord disease, then spinal cord tumor, syringomyelia, amyotrophic lateral sclerosis, and postvaccinal and postinfectious myelitis must be excluded. The differential diagnosis of optic neuritis in children includes that which occurs after immunization as well as after measles, mumps, chickenpox, and pertussis. Glioma of the optic nerve and craniopharyngioma must be excluded. Leber's optic atrophy may be associated with a familial history. Hereditary forms of cerebral, cerebellar, and spinal cord disease may be associated with optic atrophy. In these disorders the course is progressive, and there is sometimes a family history of a similar degenerative disease. The combined involvement of optic nerves and spinal cord that occurs in multiple sclerosis must be distinguished from the clinical picture of neuromyelitis optica, which is a closely associated if not identical demyelinating disorder.

Treatment. There is no specific therapy for multiple sclerosis. Steroid therapy is frequently used to treat acute optic neuritis and, infrequently, to treat exacerbations of multiple sclerosis. However, there is no conclusive evidence that steroids or ACTH affect the natural course of multiple sclerosis. Activities are usually limited during acute exacerbations, although bed rest is of no specific value. Physical and occupational therapy are of importance in retraining after motor disability has occurred.

Prognosis. In two thirds of children with multiple sclerosis, the course is characterized by exacerbations and remissions, whereas in the other third it is chronically progressive. In a few cases of acute multiple sclerosis, the initial signs are extensive and severe, resulting in death within 2 to 6 months after onset.

In the majority of patients, the first attack is usually followed by complete or nearly complete remission. Although visual acuity may be severely reduced during an acute attack of optic neuritis, it usually returns to normal or near normal. Sensory symptoms and motor findings may clear completely.

The interval between the initial episode and the second attack of multiple sclerosis may vary from a few months to as long as 30 years. The limited data available concerning prognosis in children suggest that the course is approximately the same whether it begins between 10 and 16 years of age or in adult life.

Of particular interest in relation to the prognosis of multiple sclerosis is the frequency with which optic neuritis in children is related to the subsequent development of the characteristic clinical picture of multiple sclerosis. One fourth of a group of children who had had an acute attack of optic neuritis between 5 and 15 years of age developed multiple sclerosis after an average follow-up period of 8 years. This incidence is slightly lower, although similar, to that found in adults.

When a second episode due to multiple sclerosis occurs, it is usually followed by more residual disability than that observed after the first episode. For example, a second episode of optic neuritis is frequently followed by residual defect in visual acuity. A second episode of spinal cord involvement may result in a residual spastic hemi- or paraparesis, sensory changes, or urinary incontinence. Subsequent acute attacks are then followed by increasing amounts of disability.

Because most children who develop an initial episode of multiple sclerosis late in childhood do continue to live into adult life, the data on the ultimate prognosis in multiple sclerosis, which are available for adults, are pertinent. Twenty-five years after the initial attack of multiple sclerosis, one fourth of adults are dead and one third are disabled. Some patients continue to function adequately for 30 to 40 years after the initial onset of illness. The most common cause of death is acute respiratory infection.

Injury, Tumors, and Vascular Disease of the Brain Stem

See Chapters 13, 14, and 15.

Idiopathic Facial Paralysis (Bell's Palsy)

Etiology. Idiopathic facial paralysis is due to swelling and inflammation of the portion of the facial nerve that lies in the temporal bone. The etiology of this neuropathy is not known.[101]

Symptoms. There is usually a sudden onset of weakness involving the upper and lower portions of the face on one side associated with pain in the region of the ear on the affected side. It occurs from infancy throughout childhood.

Examination. With severe involvement, the child is not able to raise the eyebrow, to close the eye (Fig. 16-5), or to smile on the affected side. Sensation of taste is usually lost on the anterior two thirds of the tongue on the same side. Facial weakness is noted on smiling and crying. The ears, nose, throat, and other systems are normal when examined for evidence of infection or tumor. Lacrimation and accumulation of food between the cheek and the teeth may be noted. In some children, the weakness is incomplete and taste sensation is preserved.

Laboratory Examination. Roentgenograms of the skull and mastoid are normal. Lumbar puncture reveals normal cerebrospinal fluid. Measurement of facial nerve conduction velocity may provide evidence of prognostic value. If there is complete denervation, the nerve becomes unexcitable after 1 week.

Differential Diagnosis. Isolated facial nerve palsies in children are usually idiopathic. Facial nerve paralysis may occasionally be due to local trauma, tumor, or, rarely, osteopetrosis. Rarely, it may be secondary to hypertension, otitis media or mastoiditis, varicella, mumps, or encephalitis. Rarely, facial paralysis may be due to infection with herpes zoster; vesicular lesions may be present on the external ear. Recurrent facial paralysis may be associated with swelling of the lips (Melkersson's syndrome).

Treatment. No specific therapy is available. With severe involvement of the orbicularis oculi muscle, the eyelid cannot be closed to protect the cornea. Therefore, an eye patch or other protective device should be worn. Solutions comparable to artificial tears are instilled every 2 hours during the day to prevent drying of the cornea. Active exercising of weak muscles in front of the mirror is of value. With partial weakness of the facial nerve, recovery is always complete or nearly complete so that no further therapy is indicated. The possible beneficial effect of early treatment with prednisolone in children with complete facial paralysis has not been thoroughly evaluated as it has been in adults. In the rare cases of complete facial paralysis in which there is no return of facial muscular function after a period of a year, surgical procedures may be considered. The ninth, eleventh, or twelfth cranial nerve can be sectioned on the ipsilateral side and transplanted to the trunk of the facial nerve. A fascial sling may be placed at the corner of the mouth beneath the skin and attached to the masseter or temporalis muscle. Patients soon use this muscle to pull the fascial sling and thereby retract the corner of the mouth. This results in cosmetic improvement in the few children in whom functional recovery does not occur.

Prognosis. In idiopathic facial paralysis, useful function returns in 90% of patients. The speed and extent of recovery depend upon whether denervation has occurred. If denervation does not occur, there is complete return of function in an average time of 2 months. If denervation does occur, there is incomplete recovery, although half of these patients obtain a satisfactory cosmetic result. Idiopathic facial paralysis recurs on either the same or the opposite side of the face in approximately 10% of children.

FIG. 16-5. Idiopathic facial paralysis. This 9-month-old boy suddenly developed paralysis of the upper and lower portions of the left side of the face.

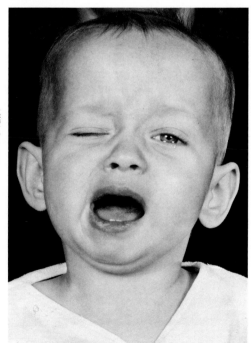

Asymmetric Crying Facies (Congenital Hypoplasia of the Depressor Anguli Oris Muscle)

Asymmetric crying facies, a relatively minor anomaly, is often confused with congenital facial paralysis during the newborn period or with Bell's palsy during infancy or childhood. The face characteristically appears normal during rest and sucking is not impaired. When the infant cries or smiles the mouth becomes asymmetric due to isolated weakness of the depressor anguli oris muscle. It is not unusual for the weakness to be ascribed to the normal side.[116] The condition may be familial and warrants examination of the parents for a similar defect. Asymmetric crying facies have been associated with other more serious anomalies of the cardiovascular,[25] genitourinary, and musculoskeletal systems.[124,126] Anatomical and electromyographic studies have not clarified the basis for this defect. Compression of the ramus marginalis of the facial nerve by obstetric trauma such as forceps or pressure of the mandible against the clavicle in utero does not seem a satisfactory explanation.[70]

Progressive Facial Hemiatrophy

Progressive facial hemiatrophy is a disorder characterized by progressive atrophy of the skin, subcutaneous tissue, bone, and, to a lesser degree, muscle of one side of the face. Neurologic complications are frequently associated with progressive facial hemiatrophy.[159] The onset may be during childhood or adolescence. Wasting usually begins with a pigmented lesion over the cheek or at the angle of the mouth. The atrophic locus may remain localized or gradually become diffuse over one side of the face. Maximum wasting is usually reached in 2 to 10 years from the time of onset. Rarely, the atrophy becomes bilateral. A characteristic lesion is a coup de sabre linear atrophic deformity over the forehead. When this lesion is present, it is necessary to differentiate the condition from scleroderma (morphea). Histologic differentiation is possible because elastic tissue is spared in progressive facial hemiatrophy. Although there is no satisfactory form of therapy, some cases are amenable to surgical reconstruction.[32]

Congenital Neural Deafness

Etiology. Congenital deafness in different families is transmitted as an autosomal dominant, autosomal recessive, or sex-linked recessive gene.[90] There are several loci for recessive deaf-mutism. In 20% of congenitally deaf children there is a history of rubella infection in the mother. Rubella infection during the first trimester of pregnancy results in deafness in the child in about 5% of cases. However, in many of these children there is also a genetic disposition to deafness.[5]

Pathology. Congenital deafness is usually due to a defect of the cochlea and sacculus. Other forms of congenital deafness are due to pathologic changes in the middle ear.[3]

Examination. Neural hearing loss is present from birth and may be uni- or bilateral, moderate, or severe. Although pure tone or speech audiometry is informative, hearing can be assessed more accurately by determining averaged brain stem auditory evoked responses.[83] Vestibular function is usually normal, although it may be decreased or absent. Bilateral congenital deafness results in deaf-mutism. In some children, deafness is total, whereas others can hear extremely loud sounds. The cries of an infant with congenital deafness have no variation in pitch, and the voice is abnormal. With increasing age, the child does not understand spoken words and does not learn to talk. Development is retarded in many spheres owing to inability to communicate with others.

Deafness may be associated with various skin changes. There may be widely spaced medial canthi with confluent eyebrows, depigmentation of the skin with leopardlike spots, atopic dermatitis, and hyperkeratosis. Deafness may be associated in different families with retinitis pigmentosa, with prolonged conduction in the myocardium and recurrent Stokes-Adams attacks resulting in sudden death, or with skeletal defects such as congenital absence of one or both tibias. In Pendred's syndrome, an autosomal recessive congenital neural deafness is associated with thyroid enlargement, which develops between infancy and adolescence and is presumably due to an inborn error in thyroxine synthesis.

Differential Diagnosis. Congenital deafness must be distinguished from congenital aphasia and from mental deficiency associated with unresponsiveness to sounds.

Therapy. Deaf-mutism requires early intensive speech training and instruction in lip-reading.

Neural Hearing Loss in Children

Autosomal dominant nerve deafness may begin during childhood and become more severe in adult life. Autosomal recessive and sex-linked recessive neural hearing loss may have its onset during early childhood with bilateral severe deafness by 6 years of age. Mumps is the most common cause of acquired neural deafness in children. Hereditary neural deafness may be associated with external ear malformation such as preauricular pits and thickened ear lobes.[90]

Benign Paroxysmal Vertigo

Etiology. The etiology of benign paroxysmal vertigo is unknown. The responsible lesion is presumed to be located in the vestibular nerve central to the labyrinth.[41] Benign paroxysmal torticollis[134] may represent an infantile form of benign paroxysmal vertigo. Other cases are thought to represent a childhood form of migraine.[46]

Symptoms. Very brief attacks of vertigo, nausea, and marked unsteadiness first occur before 3 years of age. Associated torticollis may be more prominent in infants and persists for a longer period of time than the acute attack of vertigo.[41] Attacks last for a few seconds to several minutes and may recur at intervals of several days to several months. The child remains conscious with normal speech during an attack. Over several months to several years, the attacks may cease to recur.

Examination. An attack begins suddenly without apparent precipitating factors. The child usually appears frightened and may cry in distress. To prevent himself from falling, he may seek support by clinging to his parents or to furniture. The child may appear pale, diaphoretic, and nauseated. Vomiting may occur during an episode or between attacks. Nystagmus is frequently noted and torticollis may be present. When walking, the child exhibits unsteadiness and may fall. The attack ends as abruptly as it commences, with a return of well-being. Between attacks, the neurologic examination results are usually normal.[41]

Laboratory Examination. The audiogram is normal. Caloric tests usually reveal a uni- or bilateral canal paresis.[89] Brain stem auditory evoked responses are normal, as is the electroencephalogram.

Differential Diagnosis. This disorder must be distinguished from partial complex seizures (temporal lobe epilepsy), in which there is a definite disturbance of awareness. Epilepsy may be associated with an abnormal electroencephalogram and normal caloric tests. Ménière's disease, which is rare in children, produces similar attacks; audiograms usually reveal hearing loss and recruitment.

Treatment. Dimenhydrinate (Dramamine) in a dosage of 10 to 20 mg three times daily may be of symptomatic value in children with frequently recurring attacks.[41]

Recurrent Aural Vertigo (Ménière's Disease)

Pathology. Ménière's disease, which occurs rarely in children and adolescents, is associated pathologically with edema of the membranous labyrinth.

Symptoms. Acute attacks of vertigo produce the sensation that either the patient or his surroundings are moving in one particular direction. With a severe attack, the patient lies down to avoid falling. Nausea and vomiting usually occur. The attack may subside after a few minutes or may last for several days. The frequency may vary from several times a week to once in several years. The patient notes tinnitus and decreased hearing in one ear. In 10% to 15% of patients, the disease ultimately becomes bilateral.

Examination. Examination during an acute attack reveals nystagmus in one lateral direction, which disappears after the acute attack subsides. Audiograms done between attacks reveal nerve deafness with loudness recruitment, and caloric tests demonstrate decreased vestibular function in the affected ear.

Treatment. Dimenhydrinate (Dramamine) is useful in aborting recurrent attacks. Nicotinamide, restriction of sodium intake, and the administration of oral potassium chloride have also been used.

Prognosis. Attacks continue into adult life.

REFERENCES

1. **Agamanolis DP, Greenstein JI:** Ataxia-telangiectasia. Report of a case with Lewy bodies and vascular abnormalities within cerebral tissue. J Neuropathol Exp Neurol 38:475, 1979

2. **Alexander MP, Emery ES III, Koerner FC:** Progressive bulbar paresis in childhood. Arch Neurol 33:66, 1976

3. **Alteneau MM:** Histopathology of sensorineural hearing loss in children. Otolaryngol Clin North Am 8:49, 1975

4. **Altman AJ, Baehner RL:** Favorable prognosis for survival in children with coincident opso-myoclonus and neuroblastoma. Cancer 37:846, 1976

5. **Anderson H, Barr B, Wedenberg E:** Genetic disposition—a prerequisite for maternal rubella deafness. Arch Otolaryngol 91:141, 1970

6. **Anthony JH, Ouvrier RA, Wise G:** Spasmus nutans. A mistaken identity. Arch Neurol 37:373, 1980

7. **Arnason BGW, Waksman BH:** Immunoregulation in multiple sclerosis. Ann Neurol 8:237, 1980

8. **Aron AM, Freeman JM, Carter S:** The natural history of Sydenham's chorea. Am J Med 38:83, 1965

9. **Barbeau A:** Update on the biochemistry of Huntington's chorea. Adv Neurol 23:449, 1979

10. **Barbeau A, Melancon S, Butterworth RF et al:** Pyruvate dehydrogenase complex in Friedreich's ataxia. Adv Neurol 21:203, 1978

11. **Barr AN, Heinze WJ, Dobben GD et al:** Bicaudate index in computerized tomography of Huntington disease and cerebral atrophy. Neurology (Minneap) 28:1196, 1978

12. **Bassen FA, Kornzweig AL:** Malformation of the erythrocytes in a case of atypical retinitis pigmentosa. Blood 5:381, 1950

13. **Berg RA, Kaplan AM, Jarrett PB et al:** Friedreich's ataxia with acute cardiomyopathy. Am J Dis Child 134:390, 1980

14. **Bird MT, Palkes H, Prensky AL:** A follow-up study of Sydenham's chorea. Neurology (Minneap) 26:601, 1976

15. **Bird MT, Paulson GW:** The rigid form of Huntington's chorea. Neurology (Minneap) 21:271, 1971

16. **Bittenbender JB, Quadfasel FA:** Rigid and akinetic forms of Huntington's chorea. Arch Neurol 7:275, 1962

17. **Blass JP, Gibson GE:** Studies of the pathophysiology of pyruvate dehydrogenase deficiency. Adv Neurol 21:181, 1978

18. **Bodensteiner JB, Goldblum RM, Goldman AS:** Progressive dystonia masking ataxia in ataxia-telangiectasia. Arch Neurol 37:464, 1980

19. **Boller F, Boller M, Gilbert J:** Familial idiopathic cerebral calcifications. J Neurol Neurosurg Psychiatry 40:280, 1977

20. **Brody JA, Sever JL, Henson TE:** Virus, antibody titers in multiple sclerosis patients, siblings, and controls. JAMA 216:1441, 1971

21. **Burr IM, Slonim AE, Danish RK et al:** Diencephalic syndrome revisited. J Pediatr 88:439, 1976

22. **Byers RK, Gilles FH, Fung C:** Huntington's disease in children. Neurology (Minneap) 23:561, 1973

23. **Carroll WM, Kriss A, Baraister M et al:** The incidence and nature of visual pathway involvement in Friedreich's ataxia. A clinical and visual evoked potential study of 22 patients. Brain 103:413, 1980

24. **Carroll WM, Mastaglia FL:** Leber's optic neuropathy. A clinical and visual evoked potential study of affected and asymptomatic members of a six generation family. Brain 102:559, 1979

25. **Cayler GG:** Cardiofacial syndrome. Arch Dis Child 44:69, 1969

26. **Center for Disease Control:** Rh hemolytic disease, United States, 1968–1977. Morbidity and Mortality Weekly Report. 27:487, 1978

27. **Chun RWM, Daly RF, Mansheim BJ et al:** Benign familial chorea with onset in childhood. JAMA 225:1603, 1973

28. **Cohen SR, Herndon RM, McKhann GM:** Radioimmunoassay of myelin basic protein in spinal fluid. An index of active demyelination. N Engl J Med 295:1455, 1976

29. **Cooper IS:** 20-Year followup study of the neurosurgical treatment of dystonia musculorum deformans. Adv Neurol 14:423, 1976

30. **Cotzias GC:** Levodopa in the treatment of parkinsonism. JAMA 218:1903, 1971

31. **Dancis J, Hutzer J, Rokkones T:** Intermittent branched chain ketonuria: Variant of maple-syrup urine disease. N Engl J Med 276:84, 1967

32. **Dedo DD:** Hemifacial atrophy. A review of an unusual craniofacial deformity with a report of a case. Arch Otolaryngol 104:538, 1978

33. **Dekaban A, Carr R:** Congenital amaurosis of retinal origin. Arch Neurol 14:294, 1966

34. **DeSousa AL, Kalsbeck JE, Mealy J Jr et al:** Diencephalic syndrome and its relation to opticochiasmatic glioma: Review of twelve cases. Neurosurgery 4:207, 1979

35. **Dische MR, Porro RS:** The cardiac lesions in Bassen-Kornzweig syndrome. Am J Med 49:568, 1970

36. **Dobyns WB, Goldstein NP, Gordon H:** Clinical spectrum of Wilson's disease (hepatolenticular degeneration). Mayo Clin Proc 54:35, 1979

37. **Dods L:** A diencephalic syndrome of early infancy. Med J Aust 1:222, 1967

38. **Donat JR, Auger R:** Familial periodic ataxia. Arch Neurol 36:568, 1979

39. **Dooling EC, Richardson EP Jr, Davis KR:** Computed tomography in Hallervorden-Spatz disease. Neurology (Minneap) 30:1128, 1980

40. **Dooling EC, Schoene WC, Richardson EP Jr:** Hallervorden-Spatz syndrome. Arch Neurol 30:70, 1974

41. **Dunn DW, Snyder CH:** Benign paroxysmal vertigo of childhood. Am J Dis Child 130:1099, 1976

42. **Elejalde BR, Elejalde MMJ, Lopez F:** Hallervorden-Spatz disease. Clin Genet 16:1, 1979

43. **Emery JL, MacKenzie N:** Medullo-cervical dislocation deformity (Chiari II deformity) related to neurospinal dysraphism (meningomyelocele). Brain 96:155, 1973

44. **Erdohazi M, Marshall P:** Striatal degeneration in childhood. Arch Dis Child 54:85, 1979

45. **Evans OB, Kilroy AW, Fenichel GM:** Acetazolamide in the treatment of pyruvate dysmetabolism syndromes. Arch Neurol 35:302, 1978

46. **Fenichel GM:** Migraine as a cause of benign paroxysmal vertigo of childhood. J Pediatr 71:114, 1967

47. **Fisher-Williams M, Roberts RC:** Cerebrospinal fluid proteins and serum immunoglobulins. Occurrence in multiple sclerosis and other neurological diseases: Comparative measurement of γ-globulin and the IgG class. Arch Neurol 25:256, 1971

48. **Frigoletto FD, Umansky I:** Erythroblastosis fetalis: Identification, management, and prevention. Clin Perinatol 6:321, 1979

49. **Frith CD, Johnstone EC, Joseph MH et al:** Double-blind clinical trial of 5-hydroxytryptophan in a case of Lesch-Nyhan syndrome. J Neurol Neurosurg Psychiatry 39:656, 1976

50. **Fryer DG, Winckleman AC, Ways PO et al:** Refsum's disease: A clinical and pathological report. Neurology (Minneap) 21:162, 1971

51. **Gardner E, O'Rahilly R, Prolo D:** The Dandy-Walker and Arnold-Chiari malformations. Clinical, developmental, and teratological considerations. Arch Neurol 32:393, 1975

52. **Gartner LM, Snyder RN, Chabon RS et al:** Kernicterus: High incidence in premature infants with low serum bilirubin concentrations. Pediatrics 45:906, 1970

53. **Gatti FM, Rosenheim E:** Sydenham's chorea associated with transient intellectual impairment: a case study and review of the literature. Am J Dis Child 118:915, 1969

54. **Gibberd FB, Billimoria JD, Page NGR et al:** Heredopathia atactica polyneuritiformis (Refsum's disease) treated by diet and plasma-exchange. Lancet 1:575, 1979

55. **Gilbert GJ:** Dyssynergia cerebellaris myoclonica. In Bruyn PJ, Vinken WG (eds): Handbook of Clinical Neurology, Vol 21, System Disorders and Atrophies, Part I, pp 509–518. Amsterdam, North-Holland, 1975

56. **Gilbert GJ:** Multiple sclerosis in the child of conjugal multiple sclerosis patients. Neurology (Minneap) 21:1169, 1971

57. **Gilman S, Barrett RE:** Hallervorden-Spatz disease and infantile neuroaxonal dystrophy. Clinical characteristics and nosological considerations. J Neurol Sci 19:189, 1973

58. **Gomez MR, Clermont V, Bernstein J:** Progressive bulbar paralysis in childhood (Fazio-Londe's disease). Arch Neurol 6:317, 1962

59. **Gotto AM, Levy RI, John K et al:** On the protein defect in abetalipoproteinemia. N Engl J Med 284:813, 1971

60. **Grand RJ, Vawter GF:** Juvenile Wilson disease: Histologic and functional studies during penicillamine therapy. J Pediatr 87:1161, 1975

61. **Green JB, McLeod S:** Short latency somatosensory evoked potentials in patients with neurological lesions. Arch Neurol 36:846, 1979

62. **Groothuis JR, Groothuis DR, Mukhopadhyay D et al:** Lupus-associated chorea in childhood. Am J Dis Child 131:1131, 1977

63. **Halliday AM, McDonald WI, Mushin J:** Delayed visual evoked response in optic neuritis. Lancet 1:982, 1972

64. **Herbert P, Gotto AM, Fredrickson DS:** Familial lipoprotein deficiency. Abetalipoproteinemia. In Stanbury JB, Wyngaarden JB, Fredrickson DS (eds): The Metabolic Basis of Inherited Disease, 4th ed, pp 553–565. New York, McGraw-Hill, 1978

65. **Herd JK, Mehdi M, Uzendoski DM et al:** Chorea associated with systemic lupus erythematosus: Report of two cases and review of the literature. Pediatrics 61:308, 1978

66. **Herrman C:** Head shaking with nystagmus in infants. A study of sixty-four cases. Am J Dis Child 16:180, 1918

67. **Herskovitz E, Blackwood W:** Essential (familial, hereditary) tremor: A case report. J Neurol Neurosurg Psychiatry 32:509, 1969

68. **Hill W, Sherman H:** Acute intermittent familial cerebellar ataxia. Arch Neurol 18:350, 1968

69. **Hoefnagel D, Biery B:** Spasmus nutans. Dev Med Child Neurol 10:32, 1968

70. **Hoefnagel D, Penry JK:** Partial facial paralysis in young children. N Engl J Med 262:1136, 1960

71. **Hunt JR:** Dyssynergia cerebellaris myoclonica—primary atrophy of the dentate system. A contribution to the pathology and symptomatology of the cerebellum. Brain 44:490, 1921

72. **Husby G, Rijn I, Zabriskie JB et al:** Antibodies reacting with cytoplasm of subthalamic and caudate nuclei neurons in chorea and acute rheumatic fever. J Exp Med 144:1094, 1976

73. **Hyman CB, Keaster J, Hanson V et al:** CNS abnormalities after neonatal hemolytic disease or hyperbilirubinemia. Am J Dis Child 117:395, 1969

74. **Illingworth DR, Connor WE, Miller RG:** Abetalipoproteinemia. Report of two cases and review of therapy. Arch Neurol 37:659, 1980

75. **Jason JM, Gelfand EW:** Diagnostic considerations in ataxia telangiectasia. Arch Dis Child 54:682, 1979

76. **Jayalakshmi P, Scott TFM, Tucker SH et al:** Infantile nystagmus: A prospective study of spasmus nutans, congenital nystagmus, and unclassified nystagmus of infancy. J Pediatr 77:177, 1970

77. **Jervis GA:** Early infantile cerebellar degeneration: Report of 3 cases in one family. J Nerv Ment Dis 111:398, 1950

78. **Jervis GA:** Huntington's chorea in childhood. Arch Neurol 9:244, 1963

79. **Johnson WG, Chutorian A, Miranda A:** A new juvenile hexosaminidase deficiency disease presenting as cerebellar ataxia. Neurology (Minneap) 27:1012, 1977

80. **Kanter W, Wooten GF, Eldridge R:** Dopamine β-hydroxylase and the torsion dystonias. Adv Neurol 14:303, 1976

81. **Kark RAP, Rodriguez-Budelli M, Blass JP:** Evidence for a primary defect of lipoamide dehydrogenase in Friedreich's ataxia. Adv Neurol 21:163, 1978

82. **Kaufman DB, Miller HC:** Ataxia telangiectasia: An autoimmune disease associated with a cytotoxic antibody to brain and thymus. Clin Immunol Immunopathol 7:288, 1977

83. **Kavanagh KT, Beardsley JV:** Brain stem auditory evoked response. Ann Otol Rhinol Laryngol 88(Suppl 58, Part 2):11–21, 1979

84. **Kayden HJ:** Abetalipoproteinemia. Annu Rev Med 23:285, 1972

85. **Kennedy C, Carter S:** Relation of optic neuritis to multiple sclerosis in children. Pediatrics 28:377, 1961

86. **Kilroy AW, Paulsen WA, Fenichel GM:** Juvenile parkinsonism treated with levodopa. Arch Neurol 27:350, 1972

87. **Kinast M, Erenberg G, Rothner AD:** Paroxysmal choreoathetosis: Report of five cases and review of the literature. Pediatrics 65:74, 1980

88. **Klawans HL, Goetz CG, Perlik S:** Presymptomatic and early detection in Huntington's disease. Ann Neurol 8:343, 1980

89. **Koenigsberger MR, Chutorian AM, Gold AP:** Benign paroxysmal vertigo in childhood. Neurology (Minneap) 20:1108, 1970

90. **Konigsmark BW:** Hereditary deafness in man. N Engl J Med 281:713, 774, 827, 1964

91. **Kurtzke JF, Beebe GW, Norman JE Jr:** Migration and multiple sclerosis in the United States. Neurology (Minneap) 29:579, 1979

92. **Lange H, Thorner G, Hopf A et al:** Morphometric studies of the neuropathological changes in choreatic diseases. J Neurol Sci 28:401, 1976

93. **Larroche JC:** Kernicterus. In Vinken PJ and Bruyn GW (eds): Handbook of Clinical Neurology, Vol 6, Diseases of the Basal Ganglia, pp 491–516. Amsterdam, North-Holland, 1968

94. **Leon GA, Grover WD, Huff DS:** Neuropathologic changes in ataxia-telangiectasia. Neurology (Minneap) 26:947, 1976

95. **Lesch M, Nyhan WL:** A familial disorder of uric acid metabolism and central nervous system function. Am J Med 36:561, 1964

96. **Leu ML, Strickland GT, Wang CC et al:** Skin pigmentation in Wilson's disease. JAMA 211:1542, 1970

97. **Lewis PD:** Parkinsonism—Neuropathology. Brit Med J 3:690, 1971

98. **Ling W, Oftedal G, Simon T:** Central retinal artery occlusion in Sydenham's chorea. Am J Dis Child 118:525, 1969

99. **Link H, Laurenzi MA:** Immunoglobulin class and light chain type of oligoclonal bands in CSF in multiple sclerosis determined by agarose gel electrophoresis and immunofixation. Ann Neurol 6:107 1979

100. **Lonsdale D, Faulker WR, Price JW et al:** Intermittent cerebellar ataxia associated with hyperpyruvic acidemia, hyperalaninemia, and hyperalaninuria. Pediatrics 43:1025, 1968

101. **Manning JJ, Adour KK:** Facial paralysis in children. Pediatrics 49:102, 1972

102. **Markham CH, Knox JW:** Observations on Huntington's chorea in childhood. J Pediatr 67:46, 1965

103. **Marsden CD, Harrison MJG:** Idiopathic torsion dystonia (dystonia musculorum deformans). A review of forty-two patients. Brain 97:793, 1974

104. **Martin JP:** Wilson's disease. In Vinken PJ, Bruyn GW (eds): Handbook of Clinical Neurology, Vol 6, Diseases of the Basal Ganglia, pp 267–278. Amsterdam, North-Holland, 1968

105. **Martin WE, Resch JA, Baker AB:** Juvenile parkinsonism. Arch Neurol 25:494, 1971

106. **McFarlin DE, McFarland HF:** Histocompatibility studies and multiple sclerosis. Arch Neurol 33:395, 1976

107. **McFarlin DE, Strober W, Waldmann TA:** Ataxia-telangiectasia. Medicine (Baltimore) 51:281, 1972

108. **Melchior JC, Benda CE, Yakovlev PI:** Familial idiopathic cerebral calcifications in childhood. Am J Dis Child 99:787, 1960

109. **Moskowitz MA, Winickoff RN, Heinz ER:** Familial calcification of the basal ganglions. A metabolic and genetic study. N Engl J Med 285:72, 1971

110. **Muenter MD, Whisnant JP:** Basal ganglia calcification, hypoparathyroidism, and extrapyramidal motor manifestations. Neurology (Minneap) 18:1075, 1968

111. **Muller DPR, Lloyd JK, Bird AC:** Long-term management of abetalipoproteinemia. Possible role for vitamin E. Arch Dis Child 52:209, 1977

112. **Murphy MJ:** Clinical correlations of CT scan-detected calcifications of the basal ganglia. Ann Neurol 6:507, 1979

113. **Naidu S, Narasimhachari N:** Sydenham's chorea: A possible presynaptic dopaminergic dysfunction initially. Ann Neurol 8:445, 1980

114. **Naidu S, Wolfson LI, Sharpless N:** Juvenile parkinsonism: A patient with possible primary striatal dysfunction. Ann Neurol 3:453, 1978

115. **Nausieda PA, Grossman BJ, Koller WC et al:** Sydenham chorea: An update. Neurology (Minneap) 30:331, 1980

116. **Nelson KB, Eng GD:** Congenital hypoplasia of the depressor anguli oris muscle: Differentiation from congenital facial palsy. J Pediatr 81:16, 1972

117. **Nelson RF, Guzman DA, Grahovac Z et al:** Computerized cranial tomography in Wilson disease. Neurology (Minneap) 29:866, 1979

118. **Noble KG, Carr RE:** Leber's congenital amaurosis. A retrospective study of 33 cases and a histopathological study of one case. Arch Ophthalmol 96:818, 1978

119. **Norman RM:** Primary degeneration of the granular layer of the cerebellum: An unusual form of familial atrophy occurring early in life. Brain 63:365, 1940

120. **Norton EWD, Cogan DG:** Spasmus nutans. A clinical study of twenty cases followed two years or more since onset. AMA Arch Ophthalmol 52:442, 1954

121. **Nyhan WL:** The Lesch-Nyhan syndrome. Dev Med Child Neurol 20:376, 1978

122. **Oliver J, Dewhurst K:** Childhood and adolescent forms of Huntington's disease. J Neurol Neurosurg Psychiatry 32:455, 1969

123. **Oppenheim H:** Uber eine eigenartige krampfkrankheit des kindlichen und jugendlichen alters (dysbasia lordotica progressiva, dystonia musculorum deformans). Neurol Cbl 30:1090, 1911

124. **Pape KE, Pickering D:** Asymmetric crying facies: An index of other congenital anomalies. J Pediatr 81:21, 1972

125. **Paterson MC, Smith PJ:** Ataxia-telangiectasia: An inherited human disorder involving hypersensitivity to ionizing radiation and related DNA-damaging chemicals. Annu Rev Genet 13:291, 1979

126. **Perlman M, Reisner SH:** Asymmetric crying facies and congenital anomalies. Arch Dis Child 48:627, 1973

127. **Podolsky S, Sheremata WA:** Insulin-dependent diabetes mellitus and Friedreich's ataxia in siblings. Metabolism 19:555, 1970

128. **Refsum S:** Heredopathia atactica polyneuritiformis: A familial syndrome not hitherto described. A contribution to the clinical study of the hereditary diseases of the nervous system. Acta Psychiatr Scand (Suppl 38):1, 1946

129. **Roesmann U, Schwartz JF:** Familial striatal degeneration. Arch Neurol 29:314, 1973

130. **Rosman NP, Schapiro MB, Wolf PA:** Sclerotic atrophy of the cerebellum: A clinicopathological survey. J Neuropathol Exp Neurol 37:174, 1978

131. **Russell A:** A diencephalic syndrome of emaciation in infancy and childhood. Arch Dis Child 26:274, 1951

132. **Sachdev KK, Singh N, Krishnamoorthy MS:** Juvenile parkinsonism treated with levodopa. Arch Neurol 34:244, 1977

133. **Salisachs P:** Jaw reflex in Friedreich ataxia. Neurology (Minneap) 29:1049, 1979

134. **Sanner G, Bergstrom B:** Benign paroxysmal torticollis in infancy. Acta Pediatr Scand 68:219, 1979

135. **Sarnat HB, Alcala H:** Human cerebellar hypoplasia. A syndrome of diverse causes. Arch Neurol 37:300, 1980

136. **Scanu AM:** Abetalipoproteinemia and hypobetalipoproteinemia: What is the primary defect? Adv Neurol 21:125, 1978

137. **Schwartz JF, Rowland LP, Eder H et al:** Bassen-Kornzweig syndrome: Deficiency of serum β-lipoprotein. Arch Neurol 8:438, 1963

138. **Seegmiller JE:** Inherited deficiency of hypoxanthine-guanine phosphoribosyl-transferase in X-linked uric aciduria (the Lesch-Nyhan syndrome and its variants). Adv Hum Genet 6:75, 1976

139. **Seligman JW:** Recent and changing concepts of hyperbilirubinemia and its management in the newborn. Pediatr Clin North Am 23:509, 1977

140. **Senelick RC, Bray PF, Lahey ME et al:** Neuroblastoma and myoclonic encephalopathy: Two cases and a review of the literature. J Pediatr Surg 8:623, 1973

141. **Shenker DM, Grossman HJ, Klawans HL:** Treatment of Sydenham's chorea with haloperidol. Dev Med Child Neurol 15:19, 1973

142. **Sieben RL, Hamida MB, Shulman K:** Multiple cranial nerve deficits associated with the Arnold-Chiari malformation. Neurology (Minneap) 21:673, 1971

143. **Sobrevilla LA, Goodman ML, Kane CA:** Demyelinating central nervous system disease, macular atrophy and acanthocytosis (Bassen-Kornzweig syndrome). Am J Med 37:821, 1964

144. **Steele JC, Gladstone RM, Thanasophon S et al:** Acute cerebellar ataxia and concomitant infection with *Mycoplasma pneumonia*. J Pediatr 80:467, 1972

145. **Steinberg D:** Phytanic acid storage disease: Refsum's disease. In Stanbury JB, Wyngaarden JB, Fredrickson DS (eds): The Metabolic Basis of Inherited Disease, 4th ed, pp 689–706. New York, McGraw-hill, 1978

146. **Steinberg D:** Elucidation of the metabolic error in Refsum's disease: Strategy and tactics. Adv Neurol 21:113, 1978

147. **Steinberg D, Mize CE, Herndon JH Jr et al:** Phytanic acid in patients with Refsum's syndrome and response to dietary treatment. Arch Intern Med 125:75, 1970

148. **Teplitz RL:** Ataxia telangiectasia. Arch Neurol 35:553, 1978

149. **Thiebault F:** Sydenham's chorea. In Vinken PJ, Bruyn GW (eds): Handbook of Clinical Neurology, Vol 6, Diseases of the Basal Ganglia, pp 409–434. Amsterdam, North-Holland, 1968

150. **Tyrer JH:** Friedreich's ataxia. In Vinken PJ, Bruyn GW (eds): Handbook of Clinical Neurology, Vol 21, System Disorders and Atrophies, Part I, pp 319–364. Amsterdam, North-Holland, 1975

151. **Vanasse M, Bedard P, Andermann F:** Shuddering attacks in children: An early clinical manifestation of essential tremor. Neurology (Minneap) 26:1027, 1976

152. **Waldmann TA, McIntire KR:** Serum alpha-fetoprotein levels in patients with ataxia-telangiectasia. Lancet 2:1112, 1972

153. **Wallace DC:** A new manifestation of Leber's disease and a new explanation for the agency responsible for its unusual pattern of inheritance. Brain 93:121, 1970

154. **Weiss S, Carter S:** Course and prognosis of acute cerebellar ataxia in children. Neurology (Minneap) 9:711, 1959

155. **Westmoreland BF, Goldstein NP, Klass DW:** Wilson's disease: Electroencephalographic and evoked potential studies. Mayo Clin Proc 49:401, 1974

156. **White JC:** Familial periodic nystagmus, vertigo, and ataxia. Arch Neurol 20:276, 1969

157. **Wigboldus JM, Bruyn GW:** Hallervorden-Spatz disease. In Vinken PJ, Bruyn GW (eds): Handbook of Clinical Neurology, Vol 6, Diseases of the Basal

Ganglia, pp 604–631. Amsterdam, North-Holland, 1968

158. **Winkler GF, Young RR:** Efficacy of chronic propanolol therapy in action tremor of the familial, senile or essential varieties. N Engl J Med 290:984, 1974

159. **Wolf SM, Verity MA:** Neurologic complications of progressive facial hemiatrophy. J Neurol Neurosurg Psychiatry 37:997, 1974

160. **Zeman W:** Dystonia: An overview. Adv Neurol 14:91, 1976

161. **Zeman, W, Dyken P:** Dystonia musculorum deformans. In Vinken PJ, Bruyn GW (eds): Handbook of Clinical Neurology, Vol 6, Diseases of the Basal Ganglia, pp 517–543. Amsterdam, North-Holland, 1968

Spinal Cord Disorders

17

Thomas W. Farmer

DEVELOPMENTAL DEFECTS

Spina Bifida, Meningocele, Meningomyelocele

Spina bifida occulta is the failure of closure of the bony spine at any level, most commonly in the lumbosacral area. Spina bifida may be associated with defects of the meninges and spinal cord. A meningocele, a saclike mass covered by skin and containing meninges, may protrude at the site of the spina bifida. If this mass contains meninges and neural elements of spinal cord or nerve roots, it is classified as a meningomyelocele. Sacral agenesis may be associated with meningomyelocele.[18]

Etiology. By the fourth week of intrauterine life the spinal canal closes, and by the twelfth week the bony canal closes. Thus, the etiologic factors relating to these disorders are effective early in fetal life. Spina bifida is frequently associated with other developmental defects and may be familial. Therefore, hereditary factors probably play the dominant role.

Pathology. A meningocele is covered by an outer layer of skin and an inner layer of meninges which communicate with the meninges lining the spinal subarachnoid space. Portions of the spinal cord or of the nerve roots may extend into this sac in a meningomyelocele.

Symptoms. Spina bifida occulta occurs in about one fourth of children and by itself produces no symptoms. Simple meningocele is also usually asymptomatic, whereas a meningomyelocele results in neurologic deficit. Meningocele or meningomyelocele occurs at an incidence of 1 per 1000 live births.

Examination. The sac of a meningocele or a meningomyelocele is apparent on inspection of the lower back (Fig. 17-1). A localized tuft of hair or a dimple in the skin sometimes overlies a spina bifida occulta. Subcutaneous lipomas and the bony defect produced by the spina bifida may be palpated. The head size may be increased with hydrocephaly. Shortening of the neck may be noted. With associated involvement of the cauda equina, motor weakness and atrophy, sensory and reflex loss in the legs, and bladder dysfunction occur. With meningomyelocele involving the spinal cord, the neurologic deficit corresponds to the level of the lesion.

Laboratory Examination. Radiographs of the spine at the level of a spinal meningocele reveal spina bifida with variable defects of the laminae and pedicles. Other radiographs may reveal evidence of hydrocephaly, Klippel-Feil anomaly of the cervical vertebrae, or scoliosis. Computed tomographic metrizamide myelography may reveal an associated lipoma, and at the distal level of the cord, an abnormal filum terminale, or defects in the covering of the spinal cord can be identified.[13]

Treatment. A meningocele that contains no neural tissue is corrected surgically. The vast majority of infants with meningomyeloceles are treated conservatively at home.

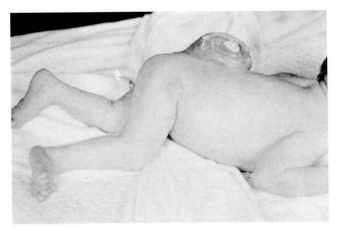

FIG. 17-1. Meningomyelocele. This 4-week-old infant was born with a large lumbosacral meningomyelocele. Complete flaccid paralysis of both legs, absence of knee and ankle jerks, and absence of anal sphincter tone were present. (Of two siblings, one had a meningomyelocele, as did an uncle of the mother.)

The meningomyelocele is washed, dressed, and suitably protected from pressure each day. Meticulous care of the skin in the perineum is essential to prevent skin infection. If weakness or paralysis in the legs is present, active or passive exercises are carried out. Periodic examinations are done with measurements of head circumference and evaluation of neurologic disability.

Surgical therapy of meningomyelocele to remove the protruding mass and to prevent infection is restricted to selected cases.[19] In infants with meningomyelocele associated with partial paralysis and partial sphincter disorder without hydrocephalus, early surgery is carried out. In infants with complete paralysis of the legs and of the sphincters, surgery is not indicated. If a child with meningomyelocele is also developing progressive hydrocephalus, surgery is contraindicated.

In those children with paraplegia who have survived on conservative therapy during infancy and who are showing normal intellectual development, excision of a meningomyelocele may be considered in order to improve nursing care and to permit efforts at ambulation. However, surgery does not decrease the extent of neurologic disability.

Prognosis. With successful closure of a simple meningocele, the prognosis is good. Most infants with meningomyelocele die from infection. In one series,[14] more than 90% of infants who were not given early surgical treatment died before they were 1 year old. An occasional child with partial neurologic deficit in whom successful repair of the sac is performed may survive into adult life with a stationary disability.

Prevention. A woman who has been delivered of a child with a neural tube defect is at 2% risk of having another similarly affected offspring in each succeeding pregnancy. Pregnancies with a neural tube defect in the fetus are also associated with increased amounts of alpha-fetoprotein (AFP) in the amniotic fluid after about 14 weeks of pregnancy. AFP is produced in the fetal liver and yolk sac. Fetal cerebrospinal fluid and fetal serum both contain high concentrations of AFP. With an open neural tube defect or with anencephaly, AFP leaks into the amniotic fluid. By 24 weeks of gestation, the amniotic fluid of 90% of fetuses with an open spina bifida contain an elevated amount of AFP. However, an elevated amniotic fluid AFP level is not specific for an open neural tube defect. Elevated levels also occur with intrauterine death, congenital nephrosis, congenital hernia into the umbilical cord, and fetal teratoma. When an elevated AFP level is found, the chances are overwhelming for either a major fetal malformation or impending demise of the fetus. The parents can then decide whether to abort the fetus or prepare for the birth of a child with a malformed spinal column or brain.[12,16]

Screening tests are available that attempt to identify neural tube defects in the fetuses of women with no previous history of neural tube defect. The initial screening tests are to determine the level of AFP in the serum. The initial serum sample is obtained in the second trimester of pregnancy, ideally during the 16th or 17th week. If the AFP level is elevated in the serum, a second serum sample is obtained 1 week later and tested. An elevation of the AFP level in the serum of a pregnant woman may be related to a neural tube defect, twin pregnancies, prematurity, or low birth weight. If two elevated levels are obtained on the serum of a pregnant woman, then ultrasound examination is done to confirm the gestational date and to check for multiple pregnancies. If the pregnant woman has a single pregnancy of the correct gestational age, then amniocentesis under sonographic surveillance with measurement of AFP in the amniotic fluid is done. If the amniotic fluid AFP is elevated, a second confirmatory amniocentesis is carried out. Further evaluation will determine the effectiveness of the screening procedures.

Diastematomyelia

Etiology. Diastematomyelia, a cleft in the spinal cord, is a congenital malformation in which the spinal cord is divided into two parts by a small, bony, cartilaginous or fibrous septum. The fibrous bands, which divide the cord in the anterior-posterior axis, prevent its normal rostral migration. At the third embryonic month, the cord and the vertebral column are equal in length. At birth, the conus medullaris is opposite the third lumbar vertebra, and at maturity it is opposite the first lumbar vertebra.

Pathology. A fibrous band transects the cord, usually in the lower thoracic or lumbar region, but sometimes in the upper thoracic cord. The cord is partly or completely divided over one or several segments. In the lower lumbar area, the septum may divide the cauda equina.

Symptoms. Although the cutaneous and skeletal anomalies are present at birth, symptoms first develop after the child starts to walk, and they may not occur until late childhood. The child may complain of low back pain aggravated by coughing and sneezing. Pain may radiate down one or both legs in a root distribution. The parents may note that the child holds his back stiff and does not stoop or play, or even that he wants to stay in bed. Bladder dysfunction or slowly progressive weakness in the legs may be noted.

Examination. Hypertrichosis characterized by long, soft hair in the midline of the back usually covering the region of the underlying spinal anomaly occurs in the majority of children with diastematomyelia. Congenital dermal sinus, lipoma, skin dimples, abnormal bony protrusions, or meningomyelocele at the same spinal level may be associated findings, and congenital anomalies of one or both feet or legs are frequently seen.[11]

Weakness, atrophy, and reflex and sensory changes in the legs and feet may develop. The tendon reflexes may be decreased or absent. Occasionally, extensor plantar responses are present. Bladder and bowel function may be altered. Indolent ulcers may develop on the feet in areas of analgesia.

Laboratory Examination. Radiographs or computerized tomography (CT) of the spine may reveal an irregularly shaped bone spur in the midline at the level of the cleft (Fig. 17-2). However, if this cord-dividing septum is cartilaginous or fibrous, it cannot be seen on radiographic study. Lumbar puncture reveals normal findings. Myelography with computed tomographic metrizamide shows a characteristic midline bony, cartilaginous, or fibrous septum that divides the cord. The column is split in two, and the septum is outlined as a filling defect. An associated radiographic finding is that of spina bifida occulta with fusiform widening of the spinal canal over several segments.

In children who have had bladder symptoms, intravenous pyelograms may reveal dilatation of the ureters and of the renal pelves. Urine cultures may be positive.

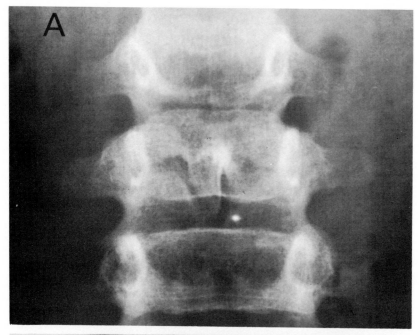

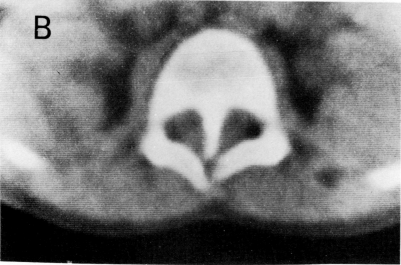

FIG. 17-2. Diastematomyelia. *A.* Radiograph of the lumbar spine of an 8-year-old boy. An irregularly shaped bone spur is present in the midline at the level of the third lumbar vertebra. This is associated with spina bifida occulta. *B.* CT scan of a section of the second lumbar vertebra of a 9-year-old girl. A bony spur is present in the midline associated with spina bifida occulta.

Differential Diagnosis. The diagnosis of diastematomyelia is suggested by the frequent presence of cutaneous and skeletal defects associated with neurologic signs involving the legs or feet. The diagnosis is established by radiologic and myelographic studies.[17]

Treatment. Surgical treatment is indicated with removal of the cord-transfixing septum.

Prognosis. Surgical therapy prevents progression of neurologic deficit if it is already present. If surgery is carried out early before significant neurologic deficit has occurred, there is normal ascent of the cord within the vertebral canal during childhood with normal neurologic function. If diastematomyelia is associated with meningomyelocele and the infant is paraplegic, the prognosis is determined by the severity of the meningomyelocele.

VASCULAR ANOMALIES

Arteriovenous Fistula

Arteriovenous fistulas usually involve the cervical enlargement anteriorly or the thoracic or lumbar cord posteriorly. This rare vascular anomaly usually results in symptoms during childhood. The child may develop an acute paraplegia related to thrombosis of vessels in the anomaly or related to hematomyelia. A gradual onset of paraplegia may be related to cord compression by the large anomaly. Motor and sensory deficit are present below the level of the lesion. Lumbar puncture may reveal evidence of subarachnoid hemororhage or evidence of subarachnoid block. Myelography may show characteristic pulsations of the column of oil under fluoroscopy, and partial or complete block may be demonstrated. Arteriovenous fistulas may be associated with cutaneous angiomas, pigmented nevi, spina bifida, and lipomas. These associated findings might suggest the diagnosis of a vascular anomaly from the clinical examination. If other anomalies are not present, the diagnosis is established by myelography. With repeated episodes of thrombosis or hemorrhage involving the cord, severe paraplegia or quadriplegia with sphincter disorder eventually results.

There has been a revival of interest in the surgical treatment of spinal cord arteriovenous malformations due to advances in arteriographic and microsurgical techniques. The arterial feeders are demonstrated by arteriography. Surgical treatment may consist of ligation of the feeding arteries or total extirpation of the malformation.[9]

Telangiectases

Telangiectases are rare vascular anomalies found at any level of the spinal cord. With bleeding, hematomyelia occurs. Acute symptoms of spinal cord deficit occur with bleeding into the spinal cord. The cerebrospinal fluid does not contain blood. Cutaneous nevi are often associated with telangiectases. These lesions must be distinguished from spinal cord tumor and syringomyelia in children. No specific therapy is available. Recurrent bleeding with progressive cord disease usually occurs.

Venous Angioma

Venous angiomas rarely produce symptoms during childhood. They occur in the thoracic and lumbar cord, and the symptoms are recurrent, acute episodes of paraplegia and root pain. These episodes may be followed by remissions in signs and symptoms. Skin nevi may be associated with these vascular anomalies. Lumbar puncture may reveal partial or complete subarachnoid block, and the protein content may be elevated. After an acute episode, the lymphocytes may be increased in the fluid. Myelography may reveal partial filling defects due to large tortuous vessels. With recurrent episodes increasing cord deficit occurs. Selective spinal angiography identifies the location and blood supply of an angioma.[8] With microneurosurgery, angiomas of the posterior part of the spinal cord can be removed. Embolization of intramedullary angiomas at the time of selective angiography may also be possible.[15]

DEGENERATIVE DISORDERS

Progressive Spinal Muscular Atrophy

Etiology. Progressive spinal muscular atrophies, familial disorders of unknown etiology, are transmitted by an autosomal recessive gene. The most severe variety is infantile progressive muscular atrophy, or Werdnig-Hoffmann disease. Intermediate forms of severity usually begin in early childhood. The mild form, Kugelberg-Welander-Wohlfart type, begins in childhood or adolescence. Because the etiology of this disorder is not known, it is reasonable to describe the clinical pictures as a continuous spectrum of spinal muscular atrophy from infancy to adult life. However, the etiology may be single or multiple.

Pathology.   Degenerative changes occur in the large anterior horn cells of the spinal cord and also in motor cells of the fifth, sixth, seventh, tenth, eleventh, and twelfth cranial nerves. Secondary changes of wallerian degeneration appear in roots and nerves, and denervation atrophy of muscle is prominent. The process is always symmetrical. Anterior horn cells show symmetrical swelling of the cytoplasm, eccentric swollen nuclei, and fragmentation of the Nissl bodies. Denervation atrophy of the skeletal muscles supplied by spinal nerves is more marked than that seen in bulbar musculature. The diaphragm is normal. All tracts within the spinal cord show normal myelination. Atrophy of the cerebellum and ventral pons has occasionally been reported in infants with progressive muscular atrophy.[10]

Examination.   The onset of muscular atrophy may occur in utero, during the first or second year of life, or in later childhood. The severity of spinal muscular atrophy usually varies directly, at least in part, with the age of onset of the disorder. The mild form, with onset in childhood and with very slow progression, is the Kugelberg-Welander-Wohlfart type.

If the disorder develops during pregnancy, the mother may note a decrease or absence of fetal movements during the last few weeks of pregnancy and the infant may appear inactive at birth. If the onset is in utero or during the first 2 postnatal months,

weakness is severe and generalized at the onset. Limited movements of the infant's arms display weakness of shoulder and arm muscles. Intercostal paralysis is frequently present, with collapse of the chest (Fig. 17-3). The diaphragm moves normally. The legs are externally rotated and abducted at the hips with flexion at the knee. Active movements are usually confined to the fingers and toes. Mild facial weakness may be present, and difficulty in swallowing may be noted. The anterior neck muscles are weak, and fasciculations of the tongue are frequent.[5]

If the onset of muscular atrophy is at 2 to 12 months of age, motor weakness occurs first in the legs and initially involves proximal musculature. Subsequently, there is involvment of the arms with associated fasciculations of the tongue and occasional additional lower cranial nerve involvement. These infants achieve the ability to sit without support between 6 and 12 months of age, and thus they represent an intermediate form of severity. Eighty percent of infants with infantile muscular atrophy are in the intermediate group. One third of the intermediate group learn to walk. Half of them develop scoliosis between 1 and 4 years of age.[3] If the disorder begins at 1 to 2 years of age, weakness is initially localized to the thighs and spreads to the shoulders. Sensory examination is normal. In mild Kugelberg-Welander-Wohlfart type, proximal limb muscle weakness begins at two to

FIG. 17-3. Infantile progressive muscular atrophy. Eight-month-old boy has bilateral facial weakness with lack of expression, marked wasting of shoulder girdle muscles, and intercostal paralysis with diaphragmatic breathing. The characteristic posture is that of abduction at the shoulder, flexion at the elbow, and flexion at the hip and knee.

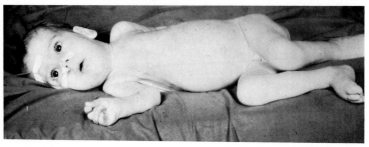

seventeen years of age and progresses over many years. Weakness of respiratory muscles with chronic hypoventilation may develop. Severe muscular weakness may not develop until 30 to 40 years of age. The muscles innervated by cranial nerves are usually not involved.

Severely affected infants are areflexic early in the course of the disorder. With onset of symptoms during the second year of life, tendon reflexes may be preserved until further progression of disability occurs. With onset late in infancy, the plantar responses remain flexor and spasticity does not develop. In atypical cases with additional involvement of supraspinal and suprabulbar structures including the cerebellum, the clinical picture of paralysis of the trunk and extremities is associated with mental retardation, spasticity, contractures, and cortical blindness.[10]

Laboratory Examination.   Electromyography and muscle biopsy reveal evidence of neural atrophy.[4] Examination of the cerebrospinal fluid yields normal results.

Differential Diagnosis.   Infantile progressive muscular atrophy must be distinguished from the hypotonia and retarded motor development seen in cerebral disease. Poliomyelitis during infancy may produce widespread muscular atrophy and loss of reflexes. Glycogen storage disease may affect anterior horn cells. Trauma to the spinal cord at birth may produce a transverse myelitis associated with limpness of the legs and trunk. Peripheral neuropathy may result in flaccid weakness in infants. The weakness in acute infectious polyneuritis is frequently greater distally than proximally in contrast with the greater proximal weakness in progressive muscular atrophy. In infectious polyneuropathy, the spinal fluid protein is frequently elevated. This disorder must be distinguished from benign congenital hypotonia in which tendon reflexes are preserved and progression of disability does not occur.

The mild Kugelberg-Welander-Wohlfart type of spinal muscular atrophy is associated with proximal limb weakness similar to that seen in limb-girdle muscular dystrophy. However, electromyography and muscle biopsy reveal findings consistent with neurogenic atrophy, and serum enzymes are normal in spinal muscular atrophy.

Treatment.   No specific therapy is available. Orthopedic measures may be of some value in aiding ambulation of those children affected late in infancy. This may delay the development of scoliosis and of contractures at the ankles and knees.

Prognosis.   The acute form of infantile spinal muscular atrophy is steadily progressive and terminates fatally. If the disorder develops during the neonatal period, death usually occurs by 1 to 2 years of age. With onset during the first year of life, death occurs within an average of 2 to 3 years. If the onset is during the second year of life, the average length of survival is 7 years. In the mild form, severe disability may not occur until 30 to 40 years of age. Death is usually due to pulmonary infection.

Prevention.   Parents who have had an infant with progressive muscular atrophy are advised that there is a one in four chance that the disorder will recur in each pregnancy of the affected marriage.

Hereditary Amyotrophic Lateral Sclerosis

Hereditary amyotrophic lateral sclerosis is a rare familial disorder of unknown etiology in which the pathologic findings are those of degeneration of the anterior horn cells in the spinal cord and of the corticospinal tracts. The onset is usually at 5 to 15 years of age either with initial spasticity or muscular atrophy. Atrophy usually begins distally in the hands and extends to involve arm and shoulder muscles. Fasciculations are usually present. With involvement of brain stem nuclei, atrophy of the tongue and weakness of the palate develop. The voice becomes nasal in quality, and difficulty in swallowing may occur. Spasticity develops in the legs and progresses to paraplegia. The signs may be initially unilateral, but subsequently they become bilateral and relatively symmetrical. The usual pattern is characterized by atrophy and fasciculations in the arms and spasticity in the legs. The tendon reflexes are hyperactive, and plantar responses are extensor. There are no sensory findings. There is no effective treatment. The disorder is slowly progressive over a period of years with death frequently resulting from pulmonary infections or respiratory failure.

Friedreich's Ataxia

Friedreich's ataxia, which involves cerebellar as well as spinal cord pathways, is discussed in the section on cerebellar disorders in Chapter 16.

Familial Spastic Paraplegia

Familial spastic paraplegia is a rare hereditary disorder occurring primarily in children. The etiology is not known. It may be transmitted by an autosomal dominant or recessive gene.

Pathology. The usual histologic changes are those of degeneration of the corticospinal tract in the spinal cord. In some cases, involvement also includes the spinocerebellar tracts, the posterior columns, and degneration of the cells in the column of Clarke. These additional pathologic findings suggest that this disorder may be related to Friedreich's ataxia.

Symptoms. The initial symptoms of weakness and stiffness in the legs may develop at any time during childhood or in early adult life. Initially, the gait becomes slow with difficulty in running. Males are affected more frequently than females.

Examination. The cranial nerves are normal. The motor system reveals a spastic gait that may become scissorlike when the disorder becomes severe. Moderate weakness may develop in the flexors of the hips and knees and of the dorsiflexors of the ankles. Response to sensory examination is normal. The knee and ankle jerks are hyperactive, and clonus may be present. The plantar responses are extensor. There is no disturbance in function of the sphincters.

One recessive form of infantile spastic paraplegia is associated with dysarthria and distal muscle wasting (Troyer syndrome).[7] Another recessive form of juvenile spastic paraplegia is associated with dysarthria and

dementia (Mast syndrome).[6] In another form, spastic paraplegia is associated with ichthyosis and mental deficiency (Sjögren-Larsson syndrome).

Laboratory Examination. Lumbar puncture reveals normal dynamics and normal cerebrospinal fluid.

Differential Diagnosis. If a similar disorder is present in other members of the family, the clinical diagnosis may be obvious. If the spastic weakness in the legs is associated with evidence of loss of position and vibration sense or with cerebellar ataxia in the patient or in a sibling, the diagnosis of Freidreich's ataxia may be the correct one. In a child with spastic paraplegia in whom no familial incidence is known, careful study should be done to exclude the possibilities of spinal cord tumor and occasionally multiple sclerosis.

Treatment. No specific therapy is available.

Prognosis. Spasticity and weakness in the legs usually progresses slowly over many years. The patient may become relatively incapacitated within 5 to 10 years (or after 20 years) or more.

Syringomyelia and Syringobulbia

Syringomyelia is a cavitation that occurs within the spinal cord. If the same type of cavitation develops within the brain stem or extends from cervical segments to the brain stem, the disorder is referred to as syringobulbia. The formation of the syrinx is most common in the cervical spinal cord, second most common in the brain stem, and next in the lumbosacral cord. Involvement may occur in one or all three of these portions of the central nervous system.

Etiology. The etiology is unknown. Syringomyelia is frequently associated with other congenital defects such as cranial malformations, hydrocephaly, Klippel-Feil syndrome, basilar impression, scoliosis, spina bifida, and clubfeet. These findings suggest that syringomyelia represents a developmental defect. The occasional association of syringomyelia with intramedullary cord tumor suggests a neoplastic etiology.

Pathology.   At the level of a syrinx, the cord may be swollen or atrophic. A syrinx usually extends over a number of segments and consists of several longitudinal cavities that may or may not connect with one another and with the central canal of the spinal cord. Similar cavitation may extend into the medulla. Here there is usually a narrow cavity extending laterally and anteriorly from the fourth ventricle. These cavities, lined with glial fibers, may be distended with fluid with resultant swelling. Solid masses of glial tissue form a definite neoplasm in approximately 15% of cases. These cavities usually involve first the gray matter near the central canal, the base of the posterior column, and the posterior horns. Subsequently, anterior horn cells and corticospinal tracts are involved. Through the medulla, the syrinx usually damages the descending root of the fifth nerve, the descending sympathetic pathways, and the nuclei of the tenth, eleventh, and twelfth cranial nerves.

Symptoms.   Syringomyelia is primarily a disorder of adults, although symptoms are frequently first noted in children at 10 to 16 years of age. The most common symptoms relating to cervical syringomyelia are painless burns of the fingers or arms and weakness of the hands. With involvement of the lumbar region, wasting and weakness of leg muscles may be noted. With bulbar involvement, the child may develop nasal speech. Familial syringomyelia occurs rarely in siblings.

Examination.   Examination may reveal loss of pain and temperature sensitivity on one or both sides of the face. Nasal speech, difficulty in swallowing, and laryngeal stridor may be present. The tongue may become atrophied and have fasciculations. There may be atrophy of the trapezius and sternomastoid muscles. Horizontal nystagmus may occur. Horner's syndrome may be present. Weakness and atrophy of the hand muscles occur frequently. With more extensive involvement, arm and shoulder muscles may also show weakness and atrophy. Weakness and spasticity may be present

in the legs, and flaccid weakness with atrophy may occur in the leg musculature.

The sensory findings are quite variable and relate to the sites and extent of the cavity formation. In cervical syringomyelia, a characteristic finding is that of segmental loss of pain and temperature sensation. This frequently extends from midcervical to upper thoracic segments, is usually bilateral, and is related to interruption of fibers passing through the central gray substance of the cord over the longitudinal extent of a syrinx. Characteristically, sensitivity to light touch is preserved in this area. Thus, there is dissociation of sensory loss with marked loss of pain and temperature and preservation of light touch sensitivity. Another common type of sensory deficit is that of loss of all sensory modalities in one or more segments due to involvement at the posterior root entry zone. A third type of sensory deficit is loss of pain and temperature sense extending from the cervical or upper thoracic level through the sacral area due to involvement of the contralateral spinothalamic tract. Loss of position and vibration sense occurs frequently due to involvement of the posterior columns.

In association with a cervical syrinx, the tendon reflexes in the arms are decreased or absent. Similarly, with a lumbar syrinx the knee and ankle jerks are diminished or absent. With cervical syringomyelia and associated involvement of corticospinal tracts, the tendon reflexes of the legs are increased with ankle clonus and extensor plantar responses.

Examination frequently reveals scars from previous burns. With severe involvement in the cervical cord and associated sensory loss in the hands, deformities of the fingers may occur and digits may be lost. Syringomyelia may also be associated with destruction of joints, usually at shoulder, elbow, hip, or knee (Charcot joints), as well as kyphosis, scoliosis, and clubfeet.

Laboratory Examination.   The cerebrospinal fluid is usually clear under normal pressure. In half of the patients there is an increase in the protein content. Rarely, a complete subarachnoid block may be present. Cervical myelography may reveal a fusiform enlargement of the cervical cord.[20] If the syringomyelic syndrome is associated with a type I Chiari malformation, myelography usually demonstrates abnormal flow through the foramen magnum and prolapse of the cerebellar tonsils.

Differential Diagnosis. Syringomyelia must be differentiated from spinal cord tumor in children. The neurologic signs associated with intramedullary tumor are similar to those seen in syringomyelia. Syringomyelia is the most likely diagnosis in a child with localized muscular atrophy, scars of old burns, dissociated sensory loss, and scoliosis. However, it is essential that myelography be done.

Sensory and motor findings similar to those seen in syringomyelia may occur in children with multiple sclerosis who have spinal cord involvement. However, severe, segmental loss of pain and temperature is unusual. The occurrence of optic neuritis or of other signs of involvement elsewhere in the nervous system differentiate multiple sclerosis from syringomyelia. Familial amyotrophic lateral sclerosis, which occurs rarely in children, is not associated with sensory findings. Basilar impression, which may produce signs similar to those seen with syringobulbia, is diagnosed by the radiologic findings.

Treatment. The two methods of therapy used to retard the progression of syringomyelia are irradiation of the affected segments of the spinal cord or medulla and operation with evacuation of the contents of the syringomyelic cavity. Neither method has been established as a successful form of therapy. The child is instructed in the prevention of burns to anesthetic areas. Surgical correction of associated abnormalities at the foramen magnum may produce benefit in some patients.[21]

Prognosis. The course is usually a slowly progressive one, although sudden exacerbations followed by minimal remissions may occur. In syringobulbia, the course may be fatal within a year owing to respiratory complications. In cervical and lumbar syringomyelia, progression with disability occurs over many years. The course may be relatively stationary for as long as 5 to 10 years.

DEMYELINATING DISORDERS

Multiple Sclerosis and Neuromyelitis Optica

See Chapter 16.

Acute Transverse Myelopathy

Pathology. Acute transverse myelopathy, a disorder of unknown etiology, is associated with edema and necrosis of the spinal cord at any level. The thoracic cord is involved in two thirds of the cases.

Symptoms. This rare disorder is occasionally preceded by a respiratory infection. The onset is frequently acute, with progressive weakness developing within 1 to 2 days in some patients. It may be associated with back and root pains. Fever, headache, and stiff neck may be present, followed by weakness that may progress to complete paralysis within 1 to 2 days or which may slowly progress over several weeks.

Examination. Fever and stiff neck may be present, and spinal tenderness may be observed. Weakness of trunk and legs is noted with a thoracic lesion. With cervical involvement, arm weakness is also present. Sensory loss is noted with a sensory level. Initially, the tendon reflexes are usually absent. The plantar responses may be absent or extensor. Urinary and fecal incontinence may be present.

Laboratory Examination. Lumbar puncture reveals clear fluid. Manometric studies in the vast majority of cases are normal, although subarachnoid block is infrequently noted. The fluid usually contains a normal cell count or a slight increase in white blood cells, although the cell count may be as high as 8000/cu mm. The protein level is usually normal, although it may be as high as 200 mg/dl.

Radiographs of the spine at the level of the cord lesion are normal. Myelography is usually normal, but rarely it shows an increased diameter of the cord at the level of the lesion or a complete subarachnoid block.[2]

Differential Diagnosis. The sudden onset of a transverse spinal cord lesion not associated with back pain, or evidence of subarachnoid block on lumbar puncture is suggestive of the clinical syndrome of transverse myelopathy of unknown etiology. It must be differentiated from spinal epidural abscess, which may be associated with a preceding bacterial infection, local back and root pains, evidence of osteomyelitis of the vertebra at the level of the lesion, or subarachnoid block on myelography. The possibility of spinal cord neoplasm must be excluded. Also, the possibility of hematomyelia associated with trauma to the spine is differentiated on the basis of history. Acute transverse myelopathy may occur in the demyelinating disorders, multiple sclerosis, and neuromyelitis optica.

Treatment. The patient is treated symptomatically with proper care of the bladder, passive and subsequently active exercise of the involved muscles, and careful skin care.

Prognosis. Complete or partial recovery may occur over several months.

INFECTIONS

Acute Spinal Epidural Abscess

Etiology. *Staphylococcus aureus* is the most frequent etiologic agent of acute spinal epidural abscess. The infection may be metastatic from a furuncle on the skin, osteomyelitis, an infected wound, empyema, perinephritic abscess, or pharyngitis.

Pathology. Epidural abscesses are most frequently located in the midthoracic and lumbar regions. A collection of pus extending over several segments is present posteriorly in the epidural space. Associated with this there may be thrombosis of arteries and veins and secondary degeneration of tracts in the spinal cord.

Symptoms. The disorder is rare, particularly in children. The history of a previous systemic bacterial infection, such as a furuncle, may be elicited. The initial symptom is severe back pain, frequently followed by root pain in the trunk or legs. This is associated with headache, fever, stiffness of the neck, and vomiting. Over a period that may be only a few days or that may extend over several weeks, progressive paralysis of the trunk and legs develops.

Examination. Temperature and pulse rate are elevated. The neck is stiff, and Kernig's sign is present. There is tenderness on palpation of the spinous processes at the level of the subjective back pain. There may be evidence of purulent infection of the skin, pharynx, or other area. Neurologic examination reveals weakness of the legs or complete paralysis. Sensory examination may reveal a decrease in one or more sensory modalities in the legs. If the sensory findings are severe, there may be a complete sensory loss to all modalities extending to the approximate level of the lesion. Associated with acute onset of weakness in the legs, the tendon reflexes may be absent. Plantar stimulation may produce no response or an extensor response. There may be urinary or fecal incontinence.

Laboratory Examination. The peripheral blood reveals a polymorphonuclear leukocytosis. Radiologic findings indicative of osteomyelitis of the vertebra at the level of cord damage is present in approximately half of the cases. An adjacent soft tissue mass may also be present.

Lumbar puncture is performed with great caution. The needle is introduced slowly. When it reaches the epidural space, pus may drip from the needle or be extracted with a syringe. This occurs if the epidural space is infected at the lumbar level where the puncture is done, but if the epidural abscess is above this level, no pus is obtained. Then the needle is advanced into the subarachnoid space. The fluid is usually clear and may be xanthochromic. Complete or partial block of the subarachnoid space is usually demonstrated by manometric studies. The fluid generally contains leukocytes, 10 to 500/cu mm. These may be predominantly lymphocytes or polymorphonuclear leukocytes. Usually the protein content is elevated, varying from 50 to 1500 mg/dl. The sugar content is normal, and cultures are sterile.

If partial or complete block is demonstrated, the needle is kept in place and ethyl iodenylundecylate (Pantopaque) is injected to demonstrate radiologically the level of the block. Myelography is always indicated prior to surgery.

Differential Diagnosis. If pus is withdrawn from the spinal epidural space in the lumbar area, the diagnosis is established. The diagnosis should also be considered in any child with an acute bacterial infection associated with severe back pain and meningeal signs associated with nonpurulent cerebrospinal fluid, and especially with evidence of partial or complete subarachnoid block. It is of the utmost importance to exclude this diagnosis in such patients as early as possible, because epidural abscess, if untreated, may be associated with the very rapid development of paralysis of the legs. Myelography outlines the lesion.

Neoplasms involving the spinal canal produce a similar transverse cord lesion associated with subarachnoid block. However, there is usually no preceding bacterial infection, and the course is characteristically slowly progressive. Hematomyelia with transverse myelopathy is usually associated with a history of trauma. Acute transverse myelopathy of unknown etiology is clinically very similar, although complete subarachnoid block is rare in this condition. Multiple sclerosis may occasionally produce a partial transverse myelopathy in a child. Signs of neurologic disease elsewhere in the central nervous system may be noted. Neuromyelitis optica produces a transverse myelopathy associated with optic neuritis.

Treatment. Immediate surgical drainage by laminectomy is necessary to prevent or restore the function of the spinal cord as well as to provide adequate drainage for the abscess. Chemotherapeutic and antibiotic drugs are administered before and after operation.

Prognosis. With early surgical drainage of an epidural abscess and with response of the infection to antibiotic therapy, complete recovery may occur with little or no neurologic deficit. If diagnosis is delayed until a complete transverse myelitis has de-

veloped at the level of the abscess, there is a complete or partial residual paraplegia that may be associated with a permanent sphincter disorder. If the infection cannot be controlled with antibiotic therapy, death may result.

Tuberculoma

Tuberculomas are now extremely rare. They may occur separately from tuberculous meningitis. If the local tuberculous infection is extramedullary, a granulomatous mass develops either intra- or extradurally and overlies several segments of the spinal cord. Rarely, intramedullary tuberculoma occurs in children (Fig. 17-4). The clinical picture produced by tuberculoma is very similar to that produced by spinal cord tumor. Usually the diagnosis is established at operation. Tuberculomas may be treated successfully by surgery and antituberculous therapy (Chap. 12, Table 12-5).

Acute Anteriior Poliomyelitis

See Chapter 12.

TRAUMA

Etiology. Trauma to the spinal cord is rare in children. It may occur at birth with breech delivery. Acquired injuries are usually the result of severe automobile accidents, falls, or diving injuries. Compression, contusion, laceration, and hemorrhage of the cord are commonly the result of compression fractures or fracture dislocations of the vertebrae.

Pathology. With severe cord damage, there may be complete transection, severe hemorrhage with hematomyelia, or edema. With permanent damage, secondary degeneration of fiber tracts occurs.

Symptoms. After a severe neck injury, the child may note paralysis and numbness of arms, trunk, and legs. Often, however, due to concomitant head injury, the patient is not aware of the initial symptoms. With a thoracic cord injury, paralysis and numbness of the legs occurs.

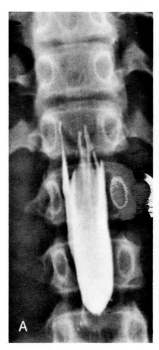
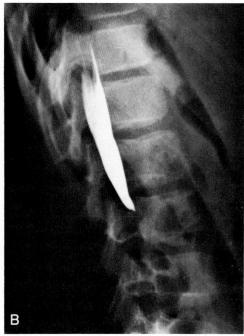

FIG. 17-4. Intramedullary tuberculoma in a 12-year-old boy. *A.* Lumbar myelogram, frontal view, reveals complete block of the column of oil at the upper level of the first lumbar vertebra. There is marked widening of the spinal cord at this level. *B.* Lumbar myelogram, lateral view.

Examination. With severe cervical cord injury, initial examination reveals flaccid paralysis of the arms, trunk, and legs. Due to intercostal paralysis, respirations are entirely diaphragmatic. There is complete loss of sensation to all modalities below the level of the injury. At first the reflexes are absent, and there is loss of sphincter control. After the initial period of spinal shock, which usually lasts a few days or a few weeks, muscle tone returns and reflex activity increases, but if the cord has been transected, function does not return. With incomplete damage, the amount of recovery is related to the severity of cord damage. When there is severe injury to the thoracic cord, similar paralysis and sensory loss occurs in the trunk and legs.

Laboratory Examination. Radiography of the spine usually reveals vertebral fracture or dislocation, although cord injury may occur with no abnormality present on radiographic examination. Rarely, fracture of the odontoid process occurs, sometimes associated with anterior dislocation of the first cervical vertebra on the second cervical vertebra (Fig. 17-5A). Laminagrams may demonstrate the fracture line better than a plain film (Fig. 17-5B). Dislocations may occur at any cervical level, although fifth and sixth cervical dislocations are most common (Fig. 17-6). Compression fractures occur in the thoracic and lumbar spine. The most common levels of fracture are the tenth, eleventh, and twelfth thoracic vertebrae (Fig. 17-7).

Diagnosis. There is nearly always a history of severe trauma. The level of the injury is established by neurologic examination and radiographs of the spine.

Treatment. Immediately after an injury, the child should be moved on a firm stretcher with adequate support to prevent movement of the spine. In cervical injury, skeletal traction with increasing weights is applied to reduce dislocation. In many instances, fusion is indicated. In thoracic and lumbar compressions, immobilization and sometimes fusion are carried out.

A child with a severe spinal cord injury requires superb nursing care. He is placed on a frame and careful daily skin care is given to prevent bedsores. Turning the patient every 2 hours prevents compression necrosis of the skin and facilitates normal expansion of the lungs. A nutritious, appetizing diet is extremely important. A child with a severe cervical cord injury requires assistance in feeding. Initially, an indwelling catheter is frequently necessary. Subsequently, the catheter is removed periodically until the patient is able to empty his bladder every 3 to 5 hours automatically or until normal bladder function returns. Early treatment of urinary tract infections is essential. Physical therapy with daily active and passive stretching exercises is important to prevent muscle contractures and to maintain a full range of joint movement. Positioning in bed is important to prevent foot drop and flexion contractures at the hips and knees. Toys and games may provide the stimulus for active exercises of the hands and arms. The child can be placed in a semierect position on the tilt table. When he is ready to stand, the degree of postural hypotension must be evaluated and syncope avoided. After initial exercises in the standing position, efforts at ambulation are begun in the parallel bars.

Prognosis.   Severe high cervical cord injury results in sudden respiratory death due to paralysis of the intercostal muscles and the diaphragm. With cervical cord injury below the fifth cervical segment, diaphragmatic function is preserved and the child is able to maintain respirations with adequate hospital care. However, if there is complete transection of the cord, death may subsequently occur due to urinary tract infection, bedsores, or respiratory infections. With incomplete transection, return of function gradually occurs and may continue for 6 months. Frequently residual weakness, sensory loss, and bladder dysfunction remain permanently. An auto-

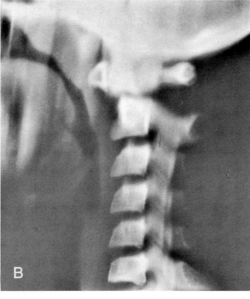

FIG. 17-5. Lateral radiograph (A) and lateral laminagram (B) of the cervical spine. There is an anterior dislocation of the first cervical vertebra on the second cervical vertebra with a separation of the odontoid process. This 14-year-old boy fell from a truck and landed on his left shoulder and neck. Neurologic examination was normal.

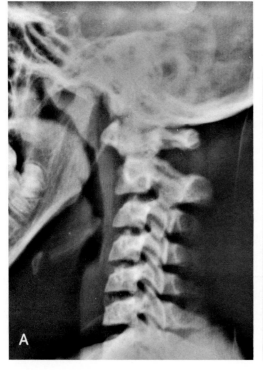

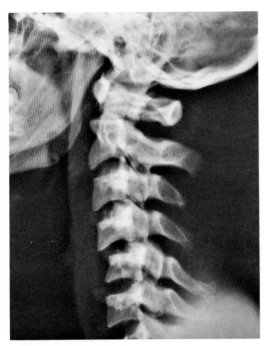

FIG. 17-6. Radiograph of the cervical spine, lateral view, of a 16-year-old boy. There is an anterior dislocation of the fourth cervical vertebra on the fifth cervical vertebra. The thickness of the soft tissues in the prevertebral space is increased. This injury, which was sustained in a high speed automobile accident, also produced a complete transverse lesion of the spinal cord at the same level.

matic bladder usually develops. Flexor and extensor spasms in the legs frequently occur. With persistent paraplegia, renal stones and pyelonephritis may develop. Complete recovery sometimes occurs with less severe cord damage.

TUMORS

Tumors of the spinal cord may be extramedullary or intramedullary. Extramedullary tumors may be intradural, extradural, or extravertebral.

FIG. 17-7. *A.* Frontal radiograph of the thoracic spine. Compression fracture of the body of the tenth thoracic vertebra with involvement of the superior surface and the pedicles. The spine is angulated to the left below the level of the fracture. Swelling of the paravertebral tissues on the left side is evident. The disk space between the ninth and tenth thoracic vertebrae is slightly narrowed. The superior cortex of the posterior part of the right tenth rib has been avulsed, and similar changes are noted in the corresponding portions of the eighth and ninth ribs. This 16-year-old boy was paraplegic immediately after a severe automobile accident. *B.* Lateral radiograph of the thoracic spine. Compression fracture of the body of the tenth thoracic vertebra.

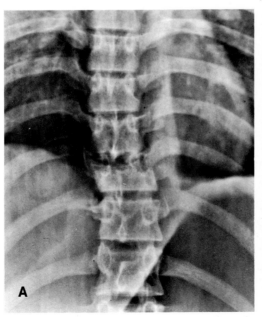

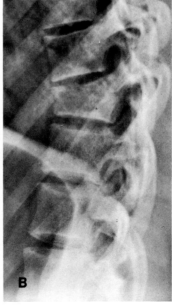

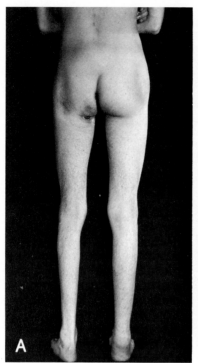

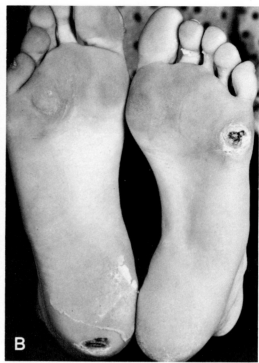

FIG. 17-8. Subcutaneous and intraspinal lipoma. *A.* A 16-year-old boy with a large bilateral mass in the lumbosacral region that had been present since birth. A trophic ulcer is present on the left buttock. Atrophy of the left gluteus maximus muscle and of the left calf is apparent. This was associated with weakness of the left leg and foot, first noted at 12 years of age. Additional findings included sensory loss from the fifth lumbar to the fifth sacral segment, hypoactive knee jerks, absent ankle jerks, difficulty in initiating micturition, and occasional rectal incontinence. *B.* Chronic ulceration of the right heel and left lateral sole secondary to anesthesia in this area. *C.* Radiograph of the lumbosacral spine (*posterior view*) reveals a wide spina bifida at the fifth lumbar and first sacral vertebrae with thinning of the pedicles and widening of the spinal canal at this level. The left lamina of the fifth lumbar vertebra and the first sacral laminae are rudimentary or absent. There is moderate scoliosis to the left centered at the fourth lumbar vertebra. *D.* CT scan of a section of the sacral spine with an area of decreased density posteriorly characteristic of a lipoma in the spinal canal.

Pathology. The most common types of spinal tumors in children are dermoid cysts, teratomas, astrocytomas, neuroblastomas, and ependymomas. Less common are lipomas, meningiomas, ganglioneuromas, and other histologic types.

Symptoms. Tumors are much less common in children than in adults. An early symptom frequently associated with extramedullary tumors is root pain. This radiating pain is the result of root involvement at the level of the tumor. The pain may radiate down the arms, around the chest or abdomen, or down the legs. Progressive weakness and numbness develop later. Urinary incontinence or retention may be noted.

Examination. In upper cervical cord tumors, weakness or wasting of the palate, trapezius, sternomastoid, tongue, or neck muscles may be present. With involvement at the fourth cervical level, paralysis of the diaphragm occurs. Shoulder girdle muscles are involved with a tumor at the fifth cervical level. At the sixth cervical level there is weakness of the triceps and of the wrist

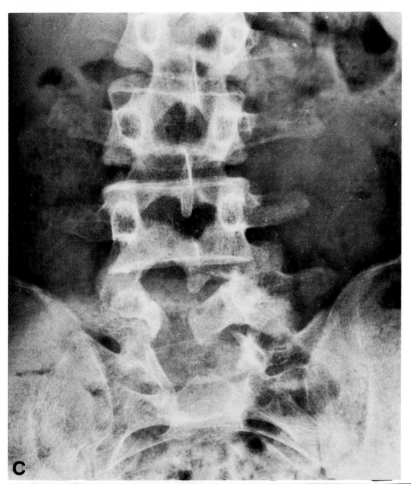

C

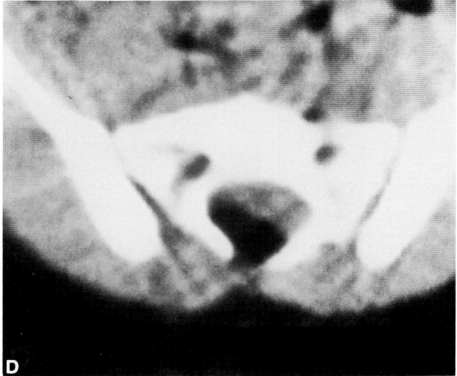

D

extensors. Weakness of hand muscles occurs with a lesion at the seventh cervical level. These findings may be associated with spastic weakness in the legs. Sensory loss may involve pain and temperature over the face with high cervical tumors. There usually develops a sensory level involving all sensory modalities with its upper border corresponding to the level of the tumor. This may develop late in the clinical course. There may be loss of reflexes in the arms at the level of the tumor. For example, at the fifth cervical level the biceps and radioperiosteal reflexes are lost, and at the sixth cervical level the triceps reflex is lost. Abdominal reflexes may be absent. The tendon reflexes in the legs are usually hyperactive, and the plantar responses are frequently extensor. Horner's syndrome with enophthalmos, meiosis, ptosis, and loss of sweating on the involved side of the face may be noted. Nystagmus may occur. Tenderness over the spinous processes at the involved level may be elicited by percussion.

FIG. 17-9. Meningioma extending from the first to the seventh cervical vertebral level. *A.* Frontal radiograph of the cervical spine of a 7-year-old boy. There is an increase in interpediculate distances from the third to the seventh cervical vertebrae. Measurements at the fifth and sixth cervical levels are 34 mm. The upper limit of normal at this age is 29 mm. *B.* Lateral radiograph of the cervical spine. The cervical spine canal is definitely enlarged in anterior-posterior dimension.

In the thoracic cord, the level of a tumor can be approximated by the upper level of motor dysfunction. There may be weakness of upper or lower intercostal muscles, or weakness of upper or lower abdominal muscles. An upper sensory level may correspond to the level of the tumor. The tendon reflexes in the legs are hyperactive, and the plantar responses are frequently extensor.

Tumors of the lumbar cord are associated with weakness in leg muscles and sensory loss in the legs. With involvement of the cauda equina there is weakness and atrophy of leg muscles (Fig. 17-8A), sensory loss, loss of knee and ankle jerks, and urinary retention. Sensory loss may result in trophic ulcers of the buttocks (Fig. 17-8A) or of the heels or soles of the feet (Fig. 17-8B). A subcutaneous lipoma (Fig. 17-8A) or an unusual growth of hair in the midline may be noted in the lumbosacral area.

Laboratory Examination. Radiographs of the spine should include the vertebrae corresponding to the highest possible level of the lesion. Plain radiographs may be normal, particularly with intramedullary tumors. However, they often reveal abnormalities indicative of tumor. There may be a spina bifida associated with a tumor of the cauda equina (Fig. 17-8C and D). The

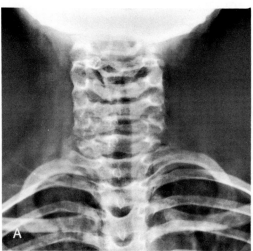

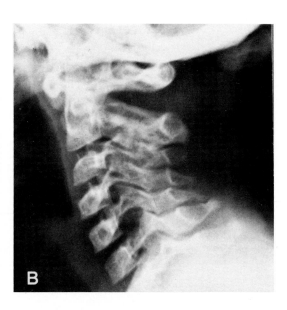

spinal canal may be widened at the level of the tumor and the interpedicular distance may be increased (Figs. 17-9) and 17-10). The pedicles may be thin or eroded (Figs. 17-8C and 17-10). Scalloping of the posterior portions of the vertebral bodies may be prominent (Fig. 17-11A).

If the radiographs of the spine are normal and if the possibility of neoplasm appears remote, lumbar puncture is done. The most important part of this procedure is to test carefully for evidence of partial or complete subarachnoid block, which frequently occurs with spinal cord tumors. Early in the course of tumor, the dynamics may be normal. The cell count is normal, and usu-

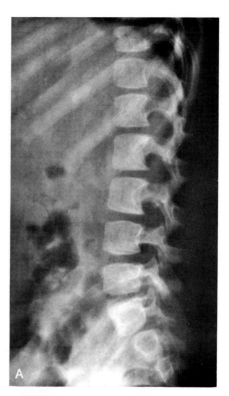

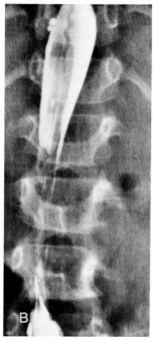

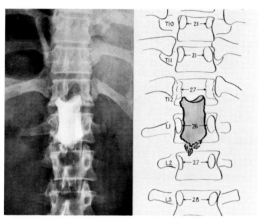

FIG. 17-10. Neurofibroma. On the plain film the increase in the interpediculate distance and the erosion of the pedicle on the right at the twelfth thoracic level are apparent. The myelogram shows complete block at the 12th thoracic level with a smoothly concave curve outlining the inferior border of the tumor. This is characteristic of extramedullary, intradural tumors.

FIG. 17-11. Paravertebral and intraspinal ganglioneuroma. *A.* Radiograph of the lumbar spine, lateral view. Posterior scalloping of all the lumbar vertebrae is present, but this is most marked at the first, second, and third lumbar vertebrae. The spinal canal is widened. *B.* Thoracic and lumbar myelogram. From the 11th thoracic to the first lumbar vertebra, the cord is displaced to the right side of the spinal canal. There is extradural compression of the lumbar subarachnoid space extending from the first to the fourth lumbar vertebra.

ally the protein content is elevated. With subarachnoid block the fluid becomes xanthochromic. If radiographs reveal evidence of probable neoplasm, it is advisable to combine lumbar puncture with myelography.

In a child with complete subarachnoid block due to an extramedullary tumor, myelography characteristically reveals a smooth, concave curve outlining the edge of the tumor (Fig. 17-10). Sometimes a double concave curve is seen. With partial subarachnoid block, myelography may show displacement of the spinal cord by an extradural mass (Fig. 17-11B). With an intramedullary tumor, myelography may reveal enlargement of the cord with a localized mass within the cord.

Differential Diagnosis. Syringomyelia may present a clinical picture very similar to that of intramedullary tumor in a child. If the clinical picture suggesting syringomyelia is associated with the finding on lumbar puncture of subarachnoid block, exploration is necessary in order to make a definite diagnosis. Multiple sclerosis occasionally occurs in children and produces a myelopathy at any level in the spinal cord. The onset is often subacute and may be associated with evidence of optic neuritis or of cerebellar or brain stem dysfunction. The cerebrospinal fluid in multiple sclerosis reveals normal dynamics. There may be an increase in cell count, total protein, or γ-globulin.

Treatment. The treatment of spinal cord tumors is surgical. Benign lesions may be completely removed. Infiltrative lesions may be partially removed with decompression and subsequent irradiation. Intramedullary gliomas may respond to irradiation.

Prognosis. If the tumor is benign and is completely removed, there may be marked improvement in neurologic signs and eventually complete recovery. If the tumor is invasive and not completely removed, irradiation may result in partial remission with subsequent recurrence of progressive weakness and sensory change. With complete paraplegia or tetraplegia, respiratory and bladder infections and decubitus ulcers are common, and these may result in death.

REFERENCES

1. **Altrocchi PH:** Acute spinal epidural abscess *vs.* acute transverse myelopathy. Arch Neurol 9:17, 1963
2. **Altrocchi PH:** Acute transverse myelopathy. Arch Neurol 9:111, 1963
3. **Benady SG:** Spinal muscular atrophy in childhood: Review of 50 cases. Dev Med Child Neurol 20:746, 1978
4. **Buchthal F, Olsen PZ:** Electromyography and muscle biopsy in infantile spinal muscular atrophy. Brain 93:15, 1970
5. **Byers RK, Banker BQ:** Infantile muscular atrophy. Arch Neurol 5:140, 1961
6. **Cross HE, McKusick VA:** The Mast syndrome: A recessively inherited form of presenile dementia with motor disturbances. Arch Neurol 16:1, 1967
7. **Cross HE, McKusick VA:** The Troyer syndrome: A recessive form of spastic paraplegia with distal muscle wasting. Arch Neurol 16:473, 1967
8. **Djindjian R:** Angiography of the spinal cord. Surg Neurol 2:179, 1974
9. **Doppman JL, Wirth FP Jr, Di Chiro G et al:** Value of cutaneous angiomas in the arteriographic localization of spinal-cord arteriovenous malformations. N Engl J Med 281:1440, 1969
10. **Goutieres F, Aicardi J, Farkas E:** Anterior horn cell disease associated with pontocerebellar hypoplasia in infants. J Neurol Neurosurg Psychiatry 40:370, 1977
11. **Guthkelch AN:** Diastematomyelia with a median septum. Brain 97:729, 1974
12. **Haddow JE, Macri JN:** Prenatal screening for neural tube defects. JAMA 242:515, 1979
13. **Harwood-Nash DCF, Fitz CR, Resjo IM et al:** Congenital spinal and cord lesions in children and computed tomographic metrizamide myelography. Neuroradiology 16:69, 1978
14. **Hide DW, Williams HP, Ellis HL:** The outlook for the child with a myelomeningocele for whom early surgery was considered inadvisable. Dev Med Child Neurol 14:304, 1972
15. **Houdart R, Djindjian R, Hurth M et al:** Treatment of angiomas of the spinal cord. Surg Neurol 2:186, 1974
16. **Milunsky A:** Prenatal detection of neural tube defects. VI. Experience with 20,000 pregnancies. JAMA 244:2731, 1980
17. **Perret G:** Symptoms and diagnosis of diastematomyelia. Neurol (Minneap) 10:51, 1960
18. **Sarnat HB, Case ME, Graviss R:** Sacral agenesis. Neurologic and neuropathologic features. Neurology 26:1124, 1976
19. **Sharrard WJ: Meningomyelocele:** Prognosis of immediate operative closure of the sac. Proc R Soc Med 56:510, 1963
20. **Wells CEC, Spillane JD, Bligh AS:** Cervical spinal canal in syringomyelia. Brain 82:23, 1959
21. **Williams B:** A critical appraisal of posterior fossa surgery for communicating syringomyelia. Brain 101:223, 1978

Disorders of Roots, Plexuses, and Peripheral Nerves

Colin D. Hall

Diseases of the peripheral nerves are not common in childhood. Most of the processes that cause neuropathies in adults can also cause them in children, but the etiologies are differently represented.[24] Acute disorders in children are usually due to postinfectious polyneuropathy, occasionally due to exposure to toxic substances. Chronic neuropathies are most commonly due to heredodegenerative diseases. Disorders of metabolism may cause progressive or episodic abnormalities of the peripheral nervous system, which may be masked by concomitant central nervous system involvement. A variety of other conditions must be considered in each case, because accurate diagnosis leads to a logical approach to treatment, prognosis, and counseling of the patients and their families.

Patients suffering from disorders of their peripheral nerves or nerve roots present with varying degrees of flaccid weakness, pain, paresthesias, or sensory loss, and show diminished or absent deep tendon reflexes. Further subclassifications are listed below. The various clinical features can be found under the different headings and possible disease entities can then be found. This method is not infallible, but may provide significant help in considering more specific tests. Appropriate laboratory tests are discussed with each disease. In general, nerve conduction studies and electromyography are helpful to confirm the presence of a neuropathy and delineate its anatomical extent, and to estimate whether the pathologic involvement is primarily that of axonal loss or segmental demyelination (see Chap. 1). Evaluation of the cerebrospinal fluid is helpful in postinfectious polyneuropathy, in some hereditary and storage diseases, and in granulomatous neuropathy, and helps to exclude other conditions, such as meningeal lymphomatosis, poliomyelitis, and multiple sclerosis.

Nerve biopsy should not be undertaken unless adequate handling and evaluation of the pathologic specimen is possible, and this should include evaluation of single teased nerve fibers and electron microscopy[3,c] (Fig. 18-1, 18-2). The findings may be diagnostic in vasculitides, storage diseases, amyloidosis, leprosy, sarcoidosis, and some of the hereditary neuropathies. No single nerve is ideal, but the sural nerve is most often used for biopsy. It has the disadvantage of having no motor fibers, but the advantages of leaving relatively little sensory loss when sectioned and of being easily approachable surgically. Occasionally, the great auricular

A Clinical Approach to the Differentiation of Diseases of the Peripheral Nerves

Extent of Involvement
Mononeuropathy: Only one nerve involved
    (trauma, pressure palsies, vascular disease,
    herpes zoster)
Mononeuropathy Multiplex: Asymmetric
    involvement of more than one peripheral nerve;
    may eventually involve enough nerves to
    become symmetric (diabetes, vasculitides,
    leprosy, hypothyroidism, lead toxicity, brachial
    neuritis)
Polyneuropathy: More or less symmetric, usually
    ascending from the feet (amyloid, Bassen-
    Kornzweig disease, diabetes, diphtheria, Fabry's
    disease, hereditary, Krabbe's disease,
    metachromatic leukodystrophy, nutritional,
    paraneoplastic, porphyria, acute inflammatory
    polyradiculoneuritis, Refsum's disease, toxic,
    Tangier disease, etc.)
Location of Nerves Involved
Most are distal first, with more proximal
    involvement as they progress
    Primarily Proximal: Porphyria, acute inflammatory
        polyradiculoneuritis
Type of Nerves Involved
Most are mixed sensory-motor, but some may show
    predominance of one or other feature.
    Primarily Motor: Diphtheria, hereditary, lead,
        porphyria, acute inflammatory
        polyradiculoneuritis
    Primarily Sensory: Amyloid, arsenic, diabetic,
        hereditary, nutritional, paraneoplastic
    Primarily Autonomic: Amyloid, diabetes, leprosy,
        porphyria, acute inflammatory
        polyradiculoneuritis
Course
Abrupt Onset: With or without subsequent
    improvement (compressive, traumatic, vascular)
Developing Over Days to Weeks: Allergic,
    paraneoplastic, acute inflammatory
    polyradiculoneuritis, toxic
Chronic: Hereditary, storage diseases
Fluctuating Course: Metabolic, toxic with repeated
    exposure, recurrent inflammatory
    polyradiculoneuritis, porphyria
Palpation of the Nerve Trunks
Clinically Enlarged Nerves: The great auricular,
    ulnar, and peroneal nerves are easily palpated
    (hereditary, leprosy, storage diseases)

nerve can be sectioned to show motor fibers, but this leaves a scar in the neck.

Muscle biopsy may confirm the diagnosis of vasculitis, amyloidosis, or granulomatous disease, but again should only be considered by those who are prepared to adequately process and examine the specimen.[18]

THE HEREDITARY NEUROPATHIES

The hereditary neuropathies account for the major group of progressive neuropathies of childhood. Research seems to indicate that they result from a number of different enzymatic and metabolic diseases, but, at present, specific defects can rarely be identified.

There are no reliable clinical, biochemical, electrodiagnostic, or pathologic "markers" that can be used to tabulate the different diseases in this group. Traditionally, hereditary neuropathies were named after clinicians who described them (Charcot, Marie, and Tooth; Roussy and Levy; Dejerinne and Sottas) or after certain outstanding clinical features (peroneal muscular atrophy; hypertrophic neuropathy; congenital indifference to pain). All the attempted classifications are, however, incomplete and will change radically as our knowledge increases.[7,20,21] The following sections give some broad differentiations based on clinical and pathologic findings and may be of some help in prognosis in individual cases.

The hereditary nature of these diseases is often difficult to establish, and careful clinical and electrodiagnostic examination of other family members is essential.

HEREDITARY MOTOR SENSORY NEUROPATHIES (HMSN)

Hereditary motor sensory neuropathies consist predominantly of motor weakness and are slowly progressive over years. There is variable sensory and autonomic dysfunction. The defects are usually but not always symmetrical and affect the lower more than the upper limbs.

HMSN, Segmental Demyelinating Type (Hypertrophic Peroneal Muscular Atrophy, Charcot-Marie-Tooth Disease, HMSN I)

Incidence. The segmental demyelinating type of HMSN is the commonest of the hereditary neuropathies. There are no

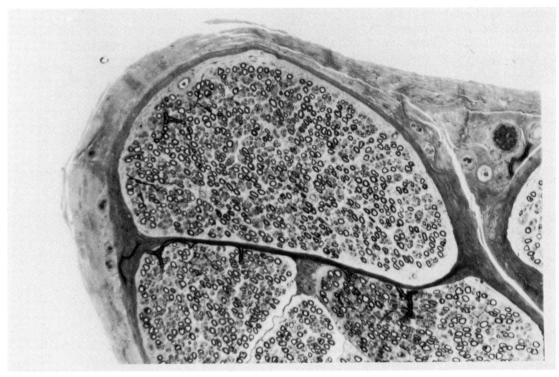

FIG. 18-1. Cross section of normal nerve fascicle. The small dense circles are myelin sheaths. Unmyelinated fibers can be seen scattered between these, without membrane around them.

FIG. 18-2. Normal teased single myelinated nerve fiber. The junction at the center of the illustration is a node of Ranvier, the junction of the myelin sheaths of two adjacent segments of the nerve.

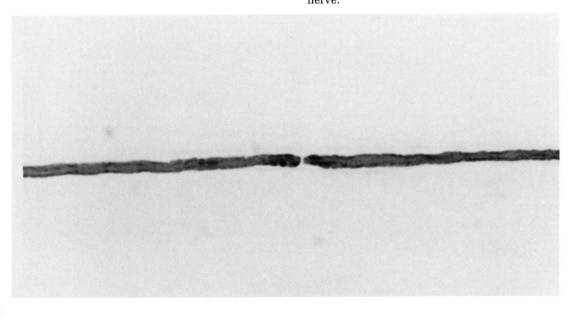

figures available for the incidence or prevalence of any of the hereditary neuropathies, but a neurologist is likely to be following several patients with this disease at any given time.

Genetics. The vast majority of families have an autosomal dominant mode of inheritance. Some autosomal recessive and X-linked recessive modes have been reported. Sporadic cases are not infrequent, and this may be partly due to incomplete family evaluation and marked intrafamily variability of findings.

Pathology. There is predominant loss of myelinated fibers in the peripheral nerves (Fig. 18-3), with repeated attempts at remyelination, which leads to abnormal thickening of the myelin sheaths around in-

dividual axons, yielding "onion-bulbs" (Fig. 18-4). There may also be abnormalities of the posterior columns of the spinal cord.

Clinical Features. There is marked variability in clinical features among different family members. Those who present with weakness generally do so during the second and third decades. There is often a history of prior foot abnormalities, such as flat feet, high arches, or hammer toes. The child becomes progressively more clumsy and has increasing difficulty with running and kicking a ball, and often complains of tripping easily and of weak ankles. The gait may be steppage and may show foot drop, with damage to the toes of shoes. Walking on toes or heels may be impossible. The small muscles of the feet and the anterior tibial compartments show wasting that gives a "stork leg" or "inverted champagne bottle" appearance (Fig. 18-5). As the disease progresses, the proximal leg muscles and muscles of the hands and forearms may become affected with the characteristic claw

FIG. 18-3. Segmental demyelination. The segments of two single teased nerve fibers when seen at the left of the illustration show normal myelination. Following the nodes of Ranvier, the fibers when seen on the right of the illustration have lost their normal myelin cover.

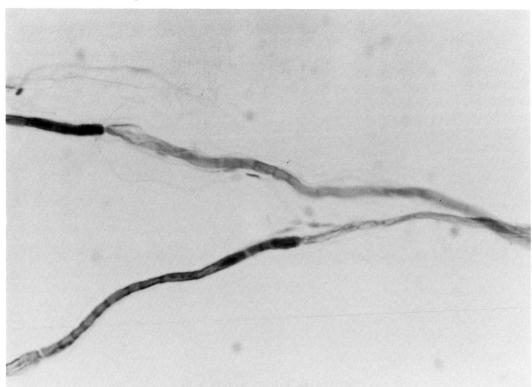

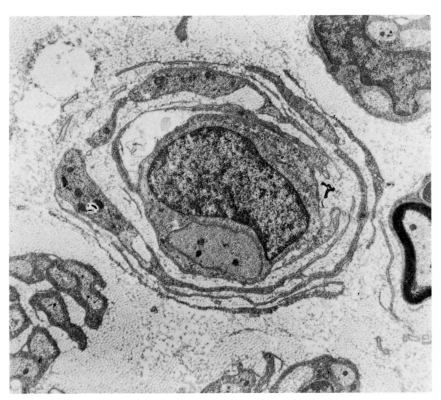

FIG. 18-4. Onion bulb formation. The nerve axon is seen in the central part of the illustration, surrounded by multiple layers of poorly formed regenerating myelin.

hand of intrinsic muscle weakness (Fig. 18-6). Involvement of paraspinal muscles may result in kyphoscoliosis. Sensory loss is usually mild and may be absent initially or throughout the course in relation to the usual standards of measurements, but more sophisticated techniques of evaluation often reveal subtle loss. Deep tendon reflexes are lost in almost all cases, starting with the ankle jerks and progressing slowly to involve the knees and finally the upper limbs. The patient may be areflexic when first seen, but usually upper limb reflexes are preserved at this stage. The peripheral nerves may be enlarged and rubbery.

Laboratory Studies. No specific studies are recommended. Diabetes, thyroid deficiency, toxin exposure, and vitamin deficiencies should be ruled out if appropriate. Nerve conduction velocities are slowed, indicating a segmental demyelinating neuropathy; this feature may often be found in otherwise unaffected parents or siblings.

Differential Diagnosis. The most important conditions to exclude are those due to chronic exposure to environmental toxins such as lead, mercury, and organic solvents. The other hereditary neuropathies and the hereditary disorders of anterior horn cells (Chap. 17) may have quite similar onset and course, but accurate differentiation of these makes little difference to prognosis or therapy. Myotonic dystrophy (Chap. 19) may present with weakness and wasting of the distal limb muscles, no sensory findings, and an autosomal dominant mode of inheritance. Ptosis and weakness of muscles supplied by the lower cranial nerves usually makes the distinction from the neuropathies clear, and this is confirmed by characteristic electromyographic findings.

Treatment. There is no specific treatment available. See section on treatment at the end of this chapter.

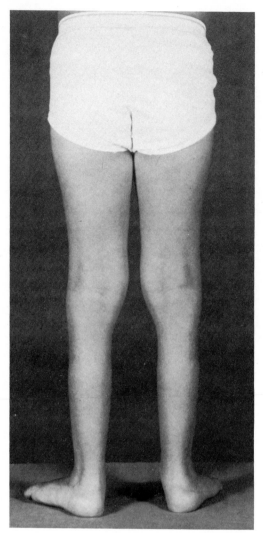

FIG. 18-5. Hereditary motor sensory neuropathy. There is loss of bulk in the gastrocnemii compared to the thigh muscles, giving an "inverted champagne bottle" appearance to the legs. The arches of the feet are poorly formed, and there is a valgus deformity at the ankles.

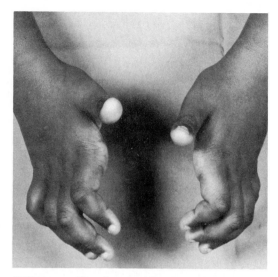

FIG. 18-6. Claw hands. The typical appearance following intrinsic muscle weakness.

Prognosis. The features are very slowly progressive. Life expectancy is probably not significantly reduced, and with suitable choice of occupation, the patient may lead a full and productive life.

HMSN, Axonal Type (HMSN II)

Incidence. The axonal type of HMSN is about one fifth as common as type I.

Genetics. Again, the usual form of inheritance is autosomal dominant.

Pathology. Pathologic changes are the main differentiating features of the two types of HMSN. The nerves show degeneration of some axons with retention of others in a relatively normal state (Fig. 18-7), and there is much less evidence of remyelination, so the nerves do not become clinically thickened.

Clinical Features. The differences between type II and type I HMSN are not great. The clinical presentation of HMSN II tends to be later, and there is more involvement of the posterior calf muscles and less of the hand muscles. Sensory involvement is more common.

Laboratory Studies. Because a significant population of axons remains unaffected, nerve conduction velocities remain normal or only slightly slowed, although there is reduction of amplitude of the compound muscle action potential and denervation on electromyography. These findings indicate an axonal neuropathy.

Differential diagnosis, treatment, and prognosis are no different from those described for type I.

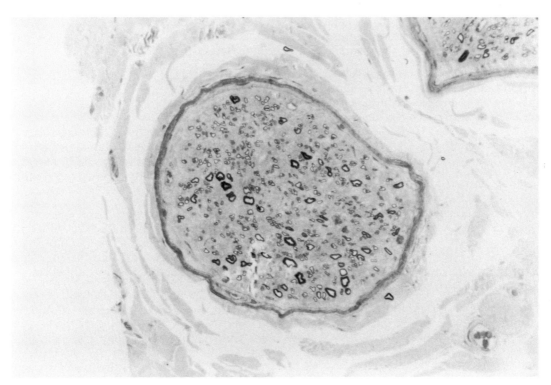

FIG. 18-7. Axonal neuropathy. When compared to Figure 18-1, the density of both mylineated and unmyelinated fibers is seen to be markedly reduced. The remaining fibers are normal in appearance.

Dejerine-Sottas Disease (Hypertrophic Neuropathy of Infancy, HMSN III)

Incidence. Dejerine-Sottas disease is considerably less common than the previous two types of HMSN.

Genetics. Inheritance is autosomal recessive.

Pathology. There is severe disruption of myelin in segments of all myelinated fibers, with marked "onion bulb" formation and nerve hypertrophy (see Fig. 18-4). The posterior columns of the spinal cord may be affected.

Clinical Features. Onset is generally earlier than with types I and II. The early developmental milestones are often delayed, and the child may walk late and may never run adequately. Weakness is more severe and diffuse, often involving proximal as well as distal limb muscles. Skeletal deformities such as pes cavus and kyphoscoliosis are common and may be severe. Sensory loss is frequent and may be marked, with accompanying spontaneous "lightning" pains in the limbs. Areflexia is usual. There may be associated ataxia of the limbs and nystagmus. Pupillary responses and the lower cranial nerves may be affected.[4] The nerves may show marked clinical enlargement, including the great auricular nerve as it courses over the posterior border of the upper sternocleidomastoid muscle.

Laboratory Studies. Cerebrospinal fluid protein values vary from normal to several hundred mg/dl in different patients. Nerve conduction velocities show marked slowing compatible with segmental demyelination.[9]

Differential Diagnosis. When clinical findings are marked in the first few years, the disease must be differentiated from metachromatic leukodystrophy and globoid cell leukodystrophy. When nystagmus and ataxia are prominent, it may be confused with the spinocerebellar degenerations, and indeed these may represent different ends of a clinical spectrum.

Treatment. For those cases that show episodic sudden deterioration, steroid therapy has been suggested, but its value has not been established.

Prognosis. These patients generally show more incapacity than HMSN type I or II patients. Activities of daily living may be severely impaired, and independent existence may be impossible in later life. Often they are wheelchair bound in the third or fourth decade. Occasionally, there is a more benign course.

Hereditary Neuropathy With Liability to Pressure Palsies

Incidence. Hereditary neuropathy with liability to pressure palsies is another rare familial neuropathy.

Genetics. Transmission is autosomal dominant.

Pathology. Biopsy of the sural nerve, whether clinically affected or not, shows characteristic sausage-shaped swellings in the teased nerve fibers,[5] leading to the name *tomaculous neuropathy* (Fig. 18-8).

Clinical Features. Generally, patients are symptom-free until they undergo trauma to the peripheral nerve; this may be only very minor compression, such as sleeping on the arm or leaning on the elbow. A motor and sensory loss develops in the distribution of the affected nerve or nerves, and there may be reflex loss and wasting of the affected muscles. Some cases present as recurring brachial plexus neuropathy.[10]

Laboratory Studies. Slowing of nerve conduction velocities is found in both affected and unaffected nerves, and may also be seen in clinically unaffected family members.

Differential Diagnosis. If there is no family history, the first attack is generally misdiagnosed as a common uncomplicated pressure palsy. A clue may be electrical slowing in clinically unaffected nerves.

Treatment. General physical therapy and supportive measures should be carried out as described under the section on treatment. The patient and identified family members should be advised on methods to avoid compression of susceptible peripheral nerves.

Prognosis. There is an excellent chance of recovery from each individual episode. Recurring involvement of the same nerve or prolonged compression may at times lead to permanent residual loss of function.

FIG. 18-8. Tomaculous neuropathy. Two sausage-shaped enlargements of teased nerve fiber can be easily seen.

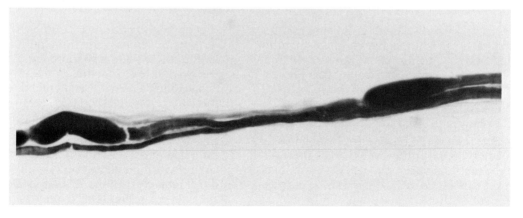

THE HEREDITARY SENSORY NEUROPATHIES (HSN)

The hereditary sensory neuropathies are very rare, poorly understood conditions, and their classification remains incomplete. The following classification is based on that of Dyck and Ohta[21] and tries to make order out of a series of terms such as *congenital indifference to pain, Denny-Brown's disease,* and *hereditary sensory radicular neuropathy.*

HSN Type 1

Genetics. HSM type 1 is an autosomal dominant disorder.

Pathology. Fiber loss is mostly of the smallest diameter unmyelinated fibers, and least of the large diameter myelinated fibers.

Clinical Features. The onset is usually insidious in the second decade or later and is usually limited to the lower limbs. There is loss of pinprick and temperature sensation, and this leads to recurring, at times unnoticed, ulcerations about the feet that may eventually lead to osteomyelitis and loss of toes or feet. Vibration and joint position senses are less affected. Foot deformities are common. Deep tendon reflexes are depressed or absent, and some degree of motor weakness may be present. Sphincter and sexual function are unaffected.

Laboratory Studies. Sensory nerve conduction responses are absent. Motor nerve conduction velocities are normal.

Differential Diagnosis. Without a family history, other neuropathies that may give perforating ulcers must be considered. These are rare in children, and include leprosy and diabetes.

Treatment. Exceptional care must be taken to avoid foot trauma. Footwear should be chosen carefully and podiatric advice sought regularly. Infections should be vigorously treated.

Prognosis. If infection is adequately treated and care is taken to avoid trauma, a normal life expectancy is the rule.

HSN Type II

Genetics. HSN type II is an autosomal recessive disorder.

Pathology. In sural nerve, there is almost total loss of myelinated fibers with relative sparing of unmyelinated fibers.

Clinical Features. The onset is in infancy or early childhood. All limbs are involved. All sensation is affected, touch and pressure more than pain and temperature. Undetected bone fractures are common. Deep tendon reflexes are depressed or absent. Some autonomic dysfunction is not uncommon.

Laboratory Studies. Sensory nerve action potentials are absent on nerve conduction studies.

Differential diagnosis is the same as that for HSN I. With hand involvement, syringomyelia and intrinsic neoplasms of the cervical cord must be considered.

Treatment is the same as that for HSN I.

Prognosis. Insufficient follow-up studies are available to know the overall prognosis.

HSN Type III (Dysautonomia, Riley-Day Syndrome)

Genetics. HSN type III is an autosomal recessive condition. Most patients are from Jewish families.

Pathology. The sural nerve shows primarily loss of unmyelinated fibers. In addition, autopsy studies may show abnormalities of the brain stem, lower cranial nerve nuclei, cerebral cortex, and spinal cord.

Clinical Features. The onset is usually in infancy. There is insensitivity to pain. Autonomic dysfunction may be marked, with decreased lacrimation, increased sweating, hypertension, hypotension, and loss of temperature control. Deep tendon reflexes are depressed or absent. Babies often feed poorly and have recurring chest infections and episodes of vomiting. There may be some mental retardation. A constant feature is the absence of fungiform papillae on the tongue.[14]

Laboratory Studies. At times there may be slight slowing of nerve conduction velocities. There may be an absent flare response to intradermal histamine. There is increased excretion of homovanillic acid and reduced excretion of vanillylmandelic acid in the urine, with normal metanephrines and normetanephrines. Serum dopamine B-hydroxylase is reduced.

Treatment. Again, trauma should be avoided and infection treated vigorously. There is no specific therapy.

Prognosis. Death within the first 5 years is common, usually secondary to aspiration pneumonia. Patients rarely live beyond the second decade.

HEREDITARY NEUROPATHIES ASSOCIATED WITH OTHER INVOLVEMENT OF THE NEURAXIS

A significant problem with the classification of the hereditary neuropathies is that the clinical features frequently vary dramatically, not only between families but even within the same family. Thus, one family member may show severe clinical evidence of disease whereas the parent or sibling may have only mildly delayed nerve conduction velocity as evidence of involvement. Also, some families show cortical, cerebellar, and spinal involvement in addition to a peripheral neuropathy, which may be a mild incidental finding or the overwhelming clinical abnormality. With the exception of Friedreich's ataxia (Chapter 16), our current level of knowledge does not make further classification of these disease processes helpful.

DISEASES BELIEVED TO RESULT FROM INBORN ERRORS OF METABOLISM

Diseases believed to result fron inborn metabolic errors probably include all the hereditary neuropathies, but certain diseases, often multisystem in their involvement, that most commonly present in childhood can appropriately be considered under this heading. Involvement of the peripheral nervous system varies from being the predominant clinical feature to being an unusual or minor additional finding.

HEREDOPATHIA ATACTICA POLYNEURITIFORMIS (REFSUM'S DISEASE)

Heredopathia atactica polyneuritiformis is one neuropathy in which we have a specific biochemical "marker," allowing a definitive diagnosis. There is a failure of phytanic acid metabolism, leading to buildup of serum levels of this substance that occurs in no other known condition.[39]

Incidence. This is one of the rarest of clinical diseases, with under 100 reported cases. Most have lived in Northern Europe.

Genetics. Inheritance is by the autosomal recessive mode.

Pathology. There is macroscopic nerve thickening. The nerves show demyelination and marked "onion bulb" formation. Electron microscopy reveals lipid granules and large crystallinelike inclusions in Schwann cells. In addition, there are focal areas of demyelination in the brain stem and increased fat deposition in the meninges.

Clinical Features. The general clinical features may vary in severity and age of onset, but the major findings are remarkably constant.[32] The eyes, skin, heart, and nervous system are almost always involved. The onset is between early childhood and the third decade, usually insidious but occasionally acute and sometimes precipitated by intercurrent infections. Night blindness may be the first feature, and all eventually show this and retinitis pigmentosa. One third of patients have had cataracts. Miosis and poor pupillary responses are not uncommon. Nystagmus is fairly frequent. Skin changes vary from slight drying to marked ichthyosis. Most patients show cardiomyopathy or tachycardia. Skeletal changes in the feet are common, and there may be epiphyseal dysplasia at the shoulders, elbows, and knees. Hearing defects are often present early and may result in complete deafness. Anosmia may occur. The neuropathy is generally symmetrical, starting in the lower limbs. Both motor and sensory fibers are affected. The disease progresses gradually or episodically, often to affect the truncal musculature as well as the limbs. There is progressive loss of deep tendon reflexes. Peripheral nerves may be palpably enlarged. There is often ataxia of the trunk and limbs which, in association with the nystagmus, may represent cerebellar involvement.

Laboratory Studies. Cerebrospinal fluid protein levels are raised and may be up to 700 mg/dl. Nerve conduction velocities may show marked slowing. There are frequent conduction defects apparent on electrocardiography. Phytanic acid levels in serum are high, representing up to 30% of serum lipid. There is phytanic acid accumulation in body organs. Skin fibroblasts in culture show marked reduction in their ability to oxidize phytanic acid.

Differential Diagnosis. The other heredodegenerative neuropathies must be considered. The cerebellar features may suggest Friedreich's ataxia or other spinocerebellar degenerations; the presence of retinitis and skin changes helps to exclude these. Bassen-Kornzweig disease must also be considered. Estimation of serum phytanic acid is a specific diagnostic test.

Treatment. Recent reports of therapy using a low phytanic acid diet plus plasmapheresis are very encouraging and suggest that the defects may be reversible and controllable.

Prognosis. It is too early to know the long-term prognosis with modern treatment methods. Untreated, the disease may progress inexorably or may show marked fluctuation. Death may result from severe neuropathy or may occur suddenly from cardiac causes.

ANGIOKERATOMA CORPORIS DIFFUSUM (FABRY'S DISEASE)

Angiokeratoma corporis diffusum is a rare multisystem storage disease in which the principal clinical symptoms are due to peripheral nerve involvement.[12]

Genetics. Transmission is by X-linked recessive mode. Female carriers may also show clinical features.

Pathology. There are crystalline inclusions of abnormal substance in many organs. The peripheral nerves show variable involvement with stored material and some reduction in unmyelinated fibers.

Biochemistry. There is increased storage of ceramide trihexoside in different body organs, due to a reduction in activity of the enzyme ceramide trihexosidase.[11]

Clinical Features. The commonest clinical presentation is of burning dysesthesias and tenderness in the feet and lower legs in boys and young men. Usually there will be a reddish-purple maculopapular rash over the abdomen, scrotum, inguinal, and gluteal areas. There may be telangiectasias of the nail beds, conjunctival membranes and oral mucous membranes. Corneal opacities are probably always present. Other features include anhidrosis, cardiomegaly, hypertenison, and cerebrovascular disease. Renal failure eventually results from deposition in the kidneys. Heterozygotic female carriers may have leg pains, but these generally come on later in life. They may have mild renal disease and corneal clouding.

Laboratory Studies. Renal function test results may be abnormal. Ceramide trihexosidase may be estimated by radioactive enzyme assay. An easier and reliable study is to demonstrate reduced alpha-galactosidase activity in cultured skin fibroblasts. Prenatal diagnosis is also possible by estimation of alpha-galactosidase activity in amniotic fluid. Nerve conduction studies are normal.

Treatment. In some cases, pain relief is obtained using phenytoin, starting with 5 mg/kg per day. Hemodialysis is of great value as a palliative therapy. There are reports of permanent benefit following renal transplantation, which appears to supply a permanent and sufficient amount of ceramide trihexosidase. A means of direct enzyme replacement is also being developed.

Prognosis. Untreated, the patient usually dies in his 40s as a result of renal failure or cerebrovascular disease. It is hoped that modern therapy will drastically improve this condition.

ABETALIPOPROTEINEMIA (BASSEN-KORNZWEIG DISEASE)

Abetalipoproteinemia is a rare multisystem disease that may show a significant peripheral neuropathy.[25]

Genetics. Transmission is by autosomal recessive mode.

Pathology. There have been very few studies of the pathology of the peripheral nerve. There is mild segmental demyelination with some axonal loss.

Clinical Features. Generally, features start in infancy with steatorrhoea and malabsorption. Affected children gradually develop weakness and areflexia. There is often a "glove-stocking" sensory loss, and scoliosis and foot deformities. There is usually central nervous system involvement, with ataxia, dysarthria, and intention tremor. Nystagmus, chorea, and extensor plantar responses may develop. Retinal depigmentation and an atypical retinitis pigmentosa develop from about age 5 years and progress to eventually give scotomas and visual deterioration. Cardiomegaly may occur.

Laboratory Studies. There are characteristic changes in blood constituents. Acanthocytes, red blood cells with spiky or thorny protruberances, are found from infancy; they are best seen in a wet preparation of fresh blood. Plasma cholesterol is low, and there is absence of plasma low density lipoproteins and chylomicrons. There may be a mild reduction in motor nerve conduction velocity.

Differential Diagnosis. Several families have been reported with acanthocytosis and a variety of neurologic abnormalities but without abnormalities in plasma lipoproteins. The relationship of these factors to this disease is unclear.

Treatment. A diet low in long-chain triglycerides with vitamin replacement is recommended.

Prognosis. The neurologic symptoms generally progress through childhood and adolescence but stabilize in early adulthood. Death may result from cardiac failure.

ANALPHALIPOPROTEINEMIA (TANGIER DISEASE)

Analphalipoproteinemia is another rare autosomal recessive disease involving abnormalities of cholesterol metabolism. Fifty percent of those involved develop peripheral neuropathy.[25]

Pathology. Multiple body organs show foam cells full of cholesteryl esters and free cholesterol. These are seen in Schwann cells of peripheral nerves. Peripheral nerves show marked loss of unmyelinated and large myelinated fibers.

Clinical Features. There is organomegaly due to deposition of cholesteryl esters. The tonsils are invariably enlarged and are yellow-orange in color. Hepatosplenomegaly is frequent. Signs of peripheral neuropathy may develop at any stage from early childhood to adulthood. This may progress as mononeuropathy multiplex, particularly involving sensory fibers carrying pain and temperature appreciation, but motor fibres are also involved. Some patients show predilection for the cranial nerves to be involved.

Laboratory Studies. There is marked reduction in plasma cholesterol and dramatic increase in high-density lipoproteins. Cerebrospinal fluid protein is occasionally mildly elevated. Biopsy of skin, rectal mucosa, or nerve will show the vacuolated foam cells.

Differential Diagnosis. The progressive, patchy mononeuropathy multiplex may resemble that found in leprosy. However, the hematologic findings and the clinical evidence of characteristic tonsillar hypertrophy are characteristic. Rare cases of similar but not identical cholesteryl ester storage disease have been reported.

Prognosis. The prognosis is variable. Tonsillar hypertrophy may lead to sudden death in childhood. Adults frequently succumb to cardiovascular complications.

SUBACUTE NECROTIZING ENCEPHALOMYELITIS (LEIGH'S SYNDROME) AND OTHER PYRUVATE DEHYDROGENASE COMPLEX DEFICIENCIES

Peripheral nerve involvement is probably present in many cases of pyruvate dehydrogenase complex deficiency, but it is an unusual clinical presentation. Occasional cases of Leigh's syndrome have been reported with clinical peripheral neuropathy and an increase in cerebrospinal fluid protein.[37]

METACHROMATIC LEUKODYSTROPHY

Metachromatic leukodystrophy is a storage disease due to deficiency of the enzyme arylsulfatase A. There is increased storage of sulfatide throughout the nervous system.

Genetics. Transmission is by autosomal recessive mode.

Pathology. Sural nerve biopsy always shows abnormality. There is a reduction in myelinated fibers with an accumulation of metachromatic granules.

Clinical Features. Most cases present in early childhood. The clinical features are predominantly due to brain involvement. After normal development for 15 to 18 months, the child shows progressive deterioration in gait, with weakness and ataxia. There will also be mental deterioration. At this time, there may be evidence of peripheral nerve involvement with hypotonia and hyporeflexia of the legs and perhaps the arms.[49] Neuralgic pain and muscle cramps are common. As the disease progresses, the central features predominate, with tetraplegia, severe mental changes, and often seizures, leading to decerebrate rigidity, blindness, and bulbar palsy.

Juvenile and adult forms of the disease occur, but these do not show clinical evidence of peripheral neuropathy.

Laboratory Studies. Cerebrospinal fluid protein is raised, generally to 100 to 200 mg/dl. Motor nerve conduction velocities are markedly delayed. There is increased sulfatide in the urine and reduced arylsulfatase A activity in the blood. Occasionally, metachromatic granules can be identified in the urine.

Differential Diagnosis. The differential is generally from the other degenerative brain diseases. The presence of hypotonia and reflex loss in this situation could suggest Krabbe's disease.

Treatment. There is no adequate therapy.

Prognosis. In the infantile form, the progress is inexorable, and death occurs in 2 to 4 years. The forms with later onset have a more protracted course.

GLOBOID CELL LEUKODYSTROPHY (KRABBE'S DISEASE)

Krabbe's disease results from deficiency of the enzyme cerebroside beta-galactosidase. Symptoms generally start in the first few months of life. There may initially be some hypotonia and hyporeflexia, indicating peripheral nerve involvement,[19] but upper motor neuron abnormalities predominate. Cerebrospinal fluid protein is frequently increased, and motor nerve conduction velocity is reduced in 50% of patients. Nerve biopsy usually shows little microscopic abnormality, but there are frequently inclusions in Schwann cells.

OTHER LEUKODYSTROPHIES

Structural abnormalities of peripheral nerves are found in adrenoleukodystrophy,[38] Canavan's disease, Cockayne's syndrome,[36] and Pelizaeus-Merzbacher disease.

These are not of significant clinical or diagnostic importance.

GIANT AXONAL NEUROPATHY

Giant axonal neuropathy is a recently described condition that presents as ataxia and peripheral neuropathy in the first years of life in children who appear to have rather typical pale reddish, tight-curly hair. Central nervous system involvement is minor but may include extensor plantar responses and abnormalities of the electroencephalogram. Sural nerve biopsy shows giant balloonlike swelling of the axons containing characteristic neurofilamentous masses.[36]

INFANTILE NEUROAXONAL DYSTROPHY (SEITELBERGER'S DISEASE)

Hypotonia and atrophy with loss of pain sensation are occasionally seen in this condition, suggesting involvement of the peripheral nervous system, and peripheral nerve biopsy has been reported to be of diagnostic value.[48]

NIEMANN-PICK DISEASE

In type A, the classic form of this disease, hypotonia and areflexia are common Demyelination of the peripheral nerves with cytoplasmic inclusions in Schwann cells has been reported in association with reduced nerve conduction velocities.[27]

THE MUCOPOLYSACCHARIDOSES

The peripheral nervous system is generally uninvolved in the mucopolysaccharidoses (see Chap. 9). In Scheie's syndrome (mucopolysaccharidosis type 5), there is a very high incidence of carpal tunnel syndrome. Morquio's disease (mucopolysaccharidosis type 4) may show nerve root compression secondary to spinal deformity, particularly in the cervical area.

ATAXIA-TELANGIECTASIA (LOUIS-BAR SYNDROME)

Features of peripheral neuropathy may occur later in the course of ataxia-telangiectasia but they are overshadowed by intellectual deterioration, disorders of eye and body movement, and cerebellar abnormalities. Nerve biopsy may show neuronal loss.

CHEDIAK-HIGASHI SYNDROME

A rare inherited disorder that usually causes death through a lymphoreticular malignancy, Chediak-Higashi syndrome is characterized by the presence of huge subcellular granules in the leukocytes and cells of other tissues. Various associated neurologic abnormalities have been described, for example, mental retardation, seizures, nystagmus, muscular weakness, and neuropathies. One child with a progressive peripheral neuropathy was described in whom the specific granules could be demonstrated in Schwann cells.[34]

THE TOXIC NEUROPATHIES

Many different chemical and industrial compounds are toxic to the peripheral nervous system. Some agents worth considering can be found in the list below. As clinical observations continue, this list will undoubtedly increase. Drug-induced neuropathies are usually established by history and by improvement on removal of the offending agent, and metal neuropathies are generally associated with toxic levels of the metal in blood and urine. Neuropathies due to industrial agents are much commoner in adults working with these substances, but occasionally may occur in exposed children. Diagnosis is difficult, and depends upon the exclusion of the other known causes of neuropathy plus painstaking detection of possible toxins in the environment.

Generally, these neuropathies cause axonal damage rather than segmental demyelination. They result in a slowly progressive loss of function, usually starting in the feet and progressing later to the hands and trunk. Sensory dysesthesias and glove- and -stocking sensory loss are usually present before motor loss. At times, heavy exposure may lead to rapid deterioration.

It is not possible to cover each of these entities. The following, however, have particular significance in childhood.

Toxic Agents That May Cause Neuropathies in Childhood

Drugs	Metals
Amitriptyline	Arsenic
Amphotericin B	Gold
Chloramphenicol	Lead
Chloroquine	Mercury
Clinoquin	Thallium
Dapsone	
Ergotamine	**Industrial Agents**
Ethambutol	Acrylamide
Ethionamide	Carbon disulphide
Glutethimide	Carbon monoxide
Hydralazine	Carbon tetrachloride
Imipramine	Gasoline
Isoniazid	Glue (sniffing)
Nitrofurantoin	Herbicides
Nitrogen mustards	Hexane
Nitrous oxide	Hexachlorophene
Phenytoin	Insecticides
Stilbamidine	Kepone
Sulfonamides	Organophosphates
Thalidomide	Trichlorethylene
Vinblastine	Triethyl tin
Vincristine	

DRUG TOXICITY

Amitriptyline and Imipramine Toxicity

Amitriptyline and imipramine are antidepressant agents occasionally used in childhood bedwetting and other conditions. A complaint of sensory dysesthesias or mild numbness of the distal limbs is not uncommon. Frank neuropathic changes are unusual.

Chloramphenicol Toxicity

A mild sensory neuropathy with diminished deep tendon reflexes has rarely been reported in patients taking high dosages of chloramphenicol. Optic nerve involvement may also occur, with diminution in visual acuity.[47] There is full recovery on terminating therapy.

Dapsone Toxicity

Dapsone is the most commonly employed agent in the treatment of leprosy. In high doses, it may cause a peripheral neuropathy that is primarily motor.[28]

Glutethimide (Doriden) Toxicity

Glutethimide may cause a primarily sensory neuropathy. Accidental or deliberate overdosage may cause pupillary areflexia and asymmetry, which is not related to the degree of coma.

Isoniazid Toxicity

Incidence and Etiology. A peripheral neuropathy, usually of mild degree, may result from administration of isoniazid for tuberculosis. Occurrence, however, is unknown before adolescence. In adults the incidence is partly dose-related, being rare when dosage is maintained at 3 to 5 mg/kg body weight per day. Children, however, tolerate 10 to 20 mg/kg without developing this complication, perhaps because of more rapid inactivation. The exact pathophysiology is uncertain, but there is evidence that isoniazid combines with pyridoxine to form a hydrazone, which is excreted in the urine. In addition, isoniazid can be shown to inhibit pyridoxine-dependent enzymatic reactions.

Clinical Features. Tingling and numbness may appear in the hands and feet within 3 weeks of the onset of treatment, but is more common after 2 to 3 months. Weakness is not prominent, but the deep tendon reflexes are reduced or absent. Convulsions and mental changes may also occur in some patients.

Prophylaxis and Treatment. Daily administration of 10 mg pyridoxine for every 100 mg isoniazid administered prevents the development of neuropathy and produces recovery in the majority of patients if neuropathy has already appeared.[41]

Ethionamide and Hydralazine Toxicity

Ethionaminde and hydralazine also appear to cause a peripheral neuropathy due to induced pyridoxine deficiency.

Nitrofurantoin (Furadantin, Macrodantin) Toxicity

Nitrofurantoin causes a symmetric sensory-motor neuropathy, occasionally associated with marked dysesthesias. Symptoms may occur early in treatment, or only after many months of medication. There may be very rapid deterioration within a few days of the onset. Impaired renal function increases the risks of peripheral neuropathy with the nitrofurantions, and is an indication for using alternative therapy. The degree of recovery depends on the severity of symptoms when medication is stopped.[44]

Nitrous Oxide Toxicity

A severe sensory-motor neuropathy has been reported with the illegal use of nitrous oxide for recreational purposes.[33]

Phenytoin (Dilantin) Toxicity

The long-term use of the anticonvulsant agent phenytoin is associated with a reduction in nerve conduction velocity and, at times, with diminution of deep tendon reflexes.[35] Other neuropathic changes are rare, and if they occur, other etiologies should be sought.

Thalidomide Toxicity

Thalidomide is of major historic importance because it did much to shape the approach to the evaluation and legalization of new therapeutic agents in the United States. Its teratogenic effects caused its withdrawal from the world market in 1961. It also caused a permanent sensory-motor neuropathy with significant dysesthetic symptoms.

Vinca Alkaloid (Vincristine and Vinblastine) Toxicity

There is a very high degree of peripheral neuropathic change with the use of the chemotherapeutic agents vincristine and vinblastine. Vincristine is the more toxic of the two. The effects are dose-related. Almost all patients show diminution of or absence of deep tendon reflexes, particularly at the ankles. Paresthesias in the hands and feet are followed by objective sensory loss and eventually motor weakness which may become severe. At times, the progression of the neuropathy is very rapid and mimics acute postinfectious polyradiculoneuropathy. Clinical recovery is usually excellent on reduction or termination of the dosage, but these children will continue to show reduced deep tendon reflexes and slowing of nerve conduction velocities, even years later. The decision on whether to stop therapy may be difficult, and requires a balance between therapeutic need and the degree of the neuropathy.[22]

METAL TOXICITY

Arsenic Toxicity

Incidence and Etiology. Arsenic poisoning is responsible for most heavy metal neuropathies. Through the centuries, arsenic has been used in many medicinal preparations, but there is now no valid reason for its therapeutic use. Poisoning is now generally from exposure to inorganic arsenites used in insecticides, rodenticides, and occasionally in paint and wallpaper preparations. This may be by accidental ingestion, inhalation, or skin exposure, but is more frequently the result of direct homicidal or suicidal attempt. In our experience, correct diagnosis is vital in homicide attempts, because there is often severe psychopathology in the attempting murderer, and other family members are also at grave risk.

Pathology. The brain and spinal cord may be involved as well as the peripheral nerves. Anterior horn cell loss is common. The nerves show an axonal neuropathy, often associated with marked interstitial fibrosis.

Clinical Features. Acute arsenic ingestion leads to a fairly characteristic picture.[30] Initially, there is severe colicky abdominal pain, thirst, nausea, vomiting, and diarrhea that may become blood stained. There is evidence of nephritis, often with hematuria. If the patient survives this stage, marrow depression may occur in a few days, with resulting anemia. The skin may show a dusky brownish discoloration, and there is frequent hyperkeratosis and sloughing of the surface of the palms and soles. Neuropathic features develop 1 to 2 weeks after the exposure. There are marked sensory symptoms, often with severe pain and dysesthesias, and motor loss in a distal stocking-glove distribution. There may also be involvement of the cranial nerves, particularly the motor 5th and 7th. The neuropathy is generally progressive for 1 to 2 weeks before stabilizing.

Chronic arsenical poisoning may be much more insidious. The patient often complains of nonspecific malaise, nausea, anorexia, weakness, and alteration in bowel habit. There may be hepatosplenomegaly. The skin again shows increased pigmentation and keratosis, and there may be chronic evidence of anemia. The neuropathy varies from mild sensory disturbances in the feet and legs to severe sensory and motor loss in all limbs. Symptoms depend on the level and duration of exposure. Significant degrees of tolerance may develop following chronic low level ingestion.

A helpful clinical sign is the appearance of transverse white lines in the beds of the fingernails and toenails (Mees' lines; Fig, 18-9), which are due to deposition of arsenic in the forming nail at the time of high tissue levels. These appear in the visible nails some 4 to 6 weeks after exposure, and grow out over the next 5 to 6 months. They may be multiple in cases of repeated intoxication. Similar lines may be seen with thallium and other heavy metal exposure.

Laboratory Studies. There may be a

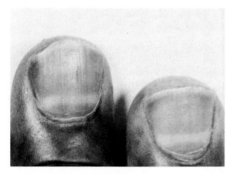

FIG. 18-9. Mees' lines in arsenical polyneuritis.

concomitant anemia. In the acute stages, blood arsenic levels are increased, and urine arsenic levels will rise within 12 hours of exposure, remaining elevated for up to 2 weeks following one administration and often for months after chronic administration. Tissue levels remain high for considerably longer periods. Arsenic deposits may be found in the hair, appearing in a few weeks in the proximal portion of the visible hair, and often remaining for years in pubic and head hair. Arsenic can be retrieved from skeletal bones after other tissues have totally degenerated. Generally, in cases of suspected poisoning, 24-hour urine collection is the most rewarding study, but occasionally nail beds or hair must be examined to confirm the diagnosis. Cerebrospinal fluid protein may occasionally be significantly elevated. Frequently, evoked nerve potentials can not be elicited, or they may show changes compatible with an axonal neuropathy.

Differential Diagnosis. Acute intermittent porphyria, lead, and thallium toxicity may present with similar abdominal pain followed by neuropathy. The chronic neuropathy may simulate many other forms of progressive sensory-motor involvement. In our experience, the initial symptoms of abdominal discomfort are often misdiagnosed in a child as a nonspecific viral infection, and the neuropathy may be confused with postinfectious acute inflammatory polyradiculoneuropathy.

Treatment. It is not clear that any form of therapy is helpful after the neuropathy has developed. There is some evidence that treatment with dimercaprol (BAL) or penicillamine may be valuable in the initial stages of exposure.

An important part of treatment is investigation of the social and family situation, with the assistance of law enforcement agencies. Unexplained or poorly explained deaths of other family members may be an indication for exhumation and evaluation for arsenic poisoning. We have seen several cases of repeated poisoning of the same patient or other family members, even after the initial diagnosis was made and (ineffective) legal action taken.

Prognosis. With mild neuropathy, recovery may be expected. With more severe loss, there is usually a significant residual defect of both motor and sensory function, and some patients continue to have marked painful dysesthetic symptoms.

Lead Toxicity

Incidence and Etiology. The primary risk of lead exposure in children was due to the use of lead in house paints. Commercial paint now contains no lead, but children living in older city areas may still be exposed owing to the ingestion of flaking old paint from the walls. Fumes from burning lead batteries, gasoline exposure, and contamination by dust carried in the clothing of parents who work in lead environments may also result in clinical disease However, children are much more liable to develop encephalopathic features, and peripheral neuropathy due to lead in this age group is very uncommon.[42]

Pathology. Despite much investigation, it is not clear whether lead damages primarily the nerve cell, axon, or Schwann cell.

Clinical Features. The commonest childhood presentation of lead toxicity is encephalopathy; neuropathy is not usually associated. When neuropathy occurs, it is more commonly a motor mononeuropathy, or mononeuropathy multiplex with little or no sensory abnormality. The nerves of the lower limb are more commonly involved, and foot drop may be the initial presentation. There may be a history of colicky abdominal pain. Lead may be deposited in the gums as a "lead line," which is a bluish linear discoloration, particularly prominent about carious teeth. A condition resembling amyotrophic lateral sclerosis, with hypotonia and fasciculations, has been reported as due to lead intoxication. This should be considered in the differential diagnosis of hypotonic infants.

Laboratory Studies. Anemia with basophilic stippling of the red cells is common with chronic intoxication. A lead line appears in the roentgenograms of long bones in children. Serum delta aminolevulenic acid and coproporphyrin levels are raised, but porphobilinogen levels are usually within normal limits, helping to differentiate this from acute intermittent porphyria. Nerve conduction velocities are frequently not significantly affected.

Treatment. Chelation with dimercaprol (BAL) or penicillamine is necessary when clinical features are associated with a high serum lead level. There is no agreed upper limit of normal for lead in childhood, but consideration should be given to chelation if the serum level is greater than 50 ug/dl. Mobilization of lead stored from bone following treatment may give a further rise in serum lead and require repeated chelation. Every effort must be made to identify and remove the source of exposure.

Prognosis. There is inadequate information as to recovery of the neuropathy following chelation in childhood.

Thallium

Thallium is no longer found in human medicinal agents. However, it is present in some insecticides and rodenticides, and rare accidental or homicidal poisoning is encountered. Clinical presentation is similar to arsenic poisoning.[16] There is initial gastrointestinal disturbance with progressive, often primarily sensory, neuropathy. There may be hyperkeratosis, and Mees' lines may be seen in the nails. A characteristic clinical picture is alopecia, which usually appears some 2 to 4 weeks after exposure. There is no treatment of proven value, although some reports suggest that sodium diethyldithiocarbamate may be of benefit.

TOXICITY OF INDUSTRIAL AGENTS

In high doses, toxic industrial agents usually result in encephalopathy and liver disease, masking any effects on the peripheral nervous system. Chronic low dose exposure may result in a progressive peripheral neuropathy.

Organophosphate Toxicity: Triorthocresyl Phosphate

The organophosphate insecticides cause acute neurologic illness due to cholinergic block. This can lead to rapid diffuse paralysis and central nervous system effects including seizures; it is rapid in onset, and is frequently fatal within 24 hours. One of these agents, triorthocresyl phosphate (TOCP), also causes a peripheral neuropathy, which has been extensively studied in the animal model.

Incidence. There have been several mass outbreaks of TOCP poisoning due to contamination of large amounts of food or drink. These include "ginger-jake" paralysis from contaminated alcohol in the United States in 1929, and an epidemic in Morocco in 1959 involving 10,000 people, 20% of whom were children. Isolated cases are uncommon.

Pathology. There is an axonal neuropathy, with the largest diameter and longest nerve fibers most affected. There are also central nervous system effects, particularly in the lateral and dorsal columns of the spinal cord.[15]

Clinical Features. High dose exposure leads to acute gastrointestinal symptoms; this appears to be uncommon in children. One to three weeks after the exposure, a peripheral neuropathy develops, with paresthesias rapidly progressing to weakness of the lower and then the upper limbs. Sensory loss is mild or absent. Unlike most neuropathies, deep tendon reflexes are frequently preserved and are often increased, accompanied by other upper motor neuron features such as spasticity and extensor plantar responses, particularly with progression of the disease.

Laboratory Studies. Electrodiagnostic studies may show the features of an axonal neuropathy without significant slowing of nerve conduction velocity.

Treatment. There is no specific therapy available.

Prognosis. The potential for recovery of significant defects is poor. Both upper and lower motor neuron defects tend to persist without significant improvement.

NEUROPATHIES ASSOCIATED WITH SYSTEMIC DISEASES

DIABETIC NEUROPATHY

Diabetic neuropathy is the commonest of the childhood neuropathies associated with systemic disease.

Incidence. If mild dysfunction (e.g., diminished deep tendon reflexes, minimal sensory symptoms in the limbs, or mild slowing of conduction velocities) is accepted as evidence of a peripheral neuropathy, then the incidence is very high, even in childhood diabetes.[26] Even when significant objective motor or sensory deficits are considered, this feature of diabetes is not uncommon, and has been seen in infancy as well as childhood.

Etiology. More than one factor appears to be involved in the development of diabetic neuropathy. The development of progressive symmetrical neuropathy suggests a metabolic precipitant. Involvement of single major nerve trunks has been attributed to ischemic changes secondary to endothelial cell proliferation in small blood vessels, the vasa vasorum. In addition, recurring episodes of hypoglycemia may cause neuropathic changes, and hyperglycemic coma may be associated with compression palsies.

Pathology. The major pathologic change is segmental demyelination. In chronic cases, it is also common to have axonal loss. The nerves, plexuses, and spinal roots are all involved. There may also be loss of anterior horn cells in the spinal cord.

Clinical Features. The ravages of diabetes on the nervous system are widespread and varied.[23] There is a tendency to increased severity with increased duration of the disease and poor control of blood sugar levels, but the symptoms and signs may also be found when or soon after the first diagnosis is made, and may even be the presenting feature. Neuropathy is commoner in poorly controlled juvenile diabetics but may occasionally be present in very young children. The following are the most frequently found clinical types. They may be present in any combination.

DISTAL SYMMETRIC SENSORY NEUROPATHY is the commonest clinical presentation. There is usually very slowly progressive sensory loss in a stocking distribution in the feet. Vibration sensation is usually the most affected, but all cutaneous sensory modalities may be involved. There is often tenderness of the calves, and there may be dysesthesias in the feet and hands that are usually mild but occasionally extremely painful. Perforating ulcers may develop in the feet due to sensory loss. The onset is usually very insidious, but occasionally remarkably rapid. Deep tendon reflexes are depressed or absent.

The neuropathy is typically sensory, but on occasion there is also mild or moderate muscle weakness in the distal extremities.

AUTONOMIC NEUROPATHY. Diarrhea that is typically nocturnal, constipation, incontinence of urine, impotence, orthostatic hypotension, and anhydrosis may all be found in diabetics in their teens.

MONONEUROPATHY AND MONONEUROPATHY MULTIPLEX. Any single nerve or combination of nerves may be involved in mononeuropathy and mononeuropathy multiplex. The onset is generally sudden with marked motor involvement. The 3rd cranial nerve is frequently involved, usually but not always with pupillary sparing. This is frequently preceded or accompanied by aching pain. Other cranial nerves, intercostal nerves, or any major nerves of the limbs may be affected singly or in combination. These are particularly prone to damage at sites where they are exposed to pressure, such as the common peroneal nerve at the knee, the femoral nerve at the inguinal ligament, or the ulnar nerve in the cubital tunnel. Pain and acute onset are the rule.

A syndrome of involvement of the major nerves around the hip girdle, generally unilateral with pain, has been described in adults and given the name *diabetic amyotrophy*. It is not clear that this is etiologically different from other multiple mononeuropathies.

Laboratory Studies. Motor and sensory nerve conduction velocities are generally delayed, and sensory nerve action potentials may be markedly diminished in amplitude, or absent. These features may be present when diabetes is initially diagnosed, and before the onset of demonstrable clinical findings. They tend to become more marked with progression of the neuropathic disease. Electromyography may show denervation in the muscles involved. Cerebrospinal fluid protein may at times be elevated, usually mildly, but occasionally up to 400 mg/dl.

Treatment. There is no specific treatment available. The evidence is that careful dietary and insulin control of diabetes may prove helpful in the control of the neuropathic features. The treatment of painful symptoms is discussed below in the section on treatment.

Prognosis. Mild sensory symptoms tend to be persistent. Severe episodes of pain, however, are generally self limiting over weeks to months. Symmetric sensory or motor loss and absent deep tendon reflexes generally persist and gradually deteriorate. Mononeuropathies and mononeuropathies multiplex have a relatively good prognosis for recovery in each individual episode, although recovery may take several weeks or months. Autonomic defects are usually persistent. Generally, the more neurologic involvement, the worse the general outlook for the patient, partly because there is usually concomitant involvement of other organs such as the retinae or kidneys.

NEUROPATHY IN HYPOGLYCEMIA

Recurring episodes of hypoglycemia may lead to damage to anterior horn cells, spinal roots, or peripheral nerves. There may be a resultant mononeuropathy multiplex or polyneuropathy. This condition is most commonly seen with insulin-secreting tumors of the pancreas, but may be associated with other causes of hypoglycemia. The development of neuropathy has been seen following the institution of insulin or other antidiabetic therapy. It is not clear whether this is a concomitant diabetic neuropathy or related to the treatment.

HYPOPITUITARISM, ACROMEGALY, AND HYPOTHYROIDISM

Mononeuropathies, entrapment neuropathies, and polyneuropathies occasionally occur in hypopituitarism, acromegaly, and hypothyroidism.

UREMIC NEUROPATHY

Incidence. The incidence of uremic neuropathy depends on the severity and duration of the renal disease. Approximately 65% of patients show some degree of neuropathy at the commencement of hemodialysis. Males are significantly more susceptible then females.

Etiology. The neurotoxic factor in uremia is not established. High levels of myoinositol, guanidine compounds, and parathyroid hormone have all been implicated.

Pathology. The defect is primarily axonal loss, most prominent in the distal segments of the nerves. There is also secondary segmental demyelination.

Clinical Features. Sensory symptoms are often an early feature. Muscle aches and pains in the lower limbs are difficult to differentiate from those found with electrolyte disturbances. The restless legs syndrome, where the patient is unable to keep the feet and legs still, is not uncommon. Eventually, burning dysesthesias develop over the feet and lower legs. Progressive motor and sensory loss with reflex loss develop as the disease progresses. Characteristically, this is extremely symmetric in both legs, eventually also appearing in the upper limbs. The auditory nerve may also be involved.[46]

Laboratory Studies. Nerve conduction velocities are generally diffusely slowed in uremia, and are a good indication of the severity of the disease. They are invariably reduced or absent with clinical neuropathic involvement. Cerebrospinal fluid protein is occasionally increased.

Differential Diagnosis. Several of the diseases that may cause uremia may also cause a peripheral neuropathy, and this must be considered in each case. The marked symmetry of uremic neuropathy is often helpful in establishing its diagnosis. Occasionally, nerve and muscle biopsy may be necessary to establish a therapeutic regimen if other etiologies are considered.

Treatment. In most cases, hemodialysis improves or reverts the neuropathy. Occasionally, the symptoms progress despite dialysis, and this is an indication for renal transplantation.

Prognosis. Most mild neuropathies completely revert. With severe disease, there is likely to be some residual defect.

HEPATIC NEUROPATHY

A mild peripheral neuropathy has been associated with chronic hepatic failure. Although there are no specific reports of this occurring in childhood, this feature has not been adequately investigated. Acute polyneuritis indistinguishable from other postinfectious polyneuropathies is occasionally encountered following viral hepatitis.

PORPHYRIA

The porphyrias are classified into two major groups: the erythropoietic form, in which there is no involvement of the nervous system, and the hepatic form, in which peripheral neuropathy is a major feature. Major types of hepatic porphyrias are variegate porphyria, which is extremely common in South Africa and rare in other parts of the world; hereditary coproporphyria, which has the same clinical manifestations as the variegate group, but somewhat different biochemical features; and acute intermittent porphyria, the commonest form seen in the United States. All types affect the peripheral nervous system, but unlike the others, acute intermittent porphyria does not have any skin manifestations. These diseases do not present until puberty.

Acute Intermittent Porphyria

Incidence. Acute intermittent porphyria is commonest in those of Scandinavian or English origin. It is rare among blacks.

Genetics. Inheritance is by the autosomal dominant mode.

Pathology. The changes are of a primarily axonal neuropathy.

Clinical Features. Most attacks are precipitated by the ingestion of either alcohol or one of a variety of pharmacologic agents. Barbiturates, estrogens including oral contraceptives, phenytoin, sulfanomides, oral antidiabetic agents, meprobamate, dichloralphenazine, and chlordiazepoxide have all been implicated in acute attacks. Barbiturates particularly must be avoided.

The usual clinical attack starts with abdominal pain that may closely mimic many acute surgical conditions. This is followed by psychological changes and, often after a period of some days, by peripheral neuropathy. If the diagnosis is not made early, and if barbiturates are used during the abdominal or psychiatric phases, then the condition is further severely exacerbated. The peripheral neuropathy is primarily motor, and may frequently start in the proximal limb muscles. It may occasionally be quite asymmetric. The cranial nerves are often involved. Occasionally, the deep tendon reflexes are preserved. There are almost invariably autonomic features, with tachycardia and changes in blood pressure, and pain is a frequent and extremely troublesome feature of the disease. Objective sensory findings are relatively uncommon.[40]

Laboratory Studies. The diagnostic feature is the presence of porphyrin metabolites in the urine. These are always present during an acute attack, but may be normal after the acute episode but before recovery of the neuropathy. On gross examination, the urine is clear when first passed, but turns dark brownish black on standing for some time, particularly in sunlight. There is an increase in delta aminolevulinic acid, porphobilinogen, and copro- and uroporphyrins in urine. Fecal metabolites are also increased.

Nerve conduction velocites show the features of an axonal neuropathy. Occasionally, there is an increase in cerebrospinal fluid proteins.

Differential Diagnosis. Lead poisoning may be confused with porphyria because of the primarily motor involvement and the fact that porphyrin metabolites are also excreted in plumbism. Delta-aminolevulinic acid levels are high, but there is little, if any, rise in porphobilinogen or uroporphyrin levels with lead poisoning. Postinfectious inflammatory polyradiculoneuropathy may present a very similar clinical picture, although pain is a less common feature, and there is no change in urinary porphyrins.

Treatment. Recently there have been reports of effective treatment of acute attacks as follows. Pain symptoms may be greatly helped by phenothiazine administration. Glucose administration is helpful, probably by suppressing porphyrin enzyme pathways. Hematin, 4 mg per kg twice a day, may be added for the same purpose. Pyridoxine, 100 mg twice a day, is also given as a cofactor to assist in metabolism.

Prognosis. Up to one third of patients with acute neurologic involvement die. Generally the manifestations reach their peak within one month, but occasionally progress for several months. In those who do not die, complete recovery is the rule, although it may take several years. Repeated attacks are not uncommon.

Prevention. Almost all attacks are drug-related, and therefore may be prevented. All drugs must be carefully checked for safety before administration. Porphyrin excretion in family members must be evaluated to identify and counsel others at risk.

POLYARTERITIS NODOSA

Polyarteritis nodosa may occur in any age group, although it is rare in childhood. Occurrence under 1 year of age may be associated with cranial nerve palsies. In other age groups, peripheral neuropathy may be a major feature. It generally presents as mononeuropathy multiplex with both motor and sensory involvement. Pain may be a predominant feature. Eventually, symptoms may progress to those of a symmetric polyneuropathy. It is generally associated with multisystem involvement. Diagnosis may be established by the demonstration of a necrotizing vasculitis in nerve or muscle. High dosage corticosteroid therapy is indicated, but the prognosis is poor. Polyarteritis with neuropathy may develop in youths who misuse methamphetamine.

SYSTEMIC LUPUS ERYTHEMATOSUS

The onset of systemic lupus erythematosus not infrequently occurs in the pediatric age group, with central nervous system involvement in about 30% of cases. Peripheral neuropathy during childhood is rare, however, and although vascular changes have been reported in patients with mononeuropathy, the etiology of the more symmetrical polyneuropathy is less certain. An acute myelopathy may mimic acute polyneuropathy in the early stages, but sphincter disturbance, extensor plantar responses, and a lymphocytic reaction in the cerebrospinal fluid may all help to differentiate this disease.

SARCOIDOSIS

Sarcoid granulomas may affect any part of the central or peripheral nervous system, or the muscles. It is a disease of adults, but rare neurologic involvement has been reported in adolescents. The commonest peripheral nerve involvement is facial palsy, which may present as a Bell's palsy. More extensive asymmetric or symmetric neuropathies may occur. Diagnosis depends on the histologic demonstration of noncaseating granulomata in biopsy tissue. These may be found in peripheral nerve or muscle. The cerebrospinal fluid characteristically shows an increase in chronic inflammatory cells and protein with a reduced sugar content. Progressive neuropathic involvement is an indication for a trial of steroid therapy, although its efficacy is not proven.

JUVENILE RHEUMATOID ARTHRITIS

Although children with rheumatoid arthritis may complain of diffuse weakness, they do not develop the neuropathy seen in the adult form.

AMYLOIDOSIS

Amyloidosis may be a hereditary disease with an autosomal dominant transmission. Neuropathy is common in this condition, but does not present until adulthood. Non-hereditary amyloidosis may be primary or may be associated with a variety of malignant or chronic suppurative condition. Peripheral neuropathy is only seen if there is a serum M component present or if there is Bence Jones proteinuria. Thus, amyloid neuropathies are not associated with juvenile rheumatoid arthritis or chronic suppurative conditions but could be seen in children who have an established monoclonal gammopathy.

NEUROPATHY ASSOCIATED WITH CANCER

Solid tumors may occasionally invade ganglia and plexuses, causing neuropathic symptoms. Pain is usually a major feature. The paraneoplastic sensory and sensory-motor neuropathies found in adults appear to be extremely rare in the nonhematologic neoplasms of childhood.

Leukemia and Lymphomas

There are several ways in which the peripheral nervous system may be involved in leukemia and lymphomas

Compression due to meningeal metastasis is the most common cause of peripheral neuropathy in children with these diseases. With increasingly effective chemotherapy, patients are surviving the systemic effects of the tumor, only to develop meningeal deposits. Tumor cells tend to grow in sheaths down the meninges, entrapping and damaging the nerves as they exit from the brain stem and spinal cord. Progressive cranial nerve palsies or radiculopathies in the trunk and limbs are common. Pain is a major feature. If the condition is untreated, the results may be devastating, with destruction of virtually all the cranial nerves, severe motor and sensory loss over the body, and eventual involvement of the spinal cord and brain stem themselves, possibly by invasion of blood vessels. Protocols for treating these tumors now include prophylactic intrathecal chemo-therapeutic agents or irradiation of the neuraxis, as most of the commonly used antineoplastic drugs do not cross the blood–brain barrier.

Endoneural Infiltration. Metastatic spread of neoplasm by endoneural infiltration is seen only with the leukemias and lymphomas. The picture may be clinically confusing, presenting as a symmetric polyneuropathy or mononeuropathy multiplex, and the pathology may show segmental demyelination without infiltration in the area sampled.

Paraneoplastic Neuropathy. Asymmetric polyneuropathy without obvious direct neoplastic involvement of the nerves has been reported. It is not clear whether this is an autoimmune phenomenon, is related to undemonstrated endoneural involvement or is a side-effect of toxic agents.

Hemorrhage in Nerve Tissue. Many leukemic mononeuropathies are due to direct hemorrhage into the nerve without any direct tumor involvement.

Neuropathy Due to Chemotherapeutic Agents

Neuropathy resulting from the use of chemotherapeutic agents is discussed in the section on toxic neuropathies.

NUTRITIONAL DISORDERS

Severe nutritional deficiencies are rare in the economically developed countries. Occasionally, they result from bizarre dietary habits or from child abuse and starvation.

In the economically underdeveloped countries, this still represents a major health problem, and its effect on the developing nervous system is obviously major but not yet fully established. There is generally inadequacy of many different nutritional constituents of the diet, and it is difficult to implicate any single vitamin or food substance in the causation of any particular clinical picture. These patients, particularly children, show abnormalities of the peripheral nerves that coexist with pathologic and clinical derangement of the spinal cord, brain, and other body organs. Therapeutic measures are aimed at providing an adequate well-balanced dietary intake with supplementary vitamins. Deficiencies of isolated vitamins do occasionally arise, and here, too, it is unusual for the peripheral nervous system to be affected without predominant central nervous system involvement. Thus, niacin deficiency results in pellagra, and vitamin B_{12} deficiency leads to the neurologic manifestations of pernicious anemia. Folate deficiency has been reported as a cause of floppy infant syndrome with hypotonia and depressed deep-tendon reflexes.[6] Special mention can also be made of the syndrome associated with thiamine deficiency.

BERIBERI

Etiology. A relatively pure picture of peripheral neuropathy may be seen in beriberi, which occurs usually in breast-fed infants when the nutrition of the mother is inadequate. Thiamine deficiency has been incriminated as the etiologic factor. Even here, however, such deficiency in infants is more likely to appear with the syndrome of Wernicke's encephalopathy—with oculomotor paralysis, nystagmus, cerebellar manifestations, and convulsions—than as a pure peripheral neuropathy.

Pathology. The changes in the peripheral nerves are nonspecific involvement of myelin and axis cylinders affecting the proximal portion of the nerves and nerve roots.

Clinical Features. A full assessment of the degree of polyneuritis is difficult in infants, but variable degrees of weakness, hypotonia, and diminished or absent deep tendon reflexes are present. Handling of the limbs may cause considerable pain.

Treatment and Prognosis. Adequate diet with supplemental thiamine in a dosage of 20 to 100 mg daily may reverse the clinical picture. Death, however, may occur from encephalopathy with convulsions if treatment is delayed.

DISORDERS ASSOCIATED WITH INTESTINAL MALABSORPTION

Malnutrition resulting from malabsorption rather than inadequate intake may rarely result in neuropathic features with celiac disease, Whipple's disease, tropical sprue, and regional enteritis, and following gastric resection. The symptoms are usually limited to paresthesias of the hands and feet with little objective change on physical examination. Pathologic changes associated with these symptoms are poorly documented. Hyporeflexia and paresthesias may also accompany the hypocalcemia and hypomagnesemia that may be encountered in these gastrointestinal disturbances.

INFECTIVE AND INFLAMMATORY DISORDERS

ACUTE INFLAMMATORY POLYRADICULONEUROPATHY

Acute inflammatory polyradiculoneuropathy is the commonest form of acute neuropathy occurring in childhood.[24] Several eponyms are used to describe what seems to be the same clinical picture, including Guillain-Barré syndrome, Landry's ascending paralysis, postinfectious, polyneuropathy, postexanthematous polyneuropathy, and postvaccinia polyneuritis. The disease presents a particular challenge to the neuromuscular team, because children who can be weathered through the severe stage, however long that may be, generally have an excellent prognosis.

Etiology and Pathogenesis. There is strong suggestive evidence that this disease results from an autoallergic attack on the myelin sheath of peripheral nerves.[2] It seems that a wide variety of different events can precipitate this attack. The commonest, presenting in about 50% of patients, is some antecedent infectious agent. Many viruses have been implicated, including the childhood exanthemata, influenza A and B, infectious mononucleosis, infectious hepatitis, and the enteroviruses. It may follow inoculation with vaccinia, particularly revaccination. An increased incidence was reported following recent swine flu inoculations. Cases have followed mycoplasma and bacterial infections. Five to ten percent of cases are associated with recent surgical procedures of one type or another. Some closely follow the development of vasculitides, and some are associated with malignant disease, particularly the lymphomas. It seems likely that in some way these traumatic events set off an autoimmune response that leads to the nerve damage and resulting clinical picture.

Pathology. The main feature is segmental demyelination associated with a marked mononuclear infiltration. There is secondary axonal loss when the disease is established. Any level of the peripheral nervous system may be involved, including the roots, ganglia, peripheral motor and sensory nerves, and the autonomic nervous system. There is also inflammatory infiltration of the intramuscular nerve endings that may actually involve the adjacent muscle and can be confused with an inflammatory myopathy on muscle biopsy.[3,a]

Clinical Features. Over 50% of patients with this disease give a history of an antecedent event as discussed above. There is usually a 1- to 3-week lapse period between infection and the onset of neuropathic symptoms, but this may at times be shorter. The clinical features are usually a combination of subjective sensory changes and muscle weakness. The onset is usually subacute over several days, with 50% of cases stabilizing within 2 weeks and 90% within 4 weeks. Continued progression after 4 weeks should put the diagnosis in some doubt. Motor weakness is generally the predominant symptom; this commonly involves the legs in an ascending fashion, and the first complaint may be of falling or inability to run. Occasionally, the proximal muscles of the thighs or the upper limbs may be involved first. With deterioration, the axial musculature is involved, with respiratory embarrassment and frequently weakness of neck flexors and extensors. Facial diplegia to some degree is present in at least half the cases, usually first seen as inability to bury the eyelashes on eye closure, or poor facial expression on laughing or crying. Severe disease may eventually involve all the motor cranial nerves, with inability to chew, swallow, or move the eyes.

Subjective sensory findings are usually present early in the disease. Rarely, they may precede motor weakness. It is then not uncommon for the condition to be misdiagnosed as hysteria or hyperventilation. The usual sensory symptoms are of vague numbness, tingling, or even itching in a glove-and-stocking distribution. Objective demonstration of sensory loss may be possible in less than 50% of cases; vibration and joint position are most likely to be involved, and may combine with motor weakness to give marked ataxia. Pain, cramping, and tenderness of the muscles are occasionally marked. Headache, papilledema, and neck stiffness are rare features, but may cause significant diagnostic difficulty.

Autonomic features appear to some degree in most cases. These include tachycardia, bradycardia, flushing, hypertension, hypotension, increased or decreased sweating, inappropriate secretion of antidiuretic hormone, and alterations in sphincter control

The deep tendon reflexes are generally absent from an early stage, and the presence of active ankle jerks makes the diagnosis very unlikely. Rarely, the plantar responses have been reported as extensor.

Laboratory Studies. The most important confirmatory finding is albuminocytologic dissociation in the cerebrospinal fluid, an increase in protein without a significant increase in cells. Generally, this does not occur during the first 1 to 2 weeks of the illness, and some patients do not show it at any time. Peak CSF protein levels are found at about 4 weeks and may be as high as 2g per 100 ml. Very high levels are associated with the patients who show papilledema.[43] Occasionally, there will be a significant increase in mononuclear cells in the cerebrospinal fluid, even up to 40 or 50 cells; this does not appear to have any significance on the outcome of the disease, but should warrant a particularly careful search for other etiologies. At times, there will be a mild rise in serum creatine phosphokinase and transaminase levels. Nerve conduction velocities usually show the changes of segmental demyelination, but may be normal in the early stages, and occasionally throughout the disease. Attempts to correlate the prognosis with the degree of alteration of nerve conduction velocities have shown no consistent pattern.

Differential Diagnosis. When pain is prominent and objective sensory findings are absent, acute poliomyelitis must be considered. Polio is associated with high fever at the onset, and more prominent meningeal signs. Generally, involvement in poliomyelitis is quite asymmetric, whereas in polyradiculoneuritis it is symmetric, but there may be exceptions to this in either direction. There is a consistent CSF pleocytosis in polio, and nerve conduction velocities remain normal or only very mildly slowed.

Acute transverse myelitis may initially give a period of "spinal shock" in which there is flaccid paralysis and absence of deep tendon reflexes. Usually, there is a discernible level of sensory loss over the trunk; sphincter involvement is profound and early, and the plantar responses are frequently extensor.

A variety of toxic neuropathies may present a similar clinical picture, and careful inquiry should be made into this possibility.

Neuromuscular junction defects, particularly botulism and tick paralysis, must be considered, and are discussed in Chapters 11 and 19.

Muscle disease associated with electrolyte imbalance, particularly the periodic paralyses, may present with progressive weakness. The deep tendon reflexes are usually preserved in the early stages, and there is no abnormality of the cerebrospinal fluid. The inflammatory myopathies are associated with massive rises in muscle enzymes in the blood.

Treatment. Hospitalization is indicated for all cases. Frequent estimations of vital capacity and blood gases are indicated until the clinical course has stabilized. The patient may deteriorate very rapidly over a few hours, and the physician must be prepared to carry out intubation and respiratory assistance at short notice. A nasal endotracheal tube may be used initially, but most cases who require ventilatory assistance will do so for significant periods of time, and early tracheostomy is indicated. Because of the good eventual prognosis, pulmonary complications should be treated aggressively, nursing care must be of the highest quality to prevent bedsores, and passive exercises of the limbs should be initiated immediately to prevent eventual contractures. Cardiovascular autonomic abnormalities may at times require appropriate medical therapy. The role of high dosage corticosteroid therapy is not established in this disease. At times, it seem to be dramatically helpful, but the disease process itself may show marked fluctuations, and there are not adequate clinical trials to show that the addition of steroids is therapeutically beneficial. They carry a significant risk of gastrointestinal bleeding and other side-effects, and at times appear to result in a steroid-dependent condition in which there is clinical exacerbation on attempts to withdraw the agents. However, in the uncommon slowly progressive form of inflammatory polyradiculoneuropathy, a trial of high dosage steroids appears indicated.

Prognosis. Various studies of acute inflammatory polyradiculoneuropathy indicated a 5% to 20% mortality rate. As respiratory support measures have improved, the mortality rate has decreased, and now the main cause of death is autonomic dysfunction with cardiac dysrhythmias or acute blood pressure changes. These may be sudden in onset and must be carefully monitored. Functional recovery is generally complete, although it usually takes months and occasionally 1 to 2 years. In about 15% of cases, there is significant residual deficit, usually in the distal muscles of the legs. It is also not infrequent for the deep tendon reflexes to remain hypoactive and the distal muscles to show mild wasting in functionally recovered patients.

RECURRENT AND RELAPSING INFLAMMATORY POLYRADICULONEUROPATHY

Less than 5% of cases of acute polyradiculoneuropathy show relapses during their convalescence, or recurrences of the disease at a later stage. Each exacerbation should be treated as above. There are no useful indicators of which cases will relapse.

CHRONIC INFLAMMATORY POLYRADICULONEUROPATHY

There is a poorly understood group of chronically progressive neuropathies that affect children and that show pathologic changes in the nerve similar to those found in the relapsing inflammatory polyradiculoneuropathies. These may at times have a history of onset with an acute systemic illness, or may have an insidious onset and progression. They may be associated with an increase in cerebrospinal fluid protein. Occasionally, there will be dramatic improvement with high dosage steroid therapy, and a one to three month trial of prednisone is worthwhile in children showing this clinical pattern. If there is no improvement at that time, steroids should be terminated. If obvious improvement occurs, the steroid therapy should be gradually reduced, usually over months, according to the clinical picture. In cases where steroids alone are of no benefit, there are reports of improvement using immunosuppressant drugs, plasmaphereses, or a combination of all three therapies. These measures are still of unproven value, but worth consideration in refractory cases.

BRACHIAL NEURITIS

The term *brachial neuritis* describes a clinical picture manifested by pain, weakness, and wasting of the muscles supplied by the brachial plexus. It has been described by a number of clinical terms, including brachial neuralgia, neuralgic amyotrophy, and the Parsonage-Turner syndrome.

Incidence. The disease is seen most commonly in adulthood, but adolescent cases are not rare. There is an approximately 3-to-1 male-to-female preponderance, and the right arm is most commonly affected.

Etiology. There are no clearly defined etiologic agents. In approximately 25% of cases, there will be some antecedent respiratory or other infection. A remarkably similar condition is seen following inoculations into the arm, and this is discussed under the neuropathy of serum sickness. In this situation, a more diffuse clinical picture is common.

Pathology. There are no adequate pathologic studies on the brachial plexus in brachial neuritis. Axonal loss has been demonstrated in the superficial radial nerve in this condition, and the clinical picture is certainly compatible with an axonal neuropathy.[45]

Clinical Features. Pain is the predominant clinical feature. It is usually described as severe, deep, and aching. It is generally centered around the shoulder girdle, but may extend into the arm and even the hand. Arm and neck movement may exacerbate the pain. Over the course of a few days to weeks, this gradually diminishes in intensity, but some degree of discomfort often persists for weeks or months. As the acute pain diminishes, evidence of muscle wasting and fasciculations becomes manifest. Muscles supplied by the upper plexus, including deltoid, supraspinatus, infraspinatus, and serratus anterior, are most commonly affected, but there may be additional or, rarely, isolated involvement of muscles supplied by the lower plexus. Deep tendon reflexes are usually lost early in the disorder. Objective sensory loss is occasionally seen, most commonly in the area of the axillary nerve.

Laboratory Studies. Electromyography shows features compatible with an axonal loss. Otherwise, there is no consistently abnormal laboratory finding, although cerebrospinal fluid protein has occasionally been reported as increased.

Differential Diagnosis. Although the clinical picture is very typical, particularly if associated with recent injections, the lack of specific tests makes this a diagnosis of exclusion. Nerve compression due to a protruded cervical disk, neoplasm, or other abnormality about the thoracic outlet must be considered. Herpes zoster may present difficulty before the evolution of the typical rash. Acute anterior poliomyelitis can usually be differentiated by the concomitant fever and cerebrospinal fluid pleocytosis.

Treatment. Adequate analgesia is required in the initial stages. Complete rest of the arm with the use of a sling is usually required. After the initial stage of severe pain, full range of motion with increasing work load should be carried out to ensure against the development of a "frozen shoulder." The role of systemic steroid therapy is not proven, but at times it seems to alleviate the initial acute pain.

Prognosis. The general prospects for recovery are excellent, although up to 2 years may be required for it to reach maximum. Less than 10% of patients are left with significant permanent residual effects. Rarely, one or more recurrences of the acute attacks will occur; these are generally less severe than the initial episode.

SERUM SICKNESS

A condition very similar to idiopathic brachial neuritis may accompany serum sickness.[1]

Etiology. This condition is seen following the injection of various forms of heterologous immune sera and vaccines. These include tetanus antitoxin and toxoid, antiserum against various bacterial infections including diphtheria, and vaccinations against typhoid, smallpox, and influenza.

Pathogenesis. Evidence suggests the defect is a vasculitis secondary to precipitation of immune complexes. This leads to secondary swelling of the nerves, and the cervical roots, with their narrow foraminal outlets, are particularly prone to involvement.

Pathology. Owing to the benign nature of the condition, there are no human pathologic studies.

Clinical Features. Initially there may be evidence of a diffuse immune complex disease, with arthralgias, skin eruptions, lymphadenopathy, crampy abdominal pain, and renal changes that may progress to frank glomerulonephritis. These may not be severe, and generally precede the onset of neuropathy by 2 or 3 days. Thus, the clinical features are very similar to those of idiopathic brachial neuritis, although there is more likely to be clinical or electrodiagnostic evidence of involvement of a more widespread nature, including diaphragmatic paralysis, dysfunction of the contralateral brachial plexus, or even a widespread peripheral neuropathy. Occasionally, there is evidence of central nervous system involvement, including headache, neck stiffness, and occasionally frank encephalopathy.

Laboratory Studies. Abnormalities of cerebrospinal fluid protein may include lymphocytic pleocytosis, increased protein, and occasionally increased pressure. There may be localized or widespread slowing of nerve conduction velocity. Proteinuria and other evidence of serum sickness may coincide.

Differential Diagnosis. Neuropathy from serum sickness must be differentiated from idiopathic brachial neuritis and the conditions discussed under its differential diagnosis.

Treatment. The treatment is that for serum sickness, including glucocorticosteroid therapy.

Prognosis. The prognosis for recovery of the neuropathy is generally excellent.

DIPHTHERIA

Incidence. Diptheria was once regarded as the commonest form of neuropathy in childhood. It is now rare in developed countries owing to aggressive programs of prophylactic inoculation, but it is still common in some parts of the world. The major serious sequelae are due to cardiac toxicity and neurotoxicity.

Etiology. The disease is due to infection with the bacillus *Corynebacterium diphtheriae*; the cardiologic and neurologic features are due to the elaboration of a toxin by the organism.

Pathology. Neuropathy due to diphtheria toxin has been studied in great detail using experimental animal models. It can be regarded as the prototype of segmental demyelinating neuropathies.[8]

Clinical Features. Primary infection is generally of the fauces, larynx, or nasal passages. However, the initial infection may also be of wounds, skin, intestines, ear, or esophagus. Infants may have primary infection of the umbilicus. After approximately 2 days' incubation, the patient develops local inflammation that may be accompanied by an exudate, and systemic illness with malaise, headache, and fever. Circulatory collapse and cardiac failure may occur early in the course. Generally, the degree of neuropathy depends on the severity of the initial attack, but at times the neuropathy may appear after minimal or no evidence of preceding illness. A nasal quality may appear in the voice within 1 week, but this is probably due to localized muscular involvement. Generally, palatal paralysis occurs at about 3 weeks, with failure of pupillary accommodation following at about 4 weeks, leading to blurring of vision. The pupillary light reflex remains intact. Within 6 weeks there may be severe paralysis of the muscles supplied by the cranial nerves and the diaphragm, leading to respiratory decompensation. Diffuse motor-sensory neuropathy appears at about 2 months; this is primarily distal, and the deep tendon reflexes are absent. When this sequence of events occurs, the diagnosis is relatively straight forward, but at times one or more of these features may not be present and their order of appearance may change. Occasionally, the picture may be mononeuritis or mononeuritis multiplex.[13]

Laboratory Studies. Early in the disease, the organism *Corynebacterium diphtheriae* may be cultured from the infection site. The cerebrospinal fluid may show some elevation of protein, cells, or both. Reports of electrodiagnostic studies are inadequate, but the underlying pathologic process would be expected to lead to severe delay in conduction velocities.

Differential Diagnosis. The history of polyneuropathy developing after an acute infectious illness suggests acute inflammatory polyradiculoneuropathy. A history of blood-stained nasal discharge should raise the possibility of diphtheria. Early bulbar signs can be confused with those found in botulism and in myasthenia gravis. The sequence of events is much more rapid in the former, and testing with edrophonium (Tensilon) should rapidly exclude the latter. Bulbar poliomyelitis must also be considered.

Treatment. The most effective treatment is to ensure inoculation of the population against the diphtheria bacillus. If the disease is contracted, the administration of antitoxins within the first 48 hours appears to be effective in reducing the incidence of cardiologic or neurologic sequelae. After 2 days, antitoxin is probably ineffective. General support measures may include tracheostomy and respiratory assistance.

Prognosis. As is general in segmental demyelinating neuropathies, the prognosis for eventual complete recovery is excellent if the patient survives the acute episode. Improvement may start within a few days to a few weeks of the paralysis, and is generally complete within a few weeks to 1 year. Occasionally, there will be some residual weakness and loss of deep-tendon reflexes.

HERPES ZOSTER (SHINGLES)

Incidence and Epidemiology. Herpes Zoster, or shingles, has been reported to involve up to five per thousand of a population. It is commoner with advancing years, but by no means rare in childhood, and is due to infection with the varicella-zoster virus. Cases are generally sporadic and rarely give evidence of recent exposure to other patients suffering from varicella or herpes zoster. On the other hand, it is not uncommon for children to develop varicella after being exposed to others with active lesions of herpes zoster. Infectivity is due to release of virus from the skin blisters. There is a significantly higher incidence in patients with malignant blood diseases, particularly lymphomas and leukemia. This group is at further risk if they have had splenectomy or chemotherapy. The incidence of herpes zoster in patients with Hodgkin's lymphoma has been as high as 25%. There may be a higher association of zoster in spinal dermatomes that are also involved with malignant disease (Fig. 18-10).

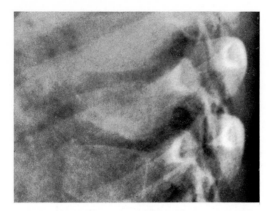

FIG. 18-10. Collapse of lower thoracic vertebra in an 11-year-old child with herpes zoster associated with lymphosarcoma.

Pathology. The dorsal root ganglia are the most commonly and severely affected areas. There are marked inflammatory changes, with neuronal cell loss and necrosis. Involvement may spread to the spinal cord, either locally or diffusely, and there may also be significant encephalopathic change.

Clinical Features. Pain and skin rash are the outstanding signs of involvement. The pain is of variable severity, and may be deep and boring or more dysesthetic in nature. It may occur up to 3 weeks before the skin eruption. Skin changes are generally of blisters in a dermatomal distribution. These are initially clear but gradually crust over within 7 to 10 days. The thoracic area is most commonly involved, usually unilaterally. Cranial nerves may also be the site of disease, particularly the trigeminal. The facial nerve ganglion may be affected, with skin changes in the external ear and additional facial paralysis, the Ramsay Hunt syndrome. Cervical, lumbar, and sacral roots may also be involved. Motor and sensory loss may occur in affected areas, but is usually mild. Generally only one dermatome shows evidence of disease, but occasionally more may be involved, and if the infection becomes disseminated, there may be spinal cord or cortical destruction.[29] This complication, along with diffuse peripheral neuropathy and autonomic dysfunction, is occasionally seen in adults, rarely if ever in childhood.

Laboratory studies are nonspecific. Viral titers have not proven helpful. The cerebrospinal fluid may show a mild rise in cells and protein. This may be marked in the face of myelitis or encephalitis.

Differential diagnosis is generally easy when the rash appears, but the misdiagnosis of other pain syndromes is common before that point. It has been suggested, but not adequately proven, that herpes zoster can give localized symptoms without a rash ever appearing.

Treatment is symptomatic. Because post-herpetic neuralgia is not a feature of childhood disease, aggressive therapy has not been undertaken in children. Localized skin measures may be required, particularly if blisters become infected owing to scratching.

Prognosis. In childhood, the prognosis is generally excellent. The residual neuralgic pain syndromes found in adults and the diffuse dissemination to spinal cord and brain are rarely if ever seen in childhood.

LEPROSY

Incidence. Leprosy is the commonest cause of treatable peripheral neuropathy in the world today. There are estimated to be between 10 and 20 million affected sufferers. Its incidence in the United States is low, and it is virtually limited to those states that abut the Gulf of Mexico and to Hawaii.

Etiology. The causative organism is *Microbacterium leprae*. The portal of entry is usually through the skin. Despite folklore to the contrary, infectivity is very low. Children are probably more susceptible to infection than are adults.

Pathology. In the tuberculoid form, localized intense granulomatosis around the nerves is common, and few, if any, bacilli are seen. In the lepromatous form, marked neuronal cell loss with little granulomatous reaction is seen, and bacilli are found in high quantities. Schwann cells of unmyelinated nerve axons appear to be particularly susceptible.

Clinical Features. The skin, cutaneous nervous system, and eyes bear the brunt of the disease. The major pathologic abnormalities are secondary to cutaneous nerve involvement. Two major categories are recognized, the tuberculoid and lepromatous forms, but intermediate cases are common. In the tuberculoid form, host resistance is high, and the disease is limited to focal areas of involvement. The lepromatous form is associated with low host resistance and is characterized by widespread involvement with minimal inflammatory response. The neuropathy starts as diminution in sensation to pin-prick and temperature, often associated with depigmentation of skin. There is a close correlation with temperature in the involved nerves; surface nerves in the coolest parts of the body are affected first, for example, the face and hands. Motor mononeuropathy multiplex eventually develops, again in nerves whose trunks run near the skin surface and therefore are subject to cooler temperatures. These include the ulnar, peroneal, facial, and median nerves. Progression is insidious. Because of sensory loss, severe deformities may eventually occur secondary to recurring unnoticed injury. At the same time, there may be progressive abnormalities owing to skin and ocular involvement. Occasionally, there may be systemic illness with high fever that lasts for days to months and usually occurs during treatment; this is called erythema nodosum leprosum and is associated with multiple painful skin nodules. The peripheral nerves may be clinically enlarged throughout the disease.

Laboratory Studies. Diagnosis depends on establishment of *Microbacterium leprae* in skin or nerve biopsies. Electrodiagnostic studies show a segmental demyelinating neuropathy.

Differential Diagnosis. Neuropathy from leprosy must be differentiated from the slowly progressive asymmetric neuropathies. Differential diagnosis may be particularly confusing in the hereditary motor-sensory neuropathies that show nerve enlargement. Generally, a history of prolonged exposure in an endemic area is necessary for the diagnosis to be considered.

Treatment. In the early stages, antibacterial agents are effective in arresting and reversing the progression of the disease. The sulfone drugs are the treatment of choice, dapsone being the most commonly used. Therapy in tuberculoid leprosy is continued for 2 years after the disease appears to have become inactive. In lepromatous leprosy, therapy is continued indefinitely. Rifampin, in the early stages of its use, shows great promise particularly for dapsone-resistant organisms. In patients with widespread disease and severe deformities, or with erythema nodosum leprosum, treatment in specialized leprosaria is necessary.

TRAUMATIC DISORDERS

DISORDERS OF CERVICAL ROOTS AND BRACHIAL PLEXUS

Etiology. The cervical roots and brachial plexus may occasionally be damaged in children by severe falls on the shoulder, traction injuries of the arm, or penetrating wounds. The commonest cause of such disorders, however, arises as a complication of childbirth. Upper plexus and root injuries (Erb type) are more common than injury of the lower plexus (Klumpke type). The former occur because of excessive traction on the shoulder during breech deliveries or to the head in cephalic presentations when the angle between the neck and shoulder may become excessively widened. Conversely, any maneuver that involves traction on the arm when it is in a hyperabducted position involves the C8 and T1 roots or the lower cord of the brachial plexus.

Pathology. Stretching the roots results in tearing the sheath, with edema and hemorrhage. The injury most commonly occurs at the junction of the fifth and sixth roots. On occasion, the roots are torn more proximally or are completely avulsed from the cord. Complete avulsion is commoner in C8 and T1 injuries. Occasionally the whole plexus is injured.

Clinical Features. Obvious paralysis exists from birth. In upper root injuries, the arm hangs limply with drooping of the shoulder girdle. It is internally rotated at the shoulder and pronated in the forearm so that the palm faces outward. Paralysis involves the spinati, deltoid, biceps, brachialis, brachioradialis, and extensor carpi radialis. A grasp response can still be elicited, but a typical Moro response is absent. The biceps and supinator jerks may be lost. Sensory loss is usually difficult to demonstrate in this age group. In lower plexus or root injuries, the T1 root suffers the major injury with lesser involvement of C8. If avulsion of the root occurs or if the injury is close to the cord, the cervical sympathetic is also injured, with a resulting Horner's syndrome. In addition, normal pigmentation of the iris on that side may be delayed. Weakness involves the intrinsic hand muscles and the long flexors of the wrist and fingers when C8 is also involved. The deep tendon reflexes are intact, but a normal grasp reflex is absent. Some sensory loss may be demonstrable over the ulnar fingers and ulnar side of the hand and forearm. Edema and cyanosis of the hand may occur if weakness is more than transient, as it usually is, and wasting may develop. Occasionally, the whole plexus may be injured, with total paralysis of the arm. Paralysis of the diaphragm on the same side may also occur if the damage involves C4. A bilateral injury may lead to gross respiratory problems and sometimes death owing to secondary respiratory infection. Posterior dislocation of the head of the radius may occur as a late complication when recovery is poor.

Differential Diagnosis. Diagnosis is usually not difficult owing to the characteristic posture of the hand and arm, particularly in the upper plexus injury. The presence of a Horner's syndrome in the lower plexus helps differentiate it from any more peripheral lesion. Poliomyelitis may be considered at times and may be hard to exclude if the patient is seen sometime after the onset and if sensory loss cannot be confidently demonstrated. In the lower plexus injury, absence of evoked sensory potentials in the ulnar nerve at the wrist with electrical stimulation of the digital nerves of the little finger may be expected if the injury involves the first sensory neuron distal to the posterior root ganglion. If the roots are avulsed from the cord, however, evoked sensory potentials may persist.

Treatment is based on usual physiotherapeutic principles. Splinting to prevent stretching of paralyzed muscles is particularly necessary in the Erb type. Various types of tendon and muscle transplant may be considered to alleviate disability in the late stages.

Prognosis. Recovery is poorer in lower plexus injuries than in those to the upper plexus, but luckily the former are less common. Degree of recovery depends largely on the initial severity of the injury, but a poor recovery may be expected in about 20% of cases. In upper plexus lesions, a late deformity of the elbow may occur and cause some disability.

THORACIC OUTLET SYNDROMES

The term *thoracic outlet syndromes* covers a variety of conditions in which there is symptomatic compression of the brachial plexus or cervical nerve roots leading to sensory or motor changes in the upper limbs. In the author's experience, these are uncommon and frequently overdiagnosed.

Etiology. There are several structures that may potentially compress the brachial plexus in the upper thorax. Accessory cervical ribs have long been implicated, but it must be remembered that approximately 0.5% of the population has cervical ribs, and their presence does not mean they are responsible for compressive symptoms. Occasionally, fibrous bands persist in this area and cause recurring and eventually symptomatic compression on various portions of the plexus. An abnormally hypertrophied scalenus anticus muscle or bad posture leading to sagging of the shoulders and continuous pressure on the plexus as it runs through this muscle may give symptoms. Fracture and subsequent abnormal callous formation in the midportion of the clavicle may lead to compression of the plexus between this bone and the first rib. Continual hyperabduction of the arm, as seen when working above the head for a protracted period or sleeping with the hands behind the head, may lead to compression of the distal part of the plexus by the pectoralis minor tendon. Neoplasms and other lesions growing up from the root of the lung may cause lower plexus symptoms and signs.

Pathology. This condition is relatively benign and there is no pathologic material available, but it can be assumed that significant compression leads to segmental demyelination in the area, at times with subsequent axonal loss, as is seen in other compressive lesions.

Clinical features may be extremely nebulous. The close proximity of nerves and major vessels in this area means that both are likely to be affected. Thus, in severe cases, ischemia of the distal arm and hand may be seen. The peripheral radial pulse may be diminished or absent at rest, or its loss may be precipitated by various maneuvers. The best known of these is that described by Adson. The patient sits with the hands on the thighs, palms upward, turns the head to the side being checked, and performs a valsalva maneuver. The radial pulse diminishes or disappears. The same effect may be obtained by forcibly pulling the arms backward or lifting them above the head. It must be remembered that a significant percentage of normal people also lose pulses under these circumstances, so this test should not be overinterpreted. Careful auscultation for bruits should be carried out around the neck and shoulders, again with the arm in various positions. The commonest neurologic feature is pain around the shoulder girdle, down the arm, or into the hand, depending on the area of the plexus involved. It is occasionally tingling and paresthetic, but more commonly described as boring, deep, and aching. It is generally worse on exercising the limbs. It may at times be reduplicated by compression in the suprascapular notch or over the scalenus anticus, or by pulling downward on the adducted arm. Objective abnormalities are frequently absent, but eventually the patient may develop varying degrees of sensory loss, reflex depression, and motor weakness and wasting. At times there may be progressive painless atrophy of muscles in the hand and arm. There may also be autonomic dysfunction with alterations in sweating, and, in very high lesions, a Horner's syndrome.

Laboratory Studies. Roentgenograms of the neck and thoracic outlet may show evidence of an anatomic abnormality. Arteriography may show compression of the subclavian or brachial vessels. Electrodiagnosis may show delay of conduction velocity across the upper plexus, but these results are not uniformly reliable. In more advanced cases, electromyography demonstrates denervation in muscles supplied by the damaged nerve.

Differential Diagnosis. This condition may prove very difficult to isolate, and it is all too easy to blame "thoracic outlet syndrome" for a whole variety of ill-defined aches and pains in the upper limbs. It should be remembered that there is a high potential for referred pain in many lesions around the neck, arm, shoulder, and hand. Myofascial syndromes are probably the commonest of these, and may be diagnosed by the localization of discrete trigger points where palpation replicates the pain, often with evidence of muscle spasms in these areas, and their ablation by injection of local anesthetics or the spraying of counterirritants on the area. Cervical spine disease with root compression may at times be suggested by plain roentgenograms of the spine, but at times may require myelography for their elucidation. Syringomyelia or spinal cord tumor can also be excluded by myelography. Patients with involvement of any of the major nerve trunks in the arm may present with shoulder pain, and nerve conduction studies may prove extremely valuable in establishing this. At times, localized forms of spinal muscular atrophy may be considered if the abnormalities are purely motor. Finally, particular care must be taken to exclude musculoskeletal disease as a cause of symptoms.

Treatment. In most cases, the initial approach must be supportive rather than aggressive. The patient should be carefully questioned about any physical activities that may be precipitating the discomfort, particularly those requiring repetitive motion around the arm and shoulder. It may be necessary to stop these for a period of several weeks to establish their role. Physical therapy may be useful in altering chronic abnormalities of posture, particularly drooping shoulders and stooping neck, which put added stress on the area of the plexus. If pain is particularly severe and intractable, and particularly if motor wasting and sensory and reflex loss develop, surgical intervention may be unavoidable. The usual operation of choice is removal of the first rib or any fibrous bands that exist.

Prognosis. Most cases will respond to conservative measures. If surgery becomes necessary, the entire first rib should be removed, as resection of only a portion of this may lead to recurring damage to the plexus from the residual stump of the rib, with further progression of the neurologic deficits.

MONONEUROPATHIES

Etiology. Whereas lesions of individual nerves may occur after prophylactic inoculation or with some systemic diseases, the majority of mononeuropathies in children, as in adults, are due to direct or indirect trauma and may occur acutely in association with fractures or dislocations or have a gradual development, as in "tardy" ulnar palsy resulting from chronic minor traumas. Dislocations are more liable to produce stretch lesions with no loss of continuity, whereas fractures may cause laceration of a nerve requiring surgical intervention.[3,a] Direct injury to nerves, particularly the sciatic and radial, may also occur as a result of badly placed injections of therapeutic material. Because of their more adequate layer of subcutaneous fat, young children seem less liable to simple pressure neuropathies, but these do occur quite commonly in older children.

Pathology. In traumatic neuropathies, transient lesions may occur owing to ischemia from pressure. More prolonged ischemia may lead to localized demyelination without any break in the continuity of the axon. More severe injuries cause distal wallerian degeneration, but if the nerve trunk remains in continuity some degree of regeneration is possible. If the nerve is lac-

erated, attempted axonal regeneration and fibrosis occurs, forming a localized swelling at the end of the nerve (a neuroma).

Clinical Features. In general, these consist only of weakness and sensory disturbance in the area served by the individual nerve. Causalgic pain occurs in about 2% to 5% of peripheral nerve injuries particularly in those involving the ulnar, sciatic, and tibial nerves, and especially as a result of gunshot or penetrating wounds. Although almost any nerve may be involved as a result of a particular injury, only those more commonly injured are described here.

SUPRASCAPULAR NERVE INJURY. The suprascapular nerve arises from the upper trunk of the brachial plexus and carries motor fibers from the C5 and C6 roots. It descends through the suprascapular notch on the scapular ridge, and supplies supraspinatus and infraspinatus muscles. Abnormalities of glenohumeral joint movements, which lead to compensatory early outward movement of the scapula on moving the arms, can lead to stretching of the nerve and compression as it goes through the notch. This is classically seen in the "frozen shoulder." Suprascapular nerve entrapment is also encountered in young athletes doing repeated weight lifting and other vigorous shoulder exercises. The most common symptom is a poorly localized, deep boring pain around the shoulder area that is worse on moving the arm, particularly on abducting it across the chest. Eventually, there may be weakness of the first 10° to 15° of abduction of the arms laterally, and of external rotation at the shoulder. The infraspinatus and supraspinatus muscles may atrophy. There is no sensory loss and no reflex abnormality. Local infiltration of anesthetic at the suprascapular notch will relieve pain temporarily. Surgical release of the nerve at the notch may occasionally be required.

LONG THORACIC NERVE INJURY. The long thoracic nerve arises from the anterior primary rami of C5, C6, and C7 and follows a relatively straight course to its termination on serratus anterior. Because of its position, it is liable to injury by stretching or direct pressure, particularly when heavy weights are carried directly on the shoulder or from straps passed over the shoulder. This nerve may also be involved as part of an "allergic" neuritis. Although no marked deformity is seen at rest, winging of the scapula is seen when the arm is elevated anteriorly.

AXILLARY (CIRCUMFLEX) NERVE INJURY. The axillary nerve passes from the posterior cord of the brachial plexus around the posterior aspect of the neck of the humerus to the deltoid muscle, which it innervates. Dislocations of the head of the humerus or fractures in this area may stretch or lacerate the nerve, and badly placed injections into the shoulder may also involve it. Weakness or paralysis of the deltoid results in limited abduction of the arm. A small patch of hypesthesia may be present over the deltoid, but in some instances is inconspicuous or absent. Involvement of the posterior cord of the brachial plexus itself may accompany such injuries and cause associated weakness in radial nerve distribution.

RADIAL NERVE INJURY. The radial nerve may be similarly involved by fractures of the shaft of the humerus or by pressure on the nerve as it emerges from the spiral groove on the lateral aspect of the humerus, at which point it is relatively superficial. Here the branches of the nerve supplying the triceps are usually spared, but there is marked weakness of brachioradialis and the extensors of the wrist and fingers. Sensory loss is mild and confined to an area on the radial aspect of the dorsum of the hand between the index finger and thumb. Involvement of brachioradialis helps to differentiate this from a root lesion of C7, which may also present with weakness of extensors of the wrist and fingers.

MEDIAN NERVE INJURY. The median nerve is occasionally damaged in anterior dislocations of the lower end of the humerus. Such an injury may be accompanied by damage to the brachial artery leading to ischemic contracture if not correctly treated. Weakness of the pronators of the forearm, long flexors of the fingers, and short abductor of the thumb are the most striking motor findings, and sensory loss is noted on the palmar surface of the thumb, index, and middle fingers, and the lateral aspect of the palm. Injury to the nerve at the wrist may occur with lunate or perilunate dislocations and only rarely with severely comminuted Colles' fracture. Here, weakness is confined to the short abductor and opponens of the thumb, and sensory disturbance is present as with more proximal lesions except that the palm of the hand is spared. The common chronic compression of the median nerve in the carpal tunnel as seen in adults is very rare in children but might be expected occasionally in association with juvenile rheumatoid arthritis and in Scheie's syndrome.

ULNAR NERVE INJURY. The ulnar nerve is most commonly injured as it passes behind the medial epicondyle at the elbow, either acutely in association with fractures and dislocations or subacutely as a late result of malalignment of the elbow in a valgus position following a fracture. The majority of ulnar palsies are chronic and result from direct pressure in this situation, perhaps precipitated by minor anatomic variations that lead to an unduly superficial position of the nerve. The clinical picture varies according to the severity, extent, and site of the lesion. Most patients show sensory disturbance in the fourth and fifth fingers, extending up the medial side of the palm to the lower forearm. Muscle weakness and wasting involve the interossei, the two ulnar lumbricals, the muscles of the hypothenar eminence, and the adductor pollicis. If the lesion is sufficiently high, flexor carpi ulnaris and flexor digitorum profundus of the fourth and fifth fingers may also be affected. In chronic and severe lesions, the hand may adopt the position of partial *main en griffe*, which is seen in a complete form when the median nerve is also involved. The ulnar nerve may be involved at or distal to the wrist with comminuted Colles' fracture, stab wounds in the palm, and occasionally from repeated trauma from pressure on the palm of the hand. In this last instance, no sensory loss is seen. Weakness and wasting are confined to the adductor pollicis and the interossei. If the lesion is at the wrist itself, the hypothenar muscles may also be involved. Such a lesion may be difficult to differentiate clinically from the early stages of syringomyelia or from the result of pressure on the brachial plexus from a cervical rib. Nerve conduction studies can be of assistance in differentiating these lesions.

INJURY TO THE SCIATIC NERVE AND ITS MAIN DIVISIONS. Damage to both sciatic nerves in the newborn has been reported to result from injection of therapeutic agents into the umbilical artery.[17] This is accompanied by evidence of vascular damage (sloughing of skin over the buttocks) and is apparently due to thrombosis of the inferior gluteal arteries. A more common danger, however, is injection of therapeutic agents, including the common antibiotics, into the buttock of young infants, particularly those who are poorly nourished. If the injection is badly sited, it may result in severe injury, which may be permanent. The sciatic nerve may also be damaged by posterior dislocations of the hip. Depending on the extent of the injury, paralysis involves all or part of the muscles supplied and may present with a drop foot or a complete flail foot. Sensory loss may be extensive below the knee, sparing only the medial aspect of the leg. The ankle jerk is usually absent. Involvement of the medial popliteal nerve in the popliteal space is relatively uncommon from dislocation or fractures. The peroneal nerve is frequently involved, not only by major injuries but also by simple compression from strapping, casts, or sitting with the legs crossed for a prolonged interval. Previous loss of weight may favor development of this lesion. Lesions of the peroneal nerve present with paralysis or weakness of the dorsiflexors and the evertors of the foot and toes, with variable sensory loss over the anterolateral aspect of the leg and the dorsum of the foot. Clinical differentiation of this lesion from partial lesions of the sciatic nerve or from root lesions involving L4 and L5 roots is sometimes quite difficult. Sciatic nerve lesions usually have a clear history of trauma, but suspected partial root lesions not associated with root pain may cause difficulty and require investigation with myelography or electromyography. Spina bifida occulta may be associated with atrophy and distal weakness in the legs, with variable sensory loss. Failure to gain normal sphincter control is often an accompanying finding, and usually the disorder is bilateral. This is discussed further in Chapter 17.

Differential Diagnosis. This was covered to some extent in the discussion of individual nerve lesions. In general, however, the diagnosis of peripheral nerve injury demands an accurate knowledge of the anatomy of peripheral nerves and their motor and sensory areas of supply. In infants and younger children, sensory testing is often difficult and unreliable, and cooperation even for motor testing may be poor. Techniques for the motor examination in this age group were well described by Johnson.[31] Information may be gained about the sensory function in certain nerves by examining evoked sensory potentials.

Treatment. A certain number of traumatic mononeuropathies are preventable, particularly those due to injection of therapeutic agents or to pressure. In the former, selection of the midanterior thigh for intramuscular injection instead of the buttock prevents sciatic nerve injuries. In pressure neuropathies, if the site of the lesion and the precipitating factor can be accurately identified, suitable advice may be given to the patient, at least to prevent recurrence of this injury. In delayed ulnar neuropathy associated with valgus deformity of the elbow, transplantation of the nerve to an anterior position relieves traction upon it and allows improvement. Transplantation may also be indicated in chronic traumatic neuropathy even when there is no obvious deformity of the elbow. Acute stretch injuries of nerves usually recover spontaneously, but active exercises of the weak muscles should be encouraged during this phase. More severe injuries, particularly where laceration of the nerve is suspected, may require surgical exploration with neurolysis, nerve suture, or occasionally nerve grafts.

Prognosis depends on the degree and site of nerve injury. The nerve may suffer a temporary and reversible conduction block (neurapraxia), or it may become narrowed over a segment or over its whole length beyond the site of injury (axonostenosis or axonocachexia). In this situation, the nerve conduction rate may be permanently slowed, but little clinical disability results. If the axon is cut (axonotmesis), wallerian degeneration occurs distally, and recovery depends on the ability of the fibers to regenerate. Separation of the cut ends or the presence of scar tissue may make this impossible. Even with surgical intervention, recovery is usually incomplete, particularly if the lesion is proximally placed. Varying degrees of injury may coexist simultaneously in neighboring nerve fibers so that it may be very difficult to give an accurate prognosis in the early stage of a nerve injury. Electrodiagnostic studies assist in this process.

TUMORS OF THE PERIPHERAL NERVOUS SYSTEM

BENIGN TUMORS

Schwannomas, and less commonly lipomas, hamartomas, and hemangiomas, may occur singly or multiply in one or more nerves of children. They generally present with pain or paresthesias, and objective motor findings are unusual. Diagnosis is not difficult when they present in surface nerves as a visible and palpable swelling, but may be extremely misleading when they occur in nonpalpable portions of the nerves. If resection is necessary, it is extremely important that they are treated by a surgeon familiar with peripheral nerve resections because using modern electrodiagnostic techniques and the operating microscope, they can usually be enucleated without sacrificing function in the nerve trunk.

By far the commonest nerve tumor found in childhood is the fibroma. This may appear as an isolated lesion, but usually is part of the clinical picture of neurofibromatosis.

Neurofibromatosis (Von Recklinghausen's Disease)

Incidence and Genetics. Neurofibromatosis is not an uncommon condition, with an autosomal dominant mode of transmission. There is frequently marked variation in involvement of different family members.

Pathology. There is involvement of multiple tissues of ectodermal origin. Peripheral nerve tumors may be from Schwann cells, fibrous tissue, or both.

Clinical Features. Symptoms and signs are varied. Skin changes include *cafe au lait* spots that tend to increase in number and size through the years, particularly at puberty and with pregnancy. Tumors of nerve terminals lead to multiple cutaneous and subcutaneous lumps, which may become huge and disfiguring. Axillary freckles are highly suggestive of the disease. Tumors adjacent to bone may lead to multiple skeletal deformities, including kyphoscoliosis and aberrant limb size. A frequent site of nerve involvement is at intervertebral foramina, compressing the cervical nerve roots; this may lead to the formation of a "dumbbell" neurofibroma with portions both inside and outside the spinal canal. However, roots and peripheral nerves may be involved at any level. As the patient grows older, there is a significant increase in benign and malignant tumors involving other elements of the neuroectoderm, including astrocytomas, meningiomas, and medulloblastomas.

Laboratory Studies. When tumors abut the meninges in the spinal canal or cranial vault, the cerebrospinal fluid may be markedly elevated. There may be electrodiagnostic evidence of involvement of individual nerves or roots. Plain roentgenograms of the cervical spine may show enlarged intravertebral foramina in the area of a dumbbell neurofibroma, and there may be widespread bony abnormalities including kyphoscoliosis, spina bifida, and hyperostosis of bone around areas of involvement.

Differential Diagnosis. When solitary lesions arise, or before the full-blown skin picture develops, examination of family members may be very helpful in differentiating these from isolated schwannomas.

Treatment. Individual tumors may need surgical extirpation when they become clinically troublesome, and this should again be done by a clinician familiar with operating on peripheral nerves.

Prognosis. The principle risk to life is the development of malignant tumors. This is unusual in the peripheral nerves, but more common in the central nervous system. Otherwise, although frequently very troublesome and disfiguring, these abnormalities do not lead to a shortening of life expectancy.

MALIGNANT TUMORS

Solitary sarcomas, neuroepitheliomas, or sarcomatous change in neurofibromas are extremely rare in childhood. Secondary malignant involvement of peripheral nerves was discussed earlier in the chapter.

TREATMENT

There are few specific treatments available for diseases of the peripheral nerves. It is important that this does not lead to a nihilistic approach, because many important nonspecific measures can make a great difference to the patient's well-being. The physician rarely has expertise in these measures, and a multidisciplinary approach leads to the best results. In centers treating a significant number of these patients, a program is usually well developed, but the physician seeing few such children may not think to seek advice from the appropriate experts. The following is a brief resume of the measures that may be taken.

Treatment of Pain

Fortunately, pain is not a frequent accompaniment of the childhood peripheral neuropathies. Acute pain may occur in acute intermittent porphyria, some toxic neuropathies, and acute inflammatory polyradiculoneuropathies. This may be relieved by massage, local heat, and hydrotherapy. Analgesics may be required, but long-term usage should be avoided if possible.

Dysesthesias may accompany regeneration of nerve in recovering neuropathies. Often, reassurance that this is a healthy sign and self-limiting is sufficient therapy.

When chronic pain does occur, it may prove a very disabling and difficult problem. Various drug therapies have been tried with rather low overall success. Analgesics are often ineffective and are potentially habit-forming. Phenytoin and carbamazepine should be tried, but have not been very helpful in my experience. A combination of a tricyclic antidepressant (amitriptyline) at night and phenothiazine (fluophenazine) three times a day has had dramatic success in some cases, although the child is then subjected to all the side-effects of these medications.

Repeated massage, heat treatment, and muscle stretching exercises may be helpful. Whirlpool baths are often a great boon. Transcutaneous nerve stimulation by low-voltage electrical current may give very significant pain relief, and all but the youngest children can learn to use this intermittently as required.

For localized nerve pain, the advice of the anesthesiologist and neurosurgeon should be sought as to sympathectomy, localized nerve block, nerve section, or tractotomy. This may be particularly helpful in post-traumatic nerve pain.

Occupational Therapy

Activities of daily living can be helped by a large variety of aids. Eating utensils, pens, combs, and other hand-held instruments may be altered to aid the person with distal muscle weakness. Velcro fasteners may be substituted for buttons; elastic shoelaces allow shoes to be put on and off without knots being tied.

Environmental aids include raised toilet seats, shower seats that allow the child to bathe in comfort and safety, mechanical hoists to lift the heavy child in and out of the bed and the bath, strategically placed handrails and trapezes in the home, and ramps as alternatives to steps.

The occupational therapist can suggest and design games and activities suited to the child's particular problem. These provide interest and entertainment and help to develop skills.

A very exciting recent development is in the use of small, inexpensive computers to allow the patient to control his environment. These can be modified for use by the most severely handicapped, with switches worked by eye blink, the tongue, or even respirations. The patient can then use them to control radio, television, stereo systems, hospital bed, room temperature, telephone, typewriter, calculator, page-turner, and any other electrical apparatus, as well as various alarm systems or methods to call for help.

Orthotic and Prosthetic Aids

Bracing is frequently necessary to prevent contraction deformities, particularly of the ankles and hands. The modern lightweight polypropylenes allow appliances to be rapidly and accurately custom made for specific needs. Braces may also offer a substitute for weakened muscles; shoe springs often allow the person with foot drop to walk without constantly tripping. Various forms of thoracic suspension orthoses and jackets are designed to prevent progressive scoliosis and to aid respiration. Specialized footwear is needed for children with foot weakness and deformity. Arm supports with ball-valve action allow the elbow to be flexed and extended and may allow the patient with upper limb weakness to feed himself. In the future, a variety of artificial limbs worked by the patient's own nerve or muscle impulses may revolutionize the care of the chronically disabled.

Physical Therapy

Evaluation. For the physician without the time or expertise to evaluate all muscle groups, the physical therapist may give great help in initially evaluating and in following progression of disease.

Prevention of Deformities. Range of motion exercises, usually carried out at least twice a day, are essential to prevent joint contractures in paralyzed limbs. These may be done regularly by the therapist or, more commonly, the patient or parents are instructed in doing them at home.

Strengthening and Reeducation. Specific programs are developed to build up strength in available muscles and to teach the use of other muscles in place of those that are paralyzed.

Transferring, lifting, and gait training can be taught to the patient or his attendants as appropriate.

Care of Skin and Nails

The paralyzed limb is particularly prone to ulceration and infection. Careful avoidance of undue pressure and trauma by heat, mechanical, or chemical agents must be taught to the patient and his attendants. Foam pads and cushions, water beds, and sheepskins may help prevent skin breakdown. Toenails should be regularly and carefully manicured, and a podiatrist may be helpful in initially instructing the patient and in later consultation.

Orthopedic Approaches

In selected cases, arthrodeses, tendon transplantations, release of contractures, thoracoscapular fixation, spinal fixation to arrest scoliosis, and other orthopedic approaches may prove beneficial.

School Intervention

Much of the child's life is spent in school, and here he or she develops the interpersonal skills necessary to relate to fellow beings, as well as the educational skills that help make up for significant physical handicaps. It is unusual for the severely handicapped child not to have trouble in school with physical barriers, school programs, and peer relationships. Individual education programs should be structured to the child's needs, and adapted physical education programs can be organized. For the child with progressive disease, early vocational counseling is essential to his development of self-reliance. Peers can be used to help in the child's physical needs, with mutual benefit. The medical team should communicate with the regular and special education teachers, with clear explanations of the child's prognosis and needs and concise instructions as to what the child should and should not do at school.

Social and Emotional Factors

These children and their families often need a great deal of emotional support. Particularly in the progressive and incurable diseases, the physician may find it difficult to discuss what may seem a very gloomy future. The patients, their parents, and their siblings should have a realistic understanding of the disease and the prognosis. Without hiding the negative features, stress must be laid on positive approaches for therapy and rehabilitation. All involved should understand that there are substitutes for physical activity that can lead to a fruitful and happy life. The patient and family should be involved in a positive fashion, and enthusiasm engendered by the medical team is a vital part of the overall therapy. Too often, parents have been denied all but the barest information and have been left to draw their own conclusions, which are frequently more depressing than the truth, or they have been told that nothing can be done, and left with an unrealistic feeling of hopelessness. A visit to a neuromuscular clinic, the formulation of a treatment plan, and, above all, obvious evidence of concern by the medical team can do a great deal to improve the lives and well being of all involved.

REFERENCES

1. **Arnason BGW:** Neuropathy of serum sickness, pp 1104–1109. In Dyck PJ, Thomas PK, Lambert EH (eds): Peripheral Neuropathies. Philadelphia, Saunders, 1975

2. **Arnason BGW:** Inflammatory polyradiculoneuropathy. In Dyck PJ, Thomas PK, Lambert EH (eds): Peripheral Neuropathies, pp 1110–1148. Philadelphia, WB Saunders, 1975

3. **Asbury AK, Johnson PC:** Pathology of Peripheral Nerves, a, pp 120–128; b, pp 178–181; c, pp 268–281. Philadelphia, WB Saunders, 1978

4. **Austin JH:** Observations on the syndrome of hypertrophic neuritis (the hypertrophic interstitial radiculoneuropathies). Medicine (Baltimore) 35:187, 1956

5. **Behse F, Buchthal F, Carlsen F, Knappeis GG:** Hereditary neuropathy with liability to pressure palsies: Electrophysiological and histopathological aspects. Brain 95:777, 1972

6. **Botez MI:** Hypotonia and folate deficiency in children. J Pediatr 96:4, 774, 1980

7. **Bouldin TW, Riley E, Hall CD, Swift M:** Clinical and pathological features of an autosomal recessive neuropathy. J Neurol Sci 46:315–323, 1980

8. **Bradley WG:** Disorders of Peripheral Nerves, pp 137–141. Oxford, Blackwell Scientific Publications, 1974

9. **Bradley WG, Aguayo A:** Hereditary chronic polyneuropathy: Electrophysiologic and pathologic studies in affected family. J Neurol Sci 9:131, 1969

10. **Bradley WG, Madrid R, Thrush DC, Campbell MJ:** Recurrent brachial plexus neuropathy. Brain 98:381, 1975

11. **Brady RO, Gal A, Bradley RM, Martensson E, Warshaw AL, Laster L:** Enzymatic defects in Fabry's disease: Ceramide trihexosidase deficiency. N Engl J Med 276:1163–1167, 1967

12. **Brady RO, King FM:** Fabry's Disease. In Dyck PJ, Thomas PK, Lambert EH (eds): Peripheral Neuropathies, pp 914–927. Philadelphia, WB Saunders, 1975

13. **Bruce AN. In Wilson SKA:** Neurology, 2nd ed, pp 738–747. London, Butterworth, 1954

14. **Brunt PW, McKusick VA:** Familial dysautonomia: A report of genetic and clinical studies, with a review of the literature. Medicine (Baltimore) 49:343, 1970

15. **Cavanagh JB:** The toxic effects of triortho-cresyl phosphate on the nervous system. J Neurol Neurosurg Psychiatry 17:163–172, 1954

16. **Chamberlain PH, Stavinoha WB, Davis H, Kniker WT, Panos TC:** Thallium poisoning. Pediatrics 22:1170–1182, 1958

17. **Curtiss PH Jr, Tucker HJ:** Sciatic palsy in premature infants—A report and followup study of 10 cases. JAMA 174:1586, 1960

18. **Dubowitz V, Brooke MH, Neville H:** Muscle biopsy: A modern approach, pp 5–33. London, WB Saunders, 1973

19. **Dunn HG, Lake BD, Dolman CL, Wilson J:** The neuropathy of Krabbe's infantile cerebral sclerosis. Brain 92:329–344, 1969

20. **Dyck PJ:** Inherited neuronal degeneration and atrophy affecting peripheral motor, sensory, and autonomic neurons. In Dyck PJ, Thomas PK, Lambert EH (eds): Peripheral Neuropathies, pp 825–867. Philadelphia, WB Saunders, 1975

21. **Dyck PJ, Ohta M:** Neuronal atrophy and degeneration predominantly affecting peripheral sensory neurons. In Dyck PJ, Thomas PK, Lambert EH (eds): Peripheral Neuropathies, pp 791–824. Philadelphia, WB Saunders, 1975

22. **Editorial:** Neurotoxicity of vincristine. Lancet 1:980, 1973

23. **Ellenberg M:** The clinical aspects of diabetic peripheral neuropathy. In Canal N, Pozza G (eds): Peripheral Neuropathies, pp 225–237. Amsterdam, Elsevier/North Holland Biomedical Press, 1978

24. **Evans OB:** Polyneuropathy in childhood. Pediatrics 64:1, 1979

25. **Fredrickson DS, Gotto AM Jr, Levy RI:** Familial lipoprotein deficiency (abetalipoproteinemia, hypobetalipoproteinemia and Tangier disease). In Stanburg JB, Wyngaarden JB, Fredrickson DS (eds): The Metabolic Basis of Inherited Disease, pp 493–530. New York, McGraw-Hill, 1972

26. **Gallia V, Massi-Benedetti F, Firenze C, Rossi A, Agostini L, Lanzi G:** Diabetic neuropathy in children. In Canal N, Pozza G (eds): Peripheral Neu-

ropathies, pp 291–301. Amsterdam, Elsevier/North Holland Biomedical Press, 1978

27. **Gumbinas M, Larsen M, Lin HM:** Peripheral neuropathy in classical Niemann-Pick disease: Ultrastructure of nerves and skeletal muscles. Neurology 25:107–113, 1975

28. **Guttman L, Martin JD:** Dapsone neuropathy: A disorder of motor axons. Neurology 26:369, 1976

29. **Hogan EL, Krigman MR:** Herpes zoster myelitis: Evidence for viral invasion of spinal cord. Arch Neurol 29:309–313, 1973

30. **Jenkins RB:** Inorganic arsenic and the nervous system. Brain 89:479–498, 1966

31. **Johnson EW:** Examination of muscle weakness in infants and young children. JAMA 168:1306–1313, 1958

32. **Kahlke W:** Heredopathia atactica polyneuritiformis (Refsum's disease). In Schettler G (ed): Lipids and Lipidoses, pp 353–381. Berlin, Springer-Verlag, 1967

33. **Layzer RB, Fishman RA, Schafer JA:** Neuropathy following abuse of nitrous oxide. Neurology (Minneap) 28(5):504–506, 1978

34. **Lockman LA, Kennedy WR, White JG:** The Chediak-Higashi syndrome: Electrophysiological and electron microscopic observations on the peripheral neuropathy. J Pediatr 70:942–951, 1967

35. **Lovelace RI, Horwitz SJ:** Peripheral neuropathy in long term diphenylhydantoin therapy. Arch Neurol 18:69–77, 1968

36. **Moosa A, Dubowitz V:** Peripheral neuropathy in Cockayne's syndrome. Arch Dis Child 45:674–677, 1970

37. **Pincus JH:** Subacute necrotizing encephalomyelopathy (Leigh's disease): A consideration of clinical features and etiology. Dev Med Child Neurol 14:87–101, 1972

38. **Powers JM, Schaumburg HH:** Adrenoleukodystrophy: Similar ultrastructural changes in adrenal cortical and Schwann cells. Arch Neurol 30:406–408, 1974

39. **Refsum S:** Biochemical and dietary aspects of Refsum's disease. In Dyck PJ, Thomas PK, Lambert EH (eds): Peripheral Neuropathies, pp 872–881. Philadelphia, WB Saunders, 1975

40. **Ridley A:** The neuropathy of acute intermittent porphyria. Q J Med 38:307–333, 1969

41. **Ross RR:** Use of pyridoxine hydrochloride to prevent isoniazid toxicity. JAMA 168:273–275, 1958

42. **Seto DSY, Freeman JM:** Lead neuropathy in childhood. Am J Dis Child 107:337–342, 1964

43. **Schaltenbrand G, Bammer H:** La clinique et le traitment des polyneurites inflammatoires on sereuses crigues. Rev Neurol (Paris) 115:783–810, 1966

44. **Toole JF, Parrish ML:** Nitrofurantoin polyneuropathy. Neurology 23:554–559, 1973

45. **Tsairis P, Dyck PJ, Mulder DW:** Natural history of brachial plexus neuropathy. Report of 99 cases. Arch Neurol (Chicago) 27:109–117, 1972

46. **Tyler HR:** Neurological disorders in renal failure. Am J Med 44:734–748, 1968

47. **Walker GF:** Blindness during streptomycin and chloramphenicol therapy. Br J Ophthalmol 45:555–559, 1961

48. **Yagishita S, Itoh Y, Nakano T, Oizumi J, Okuyama Y, Aoki K:** Infantile neuroaxonal dystrophy. Schwann cell inclusion in the peripheral nerve. Acta Neuropathol (Berlin) 41:257–259, 1978

49. **Yudell A, Gomez MR, Lambert EH, Dockerty MB:** The neuropathy of sulfatide lipidosis (metachromatic leukodystrophy). Neurology (Minneap) 17:103–111, 1967

Disorders of Muscle

19

Charles E. Morris

The problems involved in recognizing and diagnosing primary diseases of muscle in children are formidable and often perplexing. Differentiation from anterior horn cell and peripheral nerve disorders is important in terms of management of the "floppy infant" and the "weak child." There are several general considerations that serve to distinguish primary disease of muscle or the myopathies clinically and pathologically.

From an etiologic standpoint, exogenous toxins are likely to produce neuropathic disturbances, whereas certain of the myopathic disorders tend to be heredofamilial in origin. In general, the proximal and axial musculatures are often symmetrically involved early in the primary muscle disorders, whereas the distal musculature seems to be the prominent initial site of dysfunction in the spinal and neural atrophy group of disorders (Table 19-1). Varying degrees of muscle weakness and diminished muscle bulk are seen in all of these diseases. The deep tendon reflexes are diminished to absent very early in the course of the neural and spinal atrophies, whereas they may be preserved until quite late in the course of a primary degenerative disease of skeletal muscle. No deficit in any modality of sensation is encountered in the myopathies. Fasciculations are seldom encountered in the primary disorders of muscle, being most prominent in the myelogenic atrophy group. Laboratory studies helpful in differentiating these disorders include the cerebrospinal fluid examination and electrophysiologic determinations including the electromyogram and evoked nerve potentials. The muscle biopsy is often

helpful in differentiating between these disorders in that there are usually distinctive histopathologic differences; however, in some cases the so-called characteristic histopathologic features of myopathy are also observed in patients with neurogenic muscular atrophy.[20] Measurement of serum and tissue enzyme concentrations and muscle histochemistry are also of practical clinical value in distinguishing the various types of neuromuscular disorders. Recently, questions have been raised concerning the differentiation of myopathies from other neuromuscular diseases. Clinical and experimental evidence has been accumulating to suggest that the development of some disorders thought previously to be myopathies may actually be related pathogenetically to neurogenic factors. These diseases include specific forms of muscular dystrophy and chronic nonprogressive myopathy.[41,53,76] The considerable interest generated by this new concept may lead to a better understanding of the pathophysiology of the neuromuscular disorders.

DEFECTIVE DEVELOPMENT OF SKELETAL MUSCLE

Congenital absence or defect of the various skeletal muscles in the human being is an uncommon occurrence, with the exception, perhaps, of inconstant functionally unimportant muscles such as the palmaris longus, platysma, risorius, and pyramidalis abdominis. There are, however, situations in which the absence or defect of certain muscles—e.g., the pectoral muscles, dia-

TABLE 19-1. Differentiation of Disorders of Muscle, Anterior Horn Cell, and Peripheral Nerves

Clinical and Laboratory Features	Muscle	Anterior Horn Cell	Peripheral Nerves
Site of predisposition	Usually proximal and axial musculature	Proximal or distal extremity musculature	Usually distal extremity musculature
Deep tendon reflexes	Preserved until late in course	Reduced to absent early in course	Reduced to absent early in course
Sensation deficit	Rarely observed	Not observed	Usually present
Fasciculations	Usually absent	Frequently present	Occasionally present
CSF protein	Normal	Normal or elevated	Elevated or normal
Electromyography			
Interference pattern	Normal until late in disease	Reduced	Reduced
Fibrillation potentials	Not usually present	Usually present	Present
Action potentials	Short duration	Prolonged with occasional giant potentials	Prolonged with normal or polyphasic potentials
Evoked sensory and mixed nerve potentials	Normal	Normal	Absent, diminished amplitude, or prolonged conduction time

phragm, abdominal wall musculature, and muscles innervated by the various cranial nerves—assumes a great importance in terms of function.

Etiology. The etiology of congenitally absent or defective musculature has not been defined with certainty. Some authorities feel that these conditions represent defective genetic development of the embryo. Indeed, most of these defects of muscle seem to follow a hereditary pattern. Some investigators suggest that nuclear hypoplasia might be responsible, at least insofar as the cranial nerve-innervated muscles are concerned. Others feel that the congenital defects are an expression of a primary disease of muscle.

Clinical Features. A weakened or absent abdominal wall interferes with proper pulmonary and gastrointestinal function, and infants with this condition succumb to respiratory infection within a short period of time. Occasionally, a concomitant abnormality of the genitourinary system may be associated.

An isolated defect of one or both lateral rectus muscles has been termed the retraction syndrome, or Duane's syndrome. Limitation of eye abduction, retraction of the globe, and narrowing of the palpebral fissure on attempted abduction in the affected eye are the usual clinical manifestations.

The clinical absence of a pectoral or brachioradialis muscle in association with the facioscapulohumeral type of muscular dystrophy has been observed on occasion. This relationship is not well understood.

Treatment. Surgical treatment in these disorders to improve function or for cosmetic reasons is helpful in some instances.

CONGENITAL CONTRACTURES

Several deformities in infants and children are related to shortening and fibrous changes in skeletal muscle. The deformities most frequently encountered are congenital torticollis, congenital clubfoot, congenital elevation of the scapula, and congenital contractures of the extremities. The etiology of these contractures has not been definitely established. In some instances, heredity seems to play a role. Intrauterine or birth trauma may be responsible in some cases.

MUSCULAR TORTICOLLIS

Muscular torticollis (congenital torticollis, wryneck) is due to shortening of the sternocleidomastoid muscle, which may seem enlarged and abnormally firm. Occasionally, adjacent muscles such as the trapezius and deep cervical muscles may also be involved.

Etiology. Several etiologies have been proposed. Some authorities feel that there is a relationship between the so-called sternomastoid tumor and muscular torticollis, and suggest that both lesions may be due to antenatal position.[49] Others feel that birth trauma with damage to the main blood vessels supplying the sternomastoid muscle is etiologically significant. Familial factors also play a role.

Pathology. Exposure of the sternocleidomastoid muscle during surgical operation demonstrates that it is actually reduced in bulk. The upper half of the muscle retains its natural color, but the lower half is white and glistening. Histologic examination reveals partial to complete replacement of muscle by relatively acellular connective tissue.

Clinical Features. The head is tilted and the posterior aspect of the skull is slightly turned to the side of the involved muscle (Fig. 19-1). Passive movement of the head is resisted by the shortened muscle. The vertical length of the face is diminished, the eyebrow on the side of the affected muscle appears to deviate downward, and the face is broadened.

Treatment. The treatment of this contracture is not altogether satisfactory. In severe cases, surgical division of the lower attachment of the muscle has been satisfactory. Physical therapy is undertaken immedi-

FIG. 19-1. Congenital torticollis. Three-year-old child with a history of shortening of the left sternocleidomastoid muscles and tilting of the head since birth.

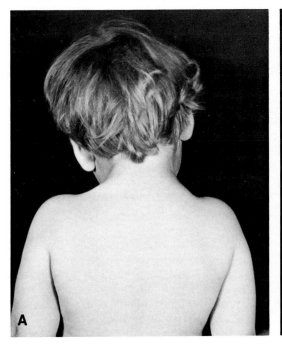

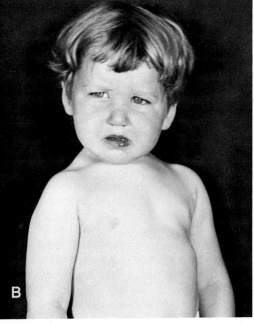

ately following operation. Most authorities feel that treatment should be started as early as possible in an attempt to prevent asymmetry, which tends to become more pronounced as the child grows.

CONGENITAL CLUBFOOT

Congenital clubfoot may assume any one of several abnormal postures. Of these, the most common type is talipes equinovarus, in which the foot is plantar flexed and inverted.

Etiology. Various possible etiologies have been proposed, including defects in the spinal cord and in muscle, damage to peripheral nerves and unusual pressures, and abnormal postures *in utero.*

Clinical Features. Congenital clubfoot is readily recognized at birth and usually involves only one extremity. If uncorrected, certain leg muscles fail to develop. There is resultant shortening of other muscle groups such as the gastrocnemius. The tendons are displaced, and the foot assumes various degrees of deformity through the unusual stress.

Treatment. Early treatment is absolutely essential; for cases diagnosed during infancy, this consists of manipulation and fixation in an overcorrected position. Surgical correction may be necessary in older children.

CONGENITAL ELEVATION OF THE SCAPULA (SPRENGEL'S DEFORMITY)

In Sprengel's deformity, the affected scapula is elevated and is usually rotated laterally, bringing the lower angle in closer proximity to the spine. The length of the scapula is diminished in the vertical and increased in the transverse dimensions.

Etiology. The etiology of this disorder is obscure. It has been suggested that the abnormality frequently appears to be related to a defect in the innervation or development of the trapezius or serratus anterior muscle.

Clinical Features. The condition is usually unilateral, producing asymmetry in the shoulders, the deformed shoulder being elevated and advanced. Scoliosis frequently accompanies this deformity, and in a small proportion of cases torticollis is present. On occasion this contracture is accompanied by a cervical spina bifida or a Klippel-Feil deformity of the spine.

Treatment. The treatment of this condition is surgical and often not very satisfactory. However, a procedure has been described in which surgical correction is obtained by moving the origins of the trapezius and rhomboid muscles downward after resection of the omovertebral bone or other fibrous bands.

CONGENITAL CONTRACTURES OF THE EXTREMITIES

Congenital contractures of the extremities (also referred to as amyoplasia congenita, multiple congenital articular rigidities, myodystrophica congenita deformans, and arthrogryposis multiplex congenita) are characterized by the immobility of one or more joints in association with absence or defective development of specific skeletal muscles.

Etiology. It is likely that this condition is a syndrome with several possible etiologies. Some authorities feel that all cases classified as arthrogryposis are not alike, but differ in etiology and in clinical picture. Adams *et al* feel that in some cases there is a developmental defect of the spinal cord with failure of innervation of skeletal muscles, whereas in others an infantile muscular dystrophy is the cause of the contracture.[1] In still other cases, a developmental defect in the joints themselves may be responsible for contractures of the limbs. Hereditary factors play a role in some cases.

Pathology. Histopathologic changes seem to vary. In some patients, lesions are confined to the muscle fibers, which on occasion are replaced by fat cells, and are extremely variable in size, exhibiting a dystrophic picture. In other cases, the anterior horn cells and intramuscular nerves exhibit the abnormal changes.

Clinical Features. Clinically, the infant presents with the so-called wooden doll appearance, the extremities assuming fixed posturing in almost any position (Fig. 19-2). The affected limbs are frequently shortened. The range of movement at the affected joints is greatly impaired. Muscular weakness and hypotonia are prominent features in most cases. The deep tendon reflexes are diminished to absent. The skin and subcutaneous tissues are wrinkled and flabby. Other congenital abnormalities are sometimes associated with arthrogryposis. As a rule, intellectual functions are not impaired. In some cases, flexor postures with flexion contractures are present, whereas in others extensor posturing predominates.

Laboratory Data. Roentgenographic alteration of the joints or joint capsules is not present, but muscle shadows frequently appear to be very small. Electromyographically, the muscle action potentials are feeble or absent, but the reaction of degeneration is not observed.

Treatment. Physical therapeutic measures including passive movement and manipulation may be of some help. In severe cases, attempts at surgical correction may be advisable.

MUSCULAR DYSTROPHY

The muscular dystrophies constitute an important group of primary degenerative diseases of skeletal muscle in children.

FIG. 19-2. Arthrogryposis multiplex congenital. Frontal (A) and lateral (B) views. Six-year-old child with a history of multiple congenital contractures of all extremities.

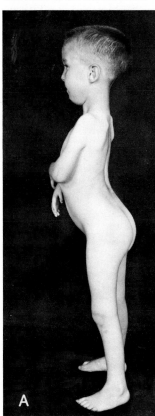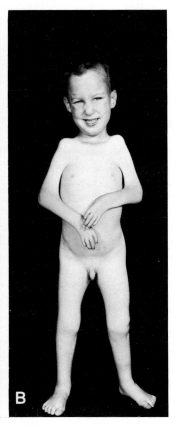

Etiology. The etiology of the muscular dystrophies is uncertain, although genetic and biochemical factors undoubtedly play an important role in the pathogenesis. Recently, clinical studies involving dystrophic patients and experimental studies on a strain of dystrophic mice suggest that certain muscular dystrophies may be related to defects within the nervous system itself, perhaps in the motoneuron.[11,53,76] Other experimental studies in animals have suggested the possibility of an autoimmune etiology.[97]

Pathology. Although the several clinical types of muscular dystrophy differ markedly in course and distribution, the abnormalities in the muscles are almost the same in all of them. On inspection at biopsy or necropsy, the muscles appear unnaturally small and have a different color from normal muscle, varying from yellowish to pinkish gray with a pale translucence. The histopathologic changes are as follows: There is disappearance of muscle fibers with apparent increase of connective tissue and fat cells, as well as marked variation in the size of individual fibers, which may be observed in adjacent muscle fibers. Homogenization or hyalinization of the muscle fiber with loss of striation may occur. The sarcolemmal nuclei of both the swollen and atrophied fibers are large and increased numerically, and seem to exhibit a wider variation in shape than normal. In some fibers, long chains of centrally placed sarcolemmal nuclei are observed; this is more characteristic of myotonic dystrophy than other types. As the myopathy progresses, the muscle fibers tend to atrophy and disappear in greater numbers. Granular degeneration is found in some fibers. The smallest fibers appear to fragment. The nuclei shrink and tend to exhibit a dark-staining character. Regenerative changes may be present early in the disease but are strikingly absent later. The motor and sensory nerve fibers are not damaged, although as the state of degeneration progresses, the motor end-plate does exhibit some atrophic changes. Muscle spindles are preserved even after all muscle fibers have disappeared. No significant changes are present within the central nervous system. In the late stages of progressive muscular dystrophy, the ultimate fate of the muscle fiber closely simulates that of a muscle fiber deprived of its innervation.

Myotonic dystrophy differs histopathologically from the other forms of dystrophy due to the presence of extensive, centrally placed sarcolemmal nuclei, sarcoplasmic masses, and ring annulets. In the Landouzy-Dejerine type of restricted dystrophy there is rather profound fibrosis, which may account for the increased frequency of contractures observed in this form of the disease.

Clinical Types. It is convenient to classify muscular dystrophy in children into the following clinical types: (1) the severe generalized familial type, (2) the mild restricted type, (3) the progressive dystrophic ophthalmoplegic type, (4) myotonic dystrophy, (5) the infantile type, and (6) the distal type (Table 19-2).

Generalized Familial Muscular Dystrophy (Pseudohypertrophic Muscular Dystrophy, Duchenne's Muscular Dystrophy). Although generalized familial muscular dystrophy is not present clinically at birth, it commences early in life, usually prior to 6 years of age. The hereditary nature of this type has been conclusively established. It appears that it is sex-linked, transmitted by an unaffected female, and seen far more frequently in males than females. Subtle symptoms, such as inability to walk at the customary age and enlargement of muscles, may be present long before the full-blown clinical picture is observed. As the disease progresses and the clinical manifestations become overt, two features are prominent: progressive alteration in muscle size and profound weakness of specific muscles. The muscles may increase or decrease in size. The muscles that exhibit enlargement most frequently are the calf muscles, the infraspinati, and the deltoids. Occasionally, the quadriceps, glutei, and triceps are similarly involved. Rarely, the hypertrophy affects almost any of the skeletal muscles of the body. The enlarged muscles possess a firm, resilient quality and are definitely weaker than uninvolved muscles of comparable size. Ultimately, the enlarged muscles become atrophied and wasted. The muscles of the pectoral and

TABLE 19-2.   Clinical Types of Muscular Dystrophy

Parameter	Severe Generalized Muscular Dystrophy	Mild Restricted Muscular Dystrophy	Progressive Dystrophic Ophthalmoplegia	Myotonic Dystrophy	Infantile Muscular Dystrophy	Hereditary Distal Myopathy
Age at onset	Prior to 6 years	Usually late in first decade, occasionally later	Infancy to age 50–55	Childhood to fourth decade	At birth or soon thereafter	Within first 2 years of life
Inheritance	Sex-linked	Simple dominant, simple recessive, or sex-linked	Simple dominant or simple recessive	Usually dominant with anticipation and potentiation	Not yet defined	Autosomal dominant
Sex incidence	More frequent in males (6:1)	Males and females equally affected	Males and females equally affected	Males and females equally affected	Not yet defined	Males and females equally affected
Muscle groups involved	Pelvic and shoulder girdle muscles involved early; periphery of limbs late	Largely confined to facial, pelvic, and pectoral girdle muscles	Confined to ocular muscles in most cases	Distal extremities often affected before proximal muscles	Generalized	Distal extremities primarily
Myotonia	Absent	Absent	Absent	Most prominent in hands, tongue, or facial musculature	Absent	Absent
Endocrine abnormalities	Not observed	Not observed	Not observed	Testicular atrophy	Not observed	Not observed
Cardiac abnormalities	Occasional minor disorders of cardiac rhythm and cardiac hypertrophy	ECG alterations, occasionally tachycardia	Not observed	Variety of ECG abnormalities	Not observed	Not observed
Prognosis	Survival rarely beyond 20 years	In most cases good; occasionally severe disability	Major deficit restricted to eye movements	Progressively disabling over many years	No survival beyond 5–6 years	Generally good, no obvious progression after age 18

pelvic girdle and lumbosacral spine appear wasted early in the course of the disorder in contradistinction to the enlarged appearance of the muscles cited previously. Quite early in the course of the disease, a waddling type of gait is seen because of instability due to weakness of the muscles about the pelvis and vertebral column. When the child attempts to arise from the squatting position, he uses his hands to support his trunk and appears to "climb up his thighs"—Gowers' sign. As the disease progresses, with increasing weakness in the flexors and extensors of the hip and the extensors of the knee, the patient has great difficulty in maintaining erect posture. Consequently, he places his feet far apart to maintain stability. Weakness of the abdominal wall, lumbar spine, and pelvic girdle musculature gives rise to prominent lordosis on standing and instability when sitting. In the later stages of the disease, muscle strength in the proximal limb and trunk musculature is markedly diminished, and the wasting and weakness spread to involve the distal extremities, with the face, jaw, laryngeal, pharyngeal, ocular, and hand muscles usually being involved very late in the course. Along with the distal involvement, shortening and contractures of the extremities appear. As the patient becomes bedridden, fixed flexion attitudes at the elbows and knees and kyphoscoliosis develop. Although the deep tendon reflexes are preserved early in the course of the disorder, later they tend to disappear as the muscles become weak and wasted. Death frequently occurs prior to age 20, usually from intercurrent infection. Disorders of cardiac rhythm, hypertrophy of the heart, and cardiac failure have been reported in these patients. Dysfunction of smooth muscle structures has not been observed.

Mild Restricted Muscular Dystrophy. Five separate forms of this type of muscular dystrophy have been described. The first is benign X-linked muscular dystrophy (Becker's form), which is clinically different from the Duchenne type described previously.[6] In this benign form, the age at onset is usually later than 8 years, and the ability to walk is retained beyond 16 years of age. Survival is prolonged beyond the age of 32. Clinically, benign X-linked dystrophy is similar to the Duchenne type except for the milder temporal progression. Weakness and wasting of the proximal limb muscles slowly progressive in character along with contractures at joints are seen in these patients. The pseudohypertrophy is not as consistently observed clinically in the benign form as in the severe generalized type.[86] Just as in the Duchenne type, benign X-linked muscular dystrophy is transmitted by an unaffected female to her male offspring. Of interest is the fact that the benign form and the Duchenne type of X-linked

muscular dystrophy do not occur in the same family.

The second form of mild muscular dystrophy is the facioscapulohumeral dystrophy of Landouzy and Dejerine. The onset of symptoms in this form usually occurs during the first or second decades of life, although rarely it has been reported to arise in the third decade. The initial clinical manifestation is weakness in the shoulder girdle musculature (Fig. 19-3). The patient has difficulty in elevating the arms above the head. This may be associated with some difficulty in eye closure due to involvement of the facial muscles observed in some patients early in childhood. As the disease progresses, the patient is unable to purse the lips. This is associated with protrusion of the lips, giving rise to the so-called myopathic facies. As this form progresses, the muscles attached to the scapulas become weak and wasted, giving rise to poor scapular fixation. Other muscles, including the sternomastoids, deltoids, latissimus dorsi, and erectors of the spine, also become weak and wasted. The triceps and biceps subsequently become involved. The bones of the shoulders and back protrude conspicuously, and the upper arm is wasted as compared to the preserved forearms, giving an "alley-oop" appearance to the upper extremities. This clinical type usually shows no further progression, although occasionally slight weakness of the pelvic girdle musculature without noticeable atrophy may be observed.

The third form of mild restricted dystrophy is termed juvenile muscular dystrophy of Erb. Clinical manifestations of this form arise late in the first decade, rarely as late as age 45. Specific shoulder girdle muscles such as the trapezii, serrati anterior, pectorals, latissimus dorsi, and rhomboids are weak and wasted in this form. As the disease progresses, the muscles of the upper arm and pelvic girdle also become involved. Facial muscle wasting occurs very late in this disorder. Just as in the facioscapulohumeral form, juvenile muscular dystrophy affects males and females equally. However, the facioscapulohumeral form follows the pattern of a simple dominant gene, whereas in juvenile dystrophy of Erb the pattern is one of a simple recessive inheritance.

The fourth form of mild restricted

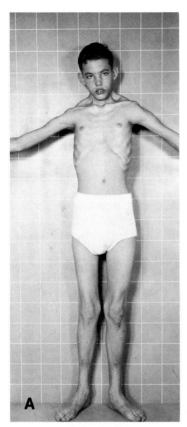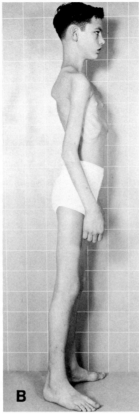

FIG. 19-3. Mild restricted muscular dystrophy. Frontal (A) and lateral (B) views. A 13-year-old boy with a 2-year history of weakness and wasting of muscles of pelvic and shoulder girdle.

muscular dystrophy is femoral dystrophy of Leyden and Moebius. The hip and thigh muscles are usually affected first, with involvement of the shoulder and upper extremity musculature occurring much later.

An additional form of mild restricted muscular dystrophy has been reported in which there is muscle weakness in the upper extremities proximally, and in the lower extremities distally. This has been referred to as the scapuloperoneal syndrome. Some families show only myopathic disturbances, which may be inherited as an autosomal recessive, autosomal dominant, or X-linked recessive trait. Occasionally the disorder may occur sporadically. Other families with this entity have clearly defined, neurogenic abnormalities.[100]

Cardiac disorders, mild in character, are often seen in the restricted muscular dystrophies. Extrasystoles and tachycardia have been reported to occur, along with cardiac hypertrophy. Cardiac failure with relatively sudden death is rare.

Progressive Dystrophic Ophthalmoplegia. Ptosis of the eyelids is the most frequent initial manifestation in this type of muscular dystrophy. Progressive weakness of the external ocular muscles develops gradually. Late in the course of this form, all extraocular movements are paralyzed, with the eyes remaining slightly divergent. The disorder is usually symmetrical. However, on occasion, involvement of one eye may precede the other, giving rise to diplopia. Just as in other patients with chronic ptosis, the forehead appears constantly wrinkled and the head is tilted backward. Facial weakness and wasting, particularly in the orbicularis oculi muscles, are observed in an appreciable percentage of cases. The muscles of mastication and of the shoulder girdle are weak and wasted in some cases. The age at onset of this disorder ranges from infancy to the sixth decade. The course is characterized by very slow progression of signs and symptoms. The disease may arrest at any stage in its evolution. Familial incidence is noted in approximately 50% of the cases. In some, inheritance is dominant; in others, the disease seems to express itself as a recessive trait. The incidence of this type of dystrophy in males and females seems to be approximately equal.

Oculopharyngeal muscular dystrophy is a familial cranial myopathy with delayed onset inherited in an autosomal dominant pattern. The main features in this disorder include ptosis of the eyelids and dysphagia. The dystrophic characteristics of this myopathy are evident on histopathologic examination. The association of total external ophthalmoplegia in some of these patients supports a relationship to progressive dystrophic ophthalmoplegia. Involvement of the extremity and girdle musculature in this disorder has also been reported.[106]

Myotonic Dystrophy (Dystrophia Myotonica, Myotonia Atrophica, Steinert's Disease).   Classical myotonic dystrophy is inherited in an autosomal dominant pattern and usually occurs in adolescence or in adult life, but may present earlier in a congenital form. Males and females alike are affected in this progressive familial disorder. In this form of dystrophy, the distal extremities in the muscles of the face, jaw, neck, and eyelids become weak and wasted early, whereas proximal extremity and axial musculature is involved considerably later in the evolution of the disease. Thus, in patients with classical myotonic dystrophy, the small muscles of the distal upper extremities and the extensor muscles of the forearm exhibit weakness and wasting. Ptosis of the eyelids, lack of facial expression, thinness of the face—the so-called myopathic facies—may be present from childhood in some cases. Wasting of the muscles in the distal lower extremities also constitutes an early sign in some families. Pronounced weakness and wasting of the masseter and the sternocleidomastoid muscles, in association with a prominent forward curvature of the neck, produce the characteristic "swan neck" appearance almost universally present in these patients. The deep tendon reflexes tend to be lost as the disorder progresses. A weak, nasal voice accompanied by dysphagia indicates weakness of pharyngeal and laryngeal musculature, which also tends to occur early. Degenerative changes in the endocrine glands and in other tissues, including cataracts, alopecia, and testicular atrophy, accompany the myopathic changes. Myotonia characterized by prolonged contraction of involved specific muscles after electrical or mechanical stimulation and by delay in relaxation following strong voluntary muscular contraction may precede the muscle wasting by 2 to 3 years. The temperature of the environment seems to play a role in this as well as in other myotonic disorders, cold tending to make the myotonia worse. Repetition of a given movement tends to enhance relaxation. Myotonia may be completely absent in some patients exhibiting the characteristic distribution of muscle wasting, endocrinopathy, and cataracts.

The congenital form of myotonic dystrophy invariably occurs in the offspring of an involved mother. Clinically, this form of the disease may be heralded in the newborn period as a "floppy baby" syndrome, characterized by generalized hypotonia with associated difficulties in sucking and swallowing. Respiratory impairment may also be a serious consequence. It is not uncommon for the mother to have noted a paucity of movement of the fetus during gestation. Clinical evaluation of the infant reveals marked facial diplegia with impairment of eye closure. Myotonia, either clinically or electrically, is not present. Associated skeletal deformities occur. The mother usually demonstrates at least some clinical features of myotonic dystrophy if examined closely. Mental deficiency may accompany the other signs and symptoms in this congenital form. Patients with this form tend to improve gradually, with increase in muscle tone and the capability of walking, although the motor developmental milestones may be delayed. Over a period of time, however, these children develop the classical form of myotonic dystrophy characterized by myotonia, muscle weakness, and wasting.[31,32,109]

Infantile Muscular Dystrophy.   A rather rare type of dystrophic myopathy is seen to develop before, at, or soon after birth with rapid progression of disability leading to death within 2 to 6 years. Familial factors seem to play a role in this type. In one such family reported, arthrogryposis was encountered in one child at birth and a simple dystrophy was present in a second child. Both children were greatly handicapped by this myopathy, which apparently had been present in utero.

Hereditary Distal Myopathy with Onset in Infancy (Distal Muscular Dystrophy). A hereditary myopathy involving primarily the distal muscles has been described, with onset during early childhood.[50,102] These patients show bilateral foot drop as an early manifestation by age 2, and weakness of the hands and wrists become apparent during childhood, with a predilection for the finger extensor muscles. No obvious progression of the disease was noted after age 18. It appears to be transmitted as an autosomal dominant trait, with males and females equally affected. This disorder is differentiated from other neuromuscular disorders by the myopathic nature of the electromyograms and the histopathology.

Laboratory Examination. As yet, no specific biochemical diagnostic studies for muscular dystrophy have been devised. Creatine metabolism is altered just as in other diseases involving muscle. A decrease in urinary creatinine content and an increase in urinary creatine associated with a mild hypercreatinemia have been reported and are observed with consistency in the dystrophies. There is impairment in creatine tolerance, indicating that functional muscle mass is reduced. Another prominent biochemical abnormality observed in the muscular dystrophies as well as in other myopathies is the elevation of serum enzyme levels. Creatine phosphokinase, aldolase, glutamic oxaloacetic transaminase, glutamic pyruvic transaminase, and lactic dehydrogenase have all been observed to be increased in the serum of patients with muscular dystrophy, especially early in the disorder. Because it has been shown that the frequency of the elevation of any particular enzyme, especially in the Duchenne type of muscular dystrophy, is not appreciably different statistically, it appears that determination of the levels of the various enzymes is of about equal value in

the diagnosis.[87] Elevated serum enzyme levels are observed in the preclinical stages in some members of a muscular dystrophy family. It has been demonstrated that serum creatine phosphokinase levels are appreciably elevated in patients with Duchenne muscular dystrophy and moderately elevated in a large percentage of patients with mild restricted muscular dystrophy, whereas only slight elevations occur in patients with myotonic dystrophy. The presence of elevated creatine phosphokinase in a number of clinically unaffected mothers and sisters of patients with severe generalized muscular dystrophy has also been observed.[29]

Electromyographic findings differ somewhat in the various types of muscular dystrophy. In the severe generalized type, there is a decrease of mean action potential voltage at full effort with an associated decrease in the duration of motor unit action potentials. In addition, an increase in polyphasic potentials in all of the muscular dystrophies may be of help in diagnosis. The electromyogram in myotonic dystrophy shows a typical myotonic "dive bomber" type of response and in this respect differs from the other muscular dystrophies. Muscle biopsy is useful in diagnosing muscular dystrophy, although there is a histologic similarity to the appearance observed late in other neuromuscular disorders.

Differential Diagnosis. The various forms of muscular dystrophy can be differentiated from other neuromuscular syndromes by the site of predilection involving the proximal and axial musculature (Table 19-2). The deep-tendon reflexes are often preserved until late in the dystrophic disorders, and deficit in sensation is not encountered. Electromyographic studies serve to distinguish the dystrophies from neuropathic and myelopathic disorders (Table 19-1). The muscle biopsy is often helpful in the diagnosis of dystrophy, although a similar histologic appearance may be observed late in the course of many of the neuromuscular disorders. Hereditary factors play a role in all the types of muscular dystrophy. The severe generalized type is transmitted as a sex-linked recessive trait, whereas the mild restricted types follow the pattern of either sex-linked recessive, autosomal dominant, or autosomal recessive inheritance. Myotonic dystrophy differs in that the inheritance tends to exhibit a dominant pattern but may be variable with features of anticipation and potentiation. Involvement of the distal musculature occurs early in myotonic dystrophy in contradistinction to other myopathies. The presence of myotonia in the distal upper extremity, the tongue, and the facial musculature, and its relative absence in other muscles serve to differentiate this from other forms of myotonia. Severe generalized dystrophy tends to present a full-blown picture at an earlier age than the mild restricted types. The elevation of the serum enzyme levels tends to be more pronounced in the active dystrophies seen in childhood than in the more chronic types observed in adults (Table 19-2).

Therapy.   Many different forms of therapy have been attempted for the muscular dystrophies. Drugs used include glycine and other amino acids, isoniazid, adenosine triphospate, and α-tocopherol phosphate. None of these has had a consistent beneficial effect in altering the progression of the disease. The anabolic synthetic steroid, 1-methyl-Δ-androstenolone, in association with a digitalis preparation, has been reported to delay the progression of the disease process in patients with restricted muscular dystrophy, although children with generalized muscular dystrophy remain unaided.[19] Physical therapy including massage may be of some help in maintaining nutrition of the muscles, and it may delay contracture development. If contractures develop, orthopedic surgical techniques may be employed. Procaine amide, 25 mg/kg/day in divided doses, and quinine hydrochloride, 5 mg/kg/day in divided doses, have been useful in relieving myotonia in patients with myotonic dystrophy, but they have no effect on the relentlessly progressive underlying dystrophic process. With increased knowledge of the basic biochemical genetic processes in the development of muscle, new methods of prevention and treatment may arise.

Prognosis.   The generalized or pseudohypertrophic type is invariably and relentlessly progressive. Deformity and debility in the end stages are extensive. Initially, the muscular weakness increases and renders the patient unable to walk. Contractures develop, especially in the lower extremities, with severe scoliosis. Death occurs as a rule before the end of the second decade and is usually due to intercurrent infection. The patient is especially vulnerable to respiratory infection because of the involvement of the respiratory muscles and the muscles of deglutition. The severe generalized type progresses more rapidly than the other clinical types. Myotonic dystrophy is more incapacitating than progressive dystrophic ophthalmoplegia and the restricted dystrophies. The myotonic patient may survive for many years, usually succumbing to an intercurrent illness during late middle age. In the restricted types, the disease process progresses to a point at which the disorder may be arrested without rendering the person disabled. Infantile dystrophy in the limited number of reported cases seems to show rapid progression and death during the first 5 years of life.

MYOSITIS

Among the primary disorders of skeletal muscle are the myositides, which involve localized or diffuse inflammatory degenerative changes. These changes may be acute, subacute, or chronic, involving a single muscle or multiple muscles. A useful classification based on etiology separates myositis into two major categories.[68] In the first, the causative agent can be identified as a virus, a bacterium, a fungus, or a parasite, whereas in the second category the etiology is obscure. The second category includes polymyositis and dermatomyositis, the interstitial myositis of the connective tissue disorders, and sarcoidosis of muscle.

VIRAL MYOSITIS

Epidemic pleurodynia, also termed devil's grip, epidemic myalgia, and Bornholm's disease (the latter relating to the Danish island of Bornholm where an outbreak of myositis occurred), is an inflammatory disorder of muscle caused by a virus.

Etiology. Coxsackie group B virus has now been established as the etiologic agent of epidemic pleurodynia, although the echo-viruses were isolated in some cases. Epidemic and sporadic outbreaks of this disorder have been seen throughout the world, usually occurring in the summer or early fall. Children between the ages of 5 and 15 are the most susceptible. Epidemiologically, the spread of this enterovirus is probably by direct contact, although water and insect transmissions have also been suggested.

Clinical Features. The disorder is usually heralded by severe pain in the chest and, less often, in the back, shoulders, abdomen, or hips. The involved muscles are exquisitely tender to pressure. Voluntary or reflex contraction produces pain. Rapid, shallow respirations owing to the intense pain on inspiration are observed. The patient may assume abnormal postures and may be unable to negotiate certain specific movements because of the muscle pain. Singultus is occasionally present. A pleural friction rub is sometimes encountered. Slight temperature elevation is often an accompaniment. The acute pain and fever last 1 to 3 days, and after initial improvement one or more relapses have been reported in almost one fourth of the cases in one series. Coxsackie B viruses also cause aseptic meningitis, acute benign pericarditis, and myocarditis in the newborn (Chapter 12).

Laboratory Examination and Diagnosis. Definitive diagnosis is made in the laboratory by isolating the virus from stools and by a rise in titer of specific complement-fixing antibodies.

Treatment. Symptomatic treatment with analgesics may be helpful, but no specific treatment has been developed.

Prognosis. The prognosis in epidemic pleurodynia is favorable for complete recovery.

BACTERIAL MYOSITIS

An acute purulent inflammation of muscle may occur with septicemia or may arise by direct extension from an infectious arthritis, a pleuritis, or a decubitus ulcer.

Etiology. A variety of pyogenic organisms may be responsible. Staphylococci and streptococci are incriminated most frequently.

Pathology. Histologic studies of biopsy material reveal a necrotic destruction with extensive infiltration of inflammatory cells in the muscle tissue. The area of reaction may become encapsulated with abscess formation.

Clinical Features. Systemic symptoms including headache, chills, temperature elevation and diaphoresis are observed acutely in some cases of local suppurative myositis. These symptoms precede the local pain and swelling of the involved individual muscle(s).

Traumatized muscle is particularly susceptible to clostridial organisms. Gas gangrene (*Clostridium welchii*) tends to develop in deep puncture wounds and is especially common in compound fractures. *Mycobacterium tuberculosis* can give rise to infection in muscle by local extension from an adjacent tuberculous focus or by hematogenous spread with isolated miliary lesions in the muscles. A generalized tuberculous polymyositis may arise.

Treatment. The treatment includes surgical incision and drainage as well as specific appropriate antibiotic therapy.

FUNGUS MYOSITIS

Actinomyces bovis is the fungus that most frequently gives rise to muscle disease. The infection is spread by direct extension from an adjacent focus such as an actinomycotic lesion of the pleura or skin.

PARASITIC MYOSITIS

Trichinosis

Etiology. Humans become infected with the nematode *Trichinella spiralis* through ingestion of poorly cooked pork or game meat.

Pathology. The gross appearance of the muscle after heavy infestation is that of a pale, soft, granular tissue. Microscopically, the characteristic spiral form becomes visible in the muscle fiber about 10 days after invasion of the muscle. The involved muscle fiber contains numerous eosinophils and exhibits a granular alteration of the sarcoplasm with loss of cross striations occurring even earlier than the appearance of the spiral form. The sarcolemmal nuclei enlarge rapidly and multiply. An intense inflammatory reaction develops in the surrounding connective tissue, with infiltration of cellular elements. The trichinae tend to survive best in skeletal muscle. Invasion of the heart, liver, brain, and other organs by these organisms is also observed. Muscle fiber regeneration may occur. The muscles most susceptible to invasion by trichinae are the diaphragm, extraocular muscles, tongue, and intercostal, back, abdominal, and limb muscles.

Clinical Features. Most cases of *Trichinella spiralis* infections are subclinical. However, when a large number of the parasites are ingested at one time, the clinical picture consists of a gastrointestinal disturbance with diarrhea, elevation of temperature, and angioneurotic edema, particularly of the upper eyelids. In several days the skeletal muscles, especially the gastrocnemii, become painful and tender. Unusually heavy infestations give rise to central nervous system signs and symptoms such as delirium, somnolence, coma, paralysis, and dysphasia. This disease seldom has a fatal result, but when death occurs, usually between the third to the eighth week, either myocardial failure or respiratory muscle paralysis is responsible. The symptoms usually subside within 8 to 10 weeks after onset.

Laboratory Examination and Diagnosis. Laboratory studies including a complete blood count, measurement of complement-fixing antibodies, flocculation, and skin tests are helpful in diagnosing this disorder after the second week. Eosinophilia is noted on the blood smear and is sometimes as high as 80%. Trichinal larvae are observed in the muscle biopsy in approximately 75% of the cases and are diagnostic. Calcified larvae may be seen after several weeks on roentgenograms of skeletal muscle.

Treatment. Treatment is largely symptomatic. It includes bed rest, adequate fluid intake, and appropriate analgesic agents to relieve headaches and muscle pain. If congestive heart failure occurs, appropriate specific measures including fluid restriction, low salt diet, diuretics, and digitalization may be indicated. Prednisone, initially 40 mg/day with a gradual decrease in the dosage as the symptoms improve, has been recommended. Adrenocorticotropic hormone has also been used successfully in alleviating symptoms. The anthelmintic agent thiabendazole has been reported to be helpful in the treatment of human trichinosis. There is evidence that this agent is capable either of sterilizing the larvae in the muscles or markedly decreasing their virulence. Oral doses of thiabendazole, 25 mg/kg every 12 hours for 2 to 7 consecutive days according to the response of the individual patient, have been recommended. The combination of steroid therapy and thiabendazole has been reported to be an effective means of treatment.[99]

Other Parasitic Myopathies

Cysticercus cellulosae, the larvae of the pork tapeworm *Taenia solium*, enter the general circulation in the human after penetrating the mucosa and muscle. They are thus distributed throughout the body, and they survive in several different organs including the skeletal muscle and the brain. The larvae tend to encyst, producing an inflammatory reaction and subsequently a granuloma with ultimate calcification. Two types of pathologic reactions in muscle have been reported. The most common response is death of the larvae and subsequent calcification. However, a rare and unusual response is the induction of a pseudohypertrophic myopathy for which there is no known treatment.[39] Symptomatic myositis with pain and tenderness of skeletal muscle results from an infection with the dog tapeworm *Echinococcus granulosus*, which is acquired by petting or handling dogs carrying the ova in their hair. Generalized muscular weakness and wasting occur in patients with schistosomiasis caused by *Schistosoma mansoni* or *Schistosoma haematobium*. An asymptomatic myositis is present in infection by the protozoan *Tox-*

oplasma gondii in children and adults. The South American form of trypanosomiasis caused by infection with *Trypanosoma cruzi* involves skeletal muscle and produces myositis in humans. The myositis, however, is usually asymptomatic.

MYOSITIS OF UNKNOWN ETIOLOGY

Primary idiopathic myositis may be classified in two groups on a descriptive basis. The term *polymyositis* refers to those cases in which the inflammatory disease process is confined to the muscles. The term *dermatomyositis* refers to the combination of muscle and skin inflammatory lesions and is the more common form observed in children.[22,66,108] Some authorities believe that there are more important differences, especially in pathogenetic mechanisms, in these two groups than the mere presence or absence of a rash.[75] When the disease evolves rapidly, the term *acute* is added to the polymyositis or dermatomyositis. *Subacute* and *chronic* apply when the course of the disease is more protracted. A recent report of pathologic and electrodiagnostic features of polymyositis in a series of patients with facioscapulohumeral muscular dystrophy suggests the possibility of a relationship between inflammatory myopathies and mild, restricted muscular dystrophy.[60]

Etiology. The etiology of this disorder has not been established with certainty. There is some evidence that an autoimmune process is involved. Several authorities recently presented suggestive evidence that a slow virus may be playing a pathogenetic role, at least in some cases of chronic polymyositis and dermatomyositis.[13,14,80,81] It has been suggested that perhaps an autoimmune mechanism triggered by a virus infection might be the pathogenetic process involved in polymyositis. Immunologic studies suggest that polymyositis may be due to lymphocyte-mediated delayed hypersensitivity.

Pathology. On gross examination, the involved skeletal muscle assumes a pale red or yellowish color and may be either soft and friable or rubbery and firm, depending on the disease. Microscopically, the cardi-

nal abnormalities observed in dermatomyositis of the adult (*i.e.*, muscle fiber necrosis, variation in fiber diameter, and regeneration) are not frequently observed in the childhood form. Instead, the most striking changes are observed in the blood vessels located in the connective tissues of the skin, gastrointestinal tract, muscles, and small nerves. Arteritis and phlebitis with perivascular collections of inflammatory cells are observed early (Fig. 19-4). Hyperplasia of the intima of the arteries and veins is noted later with resultant occlusion of many of these vessels. The occlusions appear in all stages of organization and recanalization, with resultant ulcerations and perforations of the gastrointestinal tract and infarction of muscle. Involvement of peripheral nerves and some degree of denervation atrophy of muscles have also been reported.[5]

Clinical Features. The shoulder girdle musculature and the muscles of deglutition are often involved first. Soon thereafter, the proximal muscles of all extremities become tender, edematous, firm in consistency, and weak. In a large proportion of cases, the skin overlying the affected muscles assumes a reddish brown hue. The eyelids become swollen, often with a heliotrope appearance (Fig. 19-5). An erythematous rash is observed over the face and neck. An elevated temperature may be seen in initial phases of the acute variety. Patches of pigmentation and depigmentation over the extensor surfaces of the joints are noted. When present, the skin lesions may precede or accompany the muscle symptoms. Desquamation frequently occurs. In a matter of days, other muscles of the extremities become involved, and the deep tendon reflexes are diminished to absent. As the muscles of the pharynx and upper esophagus weaken, dysphagia results in a formidable problem in feeding and in handling secretions. Abdominal pain similar to that observed in peptic ulcer is a frequent complaint in all stages of this disorder, and late in the course of the disease is often associated with hematemesis and melena. In some instances, death occurs as the result of respiratory failure in the acute phase, aspiration pneumonia secondary to dysphagia, and ulcerations of the gastrointestinal tract with sub-

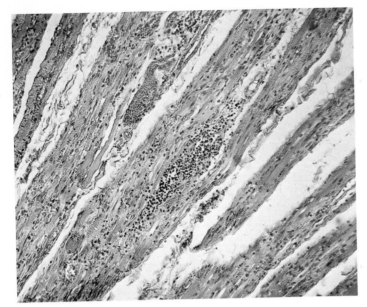

FIG. 19-4. Polymyositis. Note the diffuse degeneration and fragmentation of muscle fibers with collections of inflammatory cells.

FIG. 19-5. Eleven-year-old child with acute dermatomyositis. Note the heliotrope appearance and eyelid swelling.

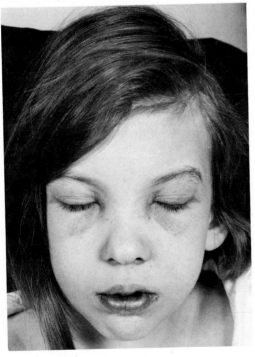

sequent perforation. In patients who survive, as the swelling and induration of the musculature subside there is much wasting and fibrotic shortening of the muscles. The resultant residual contractures in a posture of flexion and adduction are very disabling and present a serious and difficult nursing problem. The destruction of subcutaneous tissue and muscle is frequently associated with calcium deposition, which may be circumscribed or generalized. The subacute and chronic varieties of polymyositis and dermatomyositis are less common in children than in adults. In these forms, the onset is insidious and is associated with vague prodromal symptoms with weakness of the lower limbs as an early finding. As the subacute and chronic forms progress, the weakness ascends to involve the muscles of the distal upper extremities. Contracture and muscle wasting may be quite pronounced in these forms. The association of dermatomyositis and polymyositis with malignant neoplasms, which has been observed in adults, is rarely encountered in children.

Laboratory Examination. Routine hematologic studies reveal a polymorphonuclear leukocytosis with a marked elevation in the erythrocyte sedimentation rate. Electromyographic studies frequently show an increased insertion activity and a normal interference pattern with action potentials of short duration until late in the course of the disease. Occasionally, fibrillation potentials and brief flurries of high frequency discharges are observed. Serum levels of the enzymes creatine phosphokinase, transaminase, and aldolase are markedly elevated even early in the course of the disorder, tending to return toward normal levels as the patient improves. Measurement, therefore, of these enzymes is of value not only in diagnosis but in following the course of treatment. Nonspecific laboratory findings in dermatomyositis also occasionally include a mild anemia and eosinophilia. The electrophoretic pattern of the serum proteins is usually normal.

Differential Diagnosis. The progressive course in association with painful, tender, edematous muscles usually accompanied by a characteristic skin rash serves to differentiate acute polymyositis or dermatomyositis from other myopathic disorders.

Treatment. The response to treatment among patients has not been universally successful. However, steroid therapy has resulted in dramatic improvement in some cases. Prednisone, 1 to 2 mg/kg/day, usually begins to suppress the disease process within 1 to 2 weeks. As the serum enzyme levels return to the normal range, the dosage can then be reduced gradually until minimal suppressive dosage is reached—usually 2.5 to 7.5 mg/day. This maintenance dosage should be continued for approximately 1 year after the disease is in full remission. Some authorities, however, feel that endocrine therapy provides only symptomatic relief in this disease rather than any specific beneficial effect, and they employ only relatively small doses of medication, 5 to 15 mg of prednisone per day. Treatment with immunosuppressive agents was employed recently with success, and is particularly useful in those patients who do not respond to steroid therapy. Azathioprine, methotrexate, and cyclophosphamide are agents in this category that have been used successfully. Some authorities feel that oral cyclophosphamide is less toxic and more effective than the other immunosuppressive drugs and dosages of 2.5 mg/kg/day have been employed.[65]

Prognosis. Although the course of this disease is frequently rapidly progressive, on occasion it is quite protracted. Recovery has been reported to occur even after a prolonged stationary period. Occasionally, the course is characterized by remissions and exacerbations. Some authorities are of the opinion that dermatomyositis differs from polymyositis because the relatively high mortality observed in dermatomyositis is not seen in patients without the rash.[75]

SECONDARY FORMS OF MYOSITIS

A form of myositis occurs frequently in association with the other connective tissue disorders. A diffuse polymyositis is often seen in association with scleroderma. Pathologic studies of muscle in acute rheumatic fever, lupus erythematosus disseminata, and rheumatoid arthritis have demonstrated miliary inflammatory nodules in skeletal muscle. A dermatomyositis-like syndrome has been reported in children with congenital agammaglobulinemia. In these patients the skin rash is mild, if at all present. Contractures and severe induration of the tissues are noted, but the edema, which may involve face, extremities, and trunk, is the prominent aspect. In sarcoidosis, occasionally there is muscle involvement, which may be of two types: (1) a neural atrophy owing to involvement of one of several peripheral nerves, and (2) a localized inflammatory degeneration of muscle fibers. The clinical picture depends on the predominant type.

TUMORS OF SKELETAL MUSCLE

Primary neoplasms of mesodermal origin that differentiate into cells of striated muscle are very rare. Congenital rhabdomyoma of the heart is a benign tumor that presents as a multiple circumscribed mass within the wall of the heart. This tumor is probably the result of an embryogenic developmental abnormality of the heart. In some instances it is associated with tuberous sclerosis. The rhabdomyosarcoma is a tumor that develops within skeletal muscle and is extremely malignant. The only clinical features usually present is a deep-seated immobile muscle mass. The tumor is most unusual in children. Early and radical excision of the lesion is an absolute necessity. Teratomatous rhabdomyomas of the genital organs in both boys and girls may arise before birth and develop during childhood. Clinically, in the girl there is a large polypoid mass that may protrude from the vagina with hemorrhage and fetid discharge, whereas the prostatic tumor in the boy causes bladder neck obstruction. Rhabdomyoma of the testes is yet another example of this type of tumor. The teratomatous rhabdomyomas are highly malignant neoplasms. Carcinomas may rarely involve skeletal muscle in children by direct extension from a neighboring tumor or by metastasis from a distant lesion.

METABOLIC DISORDERS OF MUSCLE

MYOPATHIES ASSOCIATED WITH THE GLYCOGEN STORAGE DISEASES

Glycogen is a polysaccharide stored primarily in the liver and in skeletal muscle. It is the main source of energy for anaerobic muscular contraction. The normal synthesis and breakdown of glycogen are mediated by a number of intracellular enzymes. Biochemical dysfunction due to enzyme abnormality anywhere along these metabolic pathways may give rise to clinical disease. The various clinical expressions of abnormal glycogen metabolism are referred to as the glycogen storage diseases (the glycogenoses). The abnormal deposition of large amounts of glycogen in the liver was first recognized as a chemical manifestation of a specific disease by Von Gierke in two affected children.[107] Subsequently, Cori and Cori demonstrated that the enzyme glucose-6-phosphatase was either absent or reduced in quantity in the liver and that the inability of the liver to convert this enzyme to glucose was responsible for the accumulation of glycogen in the liver, kidney, and other tissues.[15] Because glucose-6-phosphatase is normally absent in muscles, muscles are not involved in this form of glycogenosis. Additional enzyme abnormalities involved in glycogen metabolism resulting in clinical disease have been described, and these glycogenoses involving skeletal muscle are discussed here.

Pathology. The histopathologic abnormality seen with conventional light microscopy and by using Best's carmine or Bauer's periodic acid-Schiff method include gross vacuolar changes within muscle fibers in association with an abnormal glycogen accumulation. In addition to the substantially increased glycogen in the sarcoplasm of the muscle fibers, a large number of vacuoles of all sizes can be observed by electron microscopy. Some of these vacuoles contain glycogen granules, whereas osmophilic clumps are observed in some smaller vacuoles; these are much larger than glycogen granules and probably contain complex lipids. The electron microscopic findings are different in the various types of skeletal muscle glycogenosis.

Specific Enzyme Deficiencies. *Cardiomuscular Glycogen Storage Disease (Pompe's Disease, Cori Type 2, Amylo-1,4-Glucosidase Deficiency, Acid Maltase Deficiency).* Cardiomuscular glycogen storage disease is due to a deficiency of the enzyme amylo-1,4-glucosidase (acid maltase), which can hydrolyze glycogen to glucose directly. This defect was initially described by Hers in 1963.[35] Recently it became apparent that there are two clinical forms in which this enzyme defect can express itself. The first is a rapidly progressive, fatal disease in infancy characterized by difficulty in feeding, evidence of cardiac dysfunction as manifested by respiratory distress with cyanosis and cardiac failure, a generalized hypotonic weakness of skeletal muscle, and macroglossia. This generalized form was initially described by Pompe in 1932.[71] Tissues other than cardiac and skeletal muscle, including liver, kidney, and nerve, contain variable amounts of glycogen. Because motor neurons may be disordered by glycogen deposition and sometimes show degeneration, neuronal lesions may contribute to the hypotonia and muscular weakness seen in these patients. In most cases the cardiac features predominate. In the second or mild form, the clinical and pathologic features of muscle disease play a more prominent in the overall picture. In some cases there is no evidence of tissue involvement other than skeletal muscle. In some way in the mild form, therefore, the enzyme defect is restricted primarily to skeletal muscle. These patients may demonstrate only muscular weakness and hypotonia.[38]

Limit Dextrinosis (Cori Type 3, Recant Type 4, Forbes' Disease, Debrancher Enzyme Deficiency). Limit dextrinosis is a rare type of glycogen storage disease in which the defective enzyme is amylo-1,6-glucosidase, a glycogen debrancher enzyme. The disorder occurs in both children and adults. Clinically, these patients show progressive muscular weakness with stiffness and cramping, difficulty in swallowing, and regurgitation of food. Macroglossia, cardiomegaly, and hepatomegaly have been reported.[63]

McArdle's Syndrome (Cori Type 5, Phosphorylase Deficiency). In 1951, McArdle suggested that a defective glycogen breakdown might explain the symptoms of muscular pain, stiffness, and weakness on exertion in a 30-year-old man with these complaints his entire life.[52] Hepatic glycogen breakdown was unimpaired, demonstrated by a normal hyperglycemic response to parenteral adrenaline. Two independent investigations involving histochemical studies in patients with symptoms similar to those of McArdle's patient showed the absence of any significant phosphorylase activity and an increased muscle glycogen content.[59,84] Thus, McArdle's syndrome was the first muscle glycogenosis described in which the site of the biochemical defect was precisely delineated. The clinical features usually express themselves in childhood. Muscular cramping on exertion is a prominent early symptom. Weakness of a muscle or group of muscles that are continuously or intensively exercised is also observed. Although there seems to be no specificity for any individual muscle, the muscle groups of the arms, fingers, back, and legs are involved most frequently. The disorder usually presents during childhood or early adult life,

although a late onset form has been described. The passage of reddish brown urine following intense activity is seen in some patients, the discoloration being related to the presence of myoglobin. There is no apparent explanation for its occasional occurrence in this disorder. Episodic loss of consciousness, usually related to exertion, may occur. This may be precipitated by hypoglycemia, because the energy for muscular contraction during severe exertion is dependent upon excessive glucose utilization, and glucose may enter the glycogenolytic pathway after the stage requiring phosphorylase. In some cases, there may be a genetic basis for this form of the disease with the hereditary pattern being autosomal recessive.[77,83]

Phosphofructokinase Deficiency. In another type of glycogen storage disease there is a deficiency of phosphofructokinase with impaired conversion of fructose-6-phosphate to fructose-1,6-diphosphate. The disorder frequently presents in childhood, with easy fatigability of muscles, muscular cramping, stiffness and weakness on exertion that is relieved by resting, and occasional episodes of pigmenturia after especially severe exertion.[45,98]

Other Enzyme Deficiencies. Several additional enzyme deficiencies in glycogen metabolism have been reported to account for clinical abnormalities consisting of muscle weakness and cramping. The enzymes include phosphoglucomutase and hexophosphate isomerase.[82,101]

Laboratory Diagnosis. In the above described disorders of glycogen metabolism, the normal rise of blood lactate observed in muscles after exercise is impaired in the venous blood because of the enzymatic deficiency in glycogen breakdown. The ischemic exercise test, therefore, constitutes an excellent clinical test for the skeletal muscle glycogenoses, with the exception perhaps of the generalized form of Pompe's disease. This test is performed according to the method described by McArdle.[52] The forearm muscles are made ischemic, inflating a sphygmomanometer cuff applied around the upper arm. Admixture with blood from the hand is prevented by applying a second cuff around the wrist. The forearm muscles are then exercised by the patient squeezing a sphygmomanometer bulb for 45 seconds. In normal subjects the blood lactate level rises to at least two to three times the basal level. This rise does not occur in patients with impaired glycogen breakdown.

Although failure of the blood lactate level to rise after ischemic exercise suggests defective glycogenolysis, the specific enzyme deficiency responsible is determined by biochemical analysis of biopsied muscle. Electromyography in advanced cases of skeletal muscle glycogenosis occasionally demonstrates poor insertion activity and a poor interference pattern or absence of a pattern on repeated exercise. Serum creatine phosphokinase, serum glutamic oxaloacetic acid transaminase, and serum glutamic pyruvic transaminase levels are elevated in some patients with phosphorylase deficiency.

Treatment and Prognosis. No specific treatment for the muscle glycogenoses has yet been developed. Vigorous exercise should be avoided, especially in phosphorylase deficiency. In some patients with this deficiency, the ingestion of fructose is beneficial.[26] The prognosis in phosphorylase deficiency, amylo-1,6-glucosidase deficiency, phosphofructokinase deficiency, and the muscular form of amylo-1,4-glucosidase deficiency is good because the symptoms are usually related to increased muscle activity. However, in the generalized form of amylo-1,4-glucosidase deficiency, death usually supervenes before the end of the first year of life owing primarily to intercurrent infection, although some patients are still alive at the end of the first decade.

MYOPATHIES ASSOCIATED WITH ABNORMAL LIPID METABOLISM IN SKELETAL MUSCLE

The oxidation of free fatty acids occurs within the mitochondria of the muscle cell. This reaction may occur either at rest or during periods of exercise, and contributes a significant portion of skeletal muscle energy supply. Carnitine, a compound that occurs in high concentration in skeletal muscle, is a carrier that couples with the fatty acids, enabling the fatty acids to be transported from cytoplasm into the mitochondria for oxidation. Carnitine palmityl transferase is the enzyme responsible for the combination of carnitine and fatty acids. Two forms of carnitine palmityl transferase have been described: one acting at the outer surface face of the inner mitochondrial membrane and the other acting at the inner membrane surface.[36]

Two myopathies due to defective lipid metabolism have been described: carnitine deficiency and carnitine palmityl transferase deficiency. Numerous cases documenting both of these deficiency states have been reported. Undoubtedly, additional myopathies will be described in the future.

Carnitine Deficiency. Since carnitine is synthesized in the liver and subsequently transported to other tissues, defective liver synthesis may result in reduced levels in muscles and other tissues. Thus, a syndrome of muscle weakness, with or without associated liver or central nervous system manifestations, has been reported to result from carnitine deficiency. In several case reports, muscle weakness was clinically manifested at a very early age, in one case at 18 months. Treatment of this rare myopathy with alternate-day prednisone has been reported to produce beneficial results, even after reducing the dosage. Carnitine administration has also been effective. This form of lipid abnormality seems to be inherited as an autosomal recessive gene, both parents being heterozygotes.[42,103]

Carnitine Palmityl Transferase Deficiency. Carnitine palmityl transferase deficiency was initially reported in 1973 in a patient with periodic muscle cramps and myoglobinuria without weakness of muscles. The diagnosis was verified on muscle biopsy manifested by an enzyme deficiency of carnitine palmityl transferase.[18] Subsequently, there have been additional reports of patients with myoglobinuria, recurrent muscle cramps on exercising, decreased production of ketone bodies during fasting, and, in some cases, respiratory paralysis as a result of a deficiency in the enzyme carnitine palmityl transferase.[4,7,10]

MITOCHONDRIAL MYOPATHIES

Functional mitochondrial abnormalities are seen in several disorders of myopathic origin including cases of facioscapulohumeral muscular dystrophy.[37] However, two myopathies have been reported with the primary pathology involving mitochondria.

Megaconial Myopathy

Megaconial myopathy is a heredofamilial disorder in which the pathologic ultrastructural examination demonstrates giant mitochondria with several types of inclusions. In addition, intracellular neutral lipid is present within the muscle cells and in liver and kidney cells as well. Clinically, muscle weakness and hypotonicity are noted at birth or shortly thereafter, with subsequent development of marked proximal muscle weakness evidenced by difficulty in walking, climbing stairs, and arising from a chair. The disorder, extremely rare, is very slowly progressive, and there is no known treatment.[89]

Pleoconial Myopathy

In pleoconial myopathy there are large numbers of mitochondria seen throughout the muscle cells on ultrastructural inspection. These mitochondria are only moderately enlarged. Clinically, there is hypotonia with floppy appearance at birth and subsequent development of progressive proximal weakness and wasting. In addition, a craving for salt is noted, and prolonged episodes of flaccid paralysis may be superimposed on the underlying proximal weakness. Sodium deprivation, potassium loading, and aldosterone antagonists do not precipitate the attacks of flaccid paralysis. The disease is apparently slowly progressive, and there is no known treatment.[89]

MUSCLE DISORDERS RELATED TO SYSTEMIC ALTERATIONS IN POTASSIUM METABOLISM

The association of skeletal muscle weakness and abnormalities of potassium metabolism has been observed in a number of syndromes in clinical medicine.

Secondary Hypokalemia

Muscle weakness is observed in a variety of situations in which levels of serum potassium are abnormally low, including such disease states as chronic nephritis, primary aldosteronism, chronic enteritis, idiopathic steatorrhea, and certain cases of hypothyroidism. Certain pharmacologic agents including para-aminosalicylic acid, ion exchange resins, insulin, and certain diuretics can occasionally produce hypokalemic muscle weakness. This syndrome may also be observed following partial gastrectomy. Complete paralysis is extremely rare. Serum enzyme activity is often elevated. Electrocardiographic changes including cardiac dysrhythmias, prolonged systole, and eventual cardiac arrest in systole are encountered. With treatment and subsequent return of the serum potassium level to normal, improvement occurs rapidly, with serum enzyme levels gradually decreasing to normal.[104]

Hyperkalemia (Potassium Intoxication)

Potassium intoxication may be related to impaired renal function, severe tissue trauma, a massive hemolytic reaction, severe states of sodium chloride loss such as salt-losing nephritis, and diabetic coma. Although muscle paralysis is unusual, it has been reported in a few cases and is characterized as a severe, rapidly reversible process consisting of thickness of speech, difficulty in swallowing, and subsequent weakness and paralysis of limb, trunk, and neck muscles occurring within 1 to 2 hours. Perceptible slight movements of the fingers and toes and the muscles supplied by the cranial nerves may be the only persisting muscle function. Sensation deficit, including numbness, decreased appreciation of vibration, and impairment of joint position sense with loss of deep tendon reflexes, has been reported. The skeletal muscles themselves are flaccid but may exhibit twitching in response to direct percussion. The electrocardiogram is also a sensitive indicator of potassium intoxication, with the initial feature being an elevation of the T wave with subsequent decrease in the size of the R and increase in the size of the S component. Later there is disappearance of the P wave and obliteration of the S-T segment; finally, large biphasic S-T complexes are observed. A serum potassium level of 7 to 10.5 mEq/liter is associated with this syndrome. The most effective treatment is the administration of sodium chloride and control of the underlying disease. Clinically, potassium intoxication differs from the primary potassium syndromes (which include periodic paralysis) in that in the latter, response from mechanical stimulation eventually fails and the cardiac dysfunction is usually minimal. It has been proposed that the mechanism of the disturbance in potassium intoxication is related to the inability of the end-plate structures to initiate an impulse in the membrane of the muscle fiber. Hyperkalemic muscle weakness differs from myasthenia gravis and curare poisoning in that the muscles supplied by the cranial nerves are the last to be paralyzed.

INTRINSIC DISORDERS OF SKELETAL MUSCLE RELATED TO POTASSIUM METABOLISM

The group of intrinsic disorders of episodic skeletal muscle weakness related to potassium metabolism includes familial periodic paralysis, adynamia episodica hereditaria, normokalemic periodic paralysis, and paramyotonia congenita, all four of which are apparently inherited disorders (Table 19-3). There is some evidence to suggest that an abnormality of the muscle membrane may play a role in the pathogenesis of these disorders.

Familial Periodic Paralysis

Familial periodic paralysis, also known as hypokalemic periodic paralysis, is an uncommon and unusual type of intermittent paralysis usually inherited as an autosomal dominant trait, although irregular dominant inheritance has been reported with sparing of one or more generations. The attacks usually begin during adolescence, although onset has been reported as early as 8 and as late as 31 years of age. During the fourth decade, the attacks tend to decrease in frequency and severity, and may disappear completely. The disorder is three times as common in males as in females.

Etiology. Although the pathogenetic mechanisms in this disorder are not completely understood, abnormalities in muscle membrane and carbohydrate metabolism in muscle have been reported as being etiologically significant.[51,91] More recent studies, however, raise some doubts as to the importance of these mechanisms.[16,23]

Pathology and Pathophysiology. On histologic inspection, muscle biopsies obtained during and following acute episodes of paralysis show only round to oval vacuoles in the center of some fibers. This may represent only an alteration in the quantity of intracellular fluid. Most authorities feel that periodic paralysis is related to sleep and is directly associated with carbohydrate metabolism. The serum potassium levels during an acute attack tend to be lower than the normal range of 3.5 to 5 mEq/liter. Usually, the skeletal muscle paralysis begins when a level of 3 to 3.5 mEq/liter is attained. Of interest is the fact that in hypokalemia induced experimentally in normal subjects or in patients with hyperthyroidism, muscle weakness occurs at a much lower serum potassium level. The metabolism of potassium within the fiber itself is probably the primary factor because periodic paralysis may occur at different serum potassium levels even when the concentration is normal. Most authorities hold that potassium does move into skeletal muscle fibers, although no satisfactory explanation for this movement has yet been found. It has been proposed that the potassium concentration in the muscle cell during an attack is maintained and that there is a marked increase of intracellular water; this is probably related to a defect in the glycolytic cycle as a primary disturbance, with abnormal intermediaries of high molecular weight to account for the osmotic shifts. The electric inexcitability and the shifts in potassium remain to be explained.

Clinical Features. The disorder is characterized by episodic attacks of flaccid paralysis that may recur for years without alteration in type or severity. The arms, legs, and trunk musculature are profoundly affected, with areflexia and total electrical inexcitability of the involved muscles. The

TABLE 19-3. Differentiation of Intrinsic Disorders of Muscle Related to Alterations in Potassium Metabolism

Parameter	Familial Periodic Paralysis	Adynamia Episodica Hereditaria	Normokalemic Periodic Paralysis	Paramyontonia Congenita
Age at onset	8–31 years	First decade	First decade	Infancy or early childhood
Inheritance	Autosomal dominant	Autosomal dominant	Autosomal dominant	Autosomal dominant
Sex incidence	Three times as common in males	Males and females equally affected	Males and females equally affected	Males and females equally affected
Clinical features	Episodic attacks of flaccid paralysis involving arms, legs, and trunk with areflexia lasting 1 hour to as long as 9 days; occasional cardiac dysrhythmias	Episodic weakness in extremities occasionally accompanied by paresthesias, lasting several minutes to hours; deep tendon reflexes diminished during attack	Episodic weakness frequently lasts days or weeks, occurring usually at night	Episodic weakness especially in proximal muscles; myotonia in lingual muscles and eyelids, facial muscles, and extremity muscles when patient is exposed to cold; may last as long as 24 hours
Precipitating factors	Heavy evening meal or bedtime snack	Intense physical exertion, hunger, oral ingestion of 1–7 g potassium chloride	Rest after undue exertion, alcohol, anxiety, potassium-containing compounds	Cold environment
Serum potassium levels	Usually low, 2.5–3.5 mEq/liter	Usually high-normal or elevated	Normal	Usually high-normal or elevated
Prophylactic measures	Daily potassium supplement; avoid fatigue, excessive carbohydrate consumption, emotional excitement, alcohol imbibition, exposure to cold	Avoid intense physical exertion; eat frequently	Regular meals with increased salt intake	Avoid sudden exposure to extreme cold
Treatment	Oral administration of 2–10 g potassium chloride	Ingestion of food, gentle exercise, intravenous calcium gluconate, Diuril	Oral sodium chloride, 250 mg acetazolamide, 0.1 mg 9α-fluorohydro-cortisone daily	Consistent effective treatment not available
Prognosis	Severity and frequency of attacks greatest in second and third decades; attacks usually disappear in fifth decade	Attacks short in children, tending to increase in severity, frequency, and duration after puberty; attacks lessen in frequency and severity after fourth decade, disappearing in sixth decade	Patients improve with age	Patients improve with age

onset occurs most frequently at night, at which time the patient may awaken from a sound sleep and find himself unable to move his extremities. The ability to speak and breathe are not usually impaired. A given attack may be brief, lasting 1 to 3 hours, or it may be protracted, lasting as long as 7 to 9 days with slow recovery. Incomplete paralysis may occur. A heavy evening meal or bedtime snack is likely to enhance the possibility of an attack in a susceptible person. Excessive perspiration and thirst may precede the muscle weakness. Frequently, the patient states that he is able to ward off an impending attack by exercise. Severe attacks with involvement of the cranial nerve-innervated muscles and the muscles of respiration have been reported, although they are extremely rare. All modalities of sensation are completely spared. Cardiac dysrhythmias and hypotension have been reported during an acute attack.

Laboratory Examination. The serum potassium values are usually in the range of 2.5 to 3.5 mEq/liter during an acute episode. However, as previously mentioned, serum potassium levels are sometimes normal. Electrocardiograms obtained during an acute attack demonstrate flattening of the T waves and S-T segment changes.

Treatment. Treatment consists of avoiding precipitating factors such as fatigue, excessive carbohydrate consumption, emotional excitement, alcohol ingestion, and exposure to cold. The oral administration of potassium chloride, 100 to 200 mg/kg, is effective in terminating a given attack. When the patient is unable to swallow, potassium chloride must necessarily be administered by stomach tube or by intravenous infusion of 30 to 50 mg/liter at a rate of 10 ml/kg/hour, with the usual precautions. When the individual attacks tend to occur with increased frequency, and especially at night, 2 to 10 g of potassium chloride should be ingested prophylactically before retiring. In addition, it is recommended that the sodium intake be restricted to less than 10mg/day. Daily ingestion of acetazolamide (Diamox) may help to prevent attacks.[30] Some authorities advocate the use of spironolactone, an aldosterone antagonist, 100 to 200 mg daily, as a prophylactic measure.

Prognosis. The intermittent attacks of paralysis are most frequent and severe in the adolescent and young adult. They usually diminish slowly in intensity and frequency during the third and fourth decades and tend to disappear completely by the fifth or sixth decade. However, some patients develop permanent progressive weakness and wasting.[67]

Adynamia Episodica Hereditaria

Recurrent attacks of muscular weakness characterize adynamia episodica hereditaria (periodic hyperkalemia, hyperkalemic periodic paralysis, Gamstorp's syndrome), which is clinically similar to familial periodic paralysis. It is inherited as a mendelian dominant trait with complete or almost complete penetrance. Incidence is distributed equally among the sexes. The onset is usually during the first decade of life.

Etiology and Pathophysiology. The causative factors in this disease have not been defined with certainty, although muscle membrane abnormalities are etiologically significant. The serum potassium is usually on the high side of normal or is elevated without significant increase in intracellular potassium.

Clinical Features. This disorder was initially described clinically by Gamstorp in 1956.[28] The episodic muscle weakness in these patients often begins with a feeling of heaviness in the extremities, occasionally accompanied by paresthesias. The weakness is usually first noted in the legs and spreads to involve the upper extremities. The muscles of the trunk and the muscles innervated by cranial nerves are also involved on occasion. The attacks tend to occur during the day, often after a period of intense physical exertion. Mild exercise at the onset of the initial symptoms of weakness may ward off an attack. Hunger seems to predispose the susceptible patient to an attack of weakness, and food intake at the beginning of an attack seems to hasten improvement. Individual episodes of weakness may last several minutes to many hours. In children the episodes are characteristically short; they increase in duration, severity, and frequency after puberty. The deep-tendon reflexes tend to be diminished to absent during an attack in some patients. Oral administration of 1 to 7 g of potassium chloride may precipitate an attack. The respiratory muscles are not usually affected. A permanent myopathic weakness involving primarily the proximal musculature may develop after several years of clinical disease.[67] Myotonia may be present clinically in the tongue, eyelid, face, and thenar muscles.[44] Cold weather in some cases tends to increase the frequency and severity of attacks.

Laboratory Examination. During attacks, serum potassium levels as high as 7 mEq/liter are frequently encountered, although in some patients there is no elevation of serum potassium. The electrocardiogram reveals high, sharp T waves characteristically seen in hyperkalemia. Electromyography demonstrates myotonia, mechanical irritability, and spontaneous discharges in some cases.

Treatment. Treatment consists of gentle exercise and food ingestion at the onset of episodes. When the attack is severe, the intravenous administration of 10 to 20 ml of 10% calcium gluconate usually results in a prompt beneficial response. An infusion of glucose and insulin intravenously may also be helpful. Chlorothiazide or acetazolamide administration may also be helpful in preventing recurrent attacks. Extreme exertion with undue fatigue should be avoided by susceptible patients.

Prognosis. Although the attacks usually lessen in frequency and severity after the third to fourth decade and disappear after 60 years of age, severe permanent weakness may occur after several years of clinical disease.[28,67]

Normokalemic Periodic Paralysis

Periodic paralysis has been occasionally reported in patients with normal levels of potassium during the acute attacks.[57,72] Clinically, in most cases, the features are similar to those in hypokalemic patients. The initial episode frequently occurs during the first decade of life, and subsequent attacks may

be induced by rest after undue exertion or may be due to exposure to extreme cold and damp conditions. The attacks usually occur at night. Muscle weakness is sometimes present when the patient awakes in the morning. Alcohol, anxiety, and administration of potassium-containing compounds may precipitate attacks. The episodes are reported to be more severe than those seen in the hyperkalemic variety, with complete paralysis occurring not infrequently. The incidence seems to be equal in both sexes. In some instances, attacks may last as long as days to weeks.

Treatment. Oral sodium chloride is very effective in these patients. Prophylaxis consists of regular meals with increased salt intake. Acetazolamide may also be helpful. In addition, treatment with 9α-fluorohydrocortisone has been recommended.

Paramyotonia Congenita

Paramyotonia congenita (paramyotonia of Eulenberg) is a familial disease transmitted by an autosomal dominant gene with complete or nearly complete penetrance. The incidence among males and females appears to be equal.

Etiology. The etiology in this disorder has not been established with certainty. However, there appears to be an excessive lability of serum potassium, which is either elevated or on the high side of normal. Some authorities suggest that there is a basic muscle membrane abnormality in this disorder. Histopathologically, the muscle is similar to that seen in myotonic dystrophy; sarcoplasmic masses and ring annulets are occasionally observed.

Clinical Features. There is an intermittent flaccid weakness that occurs mainly in the proximal musculature. Myotonia involving the lingual muscles is frequently present, and when the person is exposed to cold the eyelids, facial musculature, and muscles of the extremities also exhibit this sign. Myotonia often precedes weakness and may occur independently even without exposure to cold. Warming the patient tends to relieve the symptoms. Weakness may persist for several minutes or as long as 24 hours. Between attacks, only percussion myotonia of the tongue may be present. Paradoxical myotonia (myotonia aggravated rather than improved with activity) is observed in this disorder. Neither muscle wasting nor hypertrophy is commonly encountered. Some patients complain of upper gastrointestinal distress, and emotional lability has been noted in some. The myotonia and episodic flaccid weakness precipitated by exposure to cold often arise early in childhood. Total paralysis of muscle never occurs, although disability can be quite prominent. Variability in a given family is observed in this disorder; some members demonstrate intermittent paralysis without ever experiencing myotonia, whereas others in the same family have myotonia without weakness. There is increasing clinical evidence to suggest that this disorder is closely related to adynamia episodica hereditaria; perhaps they are identical.

Treatment.   Treatment consists of avoiding extreme cold. Because of the relationship between this disorder and adynamia episodica hereditaria, the same treatment measures are recommended.

Prognosis.   This condition is nonprogressive, and it tends to diminish with age.

Differential Diagnosis of Primary Potassium Syndromes

In all the primary potassium syndromes, the inheritance is by way of a single autosomal dominant gene. Hypokalemic periodic paralysis seems to be more common among males, whereas in the other two forms there is no sex preference. In hyperkalemic periodic paralysis, normokalemic periodic paralysis, and paramyotonia congenita, the disease usually has its onset during the first decade of life, frequently before the fifth year. In hypokalemic periodic paralysis, the initial attack may not occur until the late teens or even the fourth or fifth decade. In hypokalemic periodic paralysis and normokalemic periodic paralysis, the attacks are usually less frequent, occurring at intervals of weeks or months. They occur more commonly at night and are unrelated to muscular activity. In hyperkalemic periodic paralysis, daytime attacks are more common

and tend to be precipitated by exertion. The spontaneous attacks, either major or minor in degree, usually occur one or more times daily in hyperkalemic paralysis. High carbohydrate or high alcohol intake tends to provoke attacks of hypokalemic periodic paralysis. The level of serum potassium is an important point in the differentiation of these disorders. During an acute attack of hypokalemic periodic paralysis, there is, as a rule, a decreased serum potassium level associated with hypokalemic electrocardiographic changes consisting of flattening of the T waves and S-T segment changes, whereas in the other disorders there is usually a normal or increased serum potassium level. Episodes of hypokalemic periodic paralysis can be precipitated by the administration of sodium chloride, glucose and insulin, Adrenalin, or fluorohydrocortisone. In the other disorders, potassium chloride provokes attacks, and in hyperkalemic periodic paralysis, calcium gluconate and glucose have a good prophylactic effect. Myotonia occurs in paramyotonia congenita and frequently in hyperkalemic periodic paralysis but is not observed in hypokalemic periodic paralysis or normokalemic periodic paralysis.

MYOPATHIES RELATED TO ENDOCRINE DYSFUNCTION

Thyrotoxic Myopathy

Thyrotoxicosis in children is unusual. Mild weakness of muscles and easy fatigability is observed in some patients with Graves' disease and may represent a mild form of thyrotoxic myopathy. The full-blown clinical picture of thyrotoxic myopathy, consisting of proximal muscle weakness and wasting with associated difficulty in climbing stairs, is extremely rare under the age of 18. The symptoms of muscle weakness may appear prior to the other clinical features of thyrotoxicosis. The incidence in males is three times that in females.

A high incidence of periodic paralysis related to thyrotoxicosis has been observed in patients of Oriental ancestry. The disease is said to resemble hypokalemic periodic paralysis rather than thyrotoxic myopathy.[54,62]

Treatment. Improvement in the patient's thyrotoxic myopathy may be noted with successful treatment of the underlying thyrotoxicosis; frequently, no impairment is observed following return to the euthyroid state.

Hypothyroid Myopathy. Myopathic disorders have been reported in myxedema (Hoffmann's syndrome) and cretinism (Kocher-DeBre-Semelaigne syndrome). In these disorders there is proximal muscle weakness, especially of the lower limbs, but there is an occasional spread to the muscles of the distal lower extremities. Increased muscle bulk is noted in some cases, and delayed contraction and relaxation may be present. Painful muscle cramping also occurs.[94] Treatment of the hypothyroid state with restoration and maintenance of a euthyroid condition results in improvement of this myopathy.

Steroid Myopathy

It has been recognized for some time that weakness of muscles is a common finding in hyperadrenocorticism. Severe muscle weakness with associated muscle wasting has been observed in patients with various disorders unrelated to muscle disease treated with corticosteroids. The etiology of the so-called steroid myopathy has not been established with certainty. However, creatine storage is impaired, and this combined with increased creatine synthesis might account for the massive elevations of serum and urinary creatine in patients with steroid myopathy. It has also been suggested that disordered protein metabolism may play a role. Pathologic changes in muscle biopsies of these patients have been minimal, the most consistent feature being large, clear, empty vacuoles in individual muscle fibers similar to those seen in the muscles of patients with familial periodic paralysis.

Clinical Features. Generalized muscle weakness especially marked in the proximal muscles in the lower extremities is the most prominent finding. The weakness is moderately severe and is associated with noticeable muscle wasting. The deep-tendon reflexes are diminished but as a rule are not lost. The time between the initiation of steroid therapy and the onset of the weakness varies in different patients from 3 weeks to 20 months. The most frequent early symptom is difficulty in climbing stairs. Within 2 to 4 weeks after onset of muscle weakness, rising from a chair becomes difficult and walking is virtually impossible. The relationship between the amount of steroid dosage employed and the development of muscle weakness varies from patient to patient. In some patients, symptoms appear after relatively small dosages; in others, symptoms develop only after very large amounts are employed. Universally, however, return of muscle strength is noted 8 to 10 days after the steroid is reduced in dosage or discontinued, and by 2 to 3 weeks after cessation, muscle strength is usually normal.

Myopathy Associated with Metabolic Bone Disease

A myopathy has been observed in patients with osteomalacia of varying causes, including (1) gluten-sensitive enteropathy, (2) postgastrectomy syndrome, (3) distal small bowel resection, (4) nutritional osteomalacia, (5) renal tubular acidosis, and (6) vitamin D-resistant osteomalacia. It has also been observed in patients with hyperparathyroidism. The disorder is characterized by proximal muscle weakness, usually beginning in the lower extremities, with associated difficulty in arising from a chair or climbing stairs and with subsequent gait difficulties. As the disorder progresses, the trunk and arms tend to become involved. Occasionally, patients demonstrate wasting and loss of muscle bulk. Myotonia is not observed. On electromyography, short-duration polyphasic potentials in the absence of fibrillation have been recorded. Successful treatment consists of dietary measures in patients with gluten-sensitive enteropathy, surgical treatment of those with hyperparathyroidism, and vitamin D treatment (1000 USP units) in patients with myopathy and osteomalacia.[93]

MYOGLOBINURIA

Myoglobin or myohemoglobin is a sarcoplasmic protein occurring in the muscle cells between fibrils. It is reddish brown or mahogany in color. Several laboratory methods used for identification of myoglobin include spectrophotometry, electrophoresis, and immunologic techniques. Myoglobin has been found in the urine in several specific pathologic states. Among these disorders are idiopathic paroxysmal myoglobinuria, Haff disease, traumatic and crush injuries of muscle, and the anterior tibial syndrome. Myoglobinuria has also been observed incidentally in patients with dermatomyositis and in the McArdle type of glycogen storage disease with or without associated convulsions.[25] It may also be present in carbon monoxide poisoning, barbiturate poisoning, diabetic acidosis, enteritis, alcoholic myopathy, and sea snake poisoning. In addition, it has been observed in association with steroid therapy. A completely satisfactory classification of myoglobinuria has not been devised because of the large number of cases in which the basic pathogenetic mechanisms are not yet understood. The subject was comprehensively reviewed by Rowland et al.[74]

Idiopathic Paroxysmal Myoglobinuria (Meyer-Betz Disease)

Repeated episodes of muscle cramping followed by the production of a reddish brown, mahogany-colored urine characterize this form of myoglobinuria, originally described in 1911.[56] The onset may occur at any age; cases have been reported as early as age 2 and as late as 56 years of age. It is more common in males than females, in a ratio of 4:1. Familial incidence has been observed in some cases, but as a rule the disorder appears sporadically.

Etiology. The cause of this disorder has not been established. The appearance of myoglobin in the urine is but one of a number of biochemical derangements. With increased understanding of biochemical pathology, it has become apparent that fewer patients actually fall into this category of myoglobinuria.

Pathology. Histologically there is extensive damage of the contractile elements of muscle with severe coagulative necrosis similar to Zenker's degeneration. Loss of striation, hyaline necrosis, and decoloriza-tion of fiber segments are also present. Calcium deposits are observed in some necrotic fibers, and an occasional vacuolated muscle fiber is encountered.

Clinical Features. The onset of an attack is usually sudden and is characterized by severe, intense pain and muscle cramping, usually in the lower extremities. These symptoms are soon followed by transient muscle paresis or occasionally even complete paralysis. During the attack the involved muscles are edematous and firm. Tenderness to slight pressure is present. The attacks are often associated with systemic symptoms including anorexia, emesis, chills, fever, and abdominal pain. A given episode may be induced by excessive exertion. In some patients, following repeated attacks, the affected muscles are wasted and atrophied. In other patients, no signs or symptoms are present between the acute episodes. In a number of reported cases, oliguria or anuria was the ultimate result of the intrinsic renal damage from the presence of myoglobin or other substances released from the damaged muscle fibers. Death in acute renal failure has also been reported. The attacks often last for several days with the urinary findings continuing for 48 to 72 hours after clinical recovery.

Laboratory Examination. Leukocytosis is an early finding, and within a few hours after development of the muscle weakness and cramping, the urine becomes pink. After several additional hours it is deep reddish brown. In severe cases, an elevated blood urea nitrogen level is an ominous sign of impending kidney decompensation.

Differential Diagnosis. The differentiation from the muscular dystrophies can be made by the clinical picture with the associated urinary findings. Myoglobinuria can be distinguished from other forms of pigmenturia such as hemoglobinuria and porphyria by spectrophotometry, electrophoresis, or specialized immunologic techniques.

Treatment. Treatment in this disorder is symptomatic.

Haff Disease

Attacks of myoglobinuria following ingestion of fish poisoned by discarded waste products from a cellulose factory were reported and termed Haff disease, referring to the area in Germany where the disorder was initially described.[3] The exact cause of the disease has not been established.

Traumatic and Crush Injuries of Muscle

Myoglobinuria is seen in some patients who have sustained severe crush injuries. These patients rapidly develop renal failure and anuria, thought to be due to blocking of the renal tubules by the muscle pigment. Injury to muscles by high voltage currents also gives rise to myoglobinuria.

Anterior Tibial Syndrome

In the anterior tibial syndrome (traumatic necrosis of pretibial muscles), the muscles of one or both lower extremities become acutely swollen, painful, and paralyzed after vigorous exercise. Although the etiology of this disorder has not been established with certainty, it is suggested that unconditioned muscles subjected to extensive vigorous exercise tend to liberate excessive quantities of metabolites, which leads to edema. Because the pretibial muscles are confined within the rigid, anterior tibial compartment, swelling results in vascular compression with ischemic necrosis of muscles and nerves. The patient is usually a young male who is engaged in vigorous running, jumping, or marching for long distances without adequate previous conditioning or training. The pain often begins in the pretibial regions of one or both lower extremities during exercise or following exercise within several hours. Edema and paralysis in the pretibial muscles are prominent features, in addition to the severe pain. The overlying skin tends to become edematous, hot, and erythematous. Systemic manifestations include low-grade temperature elevation, polymorphonuclear leukocytosis, and albuminuria. The arterial pulsations of the foot are diminished. The affected muscles do not respond to faradic or galvanic stimulation, and electromyography reveals no electrical activity. The pain, skin manifestations, and systemic systems tend to improve after several days to a week, but the paralysis may persist. Circulatory collapse and death from renal failure, especially after attempts to manipulate the limbs during the acute phases of the illness, have been reported. Myoglobinuria is a frequent accompaniment.

Treatment. Incision of the anterior crural fascia surgically has proved beneficial when performed early in the acute phase of this disorder. Muscle paralysis often persists permanently.

MYOSITIS OSSIFICANS

Two forms of myositis ossificans are recognized. One, traumatic myositis ossificans, is a condition in which injury to the muscle results in the formation of osseous tissue The second form, generalized or progressive myositis ossificans, is a disease entity of uncertain etiology.

Traumatic Myositis Ossificans

Traumatic myositis ossificans may follow a single severe injury to a given muscle or may occur after repeated minor trauma to a muscle. Specific activities or habits are frequently associated with solitary muscle ossification. This type of myositis ossificans occurs in any age group but most frequently in young men.

Etiology. A number of theories have been proposed concerning the formation of osseous tissue in muscle, including (1) displacement of osteoblasts into muscle by trauma to adjacent bones, (2) metaplasia of connective tissue or fibrocartilage, and (3) activation by trauma of periosteal implants residing in muscle.

Pathology. Histologically extensive proliferation of intramuscular connective tissue is noted with subsequent appearance of islands of bone and cartilage arising in the thickened connective tissue septa. Individual muscle fibers do not seem to be primarily involved in the ossification but are incorporated in and compressed by the calcifying tissue.

Clinical Features. The individual muscles that usually undergo ossification are the quadriceps femoris and the brachialis anticus. At 1 to 4 weeks after the trauma, a firm, painful mass is observed in the muscle that eventually may seriously limit mobility. Because stress and strain during the early stages of injury enhance the bone formation, stretching or manipulation of that portion of the extremity should be avoided. In some cases, ossification remains asymptomatic for many years.

Laboratory Examination. Roentgenographic studies show either a feathery pattern of calcification or an irregular calcified structure varying in density.

Treatment and Prognosis. Surgical treatment is necessary when pain and tenderness are protracted. Because recurrences of the osseous tissue occur when surgical treatment is either performed prematurely or is inadequate, a wide excision is not usually undertaken until 6 months after the onset of symptoms. Specific treatment is not necessary in cases in which the ossification is asymptomatic.

Progressive Myositis Ossificans

Progressive myositis ossificans, usually encountered in young children, adolescents, or young adults, is a rare disorder wherein ossification occurs in tendons, ligaments, skin, and fascia in addition to the interstitial tissues of the muscle. Concomitant congenital anomalies consisting of microdactyly, exostoses, hallux valgus, earlobe aplasia, dental abnormalities, and spina bifida have also been observed in children with myositis ossificans. In some instances there is a family history of the disorder. On occasion, the disorder may be present at birth, but usually the onset occurs during the first 2 decades of life.

Etiology. Some authorities feel that this is a disorder of connective tissue rather than a primary disease of muscle. Others suggest an inborn defect in metabolism is the cause of this rare disorder, but the etiology has by no means been established.

Pathology. The pathologic changes are similar to those encountered in traumatic myositis ossificans.

Clinical Features. The disease is often heralded by the appearance of swelling, which may occur anywhere in the body but frequently occurs in the neck and back. The masses vary in size and shape and may entirely disappear or diminish in size prior to becoming indurated. The overlying skin is often reddened. Pain and tenderness are not common accompaniments. Ulceration, with discharge of a chalky material from the bony mass, may occur occasionally. The disease process may eventually involve all the musculature on the dorsal aspect of the trunk and of the extremities. The lingual, laryngeal, ocular, and peroneal muscles seem to be relatively immune, as do the diaphragm and the heart.

Laboratory Examination. Roentgenographic studies show widespread calcification.

Diagnosis. Incipient generalized myositis ossificans must be differentiated from congenital torticollis. The associated congenital anomalies, especially microdactyly, which occurs in the ossifying disease, can be very helpful signs.

Treatment. No specific treatment is effective, although the use of corticosteroids may be of some value.

Prognosis. As the course of the disorder progresses, entire groups of muscles may be transformed into bone. Calcifications bridging adjacent muscles and involving articulations may result in ankylosis, restriction, and immobility. The disease process eventually involves the intercostal muscles. This is an ominous development, and demise often results from intercurrent pulmonary infection.

DISORDERS OF NEUROMUSCULAR TRANSMISSION

Tick Paralysis

Tick paralysis is a disease of man and animals manifested by an acute ascending flaccid paralysis with or without change in sensation. It occurs following attachment to the skin by a member of the tick family.

Etiology. Originally it was thought that this disorder was produced by a toxin elaborated by a gravid member of *Dermacentor andersoni* (wood tick) or *Dermacentor variabilis* (dog tick), but it was subsequently observed that male tick members of *Amblyomma americanum* are also capable of producing toxin.[34] Other tick families including Ixodus, Haemaphysalis, and Ornithodoros also can produce this disorder. The exact pathogenetic mechanisms are not completely understood. However, it is believed that the tick elaborates a toxin that interferes with somatic nerve conduction, produces a depolarizing block at the neuromuscular junction, or acts at the level of the muscle itself to prevent contraction.[12]

Pathology. The majority of patients who died from this disorder demonstrated no histopathologic abnormalities.

Clinical Features. Girls are more frequently affected than boys, possibly because of their longer hair. There is usually a latent period of 5 to 6 days before the onset of restlessness and irritability, prominent early signs of the disorder. Paralysis develops, usually beginning in the lower extremities, 12 to 24 hours after the patient becomes irritable. Mild paresthesias in the lower extremities are frequently a comcomitant complaint. Pain may occur but is unusual. Weakness of the upper extremities develops after 24 hours, followed by complete paralysis of the upper extremities and the bulbar musculature. With this event, death from respiratory paralysis follows. Occasionally, isolated muscle weakness and twitching may occur in the region of the engorging tick. In some patients, a bluish discoloration occurs close to the attached tick. In others, the skin around the attachment may be edematous. Occasionally, a measles-like rash occurs. Rarely, choreiform movements, nausea, visual blurring, diplopia, severe abnormalities in sensation, and sphincter disorders may be observed.[85]

Laboratory Studies. Results of laboratory studies including white blood count, cerebrospinal fluid, and bacterial cultures are normal.

Differential Diagnosis. The presence of the tick is the major differential point. The incidence of this illness is highest during the summer months when members of the tick family are active. This disorder must be differentiated from poliomyelitis, in which asymmetrical weakness and spinal fluid pleocytosis are more common. The normal spinal fluid protein in tick paralysis also tends to exclude polyradiculoneuritis. Other polyneuropathies such as arsenic and triorthocresyl phosphate poisoning must be differentiated.

Treatment. Cautious removal of the whole tick is extremely important. Evulsion (with a hemostat) of the small area of the patient's skin containing the mouth parts of the tick ensures total removal.

Prognosis. Following tick removal, clinical improvement is noted within 30 minutes, and the strength in the lower extremities usually returns by 12 hours. Complete recovery occurs within 1 week.

Myasthenia Gravis

Myasthenia gravis (asthenic bulbar palsy without anatomic basis, myasthenia gravis pseudoparalytica, or Goldflam's disease) is a chronic disorder characterized by variable weakness of skeletal muscles following continued use. Cardiac and smooth muscles are not involved. The muscles most commonly affected include those subserving ocular movements, mastication, facial expression, deglutition, and respiration, as well as the muscles of the neck, trunk, and limbs. The onset of myasthenia may occur at any age. In most instances there is no evidence that hereditary factors play a role, although a familial incidence has been reported.[61] The incidence in girls is considerably greater than in boys.

Etiology. The primary defect in myasthenia gravis is related to dysfunction of neuromuscular transmission. During the past 20 years, evidence has accumulated to suggest that myasthenia gravis is an autoimmune disorder.[92] In this connection, it has been observed that other disorders thought to be autoimmune in character occur with increased frequency in patients with myasthenia gravis; these disorders are lupus erythematosis, thyroiditis, rheumatoid arthritis, pemphigus, sarcoidosis, pernicious anemia, and Sjögren's syndrome, as well as hemolytic anemia.[70] Muscle-binding, complement-fixing serum globulin has been reported in the serum of myasthenic patients. Muscle antibodies, as well as antibodies to purified myosin, have also been reported in these patients.[69,96] Recent experimental evidence in animals immunized with acetyl receptor protein has demonstrated striking similarities to patients with myasthenia gravis.[46] Evidence has been amassed suggesting that an antigen–antibody combination involving acetylcholine receptor protein as antigen at the postsynaptic membrane interferes with normal neuromuscular transmission.[47,48] In addition to an association of myasthenia gravis with other so-called autoimmune diseases, there appears to be a significant association with diseases of the thyroid, adrenal, and thymus glands. Hyperthyroidism is observed in approximately 5% of patients with myasthenia gravis and may occur simultaneously or at another time.[64]

Pathology. Grossly, the muscles appear normal except in severe cases in which there is loss of muscle bulk, which probably results from disuse and from frequently associated poor nutrition. Microscopically, in an occasional case, focal collections of small lymphocytes termed lymphorrhages have been observed surrounding small blood vessels in the interstitial tissues of the affected muscles. Rarely, foci of severe coagulative necrosis of isolated muscle fibers adjacent to the cellular infiltrations have been described in the upper digestive tract, heart, diaphragm, and skeletal muscles of the trunk and extremities. Recently, with special techniques, highly characteristic abnormalities in the anatomy of the motor endplate were observed.

Clinical Types. Millichap and Dodge classified myasthenia gravis in three groups based on age at onset and clinical features: (1) neonatal transient myasthenia gravis, (2) neonatal persistent (congenital) myasthenia gravis, and (3) juvenile myasthenia gravis.[58]

Neonatal transient myasthenia gravis appears in infants born to mothers with myasthenia gravis. Symptoms and signs consisting of generalized muscular weakness with little spontaneous movement, a weak Moro response, facial weakness, ptosis, respiratory weakness, and dysphagia are observed. These clinical features usually last less than a month. The transitory character of this form suggests the presence of a substance that passes the placental barrier and is slowly excreted or destroyed by the neonate. It appears that this type is both unrelated to the duration of the disease in the mother and to any forms of therapy during pregnancy. The signs and symptoms may disappear so suddenly that in some patients toxic reactions to treatment may occur as the tolerance to the medication is lost. Thymectomy performed on mothers prior to pregnancy does not seem to prevent the diseases in the infant.

Neonatal persistent myasthenia gravis, with its onset at birth, differs from the neonatal, transient form in that mothers do not have the disorder. The principal presenting clinical features are ptosis, external ophthalmoplegia, generalized weakness, and a weakened cry. Respiratory dysfunction is not common. The neonatal persistent form differs from the juvenile type in that the symptoms are much milder, the course is longer, and there is relative resistance to drug therapy, in addition to its onset at birth.

Juvenile myasthenia gravis may have its onset from 2 years of age to adolescence. Ptosis, usually bilateral but occasionally unilateral, is the commonest presenting sign (Fig. 19-6). Weakness in the arms and legs occurs with some frequency, as does diplopia, external ophthalmoplegia, weakness in mastication, weakness of facial musculature, difficulty in deglutition, and dysphonia. Respiratory difficulty is not an uncommon finding. In the morning the signs and symptoms are less severe, but as the day progresses the weakness becomes more apparent. In general, weakness of the bulbar muscles occurs considerably earlier than involvement of the extremities. Sudden, unexpected death from respiratory insufficiency may occur. The deep-tendon reflexes and sensory responses are normal. Rest during the course of the day almost

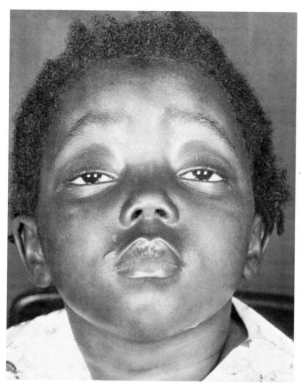

FIG. 19-6. Juvenile myasthenia gravis. Four-year-old child with a 3-week history of drooping eyelids and weakness in extremities.

invariably produces amelioration of signs and symptoms, whereas exercise of varying degrees of intensity tends to make the symptoms worse. In a significant number of female patients, the myasthenic symptoms often worsen just prior to the onset of menstruation and improve during the first or second day. Pregnancy varies in its effect on myasthenic patients; some such patients have the onset or exacerbation of symptomatology, whereas others experience marked improvement or even remission. Emotional trauma has been reported to aggravate the symptoms with a significant consistency. Systemic infections also tend to aggravate the disease; at times, a child who has been under excellent control on medication has a serious resurgence of symptoms from even a mild upper respiratory infection.

Clinical and Laboratory Diagnosis. The diagnosis of this disorder can frequently be made on the basis of the Tensilon test. Edrophonium chloride (Tensilon) is an ana-

logue of neostigmine bromide (Prostigmin). In the normal person, edrophonium chloride administration does not alter muscle strength. Cholinergic side-reactions—for example, excessive perspiration, salivation, lacrimation, epigastric distress, and fasciculations—are almost universally observed. The positive response in the myasthenic patients—a minimal cholinergic side-reaction associated with marked improvement in weak muscles—usually occurs within the first minute after injection and is generally unaccompanied by fasciculations. The beneficial effects of the drug in such a patient disappear within 5 minutes after injection, and the patient then returns to his pretest status. The intravenous test dose of edrophonium chloride in children weighing up to 75 pounds is 1 mg, and for children above this weight it is 2 mg. In the event the intravenous route is technically difficult, intramuscular injection of 2 mg in children weighing up to 75 pounds and 5 mg in children weighing more than 75 pounds is employed. Another agent that stimulates the neuromuscular junction and increases the strength of the muscle tested in the same way as edrophonium chloride is neostigmine bromide, which was formerly used as a diagnostic test. However, edrophonium chloride is the superior of the two agents because of its short duration of action and rapid excretion.

The electrical reactions of skeletal muscle in myasthenia gravis are usually quite characteristic. Faradic stimulation produces strong muscle contractions initially; as the stimulus is repeated, diminution of the contractions is noted and the muscle ultimately fails to respond (Table 19-4). In the electromyogram, action potentials from muscles stimulated with a repetitive current show a gradual diminution in amplitude as the stimulation is continued.

Differential Diagnosis. Other diagnostic possibilities include congenital external ophthalmoplegia, other myopathic disorders, polyneuropathy, poliomyelitis, brain stem neoplasms, hyperthyroidism, and psychoneurosis. The progressive weakness of muscles after exercise, the electrical reactions, and a positive edrophonium chloride test serve to differentiate myasthenia gravis from these disorders.

Treatment. Cholinesterase inhibitors, including neostigmine bromide and pyridostigmine bromide (Mestinon) have been found useful in the treatment of myasthenia gravis. Although patients are greatly improved on these medications, they do not improve to the extent seen during a spontaneous remission. The dosage of these agents is variable, and the individual case must be considered in accordance with the age of the patient and the response to medication. In infants and young children, a trial dose of 10 mg of pyridostigmine bromide orally may be given. If no sign of improvement is observed, the dose may be increased by 5-mg increments until a satisfactory result is obtained. In older children, the initial dose of pyridostigmine bromide is 30 mg. This can be increased by 15 mg increments until satisfactory results are obtained. If pyridostigmine bromide is unsatisfactory, neostigmine bromide, 1 to 10 mg orally, can be tried, with the dosage varied to fit the needs of the patient.

An additional drug used in the treatment of myasthenia gravis that may potentiate the beneficial effects of neostigmine bromide is ephedrine sulfate, 25 mg/day.

TABLE 19-4. Clinical Types of Myasthenia Gravis in Children

Parameter	Neonatal Transient	Neonatal Persistent	Juvenile
Age at onset	Present at birth	Present at birth	After age 2 years
Inheritance	Patients born of myasthenic mothers	Occasionally a familial history	Rarely a familial history
Sex incidence	Males and females equally affected	Males and females equally affected	Girls affected six times more frequently than boys
Clinical features	Generalized muscle weakness	Ptosis and generalized weakness early; external ophthalmoplegia later	Ptosis common presenting sign; weakness of extremities, external ophthalmoplegia, and dysphagia later
Electrophysiologic reactions	Faradic stimulation produces progressive diminution of muscle contraction	Faradic stimulation produces progressive diminution of muscle contraction	Faradic stimulation produces progressive diminution of muscle contraction
Laboratory diagnosis	Tensilon test	Tensilon test	Tensilon test
Prognosis	Complete recovery in less than 1 month	Disease protracted but mild	Outlook unfavorable with respiratory failure an occasional accompaniment

Germine diacetate has also been recommended as an adjunct medication, but has been observed to have limited efficacy.[27]

The importance of the thymus gland in myasthenia gravis has long been recognized, although the exact nature of the association remains uncertain. It has been shown that thymectomy, especially in young females, is beneficial in terms of producing remission or improvement. This procedure is essential, of course, in the presence of a thymic tumor, even though a favorable outcome may not occur when a thymona is present. Unfortunately, there are as yet no definite criteria to identify prior to surgery those patients in whom thymectomy will be beneficial. Although it is reported that young females are the patients who benefit the most from thymectomy, some authorities believe that this is partially an artifact of selection. Thymic irradiation has been advocated by some. The use of cholinesterase inhibitors alone is reserved for those patients whose deficits can be corrected satisfactorily with these agents. Other patients with myasthenia gravis may be given a course of oral corticosteroids, initially at high doses with subsequent tapering to maintenance low dose therapy. Some authorities suggest that cholinesterase inhibitors may be used as needed while the patient is receiving corticosteroids. Most patients should exhibit sustained improvement within the first 2 weeks, reaching significant improvement at approximately 3 to 5 months after the onset of steroid therapy. Myasthenic weakness may be exacerbated in the early phases of treatment with steroids. Such exacerbations commonly are mild, occur within 2 weeks, and have a mean duration of 5 days. Most patients have been able to tolerate an alternate day schedule of prednisone therapy when maintenance levels are achieved. In selected patients after establishment of maximal improvement, thymectomy may be considered. These patients are continued on maintenance steroid therapy after surgery for an arbitrary period of time, perhaps for as long as a year. A certain proportion of patients achieve permanent remission at this point. Should the patient relapse after the medication has been discontinued, oral steroids are reinstituted. Non-steroid immunosuppressive therapy, using antimetabolites, has also been

shown to be helpful in some refractory patients.

Plasma exchange therapy or plasmapheresis has recently been demonstrated to be of considerable benefit in managing patients who have failed to respond satisfactorily to steroid therapy. Its use thus far in children has been limited; however, any situation in which a rapid though temporary improvement in strength would be of benefit to the patient could be an indication for plasmapheresis, for example, a surgical emergency or respiratory failure potentially requiring tracheostomy. Because plasmapheresis is a relatively new procedure, its role in the overall treatment of myasthenia gravis has not yet been fully defined. In the future, it may very well be used individually or adjunctly with other forms of therapy in myasthenia gravis just as in other autoimmune disorders.[43,78,79]

Myasthenic and Cholinergic Crisis. Two types of crisis of sudden, profound deterioration occur in the patient with myasthenia gravis. Myasthenic crisis frequently occurs in association with an upper respiratory infection or with emotional or physical trauma. In some manner not yet thoroughly understood, the amount of anticholinesterase medication that had previously been effective abruptly becomes inadequate. The clinical picture is characterized by profound weakness with severe respiratory distress. The second type of crisis in these patients is due to overdosage with anticholinesterase medication and is termed cholinergic crisis. The signs and symptoms simulate myasthenic crisis in that the patient is extremely weak with profound respiratory difficulty and coma.

The differentiation between myasthenic and cholinergic crisis is extremely important. If the patient is able to give a history, the relationship of time and dosage may be helpful. In myasthenic crisis there is usually a history of an intercurrent infection, emotional trauma, irregular or incomplete medication, and even perhaps irregularities in the menstrual cycle in the female. The usual dose of drug becomes ineffective, but unlike cholinergic crisis there is no history of increased weakness or side-reactions after taking medications. The patient in cholinergic crisis presents the same marked weakness as is seen in myasthenic crisis; in addition, he generally exhibits pallor, hypertension, bradycardia, miosis of the pupils, increased salivation, diaphoresis, muscular fasciculations, and a cold, clammy skin. When all these side-effects of the cholinergic crisis are present, there is little difficulty in differentiation. However, under some circumstances an easy differentiation cannot be made. In this situation the parenteral injection of 1 mg edrophonium chloride is most valuable in the differentiation. If the symptoms improve, it can be concluded that the patient needs more anticholinesterase medication. If the symptoms worsen, the patient likely is in cholinergic crisis and all medication should be discontinued. The patient should be given respiratory assistance until such time as additional edrophonium chloride produces improvement. Then, treatment with pyridostigmine bromide, neostigmine bromide, or ambenonium chloride should be reinstituted and the patient reregulated.

Crisis occurs infrequently in children as compared with adults.

Prognosis.   The prognosis in the neonatal types of myasthenia gravis is good, provided treatment is instituted promptly. However, in juvenile myasthenia gravis the outlook in general is unfavorable; sudden severe exacerbation of symptoms with respiratory failure may arise at any time, and the outcome may be fatal. Complete remission may be expected in about 20% of patients and may occur more frequently in response to thymectomy than to medical therapy alone.

OTHER MYOPATHIES

Myotonia Congenita (Thomsen's Disease)

Myotonia congenita is an inherited anomaly of muscular contraction that is often present early in life and is characterized by delayed relaxation following voluntary muscular contraction. About one fourth of the reported cases clearly show a heredofamilial trait appearing as a mendelian dominant gene with equal distribution among the sexes. Some authorities suggest that a recessive genetic factor may play a role in some of the cases.

Etiology.   The cause of this disorder is unknown.

Pathology.   Grossly, the muscles appear large and pale. Abnormal irritability of the biopsy specimen is observed for 10 to 15 minutes after excision. The only consistent abnormality seen histopathologically is marked hypertrophy of all muscle fibers. In some fibers, a centrally placed nucleus is seen rarely, but the long chains of centrally placed nuclei, which are characteristically observed in dystrophia myotonica, are not present. The hypertrophied fibers are made up of normal-appearing myofibrils with no observable degenerative changes.

Clinical Features.   The most outstanding feature of this disorder is the phenomenon of myotonia or tonic contraction that may be present in any skeletal muscle. This phenomenon often arises during childhood and may occur even in early infancy. Motor development may be retarded. Difficulty in ambulation and movement is first noted between the ages of 6 and 8 years. The degree of myotonia differs even in a given family. Myotonia in the lower extremities is usually marked and in some cases is confined to these limbs. Movements are performed slowly. The patient often complains of difficulty in initiating any movement after rest. As the movement is carried out, there is an uncomfortable delay in relaxation. With repetitive efforts, the movement is gradually performed with greater facility and relaxation is more prompt. After a number of specific repetitions, the movement can be rapidly and freely performed with normal relaxation. After resting several minutes, renewed efforts to make the movement may provoke further myotonia. Prolonged rest, however, is necessary before severe myotonia can occur. Limbering up one set of muscles by repetitive movement does not prevent myotonia from occurring in a separate set of adjacent muscles. Thus, a patient who has walked until his limbs are loose may be immobilized by spasm as he ascends a flight of stairs. In extreme cases, myotonia of extraocular muscles may lead to convergence strabismus, and respiration may be severely disordered. The heart and abdominal viscera are not involved, and there is no evidence of associated endocrine dysfunction in this disorder.

Myotonia is readily observed when the surface of any muscle is percussed with an object such as a reflex hammer. A local contraction is initiated, and the affected area of muscle remains tightened for several seconds before relaxation. An apparent muscle weakness is probably related to difficulty in initiating movements because of inability in antagonist relaxation. The deep tendon reflexes and sensation are within normal limits. However, the abdominal and cremasteric reflexes are accompanied by myotonia.

Worsening of the myotonia on exposure to cold weather is a complaint of some patients; this difficulty is thought to be chiefly subjective. In complete relaxation, the muscles have a natural consistency, but when the myotonia is marked they are firm, hard, and tense. Myotonia is almost universally associated with pronounced muscular hypertrophy, which may give the patient a so-called Herculean appearance (Fig. 19-7).

Laboratory Examination. An increase in creatine tolerance is noted in myotonia congenita. This feature may be related to the fact that hypertrophied muscles have a greater propensity for creatine because of increased metabolism. Creatine is not excreted in the urine, and urinary creatinine levels are in the high-normal range. There are no additional metabolic abnormalities associated with this disorder. The electromyographic findings of myotonia are similar in all the myotonic disorders. Immediately after insertion of the needle electrode into the myotonic muscle, there is a rapid volley of action potentials. This shower of activity results in sounds emanating from the electromyographic loudspeaker, which exhibits a crescendo and decrescendo qual-

FIG. 19-7. Myotonia congenita. Frontal (A) and lateral (B) views. Seven-year-old child with a history of muscle cramping, difficulty in relaxation, and muscle hypertrophy since infancy.

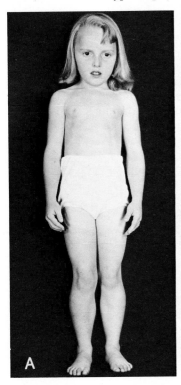
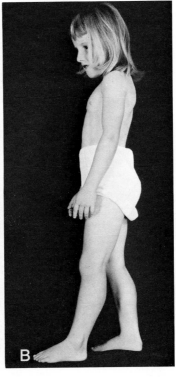

ity often likened to a diving airplane (Fig. 19-8). This type of activity tends to disappear but can easily be reactivated by tapping the electrode or by moving it further into the muscle substance. After a time, electrical silence ensues as the muscle becomes quiescent. With further muscle contraction and subsequent relaxation, some patients show an intense discharge of action potentials of high voltage greater than can be developed during normal efforts. This is termed afterspasm and is identical with the dive-bombing sounds elicited by insertion or probing with the electrode. The action potentials thus elicited are referred to as myotonic potentials.

Differential Diagnosis. It is important to distinguish myotonia congenita from the other myotonic disorders, that is, myotonic dystrophy and paramyotonia of Eulenberg. In myotonia congenita there are no dystrophic features. The myotonia is generalized rather than confined to a few muscle groups, and tends to be more severe than in the other myotonic disorders. Myotonia congenita is usually associated with a much earlier onset of symptoms than myotonic dystrophy. These various disorders cannot be differentiated by electromyography with any consistency. The creatine tolerance in myotonia congenita is increased, whereas in myotonic dystrophy it is reduced. Endocrinopathies and cardiopathies are not associated with myotonia congenita. Marked increase in myotonia on exposure to cold, muscle weakness, and paradoxical myotonia—all features of paramyotonia—are not observed in Thomsen's disease. Disturbance of serum and tissue electrolyte metabolism does not occur in myotonia congenita.

Treatment. Quinine hydrochloride and procaine amide are both effective drugs in relieving myotonia.

Prognosis. This condition rarely causes severe incapacity and tends to remain static.

Chloroquine Myopathy

Irreversible myopathy has been observed in patients treated with chloroquine, a quinilone derivative initially introduced as an antimalarial drug but widely employed in the treatment of connective tissue disease, certain skin diseases, and amebiasis. The condition is rare, and its presence is related more to individual susceptibility than cumulative toxicity. Clinically, the essential feature is that of a proximal myopathy. Improvement in this myopathy occurs within several months after discontinuing the drug.[21]

Hypertrophic Myopathy

Hypertrophic myopathy (hypertrophia musculorum vera) is a rare disorder characterized by enlargement of skeletal muscles. The muscle hypertrophy usually has its onset during childhood but may occur initially in adolescence or early adult life.

FIG. 19-8. Electromyogram in myotonia congenita. Note the rapid volley of action potentials upon insertion of the needle electrode (*arrows*).

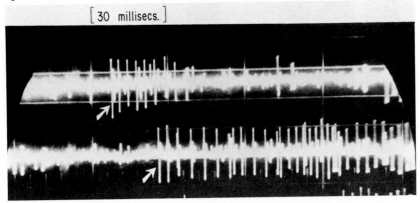

[30 millisecs.]

The incidence is greater among males than females. The muscular hypertrophy may be widespread or limited to an extremity, to half the body, or to a group of muscles. The onset is insidious with progression to a point. The condition tends toward spontaneous arrest in time. The strength of the enlarged muscles is variable. In some patients it is increased, though in some instances weakness and excessive fatigue are noted. A myotonic phenomenon is occasionally demonstrated in these patients. Sensation deficit is unusual, and vasomotor disturbance, although rare, has been reported. The deep-tendon reflexes are within normal limits as are the electrical reactions. The hypertrophy is confined to skeletal muscle. Microscopically, the only definite change is the enlargement of muscle fibers, with both myofibrils and sarcoplasm being increased in the usual proportions.

Another form of true muscular hypertrophy occurring at birth in association with extrapyramidal motor disturbances and mental deficiency is de Lange's syndrome. Death usually occurs within a few months in this disorder.

Myopathy Associated With Malignant Hyperpyrexia

A family was recently described in which there were three deaths from malignant hyperpyrexia. In this condition, general anesthesia causes a steep rise in body temperature, which is often fatal. In all there had been 10 deaths in this family attributable to general anesthesia. The finding of an abnormally high creatine phosphokinase level in symptom-free relatives in this family suggested the possibility of myopathy, and several family members were examined. Two were found to have definite clinical evidence of myopathy manifested by proximal weakness in the lower extremities; one had an associated abnormal electromyelogram.[17] The investigators suggest that perhaps other myopathic disorders may be associated with malignant hyperpyrexia. They also suggest that all relatives of patients who have had malignant hyperpyrexia should be examined clinically and their serum creatine phosphokinase levels determined so that affected persons can be warned about the dangers of general anesthesia.

Congenital Nonprogressive Myopathy

Congenital nonprogressive myopathy (central core disease, congenital nonprogressive myopathy of Shy and Magee) is a heredofamilial disorder that follows an autosomal dominant pattern; it is characterized by proximal muscle weakness hypotonia giving rise to a floppy appearance in infants, and a specific histologic change consisting of aberrant, fibrillary bundles found in the center of almost every muscle fiber. In addition to these muscle fiber abnormalities, numerous large fibers with centrally placed nuclei are also observed. Histochemical studies of the central core of the muscle fibers have revealed an absence of oxidative enzymes and phosphorylase activity. The muscles tend to be more severely involved in the lower extremities, resulting in delayed walking and retarded motor development. The extreme hypotonia seen in children with this disorder is not observed in adult patients. The deep-tendon reflexes tend to be normal. Muscle wasting is not prominent, and disturbances of sensation are not observed. No specific treatment is available. The disease is essentially benign, and the outlook is much more favorable than in the muscular dystrophies.[24,90]

Nemaline Myopathy

Nemaline myopathy (rod myopathy, Z-band myopathy) is an essentially nonprogressive, proximal myopathy with a probable autosomal dominant inheritance. Pathologically, an abnormality in skeletal muscle is noted, characterized by rodlike or threadlike structures without cross striation, occupying the entire length of the involved muscle fibers. These structures have been described as forming palisades at right angles to the normal fibrils within the muscle cell. Ultrastructurally, the rodlike forms have a fibrous structure. The appearance of rods or coils of threadlike structure gave rise to the name nemaline myopathy.[88] The specificity of the rodlike forms for this particular disease is questioned because typical rods have been produced experimentally by tenotomy in animals.[73] This disorder may actually result from a disturbance of alpha motor neuron innervation and may not be primarily a disease of skeletal muscle.[41]

Clinical Features. The clinical features of the disorder include a floppy appearance during infancy, retarded motor development, proximal limb weakness with hypotonia, muscle wasting, and diminished to absent deep tendon reflexes, all present in a slow, nonprogressive course. Recently, a progressive, nonhereditary, late-onset form of this disorder was described that was pathologically indistinguishable from the congenital form.[33] The suggestion that nemaline myopathy and central core disease may be different manifestations of one process has been raised by the diagnosis of both of these disorders in one family.[2] A variant of congenital and nemaline myopathy was reported in which the clinical course of the patient was one of extreme muscular weakness and hypotonia involving all of the skeletal muscles from birth, resulting in death at age 2 months. Pathologically, this disorder is similar to nemaline myopathy, except that crystalline intranuclear inclusions are present.[40]

Treatment. No specific treatment is available.

Prognosis. Prognosis in the congenital form usually tends to be quite good; greater incapacity is observed in the late form.

Myopathy Associated With Central Nuclei, Myotubes, and Type I Hypotrophy

In the myopathy associated with central nuclei, myotubes, and type I hypotrophy (central nuclear myopathy, familial myotubular myopathy), some authorities suggest that there is an arrest at cellular level in the development of the skeletal muscle in early life,[95] whereas others question this explanation of the pathogenesis. Pathologically the most characteristic feature in this group of myopathies is the presence of skeletal muscle fibers of small diameter with a peripheral ring of myofibrils surrounding a central granular zone containing a single nucleus or sarcoplasmic components. Recently, a family was reported with type I fiber myopathy where the most prominent histopathologic feature was the accumulation of finely granular material stained intensely with the myosin ATP-ase reaction.

Electron microscopy in these patients suggested a breakdown, or at least an accumulation, of myofibrillar fragments in the abnormal areas of muscle fibers. This disorder is slowly progressive with probably an autosomal recessive pattern of inheritance.[9]

Clinical Features. The clinical features in these patients are somewhat variable. The sexes are about equally affected. The onset of disease is at birth or shortly thereafter. The most consistent prominent findings in this group of disorders is weakness of the extraocular facial and neck muscles. Areflexia is a common accompaniment and raises the possibility of a neuropathic rather than myopathic disease process.[105]

Treatment. There is no specific treatment for this disease.

Prognosis. This myopathy is very slowly progressive.

REFERENCES

1. **Adams RD, Denny-Brown E, Pearson CM:** Congenital defects of skeletal muscles in diseases of muscle, 2nd ed, pp 299–323. New York, Harper & Row, 1962

2. **Afifi AK, Smith JW, Zellweger H:** Congenital nonprogressive myopathy: Central core disease and nemaline myopathy in one family. Neurology (Minneap) 15:371, 1965

3. **Assmann H, Bielenstein H, Habs H et al:** Beobachtungen und untersuchungen bei der Haffkrankheit. Dtsch Med Wochenschr 59:122, 1933

4. **Bank WJ, diMauro S, Bonilla E et al:** A disorder of muscle lipid metabolism and myoglobinuria: Absence of carnitine palmityl transferase. N Engl J Med 292:443–449, 1975

5. **Banker BQ:** Dermatomyositis of childhood. Trans Am Neurol Assoc 87:11, 1962

6. **Becker PE, Kiener F:** Eine neue x-Chromosomale Muskeldystrophie. Arch Psychiatr Nervenkr 193:427, 1955

7. **Bertorini T, Yeh Y, Trevisan C et al:** Carnitine palmityl transferase deficiency: Myoglobinuria and respiratory failure. Neurology 30:263–271, 1980

8. **Bradley WG, Hudgson P, Gardner-Medwin D et al:** Myopathy associated with abnormal lipid metabolism in skeletal muscle. Lancet 1:495, 1969

9. **Cancilla PA, Kalyanaraman K, Verity MA et al:** Familial myopathy with probable lysis of myofibrils in type I fibers. Neurology (Minneap) 21:579, 1971

10. **Carroll J, Brooke M, Devivo D et al:** Biochemical and physiologic consequences of carnitine-palmityl-transferase deficiency. Muscle Nerve I: 103–110, 1978

11. **Caspary EA, Currie S, Field EJ:** Sensitized lymphocytes in muscular dystrophy, evidence for a neural factor in pathogenesis. J Neurol Neurosurg Psychiatry 34:353, 1971

12. **Cherington M, Snyder RD:** Tick paralysis, neurophysiologic studies. N Engl J Med 278:95, 1968

13. **Chou SM:** Myxovirus-like structures and accompanying nuclear changes in chronic polymyositis. Arch Pathol 86:649, 1968

14. **Chou SM:** Myxovirus-like structures in a case of human chronic polymyositis. Science 158:1453, 1967

15. **Cori GT, Cori CF:** Glucose-6-phosphatase of the liver in glycogen storage disease. J Biol Chem 199:661, 1952

16. **Creutzfeldt OD, Abbott BC, Fowler WM et al:** Muscle membrane potentials in episodic adynamia. Electroencephalogr Clin Neurophysiol 15:508, 1963

17. **Denborough MA, Ebeling P, King JO et al:** Myopathy and malignant hyperpyrexia. Lancet 1:1138, 1970

18. **diMauro S, diMauro, PM:** Muscle carnitine palmityl-transferase deficiency and myoglobinuria. Science 182:929–930, 1973

19. **Dowben RM:** Treatment of muscular dystrophy with steroids: A preliminary report. N Engl J Med 268:912, 1963

20. **Drachman DB, Murphy SR, Nigam MP et al:** "Myopathic" changes in chronically denervated muscle. Arch Neurol 16:14, 1967

21. **Eadle MJ, Ferrier TM:** Chloroquine myopathy. J Neurol Neurosurg Psychiatry 29:331, 1966

22. **Eaton LM:** The perspective of neurology in regard to polymyositis. Neurology (Minneap) 4:245, 1954

23. **Engle AG, Potter CS, Rosevear JW:** Studies on carbohydrate metabolism and mitochondrial respiratory activities in primary hypokalemic periodic paralysis. Neurology (Minneap) 17:329, 1967

24. **Engel WK, Foster JB, Hughes BP et al:** Central core disease: An investigation of a rare muscle cell abnormality. Brain 84:167, 1961

25. **Farmer TW:** Glycogenosis due to deficiency of muscle phosphorylase: Recurrent myoglobinuria precipitated by grand mal convulsions. pp 70–73. In Kakulas BA (ed): Clinical studies in myology, Amsterdam, Excerpta Medica, 1973

26. **Fattah SM, Ruburis A, Faloon WW:** McArdle's disease, metabolic studies in a patient and review of the syndrome. Am J Med 48:693, 1970

27. **Flacke W, Caviness VS, Samaha FG:** Treatment of myasthenia gravis with germine diacetate. N Engl J Med 275:1207, 1966

28. **Gamstorp I:** Adynamia episodica hereditaria. Acta Paediatr Scand 45[Suppl 108]:1, 1956

29. **Goto I, Peters HA, Reese HH:** Creatine phosphokinase in neuromuscular disease. Arch Neurol 16:529, 1967

30. **Griggs RC, Engel WK, Resnick JS:** Acetazolamide treatment of hypokalemic periodic paralysis: Prevention of attacks and improvement of persistent weakness. Ann Intern Med 73:39, 1970

31. **Harper PS:** Congenital myotonic dystrophy. Britain I Clinical Aspects. Arch Dis Child 50:505, 1975

32. **Harper PS:** Congenital Myotonic Dystrophy. Britain II Genetic Basis. Arch Dis Child 50:514, 1975

33. **Heffernan LP, Rewcastle NB, Humphrey JG:** The spectrum of rod myopathies. Arch Neurol 18:529, 1968

34. **Henderson FW:** Tick paralysis. JAMA 175:615, 1961

35. **Hers HG:** Alpha glucosidase deficiency in generalized glycogen-storage disease (Pompe's disease). J Biochem 86:11, 1963

36. **Hoppel CL, Tomec RJ:** Carnitine palmityl transferase: Location of two enzymatic activities in rat liver mitochondria. J Biochem 247:832–841, 1972

37. **Hudgson P:** Muscular dystrophy—myopathy or neuropathy? In Kakula BA (ed): Clinical Studies in Myology, pp 160–171. Amsterdam, Excerpta Medica, 1973

38. **Hudgson P, Gardner-Medwin D, Worsfold M et al:** Adult myopathy from glycogen storage disease due to acid maltase deficiency. Brain 91:435, 1968

39. **Jacob JC, Matthew NT:** Pseudohypertrophic myopathy in cysticercosis. Neurology (Minneap) 18:767, 1968

40. **Jenis EH, Lindquist RR, Lister RC:** New congenital myopathy with crystalline intranuclear inclusions. Arch Neurol 20:281, 1969

41. **Karpati G, Carpenter S, Andermann F:** A new concept of childhood nemaline myopathy. Arch Neurol 24:291, 1971

42. **Karpati G, Stirling C, Engel AG et al:** The syndrome of systemic carnitine deficiency. Neurology 25:16–24, 1975

43. **LaGreca G, Sprovieri L:** Plasmapheresis on children of less than twenty kilograms weight. Proceedings of the Advanced Component Seminar, Haemonetics Research Institute, 1975

44. **Layzer RB, Lovelace RE, Rowland LP:** Hyperkalemic periodic paralysis. Arch Neurol 16:455, 1967

45. **Layzer RB, Rowland LP, Ranney HM:** Muscle phosphofructokinase deficiency. Arch Neurol 17:512, 1967

46. **Lennon VA, Lindstrom JM, Seybold ME:** Experimental autoimmune myasthenia gravis; a model of myasthenia gravis in rats and guinea pigs. J Exp Med 141:1365–1375, 1975

47. **Lindstrom J:** How the autoimmune response to acetylcholine receptor impairs neuromuscular transmission in myasthenia gravis and its animal model. Federation Proceedings 37:2828–2830, 1978

48. **Lindstrom JM, Seybold ME, Lennon VA et al:** Antibody to acetylcholine receptor in myasthenia gravis: Prevalence, clinical correlate and diagnostic value. Neur 26:1054–1059, 1976

49. **Macdonald D:** Sternomastoid tumor and muscular torticollis. J Bone Joint Surg [Br] 51b:432, 1969

50. **Magee KR, DeJong RN:** Hereditary distal myopathy with onset in infancy. Arch Neurol 13:387, 1965

51. **McArdle B:** Familial periodic paralysis. Br Med Bull 12:226, 1956

52. **McArdle B:** Myopathy due to a defect in muscle glycogen breakdown. Clin Sci 10:13, 1951

53. **McComas AJ, Sica REP, Currie S:** Muscular dystrophy: Evidence for neural factor. Nature (Lond) 226:1263, 1970

54. **McFadzean AJS, Yueng R:** Periodic paralysis complicating thyrotoxicosis in Chinese. Br J Med 1:451, 1967

55. **McFarlin DE, Engel WK, Strauss AJL:** Does myasthenic serum bind to the neuromuscular junction? Ann NY Acad Sci 135:656, 1966

56. **Meyer-Betz F:** Beobachtungen an einem eigen artigen mit muskellahmungen verbundenen fall von hamoglobinurie. Dtsch Arch Klin Med 101:85, 1911

57. **Meyers KR, Gilden DH, Rinaldi CF et al:** Periodic muscle weakness, normokalemia, and tubular aggregates. Neurology (Minneap) 22:269, 1972

58. **Millichap JG, Dodge PR:** Diagnosis and treatment of myasthenia gravis in infancy, childhood and adolescence. Neurology (Minneap) 10:1007, 1960

59. **Mommaerts WFHM, Illingworth B, Pearson CM et al:** A functional disorder of muscle associated with the absence of phosphorylase. Proc Natl Acad Sci USA 45:791, 1959

60. **Munsat TL, Piper D, Cancilla P et al:** Inflammatory myopathy with facioscapulohumeral distribution. Neurology (Minneap) 22:335, 1972

61. **Namba T, Brunner NG, Brown SB et al:** Familial myasthenia gravis. Arch Neurol 25:49, 1971

62. **Okinaka S, Shizume K, Iino S et al:** The association of periodic paralysis and hypothyroidism in Japan. J Clin Endocrinol Metab 17:1454, 1957

63. **Oliner L, Schulman M, Larner J:** Myopathy associated with glycogen deposition resulting from generalized lack of amylo-1,6-glucosidase. Clin Res 9:243, 1961

64. **Osserman KE, Tsairis P, Weiner LB:** Myasthenia gravis and thyroid disease: Clinical and immunological correlation. Mt Sinai J Med NY 34:469, 1967

65. **O'Sullivan DJ, Penny R, Ziegler J et al:** Cyclophosphamide in the treatment of neuromuscular diseases. In Kakulas BA (ed): Clinical Studies in Myology, pp 574–578. Amsterdam, Excerpta Medica, 1973

66. **Pearson CM:** Patterns of polymyositis and their responses to treatment. Ann Intern Med 59:827, 1963

67. **Pearson CM:** The periodic paralyses: Differential features and pathological observations in permanent myopathic weakness. Brain 87:341, 1964

68. **Pearson CM, Rose AS:** Myositis. Res Publ Assoc Res Nerv Ment Dis 38:422, 1960

69. **Penn AS, Schotland DL, Rowland LP:** Antibody to human myosin in man. Trans Am Neurol Assoc 94:48, 1969

70. **Penn AS, Schotland DL, Rowland LP:** Immunology of muscle disease. Res Publ Ass Nerv Ment Dis 49:215, 1971

71. **Pompe JC:** Over idiopathische hypertrophie van het hart. Ned Tijdschr Geneeskd 76:304, 1932

72. **Poskanzer CD, Kerr DNS:** A third type of periodic paralysis, with normokalemia and favorable response to sodium chloride. Am J Med 31:328, 1961

73. **Resnick JS, Engel WK, Nelson PG:** Changes in the Z disk of skeletal muscle induced by tenotomy. Neurology (Minneap) 18:737, 1968

74. **Rowland LP, Fahn S, Hirschberg E et al:** Myoglobinuria. Arch Neurol 10:537, 1964

75. **Rowland LP, Schotland DL:** Neoplasms and muscle disease: Remote effects of cancer of the nervous system. In Brain L, Norris FH Jr. (eds): Contemporary Neurology Symposia, Vol 1, pp 83–97. New York, Grune & Stratton, 1965

76. **Salafsky B:** Functional studies of regenerated muscles from normal and dystrophic mice. Nature (Lond) 229:270, 1971

77. **Salter RH:** McArdle's syndrome: A review in a preliminary report of four further cases. Postgrad Med J 43:365, 1967

78. **Sanders DB, Howard JF:** The role of plasmapheresis (plasma exchange) in the treatment of myasthenia gravis. Special Courses Syllabus, Vol II, No 8, pp 52–73. Annual Meeting, American Academy of Neurology, 1979

79. **Sanders DB, Howard JF, Johns TR:** The immunopathology and immunotherapy of myasthenia gravis. Special Courses Syllabus, Vol II, No 13, pp 30–63. Annual Meeting, American Academy of Neurology, 1979

80. **Sato T:** Myxovirus-like inclusion bodies in chronic dermatomyositis. Igaku No Ayumi Prog Med 72:639, 1970

81. **Sato T, Walker DL, Peters HA et al:** Chronic polymyositis and myxovirus-like inclusions. Arch Neurol 24:409, 1971

82. **Satoyoshi E, Kowa H:** A new myopathy due to glycolytic abnormalities. Trans Am Neurol Assoc 90:46, 1965

83. **Schmid R, Hammaker L:** Hereditary absence of muscle phosphorylase (McArdle's syndrome). N Engl J Med 264:223, 1961

84. **Schmid R, Mahler R:** Chronic progressive myopathy with myoglobinuria: Demonstration of a glycogenolytic defect in the muscle. J Clin Invest 38:2044, 1959

85. **Schmitt N, Bowmer EJ, Gregson JD:** Tick paralysis in British Columbia. Can Med Assoc J 100:417, 1969

86. **Shaw RF, Dreifuss FE:** Mild and severe forms of X-linked muscular dystrophy. Arch Neurol 20:451, 1969

87. **Shaw RF, Pearson CM, Chowdhury SR et al:** Serum enzymes in sex-linked (Duchenne) muscular dystrophy. Arch Neurol 16:115, 1967

88. **Shy GM, Engel WK, Somers JE et al:** Nemaline myopathy: A new congenital myopathy. Brain 86:793, 1963

89. **Shy GM, Gonatas NK, Perez M:** Two childhood myopathies with abnormal mitochondria. I. Megaconial myopathy. II. Pleoconial myopathy. Brain 89:133, 1966

90. **Shy GM, Magee KR:** A new congenital nonprogressive myopathy. Brain 79:610, 1956

91. **Shy GM, Wanko T, Rowley PT et al:** Studies in familial periodic paralysis. Exp Neurol 3:53, 1961

92. **Simpson JA:** Myasthenia gravis: A new hypothesis. Scott Med J 5:419, 1960

93. **Smith R, Stern G:** Myopathy, osteomalacia and hyperparathyroidism. Brain 90:593, 1967

94. **Spiro AJ, Hirano A, Beilin RL et al:** Cretinism with muscular hypertrophy (Kocher-DeBre-Semelaigne syndrome). Arch Neurol 23:340, 1970

95. **Spiro AJ, Shy GM, Gonatas NK:** Myotubular myopathy. Arch Neurol 14:1, 1966

96. **Strauss AJL:** Myasthenia gravis, autoimmunity in the thymus. Adv Intern Med 14:241, 1963

97. **Tal C, Lieban E:** Experimental production of muscular dystrophy-like lesions in rabbits and guinea pigs by an autoimmune process. Br J Exp Pathol 43:525, 1962

98. **Tarui S, Okuno G, Ikura Y et al:** Phosphofructokinase deficiency in skeletal muscle: A new type of glycogenosis. Biochem Biophys Res Commun 19:517, 1965

99. **Thibaudeau Y, Gagnon JJ:** Trichinosis, thiaben-dazol in the treatment of eleven cases. Can Med Assoc J 101:533, 1969

100. **Thomas PK, Schott GD, Norgan-Hughes JA:** Adult onset scapuloperoneal myopathy. J Neurol Neurosurg Psychiatry 38:1008, 1975

101. **Thomson WHS, MacLaurin JC, Prineas JW:** Skeletal muscle glycogenosis: An investigation of two dissimilar cases. J Neurol Neurosurg Psychiatry 26:60, 1963

102. **van der Does de Willebois AEM, Bethlem J, Meyer AEFH et al:** Distal myopathy with onset in early infancy. Neurology (Minneap) 18:383, 1968

103. **VanDyke DH, Griggs RC, Markesbery W, Mi-Mauro S:** Hereditary carnitine deficiency of muscle. Neurology 25:154–159, 1975

104. **Van Horn G, Drori JB, Schwartz FD:** Hypokalemic myopathy and elevation of serum enzymes. Arch Neurol 22:335, 1970

105. **van Wijngaarden GK, Fleury P, Bethlem J et al:** Familial ''myotubular'' myopathy. Neurology (Minneap) 19:901, 1969

106. **Victor M, Hayes R, Adams RD:** Oculopharyngeal muscular dystrophy. N Engl J Med 267:1267, 1962

107. **Von Gierke E:** Hepato-nephromegalia glykogenica (glykogenspeicher-krankheit der leber und nieren). Beitr Pathol 82:497, 1929

108. **Walton JN, Adams RD:** Polymyositis. Baltimore, Williams & Wilkins, 1958

109. **Watters GV, Williams TW:** Early onset myotonic dystrophy. Arch Neurol 17:137, 1967

Index

Page numbers in *italics* indicate illustrations. Those followed by the letter t indicate tables.